Wildlife Research in Australia

Practical and Applied Methods

Editors: Bradley P. Smith, Helen P. Waudby, Corinne Alberthsen and Jordan O. Hampton

CSIRO PUBLISHING

A catalogue record for this book is available from the National Library of Australia.

ISBN: 9781486313440 (hbk)
ISBN: 9781486313457 (epdf)
ISBN: 9781486313464 (epub)

How to cite:
Smith BP, Waudby HP, Alberthsen C, Hampton JO (Eds) (2022) *Wildlife Research in Australia: Practical and Applied Methods*. CSIRO Publishing, Melbourne.

Published by:

CSIRO Publishing
36 Gardiner Road, Clayton VIC 3168
Private Bag 10, Clayton South VIC 3169
Australia

Telephone: +61 3 9545 8400
Email: publishing.sales@csiro.au
Website: www.publish.csiro.au
Sign up to our email alerts: publish.csiro.au/earlyalert

Front cover: (top, left to right) Frog (photo by Alex Pike, DPIE), Duck (photo by Jordan Hampton), Kangaroo (photo by Jordan Hampton); (bottom) Pitfall trap (photo by Alex Pike, DPIE)

Edited by Joy Window (Living Language)
Cover design by Cath Pirret
Typeset by Envisage Information Technology
Printed by Ingram Lightning Source

CSIRO acknowledges the Traditional Owners of the lands that we live and work on across Australia and pays its respect to Elders past and present. CSIRO recognises that Aboriginal and Torres Strait Islander peoples have made and will continue to make extraordinary contributions to all aspects of Australian life including culture, economy and science. CSIRO is committed to reconciliation and demonstrating respect for Indigenous knowledge and science. The use of Western science in this publication should not be interpreted as diminishing the knowledge of plants, animals and environment from Indigenous ecological knowledge systems.

Aug22_RP_ILS

Foreword

I have had the good fortune to work on a diverse range of animals, from large mammalian carnivores to tiny passerines and much in between, using all manner of techniques to catch, tag, track and sample, in several states and territories. Many different animal ethics committees have therefore guided the proper consideration of this work and its methodological detail, and the reckoning of the work's outcomes against the costs to the individual animals involved. The oversight of animal ethics committees is critical for aligning the practice of wildlife research with community expectations, and embedding respect and care for living things.

And yet – animal ethics committees can seem idiosyncratic and confusing. I recall one committee that preferred me to voucher animals rather than pluck a few hairs for genetic analysis to determine the species. They considered the discomfort and stress of hair plucking more detrimental to the animal's welfare than humanely killing it, and were less concerned about the moral issue of causing death. (I recall thinking that the small mammals probably had the opposite view, and therefore did neither hair sampling nor vouchering.) Years later, a different ethics committee refused an application to estimate the population density of invasive black rats using kill traps, in a situation where these pest animals were causing native species to decline to extinction, and where managers were therefore killing them in large numbers with poison bait. Here, the committee considered that the welfare and rights of the individual rats prevailed over the potential benefits of the research.

Many of us who work in wildlife conservation have experienced decisions like these, that challenge us to think deeply about ethics and morality. The first section of this book sheds light on these perplexities – explaining that committees need to operate in differing state- and territory-based legislative contexts, grapple with the tension between different ethical theories, and also represent rapidly changing community perspectives. The second section of the book is an astonishingly thorough and up-to-date compendium of wildlife survey, monitoring and research techniques, even covering emerging techniques, such as drones, guardian dogs, thermal cameras and acoustic monitors. The book goes so much further than a methods manual, because it integrates this information with the specific welfare considerations each method evinces. New approaches for data gathering, such as wildlife selfies, and various citizen science initiatives, which may cause novel impacts on wildlife, are also discussed. The third section of the book comes from a different angle again, now organising methods and welfare issues into bundles that are more relevant to different animal groups. The combination of the three main book sections makes the material extremely accessible and well-structured.

The opening chapters talk about the importance of open and frequent communication between wildlife biologists and ethics committees; this book is an invaluable resource for that dialogue. It is essentially a two-way dictionary between committee members and field biologists, and will support greater consistency and higher standards across ethics committees and researchers alike. An incredible piece of collaborative work!

Professor Sarah Legge
Fenner School of Environment and Society,
The Australian National University;
Deputy Director, National Environmental Science
Program Threatened Species Recovery Hub (2015–2021)

Contents

Preface

Bradley P. Smith, Helen P. Waudby, Corinne Alberthsen and Jordan O. Hampton

Australia boasts a rich faunal assemblage, with high levels of endemism resulting from the continent's separation from Gondwana around 40 million years ago. Understanding this unique fauna, and finding ways to manage, use and conserve it, are central to most Australian wildlife research. Research and teaching related activities that involve or 'use' wildlife in Australia, are regulated and guided by national, state- and territory-based legislation, guidelines and codes, with researchers required (with few exceptions) to obtain approval from an animal ethics committee (AEC) before they commence. This process is intended to ensure that welfare outcomes for study animals, including wildlife, are in line with requirements under The Australian Code for the Care and Use of Animals for Scientific Purposes ('the Code') (see Chapter 1). This oversight is important given the number of animals used in research in Australia annually (over 6 million), and the diversity of views around the acceptable use of animals.

To a large degree, management of impacts of research on animal welfare occurs through the development and ongoing refinement of research methods, with AECs reviewing justifications from researchers for using any given method to answer a research question or meet an educational aim. In the absence of a robust foundation for evaluating animal welfare impacts, selection of one research or education method over another, and evaluation of these methods, can be subjective. Similarly, the likelihood of animal welfare impacts occurring can be difficult to evaluate for many methods, and options for replacement, reduction and refinement hard to articulate. Procedures for common approaches to wildlife monitoring and research (e.g. traditional trapping, tracking and marking techniques) are readily available, but researchers and AECs must often 'reinvent the wheel' when developing procedural documents for less commonly used wildlife research methods. Procedures for new and emerging technologies, and meeting contemporary expectations around animal welfare considerations pose further challenges for researchers and AECs alike.

This book is a practical resource for wildlife researchers and educators of all career stages, as well as AEC members and their supporting staff, to navigate animal ethics approval processes as they apply to Australian wildlife research. The book is presented in three sections. The *first* section ('Animal ethics and Australian wildlife research') addresses the administration and evaluation of wildlife research (legislative requirements, the operation of AECs, crafting and reviewing applications, and emerging and ongoing issues). The *second* section ('Research methods') details a range of wildlife research methods in the form of general operating procedures (GOPs). These GOPs are a guide to conducting these techniques in a manner that minimises negative animal welfare impacts. The *third* section ('Species profiles') focuses on taxon-specific considerations for a range of native and exotic wildlife occurring in Australia. Each GOP and species profile follows a standard template, and has been developed through extensive consultation with the Australian wildlife research community.

This guide has been compiled by over 200 researchers with considerable experience in field-based wildlife research, teaching, AEC administration, and the mentoring of other researchers. The diverse viewpoints and experiences presented here have been provided by academics, government scientists, practitioners, consultants, early career researchers and post-graduate students. The aims and methods of wildlife research are diverse, and the nature and requirements of individual research projects context specific. Consequently, this book is not intended to be prescriptive, but instead constitutes a resource for developing project-specific methods and AEC applications. It is our hope that this resource will support best practice wildlife research, the ongoing refinement of procedural documents, and assist researchers and AEC members in navigating animal ethics approval processes.

We are in gratitude to the lead authors of each chapter, and other contributing authors who provided their time and expertise. We are overwhelmed by their generosity, contributions and patience, particularly when considering that much of the book was written during a pandemic. We are indebted to Dr Damian S. Morrant for his assistance in the early conception and development of the book. Sincere thanks and gratitude to our families, friends, colleagues and mentors for their support. Thank you also to CSIRO Publishing, including Mark Hamilton, Lauren Webb and Briana Melideo for recognising the importance of the book, and guiding us through the publishing process. Finally, thank you to all of the animals that have been the subject of research; we hope this book contributes to improving the welfare of study animals in all fields of wildlife research.

About the editors

Bradley P. Smith

Dr Bradley P. Smith is a Senior Lecturer in psychology at Central Queensland University (Adelaide campus). He has a background in animal behaviour and comparative psychology, and has been actively conducting research relating to the cognition, behaviour and management of domestic and wild animals for over 15 years. Bradley has a special interest in the intersections between human and non-human animals, including strategies that help foster co-existence between humans and wildlife. Bradley serves as a Category B member of the CQUniversity Animal Ethics Committee.

Helen P. Waudby

Dr Helen P. Waudby is an Adjunct Research Fellow with Charles Sturt University, and a conservation biologist with the NSW Department of Planning, Industry and Environment (DPIE). She has over 20 years' experience in wildlife research ranging from desert rodents and marsupials, to threatened frogs and parasites, and has a particular interest in evaluating and refining wildlife research methods to achieve improved animal welfare outcomes. Helen has served as a Category B member of the DPIE Animal Ethics Committee.

Corinne Alberthsen

Dr Corinne Alberthsen is a national animal ethics coordinator and provides high-quality and contemporary professional advice, training and support to the research community on animal welfare and the ethical treatment of animals used in scientific research. She is actively involved in the evolution of animal welfare policy and procedures relating to both wildlife and laboratory animals. Corinne has participated as an animal ethics committee member or specialist advisor for over 10 years, and is currently executive officer to several animal ethics committees.

Jordan O. Hampton

Dr Jordan O. Hampton is a Research Fellow at the Faculty of Veterinary and Agricultural Sciences, University of Melbourne, and an Adjunct Lecturer with the Harry Butler Institute, Murdoch University. He is a veterinarian and wildlife biologist with almost 20 years' experience working with range of Australian wildlife including desert ungulates, marine mammals and birds of prey. He has a special interest in the management of introduced species and wildlife use. Jordan's research converges on animal welfare science, wildlife management and animal ethics.

List of contributors

Corinne Alberthsen, Biomedical Compliance Coordinator, Mater Research. corinne_hanlon@hotmail.com

Benjamin L. Allen, Senior Research Fellow, Institute for Life Sciences and the Environment, University of Southern Queensland; Research Associate, Centre for African Conservation Ecology, Nelson Mandela University. benjamin.allen@usq.edu.au

Carmen A. Amos, Assistant Programs Officer, Biodiversity, Conservation and Science Directorate, NSW Department of Planning, Industry and Environment. carmen.amos@me.com

Robert G. Appleby, Researcher, Centre for Planetary Health and Food Security, Griffith University. rob.appleby@wildspy.com.au

Asia O. Armstrong, Research fellow, University of the Sunshine Coast. ahaines@usc.edu.au

Kita Ashman, Threatened Species and Climate Adaptation Ecologist, WWF Australia. kashman@wwf.org.au

Cynthia A. Awruch, Senior Research Fellow, CESIMAR - CONICET, Argentina; Research Associate, School of Natural Sciences, University of Tasmania. cynthia.awruch@utas.edu.au

Guy Ballard, Senior Research Scientist, Vertebrate Pest Research Unit, NSW Department of Primary Industries; Associate Professor, School of Environmental and Rural Science, University of New England. guy.ballard@dpi.nsw.gov.au

Adam Barnett, Research Fellow, Marine Data Technology Hub, James Cook University. adam.barnett@jcu.edu.au

Megan Bathurst, Animal Ethics and Biosafety Advisor, Research Office, La Trobe University. m.bathurst@latrobe.edu.au

Linda Behrendorff, Ranger in Charge, Natural Resource Management, Great Sandy Area, Qld Parks and Wildlife Service, Department of Environment and Science. linda.behrendorff@des.qld.gov.au

Ian P. Bell, Senior Conservation Officer, Qld Parks and Wildlife Service. ian.bell@des.qld.gov.au

Andrew J. Bengsen, Research Scientist, Vertebrate Pest Research Unit, NSW Department of Primary Industries; Principal Vertebrate Pest Ecologist, Biosphere Environmental Consultants. andrew.bengsen@dpi.nsw.gov.au

Jocelyn Bentley, Senior Threatened Species Officer, NSW Department of Planning, Industry and Environment. joss.bentley@environment.nsw.gov.au

Karleah K. Berris, Project Officer, Kangaroo Island Landscape Board. karleah.trengove@gmail.com

Wayne Boardman, Senior Lecturer in Wildlife, Biodiversity and Ecosystem Health, School of Animal and Veterinary Sciences, University of Adelaide. wayne.boardman@adelaide.edu.au

Elise Boultby, Research Student, Future Industries Institute, University of South Australia. elisenboultby@gmail.com

Deborah S. Bower, Senior Lecturer in Zoology and Ecology, School of Environmental and Rural Science, University of New England. deborah.bower@une.edu.au

Kate J. Brandis, Senior Research Fellow, Centre for Ecosystem Science, School of Biological, Earth and Environmental Sciences, University of New South Wales. kate.brandis@unsw.edu.au

Julie Broken-Brow, Adjunct Research Fellow, Charles Darwin University. julie.brokenbrow@uqconnect.edu.au

Culum Brown, Professor, Department of Biological Sciences, Macquarie University. culum.brown@mq.edu.au

Phoebe A. Burns, Native Rodent Biologist, Wildlife Conservation and Science, Zoos Victoria. pburns@zoo.org.au

Paul A. Butcher, Principal Research Scientist, NSW Department of Primary Industries. paul.butcher@dpi.nsw.gov.au

Matthew Campbell, Senior Fisheries Biologist, Qld Department of Agriculture and Fisheries. matthew.campbell@daf.qld.gov.au

Craig Chargulaf, Senior Ecologist, FRC Environmental. craig.chargulaf@gmail.com

Simon Cherriman, Ornithologist, Insight Ornithology. aquila84@iinet.net.au

Andrew W. Claridge, Senior Research Scientist, Vertebrate Pest Research Unit, NSW Department of Primary Industries. andrew.claridge@dpi.nsw.gov.au

Jessica Clayton, Research Fellow, College of Science and Engineering, Flinders University. jess.clayton@flinders.edu.au

Nick Clemann, Senior Scientist, Arthur Rylah Institute for Environmental Research, Vic Department of Environment, Land, Water and Planning. nick.clemann@delwp.vic.gov.au

Simon Clulow, Senior Research Fellow, Centre for Conservation Ecology and Genomics, Institute for Applied Ecology, University of Canberra. simon.clulow@canberra.edu.au

Amy Coetsee, Threatened Species Biologist, Wildlife Conservation and Science, Zoos Victoria. acoetsee@zoo.org.au

Joanne H. Connolly, Senior Lecturer in Veterinary Microbiology and Discipline Lead, Captive Vertebrate Management Program, School of Animal and Veterinary Sciences, Charles Sturt University. jconnolly@csu.edu.au

Fabio Cortesi, ARC DECRA Fellow, Queensland Brain Institute, University of Queensland. f.cortesi@uq.edu.au

Graeme Coulson, Honorary Principal Fellow, School of BioSciences, University of Melbourne; Principal Consultant, Macropus Consulting. gcoulson@unimelb.edu.au

Tarnya E. Cox, Research Scientist, Vertebrate Pest Research Unit, NSW Department of Primary Industries. tarnya.cox@dpi.nsw.gov.au

Jemma K. Cripps, Senior Scientist, Arthur Rylah Institute for Environmental Research, Vic Department of Environment, Land, Water and Planning. jemma.cripps@delwp.vic.gov.au

Helen A. Crisp, Regional Ecologist South-east, Australian Wildlife Conservancy. helen.crisp@australianwildlife.org

Romane Cristescu, Research Fellow, Detection Dogs for Conservation, University of the Sunshine Coast. rcristes@usc.edu.au

Kevin Crook, PhD candidate, Science for Integrated Coastal Ecosystem Management, James Cook University. kevin.crook@my.jcu.edu.au

Jenna M. Crowe-Riddell, Research Fellow, University of Michigan. jmcroweriddell@gmail.com

Dympna Cullen, PhD candidate, University of New South Wales. dympnabcullen@gmail.com

Leanne M. Currey-Randall, Research Scientist, Australian Institute of Marine Science. l.currey@aims.gov.au

Ross K. Daley, Director, Horizon Consultancy. rossk.daley@gmail.com

Alana de Laive, Research Assistant, Herpetology, Australian Museum Research Institute, Australian Museum. alanahdelaive@gmail.com

Clare Death, Principal Consultant, WildTox Consulting; Senior Project Officer, Wildlife Health Australia. clare@wildtox.com.au

Kris Descovich, Postdoctoral Research Fellow, School of Veterinary Science, University of Queensland. k.descovich1@uq.edu.au

Chris R. Dickman, Professor in Ecology, School of Life and Environmental Sciences, University of Sydney. chris.dickman@sydney.edu.au

Zoë A Doubleday, ARC Future Fellow, Future Industries Institute, University of South Australia. zoe.doubleday@unisa.edu.au

Tegan K. Douglas, Citizen Science Project Coordinator, BirdLife Australia. tegan.douglas@birdlife.org.au

Katherine E. Doyle, Researcher, Institute for Land Water and Society, Charles Sturt University. kadoyle@csu.edu.au

Christine L. Dudgeon, Research Fellow, School of Science, Technology and Engineering, University of the Sunshine Coast. cdudgeon@usc.edu.au

J. Nicholas Dunlop, Citizen Science Project Coordinator, Conservation Council of Western Australia. tern@iinet.net.au

Judy Dunlop, Research Scientist, WA Department of Biodiversity Conservation and Attractions. judy.dunlop@gmail.com

Brendan C. Ebner, Senior Research Scientist, CSIRO Land and Water. brendan.ebner@csiro.au

Bronwyn A. Fancourt, Manager Invasive Species, Kangaroo Island Landscape Board; Adjunct Research Fellow, School of Environmental and Rural Science, University of New England. bronwyn.fancourt@une.edu.au

Luciana C. Ferreira, Postdoctoral Scientist, Australian Institute of Marine Science. l.ferreira@aims.gov.au

Lachlan Fetterplace, Environmental Assessment Specialist, Department of Aquatic Resources, Coastal Laboratory, Swedish University of Agricultural Sciences. lachlan.fetterplace@slu.se

Graeme Finlayson, SA Arid Rangelands Ecologist, Bush Heritage Australia; Visiting Research Fellow, University of Adelaide. graeme.finlayson@bushheritage.org.au

Brittany Finucci, Fisheries Scientist, National Institute of Water and Atmospheric Research. brit.finucci@niwa.co.nz

Peter J. S. Fleming, Senior Principal Research Scientist, Vertebrate Pest Research Unit, NSW Department of Primary Industries; Adjunct Professor, School of Environmental and Rural Science, University of New England. peter.fleming@dpi.nsw.gov.au

Nicole Flint, Senior Research Fellow, Coastal Marine Ecosystems Research Centre, Central Queensland University. n.flint@cqu.edu.au

J. Anthony Friend, Principal Research Scientist, WA Department of Biodiversity, Conservation and Attractions. tony.friend@dbca.wa.gov.au

Ben L. Gilby, Lecturer, School of Science, Technology and Engineering, University of the Sunshine Coast. bgilby@usc.edu.au

Matthew J. Gill, Senior Technical Officer, Faculty of Science, Charles Sturt University. mgill@csu.edu.au

Sarah J. Gill, Principal Wildlife Veterinarian, Biosphere Environmental Consultants. sarah@beconsultants.com.au

Dianne Gleeson, Professor, Environmental Genetics, Institute for Applied Ecology, University of Canberra. dianne.gleeson@canberra.edu.au

Ross L. Goldingay, Associate Professor, School of Environment, Science and Engineering, Southern Cross University. ross.goldingay@scu.edu.au

Rachael Gray, Senior Lecturer Veterinary Pathology, Sydney School of Veterinary Science, Faculty of Science, University of Sydney. rachael.gray@sydney.edu.au

Matthew J. Greenlees, Research Fellow, Macquarie University. mattg.ecology@gmail.com

Aaron Greenville, Lecturer in Spatial Agricultural and Environmental Sciences, School of Life and Environmental Sciences, University of Sydney. aaron.greenville@sydney.edu.au

Claire N. Greenwell, PhD candidate, Environmental and Conservation Sciences, Centre for Sustainable Aquatic Ecosystems, Harry Butler Institute, Murdoch University. cgreenwell@iinet.net.au

Alison L. Greggor, Senior Researcher, Conservation Science and Wildlife Health, San Diego Zoo Wildlife Alliance. agreggor@sdzwa.org

Stephen R. Griffiths, Adjunct Research Fellow, Department of Ecology, Environment and Evolution, La Trobe University. s.griffiths@latrobe.edu.au

Adrian N. Gutteridge, Fisheries Assessment Manager, Marine Stewardship Council. adrian.gutteridge@msc.org

Susannah Hale, PhD candidate, School of Life and Environmental Sciences, Deakin University. hsusa@deakin.edu.au

David G. Hamilton, Conservation Ecologist, Tasmanian Land Conservancy; Researcher, School of Natural Sciences, University of Tasmania. d.g.hamilton@utas.edu.au

Neil A. Hamilton, Consultant, Ghost Bird Consultancy. nightparrotwa@bigpond.com

Jordan O. Hampton, Research Fellow, Faculty of Veterinary and Agricultural Sciences, University of Melbourne. jordan.hampton@unimelb.edu.au

Nicole A. Hansen, Senior Project Officer, Saving our Species Program, Environment Energy and Science Group, NSW Department of Planning, Industry and Environment. nicole.hansen@environment.nsw.gov.au

David Harasti, Senior Marine Scientist, NSW Department of Primary Industries. david.harasti@dpi.nsw.gov.au

Scott A. Hardie, Adjunct Lecturer, School of Natural Sciences, University of Tasmania. scott.hardie@utas.edu.au

Sascha Healy, Senior Environmental Water Manager – Murray Darling Wetlands Working Group. sascha.healy@mdwwg.com.au

Geoffrey Heard, Adjunct researcher, Institute for Land, Water and Society, Charles Sturt University. gwheard.research@gmail.com

Jaime Heiniger, Project Officer, NSW National Parks and Wildlife Service. jaime.heiniger@environment.nsw.gov.au

Christopher J. Henderson, Lecturer, School of Science, Technology and Engineering, University of the Sunshine Coast. chenderl@usc.edu.au

Jamie Hicks, Marine Ecologist, Marine and Coastal Science Team, Science, Information and Technology Branch, Strategy, Science and Corporate Services Division, SA Department of Science and Water. jamie.hicks@sa.gov.au

Naomi Hodgens, Wildlife Detection Dog Officer, Wildlife Detection Dog Program, Wildlife Conservation and Science, Zoos Victoria. nhodgens@zoo.org.au

Bonnie J. Holmes, Lecturer, School of Science, Technology and Engineering, University of the Sunshine Coast. bholmes@usc.edu.au

Peter H. Holz, Veterinarian, Australian Wildlife Health Centre, Healesville Sanctuary, Zoos Victoria. pholz@zoo.org.au

Alan Horsup, Senior Conservation Officer, Wildlife and Threatened Species Operations, Queensland Parks and Wildlife Service and Partnerships, Qld Department of Environment and Science. alan.horsup@des.qld.gov.au

Katie Howard, Scientist, Arthur Rylah Institute for Environmental Research, Vic Department of Environment, Land, Water and Planning. katie.howard@delwp.vic.gov.au

Andrew Howe, Senior Field Ecologist, North-east Region, Australian Wildlife Conservancy. andrew.howe@australianwildlife.org

David Hunter, Threatened Species Officer, Ecosystems and Threatened Species, NSW Department of Planning,

Industry and Environment. david.hunter@environment.nsw.gov.au

Charlie Huveneers, Associate Professor, College of Science and Engineering, Flinders University. charlie.huveneers@flinders.edu.au

Christopher Izzo, Senior Research Portfolio Manager, Fisheries Research and Development Corporation. christopher.izzo@frdc.com.au

Stephen M. Jackson, Research Scientist, Vertebrate Pest Research Unit, NSW Department of Primary Industries; Adjunct Senior Lecturer, University of New South Wales, Sydney; Research Associate, Australian Museum Research Institute, Sydney. stephen.jackson@dpi.nsw.gov.au

La Toya Jamieson, Wildlife Detection Dog Officer, Wildlife Detection Dog Program, Wildlife Conservation and Science, Zoos Victoria. ltjamieson@zoo.org.au

Melissa A. Jensen, Senior Zoologist, Stantec Australia; PhD candidate, School of Biological Sciences, University of Adelaide. melissa.jensen@adelaide.edu.au

Rosalind Jessop, Deputy Chair, Victorian Wader Study Group; Committee member, Australasian Wader Studies Group. moonbird39@outlook.com

Chris J. Jolly, Postdoctoral Research Fellow, Institute for Land, Water and Society, Charles Sturt University; Research Associate, Herpetology, Australian Museum Research Institute, Australian Museum. cjolly@csu.edu.au

Darryl Jones, Professor Emeritus, Griffith University. d.jones@griffith.edu.au

Rob L. Jones, Founder and Director, The Aquarium Vet. rob@theaquariumvet.com

Neil R. Jordan, Senior Lecturer, Centre for Ecosystem Science, School of Biological, Earth and Environmental Sciences, University of New South Wales; Conservation Biologist, Taronga Institute of Science and Learning, Taronga Conservation Society Australia. neil.jordan@unsw.edu.au

Hayley Louise Jose, PhD candidate, University of Adelaide. hayley.jose@adelaide.edu.au

Gisela Kaplan, Professor Emerita in animal behaviour, School of Science and Technology, University of New England. gkaplan@une.edu.au

Shannon R. Kelleher, PhD graduate, School of Earth, Atmospheric and Life Sciences, University of Wollongong. shannonraekelleher@gmail.com

Gregory D. Kerr, Senior Ecologist, Nature Glenelg Trust. greg.kerr@natureglenelg.org.au

Alison J. King, Associate Professor, Centre for Freshwater Ecosystems, La Trobe University. alison.king@latrobe.edu.au

Roger J. Kirkwood, Senior Research Scientist, South Australian Research and Development Institute, SA Department of Primary Industries and Regions. roger.kirkwood@sa.gov.au

Gerhard Körtner, Project Officer, NSW National Parks and Wildlife Service. gerhard.koertner@environment.nsw.gov.au

Gerald Kuchling, Senior Research Scientist, Department of Biodiversity, Conservation and Attractions, Parks and Wildlife Service Swan Coastal District; Adjunct Senior Lecturer, School of Biological Sciences, University of Western Australia. gerald.kuchling@ dbca.wa.gov.au

Janet M. Lanyon, Senior Lecturer, University of Queensland. j.lanyon@uq.edu.au

Mike Letnic, Professor, Evolution and Ecology Research Centre, School of Biological, Earth and Environmental Sciences, University of New South Wales. m.letnic@unsw.edu.au

Amanda Lilleyman, Research Associate, Threatened Species Recovery Hub, National Environment Science Programme, Research Institute for Environment and Livelihoods, Charles Darwin University. amanda.lilleyman@cdu.edu.au

Lindy F. Lumsden, Principal Research Scientist, Arthur Rylah Institute for Environmental Research, Vic Department of Environment, Land, Water and Planning. lindy.lumsden@delwp.vic.gov.au

Daniel Lunney, Honorary Scientific Fellow, NSW Department of Planning, Industry and Environment; Adjunct Professor, Faculty of Science, School of Life and Environmental Sciences, University of Sydney; Research Associate, The Australian Museum, Sydney. dan.lunney@environment.nsw.gov.au

Michael Lynch, Head Veterinarian, Melbourne Zoo, Zoos Victoria. mlynch@zoo.org.au

Anna MacDonald, Project Coordinator, Oz Mammals Genomics Initiative, School of Biology, Australian National University. anna.macdonald@anu.edu.au

George Madani, Independent Wildlife Ecologist. chiro_ptera@hotmail.com

Grace Maglio, Researcher, Australasian Wader Studies Group. gracemaglio@hotmail.com

Grainne S. Maguire, Coastal Birds Program Leader, BirdLife Australia. grainne.maguire@birdlife.org.au

Helene Marsh, Emeritus Professor, College of Science and Engineering, James Cook University. helene.marsh@jcu.edu.au

Jonathan Marshall, Principal Scientist (Aquatic Ecosystems), Qld Department of Environment and Science. jonathan.marshall@des.qld.gov.au

Tyson Martin, Fisheries Scientist, Fisheries Queensland, Qld Department of Agriculture and Fisheries. tyson.martin@daf.qld.gov.au

Jasmin C. Martino, Research Associate, Future Industries Institute, University of South Australia. martino.jasmin@gmail.com

Alison Matthews, Manager Research and Professional Development, Charles Sturt University. alison@12p.consulting

Michael McFadden, Supervisor, Herpetofauna Division, Taronga Conservation Society Australia. mmcfadden@zoo.nsw.gov.au

Mel McGregor, PhD graduate, Environmental Futures Research Institute, Griffith University. mel.mcgregor@live.com.au

Rebecca McIntosh, Marine Scientist, Phillip Island Nature Parks. rmcintosh@penguins.org.au

Adam McKeown, Experimental Scientist, CSIRO. adam.mckeown@csiro.au

Donald T. McKnight, Postdoctoral Researcher, College of Science and Engineering, James Cook University. donald.mcknight@my.jcu.edu.au

Steven McLeod, Senior Research Scientist, NSW Department of Primary Industries. steven.mcleod@dpi.nsw.gov.au

Paul D. Meek, Senior Research Scientist, Vertebrate Pest Research Unit, NSW Department of Primary Industries; Adjunct Lecturer, University of New England. paul.meek@dpi.nsw.gov.au

Jane Melville, Senior Curator, Terrestrial Vertebrates, Museums Victoria. jmelv@museum.vic.gov.au

Heather Middleton, PhD candidate, Queensland Brain Institute, University of Queensland. h.middleton@uq.edu.au

Charlotte Mills, Visiting Fellow, Centre for Ecosystem Science, School of Biological, Earth and Environmental Sciences, University of New South Wales. charlotte.mills@unsw.edu.au

Jonathan Mitchell, Fisheries Biologist, Animal Science Queensland, Qld Department of Agriculture and Fisheries. jonathan.mitchell@daf.qld.gov.au

Laurie Mitchell, PhD candidate, School of Biological Sciences, University of Queensland. laurie.mitchell@uq.net.au

Jenny Molyneux, Senior Conservation Officer, Qld Department of Environment and Science. jenny.molyneux@des.qld.gov.au

Andy Moore, Adjunct Senior Research Fellow, Molecular Fisheries Laboratory, University of Queensland. andy.moore@awe.gov.au

David L. Morgan, Associate Professor, Freshwater Fish Group and Fish Health Unit, Centre for Sustainable Aquatic Ecosystems, Harry Butler Institute, Murdoch University. d.morgan@murdoch.edu.au

Damian S. Morrant, Principal Ecologist, Biosphere Environmental Consultants. damian@beconsultants.com.au

Katherine Moseby, Ecologist and Research Scientist, Centre for Ecosystem Science, University of New South Wales. katherine.moseby@adelaide.edu.au

Jenny L. Nelson, Principal Research Scientist, Arthur Rylah Institute for Environmental Research, Vic Department of Environment, Land, Water and Planning. jenny.nelson@delwp.vic.gov.au

Vere Nicolson, Veterinarian, Dreamworld. vere.nicolson@dreamworld.com.au

Samantha J. Nowland, Aquaculture Research Scientist, Aquaculture Unit, NT Department of Industry, Tourism and Trade. samantha.nowland@nt.gov.au

Lisa E. O'Neill, Project Officer, Assistant, NSW Department of Planning, Industry and Environment. lisaoneill@westnet.com.au

Joanne Ocock, Project Officer, Conservation, NSW National Parks and Wildlife Service. joanne.ocock@environment.nsw.gov.au

Penny D. Olsen, Honorary Professor, Division of Ecology and Evolution, Research School of Biology, Australian National University. penny.olsen@anu.edu.au

Jasmin G. Packer, Research Fellow, Environment Institute, School of Biological Sciences, University of Adelaide. j.packer@adelaide.edu.au

Grant C. Palmer, Senior Lecturer, Regional Futures Research Centre, School of Science, Psychology and Sport, Federation University. g.palmer@federation.edu.au

David Parker, Senior Threatened Species Officer, NSW Department of Planning, Industry and Environment. david.parker@environment.nsw.gov.au

Chris R. Pavey, Senior Research Scientist, CSIRO Land and Water. chris.pavey@csiro.au

Cara Penton, Ecological Monitoring Officer, Warddeken Land Management. ecology@warddeken.org.au

Julian Pepperell, Director, Pepperell Research and Consulting. julianp@internode.on.net

Angela J. L. Pestell, PhD candidate, Centre for Integrative Ecology, Deakin University. ajlpestell@gmail.com

Andrew Peters, Associate Professor, Charles Sturt University. apeters@csu.edu.au

Sophie Petit, Associate Professor of Wildlife Ecology, UniSA STEM, University of South Australia; Kangaroo Island Research Station. sophie.petit@unisa.edu.au

Vanessa Pirotta, Marine scientist, Department of Biological Sciences, Macquarie University. vanessa.pirotta@hdr.mq.edu.au

Benjamin J. Pitcher, Behavioural Biologist, Taronga Institute of Science and Learning, Taronga Conservation Society Australia; Research Fellow, Department of Biological Sciences, Macquarie University. bpitcher@zoo.nsw.gov.au

Anthony Pople, Senior Principal Scientist, Biosecurity Queensland. tony.pople@daf.qld.gov.au

Tim Portas, Consultant, Zoo and Wildlife Veterinary Consultancy. timp@zoovet.com.au

John L. Porter, Senior Scientist, Science, Economics and Insights Division, Environment, Energy and Science,

NSW Department of Planning, Industry and Environment; Centre for Ecosystem Science, School of Biological, Earth and Environmental Sciences, University of New South Wales. john.porter@environment.nsw.gov.au

Tarmo A. Raadik, Senior Research Scientist, Arthur Rylah Institute for Environmental Research, Vic Department of Environment, Land, Water and Planning. tarmo.raadik@delwp.vic.gov.au

Sheridan Rabbitt, PhD candidate, Schools of Biological and Social Sciences, University of Queensland. sheridan.rabbitt@uqconnect.edu.au

Cassandra L. Rigby, Research Fellow, College of Science and Engineering, James Cook University. crigby@westnet.com.au

Peggy D. Rismiller, Visiting Research Fellow, School of Biological Sciences, University of Adelaide; Senior Researcher, Pelican Lagoon Research and Wildlife Centre. rismac@internode.on.net

Euan Ritchie, Professor in Wildlife Ecology and Conservation, School of Life and Environmental Sciences, Deakin University. e.ritchie@deakin.edu.au

David T. Roberts, Senior Research Scientist, Seqwater. david.t.roberts@seqwater.com.au

Erin Roger, Citizen Science Program Lead Atlas of Living Australia, CSIRO; Chair, Australian Citizen Science Association. erin.roger@csiro.au

Troy Rogers, Senior Research Officer, Aquatic Sciences, South Australian Research and Development Institute. troy.rogers@sa.gov.au

Misha K. Rowell, PhD candidate, James Cook University. misha.rowell@my.jcu.edu.au

Nicholas Rutter, Research Scientist, Anthrozoology Research Group, School of Psychology and Public Health, La Trobe University. n.rutter@latrobe.edu.au

Laura Ruykys, Terrestrial Ecologist, Flora and Fauna Division, NT Department of Environment, Parks and Water Security. laura.ruykys@nt.gov.au

Tasmin L. Rymer, Lecturer in Zoology and Ecology, James Cook University. tasmin.rymer@jcu.edu.au

Debbie Saunders, CEO and Chief Remote Pilot, Wildlife Drones; Conservation Ecologist, Australian National University. debbie@wildlifedrones.net

Jason Schaffer, PhD Candidate, Centre for Tropical Water and Aquatic Research (TropWATER), James Cook University. jason.schaffer@my.jcu.edu.au

Lin Schwarzkopf, Professor, College of Science and Engineering, James Cook University. lin.schwarzkopf@jcu.edu.au

Jayson M. Semmens, Professor, Institute for Marine and Antarctic Studies, University of Tasmania. jayson.semmens@utas.edu.au

Melody Serena, Conservation Biologist, Australian Platypus Conservancy. melody.serena@westnet.com.au

Marcus Sheaves, Director Special Projects, Marine Data Technology Hub, James Cook University. marcus.sheaves@jcu.edu.au

Tiffany Sih, Research Fellow, Centre for Integrative Ecology, Deakin University; School of Biological Sciences, Monash University. tiffany.sih@my.jcu.edu.au

Megan Skelton, Scientific Officer, Heron Island Research Station, University of Queensland. meganskelton11@hotmail.com

Bradley P. Smith, Senior Lecturer, College of Psychology, Central Queensland University. b.p.smith@cqu.edu.au

Lysanne Snijders, Assistant Professor, Behavioural Ecology Group, Wageningen University and Research. lysanne.snijders@wur.nl

Kari Soennichsen, PhD Candidate, Institute for Applied Ecology, University of Canberra. kari.soennichsen@canberra.edu.au

Ruchira Somaweera, Principal Environmental Scientist, Stantec Australia; Adjunct Research Fellow, University of Western Australia. ruchira.somaweera@stantec.com

Jennifer A. Spencer, Senior Scientist, Science, Economics and Insights Division, Environment, Energy and Science, NSW Department of Planning, Industry and Environment; Centre for Ecosystem Science, School of Biological, Earth and Environmental Sciences, University of New South Wales. jennifer.spencer@environment.nsw.gov.au

Derek Spielman, Affiliate of the School of Veterinary Science, Faculty of Science, University of Sydney. derek.spielman@sydney.edu.au

Aditi Sriram, Project Officer, NSW Department of Planning, Industry and Environment. aditi.sriram@environment.nsw.gov.au

Colleen Cassady St. Clair, Professor, Department of Biological Sciences, University of Alberta. cstclair@ualberta.ca

Alyson Stobo-Wilson, Postdoctoral Fellow, CSIRO Land and Water; Adjunct researcher, Research Institute for the Environment and Livelihoods, Charles Darwin University. alyson.stobowilson@gmail.com

Dejan Stojanovic, Postdoctoral Fellow, Australian National University. dejan.stojanovic@anu.edu.au

Louise Streeting, PhD candidate, School of Environmental and Rural Science, University of New England. lperciv2@myune.edu.au

Deborah Sullivan, Project Officer, BirdLife Australia. deborah.sullivan@birdlife.org.au

David A. Taggart, Adjunct Associate Professor of Wildlife Biology and Conservation Research, School of Animal and Veterinary Science, University of Adelaide; Principal Scientist, FAUNA Research Alliance. david.taggart@adelaide.edu.au

Andrea Taylor, Aquaculture Research Scientist, Aquaculture Unit, NT Department of Industry, Tourism and Trade. andreal.taylor@nt.gov.au

Matthew Taylor, Principal Research Scientist, NSW Department of Primary Industries. matt.taylor@dpi.nsw.gov.au

Stephen M. Taylor, Senior Research Scientist, Department of Primary Industries and Regional Development, WA. steve.taylor@dpird.wa.gov.au

Daniella Teixeira, Research Fellow, School of Biology and Environmental Science, Queensland University of Technology. d.teixeira@qut.edu.au

Graham Thompson, Partner and Principal Zoologist, Terrestrial Ecosystems; Adjunct Lecturer, School of Biological Sciences, University of Western Australia. graham@terrestrialecosystems.com

Scott Thompson, Partner and Principal Zoologist, Terrestrial Ecosystems; Visiting Research Associate, Curtin University. scott@terrestrialecosystems.com

Ian R. Tibbetts, Associate Professor, School of Biological Sciences, University of Queensland. i.tibbetts@uq.edu.au

Jorge Tobajas, Postdoctoral Research Fellow, Instituto de Investigación en Recursos Cinegéticos (CSIC-UCLM-JCCM). jtobajas47@gmail.com

Kathy A. Townsend, Senior Lecturer, School of Science, Technology and Engineering, University of the Sunshine Coast. ktownse1@usc.edu.au

Sean R. Tracey, Associate Professor, Institute for Marine and Antarctic studies, University of Tasmania. sean.tracey@utas.edu.au

Michelle Treloar, Research Scientist, Institute for Marine and Antarctic Studies, University of Tasmania. michtailor@yahoo.com

James M. Turner, Postdoctoral Research Fellow, Institute for Land, Water and Society, Charles Sturt University. jaturner@csu.edu.au

Linda van Bommel, Postdoctoral researcher, School of Natural Sciences, University of Tasmania; Fenner School of Environment and Society, Australian National University. linda.vanbommel@anu.edu.au

Eric Vanderduys, Projects Officer, CSIRO. eric.vanderduys@csiro.au

Rebecca Vaughan-Higgins, Clinical Veterinarian, Perth Zoo, WA Dept of Biodiversity, Conservation and Attractions. rebecca.vaughan@dbca.wa.gov.au

Karl Vernes, Associate Professor in Mammalogy and Collections Manager of the University of New England Natural History Museum, University of New England. kvernes@une.edu.au

Simone Vitali, Senior Project Officer, WA Department of Biodiversity, Conservation and Attractions. simone.vitali@dbca.wa.gov.au

Daniela Waltrick, Technical Officer, WA Department of Primary Industries and Regional Development. daniela.waltrick@fish.wa.gov.au

David M. Watson, Professor of Ecology, Institute for Land, Water and Society, Charles Sturt University; Principal Scientist, FAUNA Research Alliance. dwatson@csu.edu.au

Maggie J. Watson, Lecturer in Ornithology, Institute for Land, Water and Society, School of Agricultural, Environmental and Veterinary Sciences, Charles Sturt University. mawatson@csu.edu.au

Helen P. Waudby, Adjunct Research Fellow, Institute for Land, Water and Society, Charles Sturt University. hpwaudby@gmail.com

Michael A. Weston, Associate Professor (Wildlife and Conservation Biology), School of Life and Environmental Sciences, Deakin University. mweston@deakin.edu.au

Desley Whisson, Senior Lecturer in wildlife and conservation biology, School of Life and Environmental Sciences, Deakin University. desley.whisson@deakin.edu.au

Katherine Whitehouse-Tedd, Anthrozoology research consultant, Auckland, New Zealand; Senior Visiting Fellow, School of Animal, Rural and Environmental Sciences, Nottingham Trent University. cheetah.research@gmail.com

Leanne L. Wilkinson, Executive Officer, Animal Ethics Committee, NSW Department of Planning Industry and Environment. leanne.wilkinson@environment.nsw.gov.au

Samuel M. Williams, Senior Fisheries Biologist, Animal Science Queensland, Qld Department of Agriculture and Fisheries. samuel.williams@daf.qld.gov.au

Lachlan Wilmott, Threatened Species Officer, NSW Department of Planning, Industry and Environment. lachlan.wilmott@environment.nsw.gov.au

Ian Wooden, Technical Specialist, Fisheries Research, NSW Department of Primary Industries. ian.wooden@dpi.nsw.gov.au

Leigh-Anne Woolley, Species Conservation Manager, WWF-Australia; Adjunct Research Associate, Charles Darwin University. lwoolley@wwf.org.au

Barbara E. Wueringer, Director and Principal Scientist, Sharks and Rays Australia. b.wueringer@gmail.com

Sam Young, Senior Veterinarian, Australia Zoo. sam.young@my.jcu.edu.au

Christina N. Zdenek, Research Fellow, Venom Evolution Laboratory, University of Queensland. christinazdenek@gmail.com

Frances Zewe, Doctor of Veterinary Medicine graduate, Sydney School of Veterinary Science, University of Sydney. frances.zewe@gmail.com

Mark Ziembicki, Ecological Research Consultant, Oceans without Borders, Africa Foundation. markzie@gmail.com

Section 1

ANIMAL ETHICS AND AUSTRALIAN WILDLIFE RESEARCH

Introduction

Corinne Alberthsen and Jordan O. Hampton

Australia is renowned for its diverse and unique wildlife. The importance of wildlife research to conservation, natural resource management, animal health and scientific knowledge is unquestionable. In particular, investigations on animal species, and the ecosystems that support them, are vital for the management and conservation of global biodiversity and ecosystem function. In other words, wildlife research yields important benefits. However, research also incurs costs. These costs may be economic, or impacts on people, ecosystems or the welfare of individual animals. Attempts to weigh and prioritise these costs and benefits shape how, where and why research is conducted. Questions relating to what research should be conducted and what shouldn't are outside of the reach of science; these questions are the realm of ethics. At its most basic level, ethics deals with questions about what we ought to do; ideas about what's right and wrong, or good and bad. Animal ethics is an involved field, and readers wanting to dig deeper are encouraged to explore dedicated contemporary texts such as Fischer (2019). To provide some ethical guidelines for research, an elaborate set of rules has been established to regulate how animals are studied. Researchers cannot study live animals, including wildlife, without formal approval from an animal ethics committee (AEC). This process ensures that animal-based research is constantly scrutinised to a degree that is matched by few other pursuits or activities in Australia.

In conducting contemporary wildlife research, researchers are expected to consider the welfare of any free-living, undomesticated non-human animals impacted. This includes animals they study or other wild animals inadvertently affected by their activities. 'Animals' as defined by the Australian Code for the Care and Use of Animals for Scientific Purposes (hereafter 'the Code') (NHMRC 2013) include 'all live non-human vertebrates (fish, amphibians, reptiles, birds and mammals), including domestic and purpose-bred animals, livestock and wildlife) and cephalopods' (p. 3). However, current standards exclude the vast majority of invertebrates from moral consideration. Definitions of what constitutes animal welfare are not straightforward, but current definitions converge on consideration of what animals experience and the balance between negative and positive impacts on these experiences (NHMRC 2013; Fischer 2019). Animals cannot consent to their involvement in research, and human values and attitudes around acceptable use of animals are diverse, so checks and balances have been created to structure contemporary human–animal interactions in research.

The three chapters within this section focus on the use of free-living, undomesticated native or introduced animals ('wildlife'), including those that are housed in captivity after capture from free-living populations (NHMRC 2013), for research and education purposes. 'Use' is a key concept in this discussion, and it ranges from simple observation of animals in the wild to invasive, perhaps lethal, interventions. It is the extent of the use of each individual animal, and the resulting impact on its welfare, that is pivotal in both the AEC approval process and subsequent reporting.

This section is intended for anyone undertaking wildlife research in Australia (or where Australian investigators conduct wildlife research in other countries) that requires animal ethics approval. The readers likely to gain most from this text are early career researchers and new AEC members. However, it is also intended to assist experienced individuals, to guide new recruits, and to recognise that the welfare of each animal is of central interest to the AEC. As stated in the Code, the use of animals for scientific purposes must have scientific or educational merit, and must aim to benefit humans, animals or the environment. This requirement creates a balancing act for researchers and AEC members. Researchers do not have complete freedom in conducting research, just as AECs do not have free rein over enforcing interpretations of the Code.

Throughout the section (and indeed the book), 'ethics' is used to encompass the process of obtaining approval to conduct research from an accredited AEC, operating under the Code and associated legislation. It is not the intention of this book to discuss the different ethical theories and their implications for animal use. For this perspective, see Fischer (2019). This section is based on the mainstream view that society has an imperative to conserve wildlife, but also to maximise the welfare of affected animals in every research project. The AEC is the key decision-maker in this process. Consequently, the following chapters focus on the process of seeking AEC approval as a researcher, facilitating research to proceed using best practice approaches, or developing and trialling new and improved research methods. This section provides guidance on navigating legislation, including a review of key concepts relating to animal ethics in Australia (Chapter 1); understanding the purpose and function of AECs, including the art of application writing and review (Chapter 2); and further considerations around contemporary wildlife research (Chapter 3).

REFERENCES

Fischer B (Ed.) (2019) *The Routledge Handbook of Animal Ethics*. Routledge, New York, NY.

NHMRC (National Health and Medical Research Council) (2013) *Australian Code for the Care and Use of Animals for Scientific Purposes*. 8th edn. National Health and Medical Research Council, Canberra.

1 Legislation and key concepts

Corinne Alberthsen, Helen P. Waudby, Leanne L. Wilkinson, Megan Bathurst, Daniel Lunney, Bradley P. Smith and Jordan O. Hampton

INTRODUCTION

Animal ethics frameworks in Australia (i.e. the process of a researcher submitting an application for their project to an AEC and that committee's evaluation of the protocol) have been evolving over the last four decades. To date, this framework offers the best solution to manage the expectations of stakeholders who want the use of animals in research to be constrained, and researchers who propose to use animals. Judgment on appropriate use of animals is required by both the applicant and the AEC. In some cases, the process and guidelines are not always clearly defined; this situation can result in frustration and contention for people (including administrators) involved in animal research and teaching (Lunney 2012a, b).

The laws, requirements and regulations that facilitate contemporary interactions with wildlife for researchers can initially prove difficult to navigate. This confusion is exacerbated by evolving ideas of animal welfare (especially for wildlife), plurality in animal ethics and often unstated commitments to different ethical positions, and a lack of specific guidelines for field-based wildlife research. Animal ethics frameworks in Australia (and worldwide) were historically rooted in laboratory-based studies of common laboratory species, such as rats and mice, undertaken in controlled environments (Fischer 2019). Such studies commonly focus on modelling human disease, are generally limited in the species they use, and use quantifiable numbers of animals. Conversely, wildlife research often focuses on a range of target species or communities, is undertaken in the field and uses numbers of animals that frequently cannot be predefined, usually with the aim of conserving or managing those species (Soulsbury *et al.* 2020). For example, this aim is often the case for surveys of animals in a new area or before and after an impact, such as wildfire, logging, drought, flood or building of new infrastructure.

This chapter reviews key concepts and legislation relevant to wildlife research in Australia to help all parties see the opportunities and constraints of the process, including the need for researchers to define procedures before starting a project, rather than developing them *in situ*. This chapter defines how to navigate animal research regulations and requirements. Familiarity with them is necessary for researchers and AEC members.

ANIMAL ETHICS

The field of animal ethics is engaging, challenging and rewarding, raising questions around the need to conserve and manage wildlife, how to go about it, and how to evaluate the often-competing needs and interests of the various parties (Fischer 2019). The Australian Code for the Care and Use of Animals for Scientific Purposes (the Code) defines ethics as 'a framework in which actions can be considered as good or bad, right or wrong. Ethics is applied in the evaluation of what should or should not be done where animals are proposed for use, or are used, for scientific purposes' (p. 4). How actions are determined to be right (acceptable) or wrong (unacceptable) rests on what values are recognised and what ethical theories are used to prioritise these values. At the broadest level, the three most influential ethical theories applied to animals are consequentialism (focused on outcomes), deontology (focused on the following of moral rules – including the idea of animal rights) and virtue ethics (focused on character traits) (Fischer 2019). Wildlife research is often focused on outcomes at the level of ecosystems or populations; this is hard to reconcile at times with AEC focus on individual animals. Critical reading on this subject is limited, with many writers promoting the notion of the rights of animals rather than the traditional application of consequentialism to research ethics, which evaluates the costs and benefits of research on animals (see Rose 1998 and Lunney 1998 for discussions). While some influential publications have advanced the notion that animals have the right to not be used, including for research, reaching the conclusion that animal research is morally illegitimate (e.g. see *Zoopolis* by Donaldson and Kymlicka 2011), the conservation of Australia's fauna relies on such research (Lunney 2019). Animal ethics frameworks in Australia operate under the social contract, defined in legislation and regulations as well as the Code, which rejects the notion of animal rights and advances the consequentialist view that the use of wildlife in research can be acceptable if costs and benefits are appropriately weighed and balanced.

THE CODE

The Australian Code for the Care and Use of Animals for Scientific Purposes (NHMRC 2013), referred to throughout this book as 'the Code', provides the framework and guiding principles for scientific research involving animals in Australia. In 1997, the Code was broadened from a focus on laboratory animals to encompass wildlife and ecological field studies (NHMRC 1997; Monamy and Gott 2001). That revision arose from a Wildlife Advisory Group (WAG) within the NSW Animal Research Review Panel (ARRP). It was written more to assist AEC members than researchers. It may seem sensible to AEC members initially that animals should be kept warm and dry but, on reflection, these principles, for example, do not apply to fish or frogs. In short, not all vertebrate requirements conform to the animals with which most humans are familiar. This reflects the origin of ideas of animal welfare being related to domestic mammals. Indeed, the lack of knowledge of rarely seen native Australian animals can make it difficult for AEC members to make well-considered decisions. Regardless, the applicant is responsible for providing detail and supporting justification to aid the AEC.

The Code promotes 'ethical, humane, and responsible care and use' of any living non-human vertebrate and cephalopods, for example octopuses ('animals'), used for scientific and educational purposes (NHMRC 2013, p. 1). It describes the obligations and responsibilities of all stakeholders, and the principles that guide ethical decision-making around animal use in scientific work. The Code must be understood and adhered to by anyone planning to conduct or oversee research or teaching activities involving animals. While the Code is an overarching national guideline and provides a level of detail not covered in state and territory legislation, it is not prescriptive. Consequently, the use of animals for scientific purposes relies on a model of enforced self-regulation (Whittaker 2016) or co-regulation (Timoshanko *et al.* 2016). Essentially, the Code outlines a framework, guiding principles and required outcomes around animal use, while allowing flexibility for stakeholders to determine the best means of applying these guidelines (Whittaker 2016; Timoshanko *et al.* 2016). Under the Code, institutions must establish a structure for how they will operate. Government oversight generally involves ensuring that these internal measures satisfy the requirements of the Code and any state- or territory-based legislative regulatory requirements.

LEGISLATION AND WILDLIFE RESEARCH

In Australia, animal welfare responsibilities are devolved to individual states and territories rather than being administered nationally. Each jurisdiction maintains legislation to facilitate the prevention of cruelty to animals and promote other aspects of animal welfare. Not all of these statutes deal explicitly with animal research. While they differ in their specific details, several requirements are consistent (Whittaker 2016):

1. All make provision for animals used in research and education, and refer to the Code (providing consistency at a national level), affording the Code regulatory power.

2. Institutions must obtain a licence or authorisation from the relevant regulatory body (see Table 1.1) to use animals for scientific or educational purposes; licence conditions are drawn from the Code rather than legislation.
3. Animal ethics committees (AECs) must be established to review all proposed animal use for research or education.

Ostensibly, this arrangement should provide clarity around the regulatory requirements for the use of animals for scientific purposes. However, differences in jurisdictional legislation produce complexities through variations in bureaucratic (e.g. animal ethics approval) processes, which are intended to facilitate legislative requirements for good outcomes for animal welfare. These complexities can be pronounced for wildlife research, which is often conducted in the field, and across species distributions that may span more than one state or territory. Accordingly, differing state and territory legislative requirements become complex when research occurs across multiple jurisdictions, including the definition of an 'animal'. Table 1.1 provides an overview of key legislation.

Legislative requirements are linked to the location of the animals being used rather than the location of the researcher, home institution or approving AEC. Consequently, taxa not required to be considered under the approving AEC's jurisdiction may still need to be evaluated for interstate work and sometimes by an AEC in that state. Only South Australian legislation mandates that AECs require a category E member (animal care staff) to be properly constituted. Therefore, if an applicant based in another state is applying for approval to conduct research in South Australia (partly or wholly), a

Table 1.1: Overview of Australian animal welfare legislation relevant to wildlife research, regulatory bodies and groups of animals covered by legislation.

State or territory	Governing legislation	Regulatory body	*Animals included
Australian Antarctic Territory	*Antarctic Treaty (Environment Protection) Act 1980* *Animal Welfare Act 1992* (Part 4) (Australian Capital Territory)	Department of Agriculture, Water and the Environment (Australian Antarctic Division)	As per the Code
Australian Capital Territory	*Animal Welfare Act 1992* (Part 4)	Transport Canberra and City Services	As per the Code
New South Wales+	*Animal Research Act 1985* *Animal Research Regulation 2010*	Department of Primary Industries	As per the Code
Northern Territory	*Animal Welfare Act* (section 42)	Department of Primary Industries and Resources	As per the Code
Queensland	*Animal Care and Protection Act 2001* and regulations	Department of Agriculture and Fisheries	As per the Code
South Australia	*Animal Welfare Act 1985* (Part 4)	Department of Environment Water and Natural Resources	As per the Code, excluding fish in research
Tasmania	*Animal Welfare Act 1993* (Part 4)	Department of Primary Industries, Parks, Water and Environment	As per the Code
Victoria	*Prevention of Cruelty to Animals Act 1986* (Part 3) *Prevention of Cruelty to Animals Regulations 2019* (Part 4)	Agriculture Victoria	As per the Code, plus: • lobsters • crabs • crayfish
Western Australia	*Animal Welfare Act 2002*	Department of Primary Industries and Regional Development	As per the Code, excluding fish in research

* Animals as defined by the Code are 'any live non-human vertebrate (that is fish, amphibians, reptiles, birds and mammals encompassing domestic animals, purpose-bred animals, livestock, wildlife) and cephalopods' (NHMRC 2013).

+ New South Wales and Victorian legislation is at time of writing undergoing review and reform.

category E member must be present when the application is assessed. Another idiosyncratic legislative requirement is the unique regulatory structure of New South Wales. Although all states require institutions or unaffiliated individuals to be registered as animal users, under the NSW *Animal Research Act 1985*, all individuals conducting work with animals for scientific or educational purposes must also apply for and obtain an Animal Research Authority (ARA).

PERMITS, LICENCES AND CODES OF PRACTICE

While all research or educational activities that use wildlife must be approved by an AEC, other legislative requirements may need to be considered and additional permits obtained before the commencement of work involving animals (Table 1.2). These considerations are typically outside of the remit of AECs, with responsibility residing with the principal investigator. For example, accessing wildlife in protected or managed areas (e.g. world heritage areas, national parks and reserves), land held under the Commonwealth *Native Title Act 1993*, or working with native animals, requires additional approvals and permits. These requirements are mostly state- or territory-based, rather than national, and can sometimes be addressed after attaining animal ethics approvals, but before work commences. However, in many jurisdictions, permits and authorisations will not be granted until AEC approval is obtained (see Table 1.2 for examples). Nevertheless, it is often possible to submit applications for processing simultaneously with pending ethics approvals.

Codes of practice and guidelines for research practices are also available. For example, in New South Wales the Animal Research Review Panel (ARRP) has developed guidelines for common methods used in wildlife research (ARRP 2020). The ARRP is an independent review and regulatory panel established under the *Animal Research Act 1985*. The panel comprises members across all animal research fields and provides guidance on best practice approaches to animal ethics, as well as handling disputes and complaints from researchers and the public. Similarly, the National Health and Medical Research Council (NHMRC) has developed guidelines that provide additional guidance on the use of animals in medical research and Australian native mammals (NHMRC 2013, 2014, 2017). It is important to recognise that these guidelines are not iron-clad rules and can be relatively generic in nature. The onus is on the researcher to present a protocol that fits their species, location and research objectives; if the protocol proposed differs markedly from the guidelines, an explanation is needed.

INSTITUTIONAL POLICIES AND GUIDELINES

Under the Code, institutions must develop their own policies and guidelines around animal use. They are intended to ensure that the organisation, and those employed by (or collaborating with) it, work within the confines of legislation. Research offices (or similar) provide support through compliance frameworks and policy documents. Researchers and AECs must adhere to their institutional policies, which should target the institution's particular research activities and be more prescriptive than legislation and national guidelines. While these 'in-house' policies will share commonalities, bureaucratic processes often differ. One example is the animal ethics application form. While the Code outlines the minimum information to be collected, it does not prescribe specific wording or scope. Consequently, institutions must develop forms in consultation with their AEC that meet the requirements of the Code, but also the administrative preferences and requirements of the institution. For example, questions around statistical justification of animal number, requested on animal ethics applications at different Queensland universities, range from a single request for 'statistical justification' to a six-part questionnaire that requires explanation of analysis aims, analysis methods, outcome measures, presence of independent variables and an explanation of how experimental design is appropriate for the chosen analysis (Naughtin and Alston-Knox 2019).

THE THREE RS: REPLACEMENT, REDUCTION AND REFINEMENT

The 'Three Rs' (3Rs) are the fundamental principles of modern animal research and underpin the requirement for respect for animals. Although these internationally recognised principles were originally developed with laboratory animals in mind (Russell and Burch 1959), they also apply to wildlife research. While field conditions and research aims of wildlife research differ from those of laboratory-based research, the ethical and humane use of animals is a universal requirement (Lindsjö *et al.* 2016; Zemanova 2020). The Code directs that, when designing,

Table 1.2: Additional permits that may be required in each state or territory when using wildlife for scientific purposes and associated legislation.

Governing body	Approvals and permits required in addition to AEC approval	Governing legislation
Commonwealth	Australian Bird and Bat Banding Scheme banding authority Colour marking authority Application to gain access to banding data Australian Bird and Bat Banding Scheme project approval Listed species and ecological community permits Whale and dolphin research permits Australian Marine Park permits	*Environment Protection and Biodiversity Conservation Act 1999* (EPBC Act)
	Commonwealth territories of Cocos (Keeling) Islands, Christmas Island and the Coral Sea Islands protected species permits	*Environment Protection and Biodiversity Conservation Regulations 2000* (EPBC Regulations)
	Convention on International Trade in Endangered Species of Wild Fauna and Flora (CITES) Permit	Part 13A of the EPBC Act, which incorporates Australia's obligations under the Convention on International Trade in Endangered Species of Wild Fauna and Flora (CITES)
Australian Antarctic Territory	Import licence	*Quarantine Act 1908*
	Firearm permits	*Weapons Ordinance 2001* (AAT)
	Environmental impact assessment approval and permit	*Antarctic Treaty (Environment Protection) Act 1980* *Antarctic Treaty (Environmental Protection) (Environmental Impact Assessment) Regulations 1993*
	Permit to harvest or carry out research with respect to Antarctic living marine organisms	*Antarctic Marine Living Resources Conservation Act 1981*
Australian Capital Territory	Nature conservation licence Licence relating to take/release/keep/kill/import/export animals for scientific purposes	*Nature Conservation Act 2014*
	Damage land in a reserve/remove a native tree from unleased land/interfere with nests/vehicle in a reserve Licence to take fish for scientific purposes Licence to import or export live fish into or out of the ACT	*Fisheries Act 2000*
	Boating permit to use an electric power boat on Googong Dam/Reservoir Boat licence	*Lakes Act 1976*
	Medicines or poisons research and education program licence	*Medicines, Poisons and Therapeutic Goods Act 2008* and *Medicines, Poisons and Therapeutic Goods Regulation 2008*
New South Wales	A biodiversity conservation licence (also referred to as a scientific class licence)	*Biodiversity Conservation Act 2016*, Part 2, Division 3
	Licence to harm threatened species, population or ecological community or damage habitat	*Fisheries Management Act 1994*, section 220ZW
	Import and export licences	*Biodiversity Conservation Act 2016*

Governing body	Approvals and permits required in addition to AEC approval	Governing legislation
	Boat licence	*Marine Safety Act 1998*
	Application for authority to possess or supply Schedule 8 or Schedule 9 Substances, prohibited drugs/plants for the purpose of research, instruction, analysis or treatment of animals	*Poisons and Therapeutic Goods Act 1966* *Drug Misuse and Trafficking Act 1985*
Northern Territory	Application for a permit import and export Permit to take or interfere with wildlife	*Territory Parks and Wildlife Conservation Act 2006*
	Permit to undertake scientific research on wildlife	*Territory Parks and Wildlife Conservation Act 1976*
	Application for a special permit – marine resources	*Fisheries Act 1988*, section 17
	Permit to conduct a teaching or research program involving the use or breeding of animals	*Animal Welfare Act*, Part 5, Division 3
	Possess and use a Schedule 4 or 8 substance application form	*Medicines, Poisons and Therapeutic Goods Act 2012*
Queensland	Scientific purposes or educational purposes permit	*Nature Conservation Act 1992*
	Registration as a scientific user application	*Animal Care and Protection Act 2001*, section 52
	Application to use animals for a scientific purpose	
	Wildlife movement permit Movement advice request	*Nature Conservation (Animals Regulation) 2020*, section 218
	Native animal keeping licence	Code of Practice – Aviculture Code of Practice – Captive Reptile and Amphibian Husbandry
	General fisheries permit	*Fisheries Act 1994*
	Boat licence	
	Application to the Chief Executive for an approval for animal management and/or welfare	*Health (Drugs and Poisons) Regulation 1996*
South Australia	Animal welfare research and teaching licence	*Animal Welfare Act 1985*, Part 4
	Permit to keep and sell protected animals (scientific/biological products) (Class 6)	*National Parks and Wildlife Act 1972*
	Scientific research permit	
	Import permit – wildlife (including live animals, eggs and taxidermy)	
	Euthanasia in the field	*Controlled Substances Act 1984* and regulations
	Miscellaneous research fishing permit application form	*Fisheries Management Act 2007*
	Application for a ministerial permit to possess or control noxious species	
	Application for a ministerial permit to possess or control protected species	
	Application for a ministerial permit to release aquatic resources – stage 1	
	Application for a ministerial permit to release aquatic resources – stage 2	
	Application for a ministerial permit to release fish	

(Continued)

Table 1.2. *Continued*

Governing body	Approvals and permits required in addition to AEC approval	Governing legislation
	Application for a ministerial permit to undertake activities within an aquatic reserve	*Marine Parks Act 2007*
	Application for a permit to undertake a prohibited activity in a marine park	
	Export permit – wildlife (including live animals, eggs and taxidermy)	*National Parks and Wildlife (Wildlife) Regulations 2019*
Tasmania	Requires that a veterinary surgeon must annually assess the competency of any individual undertaking microchipping in animals	*Tasmanian Veterinary Surgeon's Regulation 2012*
	Application for an interstate import permit for wildlife and wildlife products	*Animal Health Act 1995*
	Application for an interstate export permit for wildlife and wildlife products	
	Scientific permit – fauna	Issued under section 29 of the *Nature Conservation Act 2002*; regulation 4 of the *Threatened Species Protection Regulations 1996*; regulation 28 of the *National Parks and Reserves Management Regulations 2019*; section 46(1) of the *Crown Lands Act 1976*; Regulation 22 of the *Crown Lands Regulations 2001*, Part 3 of the *Wellington Park Regulations 1999*
	Fisheries permit	*Living Marine Resources Management Act 1995*
Victoria	Fisheries permits and/or authorisations	*Fisheries Act 1995*
	Wildlife research permit	*Wildlife Act 1975*
	Permit to conduct research in a national park	*National Parks Act 1975* (for research on flora, fauna, soil, water and invertebrates)
	Licences and permits to possess (and possibly supply) scheduled substances	*Drugs, Poisons and Controlled Substances Act 1981* and Drugs, Poisons and Controlled Substances Regulations 2017
	Pest animal research/education collections permit	*Catchment and Land Protection Act 1994* (CaLP)
	Marine licence	*Marine Safety Act 2010*
Western Australia	Fauna taking (scientific or other purposes) licence – Western Australia	*Biodiversity Conservation Regulations 2018*
	Fauna taking (biological assessment) licence	
	Fauna taking (relocation) licence	
	Fauna importing licence	
	Fauna exporting licence	
	Standard translocation approval	*Fish Resources Management Act 1994* (FRMA)
	Research/education permit for medicines and poisons	*Medicines and Poisons Act 2014*

conducting and evaluating research, preference is given to methods that do not involve animals. If animal involvement is essential to the research, investigators should use the minimum number of animals appropriate to their scientific goals and refine protocols so that they maximise animal health and wellbeing. The 3Rs are applied throughout the scientific process – from project conception to dissemination of findings (Monamy and Gott 2001; Lindsjö *et al.* 2016). Incorporation of these principles into wildlife research and management leads to improvements in research quality and positive animal welfare outcomes, both individually and across populations (Lindsjö *et al.* 2016; Soulsbury *et al.* 2020). Opportunities for replacing, reducing and refining animal-based research are often complementary, interconnected (see Figure 1.1 for selected examples), and continually evolving.

Replacement

Alternatives to using animals should always be preferred for research and teaching, where the same objectives can be achieved. However, animal use is often unavoidable, particularly for projects that investigate the ecology, management or conservation of wildlife or their communities, which are often the research focus. Conversely, laboratory-based studies tend to use animals as models for understanding another organism (Paul *et al.* 2016) (e.g. rodent models for investigating human cancers). Technological advances in surveillance technology, computer simulations (i.e. population movements and predictions), and genomic technology, such as environmental DNA (eDNA – see Chapter 4) (Garlapati *et al.* 2019), are examples of methods that could replace animal use in teaching and wildlife research. For example, imaging and geolocation technology has been used to replace traditional lethal methods of deep-sea faunal sampling (Green *et al.* 2019). However, for most wildlife projects that are conducted in the field, using live animals is critical. Wildlife research may necessitate observation of free-living animals, capture and temporary holding of animals in the field (e.g. when an animal recovers from anaesthetic after a tissue sample is taken for pathology or genetic research), or transportation and holding of individual animals for longer periods in suitable housing (e.g. to study reproductive behaviour for evolutionary studies). As more knowledge is gained about Australia's diverse fauna and its ecological attributes and with technological advancements, replacement opportunities will increase. Ongoing uncertainty the conservation status of most of Australia's vertebrate fauna means there is a pressing

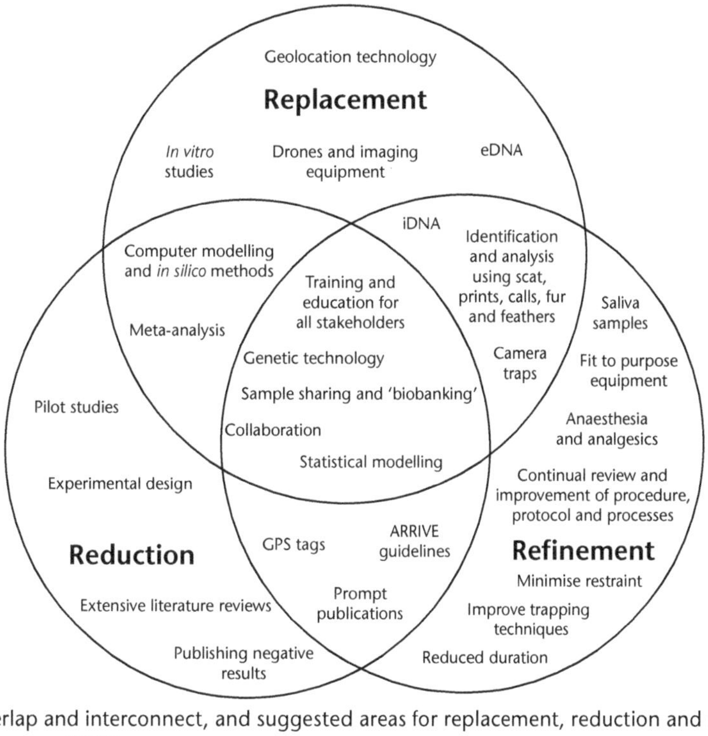

Figure 1.1: How the 3Rs overlap and interconnect, and suggested areas for replacement, reduction and refinement in wildlife research (modified from Zemanova 2020).

need for more field-based information than has been collected to date. Consider the plight of the Tasmanian devil (*Sarcophilus harrisii*); conservationists would not be as advanced in their knowledge of devil ecology and disease (Hogg *et al.* 2019) if research using animals had been denied. In many wildlife research situations, replacement is the least achievable of the 3Rs.

Reduction

The 'reduction' principle focuses on using the lowest number of animals to obtain scientifically sound and statistically meaningful data. Experimental design is key in determining the animal numbers required to answer research questions. However, it is often difficult for applicants to estimate the numbers of animals required for field-based wildlife research, particularly where the objectives are focused on creating wildlife inventories, or estimates of biodiversity or numbers of animals in a population, particularly in long-term studies that are so essential for assessing changes in population sizes (Lindenmayer 2018; Lunney *et al.* 2018; Spencer 2018). In Australia's erratic boom–bust climate, animal populations change drastically, so designs must be capable of interpreting low population sizes, not just the mean. Additionally, studies of free-ranging wildlife may use greater numbers of animals to obtain meaningful data than would laboratory-based projects because they are almost always affected by confounding variables that are difficult to control under field conditions (Soulsbury *et al.* 2020). The repercussions of poor experimental design can be catastrophic. For example, a conservation project that is informed by unrepresentative or erroneous research findings may devote precious resources to the 'wrong' work (Steidl *et al.* 1997). Poor experimental design may result in use of animals without the intended delivery of robust scientific outcomes, compromising animal welfare in the process. Further, a design that uses insufficient animals to deliver a statistically sound outcome will be invalid or require repetition. Either way, the animals used in the initial study would be wasted – an undesirable outcome, and one that does not align with the reduction principal of the Code. Researchers must clearly justify requests to use a specified number of animals in their AEC applications, and AECs should keep in mind that stipulating use of fewer animals may not deliver good research or improved welfare outcomes in the longer term.

Reduction may also include attempts to obtain additional information from the same number of animals, either by reusing those same animals over time or sharing the same animals across different projects. For example, researchers with different objectives can collaborate to gather project-specific information from one group of animals. However, while obtaining additional information from the same animals may maximise convenience and information gathering, and avoid involvement of a greater number of animals, the cumulative impact on individual animal welfare may not be acceptable. The poorer welfare outcomes for a small number of re-used animals must be balanced carefully against the better welfare outcomes for a greater number of animals used once.

Refinement

Refinement encompasses adapting, improving, changing and adopting methods that negate or minimise potential pain, suffering or distress of animals, including the development and implementation of practices and techniques that improve welfare. 'Refinement' is the most dynamic of the three principles and arguably can have the greatest effect on both scientific outcomes and animal welfare (Schuppli and Fraser 2005; Hampton *et al.* 2016). Fortunately, it is an area of active inquiry (e.g. Herbert *et al.* 2020). Better techniques benefit both the researcher and the animals being used. Researchers are encouraged to arrive at better methods, present their ideas to their AEC, and publish them.

Continual refinement of processes and procedures will reduce the risk of animals being injured or killed (Soulsbury *et al.* 2020), as would the development of 'welfare standards' that address defined thresholds for animal-based (i.e. physiological and behavioural) measures (Hampton *et al.* 2016). Reviews and ongoing assessment of operating procedures and practices within research groups (e.g. after each field trip or trapping session) and AECs (e.g. when considering requests for renewal of approval) should be undertaken. Researchers should be open to changes to 'refinement' to existing methods or practices, even where they are less convenient or more expensive. Maintaining a mantra that 'we have always done it this way' is the antithesis to refinement and will not improve animal welfare outcomes. Conversely, AEC members should be mindful that changing techniques can undermine comparisons over time, and a statistical need (i.e. to measure change) often exists for maintaining the same research protocol from year to year. For example, continuity of methods is important when assessing the long-term recovery of native animal populations after a bushfire.

The rise of non-invasive and low-impact methods (see Chapters 4 and 5) has increased opportunities for refinement. Remote monitoring (camera traps and acoustic devices) and genetic sampling via hair and faecal samples (Schnell *et al.* 2015) provide opportunities for researchers to refine their methods. However, refinements can still exert negative impacts on wildlife if used inappropriately (Jones *et al.* 2006). Parity between data collected by novel methods compared to traditional techniques is also important. Additional use of animals may be necessary in the early stages of novel technique development to determine if the method is as effective as established methods.

REPORTING GUIDELINES FOR PUBLICATIONS

Publication of research outcomes is critical to minimise the likelihood that animals will be used unnecessarily to repeat research that has already been completed (Monamy and Gott 2001). Yet publication in peer-reviewed journals is not necessarily a priority for conservationists or wildlife managers whose main goal is to inform management activities at a local or program level, where findings are commonly analysed and reported internally. Academic publication is time-consuming, may detract from the implementation of research outcomes, and is not always viewed as critical to the jurisdictional conservation or management of a species or community. Consequently, it may be relegated to a low priority or avoided entirely. Resourcing issues and the investment of time required to publish a manuscript are typically considered major constraints. In some cases, scientific publication is seen as an indulgence rather than a necessity by conservation practitioners, with employees required to work on papers in their own time. At times, government-based scientists are also discouraged or prevented from publishing controversial results (Driscoll *et al.* 2021). Nonetheless, for the protection of social licence, publication is also seen as vital for researchers to demonstrate how their research activities affect animals (McMahon *et al.* 2012). Collectively, much research is never seen by others, and is repeated by new teams and in other institutions. This situation runs counter to best practice approaches in animal research. Nevertheless, improvements in animal welfare in wildlife research can be encouraged by establishing standards for reporting on research (Osbourne *et al.* 2018; Field *et al.* 2019).

Adopting and enforcing publishing guidelines will set expectations for wildlife research and encourage compliance with standards. Some journals and publishers consider it their responsibility to ensure that manuscripts provide evidence that animal-based research was evaluated by an AEC. This aim may be done by, for example, requesting evidence of animal ethics approval (i.e. an approval document or approval number issued by an AEC) or asking that authors agree to a set of ethical guidelines (e.g. Sikes *et al.* 2016). However, the initial responsibility lies with the AEC and the researcher's affiliated institution. Journals could also ask for other supporting documentation, such as the scientific licence or permit to work in a protected area. The choice belongs to the journal; however, it may be in the interests of Australian researchers to voluntarily include an AEC approval number with their submitted manuscripts.

Other guidelines, such as the ARRIVE (Animal Research: Reporting of *In Vivo* Experiments) guidelines, can assist in the development of study designs and procedural documents on the publication of animal-based research (Kilkenny *et al.* 2010; Percie du Sert *et al.* 2020). Reliable study results and consistent reporting, including the publication of negative results (and adverse impacts; Waudby *et al.* 2019), are critical for planning and implementing evidence-based management and conservation initiatives (Lindsjö *et al.* 2016). Wildlife-specific versions of ARRIVE, such as ARROW (Animals in Research: Reporting On Wildlife) and HARRP (Harmonized Animal Research Reporting Principles) provide recommendations for minimum ethical requirements for journals who publish wildlife research (Osbourne *et al.* 2018; Field *et al.* 2019).

EXPERIMENTAL DESIGN

Wildlife research may encompass multiple species across diverse habitats, climates and contexts, and employ techniques that range from observational activities through minor conscious intervention to complex surgical or otherwise invasive procedures, and sometimes death (euthanasia, accidental death and, in rare but strongly justified circumstances, death as an endpoint) (Soulsbury *et al.* 2020). The complexity of field-based wildlife research is exacerbated by uncontrollable conditions (e.g. fire, rain, drought, rugged terrain and remoteness) and often a lack of certainty about the numbers or presence of a study species. In some cases, the statistical analyses required to address research objectives will be purely descriptive. These factors can make it difficult to articulate clearly, for example, numbers of animals required (or even expected). However, a study design that does not consider biologically and statistically relevant parameters may hinder conservation efforts. The experimental design section of an animal ethics application aims to satisfy the AEC that the research is scientifically robust and justifies the use of animals (it effectively facilitates a 'cost–benefit' analysis of the use of animals weighed against the anticipated knowledge gained).

Regardless of vagaries associated with field studies, applicants are required to explain clearly and concisely to the AEC why a research project is designed in a particular way. Additionally, researchers should justify why certain factors, which may affect animal welfare (including the numbers of animals used), cannot be controlled or defined clearly. This section of AEC applications should be completed comprehensively and written in plain English, with minimal jargon and acronyms. Ideally, applicants would treat this section of the application as a science communication exercise where they are explaining their work to a lay audience (see Chapter 2). Similarly, while it can be frustrating to receive an initial rejection or request for more information, applicants should ideally treat the situation as an opportunity to review their proposal objectively and/or modify their framing of the research.

Initial rejection and requests for resubmission, or even minor changes to a protocol, can be viewed as problematic by applicants because it usually means that the resubmission will not be considered until the next meeting of the AEC. Delay in obtaining AEC approval may compromise the research. For example, animal activity is often seasonal, so the breeding season could be missed as a result of the delay. Time frames for obtaining AEC approval can be particularly important for Honours and Masters students because their research is contained within a short window of time. Although, experienced and organised researchers submit their applications in good time to account for the process, it is not always possible given the complexities of funding, seasonal variation or co-worker availability.

AECs, the Code, laws and regulations have evolved to meet the challenge of balancing animal welfare with the need to understand Australia's fauna and its management and conservation. Given that such a large proportion of our native wildlife either is formally recognised as threatened with extinction or is declining towards being listed, such as our iconic platypus (*Ornithorhynchus anatinus*) (Bino *et al.* 2019), this evolution will continue. Interestingly, some AEC members who are concerned about threatened species may be reluctant to approve a protocol where the species to be studied is threatened, even though the research may be critical to survival of that species. Regardless of the species in question, AEC deliberations should focus on the scientific benefits and animal welfare costs of the protocol under consideration.

In wildlife research, the researcher is often a recognised species expert and AECs are not always well placed to evaluate their experimental proposals. For example, although both mammals, a world of difference exists between a dog and a bat; the decision on approving research on bats should obviously be based on species-specific knowledge and the welfare requirements of bats. When the expertise in a species, or group of species, is demonstrated clearly in the qualifications and experience of the applicant, the AEC can and should afford to place a degree of trust in the contents of the application. Regardless, AEC members are within their remit to expect better justification for a proposal than a managerial or agency directive. An AEC may struggle to determine whether a research design is justified and the onus is on the applicant to present a convincing case. AECs maintained by institutions that undertake wildlife research and teaching activities can co-opt category B members (i.e. researchers) from the relevant faculty or departments to aid the AEC during deliberations, preferably before the AEC meeting where the decision is made. Their role is to assess and explain to other committee members the scientific merit of the experimental design proposed in an application. If an AEC is struggling with understanding the value of the experimental design, the applicant is often invited to address the AEC and answer questions. What can start out looking like an impasse can often lead to improved animal welfare outcomes through collaboration and a greater rapport between the AEC and applicants.

MANAGEMENT OR RESEARCH?

Natural resource management (NRM) refers to the protection and improvement of environmental assets, including vegetation and animals, soils, water, and ecological processes and functions. Work is typically conducted to achieve a predetermined management outcome. 'Practitioners' plan and implement NRM activities, including those that potentially affect animal welfare (positively or negatively) and the status of populations (e.g. threatened species). Increasingly, and particularly where work is funded by government, practitioners are required to monitor the effect of their management activities (interventions) on the environmental assets that they are managing. Practitioners (and consultants) often study animal populations to inform government policy, mitigate project impacts, and gauge the effectiveness of on-ground management. The line between these activities and 'research' that requires animal ethics approval can be blurred, particularly when legislation is ambiguous about the definition of research (Lunney 2012a). In these cases, it is left to individual institutions and the associated AEC to define research for their applicants. For example, some management activities that involve the killing of large numbers of pest animals, while legal, do not require AEC approval (although codes of practice are typically in place) because they are not classified as research – despite the impacts on animals potentially being substantial. Once an activity that uses animals is classified as 'research', requirement is triggered for scrutiny by an AEC before that activity can commence.

Examples of AEC confusion about assessment of management and research (e.g. projects involving flying-foxes (*Pteropus* spp.) or feral horses (*Equus caballus*) are presented in Lunney (2012a). This issue is an important one for wildlife conservation agencies that conduct research and also manage land (Lunney 2012b). For example, when a research project is initiated to assess the effectiveness of a program to cull introduced species, often the managers are permitted to sign off on the cull without AEC approval, but the researchers need AEC approval. These inconsistencies are inevitable within current legislative and policy frameworks, but it is important to be acutely aware of this divide in responsibilities and ethical frameworks. Such a divide leads some in the research community (or managers whose work is classified as research) to conclude that they are unfairly targeted for ethical scrutiny, and that the approval process could be simplified and less demanding of time. Resolution of this dichotomy is not straightforward, and AEC members should be cognisant of it when assessing studies for conservation and management purposes, particularly when applicant's colleagues are permitted to trap, poison or otherwise kill animals with only limited scrutiny.

The Code defines research as 'broad and includes the creation of new knowledge or the use of existing knowledge in a new and creative way so as to generate new concepts, methodologies, inventions and understandings. This could include synthesis and analysis of previous research to the extent that it is new and creative' (NHMRC 2018, p. 5). Researchers plan and implement these activities, and while hypotheses may be explicit or implicit, no predetermined outcome is sought (as is typically the case with management-focused activities, e.g. a fauna survey in a new area as part of the preparation of a management plan).

This creates an administrative burden (if management activities are erroneously defined as research), is a potential source of friction between AECs and applicants, and is problematic for organisations that do not have a research focus. Some institutions and AECs may take a conservative approach, where any work that is seeking to answer a question (e.g. monitoring animals to answer questions about land management actions) requires approval. This conservatism can be met with resistance from practitioners who believe that, as their work is management-focused, it should be exempt from AEC approval requirements. No universal solution is available, particularly while legislation in some jurisdictions remains ambiguous about definitions of animal use and research. Ideally, the act of gaining approval should relate to not only the purpose of the activity, but also to the method being applied (and therefore the welfare implications to the species). This is why AECs develop in consultation with their various stakeholder groups, relevant policy platforms and guidelines that provide instruction and clarity on requirements and expectations. Institutions have a responsibility to engage widely within the organisations they serve, including being prepared to provide appropriate educational programs to all people involved in the care and use of animals (NHMRC 2013) to assist applicants understand and participate in the ethical review process. Practitioners should accept that AEC approval is a legislated requirement rather than a 'tick the box' exercise or inconvenience to getting work done. Animal ethics approval provides accountability for practitioners and the AEC to justify their interactions with animals, which are sometimes scrutinised by the public or interest groups (McMahon *et al.* 2012) (although approved protocols are not made public and are sometimes exempt from freedom of information requests). Accountability and transparency are particularly important for work conducted by, or on behalf of, taxpayer-funded organisations.

ASSESSING RESEARCH COMPETENCIES

The Code requires people engaged in animal-based research activities to be competent (NHMRC 2013), which is typically reflected in legislation. The Code defines competency as '[t]he consistent application of knowledge and skill to the standard of performance required regarding the care and use of animals. It embodies the ability to transfer and apply knowledge and skill to new situations and environments' (NHMRC 2013, p. 3). Competency provides a measure of confidence to all stakeholders that researchers can meet the responsibilities of animal-based research. However, the Code does not provide a framework for assessing competency (Whittaker 2016; Timoshanko *et al.* 2016). It has been a topic of discussion across institutions nationwide to determine the most practical way to assess competency. Who should be responsible for deeming another 'competent', and at what point is someone competent? The activities, techniques and procedures that scientists perform on animals may include veterinary procedures and, even though researchers working with wildlife are not necessarily veterinarians, they may be skilled physiologists, or zoologists trained in particular techniques. Many veterinarians without specialised training and skills in wildlife and research would perhaps be no more competent than an experienced researcher who has performed the procedure many times.

To adhere to the 3Rs, maintain scientific rigour and replicability, and ensure high animal welfare standards, wildlife should be handled only by suitably qualified and experienced personnel, or under their direct supervision. While 'competency' can be difficult to reconcile, institutions, in consultation with their AEC, must implement a competency assessment framework. For institutions, this framework is perhaps best addressed by providing clear policy around this requirement. In some instances, competency determination is undertaken by colleagues (i.e. referees) and provided to the AEC. However, a researcher's peers may overlook or not recognise unethical practices, which may be disseminated within research groups, and may be affected by a conflict of interest. A defined framework would increase AEC confidence that researchers are competent to perform proposed procedures involving animals. The framework should identify requirements for training, oversight and competency determination of inexperienced researchers and accommodate refresher courses for experienced persons. Ultimately the research institution must have confidence that an experienced researcher will maintain best practice standards which could be informed by an up-to-date and referenced standard operating procedure.

AEC members must also develop and maintain competency in their ability to assess research applications, and provide constructive feedback. It may be beyond the knowledge capacity of an AEC to ascertain an applicant's competence in some techniques and species-specific interventions. Inviting the applicant to meet with the AEC may help in these situations. Institutions should support AEC members attending relevant conferences and training as these events can provide exposure to best practice and cutting-edge research methods This also helps AEC members to understand the constraints and challenges that wildlife researchers contend with. Regulatory authorities could also share examples of best practice research with their registered approval holders, including adopting or developing their own comprehensive examples of best practice methods and competencies (see Section 2).

TEACHING USING ANIMALS

The Code also encompasses the use of animals for teaching and education activities that have a scientific aim or purpose consistent with curriculum or competency requirements (teaching using animals is covered in Chapter 10). Use of animals (including wildlife) for teaching and education purposes is subject to the same guiding principles as research (outlined in section 1 of the Code). Notably, animals should only be used for teaching where their use is essential to achieve a science education outcome and where suitable alternatives are unavailable. The use of wildlife in teaching can range from relatively low-impact, observation activities to high-impact work involving wild-animal handling (a common practice in some science-focused tertiary courses). This concept can become confusing for individuals seeking to undertake community engagement-type work with an educational focus, but which is not linked directly to a curriculum or competency (e.g. community events that involve spotlighting for animals, or observations of animal handling or trapping procedures). Specific requirements for undertaking any activities involving animals can be directed by the governing institution and AEC in compliance with the Code and relevant state legislation. Potential applicants are well advised to seek guidance from an AEC and obtain approval and advice in writing that are unequivocal and unambiguous.

ACKNOWLEDGEMENTS

Thank you to Damian S. Morrant and Jane DeGabriel for providing feedback on early versions of this chapter.

REFERENCES

ARRP (2020) Wildlife Research, <https://www.animalethics.org.au/policies-and-guidelines/wildlife-research>.

Bino G, Kingsford RT, Archer M, Connolly JH, Day J, Dias K, Goldney D, Gongora J, Grant T, Griffiths J, Hawke T, Klamt M, Lunney D, Mijangos L, Munks S, Sherwin W, Serena M, Temple-Smith P, Thomas J, Williams G, Whittington C (2019) The platypus: evolutionary history, biology, and an uncertain future. *Journal of Mammalogy* **100**, 308–327. doi:10.1093/jmammal/gyz058

Donaldson S, Kymlicka W (2011) *Zoopolis. A Political Theory of Animal Rights.* Oxford University Press, New York, NY.

Driscoll DA, Garrard GE, Kusmanoff AM, Dovers S, Maron M, Preece N, Pressey RL, Ritchie EG (2021) Consequences of information suppression in ecological and conservation sciences. *Conservation Letters.* doi:10.1111/conl.12757

Field KA, Paquet PC, Artelle K, Proulx G, Brook RK, Darimont CT (2019) Publication reform to safeguard wildlife from researcher harm. *PLoS Biology* **17**, e3000193. doi:10.1371/journal.pbio.3000193

Garlapati D, Charankumar B, Ramu K (2019) A review on the applications and recent advances in environmental DNA (eDNA) metagenomics. *Reviews in Environmental Science and Biotechnology* **18**, 389–411. doi:10.1007/s11157-019-09501-4

Green M, Althaus F, Williams A, Untiedt C (2019) Using complimentary imagery and targeted sampling to address 'Reduction, Replacement and Refinement' of scientific animal use: Two examples in a marine context. Annual ANZCCART Conference Proceedings: Breaking Down Laboratory Walls. 2019 Hobart, Tasmania, Australia.

Hampton JO, Hyndman TH, Laurence M, Perry AL, Adams P, Collins T (2016) Animal welfare and the use of procedural documents: limitations and refinement. *Wildlife Research* **43**, 599–603. doi:10.1071/WR16153

Herbert CA, Hutchings P, Law B, Spencer R, Predavec M (Eds) (2020) New approaches to zoology. Theme edition of *Australian Zoologist* **40**, 363–513.

Hogg CJ, Fox S, Pemberton D, Belov K (Eds) (2019) *Saving the Tasmanian Devil: Recovery through Science-based Management.* CSIRO Publishing, Melbourne.

Jones GP, Pearlstine LG, Percival HF (2006) An assessment of small unmanned aerial vehicles for wildlife research. *Wildlife Society Bulletin* **34**, 750–758. doi:10.2193/0091-7648(2006)34[750:AAOSUA]2.0.CO;2

Kilkenny C, Browne WJ, Cuthill IC, Emerson M, Altman DG (2010) Improving bioscience research reporting: the ARRIVE guidelines for reporting animal research. *PLoS Biology* **8**, e1000412. doi:10.1371/journal.pbio.1000412

Lindenmayer D (2018) Why is long-term ecological research and monitoring so hard to do? (And what can be done about it). *Australian Zoologist* **39**, 576–580. doi:10.7882/AZ.2017.018

Lindsjö J, Fahlman A, Törnqvist E (2016) Animal welfare from mouse to moose – implementing the principles of the 3Rs in wildlife research. *Journal of Wildlife Diseases* **52**, S65–S77. doi:10.7589/52.2S.S65

Lunney D (1998) The ethical zoologist. In *Ethics, Money and Politics: Modern Dilemmas for Zoology* (Eds D Lunney and T Dawson) pp. 57–61. Royal Zoological Society of New South Wales, Mosman.

Lunney D (2012a) Ethics and Australian mammalogy: reflections on 15 years on an animal ethics committee. *Australian Mammalogy* **34**, 1–17. doi:10.1071/AM10010

Lunney D (2012b) Wildlife management and the debate on the ethics of animal use. I Decisions within a state wildlife agency. *Pacific Conservation Biology* **18**, 5–21. doi:10.1071/PC120005

Lunney D (2019) Can a critical reading of *Zoopolis* by Donaldson and Kymlicka lead to advocating dialogue between animal rights theorists and zoologists? *Pacific Conservation Biology* **25**, 72–91. doi:10.1071/PC17052

Lunney D, Dickman CR, Predavec M (2018) The critical value of long-term field studies and datasets: an editorial perspective. *Australian Zoologist* **39**, 559–567. doi:10.7882/AZ.2018.045

McMahon CR, Hindell MA, Harcourt RG (2012) Publish or perish: why it's important to publicise how, and if, research activities affect animals. *Wildlife Research* **39**, 375–377. doi:10.1071/WR12014

Monamy V, Gott M (2001) Practical and ethical considerations for students conducting ecological research involving wildlife. *Austral Ecology* **26**, 293–300. doi:10.1046/j.1442-9993.2001.01111.x

Naughtin M, Alston-Knox C (2019) Sample size in animal studies. Is the justification good enough? Annual ANZCCART Conference Proceedings: Breaking Down Laboratory Walls. 2019 Hobart, Tasmania, Australia.

NHMRC (National Health and Medical Research Council) (1997) *Australian Code of Practice for the Care and Use of Animals for Scientific Purposes.* 6th edn. Australian Government Publishing Service, Canberra.

NHMRC (National Health and Medical Research Council) (2013) *Australian Code for the Care and Use of Animals for Scientific Purposes.* 8th edn. National Health and Medical Research Council, Canberra.

NHMRC (National Health and Medical Research Council) (2014) *A Guide to the Care and Use of Australian Native Mammals in Research and Teaching.* National Health and Medical Research Council, Canberra.

NHMRC (National Health and Medical Research Council) (2017) *Best Practice Methodology in the Use of Animals for Scientific Purposes.* National Health and Medical Research Council, Canberra.

NHMRC (National Health and Medical Research Council) (2018) *Australian Code for the Responsible Conduct of Research.* National Health and Medical Research Council, Canberra.

Osborne N, Avey MT, Anestidou L, Ritskes-Hoitinga M, Griffin G (2018) Improving animal research reporting standards. *EMBO Rep* **19**, e46069. doi:10.15252/embr.201846069

Paul E, Sikes RS, Beaupre SJ, Wingfield JC (2016) Animal welfare policy: implementation in the context of wildlife research – policy review and discussion of fundamental issues. *ILAR Journal* **56**, 312–334. doi:10.1093/ilar/ilv073

Percie du Sert N, Hurst V, Ahluwalia A (2020) The ARRIVE guidelines 2.0: updated guidelines for reporting animal research. *BMJ Open Science* **4**, e100115. doi:10.1136/bmjos-2020-100115

Rose M (1998) Ethical dilemmas and imperatives in a changing animal welfare mandate. In *Ethics, Money and Politics: Modern Dilemmas for Zoology*. (Eds D Lunney and T Dawson) pp. 26–31. Royal Zoological Society of New South Wales, Mosman.

Russell WMS, Burch RL (1959) *The Principles of Humane Experimental Technique*. Methuen, London.

Schnell I, Sollmann R, Calvignac-Spencer S, Siddall M, Yu D, Wilting A, Gilbert T (2015) iDNA from terrestrial haematophagous leeches as a wildlife surveying and monitoring tool – prospects, pitfalls and avenues to be developed. *Frontiers in Zoology* **12**, 24. doi:10.1186/s12983-015-0115-z

Schuppl CA, Fraser D (2005) The interpretation and application of the three Rs by animal ethics committee members. *Alternatives to Laboratory Animals* **33**, 487–500. doi:10.1177/026119290503300511

Sikes RS, Animal Care and Use Committee of the American Society of Mammalogists (2016) 2016 guidelines of the American Society of Mammalogists for the use of wild animals in research and education. *Journal of Mammalogy* **97**, 663–688. doi:10.1093/jmammal/gyw078

Soulsbury C, Gray H, Smith L (2020) The welfare and ethics of research involving wild animals: a primer. *Methods in Ecology and Evolution* **11**, 1164–1181. doi:10.1111/2041-210X.13435

Spencer R-J (2018) How much long-term data are required to effectively manage a widespread freshwater turtle? *Australian Zoologist* **39**, 568–575. doi:10.7882/AZ.2018.017

Steidl R, Hayes J, Schauber E (1997) Statistical power analysis in wildlife research. *The Journal of Wildlife Management* **61**, 270–279. doi:10.2307/3802582

Timoshanko AC, Marston H, Lidbury BA (2016) Australian regulation of animal use in science and education: a critical appraisal. *ILAR Journal* **57**, 324–332. doi:10.1093/ilar/ilw015

Waudby HP, Petit S, Gill MJ (2019) The scientific, financial and ethical implications of three common wildlife-trapping designs. *Wildlife Research* **46**, 690–700. doi:10.1071/WR19084

Whittaker A (2016) Animal research regulation in Australia – does it pass the test of robustness? *Global Journal of Animal Law* **(1)**. <https://ojs.abo.fi/ojs/index.php/gjal/article/view/1305>.

Zemanova MA (2020) Towards more compassionate wildlife research through the 3Rs principles: moving from invasive to non-invasive methods. *Wildlife Biology* **2020**. doi:10.2981/wlb.00607

2 Animal ethics committees

Corinne Alberthsen, Helen P. Waudby, Leanne L. Wilkinson, Daniel Lunney, Megan Bathurst and Bradley P. Smith

INTRODUCTION

Animal ethics committees (AECs) are established under the Australian Code for the Care and Use of Animals for Scientific Purposes (the Code) and under state and territory legislation (see Chapter 1). Effectively, an AEC is a regulatory and compliance body that oversees research and teaching activities that involve living non-human animals (see Chapters 1 and 3 for a discussion of management versus research activities). The review process undertaken by an AEC is intended to ensure that research and teaching using animals is ethically acceptable for the anticipated scientific or educational gains, that researchers and teachers are accountable for the potential animal welfare impacts of their activities involving animals, and that research and teaching is undertaken in line with the Code and organisational policies. Historically, most AECs (which were largely established in the early 1990s) focused on laboratory research (Lunney 2012). However, AECs now oversee a range of research activities, including in the areas of agriculture, ecology, field-based studies and natural-resource management that are carried out by universities, hospitals, government and not-for-profit practitioners, and environmental consultants.

Wildlife research is a specialised and nuanced science, the understanding and assessment of which will be influenced by individual values and attitudes. Even if focused on conservation outcomes, wildlife research can be controversial within the broader community and media (Lunney 2012). AEC oversight imparts a level of assurance for wildlife researchers, institutions and the community by providing an independent evaluation of the ethical aspects of animal research. Successful researcher–AEC relationships and outcomes are characterised by skilled, patient communication by applicants of their research message and well-informed, considered assessment of applications by AEC members of all categories (see below for discussion of membership categories).

THE ROLE OF ANIMAL ETHICS COMMITTEES

AECs, the Code, and state and territory legislation (Chapter 1) are the key pillars of the animal ethics framework in Australia. The Code specifies the role of AECs in regulating the ethical use of animals for scientific purposes. An AEC's primary responsibility is 'to ensure, on behalf of the institution for which it acts, that all activities relating to the care and use of animals are conducted in compliance with the Code' (NHMRC 2013, p. 25). An AEC reviews and approves activities using animals, monitors the ongoing care and use of animals, acts on adverse events and non-compliance, provides advice and recommendations regarding the care and use of animals, approves guidelines for the care and use of animals, and reports to their institution on AEC operations (NHMRC 2013).

Organisations with an AEC must establish publicly available terms of reference that describe the purpose, composition, authority and accountability of the AEC (Chapter 1) (NHMRC 2013). While the broad framework of AECs is dictated by the Code, institutional terms of reference allow for additional considerations that are not necessarily prescribed by the Code (Noonan and Williams 2008). A 'terms of reference' document provides an AEC with sufficient flexibility to operate effectively within its affiliated institution and to be shaped by the animal use activities that each committee may oversee. Terms of reference vary among institutions, but must be agreed to by all members of its AEC. It is also beneficial for employees involved in animal research to review their institutional AEC terms of reference to familiarise themselves with the committee's role and responsibilities. For example, a large university may operate multiple AECs, each with a different research focus (e.g. laboratory animals, wildlife, agricultural animals), whereas a smaller institution may have one committee that reviews applications for a variety of animal uses. AEC operating procedures provide further operational detail and an agreed framework about how AEC meetings are conducted; guidance for decision-making and monitoring approved research, records maintenance and reporting obligations; powers of executive subcommittees; conflict resolution; managing breeches or non-compliance; and quorum management (Noonan and Williams 2018). Operating procedures may be incorporated into, or separate from, the AEC terms of reference.

Historically, cultural considerations around animal welfare and wildlife research for Indigenous Australians have not been well considered in the Code or legislation, and are not currently included in animal welfare legislation. However, the development of terms of reference and operational guidelines provides an opportunity for AECs to incorporate cultural values and heritage into their decision-making. Doing so could help institutions and wildlife researchers achieve more scientifically robust (i.e. in the case of projects that are supported by traditional ecological knowledge), holistic, relevant and culturally appropriate research outcomes.

The Code criteria for AEC membership may result in most members being external to and independent of the institution. Importantly, an AEC must operate without undue influence of internal members or manipulation from within the institution (NHMRC 2013). As facilitators of ethical research and compliance with the Code, AECs define ethical 'boundaries' and help to ensure that researchers and their institutions are accountable. Committees must be well supported (administratively and financially) by their associated institution to undertake their duties effectively (NHMRC 2013). Institutions can provide support to their AEC through the employment of specialist administrators, advisors and animal welfare officers. This support is critical for the AEC to adhere to the obligations of the Code, maintain familiarity with the requirements of wildlife research and management, and ensure the best welfare outcomes for animals.

The principles of transparency and accountability in decision-making and animal use defined in the Code are intended to achieve positive animal welfare outcomes. Consequently, the performance of AECs is evaluated against these principles (Varga 2013). The Code requires institutions to review AEC operations annually via internal processes, and to organise an independent external review every 4 years. The oversight and evaluation of an AEC is especially important to the ethical review process to ensure the responsibilities set out in the Code are being met and provides assurance that the accredited organisation, through its AEC, is delivering effective oversight of the care and use of the animals in teaching and research.

ANIMAL ETHICS COMMITTEE MEMBERS

Membership of AECs is defined by the Code (Section 2.2.4). Table 2.1 reviews the categories of members that must be included, criteria for appointment and the nature of their roles. Membership should reflect a diversity of gender, age and cultural perspectives. However, recruiting and retaining members can prove difficult for institutions, as membership requires substantial time commitment for training, meeting preparation and attendance, out-of-session requests, monitoring animal-holding facilities and inspecting procedures involving animals (sometimes at remote field sites where wildlife research occurs). Membership is voluntary; however, members external to the institution are often reimbursed for expenses incurred for participation or provided with an honorarium for their service (e.g. sitting fees). While the provision of these benefits is common practice, it is not mandatory.

Whether justified or not, each category of membership can attract specific criticism from applicants seeking AEC approval to use animals. Researchers may consider category A (veterinarians) to be unqualified to assess wildlife research applications if they have no personal

Table 2.1: Key AEC committee membership categories and their roles.

Category	Description	Required	Comments
Chairperson	Impartially guides the operation of the AEC. Can meet any of the category criteria (e.g. veterinarian or researcher), but must be an appointed AEC member with equal voting rights (but not a casting vote).	Required	Usually a person who holds a senior position in the institution but can be an external person. The Code encourages the appointment of a chairperson who is 'independent of the care and use of animals for scientific purposes' (NHMRC 2013, p. 20).
Secretary	An institutionally appointed position; facilitates the AEC's administrative requirements.	Not required	Most institutions provide a secretary as part of the Code's requirement to 'ensure and support the effective operation of the AEC'. Although not mandatory, it is a highly valuable (also impartial) role. The secretary is not an appointed voting member.
A	A veterinarian.	Required	Must be eligible for registration as a veterinary surgeon in Australia (do not have to be currently registered). It is recommended that category A members either have experience relevant to the institution's animal research or teaching activities, or the ability to 'acquire relevant knowledge' to advise the committee.
B	A person with a higher research degree and experience in animal use for scientific purposes.	Required	Often a scientist employed by the governing institution, although may be external to the institution. This member can also be a qualified and experienced teacher if the sole business of the AEC 'relates to the use of animals for teaching'.
C	A person with a demonstrable commitment to animal welfare.	Required*	A category C member cannot be employed by or associated with the institution and must not be involved in the care and use of animals for scientific purposes. The Code recommends that this person be endorsed by an animal welfare organisation.
D	A lay member (or member of the wider community).	Required*	An independent representative of the broader community who 'must not fit the requirements of any other category'. The incumbent must have no background in the care and use of animals for scientific purposes (the only exception being experience gained during undergraduate studies).
Animal care staff	An institutional animal care person. Unofficially referred to as category E members (i.e. animal facility manager).	Only required in South Australia	Institutional animal care staff are only required to be included when the research is undertaken in South Australia. However, the Code recommends that all AEC include animal care staff on the committee.
Advisor	Any person with experience and knowledge deemed relevant and useful to the committee.	Not required	Examples of advisors are the institutional chief veterinary officer, animal welfare officer, or statistician. Advisors are not voting members but can provide valuable advice and assistance to the AEC.

* The Code requires that one-third of an AEC's constituted membership, and sitting members at any meeting where decisions are made, comprises category C and D members.

research or veterinary experience with the study species. Category B (researchers) can come under fire for perceived bias towards achieving research outcomes. Category C (animal welfare) and D (layperson) members are criticised because of an assumption that they are not suitably knowledgeable or qualified to evaluate the scientific value of a project against the use of animals (Tidemann and Vardon 2002; Whittaker 2016; Timoshanko *et al.* 2016). The validity of category-targeted criticism is difficult to substantiate given that votes within an AEC are confidential and AEC decisions are generally (and should be) arrived at by consensus. Applicants can assist all committee members to gain a greater understanding of the value of the research, and how potential animal welfare issues have been addressed or mitigated, by writing comprehensive applications (effectively treating the process as a science communication exercise) in plain English, avoiding or explaining jargon as appropriate. Indeed, it is both the challenge and responsibility of researchers to convince all categories of AEC membership of the worthiness of their animal research proposals, regardless of the scientific discipline and species involved.

Poorly written applications are a source of major frustration and wasted time for applicants and the AEC. Strong applications help all members to evaluate proposals objectively and efficiently, and voice questions or concerns in an informed way. Category C and D members help build accountability to the broader community into the review process – these members are intended to reflect current community values and expectations. This consideration is particularly important for demonstrating accountability in research, which is often supported by taxpayer's funds. Similarly, free-living wildlife is the property of the Crown, and communities are stakeholders in nature, including how wildlife is used and conserved across all jurisdictions. Consequently, a researcher needs a scientific licence or permit to hold or harm a native animal (as opposed to non-native laboratory animals, mostly rodents, that are purchased or bred for research by an institution or individual). The need for a licence to catch, hold, study or kill a native animal affords additional responsibilities and a duty of care by wildlife researchers. Evaluations of methods and therapeutics specific to wildlife research often require specialist knowledge. Wildlife veterinarians and animal welfare officers can assist when other AEC members have queries about these techniques. Consequently, institutions involved in wildlife research should engage category A (veterinarian) members with specific training and experience in wildlife veterinary medicine (Field *et al.* 2019).

Statistical justification for the number of animals used in research can be difficult for wildlife researchers to quantify, particularly where research is qualitative, constitutes a pilot study, or focuses on general surveys or inventories of animals (particularly for surveys or monitoring when the intent is to evaluate animal numbers and species present). Also, statistical expertise may be lacking in all AEC membership categories, making it difficult for individual members to assess and evaluate whether requested animal numbers are reasonable (Schuppli and Fraser 2005). This issue is important because a sample size that is too small to answer the research question is associated with as many welfare repercussions as one that is large, without delivery of optimal scientific outcomes. Biostatisticians or veterinary epidemiologists are not required member categories under the Code, but can be appointed to AECs as advisory members. Advisors are non-voting members who can support committee decision-making with specialist knowledge and experience, and may include animal welfare officers, research institute managers, ethics specialists, animal law professionals, veterinary epidemiologists, population geneticists and environmental managers (Table 2.1).

CRAFTING ANIMAL ETHICS APPLICATIONS (FOR RESEARCHERS)

The ethical review process is a fundamental step in wildlife research. Preparing ethics applications presents an opportunity to review and consider the justification of the study, and the methods to be used. Writing comprehensive and objective animal ethics applications is a valuable professional skill akin to science communication. Crafting a concise, considered and thorough application reduces workloads for all parties and streamlines the review process. Considerations for researchers in writing a clearly articulated and justified ethics application are detailed in Table 2.2.

Animal welfare must be considered and monitored during all steps of the study, including the end point and in response to unexpected events that escalate welfare impacts. Applicants should have clear contingency plans and mitigation options which consider the level of likely impact for these potential events (see Figure 2.1). Contingency plans should address:

- when veterinary assistance is appropriate
- how practical and accessible emergency veterinary care is
- when euthanasia *in situ* is appropriate to prevent unreasonable or unnecessary suffering, specifying investigators with the training, skill and willingness to kill an animal
- the likelihood of welfare impacts escalating
- possible unintended outcomes.

Applicants can consider approaching their AEC to request attendance at a meeting as an observer or volunteer to serve as a committee member. Doing so is particularly useful to help wildlife researchers understand how the committee operates, but also to gain an appreciation of the difficulties and complexities of the review

Table 2.2: Key considerations for crafting ethics applications.

Considerations	Details
Writing style	• Focus on readability and plain English – pitch the application to an audience that is informed, but does not have a scientific background (a requirement of the Code). Check that applications are legible. • Clearly and concisely state the aims of the project from the outset. The application should explain why the project has scientific or educational merit, and why animal use is essential to achieve the stated aims. Animal numbers must be justified. • Do not 'cut and paste' large sections of writing from a successful grant application; while this information might demonstrate the merit of the science, an AEC is primarily interested in animal welfare. Great quantities of detail are neither necessary nor welcome. This applies particularly to the plain English summary.
Application quality	• AECs have a pro forma to guide applicants. Ignoring or not completing all sections comprehensively will result in delays. • Access and submit only current application forms. Ensure contact information is up to date and all sections are properly completed. • Ideally, have subject-matter experts review applications before submission, to ensure readability and reduce the chance of errors. Avoid grammatical and copy-and-paste errors, which risk confusion and slow the approval process. • Do not submit rushed, incomplete or poorly written applications. AECs will rightly reject or seek additional information if applications are incomplete, increasing workload and frustration for all.
Level of detail	• Do the work for the reader. Define each step methodically – time lines and flow charts are invaluable when multiple procedures are proposed in one application. Increase clarity by adding well-justified numbers (including calculations) and photographs where appropriate. AECs review numerous applications at every meeting; removing ambiguity makes the process more efficient, will be appreciated by AEC members and will speed the review process. • Define acronyms and complex terminology (if it must be used). Provide detailed information about equipment (e.g. photographs and descriptions of trap design with explanation about how they work) and materials (e.g. needle gauges, medication dosages and volumes, disinfectants), clear end points (i.e. what happens to animals at the end of the study), and plans for ensuring animal welfare and dealing with emergencies.
Methods	• When detailing methods, focus on what happens to the animals at every stage of the project. • If the AEC has approved operating procedures for commonly used techniques, reference them clearly to avoid repetition or confusion. • Do not assume that because a method is common practice, or it has been approved or undertaken in the past, it will be approved again. All methods must be justified (e.g. with references) in the context of the proposal under consideration. • Develop and/or cite AEC-approved standard operating procedures for methods that are regularly used to reduce the detail and repetition in applications.
Supporting documentation	• Use tables, schematics, visual time lines and photographs wherever possible to support text and explain techniques. • Provide supporting documentation to demonstrate competencies of investigators, including training and assessment plans if training is required. • Clear monitoring sheets with appropriate intervention and end points.
General tips	• Read and adopt (where appropriate) the available AEC policies. • Seek advice: many institutions have ethics advisors on staff who provide pre-reviews, policy guidance, document and expertise referral, and a wealth of corporate knowledge from working within the system. • Remember that it is within the remit of an AEC to ask questions of applicants. It is not unusual for applications to have approval declined until further information is provided. Try not to take these situations personally. View the ethics approval process as peer review and part of the path to publication rather than a bureaucratic impediment to doing research. • Transparency is critical. Do not ignore factors that are out of researcher's control and may cause unexpected or adverse events – acknowledge them and provide a contingency plan if possible. • Questions from AECs are not unusual even when proposals are well articulated. Address these respectfully and thoroughly.

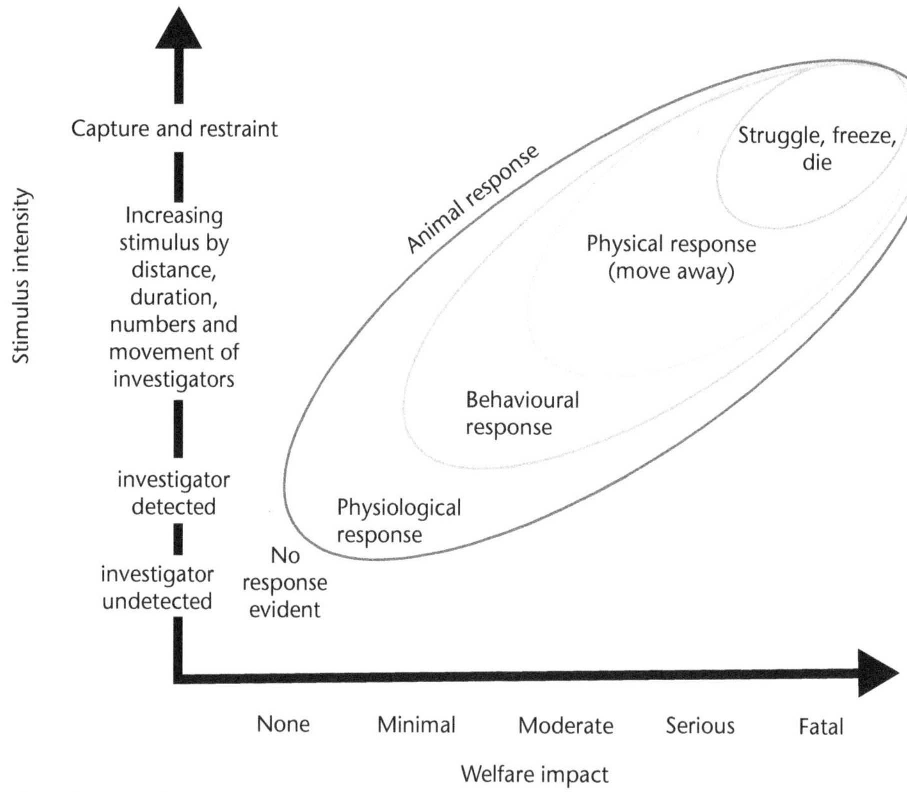

Figure 2.1: Overview of potential impacts of investigator disturbance, animal response and potential welfare impacts (modified from Wilson *et al.* 2020). Illustration by John Porter.

process. Applicants can also request to present proposals or techniques to the AEC, including bringing equipment for AEC members to view and inspect. This step can be particularly helpful where researchers are considering novel methods that could be controversial and might be difficult to explain sufficiently in an application.

REVIEWING ANIMAL ETHICS APPLICATIONS (FOR AEC MEMBERS)

Wildlife research, particularly field-based studies, generally encompasses unpredictable or uncontrollable variables, and diverse study environments and species. In a regulatory framework founded on laboratory-based studies, it is unsurprising that AEC processes and member experiences do not always align well with the needs of wildlife researchers. AEC members may not have the experience to evaluate field-based studies objectively or comprehensively (Field *et al.* 2019). Consequently, studies that do not incorporate adequate welfare measures may be approved, or conversely, an AEC may delay, or reject work or methods that would provide valuable knowledge (Tidemann and Vardon 2002).

Committee members should be open to new concepts and willing to seek advice on applications when they are unsure of proposed objectives or methods. Maintaining a level of humility is advisable, both for members and applicants. AEC members require ongoing training, and training resources and information are available to support them. The Australian and New Zealand Council for the Care of Animals in Research and Teaching (ANZCCART) provides support and advice to AEC members, including an information package that explains the roles, responsibilities and workings of an AEC (ANZCCART 2018). In addition, ANZCCART has released a series of online training modules for all animal users (ComPass, https://anzccart.adelaide.edu.au/compass). Reviewing applications thoroughly, consistently, and fairly takes experience and is influenced by the culture within each committee. Consistency and fairness in decision making is critical and supports principles of transparency and accountability. Table 2.3 provides recommendations for the operation of AEC and the review of applications.

Table 2.3: Key considerations for improved decision making by an AEC.

Embrace technology	Committee culture	Low-impact options	Processes
• Online application and data management processes, where members can review applications and submit comments and concerns before meetings, increase the efficiency of meetings, and supports more-robust discussions. • Provide in person and virtual training opportunities for researchers and committee members. • The rise of virtual meetings, as a result of COVID-19, has demonstrated the usefulness of such approaches. They support increased attendance by members and appointment of members from different geographical locations, although internet connectivity can be an issue for some members. • Online meetings and electronic application processes also benefit institutions by reducing expenditure (e.g. no catering, parking, travel expenses for members attending meetings in person; no printing and postage costs associated with hardcopy agenda packs). The resulting cost savings for institutions should be directed to member education and researcher training.	• The institutional executive should establish clear expectations regarding member roles and behaviour. Senior executives should openly and publicly demonstrate their support and commitment to the AEC process and give public recognition for the time, commitment and expertise of the AEC members. • Committees should develop a cooperative culture where members are encouraged to assist applicants to achieve the best animal welfare outcomes. • Unless there is evidence to the contrary, committee members should place some level of trust in applicants and understand that they also strive for positive animal welfare outcomes. • All committee members should be encouraged to question applications and share their views. In particular, the Chair and other members should ensure that category C and D members are not alienated or intimidated by category A and B members who may have a better understanding of the scientific nuances of a particular project (Schuppli and Fraser 2005). Conversely, less-experienced members should be open to the knowledge of more-experienced members. • Some AECs with a high number of applications delegate review to a subset of members who then speak to the application and brief others at the meeting when it is assessed. This practice is not ideal as it risks diminishing the objectivity of the ethical review system for perceived gains in administrative efficiency. However, the advantage of a member, or a subset of members, undertaking a review before the meeting is that the member can ask the applicant to clarify points that may be clear to the applicant, but would be obscure in an AEC meeting. That not only saves time, but also avoids frustration in a meeting when the subject matter, the species, or the methods are too brief or little-known. Regardless, all AEC members should have access to and the ability to read and comment on all applications.	• Developing options for expedited approval process for low-risk, low-interaction and low to nil impact projects is prudent. • Providing an abbreviated application process for projects with low or negligible impacts reduces workload for both applicants and the committee and encourages the implementation of such techniques.	• Develop systems for ensuring that questions and comments from the AEC are concise and targeted before the AEC secretary passes them on to applicants. • Encourage the development of standardised procedural documents that are reviewed and approved by the committee for commonly used techniques. • If possible, provide opportunities for researchers to mentor other researchers, and the ability to have application drafts reviewed before submission. • Committees should develop an agreed stance or policy on potentially contentious issues. These views must be reviewed frequently to ensure alignment with current best practice, new knowledge and shifting community values. Policies should be unambiguous and made readily available to applicants. • Focus on animal welfare considerations when assessing applications. If an application has an issue relating to bureaucratic process that does not affect welfare of animals, this issue can be noted, but should not affect the approval process *per se*.

ONGOING MANAGEMENT OF APPROVED PROJECTS

Under the Code, institutions licensed to undertake animal research activities must establish institutional processes and procedures to facilitate the animal ethics approval and review process. Once AEC approval is granted (and additional permit and approval requirements are met – discussed in Chapter 1), work with animals may commence. However, interaction with the AEC does not end at this point. Ongoing oversight and management of projects are required, with any changes to the approved protocol submitted to the approving AEC as amendments or modifications. Additionally, annual and final reports must be lodged with the approving AEC, and adverse events reported as soon as reasonably possible, and in line with institutional requirements. The institutional secretariat usually provides guidance on expected reporting timelines for a range of scenarios.

Amendments

Research is rarely linear, and the ethics application process often requires applicants to make educated assumptions about how projects will progress and develop, especially for complex or long-term projects. Amendment or modification of approved applications provides flexibility for investigators to achieve improved scientific or animal welfare outcomes (Jones *et al.* 2012). Amendment requests must be evaluated and approved by the original approving AEC. Amendments can include, for example, changes to personnel participating in the project, therapeutic administration, equipment, animal numbers, study sites, or the addition of an entirely new experiment linked to the overall aims of the original application. Differentiating between an amendment to an existing project and a new project can be difficult. If a proposed change to an existing project is clearly linked to the original aim, then it should reasonably be considered an amendment. However, an entirely new line of enquiry that is tenuously linked to an original aim should be considered a new project requiring separate ethical review. Researchers occasionally labour under the erroneous assumption that amendments require less work than a new protocol but amendments must be subject to the same scrutiny as new protocols.

Applicants should not assume that the AEC will remember details of the original project or have re-read the original application. Ideally, the amended submission should include the original application with tracked changes or other version control methods. Amendments should explain which protocols have already been approved and the proposed changes. Amendments can be numerous over the course of a project (but some AECs set limits such as a maximum of three) so it is critical that any personnel named on the project are familiar with not only the original application, but also with all other additions, changes, reports and correspondence. A word of caution for applicants applying for numerous amendments – doing so can create an impression, particularly among AEC members who are not versed in the mutable nature of scientific research, that the project is poorly planned and executed.

Unexpected and important research opportunities may occasionally occur in the field where it is impossible to contact the AEC for approval. An example of this is a fauna survey when an unknown or threatened species is trapped in an area where it was not thought to exist. An example is the accidental rediscovery of the Gilbert's potoroo (*Potorous tridactyylus*) in Western Australia during a study targeting quokkas (*Setonix brachyurus*) (Sinclair *et al.* 1996). A researcher may decide that opportunistically recording data about that species using low-impact techniques is critical to inform further study and conservation outcomes. Researchers should familiarise themselves with their state, territory and institutional policies on opportunistic research before commencing their approved fieldwork.

Reporting

Animal use reports are required at least annually, when renewal of AEC approval is sought, at the completion or termination (for any reason) of a project and at any other time commensurate with the approving AEC's requirements (usually dependent on the AEC's assessment of the project's animal welfare impact or other risks). Reports detail the numbers of animals used, and any issues, successes and progress of the research. While much of this information must be reported under the requirements of the Code, providing comprehensive reports is valuable for informing and educating the AEC, particularly for long-term projects. Typically, AEC members are dedicated and committed individuals, who put considerable effort into the evaluation process and they are genuinely interested in supporting research objectives. Seeing the outcomes, publications and other information from approved projects (e.g. photographs and videos of field sites) is rewarding and provides the approving AEC with an additional level of assurance that research being undertaken under their remit is achieving credible scientific and conservation outcomes.

Researchers are well advised to understand and adhere to all reporting obligations (including adverse events – see below) to avoid charges of non-compliance with their AEC approval and potential disciplinary action by their institution or statutory regulator. Accredited institutions must establish procedures for documenting, managing and reporting instances of non-compliance with AEC approvals. Consequences for non-compliance with the Code or governing legislation are serious and can result in far reaching implications including legal penalties.

Adverse events

An adverse event is an unexpected event (i.e. an outcome that is not foreseen and approved in the original application) that has a negative impact on animal wellbeing (NHMRC 2013; Hampton *et al.* 2019). Under the Code, adverse events must be reported to the approving AEC as soon as reasonably possible. Examples of adverse events provided in the Code include the unexpected death of an animal or group of animals, negative unanticipated effects following a procedure or treatment, adverse effects in a larger number of animals than predicted during the planning of the research (based on number used), a greater level of pain or distress than was predicted during the planning of the project, equipment failure or malfunction, and emergency situations or accidents (Jones *et al.* 2012; Hampton *et al.* 2020).

In animal research, adverse events occur even when researchers follow good practices and maintain high welfare standards. For example, trap-related deaths may occur in field-based wildlife research where large numbers of animals are trapped, and when factors such as weather and predator occurrence are difficult to control. Researchers must refine and review their methods and equipment to minimise negative effects on study animals (Putman 1995; Powell and Proulx 2003), but doing so requires honest evaluations of adverse events, including mortality. Honestly reporting mortality rates for capture programs assists other researchers to improve welfare standards for study animals (e.g. identifying methods that 'don't work'), and provides the approving AEC with context for their evaluations and decision-making (e.g. realistic expectations for adverse event frequency, which is rarely zero) (Waudby *et al.* 2019). Some events, which would be regarded by some AEC members as adverse, can be expected. For example, the male *Antechinus* species die-off post-mating is a documented biological phenomenon (Wilson and Bourne 1984). When trapping is undertaken near the beginning of the *Antechinus* breeding season, male deaths in traps can be expected. These situations should not be regarded as adverse events, and applicants should foreshadow in the original application that some animals will die in traps due to species-specific considerations. This concept can be applied more widely, especially during climate extremes or following drastic habitat disturbance, where old, weak and sick animals will die, regardless of the care that is exercised by the researcher.

ACKNOWLEDGEMENTS

Thank you to Dr Damian S. Morrant and Dr Jane DeGabriel for providing feedback on early versions of this chapter and to the University of Queensland Animal Ethic Committee – Native/Exotic Wildlife and Marine Animals (UQ AEC – NEWMA) for generously allowing attendance and observation of committee meetings. Thank you also to Dr John Porter and Dr Jennifer Spencer for allowing us to use the modified diagram depicted in Figure 2.1.

REFERENCES

ANZCCART (2018) Information package for members of animal ethics committees. University of Adelaide, South Australia. <https://anzccart.adelaide.edu.au/system/files/media/documents/2019-07/aec-induction-package2018-9-1.pdf>.

Field KA, Paquet PC, Artelle K, Proulx G, Brook RK, Darimont CT (2019) Publication reform to safeguard wildlife from researcher harm. *PLoS Biology* **17**, e3000193. doi:10.1371/journal.pbio.3000193

Hampton JO, Amos M, Pople A, Brennan M, Forsyth DM (2020) Minimising mortalities in capturing wildlife: refinement of helicopter darting of chital deer (*Axis axis*) in Australia. *Wildlife Research.* doi:10.1071/WR20106

Hampton JO, MacKenzie DI, Forsyth DM (2019) How many to sample? Statistical guidelines for monitoring animal welfare outcomes. *PloS One* **14**, e0211417. doi:10.1371/journal.pone.0211417

Jones M, Hamede R, McCallum H, Banks P, Lunney D, Dickman C (2012) The devil is in the detail: conservation biology, animal philosophies and the role of animal ethics committees. In *Science Under Siege: Zoology Under Threat.* (Eds P Banks, D Lunney and C Dickman). Royal Zoological Society of New South Wales, Sydney.

Lunney D (2012) Ethics and Australian mammalogy: reflections on 15 years (1991–2006) on an animal ethics committee. *Australian Mammalogy* **34**, 1–17. doi:10.1071/AM10010

NHMRC (National Health and Medical Research Council) (2013) *Australian Code for the Care and Use of Animals for Scientific Purposes.* 8th edn. National Health and Medical Research Council, Canberra

Noonan D, Williams V (2018) Chapter 12 – Laboratory animals regulations and recommendations: Australia and New Zealand. In *Laboratory Animals*. 2nd edn. (Ed. J Guillén), Academic Press. doi:10.1016/B978-0-12-849880-4.00012-X

Powell RA, Proulx G (2003) Trapping and marking terrestrial mammals for research: integrating ethics, performance criteria, techniques, and common sense. *Institute for Laboratory Animal Research* **44**, 259–276. doi:10.1093/ilar.44.4.259

Putman RJ (1995) Ethical considerations and animal welfare in ecological field studies. *Biodiversity and Conservation* **4**, 903–915. doi:10.1007/BF00056197

Schuppli CA, Fraser D (2005) The interpretation and application of the Three Rs by animal ethics committee members. *Alternatives to Laboratory Animals* **33**, 487–500. doi:10.1177/026119290503300511

Sinclair EA, Danks A, Wayne AF (1996) Rediscovery of Gilbert's potoroo, *Potorous tridactylus*, in Western Australia. *Australian Mammalogy* **19**, 69–72.

Tidemann CR, Vardon MJ (2002) Animal welfare v wildlife research? *Pacific Conservation Biology* **8**, 71–72. doi:10.1071/PC020071

Timoshanko AC, Marston H, Lidbury BA (2016) Australian regulation of animal use in science and education: a critical appraisal. *ILAR Journal* **57**, 324–332. doi:10.1093/ilar/ilw015

Varga O (2013) Critical analysis of assessment studies of the animal ethics review process. *Animals (Basel)* **3**, 907–922. doi:10.3390/ani3030907

Waudby HP, Petit S, Gill MJ (2019) The scientific, financial and ethical implications of three common wildlife-trapping designs. *Wildlife Research* **46**, 690–700. doi:10.1071/WR19084

Wilson BA, Bourne AR (1984) Reproduction in the male dasyurid *Antechinus minimus maritimus* (Marsupialia: Dasyuridae). *Australian Journal of Zoology* **32**, 311–318.

Wilson MW, Ridlon AD, Gaynor KM, Gaines SD, Stier AC, Halpern BS (2020) Ecological impacts of human-induced animal behaviour change. *Ecology Letters* **23**, 1522–1536. doi:10.1111/ele.13571

3 Emerging and evolving dilemmas in wildlife research

Helen P. Waudby, Corinne Alberthsen, Daniel Lunney, Bradley P. Smith, Leanne L. Wilkinson, Jordan O. Hampton, Damian S. Morrant and Erin Roger

INTRODUCTION

The importance of wildlife research to the conservation and management of animals and their ecosystems is undeniable. However, the use of animals in wildlife research, like their use in other research fields (e.g. laboratory-based studies focused on medical research), is not without contention. For example, the efficacy and animal welfare impacts of marking methods such as toe clipping (see the discussion in Chapter 8) and branding, continue to be debated, sometimes to the point of halting conservation research (McMahon *et al.* 2006). Similarly, research on lethal animal control methods continue to be scrutinised intensely (see discussions in van Eeden *et al.* 2017, 2020) and are often the subject of traditional and social media interest (e.g. Pickering and Norman 2020). These aspects of wildlife research, and others, have been discussed relatively comprehensively elsewhere (e.g. McMahon *et al.* 2006; van Eeden *et al.* 2017, 2020). This chapter focuses on selected issues relevant to the decision making of animal ethics committees (AECs and wildlife researchers). Some are emerging issues (e.g. social media) that have received little attention to date and are not well explored in the literature.

Novel techniques, technologies, and modes of communicating and interacting (i.e. through social media) with global audiences create opportunities, but also challenges for wildlife researchers responsible for the welfare of their study animals. While the animal welfare impacts associated with some aspects of social media are of lesser veterinary concern than, for example, toe clipping, social media's influence on the way animals are used and portrayed in research is an issue with which researchers and AECs will have to become familiar. Similarly, technological advancements, including low- or nil-impact tools, such as camera traps, acoustic recorders and smartphone applications, have led to ambiguity around AEC and researcher evaluations of 'impact' and definitions of animal 'use', including whether they should be subject to AEC approval at all. The rise of the citizen scientist brings advances in the temporal and spatial scales over which research can be conducted. This groundswell of community participation in research provides considerable opportunities for data collection, as well as education and engagement of people in wildlife research and management, but it is associated with its own suite of animal welfare and regulatory considerations that have not been addressed well to date, particularly in the context of AEC oversight of research. The topics examined here are not exhaustive, but include those that are emerging or have specific implications for AEC approval processes. This chapter provides recommendations to assist researchers and AECs with planning and decision-making.

SOCIAL MEDIA AND THE WILDLIFE 'SELFIE'

Social networking platforms (e.g. Facebook, Twitter, Instagram and TikTok) are recent phenomena that began to arise in the late 1990s (Sugimoto *et al.* 2017). These platforms have become tools for promoting wildlife research and conservation (Parsons *et al.* 2014; Wu *et al.* 2018), for closing knowledge gaps beyond the scope of traditional science communication, and for promoting interdisciplinary research collaborations (Brossard and Scheufele 2013; Sugimoto *et al.* 2017). The animal welfare implications of social media and its influence on public perceptions of research and management are potentially far reaching (e.g. see discussion in Pickering and Norman 2020 on the impacts of Tweeting about the management of introduced horses in national parks). Indeed, effective use of social media can increase the profile of threatened species, although probably disproportionately for charismatic species (Roberge 2014; Kidd *et al.* 2018). However, the recent advent of social media means that animal welfare is not necessarily well catered for in evaluations of 'use' or 'impact' by AECs or researchers, or well accommodated in legislation governing animal research. This discussion focuses on a specific aspect of researchers' use of social media that influences animal welfare outcomes on a number of levels: the recording of photographs and videos of study animals to share through online profiles.

'Selfies' are images that people take of themselves and share with global audiences through social media, or privately with friends and family. Wildlife selfies are images that include wild animals and a human subject posed in a manner that is not related to the research objectives (e.g. recording of morphological characteristics, documentation or demonstration of procedures or an animal's condition). The wildlife selfie, which typically requires closeness to wild animals, is popular among the public broadly (Pagel *et al.* 2020). The influence of social media and the likely effects of wildlife 'selfie' tourism on animals, including the use of food incentives to attract or keep wildlife in an area and foster interaction (e.g. Orams 2002; Meyer *et al.* 2020), have been acknowledged (e.g. Carder *et al.* 2018; Pagel *et al.* 2020). Indeed, at least one social media platform (Instagram) has acknowledged the potentially exploitative and dangerous outcomes of wildlife selfies for wildlife and humans, introducing warning systems for searches on certain hashtags (Mills 2017). However, in general the animal welfare impacts of selfies recorded specifically by wildlife researchers (or photographs of researchers with wildlife), are given scant consideration. Wildlife researchers are in a privileged position of having access to free-living animals and locations. While photographs and videos are useful for documenting research outcomes, public outreach, promotional material and education, they can also send mixed signals to the public about the nature of wildlife research and the acceptable use of animals (Hasanah Abd Mutalib 2018) if recorded in a certain way or viewed out of context.

Photographs of researchers conducting their research, including the processing and handling of animals, and quick photographs of animals in the hand, for posterity and future identification or study, probably create little to no additional stress to study animals and are a useful, often vital, record of research activities. Similarly, photographs of researchers handling captive-bred or habituated wildlife are less controversial than those featuring wild animals (but can be misconstrued). Indeed, such images are important for science communication and presentation of results (e.g. during conferences or in publications). These images are also useful for other researchers and AECs to demonstrate research methods or as evidence (or absence) of adverse impacts on animal welfare. For surveys where no or few voucher specimens are collected, a photograph is the next best thing for obtaining a permanent record of the animal. In these cases, photography of an animal (often in the hand) just before release is an essential activity if the study is required to have any permanence. Additionally, it is often impractical for AECs to undertake site visits to remote areas; in these cases, images of researcher's handling and treatment of wildlife in photographs or videos can be provided to AECs. Such photos are also important for scientific seminars, publications and reports to agencies.

Photographs where researchers are posed with a wild animal (rather than conducting a research procedure *per se*), or where the animal has to be manipulated more than required to conduct the approved research, are undesirable and may cause unnecessary distress to study animals. Such images may also send inappropriate messages to the public about the nature of wildlife research, and mixed messages about acceptable treatment and handling of wild animals, and the threat they pose to humans if not handled correctly. Perhaps the most obvious possible negative implication of wildlife-image sharing by researchers is the potential for others to use location information (either features in the photograph itself or location data attached to it) to locate and interfere with wild animals, some of which may be sensitive to disturbance or threatened. Indeed, the rise of smartphones and digital platforms (which geotag images and posts) has probably increased the desire and ability of some enthusiasts to observe, photograph and occasionally remove wildlife (Lindenmayer and Scheele 2017). However, to date, clear evidence of the threats to wildlife from sharing biodiversity data through social media appear limited (see the review in Tulloch *et al.* 2018).

Promoting wildlife research through photographs and videos provides opportunities for greater discourse about scientific process and outcomes, and increases public appreciation of wildlife and support for conservation. In general, images intended to be shared on social media should exclude geotagged location data, features or captions that reveal the location of species of interest (less important for very common and widespread species), be associated with a clear message promoting knowledge of a species, its environment or conservation, and not be focused on promoting research programs or individuals. Typically, researchers care for the animals they study and have no desire to cause unwarranted distress. Researchers need to make a considered judgement before photographing or filming wildlife during their research, asking:

1. What is the benefit of the image to conservation or wildlife research?
2. What level of distress is the animal reasonably expected to experience, and is it likely to be greater than that expected as part of the approved research?
3. What message does the image send to viewers?
4. Will the audience for this image understand the context?

AECs could consider the following points when developing a position or making decisions on such activities:

- Where applicants intend to record photographs or videos during their research, doing so must not cause distress to animals over and above that likely to be experienced during the approved research activities.
- Photographs or videos taken while documenting approved research procedures are useful records of research, including where voucher specimens are not being collected.
- High-quality images will require adequate lighting. Artificial lighting (such as flash photography) should generally be avoided, but will be required sometimes to record a good-quality image. Collection, holding and handling associated with taking the photographs or videos should not place an unnecessary imposition on the animal.
- Habitat should not be altered to accommodate images, including using food lures other than for legitimate and approved scientific reasons.
- The sensitivities of photographing or filming animals during their breeding season should be considered.

RESEARCH IN PERI-URBAN AND URBAN AREAS

Most of the world's population resides in urban areas (Moll *et al.* 2019). The peri-urban interface comprises the sprawling areas of relatively low-density settlement surrounding the periphery of more-populated, high-density urban areas (Amirinejad *et al.* 2018). These zones are typically transitioning towards increasing urbanisation and are often multi-use areas used for cropping, outdoor recreation, hobby farming, and industrial and residential zones. They are also used by wildlife, facilitating human–wildlife interactions. Increasing rates of global urbanisation create a need to understand and manage human–wildlife interactions in urban areas (Soulsbury and White 2015). The interest in and study of urban and suburban wildlife is growing in Australia as a subject for research and as a major contributor to wildlife conservation programs (Lunney and Burgin 2004; Lunney *et al.* 2010). Wildlife research in urban areas is associated with specific challenges, including the increased likelihood that humans will inadvertently or purposely interact with the research. These incidents may affect welfare outcomes for study and non-target animals (e.g. non-target captures of pets or livestock or people interfering with equipment or trapped animals, such as pet dogs becoming caught in traps intended for red foxes (*Vulpes vulpes*) (J. Hampton, pers. comm.). These risks tend to be little documented in peer-reviewed literature, being largely anecdotal, although tampering with wildlife monitoring cameras is a common issue (Meek *et al.* 2013). For example, one of the authors of this chapter left a captured and bagged mammal in an apparently secure location while clearing other traps (< 5 min), to find that it had been taken by local children who were observing the work. Other issues include the potential to attract predators to populated areas if using lures or poison baits, which pose risks to the predators, domesticated animals and people. Persistent use of attractants may result in the species becoming habituated (Appleby *et al.* 2018).

Human perceptions of research also create challenges for researchers and AECs, and for animal welfare outcomes, both from a population conservation perspective and an individual animal welfare context. These challenges are exemplified by the incident described by Jones *et al.* (2012) where an AEC withdrew approval for research on disease transmission in Tasmanian devils (*Sarcophilus harrisii*), which was triggered by a complaint from an external individual. Other examples include experiences of some of the authors of this chapter, involving dingo (*Canis dingo*) research. One author spent many days traversing bushland and deploying camera traps because a community member reported to the AEC that a satellite-tracking collar was reducing a collared dingo's ability to hunt. Images of the dingo, a naturally lean species in the wild, showed that the animal's condition had not changed since initial capture. As most wildlife researchers and communicators realise, the species that the public tends to feel strongly about is also often characterised by conflict. Similarly, various research techniques are sometimes distressing to the public, because of their perceived impacts on individual animals, such as collars on animals for radio tracking, ear tags or wing tags, cage trapping (e.g. for the urban brushtail possum, *Trichosurus vulpecula*), and traps in general. However, local wildlife studies, even in inner-city areas, are gaining in popularity, and councils are employing wildlife scientists to study local fauna and educate residents. For example, Inner West Council's website in 2021 opened with the appeal: 'Council needs your help as citizen scientists to track populations of fauna in the Inner West such as birds, microbats, and long-nosed bandicoots.'

Research in peri-urban and urban areas can draw the attention of residents, potentially with negative consequences for the study species. For example, in a study of peri-urban dingoes in Queensland, residents became aware that dingoes were being trapped and tracked locally. They requested that the tracked animals be killed by the local council. Similarly, a local landholder was convinced (erroneously) that a researcher had trapped dingoes in western Queensland and released them onto their property. After extensive debate with the local council, the dingoes were allowed to live and the study continued, but the process created an unexpected time delay and administrative burden (D. Morrant, pers. comm.). Conversely, the presence of high densities of people also creates opportunities to engage with communities on wildlife research (e.g. Awasthy *et al.* 2012) and raise awareness and dispel fears about wildlife. Similarly, local communities can also be engaged to assist with research projects (e.g. Mulder *et al.* 2010) as citizen scientists (see Chapter 10), including for projects where researchers are compiling databases of animal sightings (e.g. Mulder *et al.* 2010; Scott *et al.* 2014; Davis *et al.* 2017).

Urban wildlife research is a burgeoning field of study, reflecting the similarly rapid expansion of urban and peri-urban areas (Magle *et al.* 2012). It is characterised by specific challenges around maintaining high standards of animal welfare. We recommend the following principles when planning urban wildlife research in the context of animal welfare:

- Transparency is critical in all aspects of urban wildlife research. Ideally, researchers should keep local communities informed by direct contact, signage, regular newsletters, workshops or similar. Include time frames for research in these communications. The level and nature of communication should reflect the complexity and potentially controversial nature of the study or techniques being used.
- It is helpful for researchers to assure communities that research protocols are scrutinised through a statutory and independent ethical review process (i.e. AEC). Members of the public may have greater confidence knowing researchers are accountable for the project's animal welfare standards through this process, and may be inspired to participate in the AEC process as lay committee members.
- Ask for community assistance if practical. For example, ask people to record sightings of target species (including tagged individuals), observe activity around nest boxes (without interfering with the nest box or its occupants), or replace batteries in monitoring cameras.
- Preferentially use detection techniques with the lowest anticipated impact on animals, such as camera traps, acoustic recorders, or tracks, scats and other traces. Ensure equipment is positioned securely.
- Deactivate or cover traps adequately when not in use, and erect signage to warn residents of potential risks.

COLLECTION OF VOUCHER SPECIMENS

Animals may be killed during approved research activities as voucher specimens (an animal killed and preserved as a permanent record or type specimen of the species).

This subject is covered in the Australian Code for the Care and Use of Animals for Scientific Purposes (the Code) (NHMRC 2013). Some traditional conceptions of animal welfare do not place any moral weight on death, aside from any pain caused during the process of killing; it is the individual animal's experience and treatment leading up to death that are matters of concern. Nevertheless, the view that death *is* an animal welfare issue has been around for some years (Yeates 2010), with an increasing sentiment that the age at which animals die (or are killed) has implications for their welfare (Hecht 2021). Hence, the collection of voucher specimens can be viewed negatively, particularly if conservation or scientific outcomes are not immediately obvious or tangible, the collected species is threatened or rare, if a perceived excessive number of specimens are collected, or an ethical position that rejects killing of animals is held. Protocols around collecting vouchers vary among states and territories and are influenced by scientific licences, relationships with museums and, probably, the skills and values of researchers. A decision on the number of individuals that may be taken is a matter for the state or territory authority issuing the scientific licence to conduct the research, and all wildlife researchers must hold a scientific licence concurrent with their AEC approval. Referring to a museum (or the Atlas of Living Australia) before field work begins will establish what species are represented by specimens from the survey area and the time since they were recorded, which might influence decisions to collect voucher specimens.

In recent decades, fewer mammal voucher specimens have been collected globally because of assumptions that most mammal species are described. However, examples of the role of voucher specimens for evaluating the presence and conservation status of cryptic species do exist. For example, the grey-bellied dunnart (*Sminthopsis griseoventor*) was confirmed as occurring in South Australia, and its pre- and post-European settlement distributions were assessed following the collection of voucher specimens (Kemper *et al.* 2011).

Museum collections provide baseline information for investigations on spatial and temporal changes in species occurrences. Discoveries of new species are mostly made through evaluation of museum collections rather than in the field (M. Hutchinson, pers. comm.). A lack of specimens will result in fewer opportunities to establish the existence of previously unknown species or will need to be followed up by field work to gather specimens to fill gaps in information. Consequently, the cost of not collecting can be high given the difficulty of catching many species and the remote locations from which specimens are needed to solve speciation problems (e.g. Parnaby 2009 evaluated voucher specimens collected from a range of remote locations to split *Nyctophilus timoriensis*, a long-eared forest bat, into four species).

The advent of new technologies has reduced the need for the numbers of voucher specimens that were once collected (Clemann *et al.* 2014; for an explanation of 'refinement' see Chapter 1). Genetic variation is such that typically fewer than five individuals will provide 95% of the likely genetic diversity of a population. Historically, researchers relying on morphology only would have aimed to collect around 20 to 30 individuals to generate statistically significant morphometric data. Where multiple populations are included in a study, many of the populations would require a single individual if a genetic marker is available that will assign them unambiguously to a particular prospective species. Once a study has established the existence of reliable genetic markers, which correlate with species boundaries, then one individual is sufficient to provide that information. For some taxa (e.g. frogs, which frequently show sexual dimorphism), one male and one female may be the minimum number of specimens needed to assign them to a species and to check that the dimorphism (often variable among populations) can be described (M. Hutchinson, pers. comm.).

Clemann *et al.* (2014) proposed a decision framework for the collection of voucher specimens in wildlife research, which focuses on four key criteria:

1. Do knowledge gaps exist for the species?
2. Do sufficient voucher specimens already exist to address these knowledge gaps?
3. Will collecting voucher specimens affect the target population negatively?
4. Can the individuals be killed humanely?

Vouchering raises the proposition that AEC deliberations could include species- and population-level considerations as well as the welfare of individual animals, although it must be kept in mind that the relevant state or territory authority issues scientific licences to researchers authorising research on particular species, numbers of individuals and locations. Since methods that minimise negative animal welfare impacts are available for killing animals (and putting aside concerns about the importance of death to welfare), the debate is largely a philosophical one about acceptable 'use' of animals. Our recommendations to AECs are that (1) collection of voucher specimens is at the discretion of the researcher and approval by the relevant state or territory wildlife authority and (2) where collection of voucher specimens is proposed, decisions to approve these activities should include the general principles outlined by Clemann *et al.* (2014), as well as the scientific licence conditions, to decide when to collect. Additionally, while approval processes have historically tended to focus on the welfare of individuals (Fraser 1999), where research is focused on conservation or management aims, AECs should also give consideration to its benefits at the species and population levels (Clemann *et al.* 2014).

CITIZEN SCIENCE

Citizen science initiatives enlist volunteers in planning or implementation of research. Citizen science projects often proceed under supervision from professional scientists (Roger *et al.* 2020), although not always, particularly for programs that have broad objectives and geographical scopes, and do not include direct interaction with animals (e.g. some initiatives simply require citizens to help code existing datasets). For examples, see the 'Australian Citizen Science Project Finder' (www.biocollect.ala.org.au) and the NSW SEED Citizen Science (https://citizen-science.seed.nsw.gov.au). Often, citizen science-based programs do not seek to answer hypothesis-driven and experimental research. Instead, they are applied as complementary approaches to more-traditional scientific formats (Dickinson *et al.* 2010). Citizen science also taps into what has been called 'community wisdom' and is now accepted in refereed scientific journals as a valid scientific approach (Predavec *et al.* 2016). The rise of citizen science and associated technologies (e.g. data collection through smartphones and smartphone-based applications, and via social media platforms) has increased the spatial and temporal scale over which research can be conducted with relative efficiency. However, several facets (e.g. lack of direct supervision of participants, often broad geographical scale and gamification) of some types of citizen science programs present a set of challenges for evaluating and managing impacts on animal welfare, which have been given scant consideration to date.

Animal ethics committees are faced with ambiguities around approvals for citizen science projects that involve wildlife. Geographically broad programs, projects where participants are not under direct supervision of investigators, those that include public engagement aims rather than purely research objectives, transparency around data collection, including publishing of locations of sensitive species and habitats (Quinn 2021), and programs using nil-impact data collection methods all present complexities in terms of evaluating likely impacts on animal welfare and compliance with legislation, which varies across states and territories. In these situations, traditional triggers for animal ethics approval requirements (e.g. a clearly defined research question that necessitates animal use to answer it) are less obvious. Coincidentally, data collected 'third hand' (e.g. citizen science data deposited within repositories and then accessed by investigators or records obtained from wildlife rehabilitation groups) and assessment of dead animals (i.e. animals not killed for a research purpose, e.g. roadkill surveys) do not require AEC approval (although studies collecting dead native animals do require a scientific licence).

Gamification is the application of characteristics of game playing (competition, game rules, scoring and prizes) to an activity. The concept is used to engage and motivate people as a low-cost tool for recruiting and retaining participants (Newman *et al.* 2012). Examples are many, and include programs such as QuestaGame©, which encourages participants to photograph plants, animals and fungi in the wild and upload data via a smartphone application or the dedicated website (https://questagame.com). Participants score 'gold' for each sighting they upload and accumulate more gold if they can identify the species. Records of rare or interesting species win more gold. Participants can also create and participate in 'bioquests', with groups participating against one another in competitions. Data are provided to national and global databases, unless participants choose not to provide their data. Other programs, such as the Australian Museum's FrogID program (where participants upload audio recordings of calling frogs) are not inherently based on competition among participants, but do have elements of gamification where groups and individuals can compete for a place on the national 'leaderboard' based on the number of calls they submit (www.portal.frogid.net.au). A characteristic of these programs, unlike more-localised and specific projects, is that participants are not generally supervised directly by investigators. Gamification is not inherently negative for animal welfare. Indeed, programs like FrogID have produced important conservation and scientific outcomes for Australia's frog fauna (e.g. Rowley *et al.* 2019).

The effects of gamification and lack of direct supervision on animal welfare in citizen science are not well understood and warrant further attention. However, several issues should be considered by investigators and AECs. Undoubtedly, competition that relies on people finding and recording animals, including sensitive species, encourages at least some participants to increase their efforts to find and locate these species. Inadvertently (or purposefully), participants may disturb animals and habitat, although this risk may be reduced for programs with clearly communicated protocols. As participants are rarely under the direct supervision of a primary investigator for projects conducted at national, if not global, scales, identifying and mitigating these risks directly is virtually impossible. Where projects do employ gamification, but participants are supervised, the potential impacts may be lesser. Opportunities exist to build supervision into the structure of broader-scale projects through the formation of local groups under the supervision of more-experienced personnel.

General operating principles for the assessment and management of animal welfare related to citizen science projects are provided in Chapter 10. Ultimately, as with all wildlife research projects, some level of risk with respect to animal welfare that cannot be managed by investigators remains even when projects employ low-impact methods (Fraser and MacRae 2011). Smaller-scale projects, where participants are more or less under the direct supervision of experienced personnel (e.g. participants assist with checking nest boxes or monitoring nesting turtles), can simply be evaluated as per normal research project protocols. Effectively, in these cases, the citizen scientists are participating individuals, under the direct supervision of primary and associate investigators, who are named in applications if they are to be involved in the use of animals. For broader programs, AECs may need to consider the specific facets proposed for that program. For example, a project may encourage citizen scientists to record and submit animal signs or traces (scats, tracks or call data) via a smartphone application. The investigators will not supervise participants in the field directly, but will provide some training (i.e. through a workshop or provision of project materials and guides). Direct involvement of participants with animals is not proposed, and investigators discourage participants from actively seeking or handling animals, or disturbing habitat in their guiding materials and workshop. Some elements of gamification are involved (i.e. point scoring based on numbers of submissions), but no emphasis is placed on records of any particular species. In this case, an AEC might determine that negative effects on animal welfare are possible given that unsupervised participants may choose to seek out and disturb animals, but the short- and long-term consequences of these potential interactions and the controls (e.g. clear protocols) proposed by the investigators mean that negative effects are likely to be negligible.

The process for approving research can be slow and not always clear to citizen scientists; this situation is problematic when citizen scientists can also design their own research projects. Indeed, the entire process of AEC approvals remains in the domain of researchers. However, the rate of biodiversity loss and the need to scale up efforts to document and monitor biodiversity is immense (small teams of professionals can survey deeply or broadly, but not both). A balance needs to be achieved between the requirement for AEC approval (often only possible to obtain via academic and government institutions) and enabling the public to have a greater involvement in science. Procedural barriers to citizen science projects would be a deterrent to work that could genuinely affect real change. In general, AECs should have an informed discussion around issues relating to citizen science programs, provide clear advice to applicants and recognise that a 'one-size-fits-all' approach is unlikely to cater for the diversity of forms that such projects take. Ultimately, legislation and the Code may need to be amended to cater for such programs.

EVALUATING NIL- AND LOW-IMPACT METHODS

Assessments of animal welfare impacts in AEC evaluation processes are effectively cost–benefit analyses balancing costs: the likelihood of an adverse event occurring multiplied by its potential consequences and benefits: scientific value. These decisions are sometimes made with limited direct evidence of animal welfare impacts and are inferred through assumptions made in the formulation of procedural documents (Hampton *et al.* 2016). Researchers are increasingly finding technological solutions to the challenges of studying complex ecosystems (resulting in the emergence of sub-disciplines, such as 'technoecology' (Allan *et al.* 2018)). Automated and remote technologies (e.g. modern wildlife monitoring cameras and remote acoustic recording devices – see Chapters 4 and 5, as well as remotely piloted aircraft – see Chapter 6) have provided opportunities for wildlife researchers to replace or complement comparatively higher-impact methods (e.g. direct trapping and handling of animals). Two key issues arise from the employment of these types of methods. First, do they constitute animal 'use'? Second, should they require approval from an AEC?

The concept of animal 'use' and how it is applied is fundamental to the requirement for AEC evaluations and approvals. For example, the concept clearly applies differently to laboratory-based studies that use quantifiable numbers of animals under tightly controlled experimental conditions than in field-based wildlife research employing low-impact methods to evaluate animal populations or communities. The concept is at the heart of most arguments around the need for AEC approvals. Arguably, an animal's call recorded remotely on an acoustic device barely constitutes use. The collection of a recording itself does not affect animals, and recorder placement typically requires little to no disturbance, although exceptions may include where recorders are installed near nests, dens or roosting animals (Chapter 5). Studies of birds that rely on observers using binoculars to watch them from a distance are a similar example. The decision to subject such studies to AEC scrutiny or not is dependent on the interpretation of 'animal use' and definition of 'animal research', which are influenced by relevant state and territory legislation, and by policies of the governing institution (see Chapter 1). For example, in Queensland, some activities are exempt from AEC approvals, providing that they will not cause abnormal disruption to habitat or animals (Queensland Government 2020). Similarly, Queensland applicants may submit an 'Application Not Requiring Full Application' for observational studies and the use of biological samples or tissue from animals euthanised before the study. Under Victoria's animal welfare legislation administered by the Royal Society for the Prevention of Cruelty to Animals (RSPCA), passive recording is not deemed to be research, so AEC approval is not legally required.

When evaluating nil- and low-impact methods (several of these methods are covered in Chapters 4 and 5), a conservative AEC might assume that any animal involvement (even indirect) for research purposes should require evaluation. Tangentially, obtaining AEC approval provides an additional level of assurance to the public that the research is justified and being conducted in a manner likely to cause the least harm to affected animals. Demonstrating that an AEC approval has been granted can be a requirement of journals before publication of research involving animals. Indeed, journals have a potentially important role to play in improving animal welfare standards in wildlife research and management by requiring publication of AEC approvals and adherence to animal welfare standards more generally (e.g. Field *et al.* 2019), which have corresponding implications for scientific process (Brook *et al.* 2015; Field *et al.* 2019).

One matter that can cause delays and misunderstanding is when an AEC adopts an inflexible approach to defining 'use' and 'low impact', potentially placing an administrative burden on researchers, AECs and governance officers, without facilitating real improvements in animal welfare, unless iterative refinement processes are followed – see Hampton *et al.* (2021) for an example. Institutions and AECs should be clear to applicants about their accepted definition of 'use' and expedited approval processes should be developed for projects that solely use nil- or low-impact methods (see Chapter 2). Ultimately, to keep abreast of emerging techniques and issues in contemporary wildlife research, institutions, AECs and researchers should work collaboratively to establish clear policies to negate confusion between stakeholders, reduce administrative burdens, and support ongoing replacement, reduction and refinement technology and techniques for wildlife research in Australia. It is useful if AECs invite researchers to meetings to discuss emerging technologies and methods; doing so is an effective way of helping AEC members learn about new methods and helps to build rapport between researchers and AEC members.

THE ETHICAL DEBATE

Once conversations progress to what *should* or *should not* be done, the realm of ethics is entered. The values at play in these deliberations include animal welfare, the value of scientific knowledge, benefits or costs to biodiversity, economic impacts and concepts of justice or fairness. What constitutes 'ethical' research will be a product of how these values are prioritised and what ethical theory is used to guide this prioritisation. Traditionally, research has followed a consequentialist approach by means of cost–benefit analyses; see Brønstad *et al.* (2016) for an in-depth discussion. The debate on what constitutes 'ethical' use of animals in research, including wildlife research, will and should continue – in part, because of the wider community's discussion and shifting values (see van Eeden *et al.* 2017) relating to the fair treatment of wildlife and animals more broadly, and the need for increased knowledge about how to address these ever-changing and evolving issues.

It would be a devastating loss to global biodiversity if Australia's unique native fauna was allowed to fade away because of a devaluing of the role of wildlife research and conservation management. Wildlife research is a legitimate, socially accepted activity, made more so by its regulation by AECs and scientific licences provided by state and territory wildlife authorities. For example, in New South Wales, licences to study wildlife were first introduced in 1974, so the concept of oversight of research activities is relatively recent. However, AECs and wildlife research are not isolated activities in society, and the way wildlife researchers and AECs conceive and contribute to the debate matters a great deal for the future of wildlife research and the conservation of our native wildlife.

Researchers are encouraged to engage with the public to explain the value of wildlife research. As few publications have been written by authors writing as members of an AEC to explain procedures and decisions, AEC members are encouraged to address this shortcoming. The AEC process is currently the best, if imperfect, model for addressing concerns for the wellbeing of all animals used in research, while accommodating the shifting moods in society. For successful wildlife conservation outcomes, this process requires participants who value knowledge, research, animal welfare and the need to reverse the decline of native wildlife.

ACKNOWLEDGEMENTS

Thank you to Megan Bathurst, Jane DeGabriel and Mark Hutchinson for providing feedback on early versions of this chapter.

REFERENCES

Allan BM, Nimmo DG, Ierodiaconou D, VanDerWal J, Pin Koh L, Ritchie EG (2018) Futurecasting ecological research: the rise of technology. *Ecosphere* **9**, e12163. doi:10.1002/ecs2.2163

Amirinejad G, Donehue P, Baker D (2018) Ambiguity at the peri-urban interface in Australia. *Land Use Policy* **78**, 472–480. doi:10.1016/j.landusepol.2018.07.022

Appleby R, Mackie J, Smith B, Bernede L, Jones D (2018) Human-dingo interactions on Fraser Island: an analysis of incident reports. *Australian Mammalogy* **40**, 146–156. doi:10.1071/AM16026

Awasthy M, Popovic AZ, Linklater WL (2012) Experience in local urban wildlife research enhances a conservation education programme with school children. *Pacific Conservation Biology* **18**, 41–46. doi:10.1071/PC120041

Brønstad A, Newcomer CE, Decelle T, Everitt JI, Guillen J, Laber K (2016) Current concepts of harm–benefit analysis of animal experiments – report from the AALAS–FELASA working group on harm–benefit analysis – part 1. *Laboratory Animals* **50**, 1–20. doi:10.1177/0023677216642398

Brook RK, Cattet M, Darimont CT, Paquet PC, Proulx G (2015) Maintaining ethical standards during conservation crises. *Canadian Wildlife Biology and Management* **4**, 72–79.

Brossard D, Scheufele DA (2013) Science, new media and the public. *Science* **339**, 40–41. doi:10.1126/science.1232329

Carder G, Plese T, Machado FC, Paterson S, Matthews N, McAnea L, D'Cruze N (2018) The impact of 'selfie' tourism on the behaviour and welfare of brown-throated three-toed sloths. *Animals* **8**. doi:10.3390/ani8110216

Clemann N, Rowe KMC, Rowe KC, Raadik T, Gomon M, Menkhorst P, Sumner J, Bray D, Norman M, Melville J (2014) Value and impacts of collecting vertebrate voucher specimens, with guidelines for ethical collection. *Memoirs of the Museum of Victoria* **72**, 141–153. doi:10.24199/j.mmv.2014.72.09

Davis A, Major RE, Taylor CE, Martin JM (2017) Novel tracking and reporting methods for studying large birds in urban landscapes. *Wildlife Biology* **2017**. doi:10.2981/wlb.00307

Dickinson JL, Zuckerberg B, Bonter DN (2010) Citizen science as an ecological research tool: challenges and benefits. *Annual Review of Ecology, Evolution, and Systematics* **41**, 149–172. doi:10.1146/annurev-ecolsys-102209-144636

Field KA, Paquet PC, Artelle K, Proulx G, Brook RK, Darimont CT (2019) Publication reform to safeguard wildlife from researcher harm. *PLoS Biology* **17**, e3000193. doi:10.1371/journal.pbio.3000193

Fraser D (1999) Animal ethics and animal welfare science: bridging the two cultures. *Applied Animal Behaviour Science* **65**, 171–189. doi:10.1016/S0168-1591(99)00090-8

Fraser D, MacRae AM (2011) Four types of activities that affect animals: implications for animal welfare science and animal ethics philosophy. *Animal Welfare* **20**, 581–590.

Hampton JO, Amos M, Pople A, Brennan M, Forsyth DM (2021) Minimising mortalities in capturing wildlife: refinement of helicopter darting of chital deer (*Axis axis*) in Australia. *Wildlife Research* **48**, 304–313. doi:10.1071/WR20106

Hampton JO, Hyndman TH, Laurence M, Perry AL, Adams P, Collins T (2016) Animal welfare and the use of procedural documents: limitations and refinement. *Wildlife Research* **43**, 599–603. doi:10.1071/WR16153

Hasanah Abd Mutalib A (2018) The photo frenzy phenomenon: how a single snap can affect wildlife populations. *Biodiversity* **19**, 237–239. doi:10.1080/14888386.2018.1544931

Hecht L (2021) The importance of considering age when quantifying wild animals' welfare. *Biological Reviews* **96**, 2602–2616. doi:10.1111/brv.12769

Jones M, Hamede R, McCallum H (2012) The devil is in the detail: conservation biology, animal philosophies and the role of animal ethics committees. In *Science under Siege: Zoology under Threat* (Eds P Banks, D Lunney and C Dickman.) pp. 79–88. Royal Zoological Society of New South Wales, South Mosman. doi:10.7882/FS.2012.040

Kemper CM, Cooper SJB, Medlin GC, Adams M, Stemmer D, Saint KM, McDowell MC, Austin JJ (2011) Cryptic grey-bellied dunnart (*Sminthopsis grisoventor*) discovered in South Australia: genetic, morphological and subfossil analyses show the value of collecting voucher material. *Australian Journal of Zoology* **59**, 127–144. doi:10.1071/ZO11037

Kidd LR, Gregg EA, Bekessy SA, Robinson JA, Garrard GE (2018) Tweeting for their lives: visibility of threatened species on Twitter. *Journal for Nature Conservation* **46**, 106–109. doi:10.1016/j.jnc.2018.10.001

Lindenmayer D, Scheele B (2017) Do not publish: limiting open-access information on rare and endangered species will help to protect them. *Science* **356**, 800–801. doi:10.1126/science.aan1362

Lunney D (2017a) Dangerous? Necessary: we must conserve all our native fauna. *Australian Zoologist* **38**, 281–288. doi:10.7882/AZ.2017.005

Lunney D (2017b) A dangerous idea in action: the hegemony of endangered species legislation and how it hinders biodiversity conservation. *Australian Zoologist* **38**, 289–307. doi:10.7882/AZ.2017.015

Lunney D, Burgin S (Eds) (2004) *Urban Wildlife: More than Meets the Eye*. Royal Zoological Society of NSW, Mosman.

Lunney D, Hutchings P, Hochuli D (Eds) (2010). *The Natural History of Sydney*. Royal Zoological Society of NSW, Mosman.

Magle SB, Hunt VM, Vernon M, Crooks KR (2012) Urban wildlife research: past, present and future. *Biological Conservation* **155**, 23–32. doi:10.1016/j.biocon.2012.06.018

McMahon CR, Bradshaw CJA, Hays GG (2006) Branding can be justified in vital conservation research. *Nature* **439**, 392. doi:10.1038/439392c

Meek PD, Ballard G-A, Fleming PJS (2013) A permanent security post for camera trapping. *Australian Mammalogy* **35**, 123–127. doi:10.1071/AM12014

Meyer L, Whitmarsh SK, Nichols PD, Revill AT, Huveneers C (2020) The effects of wildlife tourism provisioning on non-target species. *Biological Conservation* **241**, 108317. doi:10.1016/j.biocon.2019.108317

Mills G (2017) Social media giant takes action on wildlife 'selfies'. *The Veterinary Record* **181**, 672–673. doi:10.1136/vr.j5899

Moll RJ, *et al.* (2019) What does urbanization actually mean? A framework for urban metrics in wildlife research. *Journal of Applied Ecology* **56**, 1289–1300. doi:10.1111/1365-2664.13358

Mulder RA, Guay P-J, Wilson M, Coulson G (2010) Citizen science: recruiting residents for studies of tagged urban wildlife. *Wildlife Research* **37**, 440–446. doi:10.1071/WR10007

Newman G, Wiggins A, Crall A, Graham E, Newman S, Crowston K (2012) The future of citizen science: emerging technologies and shifting paradigms. *Frontiers in Ecology and the Environment* **10**, 298–304. doi:10.1890/110294

NHMRC (National Health and Medical Research Council) (2013) *Australian Code for the Care and Use of Animals for Scientific Purposes*. 8th edn. National Health and Medical Research Council, Canberra.

Orams MB (2002) Feeding wildlife as a tourism attraction: a review of issues and impacts. *Tourism Management* **23**, 281–293. doi:10.1016/S0261-5177(01)00080-2

Pagel CD, Orams MB, Lück M (2020) Experienced photographer's behaviour during commercial swim-with-wildlife tours: comparative case studies of three operations in the South Pacific. *Current Issues in Tourism* **24**, 2312–2324. doi:10.1080/13683500.2020.1828312

Parnaby HE (2009) A taxonomic review of Australian greater long-eared bats previously known as *Nyctophilus timoriensis* (Chiroptera: Vespertilionidae) and some associated taxa. *Australian Zoologist* **35**, 39–81. doi:10.7882/AZ.2009.005

Parsons ECM, Shiffman DS, Darling ES, Spillman N, Wright AJ (2014) How Twitter literacy can benefit conservation scientists. *Conservation Biology* **28**, 299–301. doi:10.1111/cobi.12226

Pickering CM, Norman P (2020) Assessing discourses about controversial environmental management issues on social media: tweeting about wild horses in a national park. *Journal of Environmental Management* **275**, 111244. doi:10.1016/j.jenvman.2020.111244

Predavec M, Lunney D, Hope B, Stalenberg E, Shannon I, Crowther M, Miller I, Turbill J, Faulkner B (2016) What can community wisdom contribute to conservation biology? *Conservation Biology* **30**, 496–505. doi:10.1111/cobi.12698

Queensland Government (2020) Activities Requiring Approval from an Animal Ethics Committee. Queensland Government. <https://www.business.qld.gov.au/industries/farms-fishing-forestry/agriculture/livestock/animal-welfare/animals-science/activities>.

Quinn A (2021) Transparency and secrecy in citizen science: lessons from herping. *Studies in History and Philosophy of Science* **85**, 208–217. doi:10.1016/j.shpsa.2020.10.010

Roberge J-M (2014) Using data from online social networks in conservation science: which species engage people the most on Twitter? *Biodiversity and Conservation* **23**, 715–726. doi:10.1007/s10531-014-0629-2

Roger E, Tegart P, Dowsett R, Kinsela MA, Harley MD, Ortac G (2020) Maximising the potential for citizen science in NSW. *Australian Zoologist* **40**, 449–461. doi:10.7882/AZ.2019.023

Rowley JL, Callaghan CT, Cutajar T, Portway C, Potter K, Mahony S, Trembath DF, Flemons P, Woods A (2019) FrogID: citizen scientists provide validated biodiversity data on frogs of Australia. *Herpetological Conservation and Biology* **14**, 155–170.

Scott DM, Berg MJ, Tolhurst BA, Chauvenet alM, Smith GC, Neaves K, Lochead J, Baker PJ (2014) Changes in the distribution of red foxes (*Vulpes vulpes*) in urban areas in Great Britain: findings and limitations of a media-driven nationwide survey. *PLoS One* **9**, e99059. doi:10.1371/journal.pone.0099059

Soulsbury CD, White PCL (2015) Human-wildlife interactions in urban areas: a review of conflict, benefits and opportunities. *Wildlife Research* **42**, 541–553. doi:10.1071/WR14229

Sugimoto CR, Work S, Larivière V (2017) Scholarly use of social media and altmetrics: a review of the literature. *Journal of the Association for Information Science and Technology* **68**, 2037–2062. doi:10.1002/asi.23833

Tulloch AIT, Auerbach NA, Avery-Gomm S, *et al.* (2018) A decision tree for assessing the risks and benefits of publishing biodiversity data. *Nature Ecology & Evolution* **2**, 1209–1217. doi:10.1038/s41559-018-0608-1

van Eeden LM, Dickman CR, Ritchie EG, Newsome TM (2017) Shifting public values and what they mean for increasing democracy in wildlife management decisions. *Biodiversity and Conservation* **26**, 2759–2763. doi:10.1007/s10531-017-1378-9

van Eeden LM, Newsome TM, Crowther MS, Dickman CR, Bruskotter J (2020) Diverse public perceptions of species' status and management align with conflicting conservation frameworks. *Biological Conservation* **242**, 108416. doi:10.1016/j.biocon.2020.108416

Wu Y, Xie L, Huang S-L, Li P, Yuan Z, Liu W (2018) Using social media to strengthen public awareness of wildlife conservation. *Ocean and Coastal Management* **153**, 76–83. doi:10.1016/j.ocecoaman.2017.12.010

Yeates JW (2010) Death is a welfare issue. *Journal of Agricultural & Environmental Ethics* **23**, 229–241. doi:10.1007/s10806-009-9199-9

Section 2

RESEARCH METHODS

Introduction

Helen P. Waudby

'Research methods' details general operating procedures (GOPs) for a range of techniques used in Australian wildlife research. The GOPs presented in this section have been developed by people with extensive practical experience in wildlife research, including practitioners, early career researchers and post-graduate students, environmental consultants, and government and academic scientists. These GOPs can be provided to animal ethics committees (AECs) in any jurisdiction, or used as the basis for preparing detailed standard operating procedures (SOPs). Throughout this section, terms such as researchers, investigators, personnel, operators, practitioners and field workers are used interchangeably to indicate people who may use these GOPs. The intention is not to duplicate existing SOPs or guidelines, but to establish a basic set of practices deemed acceptable by experts on wildlife research practices in Australia, which may help investigators and AECs avoid confusion when faced with a range of protocols. These GOPs may be particularly useful to institutional AECs that are lacking detailed procedures for key research methods.

Wildlife research methods are diverse and constantly evolving, with increasingly low-impact methods being developed. This section provides GOPs for common and emerging techniques in Australia, including a range of low-impact methods. These GOPs are 'high-level' guides that should be reviewed in conjunction with species- or taxon-specific considerations when planning research and applying for animal ethics approvals (see Section 3). Additionally, the development of best practice procedures is valuable for ensuring consistency in implementation of methods. However, these procedures should be evaluated regularly in view of animal welfare outcomes (as best as they can be known) for study animals and non-target species that may be adversely affected.

The GOPs detailed here outline key considerations and best practice principles for techniques as they currently relate to animal welfare. Each GOP provides general procedures for undertaking the activity, specific competencies, potential alternative or complementary techniques, and workplace, health and safety (WHS) considerations. Since these GOPs are intended to be standalone documents, some repetition was unavoidable. To avoid excessive repetition, readers are sometimes referred to considerations detailed elsewhere in the chapter or book.

Importantly, contributors to these GOPs were asked to describe clearly the expected and potential effects of the method on the welfare of study animals. This information is a standard requirement of animal ethics applications and can be difficult to address, particularly where published evidence of impacts is lacking. Investigators and AECs have a requirement to consider potential impacts, even where experimental evidence is lacking. However, as pointed out by Hampton *et al.* (2016) the relationship between what is done to animals and how animals experience the method (i.e. its actual impact on them) has received little attention. This section aims to help researchers identify key potential animal welfare impacts and where available, GOPs reference published work to demonstrate the likelihood of impacts occurring. In circumstances where potential impacts have not been investigated, the GOPs note as such and infer the likelihood and consequence of the impact occurring based on the experience and knowledge of the experts who have prepared them. Investigators undertaking the described procedures may need to incorporate their own specific research parameters, requirements and limitations. These GOPs also establish likely triggers for treatment or intervention for each method.

Each GOP provides WHS considerations specific to the method. However, these considerations are general in nature and not intended to replace detailed context, project, or species-specific safe work methods statements or job safety analyses. Considerations that are common to wildlife research, such as working in remote areas, injury from animals, and the potential for transmission of zoonoses, anthropozoonoses or parasites, and spreading of other pathogens (e.g. phytophthora and myrtle rust) should be addressed by investigators before research commences. In general, investigators should maintain a high standard of hygiene practices, review their capture and handling protocols regularly in view of potential disease risks, and be aware of the risk of transmission of infectious pathogens, including in field situations, for the health of themselves and their study species. Other resources are available to help researchers evaluate the likely biosecurity risks of their research and develop protocols to mitigate them (e.g. Wildlife Health Australia 2018).

REFERENCES

Hampton JO, Hyndman TH, Laurence M, Perry AL, Adams P, Collins T (2016) Animal welfare and the use of procedural documents: limitations and refinement. *Wildlife Research* **43**, 599–603. doi:10.1071/WR16153

Wildlife Health Australia (2018) *National Wildlife Biosecurity Guidelines*. Wildlife Health Australia, Sydney.

4 Observing wildlife and its signs

Bradley P. Smith, Helen P. Waudby, Chris R. Dickman, Kari Soennichsen, Charlotte Mills, Andrew Howe, Leigh-Ann Woolley, Stephen R. Griffiths, Tarnya E. Cox, Jessica Clayton, Cara Penton, Damian S. Morrant, Mike Letnic, Dympna Cullen, Alyson Stobo-Wilson, David A. Taggart, Dianne Gleeson, Jemma K. Cripps, Matthew J. Gill and Anna J. MacDonald

INTRODUCTION

Information about the biology and behaviour of a species can be gained from direct observation, and from the secondary signs and traces that they leave behind. Typically, these methods do not involve capturing or handling animals and can be performed without disturbing them. Observing and identifying secondary animal signs are often done opportunistically during survey and monitoring activities, or while travelling between sites. However, systematic collection of scats or sand plots can help derive abundance estimates, and determine species' presence/absence. This chapter presents general operating procedures (GOPs) for direct detection survey methods, including visual observations of animals, spotlight surveys, and the use of artificial cavities (nest boxes and hollows) to study animals. It also details several forms of indirect detection based on the evaluation of distinguishing characteristics and signs of animal activity (signs or traces), including hair and scats, tracks and scratches, dens and burrows, and DNA that is shed into the environment. These methods are typically classified as low impact. They rely on the experience of the observer or identifier to conduct observations, and make accurate and reliable assessments of the animal sign. Ideally, investigators identify the best times, locations and techniques specific to the target species before commencing a study (see Section 3 of this book for species profiles). While stress is likely to be minimal, animals may still be disturbed depending on how these methods are implemented, so investigators should consider potential impacts of their specific study and clarify requirements for animal ethics approval with a relevant animal ethics committee (AEC).

VISUAL OBSERVATIONS

Bradley P. Smith and Helen P. Waudby

Target taxa

The procedures in this GOP can be applied to all free-living taxa, but particularly to mammals. For observational methods for marine mammals and reptiles, see Chapter 12, and for fishes, see Chapters 13 and 14. For avian-specific methods, see Chapter 15.

Context and scope

This GOP describes general techniques and considerations for observation of free-living wild animals by researchers, with or without visual aids. It does not include observation of animals at night with a spotlight (covered later in this chapter), or in concert with call playback (Chapter 5), planes or drones (Chapter 6), from vehicles (covered later in this chapter) and boats (Chapters 12, 13 and 14) or of animals in captive enclosures. Nor does it include the use of baits or lures that may alter behaviour (e.g. attract the animal to the observer or encourage them to remain in the area).

Observations of animals on transects, from a vantage point, or from observation stations (Engeman *et al.* 2013) are often used in studies of behaviour and abundance, and to gauge a species' presence or absence in a defined area. Observation of free-living animals can also provide a useful method for the investigation of behaviours in the context in which they evolved. This may be used as a once-off technique, or repeatedly, depending on the research objectives. Natural history observations may be opportunistic or unplanned. For example, while undertaking fieldwork an unexpected behaviour or novel event may be observed that warrants reporting (e.g. Appleby *et al.* 2013).

Animal welfare considerations

Visual observation is typically a very low impact technique if undertaken with consideration for the sensitivity and ecology of the study and non-target species. However, an observer's presence could cause unintended fear, distress or other harm to study animals depending on how it is used (see Knight 2009 for a discussion about the potential effects of recreational wildlife watching). Observer presence may also affect data collection, for example by influencing or altering the behaviour under investigation (Animal Behaviour Society 2012), or affecting detectability of the subject (Robinson *et al.* 2018).

Habituation

Reported effects of research-based observation on animals in the wild are relatively few. Studies of visitor effects on zoo animals or of tourist–wildlife interactions indicate that the extent and nature of the impact depends on (for example) noise levels and group size, and may include changes in the behaviour and physiology of observed animals, particularly during their breeding seasons (de la Torre *et al.* 2000; Birke 2002; Davey 2007; Choo *et al.* 2011). While habituation is often used by researchers to minimise observer effects on study animals, particularly primates (Jack *et al.* 2008), it may reduce the natural behaviour exhibited by a study animal, interfering with its ability to undertake its normal activities (including social interactions), and may modify an animal's behaviour in ways that are difficult to detect (Knight 2009; Crofoot *et al.* 2010).

Disruptions to normal activities

Observation of animals in the wild may disrupt their normal activities (e.g. feeding and foraging, reproduction and social interactions) as a result of the presence (including scent) of the observer. Factors likely to influence the magnitude of this impact include the duration of observation, whether the animal is being pursued continually, if the observer's location is impeding access to a resource (e.g. a watering point or food source), seasonality (e.g. if observation occurs at a critical point in the animal's breeding season), and territoriality or habitat use (e.g. if the animal follows the same route regularly). For some species, observations that occur close to denning sites or around young could lead to the relocation or abandonment of the young, although reports are few. It may also cause physiological stress resulting from the observer's presence and may increase levels of a suite of hormones used by animals to respond to stressful situations (Fardell *et al.* 2020). Remaining as far as practical from such sites, avoiding observations during the breeding season for sensitive species (unless breeding behaviour is the subject of the study), or using camera trap technology for longer-term observations (see Chapter 5) will help mitigate these risks.

General procedures

Familiarisation with the study animal

The researcher should identify key biological and ecological characteristics that may influence study animals (or sensitivity of the species), results and their own safety. These characteristics may include feeding strategies; movement and land-use patterns; known predators; shelter sites (dens, burrows or nests); social structure (e.g. solitary species versus those that live in packs); diel behaviour patterns (nocturnal; diurnal; crepuscular) and seasonality; and the level of risk that the species poses to the observer if they become distressed.

Selecting a vantage point and concealment

Typically, researchers conceal themselves (e.g. in a natural or artificial hide, behind a shrub or rock, or with camouflaged equipment and clothing) or by maintaining a suitable distance (which will vary depending on taxa and study objectives) from study animal(s). Selected distance and location of the observer may also include consideration of scent and wind direction. Researchers may choose to reduce their use of scented soaps, deodorants, perfumes, insect repellent and washing liquids to minimise the effect of their scent on the behaviour of study animals. Where the observer is not aiming to conceal themselves from the study animal, they should still aim to minimise the effect of their presence.

Observation of animals

The observer should watch animals from an appropriate distance and vantage point, with or without visual aids, for a predefined duration. During observation periods, movements that may alert, startle or alter the animal's behaviour should be avoided, and verbal discussions between observers minimised. The optimum number of observers is typically two, so that one observer can record field notes while the other monitors the study animal. Alternatively, if only one observer is available, video could be recorded or a voice recorder used to dictate observations quietly for later transcription. Animals should be monitored continuously for behavioural changes that may indicate signs of stress. On completion of the observation period, the observer should quietly gather all equipment and personal items, and leave the site. Ideally, the observer should wait until all animals have left the site.

Details, including date, time, location, weather conditions (e.g. temperature, wind speed and precipitation) and people present can be recorded, as this information may influence the behaviour of the species being observed and be important for analyses (Lehner 1996). For systematic observational studies, pre-designed ethograms and data-coding sheets can be used for note taking and data recording for behavioural studies (Lehner 1996). Studies using visual observation in concert with ethograms should be specific to both the species and the aims or goals of the research, and remain free from intrinsic bias (Altmann 1974). Observation time and sampling intervals should be considered and optimised according to the species and context (Kawanaka 1996). Seminal sources for developing, conducting and analysing visual behavioural observations include those by Altmann (1974), Martin and Bateson (1993) and Lehner (1996).

Animal treatment, withdrawal and euthanasia

The risk of injuring an animal directly through observation is low. Injuries may occur if study animals become panicked by the presence of observers, or if the presence of predators increases as a result of the observer's presence (e.g. if near an active dingo (*Canis dingo*) den; B. Smith, pers. obs.). In the unlikely event of euthanasia, suitably trained and experienced researchers should use a technique appropriate to their study animal(s) or seek veterinary advice. Factors that may result in a decision to withdraw from the study at any given point include obvious changes in the behaviour of the study species. The nature and intensity of these changes will vary depending on the species, but general considerations include behavioural signs of stress (e.g. pacing, rocking, shaking or raising hackles); alarm or distress calls; or the arrival or increased presence of predators.

Equipment and maintenance

Equipment will vary depending on the species or taxon, and the nature of the study. Typical equipment may include:

- note-taking equipment (e.g. notebook, laptop, tablet, voice recorder, or clipboard)
- navigational equipment (e.g. global positioning system, GPS; compass; maps; field guides)
- binoculars with a rangefinder or spotting scope
- visual recording equipment (e.g. camera with telephoto lens, head/body mounted cameras or handheld video camera)
- night- or thermal-vision equipment
- tripod or monopod
- personal protective equipment (PPE)
- seating for the observer
- artificial or natural hides (or observation blind)
- camouflage equipment (including clothing)
- spare batteries for electronic devices
- for remote fieldwork, and where mobile phone towers and VHF radio are unavailable, a personal locator beacon (PLB) or an emergency position indicating radio beacon (EPIRB).

Specific qualifications, experience and training

The qualifications and experience required to perform the procedure will vary depending on the sensitivity of the study species or taxon to the presence of humans, and the nature of the study, and should 'scale up' accordingly. Animal observation experience is important, but generally not critical. Having a good working knowledge of any equipment being used is important. Personnel should be competent with the technique proposed and familiar with the species, having undertaken similar work, or propose to be trained or supervised by someone who is suitably qualified. Personnel should state clearly the nature of their previous experience (including species or taxa worked with and approximate months or years). Personnel should be able to recognise signs of distress in study animals.

Workplace health and safety

Aggressive or panicked animals

The observer should select a vantage point that would allow them to escape relatively easily or seek shelter from an aggressive encounter or panicked animals. The observer should monitor animals continually for signs of aggression or uneasiness (e.g. constantly looking in the direction of the observer, unusual 'starting' behaviours, movements or vocalisations, or deliberate movement towards the observer), and for the presence of other animals that may enter the area unexpectedly (as may be the case for social animals that form herds or packs) and present an increased risk to the observer. Appropriate first aid provisions should be kept nearby in case of an injury.

Ideally, observers should avoid working alone with animals that could cause serious harm or death. In some cases, observers may wear or employ protective equipment, or develop strategies to defend themselves if attacked (e.g. using trees, backpacks and jackets). For some species it will be important for researchers to conduct visual observations in pairs (at least) to minimise the risk of injury to researchers. For example, this precaution should be taken when observing large predators, such as dingoes and crocodiles, or large and potentially aggressive animals, such as some ungulate species. Species-specific risks are detailed in Section 3.

Alternative procedures

While visual observations are inherently low impact compared with many techniques, researchers should consider if study questions could be answered with, for example, remote monitoring equipment (e.g. acoustic recorders and camera traps, Chapter 5), or other technologies (e.g. drones, Chapter 6; tracking methods, Chapter 9), which may negate the need for an observer at all.

SPOTLIGHTING FOR TERRESTRIAL AND ARBOREAL ANIMALS

Charlotte Mills, Andrew Howe, Dympna Cullen, Damian S. Morrant, Tarnya E. Cox, Mike Letnic, Jemma K. Cripps, Helen P. Waudby and Matthew J. Gill

Target taxa

This GOP applies to all terrestrial and arboreal animals, including dasyurids (Chapter 18), wombats, bandicoots, bilbies, possums and gliders (Chapter 19), koalas (Chapter 20), macropods (Chapter 21), and lagomorphs, ungulates and rodents (Chapter 24). Spotlighting techniques for birds, including ground-nesting birds, are detailed in Chapter 15.

Context and scope

This GOP describes the observation of terrestrial and arboreal wildlife on foot or from a vehicle at night, with the use of a light (spotlighting). Spotlighting (with a head torch or handheld light) is typically used to target nocturnal animals, although diurnal animals at rest may also be observed. Spotlighting is one of the most widely used field survey techniques for detecting nocturnal arboreal mammals, particularly possums and gliders (Lindenmayer *et al.* 2001). It is also a common education-focused activity that lends itself well to community-focused activities because it is relatively easy to perform. Nocturnal animals have well-developed night vision because of a layer of tissue (the tapetum) in their eyes that reflects light back onto the retina. This reflection is visible with a spotlight, although observers may also detect movement or the animal's body outline against background vegetation (e.g. Crome *et al.* 1994; Morrant and Petit 2012; Wilmott *et al.* 2019). The effectiveness of spotlighting is influenced by observer skill, weather conditions and the (often cryptic) behaviour of many nocturnal species (Wayne *et al.* 2005). Spotlighting is usually performed along predetermined transects or, when using a vehicle, along access tracks. The length and number of transects are determined by the survey objectives and analysis requirements. The technique may vary depending on habitat type and requirements of the project or study site. Terrestrial animals are easiest to observe via spotlighting in open habitats. The method can also be used effectively in closed habitats, but the total area surveyed will be lower because of reduced visibility from dense vegetation.

Animal welfare considerations

Light exposure and loss of night vision

Nocturnal mammals' eyes are sensitive to light. Exposure to bright light sources can affect their vision and ability to move through the landscape (Morrant and Petit 2012). Observations should be kept to the minimum time needed to collect adequate data. The spotlight beam should never be pointed directly at an animal's face for extended periods. After the initial sighting – the dimmer switch should be used, or the beam shifted so that its less-intense outer edge is trained on the animal. Alternatively, a red-light filter placed over the spotlight may reduce the temporary blindness induced by white light. Using relatively narrow beams can also reduce the blinding effect of spotlighting on wildlife (DSEWPC 2011a).

Disruption to normal activities and increased predation

Few studies have tested the effects of spotlighting on animal behaviour, with most reported effects being anecdotal and short term. Species may move away from lights or turn their heads while feeding (Goldingay and Sharpe 2004). Affected animals may experience temporarily reduced food consumption and vocalisations, social disruption and increased predation risk, and may avoid future spotlight attempts (Eyre *et al.* 2018). Goldingay and Sharpe (2004) spotlighted squirrel gliders (*Petaurus norfolcensis*) once per month for 1 year and found that a few individuals stopped feeding while illuminated, although the authors concluded that the frequency of surveys was unlikely to result in strong avoidance of the light by animals. The risk can be managed by minimising exposure of animals to illumination and using the direct beam to locate the animal only rather than for extended observation. If longer observation times are required, personnel should dim the light, point the direct beam away from the animal or use a red filter (Eyre *et al.* 2018). Spotlighting potentially increases predation risk because of increased visibility of the animals, noise and distraction, although this occurrence has not been reported in the literature. To reduce this risk the time spent directing any light onto individual animals should be minimised. Spotlights and car headlights should be turned off when not in use, and vehicles should not linger in one place with the engine idling. Typically, a transect should only be surveyed during the outbound journey and, where possible, consecutive nights of spotlighting in the same location avoided.

Collision with vehicles or other objects

Perhaps the greatest threat to animals during spotlighting is collision with a vehicle or another object when disturbed, especially if the survey is undertaken along a track. This risk is increased by the blinding effect of light. It can be reduced through effective communication between the observers (or the driver or passengers), tactical use of the spotlight and vehicle headlights, and the use of a red filter on the spotlight. If an animal retreats under the vehicle when spotlighting or appears disoriented on the track ahead, observers should stop the car and turn the engine and headlights off until the animal moves out of the path of the vehicle.

General procedures

Planning and study design

Surveys should be designed to collect appropriate data to answer the research questions. Data analysis methods (e.g. occupancy modelling, distance sampling) and data requirements (Wayne *et al.* 2005; Letnic and Koch 2010; Buckland *et al.* 2015; Einoder *et al.* 2018) should be determined before commencing the survey (noting that these considerations are typically less relevant to education-focused spotlighting activities). Knowledge of the target animals' behaviour and preferences (e.g. diet and habitat use) and of the study site can be used to plan transect locations. Survey transects should be planned to ensure that travel time is minimised before and after surveys to reduce disruption to animals. Spotlighting transects generally need to be repeated to account for imperfect detection of species and are sometimes conducted in tandem with other survey methods to improve detectability (e.g. Heard *et al.* 2006). Wintle *et al.* (2005) provide detection curves for some arboreal mammals, which may assist in deciding how many visits are required per site to confirm a species' presence. Data that could be recorded during spotlighting are listed in Table 4.1.

Survey timing

Spotlighting start times may reflect the ecology of the species being surveyed. Many arboreal mammal species are active at different times of the night. For example, the western ringtail possum (*Pseudocheirus occidentalis*) generally emerges shortly after dark whereas its close relative, the common ringtail possum (*Pseudocheirus peregrinus*), is often the last possum species to emerge after dark and is most active before midnight (Wayne *et al.* 2005). In tropical north Queensland, coppery brushtail possums (*Trichosurus johnstonii*) are most active in the first 6 hours after dark compared to green ringtail possums (*Pseudochirops archeri*), which are most active in the 2 h before dawn (Wayne *et al.* 2005). In Victoria's temperate forests, smaller species with a high field metabolic rate emerge from their dens first, so ideally spotlighting should not commence until 1 h after dusk to allow the full assemblage of arboreal species to emerge (Lindenmayer *et al.* 1991). Such ecological information will help determine the spotlighting schedule and repeatability to maximise species detection rates and reduce data variation.

Table 4.1: Considerations for spotlighting-based studies.

Variable	Description and procedures
Taxon/species	The species observed can be noted; binoculars can be used if necessary. Experienced observers will recognise eyeshine colour and movement particular to some species.
Individual specifics	Sex and age may be recorded; some species exhibit clear sexual dimorphism and social tendencies in adults (e.g. red kangaroos, *Osphranter rufus*). Evidence of breeding may be recorded (e.g. young-at-foot or pouch young). Coat colour, other distinguishing features and behaviour may also be recorded.
Clusters	Personnel can record the number of individuals in each group.
Environmental variables	Cloud cover, moon phase, wind, rain and temperature can be scored for each transect to account for the influence of environmental variables on population estimates.
Total transect length	The length of transect (survey effort) or area surveyed should be recorded. For driven transects, the odometer reading and average speed of the vehicle can be recorded. For walking transects, a GPS can be used to record transect length.
Distance along transect	Some data analysis methods may require the point along the transect at which each individual was sighted. For driven transects, personnel can use the odometer reading for each sighting. For walking transects, a GPS can be used to record the distance to the starting point.
Strip width	Strip width refers to the maximum distance either side of the track or road where animals can be observed reliably with illumination. Personnel can record the point on the transect where strip width changes (e.g. if travelling from open mulga woodland into dense mallee). Maximum strip width can differ by species. Predators that have very bright eyeshine (e.g. dingoes; foxes, *Vulpes vulpes*; and cats, *Felis catus*) usually have the longest detection distance (200 m or more), while European rabbits (*Oryctolagus cuniculus*) or bettongs (*Bettongia* spp.) may only be reliably spotted within 20 m of either side of the vehicle. Walking transects are generally much shorter in length compared to vehicle transects, so strip width is likely to remain the same throughout if vegetation structure is consistent. If not, an index of vegetation density can be recorded or the point along the transect at which vegetation width changes noted.
Perpendicular distance from the transect at first sighting	Measured using a rangefinder when the observer or vehicle is perpendicular to the point at which the animal/cluster was first sighted.

Unfavourable weather

Spotlighting surveys should not be undertaken during extreme or inclement weather, including rain or extreme heat, unless necessary to meet survey objectives. Animal activity and detectability are typically low at these times (Davey 1990; Wayne *et al.* 2005; Eyre *et al.* 2018).

Light intensity

Light intensity is often a source of confusion for personnel when selecting an appropriate spotlight. Light intensity refers to the power of a light source and the direction it is being emitted. Light sources created from a light emitting diode (LED) are measured in lumens (lm), an estimate of the maximum amount of light emitted by the diode. The amount of light that reaches an animal is measured in lux. The geometry of the light reflector in the spotlight (e.g. focused beam versus broad beam) will determine the concentration of light being emitted in a particular direction, and ultimately the amount of light that reaches an animal. The combination of reflector geometry and lm determines light intensity, which is measured in candela (cd). Candle power and wattage (used to measure the intensity and power of incandescent lights, respectively) are increasingly less common measures of light output because these types of spotlights are progressively being replaced in favour of LED spotlights. While cd is the true measure of light intensity, manufacturers tend to use lm to describe output of a spotlight.

Ultimately, the detectability of an animal using a torch or spotlight is influenced by torch/spotlight design, light intensity, distance to the animal, focus of the beam and spotlighting technique. Other factors, such as vegetation density and animal size, can also affect animal detectability, and subsequently, choice of light intensity. Consequently, it is difficult to prescribe thresholds for minimum and maximum light outputs. However, a low light intensity (i.e. around 300–600 lm) with a broad beam is generally useful for detecting eyeshine of arboreal marsupials in forested areas. A greater light intensity (i.e. 700 to ≥ 1000 lm) could be used to illuminate the whole animal for observation, if necessary. In dense forests of eastern Victoria, 600 lm LED spotlights with a beam distance of around 1000 m are used to detect arboreal marsupials (J. Cripps, pers. obs.). Ideally, personnel should use equipment with different settings that allow light output to be adjusted readily in response to changed conditions, technique or animal response. Greater illumination may be required for small and cryptic species, such as feathertail gliders (*Acrobates* spp.) and pygmy possums (*Cercartetus* spp.). Lower light illumination might be appropriate in very open habitats (e.g. open woodland, grasslands, sand dunes, chenopod shrublands). The value of red filters to reduce disturbance or change the detectability of individual animals is yet to be verified in the published literature, although Wayne *et al.* (2005) found no difference in detection rates for common brushtail possums (*Trichosurus vulpecula*) or western ringtail possums when using red filters or white light. Nevertheless, their use is still a standard protocol for spotlighting studies, and the absence of experimental evidence for their benefits should not preclude their use.

Spotlight technique

A light handheld spotlight that is easily held above shoulder level is ideal. An animal's eyeshine is most visible when the light source is held close to the observer's eyes. A low light intensity head torch is often suitable for animal eyeshine detection. A more-powerful spotlight can then be used for observing the animal. The observer should sweep the landscape with the torch in an arc in the direction of travel, ensuring that both sides of the transect are included in the sweep. The light should be moved at a slow and consistent speed, as appropriate to the conditions. Binoculars can be used once an animal has been detected to confirm the species' identity and record distinguishing features. Surveys should be conducted quietly to minimise disturbance to the target species, and to increase the chance of hearing calls or noises that may indicate species' presence and location (DSEWPC 2011a).

Walking (pedestrian) transects

Walking allows observers to conduct the survey at a slower pace than during vehicle-based surveys and detect species that are cryptic or at lower densities, including vocalisations. Walking transects also enables access to off-road areas. However, as less area can be covered on foot than in a vehicle, more person hours are required and the proportion of the population of target fauna that is surveyed will be less. The direction of travel should be decided in advance, by locating a track, following a GPS or by marking out a transect with flagging tape or pickets to ensure that the planned survey effort is achieved (DSEWPC 2011a) and to assist with direction at night. Monitoring time and distance with the aid of markers may help observers maintain a consistent speed. An appropriate (and conservative approximate) walking speed is 10 m per min walking, such that it would take 100 min to complete a 1000 m transect (van der Ree and Loyn 2002). However, if walking off-track in dense vegetation this speed will probably need to be reduced. Depending on the species, habitat and study objectives, schedules may need to allow time for stationary pauses to conduct detailed searches or use call playback (see Chapter 5).

Pedestrian spotlighting is best conducted in pairs, where each person searches either the left- or right-hand side of the spotlighting transect, each covering a view of 90–180°. Doing so reduces the risk of shining light beams in the face of the other observer and also ensures consistent coverage of the whole transect. Alternatively, the pair could undertake a survey of a transect on the same night, but separated by 100 m, providing that repeat observations of individuals can be identified (Cripps *et al.* in press).

Driven transects

Vehicle-based spotlighting is generally suitable for surveys that must cover large distances or in sparsely vegetated habitats where animal abundance or detectability is very low, but visibility is good. Researchers should use their knowledge of the study site and taxa to determine appropriate transect lengths and vehicle speed. Personnel should drive transects in daylight, identifying or removing any hazards, such as overhanging branches, potholes, or patches that may become boggy when wet.

Observer safety must be managed carefully when conducting vehicle spotlighting and surveys only conducted on roads with limited vehicular traffic. The driver must not be one of the observers and should focus on driving and effective communication with observers. Typically, two observers either stand on the back of a utility tray or are seated in the back seat. When standing on the back of a moving vehicle it is important to have at least three points of contact with the vehicle at any time. A clear communication system between the driver and the observers must be discussed and understood before the survey starts. The observer should have an unobstructed vantage point in the vehicle, preferably standing on a vehicle tray with a rail to hold onto, and ensuring that one arm can remain free to hold the spotlight. Two observers with torches of equal light intensity may be used. However, the number and positioning of observers should be consistent between participating vehicles and survey nights or survey occasions. The same observer(s) should be used for any/all subsequent surveys to reduce observer effects.

Before commencing the transect, the odometer should be set to zero. Observer safety should always be the most important consideration when deciding on survey speed. Ideally, the driver drives at 5–15 km/h (Letnic and Koch 2010; Eyre *et al.* 2018) with windows down and any distractions or noise removed. If surveying for small mammals (or ground-nesting birds – see Chapter 15), a slower speed of 5–8 km/h is recommended (Baker-Gabb *et al.* 2016). Vehicle speed will vary with vegetation density and size of the target species. For example, dense vegetation and small target species may require slower speeds. Generally, the vehicle should stop when eyeshine is detected to allow data to be recorded by a passenger.

Animal treatment, withdrawal and euthanasia

Spotlighting carries a very low risk of animal injury. However, collision with a vehicle or object is the most likely source of injury to animals. Animals with serious injuries should be taken to a veterinarian or euthanased appropriately by experienced personnel (see Section 3 for species-specific considerations).

Equipment and maintenance

Equipment required for spotlighting surveys is generally standard across taxa. Essential items include:

- one handheld spotlight per observer (ideally with a dimmer switch) and:
  - spare batteries (unless powered by the vehicle)
  - spare globes
  - red filter
- rangefinder
- head torch
- binoculars (8 × 42 magnification are suitable for most projects)
- handheld GPS unit
- identification field guides for target taxa
- data sheets or electronic data collection device (e.g. tablet or mobile phone)
- waterproof notebook, clipboard, pen and pencil
- suitable clothing for changing conditions (wet weather gear; warm layers)
- personal first aid kit
- emergency communication device (e.g. mobile phone; satellite safety device).

For walking transects, the following additional equipment is required:

- timing device (e.g. watch, mobile phone or tablet)
- star pickets or flagging tape to mark start, end or centre points of transects
- compass.

For driven transects, the following additional equipment is required:

- vehicle (utility vehicle with an open tray is best)
- something to hold onto (e.g. railing).

Specific qualifications, experience and training

As spotlighting does not require any animal-handling skills, most people are able to participate in this activity without having extensive prior experience. Survey participants should demonstrate competency with the 'sweep' method, animal spotting, and using a rangefinder and binoculars simultaneously with a spotlight before conducting surveys independently from other more-experienced observers. For driven spotlighting transects, drivers should demonstrate an ability to operate a vehicle safely while observers are on the tray. Participants should be familiar with the species which occur in the survey area and be able to correctly identify target species from torchlight and eye shine. For inexperienced staff or volunteers, training can be provided at the beginning of the survey (especially where only one species is the target) and the survey conducted under supervision of experienced personnel. However, a baseline knowledge of wildlife observation and identification is preferable. Additional knowledge is necessary to design spotlighting surveys adequately to answer research questions and improve detectability of the target species.

Workplace health and safety

Conducting nocturnal surveys in bushland on foot

Working at night amplifies the existing hazards and challenges of working in bushland. Simple tasks can become increasingly difficult as light and visibility decrease. Unseen tree limbs or debris at face level can cause injury to the eyes and face. Observers must be aware of their footing on uneven and slippery ground, and the location of hazards such as cliffs or steep slopes, and avoid trip hazards. Avoiding these hazards is made more difficult during surveys of arboreal species because spotlighting requires observers to spend most of their time looking up at tree trunks and canopies.

Disruptions to sleep cycles

Night work interferes with people's natural sleep cycles and fatigue must be managed accordingly. Strategies to mitigate risk associated with night and shift work should be addressed in risk management plans, safe work methods statements, job safety analyses or similar, including planning for appropriate breaks between bouts of spotlighting.

Becoming lost or disorientated

It can be easy to become lost and disoriented during the night when unfamiliar with the environment, and when familiar landmarks are not visible. During vehicle-based surveys, mechanical issues or accidents may leave personnel in need of assistance, but far from their base. Satellite-based safety equipment and GPS can be enabled to record routes. Risk assessments or similar should be undertaken before commencing work and appropriate controls put in place.

Vehicle-based surveys

Vehicle spotlighting should only be conducted in areas with minimal vehicle traffic. A survey vehicle driving slowly and constantly stopping and starting creates a hazard for observers and other road users. Spotlights may also distract and impede the vision of other drivers. Where personnel propose to stand on the tray of a utility vehicle to spotlight animals, all legal requirements should be clarified before the study is undertaken. Personnel must ensure that appropriate controls are in place to ensure to reduce the risk of injury. Institutions should develop their own detailed protocols. However, controls may include the installation of appropriate handles for observers to hold on to and a safety rail fitted at waist height. The risk of being hit by overhanging branches is minimised by driving the road during daylight and noting or removing hazards before survey, and through continuous observation of the road ahead by the driver, passenger and observers. Safety glasses can be worn to reduce the risk of eye injury. Unsealed roads present additional risks, particularly after rain.

Alternative procedures

Spotlighting is an efficient and low-impact method for capturing data on species abundance, occupancy, distribution and population dynamics. Potential alternative methods include camera traps (Chapter 5) or thermal cameras placed at ground level or in trees, depending on the ecology of the target species. These methods are used widely for cryptic arboreal species, such as phascogales (*Phascogale* spp.) and tree-rats (*Mesembriomys* spp.). Live trapping, including box and cage traps (Chapter 7), may be used for taking a census of small mammals or arboreal species, but these methods may expose animals to greater stress and are typically more labour intensive for the researcher.

VISUAL SIGNS, SCAT COLLECTION, SAND PLOTS AND EDNA

Bradley P. Smith, Chris R. Dickman, Kari Soennichsen, Dianne Gleeson and Anna J. MacDonald

Target taxa

This GOP applies to all free-living taxa. The collection of environmental DNA (eDNA) focuses on waterways and aquatic species, including monotremes (Chapter 17), amphibians (Chapter 27) and freshwater fishes (Chapter 32).

Context and scope

This GOP describes the detection of animals or their activity from observation of species-specific marks, signs and traces (Table 4.2). These signs include bodily remains and excretions, scratch marks, and tracks or prints left behind in the soil or water. Often, these signs are detected more readily than the species themselves, providing useful information about their presence and habitat use, which can also be used for selecting additional survey methods. For example, signs of nocturnal animals detected during the day can increase success rates of survey methods used at night. The method selected largely depends on the study's objectives and target species' characteristics, behaviour and habitat. For example, an index of activity, incidence or abundance can be derived if systematic methods are used,

Table 4.2: Common signs and traces used for indirect detection of wildlife.

Signs	Description	Detection method
Tracks	Marks or imprints in the ground left by an animal's feet, tail or both.	Observation, although tracks can be surveyed in a targeted manner with soil or sand plots (see later details in this GOP).
Scats	Animal faeces; scats may be observed or collected from wherever an animal defecates or directly from the animal. Typically used for dietary, genetic or parasite analyses.	Targeted searching or incidental observations, and sometimes collection (see later details in this GOP).
Rub marks and snagged hair/fur	Polished areas in the landscape where an animal rubs against an object (e.g. a tree trunk), or leaves behind snagged fur or feathers.	Targeted searching or incidental observations.
Gnaw and chew marks	Where plants, bones or sticks have been chewed or broken, leaving behind teeth marks and saliva.	Targeted searching or incidental observations.
Diggings	Where animals dig into the ground for food, such as fungi or invertebrates. Such diggings can usually be distinguished between species (Triggs 2004).	Targeted searching or incidental observations.
Signs of foraging (arboreal species)	Marks or scratches caused by claws or gnawing on the trunks of trees are often left by arboreal species searching for sap.	Targeted searching or incidental observations.
Shelter sites (nests or scrapes on the ground or trees)	Where a nest is constructed either on the ground or in a tree. Some species make temporary scrapes in the ground under trees, grasses, shrubs or in channels as resting sites.	Targeted searching or incidental observations.
Shelter sites (dens and burrows)	Sites where animals seek shelter underground, or in caves or rock overhangs.	Targeted searching or incidental observations (covered later in this chapter).
eDNA	DNA extracted from water samples to identify the presence of a particular species or group of species.	Targeted collection of water samples from inland water bodies for extraction of DNA (see later details in this GOP).

such as scat counts and sand plots. Observations of signs (e.g. diggings of bandicoots, *Isoodon* and *Perameles* spp., and potoroos, *Potorous* spp.), coupled with collection of other environmental data (e.g. temperature, time-since-fire, vegetation characteristics) can be used to develop multivariate statistical models (e.g. Claridge and Barry 2000). The methods described in this GOP (visual signs, the collection of scats, use of sand plots and collection of eDNA), are considered 'low impact' because they do not involve direct interaction with wildlife and require little to no disturbance to habitat. The collection of animal remains is not covered in this GOP as animal ethics approval is not required when no aspect of the animal's life and death were altered as part of the research or study. The collection of animal voucher specimens (see Chapter 3) requires approval if the animal is trapped and killed for that purpose.

Animal welfare considerations

Increased predation and changed behaviours

The collection and inspection of secondary signs and traces do not involve handling or trapping animals. Consequently, these methods are generally considered to have minimal direct effects on target and non-target species. However, searching for indirect signs of activity (e.g. searching for tracks and other animal signs, scat collection, monitoring dens and burrows, and raking sand plots) may result in an animal being 'flushed' from its cover or shelter if disturbed. This risk should be considered if potential predators are present (e.g. wedge-tailed eagles *Aquila audax*, which may capture a flushed animal; DSEWPC 2011a).

Interference with social interactions

For scat collection, the minimum number of samples required for analyses should be collected as the removal of the scats of species that use them for communication and signalling could affect animal behaviour or movements. For example, some quoll (*Dasyurus* spp.) species use latrines as scent stations to mark home range or territory boundaries (e.g. Kruuk and Jarman 1995). Dingoes use scent for territory maintenance and at rendezvous sites (Robley *et al.* 2015). European rabbits use latrines or buck heaps as a form of communication and territorial marking (Mutze *et al.* 2014). The oversampling of these sites could affect behaviour, although no experimental work has been undertaken to suggest that this risk is substantial.

General procedures

Visual signs and surveys

For systematic observation and recording of signs of animals at smaller sites, it may be best to search along transects (e.g. spaced at 50–100 m intervals), in quadrats or partitioned using landscape features to ensure the area is searched systematically. Survey effort will depend on the nature of the species and location. Survey site and visual sign locations should be documented (e.g. using photos, GPS coordinates, records of material or signs, measurements, habitat types or maps); doing so is particularly important for temporal sampling where repeated sampling occurs over many years (DSEWPC 2011a). DSEWPC (2010, 2011a, b) provides guidelines for threatened mammals, reptiles and birds.

Accurate observation and identification of animal signs (tracks, scratch marks or scats) is aided by species-specific field guides, including, for example, Menkhorst and Knight (2001), Triggs (2004) and Kelly *et al.* (2012). Where signs are detected, but insufficient to distinguish between species (e.g. wallaby and potoroo track profiles are almost indistinguishable; Catling *et al.* 1997), alternative survey methods (e.g. direct observation, camera traps or hair traps) may be required (DSEWPC 2011a).

Several biological and ecological factors influence a species' visibility and likelihood of detection (DSEWPC 2011a) and should be considered when planning surveys of tracks and traces. These factors may include body size; behaviour (e.g. diet and foraging activity, use of dens and nests); sociability (solitary or social); activity patterns; habit (e.g. ground-dwelling or arboreal); habitat (e.g. density of vegetation or physical attributes of the topography); and abundance. The time that tracks and traces can remain detectable in the environment should also be considered (Brown *et al.* 2015). The chances of detecting visual signs can be increased by reviewing vegetation maps and aerial photographs, and consulting those with specific local knowledge, such as Traditional Owners, landowners and park rangers. Soil plots and sand trays or predator pads can be used to facilitate detection of footprints (see 'Soil plots, sand trays and predator pads' within this GOP). Nocturnal searches can be aided with spotlights (see 'Spotlighting for terrestrial and arboreal animals' in this chapter).

Scat collection

Scats can be used to identify species, their presence at a location, sex, age, size/mass, diet, hormones, metabolites and the microbiome of the depositor (e.g. Bluff *et al.* 2011; Eisenhofer *et al.* 2021). Bones and hairs found in predator scats can provide valuable information on the presence of other vertebrate species (e.g. O'Connor *et al.* 2020). Fresh scats can reveal what species have passed by, and how recently, and indicate the presence of endoparasites (see Yoder *et al.* 2006 for methods – the use of ethanol to preserve scats will destroy soft-bodied parasites). Systematic searches of scats in a specified area (e.g. scat plots or transects) can be used to estimate a species' relative abundance over time (DSEWPC 2011a). Examples are koalas (*Phascolarctos cinereus*) (Jiang *et al.* 2020) and red foxes (Sarre *et al.* 2013). Typically, scats are collected during targeted visual searches while personnel walk transects. Searches over large areas or of elusive species can be aided by trained scat detection dogs (see Chapter 5). The location and ease with which scats are located depends on the species and its habit. For example, scats of arboreal species may be found underneath trees/roost sites; at the entrance to dens and burrows for ground-dwelling species; along tracks and landmarks for territorial animals, such as dingoes and quolls (*Dasyurus* spp.); at latrine sites for European rabbits and some other dasyurid species; and along runways through the vegetation (e.g. broad-toothed rats, *Mastacomys fuscus*). Presence and characteristics of scats may vary seasonally because of changes to diet, weather conditions, or as animals migrate (McInnes *et al.* 2017).

Scats can be identified according to size, number, colour, texture, scent, and presence of bone, hair or undigested food. Identification of scats by morphology can be difficult for some species. It is useful to know what species occur in the target area and to bring a field guide to assist in identifying scats. The use of other signs might be useful in identification, including tracks, hairs, scrapes, nests, latrines, and kills (Triggs 2004). Scat identification can also be achieved through direct observation of defecation or post-collection (e.g. using DNA).

Scats should be treated as a record of an individual. Consequently, each scat should be placed in a uniquely identified bag (for terrestrial animals) or tubes/vials (for aquatic animals) to prevent contamination with other samples. For terrestrial animals, ideally, the selected parts of the scat should be placed into a paper bag or sealable plastic bag, making sure to prevent moisture and mould. When labelling bags, tubes or other containers, all details, including suspected species, placement (e.g. on ground, log or grass), location, date of collection, collecting person's name, and any details of habitat if relevant (e.g. near den or under a tree canopy) should be noted. Photographs of each scat sample taken *in situ* with a scale (e.g. a ruler, pen or coin) may also be useful. Gloves should be used when handling scat samples, and changed between each sample to avoid cross-contamination. When collecting scats, if no gloves are available, disposable forceps or clean wooden sticks or even leaves, rocks or twigs may be used. If the scat is fresh and moist, the collector can consider adding a silica desiccant to the plastic bag or outer container that houses the paper bag, in an approximate ratio of 4 parts silica to 1 scat. Care should be taken to ensure that the silica desiccant does not come into direct contact with the scat. Handling should ensure minimal damage occurs to scat morphology and other elements that might be attached to it (grass, twigs, sand or dirt). Bags or containers can be stored in a cool and dry location. For long-term storage, samples should be maintained in cool, dry conditions (e.g. at 4°C). It is important to prevent mould, and insects that will eat stored scats.

For dietary studies, scats can be used to identify prey items through the presence of hair, bones and other remains. This method is fairly straightforward and cost-efficient, and requires little specialised equipment other than a microscope and taxonomic keys. However, a suitable reference collection or comparative material (e.g. from a museum) and experience with accurate identification of prey items are critical. For example, the identification of Australian mammalian hair can be aided by the 'Hair ID' database (Triggs and Brunner 2002; see also Chapter 5 for details on using hair traps). The number of scats collected and analysed must be sufficient for the purpose and statistical power required.

Scat collection for studies involving DNA

For genetic and microbiome studies, the sampling and storage approaches to scat collection depends on the downstream methods to be used. Initially a decision needs to be made about the most appropriate sampling method (e.g. the whole scat, part of scat, or a swab of the scat), followed by a decision about its storage in the short and long terms (e.g. dry, frozen or liquid buffer). Some applications (e.g. characterisation of scat microbiomes) require high-quality samples in the form of fresh scats (ideally < 5 days old; Panasci *et al.* 2011) from surfaces with minimal contamination. Fresh scat samples are also recommended for predator diet DNA analysis (McInnes *et al.* 2017). However, genetic methods that use short DNA fragments as markers (e.g. DNA mini-barcodes) work relatively well on degraded DNA, and in these cases older or less well-preserved scat samples can still provide valuable information. Preservation and processing methods may also depend on the weather (climate and environmental exposure) and diet of the species. Aged and contaminated samples can still yield DNA. However, these samples may require additional time and laboratory resources, and can produce less-reliable results. Nonetheless, sufficient DNA for species identification may be obtained from scats that are weeks or months old (e.g. Ramsey *et al.* 2015).

Moisture in collected scat samples should be avoided as the samples may become mouldy before they reach the laboratory. Consequently, samples should be dried if possible (e.g. Sarre *et al.* 2013); or use made of paper bags, which can then be sealed with tape, refrigerated and frozen as soon as possible (McInnes *et al.* 2017; Eisenhofer *et al.* 2021) to avoid degradation of DNA. Temperature extremes should be avoided, including repeated freeze–thaw (including household freezers with self-defrost). If freezing is not possible, other preservation methods are available (see Song *et al.* 2016). If scats are to be dried, this should be done as soon as possible by allowing them to air dry (e.g. on wire racks, with scats separated at first to avoid leakage of wet samples). Once dried, they can be stored in cardboard boxes, or plastic tubs with some ventilation, in a cool, dry location (e.g. 20°C). Properly dried, DNA can still be extracted after several years (A. MacDonald, pers. obs.).

Scat analysis methods should be selected with the species and sampling context in mind. Genetic information on the identity and sex of the animal that left the scat can be derived from the whole scat. However, it is simpler to obtain samples by shaving a piece from the outside of the scat, or from swabbing the outside of the scat and targeting the mucous coat. Choice of what part of the scat to sample can be important (e.g. Walker *et al.* 2009). Swabbing is a straightforward procedure for scats from terrestrial animals, and is generally cost-efficient (see Quasim *et al.* 2018). Shed epithelial cells can be collected and stored in a buffer solution in the field. Liquid storage techniques, such as ethanol (> 95%) and DET buffers (at 5–10 parts per part of sample) are excellent for DNA preservation. However, liquid storage options are not always practical (e.g. when sampling in alcohol-dry areas, or when postal or air transport regulations limit liquid volumes or the transport of dangerous goods). Using screw-top vials with ring seals effectively prevents leakage (Kelly *et al.* 2012). For characterising diet and microbiome, the complete scat is required so that all contents are analysed. However, this form of analysis may require the use of blocking primers in order to reduce the amount of DNA belonging to the animal that deposited the scat (Vestheim and Jarman 2008).

For planned DNA analysis from scats, collection and storage should be discussed with the laboratory conducting the sequencing before conducting field work. For technical guides for extracting DNA from scats in the laboratory, see, for instance, methodological papers by Piggott and Taylor (2003), Eggert *et al.* (2005) and Ramon-Laca *et al.* (2015). Species- or taxa-specific methodological guides are often available and should be consulted.

Soil plots, sand trays and predator pads

Terrestrial animals can be detected if they move over substrates that are soft enough to retain their footprints. Researchers can detect this activity by installing sand plots over which the animals may walk. If standardised plots are swept clear and checked regularly, they can provide an indication of what species are present and, if plots are set up and checked at different places in the landscape over time, they can provide insight into spatial and temporal changes in animal activity.

Unless a very general indication of mammal activity is desired, it is crucial that different species can be distinguished by their footprints (e.g. heel pad, toes, claws, straddle, pitch, track width and stride length), locomotion (diagonal, bound or gallop walkers). Reliable identifications of prints can be made by observing animals walking on suitable substrates, taking photographs and developing a photographic reference catalogue. Guides to the key features of mammal feet (Menkhorst and Knight 2001) and photographic keys to footprints are also available (Triggs 2004; Moseby *et al.* 2009).

Small plots (e.g. 1–5 m^2) may be most useful for small mammal species, whereas transects may be more appropriate for wide-ranging species, such as dingoes, red foxes and cats. In one study of predator activity, 40- × 0.75-m transects were installed in random locations in a sand dune environment to detect potential differences in predator habitat use (Mahon *et al.* 1998). In another, 2- × 3-m transects were set regularly, 1 km apart, across low-use dirt roads to build a general index of predator activity (Letnic *et al.* 2011). The design and number of sand plots will vary depending on the questions that are posed by the researcher. However, in almost all examples, plots are swept before the expected period of activity of the target species (most will be nocturnal) and then checked when that period has concluded. Sand plots can also be used in heath, woodland and forest habitats on harder soils, but in this situation, it is usually necessary to rake and smooth the soil surface to ensure that footprints will be captured, or to import and spread sand on the ground for this purpose (e.g. Saunders and McLeod 2007).

Soil plots are simple and inexpensive to install and monitor, and can be operated with a minimum of training to recognise the footprints of target species. However, interpretations of soil plot data are limited. For example, it is sometimes assumed that differences in the numbers of prints that are left on plots over time or space reflect differences in the abundance or density of the target species. This assumption may be correct, but it is also likely that such differences in numbers of footprints reflect variation in activity levels of the target species, its responses to local habitat or weather conditions, or the presence of other species that may alter where the target species is active (e.g. see Engeman 2005 for further discussion). If researchers wish to use plot-based counts of footprints to gauge animal abundance, the counts must be compared with other independent methods to achieve this estimate. Independent validation is needed under other circumstances too, such as when scents or lures have been applied to soil plots to increase the chance of detecting rare or elusive species. Regular use of lures may attract individuals to soil plots and result in an overestimation of their true abundance. Despite these caveats, soil plots are simple to establish and non-invasive, and provide basic information, at a minimum, on animal presence.

Environmental DNA (eDNA)

eDNA sampling is a highly sensitive technique that detects extra-organismal DNA, such as skin cells, mucus, faeces and hairs from environmental samples (e.g. water, snow, soil and the air) that do not contain obvious biological material. eDNA can be used as a species- or community-level survey tool to determine presence or absence, which can help establish baseline data on species distributions and routine monitoring programs that track species distributions over time and space, and also be used to direct targeted searches for further study and capture of individuals (McColl-Gausden *et al.* 2020). However, it is a new survey technique, with standard approaches and methodological considerations continuing to evolve (see discussions and advice in Rees *et al.* 2014; Goldberg *et al.* 2016; Cristescu and Hebert 2018; McColl-Gausden *et al.* 2020). It is assumed investigators collecting the field samples work in collaboration with a genetics laboratory that will undertake the highly technical analysis (see Freeland 2017 for advice on DNA extraction, gene regions, primer selection and marker specificity). McColl-Gausden *et al.* (2020) highlight five key methodological considerations to be made when planning to sample eDNA (Table 4.3).

Generally, sampling eDNA from aquatic sources is best undertaken from spring to autumn as eDNA detection rates typically decrease during winter. The breeding cycle of the species, or groups of species, being targeted will also affect detection rates because some species will shed large amounts of eDNA into the environment during those periods. Personnel should avoid potential field contaminants, such as blue-green algae blooms that may inhibit polymerase chain reaction (PCR) methods in the laboratory. The volume of water collected will depend on the species being targeted and the aim of the research. For detection of rare species or those with low abundance, many samples are required compared to species with high abundances (Furlan *et al.* 2019).

Filtration is the most common method of eDNA capture from water, followed by chilling, freezing or addition of a preservative and then extraction with a commercial DNA kit. DNA degrades rapidly in water (Thomsen *et al.* 2012). Consequently, best practice is to filter water samples on site and preserve filters immediately. This practice is used most often and particularly with the eDNA backpack sample and self-preserving filter housing (Thomas *et al.* 2020). However, sometimes on-site filtration cannot be done, such as when sampling time is limited, filtration equipment is unavailable or in cases when on-site filtration is difficult because of terrain, adverse weather or turbid water (Kumar *et al.* 2020). In these cases, preservation by chilling, freezing, desiccation or addition of a preservative is required to minimise or delay degradation during transport and before DNA extraction. The choice of methods generally depends on the researchers' skillset, resources and budget. The best approach is to choose methods that maximise the amount of DNA captured and extracted while limiting degradation and contamination.

For detection of targeted or single species, filtration obtains higher yields of eDNA than precipitation or

Table 4.3: Key methodological considerations when planning to sample eDNA.

Table adapted from McColl-Gausden *et al.* (2020).

Single or multi-species	Spatial and temporal considerations	Water volume	Number of samples	Sources of false positives
• Determined by the study's objective (e.g. whether monitoring communities or the occurrence of an invasive species). • Differences relate to primer/probe development; bioinformatic processing involved; sensitivity; ability to estimate abundance; cost.	• Varies according to species phenology and habitat use; and likelihood of eDNA retention and transportation. • Periods of high density or activity (e.g. breeding season). • Preferred habitat and sample location (e.g. water column versus sediment). • Flows can affect optimal timing and location. • Environmental conditions can affect eDNA detectability (e.g. solar radiation; alkalinity; biofilm).	• Dependent on capture method (e.g. filtration *v.* precipitation methods require different water volumes). • Filter type and pore size can influence water volume. Optimal pore size may depend on site conditions.	• Consider the species density and habitat type, and efficiency of capture; eDNA extraction method; sample inhibition; primer sensitivity. • Replicates are needed because of heterogeneity between samples. • Collection of samples on multiple visits may increase detection probability.	• Dependent on hygiene protocols; likelihood of natural eDNA transport to unoccupied sites; eDNA persistence. • Assess laboratory contamination via the use of negative controls during DNA extraction and PCR.

centrifugation (Deiner *et al.* 2015; Doi *et al.* 2017). Large volumes can often be processed using filtration, whereas precipitation and centrifugation methods often limit sample volumes to ≤ 100 mL (Doi *et al.* 2017). The volume of water sampled is positively correlated with DNA yield (Hinlo *et al.* 2017; Muha *et al.* 2019), so increasing sample volume could enhance detection of eDNA and potentially limit false negatives (Geerts *et al.* 2018). When collection of large volumes of water is impractical, a combination of ethanol–sodium acetate precipitation with filtration may be a suitable alternative (Muha *et al.* 2019).

Different filter paper types have been compared across studies over the years. Despite varying levels of replications and sometimes conflicting results across studies, cellulose-based filter papers (i.e. cellulose nitrate or mixed cellulose ester) have shown consistently good performance for targeted species detection (Deiner *et al.* 2015; Hinlo *et al.* 2017; Kumar *et al.* 2020). Increased yields of eDNA have also been obtained from filter papers with smaller pore sizes (≤ 0.8 µM), but their use limits the amount of water filtered, especially in turbid waters (Minamoto *et al.* 2016), reducing the probability of detection. For eDNA preservation, chilling during transport and freezing soon after collection is effective for preserving DNA. If freezing or refrigeration is difficult, ambient temperature preservation through the addition of Longmire's solution directly to water samples (1:3 ratio) or filters is as effective as freezing for up to 2 weeks (Wegleitner *et al.* 2015; Williams *et al.* 2016). Another option is to use ambient temperature preservative, DNA/RNA Shield™ to preserve filter papers and buffer ATL (Majaneva *et al.* 2018). Drying filters by using silica gel or a hydrophilic filter housing is another good alternative, even outperforming more-typical preservation methods, such as ethanol immersion (Thomas *et al.* 2020).

Several publications compared various types and sizes of filter papers to determine the effect of filtration method on eDNA metabarcoding results for multi-species detection. Majaneva *et al.* (2018) found that eDNA filtration techniques affected the amount of recovered biodiversity, and that mixed-cellulose ester (MCE) filter papers yielded a more-consistent community composition than polyethersulfone (PES) filter papers. When filtering in the field, preservation of the filter papers dried in silica gel or in lysis buffer (Qiagen's buffer ATL) outperformed preservation in ice or ethanol (Majaneva *et al.* 2018). Li *et al.* (2018) recommended 0.8 µM pore filters as best for DNA yield, probability of species detection, repeatability, consistency and filtration time in eutrophic high-density ponds.

Generally, filters with smaller pore sizes appear to perform better than filters with larger pore sizes, although trade-offs with filtration time and turbidity should be considered. For example, 5 µm filters yielded significantly more total eDNA than 1 µm filters because of larger filterable water volume before clogging in a study targeting the invasive mudsnail (*Potamopyrgus antipodarum*) (Thomas *et al.* 2018). Enclosed filters (e.g. Sterivex™ filters) also compared reasonably well in terms of performance with other filter papers, with the benefit of on-site filtration and less opportunity for contamination (Li *et al.* 2018), although the total filterable volume using these types of filters is limited.

Animal treatment, withdrawal and euthanasia

Scat collection, sand plots, collecting water samples (eDNA) and the inspection of secondary signs of fauna do not involve handling or trapping animals. Consequently, these methods are unlikely to have any direct effects on animals. Treatment or euthanasia would not be needed in any scenario.

Equipment and maintenance

General equipment required for all methods covered in this GOP (for surveys, visual signs and collection) might include:

- data recording equipment (notebooks, pens, GPS and digital camera)
- field guide to help identify scats and tracks.
  In addition, when collecting samples:
- disposable gloves
- sealable plastic and/or paper bags
- permanent marker pens for labelling samples
- silica desiccant gel or beads (optional)
- rubbish bags
- hand sanitiser.

For studies involving eDNA, specific equipment needed in addition to the above for water sampling in the field and transporting to the laboratory may include:

- data logger conductivity meter
- water-resistant notebooks and camera
- boots, chest waders
- cooler box/esky
- water sampling bottles (recommend Nalgene®) (with a volume of 1 L or more, pre-bleached)

- water sampling bottles (containing 1 L of sterilised water) – 1 bottle per day
- sodium hypochlorite cleaner spray (1 bottle)
- paper towels.

When using soil plots/sand trays/predator pads, equipment required may include:

- measuring tape of suitable length
- rake suitable for substrate
- species-specific lure.

Specific qualifications, experience or training

These methods are relatively simple to employ and to standardise. Field experience and skills are needed to be able to identify the species that the secondary sign belongs to, but inexperienced personnel can be trained easily in the field under supervision. A basic level of knowledge regarding the safe handling, collection and storage of scats and water samples is required. An understanding of the effects (direct or indirect) that may result from disturbing areas that animals frequent is important for walking transects, visual searching, and collection. Identifying species accurately based on scats, tracks or fur samples can be difficult for some species; specialist advice may need to be sought.

Workplace health and safety

Researchers should complete standard risk assessment procedures depending on how and where work is to be performed (e.g. in remote areas, in challenging terrain, near nesting/denning animals, near water). Collecting samples from the water comes with an inherent risk of drowning; investigators should have appropriate risk management procedures in place to mitigate the risk. Handling of scats is associated with a risk of zoonosis (a range of pathogens may be passed between animals and humans), so gloves should be worn, equipment kept clean and good personal hygiene practised.

Alternative procedures

Searches for indirect signs require far less effort and have less impact on animal welfare than alternative methods, such as trapping (Chapter 7). Consequently, they are preferred for many medium- and large-sized mammals, depending on the research question, as long as they are conducted at times when predators are not in the immediate vicinity (DSEWPC 2011a). Inherent problems with using convenience sampling and index values (raw counts) mean that visual signs and soil plots should not be used as stand-alone methods for determining population estimates (see Anderson 2001 2003), but as a supplement to other methods, such as camera traps (Chapter 5) and mark–recapture (Chapter 8). Collection of scats and eDNA from water samples are high-yield and low-impact methods of sampling.

INSTALLATION AND OBSERVATION OF NEST BOXES AND HOLLOWS

Leigh-Ann Woolley, Stephen R. Griffiths, Alyson Stobo-Wilson, Cara Penton and Damian S. Morrant

Target taxa

These methods apply to small dasyurids (Chapter 18), possums and gliders (Chapter 19), bats (Chapter 23), and rodents (Chapter 24). Nests and hollows for birds are covered in Chapter 15.

Context and scope

Many arboreal species rely on tree hollows for shelter and breeding sites. The installation of artificial hollows (nest boxes or hollows carved directly into the trunks or branches of live trees) is a useful research tool for targeting tree cavity-dependent wildlife (Goldingay *et al.* 2020a), and can be an effective conservation tool for some arboreal mammal species (Goldingay *et al.* 2018; Macak 2020). Nonetheless, nest boxes are not an alternative to retaining hollow-bearing trees (Lindenmayer *et al.* 2017). Evidence for the effectiveness of artificial tree hollows for conserving hollow-dependent mammals at the population or community level is equivocal (Lindenmayer *et al.* 2016; Griffiths *et al.* 2017a, 2020a), particularly for hollow-roosting Australian microbats (Chapter 23). Most bat box studies have reported relatively low rates of use, with the number of species using boxes comprising a small proportion of the local bat community; the species that do use boxes are typically common, widespread taxa (Griffiths *et al.* 2020a). Consequently, while several bat species have been recorded from boxes (e.g. Griffiths *et al.* 2019), quantifying the conservation value that bat boxes provide for Australian bat communities in areas with reduced hollow availability remains problematic (Griffiths *et al.* 2017a). Knowledge of preferred cavity characteristics is essential to ensuring that the target taxa are sampled and to improving habitat restoration for cavity-using mammals. However, for most free-ranging hollow-dependent wildlife in Australia, little is known about the specific physical characteristics of the natural tree hollows that they choose to use. Ongoing experimental research, monitoring and reporting are critical in assessing the effectiveness of conservation-focused nest-box programs.

Artificial cavities can be carved into logs, or constructed from timber or other materials, and erected on raised surfaces (Griffiths *et al.* 2018; Figure 4.1).

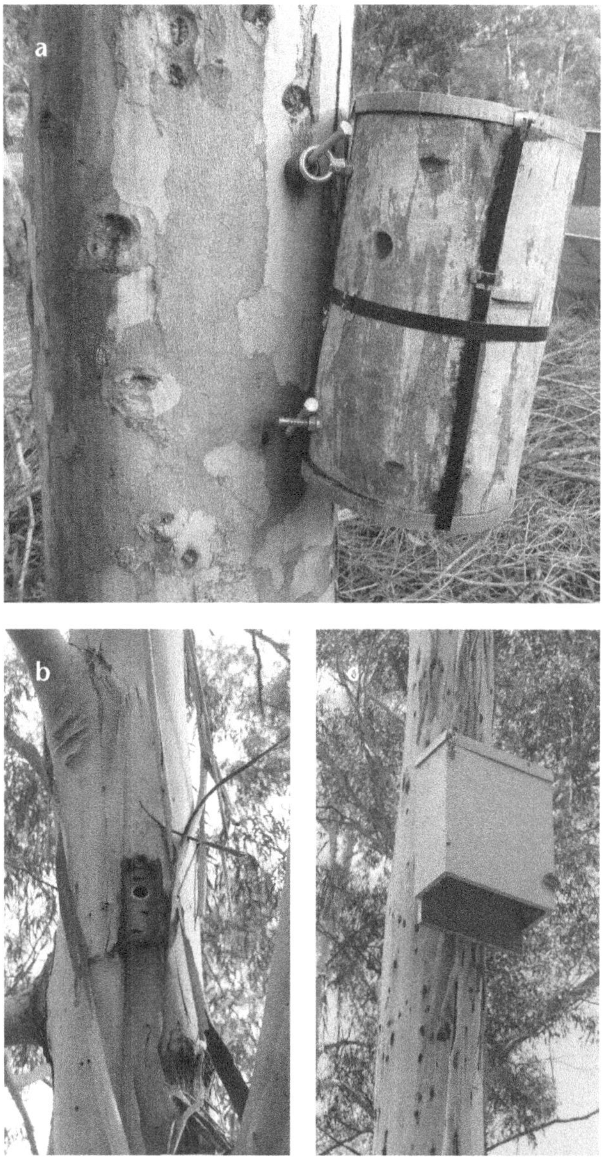

Figure 4.1: Three types of artificial cavities. (a) A salvaged log hollow, capped top and bottom with recycled high-density polyethylene plastic and a 40 mm entrance hole designed for small marsupial gliders. (b) A chainsaw hollow carved into a live eucalypt, with a 65 mm entrance hole designed for eastern rosellas (*Platycercus eximius*). (c) A four-chamber Bat Conservation International 'fissure-type' bat box. Photos by Stephen Griffiths.

Hollows can also be carved into trees directly or existing cavities modified (Griffiths *et al.* 2020b). Internal dimensions, thermal properties, and entrance size, orientation and protection are of particular importance for attracting target species and creating suitable shelter conditions (Goldingay *et al.* 2015, 2020a). Box attrition from weathering and decomposition of boxes made from plywood or timber, and loss of boxes as growing trees engulf or break the fixings used to attach boxes, (Bender 2011; Lindenmayer *et al.* 2009, 2016) can be problems. However, with regular maintenance nest boxes can remain available to wildlife for several decades (Goldingay *et al.* 2018; Griffiths *et al.* 2019). Recent efforts have tested various nest-box materials and designs to maximise longevity of the nest boxes, including fire-resistant nest boxes made from aerated concrete for greater gliders (*Petauroides volans*) (Greening Australia, pers. comm.).

It may take up to a year following installation for some species to start using artificial hollows (S. Petit, pers. comm.). Thus, researchers should be mindful of project time frames when planning to use nest boxes for population monitoring or recovery projects. Additionally, as per their natural denning behaviour, many arboreal mammal species use multiple dens, including squirrel glider (Crane *et al.* 2010), brush-tailed phascogale (*Phascogale tapoatafa*) (van der Ree *et al.* 2006) and black-footed tree-rat (*Mesembriomys gouldii*), brush-tailed rabbit-rat (*Conilurus penicillatus*) and northern brushtail possum (*Trichosurus vulpecula arnhemensis*) (Penton *et al.* 2020). Consequently, researchers should install sufficient boxes such that multiple nest boxes are available per individual, depending on the community context and the preferences of the targeted species.

Animal welfare considerations

Heat stress and thermoregulatory costs of artificial hollows

Artificial nest cavities generally experience more variable and extreme temperatures than tree hollows (Maziarz *et al.* 2017; Strain *et al.* 2021) and chainsaw-carved tree cavities (Griffiths *et al.* 2018). Temperature variation can cause a higher cumulative energy cost for species and high day-time temperatures can result in acute heat stress and dehydration (Flaquer *et al.* 2014; Rowland *et al.* 2017; Griffiths 2021). The dimensions, colour and material of artificial nest cavities can influence internal temperature and humidity profiles (Griffiths *et al.* 2017b; Larson *et al.*

2018). Yearly climatic conditions should be considered to inform the best materials for artificial cavities. Alternatively, a range of colours and materials can provide a diversity of thermal profiles suitable across seasons (Griffiths *et al.* 2017b; Rowland *et al.* 2017). Nest-box placement can also be important as the interplay between aspect and canopy cover may affect temperature extremes (Griffiths *et al.* 2017b). For example, south-east–facing artificial cavities were slightly cooler during the hottest times of the day in a temperate woodland (Goldingay 2015), while day time temperatures in north- and west-facing boxes often exceeded critical thermal tolerance limits (e.g. 40°C) of many arboreal mammal species during hot weather (Griffiths *et al.* 2017b; Rowland *et al.* 2017).

Disturbance to individuals and young

If animals, particularly those with young, are encountered in a nest box or tree hollow, disturbance should be kept to a minimum. Observation via telescopic camera rather than physical inspection is generally preferable. Ideally, measuring hollow dimensions or checking nest-box contents should be avoided if they are occupied. Some species (e.g. gliders and microbats) pose a flight risk and will often leave the hollow or nest box when it is checked physically (S. Griffiths, pers. obs.). This response can heighten individual stress and increase predation risk. If the animal does not flee immediately, disturbance may also affect natural denning behaviour by prompting the animal to vacate that hollow or nest box permanently, or use it less frequently.

Ecological impacts

The potential ecological effects of artificial nests should be considered, particularly where they could exacerbate the effects of exotic or overabundant native species (Griffiths *et al.* 2020a). For example, introduced honey bees (*Apis mellifera*), common mynas (*Acridotheres tristis*) or brushtail possums use nest boxes, and may pose predatory or competitive threats to local flora and fauna in some contexts (Grarock *et al.* 2012; Lindenmayer *et al.* 2016; Le Roux *et al.* 2016). Sometimes shelters can be designed to exclude or be unattractive to certain taxa, for example, by reducing the entrance size (Goldingay *et al.* 2020a). In particular, the establishment of introduced honey bees in nest boxes is a concern for researchers (i.e. Goldingay *et al.* 2015 reported that this situation occurs in < 10% of boxes), although two long-term artificial hollow studies have shown that hives are often abandoned after ≤ 12 months and the remnant hive removed by future artificial hollow inhabitants (Goldingay *et al.* 2015). However, in other landscapes ongoing infestation of nest boxes by honey bees can be a long-term problem (e.g. Irvine and Bender 1997).

Recently, feral cats have been recorded waiting for Leadbeater's possums (*Gymnobelideus leadbeateri*) to emerge from nest boxes (McComb *et al.* 2019). Nest boxes may be more conspicuous to predators than natural hollows and an increase in predation rates at nest boxes over time would indicate that predators identify nest boxes as a prey resource. Mitigation techniques may include placing nest boxes at greater heights (> 3 m), designing targeted predator guards and using tree collars in some situations.

General procedures

Installing artificial cavities

Prior to installing nest boxes or 'chainsaw hollows' carved directly into the trunks or branches of live trees, researchers should ensure that they are using an appropriate nest-box design or hollow dimensions known to be optimal for their target species (specifically entrance size and location of entrance) (Goldingay *et al.* 2020b). Doing so will increase the rate of use and reduce uptake by non-target species. Artificial hollow placement should also be considered carefully, depending on the ecology and behaviour of the target species or community, and potential interspecific competition for den sites that may occur.

Observing from the ground ('stagwatching')

Most arboreal mammals are nocturnal. Stagwatching is used to detect, observe and count nocturnal animals, such as owls, bats and arboreal mammals, emerging from tree hollows at night (Smith *et al.* 1989). Observations often occur at dusk and involve observers being stationary near shelter sites (see 'Visual observations' earlier in this chapter). Observers scan the crown of the tree or watch a targeted hollow for 20 min before dusk and around 40–60 min after dusk. Because nocturnal mammals seek shelter during the day, daytime searches can be conducted to locate suitable shelter sites or current dens. Stagwatching can complement radio-tracking studies (Chapter 9) focused on den tree use to confirm the accuracy of daytime tracking methods and identify specific tree hollows used by individuals (Penton *et al.* 2020).

Animals can be identified from their outline, individual markings and behaviour visible in the remaining light (aided by binoculars), or by their calls. Spotlights may be used to aid observation, but may disturb the animals (see Chapter 5). Thermal cameras can also be used and may reduce disruption.

Inspecting artificial and natural tree hollows

A telescopic pole and camera can be used to inspect the contents of a tree hollow or nest box from the ground, or via a ladder or other climbing equipment (Figure 4.2). It is important to limit disturbance, especially during breeding seasons; this factor should be considered when confirming techniques to be used and the frequency of checks to be conducted. Measuring hollows can provide insight into the dimensions or types of hollows used most frequently by a species. Horizontal and vertical entrance diameter, hollow depth, position on the tree (branch/trunk), height from ground and internal width can be measured with regular tape measures (or weighted tapes) after accessing the hollow via a ladder or by tree climbing. Evidence of hollow or nest-box use, besides the presence of an animal, can include the presence of fresh nest material, scratch marks around the hollow or nest-box entrance or on the tree trunk nearby, and sometimes traces of hair caught in the bark around a hollow or nest-box entrance (see 'Visual signs, scat collection, sand plots and eDNA' in this chapter).

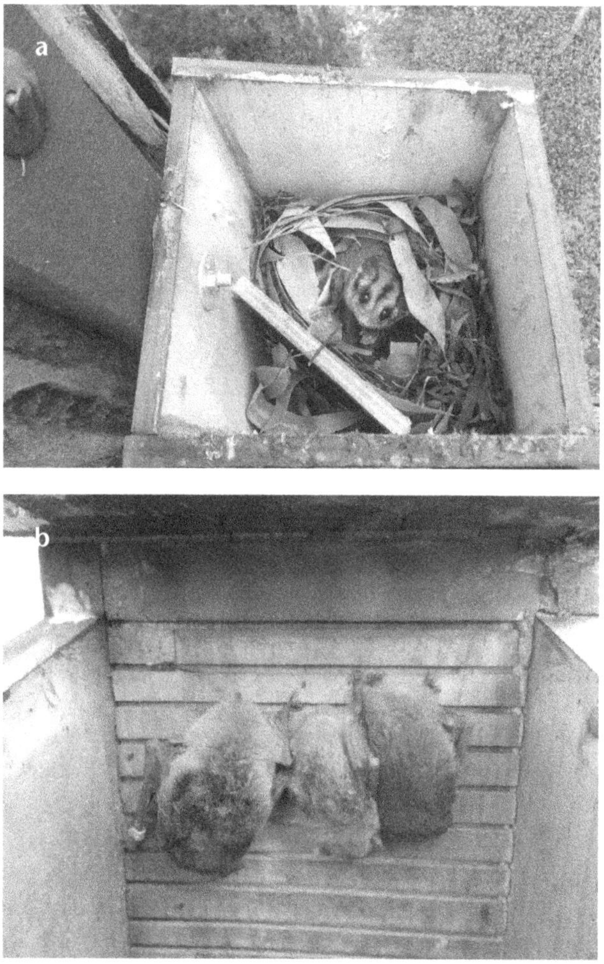

Figure 4.2: (a) A Krefft's glider (*Petaurus notatus*) in a nest constructed from eucalypt leaves in a nest box. (b) Two Gould's wattled bats (*Chalinolobus gouldii*) and one eastern broad-nosed bat (*Scotorepens orion*) roosting together in a bat box. Photos by Stephen Griffiths.

Long-term monitoring of artificial and natural hollows

Physical inspections provide a snapshot in time and while they are useful for determining the proportion of hollows or artificial hollows used at any one time, they cannot capture the frequency or duration of multi-den use behaviour. Most arboreal species use several dens within their home range. Long-term monitoring of artificial cavities or tree hollows with camera traps (Chapter 5) can provide a more-accurate representation of use (Rueegger *et al.* 2017), predation rates (McComb *et al.* 2019) and interference or competition (Davis *et al.* 2013). Cameras can be deployed via ladders or tree-climbing techniques, depending on the height of the target hollow or artificial cavity. Cameras can be attached to the tree with a bracket or on a neighbouring tree facing the entrance (e.g. Griffiths *et al.* 2020b). Cameras should not impede access to artificial or natural hollows. Bait stations can be attached to a nest box or near a hollow entrance to encourage use or provide an indication of arboreal species occurrence in the area. However, baiting may affect natural denning behaviour and should be well considered depending on research objectives.

Considerations for microbats

Bat boxes typically have a slit entrance located at the bottom of the box. When inspecting a bat box manually and removing bats (e.g. to take morphometric measurements, tag individuals or record mark–recapture data), the slit entrance should be blocked with a cloth before opening the lid to prevent bats from escaping. This procedure is particularly important during spring and summer when bats are likely to evacuate the box if disturbed, making them vulnerable to predatory birds (Speakman *et al.* 1994). For surveys conducted during the breeding season (typically October–December), pregnant and lactating adult female bats and their non-volant young should be placed back in the box manually. To stop returned bats from immediately evacuating boxes, the slit entrance can be blocked with a cloth attached to a length of cord; once all bats have been returned to the box and the ladder removed, personnel should allow them to settle for 15–20 min, then remove the cloth (i.e. from ground level) by gently pulling on the cord. See Chapter 23 for specific capture and handling considerations for microbats.

Considerations for possums and gliders

Sugar and squirrel gliders and pygmy possums breed in nest boxes and may use the same boxes over long time periods (> 5 years for gliders) if the nest boxes remain in good condition. Albeit less frequently, other threatened species, such as the yellow-bellied glider (*Petaurus australis*) and greater glider will also use nest boxes (Goldingay *et al.* 2020b). Nest-box uptake by possums and gliders may vary with the availability of hollow-bearing trees, local topography, surrounding vegetation and population abundance of the target species (Durant *et al.* 2009; Goldingay *et al.* 2020a). Animals tend to prefer particular nest types, which should be considered during design, construction and placement of artificial nests. For example, eastern pygmy possums (*Cercartetus nanus*) show a strong preference for plywood nest boxes over horizontal, capped polyvinyl chloride (PVC) pipes (Goldingay *et al.* 2015). Where abundant, smaller gliders, such as the sugar glider (including here the recently recognised Krefft's glider, *Petaurus notatus*) and savanna glider (*P. ariel*) will readily use nest boxes with an entrance diameter of 3–5 cm (Goldingay *et al.* 2015, 2020b). Sugar gliders have been recorded using both rear- and front-facing entrances, with some preference for rear-facing entrances (Goldingay *et al.* 2015). Larger possums (i.e. common brushtail and common ringtail possums) will typically use an entrance size of 8–10 cm (Goldingay *et al.* 2015, 2020b). However, some glider and possum species will increase the entrance size of nest boxes (most commonly made of plywood) by gnawing at the nest-box entrance. Typically, nest boxes should be installed > 3 m above ground.

Gliders pose a strong flight risk if nest boxes are disturbed, and are particularly vulnerable to birds and predators during daylight. Consequently, the use of a pole camera to inspect nest boxes is strongly encouraged. However, if direct inspection is required and animals are likely to be disturbed, the nest-box entrance should be concealed for 15–20 min following disturbance to reduce the likelihood of individuals abandoning the nest box. Often nest-box use by a glider can be identified by examination of nest shape and material inside the nest box. Feather-tail glider use can be inferred by the presence of ball nests (6–8 cm spheres), while other gliders will often leave a leaf nest. The presence of scats can also be used to identify species use. Manual removal from hollows and artificial cavities can be highly stressful for western pygmy possums (S. Petit, pers. comm.) and should be kept to a minimum.

Considerations for rodents and small dasyurids

Most small dasyurid species can use narrow entrances in artificial cavities (< 5 cm entrance diameter) and some studies report higher uptake for rear-facing entrances facing the tree trunk, possibly through elimination of competition with birds or larger-bodied mammals (Goldingay *et al.* 2018). Animals tend to prefer particular nest types, which should be considered during artificial cavity design, construction and placement. For example, brown antechinuses (*Antechinus stuartii*) show a strong preference for large-volume plywood nest boxes compared to smaller plywood boxes and horizontal, capped PVC pipes (Goldingay *et al.* 2015). Both phascogales and antechinuses are reported to use nest boxes between 4–8 m in height, with antechinus species more frequently visiting boxes closer to the ground (Menkhorst 1984; Soderquist 1993; Goldingay *et al.* 2015). Nest boxes have been reported to be most effective for capturing brush-tailed phascogales (Rhind and Bradley 2002), which typically construct bowl-shaped nests made of loose material, such as bark, fur, feathers or leaves (Soderquist 1993). Red-tailed phascogales (*Phascogale calura*) construct similar nests in tree hollows, often close to the ground (3–7 m), and can be readily trapped at ground level (Dickman 1991).

Recent nest-box research in coastal regions of the Northern Territory and the Kimberley has recorded arboreal rodents, such as the golden-backed (*Mesembriomys macrurus*) and black-footed tree-rat, using artificial cavities with large 9–10 cm entrance diameters (relative to their availability in tropical savanna woodlands) (L. Woolley, unpublished data). Although smaller-bodied, the brush-tailed rabbit-rat also used nest boxes with a large entrance diameter (9–10 cm) as frequently as it used nest boxes with a small entrance diameter (4–5 cm), suggesting that body size may not be as strong a determinant of nest box or hollow use for this tropical rodent as it is for taxa in temperate zones (L. Woolley, unpublished data). Brush-tailed rabbit-rats prefer dens < 8 m from the ground. Consequently, artificial hollows should be installed at a height between 3 and 8 m to target this species (Penton *et al.* 2020). Although rodents will bring nest material into artificial cavities and hollows (grasses and eucalyptus leaves), using nest material as an indication of use is not recommended as the behaviour is not consistent among these taxa. For example, tree-rats were often observed using artificial cavities devoid of nest material (L. Woolley, unpublished data). Manual removal of animals from hollows and nest boxes can be highly stressful for rodents (C. Penton, pers. obs.) and is strongly discouraged.

Animal treatment, withdrawal and euthanasia

By using well-constructed and installed species-specific boxes and cavities, and taking care when observing and monitoring artificial cavities, impacts on animal welfare should be minimal. Both initial and long-term visual inspection and monitoring of boxes or cavities are recommended (Griffiths *et al.* 2019). Researchers should be familiar with signs of extreme stress in their study and non-target species, and re-evaluate methods if these signs are observed.

Equipment and maintenance

Typical items may include:

- artificial hollow suitable for target species, including a unique identification, which can be printed on nest box or tagged carved hollow
- cordless drill, screws and mounting bracket
- GPS, camera, notebook for recording location of hollow, observations of contents and site characteristics
- climbing equipment:
  - ladder, or
  - climbing equipment and harness
  - additional safety equipment, such as helmet, chain to secure ladder to tree, tool belt or backpack to carry equipment while climbing
- telescopic pole and camera
- calico bags and animal processing equipment
- night vision goggles and thermal cameras.

Specific qualifications, experience or training

Nest-box and tree-hollow monitoring often occur at heights that are inaccessible via ladders, requiring an individual to climb the tree using rope systems or elevated platforms (Anderson *et al.* 2015). Researchers should contract qualified arborists to complete the work required (e.g. creating artificial hollows with chainsaws at heights; Griffiths *et al.* 2018). If researchers intend to complete this work themselves, they should complete the relevant technical training required to perform these activities.

Workplace health and safety

Animal bites and stings

Occupants of artificial cavities and hollows may inflict bites, stings or scratches. Spiders, bees, wasps and other invertebrates may inhabit artificial cavities or hollows; caution should be taken when inspecting the contents and researchers should wear appropriate PPE.

Working at heights

Falling from a height poses a risk of injury or fatality. Portable ladders must be compliant with Australian standards and inspected regularly to ensure they are safe to use. Personnel should follow appropriate guidelines for working at heights and ladder use, including wearing appropriate PPE.

Safety access and tree climbing

Tree-climbing procedures should be carried out as outlined by accepted standards (e.g. Work Safe Australia 2016). All gear must be compliant with Australian standards, regularly maintained and assessed visually before every use. Before attempting to climb it, visual assessment of the tree and surrounds should be carried out by a competent person, including potential hazards, condition, weather, structural integrity and location.

Alternative procedures

Artificial dens and cavities are an effective means of investigating the distribution and ecological requirements of many tree cavity–dependent taxa. Alternative or complementary methods may include monitoring with camera traps or acoustic devices (Chapter 5) rather than direct inspection of nests.

MEASURING DENS AND BURROWS

Kari Soennichsen, Chris R. Dickman, Jessica Clayton, Bradley P. Smith, Tarnya E. Cox and David A. Taggart

Target taxa

This GOP is appropriate for species that use dens and burrows, including monotremes (Chapter 17), some dasyurid species (Chapter 18), wombats, bandicoots and bilbies (Chapter 19), eutherian carnivores (Chapter 22), rabbits (Chapter 24) and lizards (Chapter 26).

Context and scope

This GOP describes methods for measuring and documenting the characteristics of shelters used by animals (either daily or seasonally) in the form of dens (a hollow or cavern often found in logs, bases of trees, stream banks, rock piles, dense shrubs or the side of hills) and burrows (a hole or tunnel excavated into the ground). Den and burrow measurements can also be useful when studying the ecology and behaviour of burrowing or burrow-dwelling animals. For many species, dens and burrows play an important ecological role, as their structures provide shelter (from predators and the weather), and offer an environment for resting, hibernation or aestivation, rearing young, foraging and food storage (Reichman and Smith 1990). Dens and burrows can range from simple shelters to elaborate constructions. Some species (such as rabbits) establish a series of connecting underground passages and holes, which are referred to as warrens. Animals can dig and construct their own burrow, modify a burrow made by another species, or live in or use a burrow established by another species. Burrows can be constructed in a variety of substrates and for a range of purposes. Consequently, their architecture varies in complexity (e.g. diameter, depth, slope, number and orientation of openings, number of chambers, active and inactive tunnels), and may be modified and made more complex by occupants over time (Kinlaw 1999).

Animal welfare considerations

Disturbance to animals and shelter destruction

Disturbance or destruction of active dens can disrupt an animal's natural activity patterns, alert predators to their presence, or induce physiological stress (see Reichman and Smith 1990). In some cases, disturbance may lead to abandonment of dens by parents, or relocation of dens (see species-specific summaries under 'General procedures'). Disturbance or destruction of inactive dens should also be considered because of the potential impact on habitat, the energetic expense to the animal of establishing burrows and the loss of available future sites for target and non-target species. For example, tunnel systems in small burrows can be mapped with expanding foam, but the burrow is destroyed to retrieve the foam mould (Felthauser and McInroy 1983).

Effects on non-target species

At times, dens and burrows of one species may be occupied or used by other species. For example, it is not uncommon to find echidnas (*Tachyglossus aculeatus*), goannas (*Varanus* spp.) and common brushtail possums using European rabbit warrens (T. Cox, pers. obs.). Echidnas, quolls, bettongs, brush-tailed possums, bandicoots, rock wallabies (*Petrogale* spp.), penguins (*Eudyptula* spp.), European rabbits, introduced red foxes, feral cats and many other species have been reported using wombat warrens (Ostendorf *et al.* 2016; Thornett *et al.* 2017). As such, any work associated with monitoring den, burrow or warren entrances should take into account the fact that non-target species may use the entrance. This consideration is particularly important when research requires the modification or destruction of the burrows, dens or warrens (such as for the placement of traps, and during den/warren ripping) of introduced species, such as European rabbits and red foxes.

General procedures

Excavation

While measurement of external burrow characteristics is straightforward, obtaining measurements from within burrows without damaging the structure or disturbing animals is more challenging and often involves specialised tools. Traditionally, burrow measurements were performed via excavation of one or more (preferably abandoned) burrows. While allowing documentation of dimensions, depth, and other characteristics of the burrows, this invasive method has great potential to disturb target and non-target species, and destroy habitat.

Remote sensing and geophysical techniques

Researchers have used remote sensing and geophysical techniques to detect and map burrows and tunnel networks of a variety of taxa (Stott 1996; Nichol *et al.* 2003; Swinbourne *et al.* 2015). Several techniques employ electric currents or electromagnetic radiation to identify near subsurface anomalies, such as air-filled cavities, by detecting differences in emitted and received electrical signals. While relatively cost-efficient, these techniques require a comprehensive understanding of the underlying geophysical calculations, so the assistance of an expert may be beneficial when conducting these types of surveys.

Ground-penetrating radar

The most frequently implemented remote sensing tool is ground-penetrating radar (GPR), which transmits constant electrical pulses and then detects the timing and amplitude of the reflected signal. Electrical permittivity of the medium affects penetration depth, which is reduced in sandy or wet clay soil, and in soil with high salt content. Interference by certain substrate types, and the inverse relationship between resolution and maximum depth, are the main limitations of GPR. Nevertheless, GPR has been used to detect burrows of a variety of taxa, including European rabbits and badgers, *Meles meles* (Stott 1996; Nichol *et al.* 2003), gopher tortoises, *Gopherus polyphemus* (Kinlaw *et al.* 2007), maritime pocket gophers, *Geomys personatus maritimus* (Cortez *et al.* 2013), and southern hairy-nosed wombats, *Lasiorhinus latifrons* (Swinbourne *et al.* 2015).

Electrical resistivity tomography

Another electromagnetic remote sensing approach is electrical resistivity tomography (ERT), where several electrodes are placed into the ground and the potential difference between electrodes is used to measure soil resistivity. This technique has been used infrequently – perhaps because it has led to mixed results when detecting and measuring animal burrows (Borgatti *et al.* 2017). Thermal imaging has also been used to detect and observe the behaviour of endotherms in their burrows or dens (e.g. Arctic ground squirrels; *Urocitellus parryii*; Boonstra *et al.* 1994). However, results of thermal imaging can be limited by environmental conditions, including direct intense sunlight and heavy rain or fog (Karp 2020).

Observational methods

Low-impact measures, such as surveys or camera traps (Chapter 5), are commonly employed to collect capture–recapture data and assess burrow usage or occupancy (Qi *et al.* 2012; Swinbourne *et al.* 2018; Treilibs *et al.* 2019). If qualitative observation of internal burrow properties suffices and quantitative measurements are unnecessary, burrows can often be inspected with an articulating optic fibrescope (e.g. Clayton *et al.* 2020).

Planning and implementation

A method suited to objectives, budget, target species and environmental conditions should be selected. Considerations should include species behaviour, data requirements, number of burrows to be examined, soil type and properties, accessibility of the site and access to specialised equipment. These criteria may quickly reduce the number of viable options for den or burrow measurement. For electromagnetic methods, it may be useful to perform a rapid electromagnetic survey to assess soil conductivity and ensure that conditions are suitable for the chosen method. The frequency of the antenna can then be modified to optimise detection for the selected site.

Prior to measurement, the target site should be mapped externally. Ideally, geophysical measurements should be complemented with a digital surface model via drone imagery, or coupled with positional data from a differential GPS. Depending on the method selected, timing and duration of measurements should be planned to avoid interference via environmental conditions and disturbance of animals. Access to appropriate processing software for geophysical methods is also crucial to transforming measurements to two-dimensional or three-dimensional images or maps of burrows.

The survey area should be set up as transects or divided into sections. For electromagnetic methods, measurement generally includes the setup of a tricycle survey cart, which houses the antenna, battery, control unit and screen display. After confirming that the antenna is detecting the emitted signal, the cart is pushed along the survey line systematically until the entire area has been covered. Alternatively, if using ERT, electrodes are inserted into the ground at a set interval or in an array and connected to the resistivity meter. Upon completion of the surveys, two-dimensional images can be processed and stitched together to create a three-dimensional diagram of the survey area.

Considerations for small ground-active mammals

Many small rodents and dasyurids use burrows that they create for themselves or usurp from other creatures, while others make dens among tangles of tree roots, piles of bark, logs or piles of rocks (Dickman 1991). Burrow entrances are sometimes obvious as small (1–5 cm diameter) and usually round holes in the ground or banks of soil. The identity of burrow users can be confirmed if footprints, scats, spoil heaps or, in the case of pebble-mound mice (*Pseudomys chapmani*), rings of small rocks that the mice have arranged around the entrance hole are present. Several helpful guides are available to assist in recognising signs of burrow-dwellers (e.g. Paltridge and McAlpin 2002; Triggs 2004; Moseby *et al.* 2009). However, small mammals generally have hidden or cryptic entrances to burrows or dens, which can be challenging to locate. It may be possible to identify animals den by observing them directly or setting camera traps in places where dens or burrows are suspected to be present (Swann and Perkins 2014; Diete *et al.* 2015). If a researcher is undertaking a live capture study (see Chapter 7 for methods), it is often feasible to attach radio tags or other tracking devices (Chapter 9) to animals so that their whereabouts can be determined after they have been released. In using any of these methods, researchers need to take care not to disturb animals in their burrows or dens. Measurements of these refuge sites and their surrounds are best made when animals have vacated them (usually at night). In one study, researchers sat 5–8 m away from the burrow openings of spinifex hopping-mice (*Notomys alexis*) and sandy inland mice (*P. hermannsburgensis*) after darkness had fallen, and observed animals emerging to begin their nightly foraging activities before attempting to measure attributes of the burrows and their locations (Dickman *et al.* 2010). Although laborious, this protocol minimised disturbance to the animals and provided an insight into how the numbers of animals using burrows changed between wet and dry periods.

When burrows or dens have been located, external measurements of openings, entrance angles, features of the location and other characteristics can be measured. However, unlike the burrows or dens of large mammals, options to assess internal burrow attributes of small mammals are relatively limited. Geophysical, thermal and remote sensing techniques are likely to return results that are too coarse to be useful. If the researcher wishes to measure physical attributes of burrows or dens, such as temperature or humidity, then data loggers or other sensing devices can be placed inside provided that they do not impede animal ingress or egress, or otherwise cause disturbance (Waudby and Petit 2017).

If a closer view of the burrow or den structure is needed, an articulating optic fibrescope can be inserted into burrows for 1 m or more to observe the burrow's interior and contents. The operator should take care to ensure that animals are not present when the scope is used (or have room to move past it if the burrow is unexpectedly occupied), and to ensure that the burrow itself is not damaged. This manoeuvre can be especially challenging if the burrow turns out to have an unexpected structure (e.g. some dunnarts, *Sminthopsis* spp., in arid Australia den temporarily in the spiral burrows of scorpions), if the scope gets tangled (e.g. dunnarts sometimes use spider burrows that have sticky trip wires and silken threads), or if the burrow dimensions are especially narrow. Nonetheless, patient threading of the articulating tip of a fibrescope can provide an unprecedented view of the interior of burrows and dens.

The second technique that has been used to explore burrow structure is excavation (Steele and Temple-Smith 1998). Although venerable, this technique is destructive and should be used only under restricted conditions. The burrow builders should be known to have vacated their structure and other organisms not moved in. Excavating the burrow should also have no negative effects on the local environment and minimal effects on edaphic processes, such as nutrient or water cycling. Predavec and Dickman (1994) excavated a burrow system of the long-haired rat (*Rattus villosissimus*) in the wake of an irruption of this species in central Australia. The site of this study had been colonised temporarily by long-haired rats following a heavy rainfall event and, after 18 months, all rats disappeared. During their tenure at the study site the rats dug extensive burrows in sandy soils, leaving the landscape pock-marked by spoil heaps of sand and honeycombed by burrows. Prior to excavating a representative burrow, the researchers confirmed that no rats or other animals were present by inspecting the sand around the burrow entrances for footprints over several days. The burrow structure was then measured, mapped and photographed as layers of sand were removed, and a model of the burrow system reconstructed using these measurements (Figure 4.3). The sand was replaced at the conclusion of the excavation. Within a year of the disappearance of the long-haired rats, all 'rat town' structures had collapsed, and the site of the burrow excavation appeared no

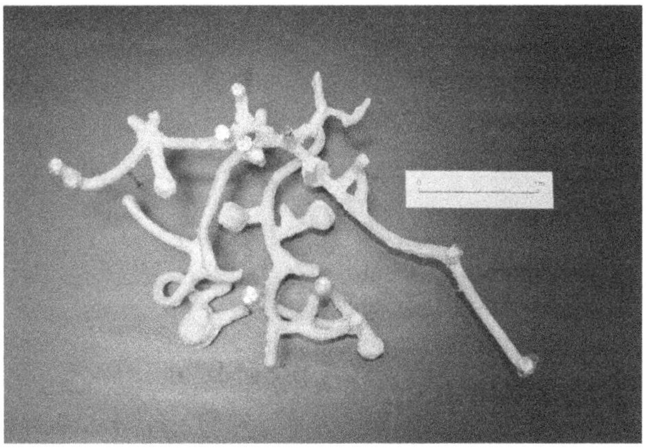

Figure 4.3: Model of a long-haired rat (*Rattus villosissimus*) burrow (top view). The burrow was measured in the field in the Simpson Desert and reconstructed as a scale model using flexible wire overlain by plaster. The burrow was first depicted in Predavec and Dickman (1994), and is re-photographed here. Photograph by Chris Dickman.

different from other sites that rats had previously occupied.

Considerations for bilbies, bandicoots and quolls

To some degree, the methods described above for small ground-active mammals can be used also to measure the burrow and den structures of larger species, such as bandicoots, bilbies (*Macrotis lagotis*) and, when they are not denning above-ground in trees, quolls. Bandicoots seldom burrow and instead nest at ground level or in a shallow scrape that is covered by a dome of vegetation and sometimes also by soil (Dickman 2015). Although these structures are often hidden under debris or dense vegetation, they can be easily studied once located. Remote cameras can readily record when animals enter and leave their nests, and an articulating optic fibrescope can be used to visualise the interior of the nest after it has been vacated by the owner. Quolls sometimes construct rudimentary nests like those of bandicoots, but more often exploit structures such as logs, hollow tree bases, crevices in rocks and underground dens. Except if quolls have commandeered the burrow of an echidna, wombat or other proficient excavator, these animals occupy shallow burrows and may use several within their home ranges. The simplicity of most quoll dens and burrows means that it is often possible to quantify the external attributes of these refuges and even see inside them. In one study, the interior chambers of three of 38 dens of the spotted-tailed quoll (*Dasyurus maculatus*) could be seen from the outside (Glen and Dickman 2006). As with bandicoots, remote cameras and articulating optic fibrescopes are probably the most useful tools to visualise quoll activity and describe the interior of quoll refuge places.

The bilby differs dramatically from bandicoots and quolls in its use of burrows and nest sites, digging deep (1.8–2.0 m) and complex structures in both sandy and hard clay soils. The burrow entrances are often set against a spinifex hummock, termite mound or other structure, and are left open. In open habitats, such as the gibber plains of the Channel Country, the burrow entrances and the soil that bilbies scatter around them are visible from the air, making aerial survey (Chapter 6) a useful way to monitor this elusive marsupial (McRae 2004). Remote cameras are valuable for detecting bilby activity at burrow systems, and articulating optic fibrescopes or borescopes again may be used to gain insight into the burrow structure and contents of the nest. However, because bilby burrows are relatively wide (12–15 cm), other techniques potentially can be used to determine their structure and dimensions. These include GPR and ERT, as described earlier in this chapter. Of these two techniques, GPR probably has the widest applicability. Although its efficacy may be reduced in the sandy and heavy clay soil habitats where bilbies now occur, GPR technology is improving rapidly. It has been used, for example, to map the tunnels of mammals as small as European moles (*Talpa europaea*; ~100 g); these animals construct deep and geometrically complex tunnels that may be no more than 5 cm in width (Allroggen *et al.* 2019). GPR is safe to use even when animals are present in their burrow systems (Cortez *et al.* 2013; Swinbourne *et al.* 2015). Despite its potential, GPR has not been used yet on marsupial species smaller than wombats (Swinbourne *et al.* 2015).

Considerations for wombats

All wombat species construct and use extensive burrow and warren networks (Wells 1989), with species such as southern hairy-nosed wombats using 1–10 warrens in an animal's home range (Finlayson *et al.* 2005). Southern hairy-nosed wombat warrens can contain > 80 burrows and cover more than 1 ha (Steele and Temple-Smith 1998; Shimmin *et al.* 2002). These massive structures are typically supported by soil type, rock and tree roots. Blind ending tunnels can extend 5–20 m and be up to 4.5 m in depth, depending on soil type. Burrow complexity increases over time with very old warrens characterised by many interconnecting burrows (Shimmin *et al.* 2002). Like the burrows of many other species (Read *et al.* 2008), wombat burrows are used by many non-burrowing vertebrate species (from brown snakes, *Pseudonaja* spp., to quolls), which use them to avoid predation, dehydration and environmental extremes (Thornett *et al.* 2017; Taggart *et al.* 2020). Thus, warrens are an important resource for all warren occupants. Disturbance of wombats when above ground can result in the animals retreating to their burrows for short periods, until the disturbance is over.

Ripping of wombat burrows for research or management purposes is ethically challenging because of (1) the difficulties in ensuring that the warrens are empty of their occupants, and (2) the removal of an important resource in the landscape protecting wildlife from a variety of threats. Current best practice methods before collapsing a warren suggests that a combination of (1) disturbance to the burrow entrance to encourage animals to leave the burrows and seek shelter in an alternative warren, and (2) use of remote cameras to monitor burrow occupancy following disturbance (O'Brien *et al.* 2020) are necessary. However, wombats can remain underground for considerable periods of time (up to 10 days), so care must be taken to ensure that warrens/burrows are vacated. If deemed necessary, warren ripping should be undertaken at a depth of at least 1 m and cross-ripping is recommended. The optimal period to engage in warren destruction is spring when weather conditions are milder and risks of dehydration are minimal.

Considerations for lizards

Small lizards will occupy arthropod burrows (e.g. Milne *et al.* 2003; Stevens *et al.* 2010). Some species, such as the pygmy bluetongue lizard (*Tiliqua adelaidensis*), occupy these burrows exclusively and show long-term fidelity to individual burrows (Bull *et al.* 2015). The same species will also use artificial burrows with a concomitant increase in lizard numbers (Souter *et al.* 2004). Interestingly, in this study, adding artificial burrows also increased the presence of a burrow-dwelling centipede that may prey on pygmy bluetongues, although no evidence of predation was observed (Souter *et al.* 2004). Arthropod burrows exploited by lizards often have one entrance and can vary in depth and morphology. If an inspection is being performed to determine a burrow's occupancy or depth, an articulating optic fibrescope or borescope with an attached light source is suitable for inspecting the burrow. The articulating end allows the observer to navigate the burrow without damaging the fragile burrow walls. Preference should be given to smaller scope diameters that allow the occupant to move past the optic fibrescope (e.g. a diameter of ~5 mm or less).

Large lizards (e.g. goannas) tend to live alone in self-constructed burrows or in dens and warrens of other burrowing species, such as rabbits (King and Green 1999) and bettongs (K. Soennichsen, pers. obs.). While lizard burrows are primarily characterised by one main entrance, bettong and rabbit warrens frequently exhibit numerous entrances, which should be considered when planning and measuring these structures. Special consideration of timing should also be taken with communally nesting goannas, such as yellow-spotted monitors (*Varanus panoptes*) and sand goannas (*V. gouldii*). Often, several females will use the same warren system for nesting (Doody *et al.* 2018a, b). Care should be taken to minimise disturbance, particularly during egg laying months, as researcher presence may deter other gravid females that would normally use the same communal warren.

Optic fibrescopes can be useful in determining burrow occupancy and examining broad internal characteristics, such as burrow orientation and the presence of branching tunnels. However, as is the case with perenties (*V. giganteus*), tunnels may exceed lengths of 7–8 m (Pianka 1982), making the available length of fibrescope a limitation for the extent of observation, and necessitating alternative methods for assessing burrow structure and dimensions. Provided they do not disturb animals or impede movement, data loggers or other sensing devices can be placed in burrows or dens to measure physical attributes, such as temperature or humidity. Because burrows are fairly wide, GPR and ERT have the potential to be effective tools to map burrow structure, although successful detection of structures may prove challenging in areas with sandy and heavy clay soil habitats. These tools can even be employed and remain low impact when animals are in their burrow systems. Despite GPR being recognised by Stott (1996) as a useful tool to measure burrows of European rabbits in South Australia, neither GPR nor ERT has been used to examine the burrow structures of large lizards to date.

Considerations for European rabbits

European rabbits often construct large warren complexes, with some older warrens containing over 50 entrances and having diameters over 20 m (T. Cox, pers. obs.). Not all warren entrances are often used and the number of active entrances usually relates to the density of rabbits in the warren (Mitchell and Balogh 2007). Entrances to warrens may be obscured by vegetation and some entrances can be located well away from the main area of the complex, often appearing as a single entrance to a different warren on the surface, but are connected to the warren complex underground. The entrances of active rabbit warrens can be detected with thermal imaging technology more effectively than they can be with visual observation (Cox *et al.* 2021). The entrances of inactive rabbit warrens can be detected through the use of a smoker. However, care should be taken when using this method as non-target species may be present. Depths of warrens are dependent on soil type and the height of the water table, but can be as shallow as 30 cm in granite/tablelands environments, or as deep as 200 cm in arid sandy environments. A variety of other species have been observed using rabbit warrens, including echidnas, brushtail possums, feral cats, red foxes and various reptile species. Consequently, any research that involves warren excavation or destruction should consider the presence of other taxa.

Considerations for dingoes and red foxes

Most of what is known about the denning and reproductive behaviour of dingoes is limited to a handful of *ad hoc* observational studies (the most comprehensive being by Thomson (1992) and Smith and Vague (2017)). Dingoes are annual breeders, with pups born in dens in the winter months (June to August; Smith 2015). As such, dens will be most active during these times. Average litter size is four or five pups, ranging from one to 10. Generally, only one bitch has a litter per territory. However, several breeding females raising litters in the same general area or territory, as well as communal denning, do occur when conditions are favourable (Smith and Vague 2017). During the first 3 weeks post-partum, mothers and pups occupy the dens almost exclusively during the night, and less so during the day. Males and relatives often remain outside the den (Hudson *et al.* 2019).

Den site choice mirrors the local conditions, with dens found in hollow logs, enlarged rabbit warrens, at the base of large trees and under large tussocks of spinifex. Dingoes prefer elevated sites, proximity to water, and den openings that limit excessive midday sun. Most often, dens only have one chamber and entrance, although multiple entrances have been found. Most openings can fit a human (~45 cm wide and 45 cm in height) with depths around 1 m (but they can be deeper) (Thomson 1992; Smith and Vague 2017). Therefore, the measurement of dens is rather straightforward and can be achieved using a tape measure and compass. High levels of dingo activity around the dens (footprints, pathways, pads/beds, scats and anthropogenic objects) can be noted. Although wild canids tend to establish den sites away from roads or areas of high human activity, they are resilient and can persist and even thrive in highly disturbed landscapes. They may occupy and change den sites within and between each season. Pups are regularly moved between dens within the territory (e.g. to a more-open den as pups mature), especially if disturbed by humans, predators or environmental conditions.

Dingoes are highly sensitive to human encroachment. Adult dingoes are likely to leave the den area when humans are present, but likely to return once they have vacated. If the site is disturbed dingo parents are likely to relocate pups to another den, and may even abandon the den and pups within (Thomson 1992; Smith and Vague 2017). As such, care should be taken when approaching dens during breeding season, the time spent at the dens should be minimised, and disturbance to the site and pups minimal. Dens and pups should only be handled if pertinent to the research. Where possible, den sites should be measured when the den is unoccupied. Considerations for monitoring red fox dens are similar to dingoes. However, some key differences include the timing of whelping (August and September) and the fact that red foxes are known to utilise dens outside of the breeding season as resting sites (see Gentle 2006 and Carter *et al.* 2012).

Animal treatment, withdrawal and euthanasia

This GOP is intended to cover the measurement of dens and burrows rather than direct interactions with animals, so disturbance should be minimal. In the event that den occupants are found to be unwell or injured, they should be left alone (unless intervention or handling is part of the study).

Equipment and maintenance

Specific equipment will vary depending on the selected method. However, basic items may include:

- recording sheet or notepad for details
- compass for determining den opening orientations
- GPS for locating and recording location
- measuring equipment (e.g. tape or callipers)
- camera and telephoto lens
- thermal/night vision scope for observing animals around the burrows or detecting whether entrances are active
- optic fibrescope or borescope.

Specific qualifications, experience and training

Monitoring dens and burrows is a relatively simple activity depending on the technique selected. However, experience with the species and equipment will probably lessen the potential impact on the target species and time in the area. Inexperienced people can be trained via manuals, and from mentoring and shadowing experienced personnel. Ideally, if personnel are monitoring and recording dens and burrows, then at least one member of the team should be familiar with the species and equipment being used.

Workplace health and safety

Large burrows can present trip or injury risks. Entrances can be obscured by vegetation, so care should be taken to ensure that all entrances are identified before conducting any work around burrows, particularly at night. When conducting night work, entrances should be mapped during the day. Observation points should be established suitable distances away from entrances to ensure normal species-specific behaviours and to reduce risk of injury to the observer when entering and leaving the area. Burrow occupants can also pose a risk to researchers. Although rarely reported, if disturbed, occupants (particularly when young are present) may bite, scratch or approach researchers aggressively. Potentially dangerous invertebrates (e.g. spiders, scorpions, centipedes, ants) may occupy smaller dens and can inflict a bite or sting if disturbed. Snakes may occupy larger burrows. Caution should be used when inspecting burrows to avoid close encounters.

Alternative procedures

The seasonal, reproductive and daily activity pattern of the study species should be considered when measuring to minimise impact. For example, if animals are mainly active in the early morning and late afternoon, researchers should measure sites at midday. Preferably (and if feasible), measurements should occur when dens are not active. Visualisation of the dens with borescopes, sonography and electrical resistivity tomography is preferred because they limit disturbance. Other methods, such as acoustic monitoring and camera traps (Chapter 5), can be useful in assessing activity at dens or burrows. Placement of these devices or additional equipment, such as data loggers, should be such that they do not impede animal movement. If dens are located in areas with sand or soft soil, examination of tracks may also help to confirm that an animal has left the area.

REFERENCES

Altmann J (1974) Observational study of behavior: sampling methods. *Behaviour* **49**, 227–266. doi:10.1163/156853974X00534

Allroggen N, Booth AD, Baker SE, Ellwood SA, Tronicke J (2019) High-resolution imaging and monitoring of animal tunnels using 3D ground-penetrating radar. *Near Surface Geophysics* **17**, 291–298. doi:10.1002/nsg.12039

Anderson DR (2001) The need to get the basics right in wildlife field studies. *Wildlife Society Bulletin* **29**, 1294–1297. https://www.jstor.org/stable/3784156

Anderson DR (2003) Response to Engeman: index values rarely constitute reliable information. *Wildlife Society Bulletin* **31**, 288–291. http://www.jstor.org/stable/3784387

Anderson DL, Koomjian W, French B, Altenhoff SR, Luce J (2015) Review of rope-based access methods for the forest canopy: safe and unsafe practices in published information sources and a summary of current methods. *Methods in Ecology and Evolution* **6**, 865–872. doi:10.1111/2041-210X.12393

Animal Behaviour Society (2012) Guidelines for the treatment of animals in behavioural research and teaching. *Animal Behaviour* **83**, 301–309. doi:10.1016/j.anbehav.2011.10.031

Appleby R, Smith B, Jones D (2013) Observations of a free-ranging adult female dingo (*Canis dingo*) and littermates' responses to the death of a pup. *Behavioural Processes* **96**, 42–46. doi:10.1016/j.beproc.2013.02.016

Baker-Gabb D, Antos M, Brown G (2016) Recent decline of the critically endangered plains-wanderer (*Pedionomus torquatus*), and the application of a simple method for assessing its cause: major changes in grassland structure. *Ecological Management & Restoration* **17**, 235–242. doi:10.1111/emr.12221

Bender R (2011) Bat roost boxes at Organ Pipes National Park, Victoria: seasonal and annual usage patterns. In *Biology and Conservation of Australasian Bats*. (Eds B Law, P Eby, D Lunney, and L Lumsden) pp. 443–459. Royal Zoological Society of New South Wales, Mosman.

Birke L (2002) Effects of browse, human visitors and noise on the behaviour of captive orangutans. *Animal Welfare (South Mimms, England)* **11**, 189–202.

Bluff LA, Clausen L, Hill A, Bramwell MD (2011) A decade monitoring the remnant Victorian population of the brush-tailed rock wallaby (*Petrogale penicillata*). *Australian Mammalogy* **33**, 195–201. doi:10.1071/AM10037

Boonstra R, Krebs C, Boutin S, Eadie J (1994) Finding mammals using far-infrared thermal imaging. *Journal of Mammalogy* **75**, 1063–1068. doi:10.2307/1382490

Borgatti L, Forte E, Mocnik A, Zambrini R, Cervi F, Martinucci D, *et al.* (2017) Detection and characterization of animal burrows within river embankments by means of coupled remote sensing and geophysical techniques: lessons from River Panaro (northern Italy). *Engineering Geology* **226**, 277–289. doi:10.1016/j.enggeo.2017.06.017

Brown WE, Ramsey DSL, Gaffney R (2015) Degradation and detection of fox (*Vulpes vulpes*) scats in Tasmania: evidence from field trials. *Wildlife Research* **41**, 681–690. doi:10.1071/WR14152

Buckland ST, Rexstad EA, Marques TA, Oedekoven CS (2015) Distance sampling: methods and applications. In *Series: Methods in Statistical Ecology*. (Eds AP Robinson, ST Buckland, P Reich and M McCarthy). Springer, Switzerland.

Bull CM, Godfrey SS, Ebrahimi M, Fenner AL (2015) Long and short term residence in refuge burrows by endangered pygmy bluetongue lizards. *Amphibia-Reptilia* **36**, 119–124. doi:10.1163/15685381-00002984

Carter A, Luck GW, Wilson PB (2012) Ecology of the red fox (*Vulpes vulpes*) in an agricultural landscape. 1. Den-site selection. *Australian Mammalogy* **34**, 145–154. doi:10.1071/AM11038

Catling PC, Burt RJ, Kooyman R (1997) A comparison of techniques used in a survey of ground-dwelling and arboreal mammals in forest of north-eastern New South Wales. *Wildlife Research* **24**, 417–432. doi:10.1071WR96073. doi:10.1071/WR96073

Choo Y, Todd PA, Li D (2011) Visitor effects on zoo orangutans in two novel, naturalistic enclosures. *Applied Animal Behaviour Science*. **133**, 78–86. doi:10.1016/j.applanim.2011.05.007

Claridge AW, Barry SC (2000) Factors influencing the distribution of medium-sized ground-dwelling mammals in southeastern mainland Australia. *Wildlife Research* **25**, 676–688.

Clayton J, Gardner MG, Fenner AL, Bull M (2020) Co-occupancy of spider-engineered burrows within a grassland community changes temporally. *Austral Ecology* **45**, 454–459. doi:10.1111/aec.12714

Cortez JD, Henke SE, Redeker E, Fulbright TE, Riddle R, Young J (2013) Demonstration of ground-penetrating radar as a useful tool for assessing pocket gopher burrows. *Wildlife Society Bulletin* **37**, 428–432. doi:10.1002/wsb.279

Cox TE, Matthews R, Halverson G, Morris S (2021) Hot stuff in the bushes: thermal imagers and the detection of fossorial burrows in vegetated sites. *Ecology and Evolution* [Online early]. doi:10.22541/au.160027530.08798648

Cripps J, Nelson J, Scroggie M, Durkin L, Ramsey D, Lumsden L Double-observer distance sampling improves the accuracy of density estimates for a threatened arboreal mammal. *Wildlife Research*, (In press).

Crane M, Lindenmayer DB, Cunningham RB (2010) The use of den trees by the squirrel glider (*Petaurus norfolcensis*) in temperate Australian woodlands. *Australian Journal of Zoology* **58**, 39–49. doi:10.1071/ZO09070

Cristescu ME, Hebert PDN (2018) Uses and misuses of environmental DNA in biodiversity science and conservation. *Annual Review of Ecology, Evolution, and Systematics* **49**, 209–230. doi:10.1146/annurev-ecolsys-110617-062306

Crofoot MC, Lambert TD, Kays R, Wikelski MC (2010) Does watching a monkey change its behaviour? Quantifying observer effects in habituated wild primates using automated radiotelemetry. *Animal Behaviour* **80**, 475–480. doi:10.1016/j.anbehav.2010.06.006

Crome F, Isaacs J, Moore L (1994) The utility of birds and mammals of remnant riparian vegetation and associated windbreaks in the tropical Queensland uplands. *Pacific Conservation Biology* **1**, 328–343. doi:10.1071/PC940328

Davey SM (1990) Methods for surveying the abundance and distribution of arboreal marsupials in a south coast forest of New South Wales. *Australian Wildlife Research* **17**, 427–445. doi:10.1071/WR9900427

Davey G (2007) Visitors' effects on the welfare of animals in the zoo: a review. *Journal of Applied Animal Welfare Science* **10**, 169–183. doi:10.1080/10888700701313595

Davis A, Major RE, Taylor CE (2013) Housing shortages in urban regions: aggressive interactions at tree hollows in forest remnants. *PLoS One* **8**, e59332. doi:10.1371/journal.pone.0059332

de la Torre S, Snowdon CT, Bejarano M (2000) Effects of human activities on wild pygmy marmosets in Ecuadorian Amazonia. *Biological Conservation* **94**, 153–163. doi:10.1016/S0006-3207(99)00183-4

Deiner K, Walser JC, Mächler E, Altermatt F (2015) Choice of capture and extraction methods affect detection of freshwater biodiversity from environmental DNA. *Biological Conservation* **183**, 53–63. doi:10.1016/j.biocon.2014.11.018

Dickman CR (1991) Use of trees by ground-dwelling mammals: implications for management. In *Conservation of Australia's Forest Fauna*. (Ed. D Lunney) pp. 125–136. Royal Zoological Society of New South Wales, Sydney.

Dickman CR, Greenville AC, Beh C-L, Tamayo B, Wardle GM (2010) Social organization and movements of desert rodents during population 'booms' and 'busts' in central Australia. *Journal of Mammalogy* **91**, 798–810. doi:10.1644/09-MAMM-S-205.1

Dickman CR (2015) Family Peramelidae (bandicoots and echymiperas). In *Handbook of the Mammals of the World – Volume 5. Monotremes and Marsupials*. (Eds DE WIlson and RA Mitermeier) pp. 362–398. Lynx Edicions, Barcelona, Spain.

Diete RL, Adamczyk SM, Meek PD, Dickman CR, Leung LK-P (2015) Burrowing behaviour of the delicate mouse (*Pseudomys delicatulus*) and the management implications for a threatened sympatric rodent (*Notomys aquilo*). *Australian Mammalogy* **37**, 260–263. doi:10.1071/AM14028

Doi H, Uchii K, Matsuhashi S, Takahara T, Yamanaka H, Minamoto T (2017) Isopropanol precipitation method for collecting fish environmental DNA. *Limnology and Oceanography, Methods* **15**, 212–218. doi:10.1002/lom3.10161

Doody JS, McHenry CR, Durkin L, Brown M, Simms A, Coleman L, *et al.* (2018a) Deep communal nesting by yellow-spotted monitors in a desert ecosystem: indirect evidence for a response to extreme dry conditions. *Herpetologica* **74**, 306–310. doi:10.1655/Herpetologica-D-18-00004.1

Doody JS, McHenry C, Brown M, Canning G, Vas G, Clulow S (2018b) Deep, helical, communal nesting and emergence in the sand monitor: ecology informing paleoecology? *Journal of Zoology* **305**, 88–95. doi:10.1111/jzo.12543

DSEWPC (2010) *Survey Guidelines for Australia's Threatened Birds: Guidelines for Detecting Mammals Listed as Threatened under the* Environment Protection and Biodiversity Conservation Act 1999. Australian Government, Canberra.

DSEWPC (2011a) *Survey Guidelines for Australia's Threatened Mammals: Guidelines for Detecting Mammals Listed as Threatened under the* Environment Protection and Biodiversity Conservation Act 1999. Australian Government, Canberra.

DSEWPC (2011b) *Survey Guidelines for Australia's Threatened Reptiles: Guidelines for Detecting Mammals Listed as Threatened under the* Environment Protection and Biodiversity Conservation Act 1999. Australian Government, Canberra.

Durant R, Luck GW, Matthews A (2009) Nest-box use by arboreal mammals in a peri-urban landscape. *Wildlife Research* **36**, 565–573. doi:10.1071/WR09058

Eggert LS, Maldonado JE, Fleischer RC (2005) Nucleic acid isolation from ecological samples – animal scat and other associated materials. *Methods in Enzymology* **395**, 73–82. doi:10.1016/S0076-6879(05)95006-4

Einoder LD, Southwell DM, Lahoz-Monfort JJ, Gillespie GR, Fisher A, Wintle BA (2018) Occupancy and detectability modelling of vertebrates in northern Australia using multiple sampling methods. *PLoS One* **13**, e0203304. doi:10.1371/journal.pone.0203304

Eisenhofer R, Helgen C, Taggart DA (2021) Signatures of landscape and captivity in the gut microbiota of southern hairy-nosed wombats (*Lasiorhinus latifrons*). *Animal Microbiome* **3**, 4. doi:10.1186/s42523-020-00068-y

Engeman RM (2005) Indexing principles and a widely applicable paradigm for indexing animal populations. *Wildlife Research* **32**, 203–210. doi:10.1071/WR03120

Engeman RM, Massei G, Sage M, Gentle MN (2013) Monitoring wild pig populations: a review of methods. *Environmental Science and Pollution Research International* **20**, 8077–8091. doi:10.1007/s11356-013-2002-5

Eyre TJ, Ferguson DJ, Hourigan CL, Smith GC, Mathieson MT, Kelly AL, Venz MF, Hogan LD, Rowland J (2018) *Terrestrial Vertebrate Fauna Survey Assessment Guidelines for Queensland*. Queensland Department of Environment and Science, Brisbane.

Fardell LL, Pavey CR, Dickman CR (2020) Fear and stressing in predator-prey ecology: considering the twin stressors of predators and people on mammals. *PeerJ* **8**, e9104. doi:10.7717/peerj.9104

Felthauser M, McInroy D (1983) Mapping pocket gopher burrow systems with expanding polyurethane foam. *The Journal of Wildlife Management* **47**, 555–558. doi:10.2307/3808536

Finlayson GR, Shimmin GA, Temple-Smith PD, Handasyde KA, Taggart DA (2005) Burrow use and ranging behaviour of the southern hairy-nosed wombat (*Lasiorhinus latifrons*) in the Murraylands, South Australia. *Journal of Zoology* **265**, 189–200. doi:10.1017/S095283690400620X

Flaquer C, Puig-Montserrat X, López-Baucells A, Torre I, Freixas L, Mas M, *et al.* (2014) Could overheating turn bat boxes into death traps? *Barbastella* **7**, 46–53. doi:10.14709/BarbJ.7.1.2014.08

Freeland JR (2017) The importance of molecular markers and primer design when characterizing biodiversity from environmental DNA. *Genome* **60**, 358–374. doi:10.1139/gen-2016-0100

Furlan EM, Gleeson D, Wisniewski C, Yick J, Duncan RP (2019) eDNA surveys to detect species at very low densities: a case study of European carp eradication in Tasmania, Australia. *Journal of Applied Ecology* **56**, 2505–2517. doi:10.1111/1365-2664.13485

Geerts AN, Boets P, Van den Heede S, Goethals P (2018) A search for standardized protocols to detect alien invasive crayfish based on environmental DNA (eDNA): a lab and field evaluation. *Ecological Indicators* **84**, 564–572. doi:10.1016/j.ecolind.2017.08.068

Gentle MN (2006) *Red Fox: Pest Status Review.* Queensland Department of Natural Resources and Water, Brisbane.

Glen AS, Dickman CR (2006) Home range, denning behaviour and microhabitat use of the carnivorous marsupial *Dasyurus maculatus* in eastern Australia. *Journal of Zoology* **268**, 347–354. doi:10.1111/j.1469-7998.2006.00064.x

Goldberg CS, Turner CR, Deiner K, Klymus KE, Francis P, Murphy MA, *et al.* (2016) Critical considerations for the application of environmental DNA methods to detect aquatic species. *Methods in Ecology and Evolution* **7**, 1299–1307. doi:10.1111/2041-210X.12595

Goldingay RL (2015) Temperature variation in nest boxes in eastern Australia. *Australian Mammalogy* **37**, 225–233. doi:10.1071/AM14040

Goldingay RL, Rueegger NN, Grimson MJ, Taylor BD (2015) Specific nest box designs can improve habitat restoration for cavity-dependent arboreal mammals. *Restoration Ecology* **23**, 482–490. doi:10.1111/rec.12208

Goldingay RL, Sharpe DJ (2004) How effective is spotlighting for detecting the squirrel glider? *Wildlife Research* **31**, 443–449. doi:10.1071/WR03010

Goldingay RL, Thomas KJ, Shanty D (2018) Outcomes of decades long installation of nest boxes for arboreal mammals in southern Australia. *Ecological Management & Restoration* **19**, 204–211. doi:10.1111/emr.12332

Goldingay RL, Quin DG, Talamo O, Mentiplay-Smith J (2020a) Nest box revealed habitat preferences of arboreal mammals in box-ironbark forest. *Ecological Management & Restoration* **21**, 131–142. doi:10.1111/emr.12412

Goldingay RL, Rohweder D, Taylor BD (2020b) Nest box contentions: Are nest boxes used by the species they target? *Ecological Management & Restoration* **21**, 115–122. doi:10.1111/emr.12408

Grarock K, Tidemann CR, Wood J, Lindenmayer DB (2012) Is it benign or is it a pariah? Empirical evidence for the impact of the common myna (*Acridotheres tristis*) on Australian birds. *PLoS One* **7**, e40622. doi:10.1371/journal.pone.0040622

Griffiths SR (2021) Overheating turns a bat box into a death trap. *Pacific Conservation Biology* Online early. doi:10.1071/PC20083

Griffiths SR, Bender R, Godinho LN, Lentini PE, Lumsden LF, Robert KA (2017a) Bat boxes are not a silver bullet conservation tool. *Mammal Review* **47**, 261–265. doi:10.1111/mam.12097

Griffiths SR, Rowland JA, Briscoe NJ, Lentini PE, Handasyde KA, Lumsden LF, Robert KA (2017b) Surface reflectance drives nest box temperature profiles and thermal suitability for target wildlife. *PLoS One* **12**, e0176951. doi:10.1371/journal.pone.0176951

Griffiths SR, Lentini PE, Semmens K, Watson SJ, Lumsden LF, Robert KA (2018) Chainsaw-carved cavities better mimic the thermal properties of natural tree hollows than nest boxes and log hollows. *Forests* **9**, 235. doi:10.3390/f9050235

Griffiths SR, Lumsden LF, Bender R, Irvine R, Godinho LN, Visintin C, *et al.* (2019) Long-term monitoring suggests bat boxes may alter local bat community structure. *Australian Mammalogy* **41**, 273–278. doi:10.1071/AM18026

Griffiths SR, Lumsden LF, Robert KA, Lentini PE (2020a) Nest boxes do not cause a shift in bat community composition in an urbanised landscape. *Scientific Reports* **10**, 6210. doi:10.1038/s41598-020-63003-w

Griffiths SR, Semmens K, Watson SJ, Jones CS (2020b) Installing chainsaw-carved hollows in medium-sized, live trees increases rates of visitation by hollow-dependent fauna. *Restoration Ecology* **28**, 1225–1236. doi:10.1111/rec.13191

Heard GW, Robertson P, Scroggie MP (2006) Assessing detection probabilities for the endangered growling grass frog (*Litoria raniformis*) in southern Victoria. *Wildlife Research* **33**, 557–564. doi:10.1071/WR04080

Hinlo R, Gleeson D, Lintermans M, Furlan E (2017) Methods to maximise recovery of environmental DNA from water samples. *PLoS One* **12**, e0179251. doi:10.1371/journal.pone.0179251

Hudson R, Elizalde M, Kennedy G, Rödel H, Smith B (2019) Diurnal pattern of pre-weaning den visits and nursing in breeding pairs of captive dingoes (*Canis dingo*). *Mammalian Biology* **94**, 86–91. doi:10.1016/j.mambio.2018.07.002

Irvine R, Bender R (1997) Introduction of the sugar glider *Petaurus breviceps* into re-established forest of the Organ Pipes National Park, Victoria. *Victorian Naturalist* **114**, 230–239.

Jack KM, Lenz BB, Healan E, Rudman S, Schoof VAM, Fedigan L (2008) The effects of observer presence on the behavior of *Cebus capucinus* in Costa Rica. *American Journal of Primatology* **70**, 490–494. doi:10.1002/ajp.20512

Jiang A, Tribe A, Murray P (2020) The development of an improved scat survey method for koalas (*Phascolarctos cinereus*). *Australian Journal of Zoology* **67**, 125–133. doi:10.1071/ZO20006

Karp D (2020) Detecting small and cryptic animals by combining thermography and a wildlife detection dog. *Scientific Reports* **10**, 5220. doi:10.1038/s41598-020-61594-y

Kawanaka K (1996) Observation time and sampling intervals for measuring behavior and interactions of chimpanzees in the wild. *Primates* **37**, 185–196. doi:10.1007/BF02381406

Kelly MJ, Betsch J, Wultsch C, Mesa B, Mills LS (2012) Noninvasive sampling for carnivores. In *Carnivore Ecology and Conservation: a Handbook of Techniques.* (Eds L Boitani and R Powell) pp. 47–69. Oxford University Press, London, UK.

King D, Green B (1999) *Monitor: The Biology of Varanid Lizards.* NSW University Press, Sydney.

Kinlaw A (1999) A review of burrowing by semi-fossorial vertebrates in arid environments. *Journal of Arid Environments* **41**, 127–145. doi:10.1006/jare.1998.0476

Kinlaw AE, Conyers LB, Zajac W (2007) Use of ground penetrating radar to image burrows of the gopher tortoise (*Gopherus polyphemus*). *Herpetological Review* **38**, 50–56.

Knight J (2009) Making wildlife viewable: habituation and attraction. *Society & Animals* **17**, 167–184. doi:10.1163/156853009X418091

Kruuk H, Jarman PJ (1995) Latrine use by the spotted-tailed quoll (*Dasyurus maculatus*: Dasyuridae, Marsupialia) in its natural habitat. *Journal of Zoology* **236**, 345–349. doi:10.1111/j.1469-7998.1995.tb04501.x

Kumar G, Eble JE, Gaither MR (2020) A practical guide to sample preservation and pre-PCR processing of aquatic environmental DNA. *Molecular Ecology Resources* **20**, 29–39. doi:10.1111/1755-0998.13107

Larson ER, Eastwood JR, Buchanan KL, Bennett ATD, Berg ML (2018) Nest box design for a changing climate: the value of improved insulation. *Ecological Management & Restoration* **19**, 39–48. doi:10.1111/emr.12292

Lehner PN (1996) *Handbook of Ethological Methods.* 2nd edn. Cambridge University Press, Cambridge, UK.
Le Roux DS, Ikin K, Lindenmayer DB, Bistricer G, Manning AD, Gibbons P (2016) Effects of entrance size, tree size and landscape context on nest box occupancy: considerations for management and biodiversity offsets. *Forest Ecology and Management* **366**, 135–142. doi:10.1016/j.foreco.2016.02.017
Letnic M, Koch F (2010) Are dingoes a trophic regulator in arid Australia? A comparison of mammal communities on either side of the dingo fence. *Austral Ecology* **35**, 167–175. doi:10.1111/j.1442-9993.2009.02022.x
Letnic M, Greenville A, Denny E, Dickman CR, Tischler M, Gordon C, Koch F (2011) Does a top predator suppress the abundance of an invasive mesopredator at a continental scale? *Global Ecology and Biogeography* **20**, 343–353. doi:10.1111/j.1466-8238.2010.00600.x
Li J, Lawson Handley LJ, Read DS, Hänfling B (2018) The effect of filtration method on the efficiency of environmental DNA capture and quantification via metabarcoding. *Molecular Ecology Resources* **18**, 1102–1114. doi:10.1111/1755-0998.12899
Lindenmayer DB, Crane M, Blanchard W, Okada S, Montague-Drake R (2016) Do nest boxes in restored woodlands promote the conservation of hollow-dependent fauna? *Restoration Ecology* **24**, 244–251. doi:10.1111/rec.12306
Lindenmayer DB, Crane M, Evans MC, Maron M, Gibbons P, Bekessy S, Blanchard W (2017) The anatomy of a failed offset. *Biological Conservation* **210**, 286–292. doi:10.1016/j.biocon.2017.04.022
Lindenmayer DB, Cunningham RB, Donnelly CF, Incoll RD, Pope ML, Tribolet CR, Viggers KL, Welsh AH (2001) How effective is spotlighting for detecting the greater glider (*Petauroides volans*)? *Wildlife Research* **28**, 105–109. doi:10.1071/WR00002
Lindenmayer DB, Cunningham RB, Tanton MT, Nix HA (1991) Aspects of the use of den trees by arboreal and scansorial marsupials inhabiting montane ash forests in Victoria. *Australian Journal of Zoology* **39**, 57–65. doi:10.1071/ZO9910057
Lindenmayer DB, Welsh A, Donnelly C, Crane M, Michael D, Macgregor C, *et al.* (2009) Are nest boxes a viable alternative source of cavities for hollow-dependent animals? Long-term monitoring of nest box occupancy, pest use and attrition. *Biological Conservation* **142**, 33–42. doi:10.1016/j.biocon.2008.09.026
Macak PV (2020) Nest boxes for wildlife in Victoria: an overview of nest box distribution and use. *Victorian Naturalist* **137**, 4–14.
Mahon PS, Banks PB, Dickman CR (1998) Population indices for wild carnivores: a critical study in sand-dune habitat, south-western Queensland. *Wildlife Research* **25**, 11–22. doi:10.1071/WR97007
Martin P, Bateson P (1993) *Measuring Behaviour: An Introductory Guide.* 2nd edn. Cambridge University Press, Cambridge, UK.
Majaneva M, Diserud OH, Eagle SH, Boström E, Hajibabaei M, Ekrem T (2018) Environmental DNA filtration techniques affect recovered biodiversity. *Scientific Reports* **8**, 4682. doi:10.1038/s41598-018-23052-8
Maziarz M, Broughton RK, Wesołowski T (2017) Microclimate in tree cavities and nest-boxes: implications for hole-nesting birds. *Forest Ecology and Management* **389**, 306–313. doi:10.1016/j.foreco.2017.01.001
McColl-Gausden EF, Weeks AR, Tingley R (2020) A field ecologist's guide to environmental DNA sampling in freshwater environments. *Australian Zoologist* **40**, 641–651. doi:10.7882/AZ.2019.025
McComb LB, Lentini PE, Harley DKP, Lumsden LF, Antrobus JS, Eyre AC, Briscoe NJ (2019) Feral cat predation on Leadbeater's possum (*Gymnobelideus leadbeateri*) and observations of arboreal hunting at nest boxes. *Australian Mammalogy* **41**, 262–265. doi:10.1071/AM18010
McInnes JC, Alderman R, Deagle BE, Lea MA, Raymond B, Jarman SN (2017) Optimised scat collection protocols for dietary DNA metabarcoding in vertebrates. *Methods in Ecology and Evolution* **8**, 192–202. doi:10.1111/2041-210X.12677
McRae PD (2004) Aspects of the ecology of the greater bilby, *Macrotis lagotis*, in Queensland. Master of Science thesis. The University of Sydney, Australia.
Menkhorst P (1984) Use of nest boxes by forest vertebrates in Gippsland: acceptance, preference and demand. *Wildlife Research* **11**, 255–264. doi:10.1071/WR9840255
Menkhorst P, Knight F (2001) *A Field Guide to the Mammals of Australia.* Oxford University Press, Melbourne.
Milne T, Bull CM, Hutchinson MN (2003) Use of burrows by the endangered pygmy blue-tongue lizard, *Tiliqua adelaidensis* (Scincidae). *Wildlife Research* **30**, 523–528. doi:10.1071/WR02087
Minamoto T, Naka T, Moji K, Maruyama A (2016) Techniques for the practical collection of environmental DNA: filter selection, preservation, and extraction. *Limnology* **17**, 23–32. doi:10.1007/s10201-015-0457-4
Mitchell B, Balogh S (2007) *Monitoring Techniques for Vertebrate Pests – Rabbits.* New South Wales Department of Primary Industries, Orange.
Morrant DS, Petit S (2012) Strategies of a small nectarivorous marsupial, the western pygmy-possum, in response to seasonal variation in food availability. *Journal of Mammalogy* **93**, 1525–1535. doi:10.1644/12-MAMM-A-031.1
Moseby K, Nano T, Southgate R (2009) *Tales in the Sand: A Guide to Identifying Australian Arid Zone Fauna Using Spoor and Other Signs.* Ecological Horizons, South Australia.
Muha TP, Robinson CV, Garcia de Leaniz C, Consuegra S (2019) An optimised eDNA protocol for detecting fish in lentic and lotic freshwaters using a small water volume. *PLoS One* **14**, e0219218. doi:10.1371/journal.pone.0219218
Mutze G, Cooke B, Lethbridge M, Jennings S (2014) A rapid survey method for estimating population density of European rabbits living in native vegetation. *The Rangeland Journal* **36**, 239–247. doi:10.1071/RJ13117
Nichol D, Lenham J, Reynolds J (2003) Application of ground-penetrating radar to investigate the effects of badger setts on slope stability at St Asaph Bypass, North Wales. *Quarterly Journal of Engineering Geology and Hydrogeology* **36**, 143–153. doi:10.1144/1470-9236/2002-42
O'Brien C, Sparrow EE, Ostendorf B, Taggart D (2020) Evaluating olfactory and visual cues to deter southern hairy-nosed wombats (*Lasiorhinus latifrons*) from their burrows. *Australian Mammalogy* **43**, 110–119. doi:10.1071/AM20007
O'Connor JM, Srivastava SK, Tindale NW, Burnett SE (2020) From carrion to Christmas beetles: the broad dietary niche of the red fox in a hybrid coastal ecosystem in south-eastern Queensland. *Australian Journal of Zoology* **67**, 82–93. doi:10.1071/ZO19059
Ostendorf B, Boardman W, Taggart DA (2016) Islands as refuges for threatened species: multispecies translocation and evidence of species interactions four decades on. *Australian Mammalogy* **38**, 204–212. doi:10.1071/AM15018
Paltridge R, McAlpin S (2002) *A Guide to Rare and Threatened Animals in Central Australia.* WWF-Australia, Sydney.
Panasci M, Ballard WB, Breck S, Rodriguez D, Densmore LD, III, Wester DB, Baker RJ (2011) Evaluation of fecal DNA preservation techniques and effects of sample age and diet on genotyping success. *The Journal of Wildlife Management* **75**, 1616–1624. doi:10.1002/jwmg.221
Pianka EM (1982) Observations on the ecology of *Varanus* in the Great Victoria Desert. *Western Australian Naturalist (Perth)* **15**, 37–44.
Penton CE, Woolley LA, Radford IJ, Murphy BP (2020) Overlapping den tree selection by three arboreal mammal species in an

Australian tropical savanna. *Journal of Mammalogy* **101**, 1165–1176. doi:10.1093/jmammal/gyaa074

Piggott MP, Taylor AC (2003) Extensive evaluation of faecal preservation and DNA extraction methods in Australian native and introduced species. *Australian Journal of Zoology* **51**, 341–355. doi:10.1071/ZO03012

Predavec M, Dickman CR (1994) Population dynamics and habitat use of the long-haired rat (*Rattus villosissimus*) in south-western Queensland. *Wildlife Research* **21**, 1–10. doi:10.1071/WR9940001

Qi Y, Noble DWA, Fu J, Whiting MJ (2012) Spatial and social organization in a burrow-dwelling lizard (*Phrynocephalus vlangalii*) from China. *PLoS One* **7**, e41130. doi:10.1371/journal.pone.0041130

Quasim S, MacDonald AJ, Sarre SD (2018) Towards more efficient large-scale DNA-based detection of terrestrial mammal predators from scats. *Mammal Research* **63**, 387–393. doi:10.1007/s13364-018-0369-x

Ramón-Laca A, Soriano L, Gleeson D, Godoy JA (2015) A simple and effective method for obtaining mammal DNA from faeces. *Wildlife Biology* **21**, 195–203. doi:10.2981/wlb.00096

Ramsey DS, MacDonald AJ, Quasim S, Barclay C, Sarre SD (2015) An examination of the accuracy of a sequential PCR and sequencing test used to detect the incursion of an invasive species: the case of the red fox in Tasmania. *Journal of Applied Ecology* **52**, 562–570. doi:10.1111/1365-2664.12407

Read JL, Carter J, Moseby KM, Greenville A (2008) Ecological roles of rabbit, bettong and bilby warrens in arid Australia. *Journal of Arid Environments* **72**, 2124–2130. doi:10.1016/j.jaridenv.2008.06.018

Rees HC, Maddison BC, Middleditch DJ, Patmore JRM, Gough KC (2014) The detection of aquatic animal species using environmental DNA - a review of eDNA as a survey tool in ecology. *Journal of Applied Ecology* **51**, 1450–1459. doi:10.1111/1365-2664.12306

Reichman OJ, Smith SC (1990) Burrows and burrowing behavior by mammals. In *Current Mammalogy*. (Ed. HH Genoways) pp. 197–244. Plenum Press, New York, NY.

Rhind SG, Bradley JS (2002) The effect of drought on body size, growth and abundance of wild brush-tailed phascogales (*Phascogale tapoatafa*) in south-western Australia. *Wildlife Research* **29**, 235–245. doi:10.1071/WR01014

Robinson WD, Lees AC, Blake JG (2018) Surveying tropical birds is much harder than you think: a primer of best practices. *Biotropica* **50**, 846–849. doi:10.1111/btp.12608

Robley A, Lindeman M, Cook I, Woodford L, Moloney P (2015) 'Dingo semiochemicals: towards a non-lethal control tool for the management of dingoes and wild dogs in Australia'. Technical Report Series No. 263. Arthur Rylah Institute for Environmental Research, Department of Environment, Land, Water and Planning, Heidelberg, Victoria.

Rowland JA, Briscoe NJ, Handasyde KA (2017) Comparing the thermal suitability of nest-boxes and tree-hollows for the conservation-management of arboreal marsupials. *Biological Conservation* **209**, 341–348. doi:10.1016/j.biocon.2017.02.006

Rueegger NN (2017) Artificial tree hollow creation for cavity-using wildlife – trialling an alternative method to that of nest boxes. *Forest Ecology and Management* **405**, 404–412. doi:10.1016/j.foreco.2017.09.062

Sarre SD, MacDonald AJ, Barclay C, Saunders GR, Ramsey DS (2013) Foxes are now widespread in Tasmania: DNA detection defines the distribution of this rare but invasive carnivore. *Journal of Applied Ecology* **50**, 459–468. doi:10.1111/1365-2664.12011

Saunders G, McLeod L (2007) *Improving Fox Management Strategies in Australia*. Bureau of Rural Sciences, Canberra.

Shimmin GA, Skinner J, Baudinette RV (2002) The warren architecture and environment of the southern hairy-nosed wombat (*Lasiorhinus latifrons*). *Journal of Zoology* **258**, 469–477. doi:10.1017/S0952836902001620

Smith AP, Lindenmayer D, Begg RJ, Macfarlane MA, Seebeck JH, Suckling GC (1989) Evaluation of the stag-watching technique for census of possums and gliders in tall open forest. *Wildlife Research* **16**, 575–580. doi:10.1071/WR9890575

Smith B (2015) Biology and behaviour of the dingo. In *The Dingo Debate: Origins, Behaviour and Conservation*. (Ed. B Smith) pp. 25–53. CSIRO Publishing, Melbourne.

Smith B, Vague AL (2017) The denning behaviour of dingoes (*Canis dingo*) living in a human-modified environment. *Australian Mammalogy* **39**, 161–168. doi:10.1071/AM16027

Soderquist TR (1993) Maternal strategies of *Phascogale tapoatafa* (*Marsupialia: Dasyuridae*). I. Breeding seasonality and maternal investment. *Australian Journal of Zoology* **41**, 549–566. doi:10.1071/ZO9930549

Song SJ, Amir A, Metcalf JL, Amato KR, Xu ZZ, Humphrey G, Knight R (2016) Preservation methods differ in fecal microbiome stability, affecting suitability for field studies. *mSystems* **1**, e00021-16. doi:10.1128/mSystems.00021-16

Souter NJ, Bull CM, Hutchinson MN (2004) Adding burrows to enhance a population of the endangered pygmy blue tongue lizard, *Tiliqua adelaidensis*. *Biological Conservation* **116**, 403–408. doi:10.1016/S0006-3207(03)00232-5

Speakman JR, Lumsden LF, Hays GC (1994) Predation rates on bats released to fly during daylight in south-eastern Australia. *Journal of Zoology* **233**, 318–321. doi:10.1111/j.1469-7998.1994.tb08593.x

Steele VR, Temple-Smith PD (1998) Physical structure of warrens of a small colony of southern hairy-nosed wombats *Lasiorhinus latifrons*. In *Wombats in Australia*. (Eds RT Wells and PA Pridmore) pp. 113–124. Surrey Beatty and Sons Ltd, Chipping Norton.

Stevens TA, Evans MC, Osborne WS, Sarre SD (2010) Home ranges of, and habitat use by, the grassland earless dragon (*Tympanocryptis pinguicolla*) in remnant native grasslands near Canberra. *Australian Journal of Zoology* **58**, 76–84. doi:10.1071/ZO09076

Stott P (1996) Ground-penetrating radar: a technique for investigating the burrow structures of fossorial vertebrates. *Wildlife Research* **23**, 519–530. doi:10.1071/WR9960519

Strain C, Jones C, Griffiths SR, Clarke R (2021) Spout hollow nest boxes provide a dryer and less stable microclimate than natural hollows. *Conservation Science and Practice* **3**, e416. doi:10.1111/csp2.416

Swann DE, Perkins N (2014) Camera trapping for animal monitoring and management: a review of applications. In *Camera Trapping: Wildlife Management and Research*. (Eds P Meek and P Fleming) pp. 3–11. CSIRO Publishing, Melbourne.

Swinbourne M, Sparrow E, Hatch M, Bowden T, Taggart D, Ostendorf B (2015) Ground penetrating radar as a non-invasive tool to better understand the population dynamics of a fossorial species: mapping the warrens of southern hairy-nosed wombats (*Lasiorhinus latifrons*). *Wildlife Research* **42**, 678–688. doi:10.1071/WR15068

Swinbourne M, Taggart DA, Ostendorf B (2018) A comparison between video and still imagery as a methodology to determine southern hairy-nosed wombat (*Lasiorhinus latifrons*) burrow occupancy rates. *Animals (Basel)* **8**, 186. doi:10.3390/ani8110186

Taggart DA, Finlayson GR, Sparrow E, Dibben R, Dibben J, Campbell E, *et al.* (2020) Environmental factors influencing hairy-nosed wombat abundance in semi-arid rangelands. *The Journal of Wildlife Management* **84**, 921–929. doi:10.1002/jwmg.21858

Thomas AC, Howard J, Nguyen PL, Seimon TA, Goldberg CS (2018) eDNA Sampler: a fully integrated environmental DNA sampling system. *Methods in Ecology and Evolution* **9**, 1379–1385. doi:10.1111/2041-210X.12994

Thomas AC, Tank S, Nguyen PL, Ponce J, Sinnesael M, Goldberg CS (2020) A system for rapid eDNA detection of aquatic invasive species. *Environmental DNA* **2**, 261–270. doi:10.1002/edn3.25

Thomsen PF, Kielgast J, Iversen LL, Møller PR, Rasmussen M, Willerslev E (2012) Detection of a diverse marine fish fauna using environmental DNA from seawater samples. *PLoS One* **7**, e41732. doi:10.1371/journal.pone.0041732

Thomson P (1992) The behavioural ecology of dingoes in north-western Australia. II. Activity patterns, breeding season and pup rearing. *Wildlife Research* **19**, 519–530. doi:10.1071/WR9920519

Thornett E, Ostendorf B, Taggart DA (2017) Interspecies co-use of southern hairy-nosed wombat (*Lasiorhinus latifrons*) burrows: implications for wildlife conservation and management. *Australian Mammalogy* **39**, 205–212. doi:10.1071/AM15052

Treilibs CE, Pavey CR, Gardner MG, Ansari MH, Bull CM (2019) Spatial dynamics and burrow occupancy in a desert lizard flood-plain specialist, *Liopholis slateri*. *Journal of Arid Environments* **167**, 8–17. doi:10.1016/j.jaridenv.2019.04.004

Triggs B (2004) *Tracks, Scats, and Other Traces: A Field Guide to Australian Mammals*. Oxford University Press, Oxford, UK.

Triggs B, Brunner H (2002) 'Hair ID: an interactive tool for identifying Australian Mammalian hair' [CD-ROM]. CSIRO Publishing, Melbourne.

van der Ree R, Loyn RH (2002) The influence of time since fire and distance from fire boundary on the distribution and abundance of arboreal marsupials in *Eucalyptus regnans*-dominated forest in the Central Highlands of Victoria. *Wildlife Research* **29**, 151–158. doi:10.1071/WR98055

van der Ree R, Bennett AF, Soderquist TR (2006) Nest-tree selection by the threatened brush-tailed phascogale (*Phascogale tapoatafa*) (Masupialia: Dasyuridae) in a highly fragmented agricultural landscape. *Wildlife Research* **33**, 113–119. doi:10.1071/WR05007

Vestheim H, Jarman SN (2008) Blocking primers to enhance PCR amplification of rare sequences in mixed samples–a case study on prey DNA in Antarctic krill stomachs. *Frontiers in Zoology* **5**, 12. doi:10.1186/1742-9994-5-12

Walker FM, Horsup A, Taylor AC (2009) Leader of the pack: faecal pellet deposition order impacts PCR amplification in wombats. *Molecular Ecology Resources* **9**, 720–724. doi:10.1111/j.1755-0998.2009.02582.x

Waudby HP, Petit S (2017) Thermoregulatory value of cracking-clay soil shelters for small vertebrates during extreme desert conditions. *Integrative Zoology* **12**, 237–249. doi:10.1111/1749-4877.12225

Wayne AF, Cowling A, Rooney JF, Ward CG, Wheeler IB, Lindenmayer DB, Donnelly CF (2005) Factors affecting the detection of possums by spotlighting in Western Australia. *Wildlife Research* **32**, 689–700. doi:10.1071/WR04089

Wegleitner BJ, Jerde CL, Tucker A, *et al.* (2015) Long duration, room temperature preservation of filtered eDNA samples. *Conservation Genetics Resources* **7**, 789–791. doi:10.1007/s12686-015-0483-x

Wells R (1989) Vombatidae. In *Fauna of Australia Volume 1B Mammalia*. (Eds BW Walton and BJ Richardson) pp. 755–768. Australian Government Publishing Service, Canberra.

Williams KE, Huyvaert KP, Piaggio AJ (2016) No filters, no fridges: a method for preservation of water samples for eDNA analysis. *BMC Research Notes* **9**, 298. doi:10.1186/s13104-016-2104-5

Wilmott L, Cullen D, Madani G, Krogh M, Madden K (2019) Are koalas detected more effectively by systematic spotlighting or diurnal searches? *Australian Mammalogy* **41**, 157–160. doi:10.1071/AM18006

Wintle BA, Kavanagh RP, McCarthy MA, Burgman MA (2005) Estimating and dealing with detectability in occupancy surveys for forest owls and arboreal marsupials. *The Journal of Wildlife Management* **69**, 905–917. doi:10.2193/0022-541X(2005)069[0905:EADWDI]2.0.CO;2

Work Safe Australia (2016) *Guide to managing risks of tree trimming and removal work*. Canberra, Australia. <https://www.safeworkaustralia.gov.au/doc/guide-managing-risks-tree-trimming-and-removal-work>.

Yoder M, De Ly IT, King IW, Mundo-Ocampo M, Mann J, Blaxter M, Poiras L, De Ley P (2006) DESS: a versatile solution for preserving morphology and extractable DNA of nematodes. *Journal of Nematology* **8**, 367–376. doi:10.1163/156854106778493448

5 Detecting and monitoring wildlife remotely

Lindy F. Lumsden, Helen P. Waudby, Paul D. Meek, Helen A. Crisp, Jemma K. Cripps, Romane Cristescu, La Toya Jamieson, Jenny L. Nelson, Daniella Teixeira, Naomi Hodgens, Nicholas Rutter, Damian S. Morrant, Deborah S. Bower, Chris R. Dickman and Kari Soennichsen

INTRODUCTION

A range of methods that do not involve capture or handling is available for the indirect detection of wildlife. This chapter details general operating procedures (GOPs) for a range of common detection methods. Many of the GOPs described here (i.e. acoustic recorders, camera traps and call playback) are likely to present little to no animal welfare risks to wildlife depending on the target species and context in which they are used. In some circumstances these methods may not require approval by an animal ethics committee (investigators should always seek clarification). In these GOPs, animal welfare evaluations focus on the risks that are most important to consider when using these methods based on the collective experience of the authors and available literature.

ACOUSTIC RECORDERS

Helen P. Waudby, Lindy F. Lumsden, Daniella Teixeira, Chris R. Dickman and Kari Soennichsen

Target taxa

Acoustic recorders are used to study species that vocalise at a range of frequencies. This GOP focuses on their use for bats (Chapter 23), frogs (Chapter 27) and birds (Chapters 33–36), but may also apply to koalas (Chapter 20). Acoustic tagging and monitoring for marine and freshwater mammals are reviewed in Chapters 12 and 13, respectively.

Context and scope

This GOP describes the use of acoustic devices (e.g. Figure 5.1) for collecting call data from frogs, birds, and mammals, including ultrasonic calls emitted by microbats as they echolocate. Acoustic recorders are employed for monitoring soundscapes, or the status and activity of vocalising animals (Crump and Houlahan 2017). They comprise static or passive (Sugai *et al.* 2020) devices fixed to a solid substrate (e.g. a tree or pole) or handheld devices used to collect call data actively (e.g. while walking through target habitat). Groups of devices (arrays) may be deployed to examine calling directionality or to track animals (Blumstein *et al.* 2011). Acoustic recorders can collect large volumes of data (e.g. Griffiths *et al.* 2020), be used in remote locations, detect uncommon or cryptic species (e.g. Measey *et al.* 2017), and enable estimates of abundance, population size, relative activity, species richness or occupancy (e.g. Duffy *et al.* 2000; Milne *et al.* 2004; Measey *et al.* 2017; Pérez-Granados *et al.* 2019).

Typically, acoustic recorders record data continuously or during scheduled time periods. Call data are analysed manually by personnel listening to recordings or viewing sonograms, or with audio recognition software (Figure 5.2; e.g. Adams *et al.* 2010). The decision to use either analysis method depends on study objectives, volume of data to be analysed, availability of reference calls, and keys or recognisers for automated systems. Remote acoustic data collection often complements traditional

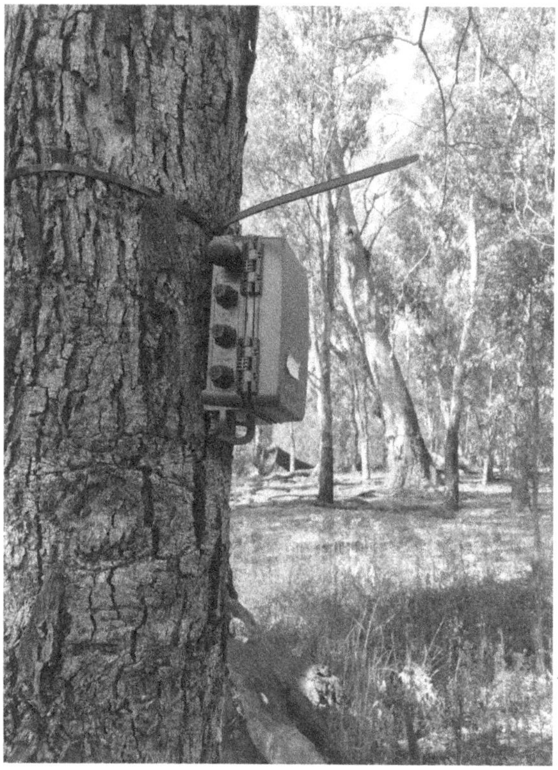

Figure 5.1: Acoustic recorder attached to a tree with cable ties. Photo by Helen P. Waudby.

forms of survey and monitoring, such as harp trapping for bats or targeted visual-encounter surveys for frogs (Chapter 7), or bird observation studies (Chapter 15). Acoustic recorders are relatively non-invasive, typically straightforward to install, and can be deployed for extended periods of time. The diversity of monitoring devices and audio recognition software creates opportunities for long-term and high-volume acoustic data collection. However, data processing can be time-consuming and the cost–benefit balance of the method relative to the study objective is an important consideration.

Animal welfare considerations

Collecting call data with acoustic recorders is a low-impact method depending on where and how devices are installed. The recording equipment itself is unlikely to affect animals and, typically, placement requires little to no disturbance to target and non-target species or their habitat.

Disturbance to target and non-target species

Impacts may arise from installation of devices in the habitat of species that are sensitive to disruptions, including (for example) near nesting sites. Personnel should consider if habitat will be disturbed during deployment (e.g. if a path must be made through thick vegetation to reach sites or vegetation removed to improve data collection) and the likely effect of this disturbance on animals. If devices are to be installed near nesting or roosting sites, or breeding colonies, personnel should consider the sensitivity of their target species to this disturbance. Mitigation methods may include installing devices before animals arrive, while nests or hollows are unattended, or ensuring that devices are not located too close to these areas. Personnel may consider installing camera traps (see 'Camera trapping' later in this chapter) along with acoustic recorders to monitor potential impacts, where the collection of camera data does not increase impacts over and above those introduced by acoustic recorders. For example, some cameras emit ultrasonic noise (Meek *et al.* 2014), which may affect bat behaviour.

Protection from animals and exposure

Microphones can be damaged (chewed) by animals, which may affect the integrity of data collection. Personnel could consider placing guards around the microphone and should maintain a supply of spare microphones or covers. Non-target species' calls may also influence data integrity. For example, some frog species (e.g. Peron's tree frog, *Litoria peronii*) can shelter behind devices attached to trees and call loudly from these positions (i.e. in proximity to microphones), affecting the audibility of other species' calls (H. Waudby, pers. obs.). Avoiding affixing devices to obvious perching points may reduce the risk of microphone damage and degradation from the excretions of perching birds. Microphones can also degrade over time through exposure, so personnel should check microphone sensitivity regularly to ensure that all units are comparable.

General procedures

Planning

Experimental design should be determined before deployment of devices, including spatial scale and distribution, number of devices required, and rotation of recorders between or within sites (i.e. Sugai *et al.* 2019, 2020). Recorders are available in a variety of brands, sizes, and programmable and recording capacities. Researchers should evaluate the features of different models (costs and capabilities vary considerably) before selecting a particular

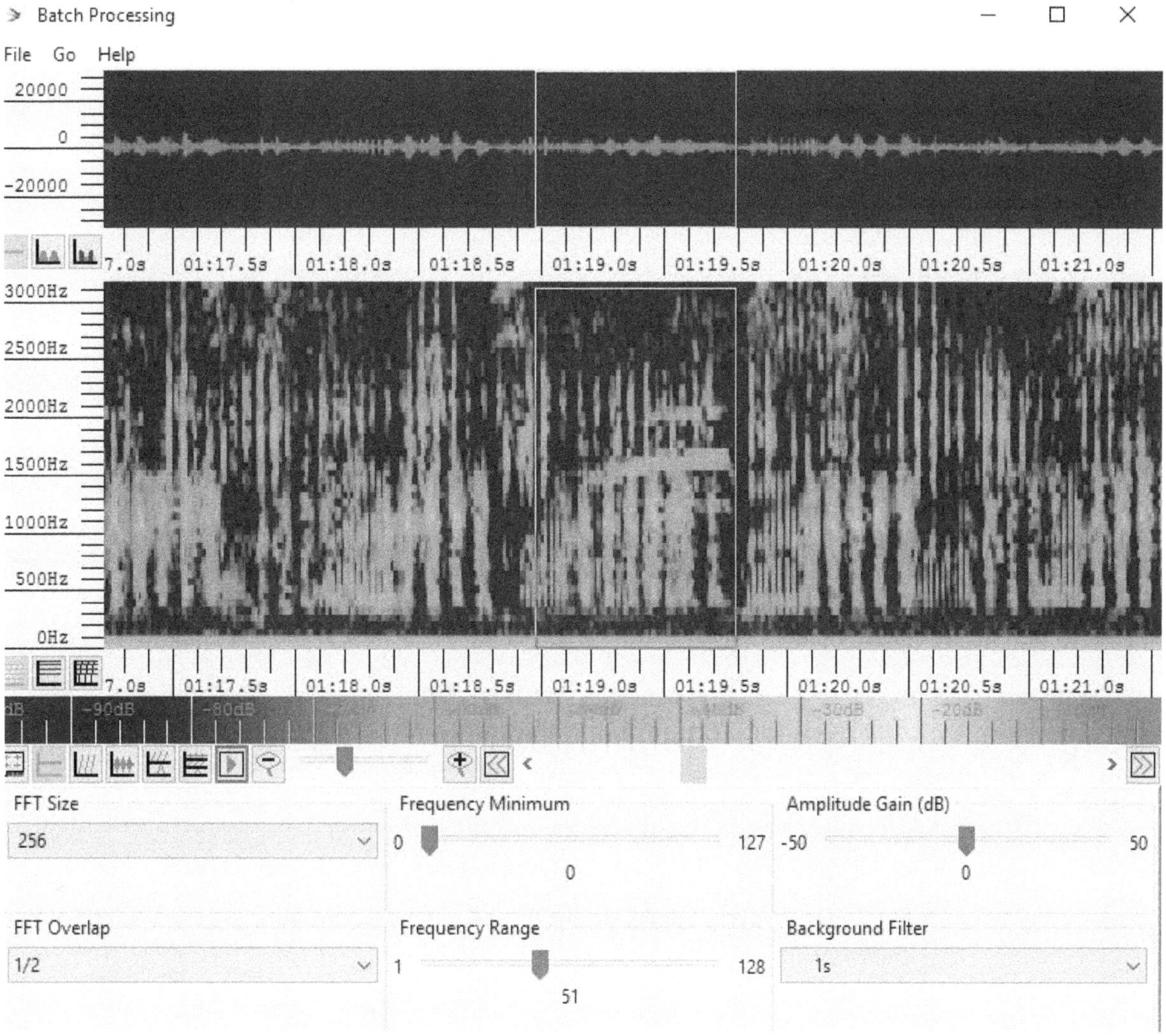

Figure 5.2: Example of a sonogram output from analysis of frog call data; the audio recognition software (in this case, Song Scope) has detected the target species' (southern bell frog, *Litoria raniformis*) call. Photo by Helen P. Waudby.

type for their study. Bat call detection typically requires specialised devices. Personnel select a type appropriate to their objectives, budget, target species and environmental conditions. Considerations include robustness, recording quality, size (i.e. larger models (~30 × 20 × 5 cm) to units around the size of a matchbox are available), visibility, battery life, microphones (single or stereo), scheduling capabilities, and capacity to record at the target species' calling frequency. For example, frogs call from approximately < 200 Hz–4 kHz; birds mostly call between ~500 Hz and 10 kHz (but can call from 0–20 kHz); and microbats echolocate from ~10 to 160 kHz. Ideally, personnel should determine the effective detection distance of their chosen device before deployment by, for example, playing recorded calls of the target species at staggered distances and confirming detection of these calls (Sugai *et al.* 2020). The variability of species' calling intensity should be considered in multi-species analyses.

An appropriate sampling schedule should be confirmed before deployment. Longer recording schedules require greater battery life and fill data storage devices more quickly than shorter ones. Personnel should consider under what conditions their species is most likely to be active and vocalise. For some species, it may be appropriate to record at certain times (e.g. night for calling frogs, sunrise and twilight for birds, during warmer weather for bats). Recording schedule and other programmable parameters should be noted. Batteries and data storage devices appropriate to the duration and likely volume of data to be collected should be selected. For lengthy deployment periods, large-capacity batteries charged by solar panels may be appropriate. Large volumes of data can amass quickly, so personnel need to plan for how they will analyse these data (i.e. manually or with audio recognition software).

Deployment

Single or multiple devices are deployed where animals (including humans) cannot interfere with them, but where data collection will not be impeded. Locations depend on the target species and effective distance at which the recorder detects that species' calls. For example, if sampling nesting birds, the device may need to be installed near nest sites. Ideally, the device is placed where it will be protected from the elements, although some devices are weather resistant. The deployment location should be free of branches, shrubbery, or other substrates that may brush against the microphone and interfere with recordings. Installing bat detectors inside possum boxes (with the microphone pointing out the entrance hole) has been successful in protecting the equipment from the elements as well as in reducing the risk of theft and vandalism (e.g. Griffiths *et al.* 2020). Deployment locations should be carefully recorded (ideally with a GPS). Photographing the device location can assist with relocation, particularly if different individuals will be servicing it.

Considerations for detecting frog calls

Male frogs of most species emit species-specific calls to attract females; their calls are often used by researchers as a proxy to identify attempted breeding (Crouch and Paton 2002). Consequently, acoustic recorders can be used to detect and monitor frogs and breeding activity via their advertising calls. Frog-calling phenology is highly variable, being influenced by season and inter-annual environmental variability (e.g. Measey *et al.* 2017), including temperature, rainfall, and water level fluctuations. Often, calling activity is greatest at night, or after seasonal rainfall and inundation of wetland habitat. Devices can be configured to capitalise on those times. Device placement will depend on the species' habitat and calling behaviour. For example, to detect frogs that call from water bodies, recorders can be placed at the edge or in the middle of the water body at about breast or head height.

Considerations for detecting echolocating bats

The high-frequency echolocation calls emitted by microbats require the use of specialised ultrasonic acoustic recorders (or detectors). Detectors may have directional or omni-directional microphones, and record in either zero crossing or full spectrum modes, or both. Devices should be placed > 1 m from any surface, at a height above 0.5 m. Extension leads (e.g. 50 m long) enable microphones to be set high above the ground, such as on wind turbines. If devices are installed in caves, detectors are typically placed in the entrance chamber, but out of the flight path of the bats. To reduce disturbance, personnel working in caves should service the units at night after bats have left to forage, if the servicing of units during the day would be audible to the roosting bats. All lights and sounds on the detector should be turned off once the unit is set. Typically, bat surveys are undertaken during the warmer months of the year, and avoid unsuitable weather conditions (e.g. cool temperatures, strong winds, heavy rain). High levels of variability in the number of calls recorded between nights are typical, even when the weather appears to be suitable, so detectors are usually set for weeks or months at a time, depending on the study objectives.

Considerations for detecting bird calls

Acoustic recorders are often used to detect and monitor bird species or assemblages. Applications include, but are not limited to, assessing species abundance, behaviour and population density. Recorders should be placed so as to minimise disruption to their target species – particularly if they are being used to monitor (for example) nesting behaviour. Recording schedules consider temporal variation in call activity of the target species. Many species will call during the dawn chorus, but other, less-noisy times of day may improve detectability of target species. Some birds have large and complex vocal repertoires. Personnel should consider the call types relevant to the study's objectives and the contexts in which these occur. Soft and infrequent calls may require more-sensitive sound recorders or programs. Automated post-processing may be challenging for highly variable call types.

Identifying calls and post-processing of call data

Personnel can analyse data by listening to or viewing sonograms of target calls, or with automated sound recognition software, or a combination of both (semi-automated post-processing). Vocalisations may vary within species

Table 5.1: Suggested equipment and materials required for deployment of acoustic recorders and processing of call data.

Installation	Data collection	Post-processing
• Suitable acoustic recording device with appropriate housing • Microphone with appropriate cover (i.e. a fur cover may be required in windy environments, a waterproof cover in wet/humid environments, or a physical barrier to protect from animal chewing) • SD cards or other storage device depending on unit requirements • Batteries of a sufficient type, quality and duration (may be solar powered), including spares • Means of attaching the device (cable ties can be useful) • Locking device to prevent theft • GPS and camera to record deployment location • Silica gel desiccant	• Containers to house collected SD cards and old batteries; SD cards to be kept separate and labelled for each device • Battery charger • Spare batteries • Spare microphone covers • Instrument to detach units	• Computer with headphones • Software to view sonograms • Audio recognition software • Reference calls (particularly if developing call recognisers) • Hardware with storage capacity for large volumes of data

for certain taxa, including frogs and bats (e.g. Duffy *et al.* 2000), and depending on the species' abundance or behaviour at the time of recording (e.g. Teixeira *et al.* 2019). For bats, a high level of variability can occur based on where individuals are flying in relation to clutter in the environment; calls of the same individuals may differ markedly in open environments compared to those recorded when they are close to vegetation. Some species also show geographical variation in their calls (e.g. Law *et al.* 2002).

If using automated software, call libraries or models should be comprehensive, geographically and species relevant, cover the full range of types of calls produced, and produce accurate identifications. Keys are ideally tested against an independent set of reference calls and error rates are documented (e.g. Lumsden and Bennett 2005; Adams *et al.* 2010). Depending on study objectives, personnel may also need to quantify false-positive and false-negative detections by manually verifying all or a subset of positive detections made by the software. Importantly, personnel should ensure that the sensitivity of the recognition algorithm aligns with the study's objectives. Less-sensitive recognisers will return fewer detections, reducing false positives, which may be useful where very high recall rates are unwarranted (i.e. where it is unnecessary to detect every instance of a species' calling). Acoustic indices and long-duration false colour spectrograms may be useful for visualising large volumes of sound data (Dema *et al.* 2020).

When interpreting data collected from bat acoustic surveys, personnel need to be aware that bat species call at different intensities and have differing levels of identifiability. For some species, most of their calls can be identified correctly most of the time, but for species whose call characteristics overlap extensively with other species, only a relatively small proportion of their calls may be identified correctly, with most calls recorded as 'unknowns' or species complexes. This variability should be considered in multi-species analyses with comparisons restricted to between treatments for individual species, rather than comparing relative activity between species within a treatment (e.g. Lumsden and Bennett 2005).

Animal treatment, withdrawal and euthanasia

Acoustic recorders are typically low-impact. For devices that are deployed close to sensitive sites, personnel should observe the target animals for a period of time. If signs of disturbance are noted, such as nest abandonment or changed behaviours, then personnel should consider removing the device or placing it at a greater distance from the target animals.

Equipment and maintenance

Any reasonable quality recorder can be used (except for detection of bat calls, which requires high-frequency detectors). However, commercially available devices designed specifically for wildlife surveys are typically weatherproof and programmable. General equipment for deployment and data analysis is listed in Table 5.1.

Specific qualifications, experience and training

Deploying acoustic recorders is relatively simple and can be standardised. However, selection of an appropriate device, location and position of the recorder, and calibration of recording settings (e.g. sampling frequency) require species-specific knowledge. Call analysis requires knowledge of the target species' calls and sources of variation. Inexperienced personnel can be trained via manuals and by experienced personnel, or data analyses can be outsourced to experienced personnel.

Workplace health and safety

No specific safety concerns are associated with this method. Standard risk assessment procedures should be undertaken, the specifics of which will depend on how and where devices are to be installed (e.g. in remote areas, in and around wetlands, at high points, near nesting or denning animals).

Alternative procedures

Acoustic recorders provide a low-impact method for sampling species and populations, depending on where and how the device is installed and the nature of monitoring (active or passive). The method sometimes negates the need to interact with animals at all.

CALL PLAYBACK FOR ARBOREAL MAMMALS AND AMPHIBIANS

Jemma K. Cripps, Lindy F. Lumsden, Jenny L. Nelson, Deborah S. Bower and Helen P. Waudby

Target taxa

This method has applications for any species that vocalise and respond to conspecific calls, but particularly possums and gliders (Chapter 19), koalas (Chapter 20) and frogs (Chapter 27). Call playback for birds is reviewed in Chapter 15.

Context and scope

This GOP describes the use of call playback for eliciting a vocal response from mammals and amphibians to determine species presence at a location. Vocalisations are important for animal communication and are often employed during territorial activities (Goldingay 1994) or to attract mates (Crouch and Paton 2002; Ellis *et al.* 2011). Call playback has traditionally been used to monitor or detect birds, especially wide-ranging species, such as large forest owls (see Chapter 15). Although some Australian arboreal marsupials have well-developed vocal behaviours, few detailed studies are available on call playback as a survey technique for this group. The key mammal species for which it appears to be a reliable method are yellow-bellied glider (*Petaurus australis*; Goldingay 1994), Leadbeater's possum (*Gymnobelideus leadbeateri*; Harley 2015) and koala (*Phascolarctos cinereus*; Barrott 1999). The technique does not appear to be effective for eliciting response calls from squirrel gliders (*Petaurus norfolcensis*; Sharpe and Goldingay 2009).

Call playback is used to increase the number of individuals vocalising or the intensity of vocalisations in a target population. These vocalisations can assist researchers to estimate the distribution, occupancy or relative abundance of the target species (Eyre and Buck 2005; Harley 2015), their breeding status or species richness in a sample area in the case of frogs (Lemckert and Mahony 2008), or as an aide to determine the exact position of an individual. Surveys typically involve broadcasting pre-recorded calls of the target species interspersed with periods of active listening for calls. In some mammal species, playback of owl calls is used because this predatory cue elicits a response from potential prey (McNabb 1994; DSEWPC 2011). For amphibians, call playback usually amplifies a species-specific call or chorus emitted by male frogs. Call playback is often conducted in tandem with spotlighting (see Chapter 4).

Animal welfare considerations

Disruptions to behaviour or social interactions

Call playback is generally considered a low-impact method, provided that the technique is conducted to avoid exposing animals to prolonged playback periods. The key animal welfare consideration for this technique is the potential for disruption to animal behaviour and social interactions, although strong evidence for either is lacking. Nevertheless, call playback elicits a behavioural response by the target species, so prolonged call playback could disrupt breeding, territorial or defensive behaviours or social interactions. Interestingly, frogs may move towards the source of call playback (e.g. green and golden bell frogs, *Litoria aurea*); this characteristic may be useful for encouraging movement into newly created habitat (James *et al.* 2015). Call playback experiments using calls of invasive cane toads (*Rhinella marina*) produced shorter and more-intense periods of calling by marbled frogs (*Limnodynastes convexiusculus*) during the silent gaps between blocks of calling (Bleach *et al.* 2015). Some frog species may also increase the amplitude of their calls in response to increasing noise levels generally (e.g. the 'Lombard effect'; Halfwerk *et al.* 2016). However, it is unclear what welfare impacts such interruptions might have on frogs, although it seems unlikely that they would be substantial, providing that continuous call playback is avoided and sites are not targeted on several successive nights.

Leadbeater's possums have also shown observable responses where they approach rapidly to within < 10 m of an observer playing calls (Harley 2015). Stress may be heightened if the animals are responding constantly to playback and disrupted from their normal activities for multiple nights; this risk is why only a few repeat visits to sites are recommended over short periods. Personnel can implement mitigation methods to minimise impacts on target animals. For example, surveys can begin with a passive listening period, followed by spotlighting, which may provide evidence of the target species without having to undertake any call playback. If the targets are not detected during this listening period, call playback can then be used.

General procedures

Planning

Investigators should determine their objective or experimental design before undertaking surveys. The probability of recording false negatives varies with weather conditions at the time of the survey (e.g. strong wind), available foraging resources and observer experience (Wintle *et al.* 2005; Ellis *et al.* 2011). Repeat surveys increase the probability that the target species will be detected.

Investigators should consider the changing detectability of the target species in response to environmental conditions (temperature or rain), diel cycles of activity (e.g. nocturnal species) or breeding seasons. For example, yellow-bellied gliders call throughout the night, but calling is most common during the first 3–4 h of their foraging period (Goldingay 1994). The seasonal pattern of calling frequency, or the seasonal response of the target species to calls of conspecifics, should also be considered before embarking on surveys. For example, koalas emit bellows almost exclusively during the peak mating season (Ellis *et al.* 2011), so call playback outside this period is unlikely to elicit a response. Similarly, Leadbeater's possums vary in their response rates to call playback over different seasons (Lumsden *et al.* 2013; Harley 2015) and many frogs have highly seasonal calling periods. This variability will influence survey design and seasonal timing of surveys.

Area of detectability should also be considered. Higher-frequency acoustic signals attenuate faster; therefore, different calls vary in their detectability by distance. The area of detection will ultimately determine the sampling area and inform the minimum distance between sampling sites. The minimum distance may also change with wind, habitat complexity and the sensitivity of the observer's hearing. In general, yellow-bellied glider calls can be heard from up to 400 m away (Kavanagh and Rohan-Jones 1982), while Leadbeater's possum vocalisations are detectable over only short distances (< 50 m; Harley 2015).

Some species may respond differently to different sound signals (i.e. social versus alarm calls). The call frequency can also produce variations in response. For example, male koalas are slower to reply to playbacks of deeper bellows, possibly because they are less willing to engage in vocal exchanges with larger males that represent more-dangerous rivals (Charlton *et al.* 2013). In such cases, it may be necessary to undertake call playback for longer periods or include longer listening periods.

Conducting call playback surveys

General procedures include the following:

- Personnel should arrive at their site (or a predetermined location) and quietly set up the equipment before commencing surveys.
- Personnel can undertake an initial listening period: for mammals 10–15 min and for frogs 3–5 min.
- Personnel then undertake a spotlight search for 10 min (optional, and exact timing will depend on the target species; frogs are typically searched for within 30 min blocks).
- Personnel broadcast the signal that will elicit a response from the target species through a speaker or megaphone, playing it intermittently for a short period (e.g. 2–5 min), with each call followed by a listening period of equivalent length.
- At the end of the final listening period, personnel can spotlight (for mammals around 10 min is appropriate) and listen to determine if the target species has been attracted to the area.

Considerations for mammals

Several recommended methods for mammal call playback surveys are available (e.g. DSEWPC 2011). To reduce disturbance to terrestrial mammals, a maximum of 2 h should be spent surveying a site using call playback. Within that time only short bursts of call broadcasting should be undertaken; this activity could comprise playing the calls of multiple species (e.g. if undertaken in conjunction with owl surveys) or focused on a single species. Generally, surveys should not be undertaken for more than three consecutive nights. Wintle *et al.* (2005) provide detection curves for some arboreal mammals that may assist in deciding how many visits are required per site to confirm presence. Personnel can also mimic the call of the target species. While the call does not project as far, this approach can be effective, especially for species such as Leadbeater's possum, with inquisitive animals often drawn to within metres of the observer.

Considerations for frogs

Many frog species will respond to call playback, although for some (e.g. *Pseudophryne* spp.), calling may also be stimulated if investigators simply shout loudly at a certain pitch (DECC 2009). Call surveys are used extensively to record frog species diversity, and the presence or absence of individual species (Lemckert and Mahony 2008), although some species have calls that are largely indistinguishable from one another (DECC 2009). Male frogs vocalise to advertise for females and as a threat display to other males; calling is influenced strongly by environmental conditions (e.g. temperature, rainfall) and season. Consequently, call-based surveys target species' breeding seasons and optimal environmental conditions for calling (Lemckert and Mahony 2008). Calling mostly occurs at night, but decreasingly so as the night progresses (i.e. as temperature drops), so surveys are timed accordingly. Call playback can be undertaken in conjunction with transect surveys (listening to and noting calls along a transect), static or point surveys (undertaken from a fixed point) and active searches as part of visual encounter surveys (DECC 2009; DEWHA 2010). Personnel should document the time spent searching and playing calls, survey method and area searched.

Animal treatment, withdrawal and euthanasia

For surveys that are undertaken during the breeding season, if signs of disturbance are observed (i.e. species-specific behaviours indicating substantial stress) then personnel should cease the survey, end playback and remove themselves from the area. Detecting stress in free-living frogs is difficult, but as long as it is not prolonged, call playback is highly unlikely to cause appreciable stress to frogs.

Equipment and maintenance

Personnel should ensure that they have appropriate equipment. Audio recordings of the target species can be pre-recorded or purchased, on CD, in MP3 format or via smartphone applications. Typical items may include:

- loud-speaker or megaphone
- mobile phone or MP3 player, with audio-recordings in a pre-arranged sequence of the target species' calls (and/or owl calls) and silence tracks (listening periods)
- white-light (plus optional red-light) spotlight or high-power headlamp
- binoculars, GPS, handheld compass and time-keeping device
- batteries for all equipment.

Specific qualifications, experience and training

Personnel must be capable of visually and audibly identifying the species that are likely to respond within a study area. Ideally, the technique should be undertaken by or under the direct supervision of a person with previous experience in this technique. This survey technique is relatively simple and can be standardised easily. The volume of the playback will depend upon the quality of the recording, background noise and habitat density, and should be adjusted accordingly. Personnel avoid excessive use of playback at single sites when targeting mammal species, as repeated playback can cause disturbance, especially to territorial species.

Workplace health and safety

For mammal surveys, a field survey team of minimum two people is generally recommended for safety purposes, but also to increase the chance of detecting any animals drawn into the call or faint response vocalisations from animals located far away. Personnel should undertake standard workplace risk assessment procedures before undertaking work at night or when working in remote places.

Alternative procedures

For some species, more-effective survey methods are available that may be less intrusive to the animals. For example, for Leadbeater's possums, remote cameras (see 'Camera trapping' in this chapter) have a higher detection probability and are more reliable for detecting the species (Harley *et al.* 2014; Nelson *et al.* 2017) than call playback, which may result in false negatives under some circumstances because of variation in response rates (Harley 2015). For frogs, passive acoustic recorders are a useful alternative for assessing occupancy and species' presence (see 'Acoustic recorders' earlier in this chapter).

Thermal imaging cameras can be effective if used in conjunction with call playback. Thermal imaging cameras detect the heat signature of animals, which is visible against the cooler background vegetation. Used alongside call playback, thermal imaging can assist with the detection of cryptic arboreal mammals that occur in dense vegetation where detection via spotlighting is difficult (Vinson *et al.* 2020). The in-built red laser can be useful in pinpointing the location of the animal in the dark, so a spotlight can then be used to confirm species identification. Care must be taken to point the laser just below the animal to avoid the risk of shining it directly into the animal's eyes.

CAMERA TRAPPING

Paul D. Meek, Lindy F. Lumsden and Jemma K. Cripps

Target taxa

Camera trapping methods can be used to study all mammals (Chapters 17–25), reptiles (Chapter 26), amphibians (Chapter 27) and birds (Chapters 33–36). Camera trapping and video monitoring methods for aquatic animals are described in Chapter 14.

Context and scope

Camera trapping is widely used throughout Australia as a wildlife monitoring and research tool (Meek *et al.* 2015). Camera trapping is considered a surrogate survey method for many earlier animal survey tools because it is more cost-effective than these methods (Cutler and Swann 1999; De Bondi *et al.* 2010). Additionally, camera trapping is considered relatively non-invasive (O'Connell *et al.* 2014) because it does not involve capturing and handling animals. However, behavioural effects of camera traps on animals have been recorded (Cutler and Swann 1999; Meek *et al.* 2014; Meek *et al.* 2016), and appear to vary between and within species (Wegge *et al.* 2004; Meek *et al.* 2016; Taggart *et al.* 2020). Camera traps can be used with or without bait to lure animals to the camera (Meek *et al.* 2012). Cameras can be detected by animals and can cause either positive (attraction) or negative (avoidance) behaviours (Meek *et al.* 2014). The latter is the focus for addressing animal welfare concerns. Other resources that describe methodological and technical considerations (including data management and analysis) in detail are available (e.g. Meek *et al.* 2012; O'Connell *et al.* 2014; Zimmerman and Rovero 2016).

Animal welfare considerations

Compared to many wildlife sampling methods, camera trapping presents few major animal welfare risks. The effects of attraction to or avoidance of camera traps by animals are more likely to influence the collection of scientific data than present a welfare concern. Although changes to resource-use around camera traps placed at focal resources may occur, no empirical data are available to confirm any negative or positive effects on target or non-target species. Some species show varying levels of acceptance of camera traps over longitudinal studies (Karanth *et al.* 2006; Lincoln *et al.* 2020) and some are attracted to the illumination emitted by them (Meek *et al.* 2016; Taggart *et al.* 2020). Nevertheless, camera trapping is a low-risk method; survey design should recognise the limitations of the survey method and the possible effects on data quality if animals modify their behaviour in the presence of camera traps (Larrucea *et al.* 2007).

Camera traps can change the behaviours of some mammals. For example, animals may change their path of travel to avoid illumination or to access bait (Meek *et al.* 2016) and, in some cases, to avoid the device through its association with humans (Séquin *et al.* 2003). Potential causes of behavioural change (Meek *et al.* 2014) include auditory, olfactory, learned association and visual (day and night) cues. In these cases, animals change behaviour because they hear, see or smell the device. In general, these disturbances to behaviour are short term and low risk, can be easily adapted to by animals, and have negligible or minor effects on animal welfare.

Disturbance of feeding or roosting animals

Camera traps placed at focal resources such as water points may cause minor changes in an animal's behaviour. For example, animals may change their normal path of access to avoid the camera. However, no evidence is available to suggest that this scenario is a realistic one and the long-term effect of such changes is unlikely to be substantial. Similarly, the variability of behaviours within and between individual animals suggests that this hazard is unlikely to be a realised risk.

Where camera traps are baited with lures, animals are attracted to the scent and may expend energy seeking access to the food. However, no studies have investigated the point of giving up by animals when food provided in bait canisters cannot be accessed. Some mesopredators do not appear to avoid food lures contaminated with human scent (Heinlein *et al.* 2020).

Most camera traps emit ultrasonic outputs (Meek *et al.* 2014), which might interfere with echolocation in bats or cause stress (affecting foraging and roost access). If these outputs are expected to disturb animals or influence study results, camera traps should be tested before being used near bat roosts (i.e. a bat detector can be used to confirm if the camera is producing ultrasonic sounds). Where camera traps are placed to monitor nests or roosts of birds, care must be taken not to place them in locations where adults will be disturbed and continually flushed, leaving fledglings unprotected.

Increasing predation risk

Predation risk could be increased if animals spend lengthy amounts of time at bait stations trying to access food, increasing their exposure to predation relative to normal foraging or movement. However, no evidence is available to suggest that this risk is a realised one. The overall impact would be temporary and minor at a population level and should be considered on a case-by-case basis.

Route of passage

Camera traps placed on posts, tunnels, logs and tracks (Fiehler *et al.* 2007; Goldingay *et al.* 2013; Ballard *et al.* 2014) could create a minor barrier to an animal's line of passage. However, unless these structures are literally excluding the animal, the impact is expected to be minor.

General procedures

Ecology of the study animal

Personnel must consider the ecology of the target species, and design monitoring procedures and camera trap placement to minimise risk and avoid restrictions to movement and activity. Placing cameras in locations that impede normal behavioural access to habitat and resources should be avoided.

Selecting appropriate illumination type and camera trap orientation

Camera trap illumination comes in two forms: white and infrared. Infrared flash is the most commonly used type, although white flash is required to identify some species (e.g. smoky mouse, *Pseudomys fumeus*; Burns *et al.* 2018), and to produce colour night images for unique identification of individuals. Behavioural responses to these illumination types vary with species and individuals. Choosing the flash type that minimises effects on animal behaviour while not compromising identification is essential. Placement and orientation are critical factors in effective use of camera traps, but personnel must avoid directly restricting normal movement patterns and activity of species. In some cases, behavioural responses in some species can be avoided by placing camera traps above the animal's field of view. Camera traps can be deployed high in trees using arborists, with this technique proving very effective for surveying threatened arboreal mammals such as Leadbeater's possum (Harley *et al.* 2014; Nelson *et al.* 2017).

Baiting

The use of bait to attract animals to camera traps is an important adjunct to camera trapping (Claridge and Paull 2014). Different baits are often used to target carnivores (e.g. chicken, tuna oil or pilchards), herbivores (e.g. peanut butter and oats) or arboreal mammals (e.g. creamed honey). Commonly, bait is encased in some form of canister to inhibit or prevent removal and reduce rate of degradation by weather (Claridge *et al.* 2010). Bait attractiveness mostly degrades with time-since-deployment and from climatic factors, such as ambient temperature, humidity and rainfall. Where possible, bait stations should be placed near logs and other structures so that prey animals can seek cover quickly if they detect a predator.

Animal treatment, withdrawal and euthanasia

The risk of injury to animals being monitored with camera traps is low. In long-term studies or where repeat sampling over time occurs, reviewing camera trap image data regularly for each camera trap site can provide a useful means of monitoring any behavioural effects on individual animals. These data will also provide an indication of predator visitation and, in rare cases, hunting success. Assessment of these data can inform survey design, such as where risk to individuals is exacerbated by the presence of the camera trap or baits. Analysis of image data from surrounding clusters of camera traps may also provide an insight into whether individual animals are becoming conditioned to or avoiding camera trap sites. It is extremely unlikely that euthanasia would be necessary as a result of camera trapping, although image data may provide evidence of disease outbreaks or severe injuries of an animal from unrelated causes that may initiate euthanasia actions.

Equipment and maintenance

Equipment required for studying animals with camera trapping has been summarised elsewhere (Kays and

Slauson 2008; Meek *et al.* 2012; Zimmerman and Rovero 2016). An adequate number of camera traps is necessary for robust data collection. Fixing devices, such as straps, brackets and posts will be necessary depending on the site and survey design. Two sets of rechargeable batteries and SD cards per camera trap are preferred. An image viewer will help with camera trap placement and orientation, and a GPS is necessary for relocating and servicing the devices. Bait stations should exclude access to the bait by vertebrates, be tethered to prevent removal by animals, and designed and located to prevent incursion by water and, to the extent possible, by invertebrates.

Specific qualifications, experience and training

Personnel need to be aware of how camera traps and passive infrared sensors work to optimise detection and minimise inappropriate or inefficient use of the equipment. Experience in using camera traps or completion of a camera trapping course will improve deployment and use of the device (although is not essential). Mentoring by a scientist experienced in camera trapping is advisable or at least advice should be sought in the planning phase. Familiarity with image data management and animal identification is imperative, as is the ability to recognise behavioural issues that indicate an animal welfare concern.

Workplace health and safety

Camera trap data download frequency varies depending on study objectives, but can be as short as a 2 week interval and up to many months depending on camera trap settings, battery life and activity at the site (Claridge and Paull 2014). Camera traps themselves pose little hazard to workers, but installing and servicing, particularly on vehicular tracks, require care.

Alternative procedures

Camera trapping methods typically have nil to very low impacts on animals. Adverse behaviours by animals, which are unlikely, will be discovered *post hoc* and, unless significant and changeable after the fact, they cannot be acted upon. Consistent observations of predators focusing their attention on bait stations (and evidence of increased predation success) could require modification to the placement to mitigate or preclude further predation, or complete removal. However, camera traps are often an alternative or surrogate approach to more-intrusive methods, such as physical capture (Swann *et al.* 2004; see Chapter 7 for a range of capture methods).

HAIR TRAPS

Helen A. Crisp and Damian S. Morrant

Target taxa

This GOP applies to most small terrestrial mammals, including dasyurids (Chapter 18), wombats, bandicoots, bilbies, possums and gliders (Chapter 19), koalas (Chapter 20), small potoroids (Chapter 21), eutherian carnivores (Chapter 22) and rodents (Chapter 24).

Context and scope

This GOP describes general techniques and considerations for using hair traps to detect mammals and collect biological (hair) samples from them. It does not include analysis of the hair samples to determine species (see Brunner and Coman 1974) or additional analyses (e.g. DNA, stable isotopes). Hair traps comprise several forms; despite their name, they are not designed to trap animals, just their hair. Hair tubes are generally made from lengths of polyvinyl chloride (PVC) pipe (e.g. Scotts and Craig 1988), hair funnels consist of moulded plastic (Figure 5.3), hair tunnels are generally constructed from a lightweight Perspex® (Murray 2005), and hair snares are usually constructed from wooden stakes or boards (Hanke and Dickman 2013). The target animal is often attracted to the hair trap using a lure, which can be food- or pheromone-based. Hair is captured on strategically placed adhesive or another hair-collecting substrate. Hair can also be collected without lures using the sticky-wicket method or similar (Berry *et al.* 2012). Hair is then removed and analysed to identify the species that visited the device. In some instances, additional analyses may be undertaken, such as DNA or stable isotopes (e.g. Morrant *et al.* 2017). In the case of hair snares, hairs are often caught in the wood fibres or on an affixed substrate, such as VELCRO®, coarse carpet or artificial turf rather than with adhesive.

Hair traps have been used across a variety of habitats, including sandstone caves (Harris and Nicol 2010), arid environments (Crisp *et al.* 2018), forests (Mills *et al.* 2002) and even snow (Sanecki and Green 2005). Hair tubes, funnels and tunnels have been used to detect a range of species, including arboreal mammals (Suckling 1978), long-footed potoroos (*Potorous longipes*) (Scotts and Craig 1988) and spotted-tailed quolls (*Dasyurus maculatus*) (Nelson 2006). Hair snares have been used for feral cats (*Felis catus*) (Hanke and Dickman 2013), red foxes (*Vulpes vulpes*) (Vine *et al.* 2009) and dingoes (*Canis dingo*) (Morrant *et al.* 2017). Hair traps can be useful for detecting cryptic species and, unlike more traditional trapping methods, are relatively low cost and can be deployed in the field for several days, or even weeks, without daily servicing. This capacity can be advantageous when surveying large areas. Hair traps are often used with other types of trapping or detection methods, particularly when evaluating species assemblages (Garden *et al.* 2007). Researchers should use hair traps in a manner that is appropriate for the target species or taxa, minimises negative effects on other vertebrates, and optimises the functionality of the traps. Personnel should also ensure that they have the capacity to analyse the collected hair accurately.

Animal welfare considerations

Reported impacts of hair traps on animals in the wild are relatively few. The most notable risk is that of smaller vertebrates becoming trapped on the adhesive. For example, Mills *et al.* (2002) observed that skinks were inadvertently 'caught' on the adhesive in hair funnels and tubes and subsequently died. The floor and lower parts of the hair tube, funnel or tunnel should be free of adhesives to reduce the risk of small reptiles, birds and frogs becoming stuck. Hair trap surveys should generally be discontinued in areas where non-target species have been captured.

General procedures

Know the target species (and presence of non-targets)

The researcher should identify key biological and ecological characteristics that may negatively affect study animals, other taxa and survey results. These characteristics may include feeding strategies, diet, size (juveniles and adults), movement and land-use patterns, known predators, shelter sites (e.g. dens, burrows or nests), social structure (e.g. solitary or communal species), diel behaviour patterns and seasonality. Animals that use olfaction to locate subterranean foods may be particularly sensitive to the smell of certain types of adhesives.

Selecting the appropriate hair trap and hair-collecting substrate

The type and size of hair trap, and placement and type of hair-collecting substrate within the trap are important considerations for successful hair collection. An appropriate substrate should be chosen in consideration of the target species. Hair-collecting substrates can consist of a range of materials, including double-sided tape (e.g. carpet tape), cloth and duct tape, VELCRO®, artificial turf, marine carpet, and styrene cards coated with adhesive (i.e. 'Faunagoo Wafer').

Placement and collection in the field

Hair tubes should be angled with the entrances pointing slightly downwards or upwards to ensure adequate drainage if conditions become damp. In very hot conditions, hair traps should be placed in the shade where possible to preserve the adhesive. If hair is present on tape or adhesive when traps are checked it should be removed and stored on a sheet of paper (separated by pieces of baking paper or paper bags) or in a small specimen jars, and labelled with appropriate information, including date collected, hair trap number or other identification, location of the adhesive (e.g. top or side). Hair caught via other substrates should be collected with forceps and stored and labelled similarly. Ready-made funnels (i.e. Figure 5.3a, b) contain a small mesh screen that protects bait and reduces the rate of disintegration; purpose-made traps can be fitted readily with similar screens (Scotts and Craig 1988). Bait should be selected to sample the target species. Honey should be avoided to reduce the trap's attractiveness to ants.

Animal treatment, withdrawal and euthanasia

The risk of injuring target taxa with hair tubes is typically very low. Injuries may occur if predator activity increases because of the hair trap's presence. Mortalities and injuries may occur to non-target taxa, particularly small reptiles, birds and frogs, which may become stuck on the hair-collecting substrate. If euthanasia is required, suitably trained and experienced personnel should use a technique appropriate to the animal (see Section 3). Factors that may result in a decision to withdraw from the study at any given point include when the likelihood of capturing non-target taxa is greater than capturing the target species or taxa, when the risk of mortality or injury to non-target taxa is deemed unacceptably high, or where weather conditions would increase the presence of non-target taxa or reduce the functionality of the hair trap (e.g. heavy rainfall).

Equipment and maintenance

Equipment will vary depending on the target species, hair trap design, and location of field site. Where possible or practical, hair traps should be prepared before deployment. Typical equipment may include:

- note-taking equipment (e.g. notebook, laptop, tablet, smartphone, voice recorder, clipboard or datasheets)
- navigational equipment (e.g. GPS, tablet, compass or maps)

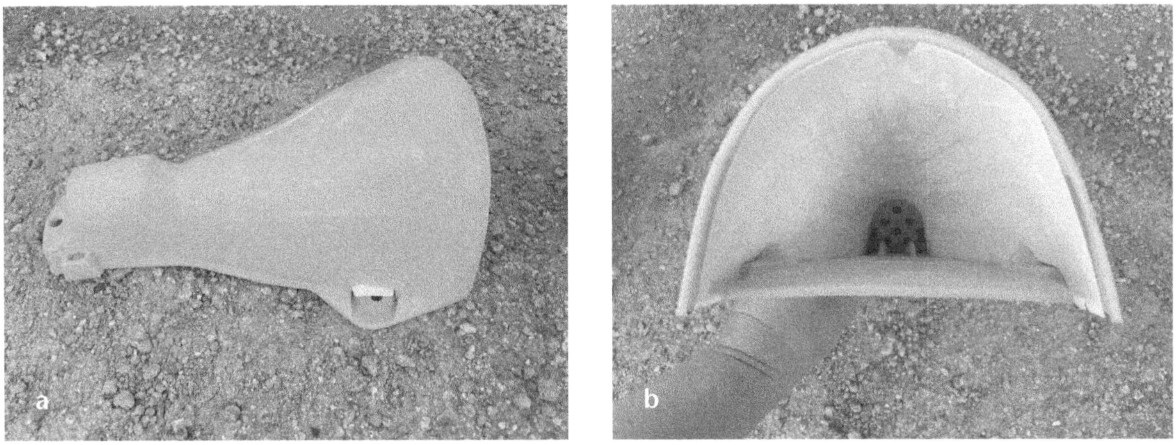

Figure 5.3: Example of a hair trap, including (a) side view of a hair funnel and (b) internal view of a hair funnel (bait is placed behind the metal grate and double-sided tape or a similar adhesive substance placed on the inside of the arch). Photos by Helen P. Waudby.

- site-marking equipment (e.g. flagging tape and permanent markers)
- hair trap and accessories (e.g. PVC pipes, hair funnel, stake, double-sided tape, VELCRO®, forceps, scissors and bait/lure container)
- bait or another attractant
- pegs or wire to secure the hair trap
- hair collection equipment (e.g. baking paper, paper bags or envelopes, plastic bags, sample jars, forceps and permanent marker)
- spare batteries for electronic equipment
- personal protective equipment (e.g. disposable gloves).

Maintenance of equipment includes the removal of all adhesive materials after the study has been completed, disinfecting the traps before reuse, thorough cleaning of bait holders and storage of equipment out of the weather and elements.

Specific qualifications, experience and training

Qualifications and experience required to undertake the procedure are minimal. Subsequent analyses of the collected hairs (e.g. species identification and genetics) should be undertaken by trained and experienced personnel.

Workplace health and safety

A range of zoonoses may be contracted via hair traps that have been in contact with animals (e.g. hydatidosis, sarcoptic mange, leptospirosis). Personnel handling hair traps should implement appropriate hygiene and protective measures, including wearing gloves and handwashing.

Alternative procedures

Hair traps are inherently low impact compared with many other survey techniques. Researchers should consider if study questions will be reliably answered using hair traps or if they could be answered via other means. For example, remote monitoring equipment (e.g. wildlife monitoring cameras – see 'Camera trapping' earlier in this chapter) could have less impact on non-target species and may suffice to answer research questions.

CONSERVATION DETECTION DOGS

Romane Cristescu, La Toya Jamieson, Naomi Hodgens and Nicholas Rutter

Target taxa

The procedures described in this GOP can apply to the detection of all free-living taxa, including terrestrial and aquatic species. The use of guardian dogs in conservation is covered in Chapter 11.

Context and scope

Detection dogs can be more accurate and efficient at finding target species and survey results less biased than some alternative methods (Smith *et al.* 2001; Cristescu *et al.* 2015; Thompson *et al.* 2020). For example, scat detection dogs are reported to show detection rates 5–20 times greater than camera trapping in a tropical savanna landscape (for maned wolf, *Chrysocyon brachyurus*, puma, *Puma concolor*, giant anteater, *Myrmecophaga tridactyla*, and giant armadillo, *Priodontes maximus* in Vynne *et al.* 2011). Detection dog surveys are also useful for detecting the presence of low-density species, such as northern (*Dasyurus hallucatus*) or spotted-tailed quolls

(*D. maculatus*), where alternative methods have been unsuccessful (Jamieson *et al.* 2021) or alternative methods are unavailable, such as for North Atlantic right whales (*Eubalaena glacialis*) (Rolland *et al.* 2006). Detection dogs have been deployed for (1) threatened species detection; (2) locating invasive plants and animals, including confirming eradication; (3) biological sample collection, including scats and guano, urine and latrines, eggs, reject pellets, nests and lairs; (4) carcass detection; and (5) non-invasive disease monitoring (see specific papers in Cristescu *et al.* 2020). In principle, detection dogs can be trained to detect any odour and almost everything has an odour. Dogs have been deployed to detect terrestrial and aquatic vertebrates and invertebrates, and plant species in land or boat-based search applications. Detection dogs are also useful for detecting targets that are challenging to locate or visually observe (e.g. underground tubercules or insect eggs).

Animal welfare considerations

Dog welfare

Many welfare factors must be considered before sourcing, training and deploying a detection dog, all of which will affect training and working outcomes (Cobb *et al.* 2015). Training methods employed will not only influence a dog teams' relationship and working success (Cobb *et al.* 2015), but can also negatively impact and compromise dog welfare (Fernandes *et al.* 2017). In addition, husbandry and welfare need to be maintained year-round, not simply during the field season, and must be tailored to the individual dog. Retirement or whole-of-life plans must also be developed. Ensuring that these high animal welfare standards are followed underpins the sustainability and productivity of the working dog industry (Cobb *et al.* 2013).

Risks to the dogs during training and field deployment can include snake bite, poison ingestion, infectious diseases, animal attacks (e.g. by large carnivores), dehydration, hyperthermia or hypothermia. Dogs may require personal protective equipment (e.g. dog boots, muzzle), which should be introduced to the dog appropriately to ensure a positive association. No nationally accepted protocols exist that detail standards for the care and welfare of Australian wildlife detection dogs, but general state standards exist (e.g. Queensland *Animal Care and Protection Act 2001* and *Animal Management (Cats and Dogs) Act 2008*). Organisations that use detection dogs regularly should develop detailed protocols.

Special provisions should be made in case of illness or accident (i.e. insurance). Safety during deployment should include specific canine risk assessment (see 'Workplace health and safety'). Conflict of interests might arise between what is best for the dog versus project delivery. Consequently, protocols should be in place to ensure that dog safety and welfare are maintained regardless of project constraints (e.g. budget, timelines).

Wildlife welfare

Little research is available to indicate the direct or indirect effects of detection dogs on target and non-target wildlife, or ecosystems more generally. It has been proposed that dog presence may cause behavioural changes in free-living wildlife (Whitehouse-Tedd *et al.* 2021). Research on the Mojave desert tortoise (*Gopherus agassizii*) determined no significant difference in tortoise or predator activity after surveys with detection dogs, compared to surveys with humans (Heaton *et al.* 2008). Nonetheless, using detection dogs in fragile ecosystems may warrant additional care. For example, we recommend dog faeces be removed from the environment to prevent introduction of parasites, pathogens or nutrients (Whitehouse-Tedd *et al.* 2021).

Detection dogs need to be exposed to a variety of taxa during controlled training sessions, conducted in simulated and field conditions, to minimise risks should wildlife or domestic animals be encountered during deployment. For example, a detection dog that chases and harms target or non-target species (e.g. kangaroos, *Macropus* and *Osphranter* spp.) that are encountered during a survey poses an unacceptable risk to wildlife welfare. How a detection dog is trained and deployed also depends on the target species. Dogs can be separated into 'general trace/scat detection dogs' and 'live animal detection dogs', yet all dogs searching in field environments should be able to reliably demonstrate safe behaviour around the wildlife they may encounter. It is the dog handler's responsibility to monitor their dogs throughout surveys and ensure that if the dogs become unresponsive to safety cues, possibly because of tiredness or low reinforcement rates, then they cease surveying that day to minimise risk of incident.

General trace or scat detection dogs

Dogs can be trained to detect traces of target species, including scats (Thompson *et al.* 2020), pellets, nests/burrows/roosts (Chambers *et al.* 2015) and carcasses

(Smallwood *et al.* 2020). These dogs must be trained to perform passive alert behaviours (such as a sit and stare) that are appropriate to the target species and survey goals. Ideally, passive alert training should ensure that dogs do not make contact with the target to avoid contaminating samples. Consultation with target species experts is recommended to confirm factors such as likely habitat and seasonality, and inform trace sample collection and storage. Dog muzzles and long leads can be incorporated into these detection roles, if the environment is suitable.

Live animal detection dogs

Dogs trained to detect live animals (e.g. Robertson and Fraser 2009; Duggan *et al.* 2011) should not chase the target (or non-target) species and must be trained to perform an alert behaviour that reveals the presence of the target animal without the need for interacting with it physically (e.g. 'sit/stand and stare'). In general, this alert behaviour should be performed at a distance that is deemed safe for the target species. Determining appropriate alert behaviours and safe distances should be specific to the target species and developed in consultation with target species experts. For example, a safe distance for a dog to alert to an insect may be 10 cm from the animal, while a safe distance for a ground-dwelling bird may be ~5 m from the target animal. As is the case for passive alert training, long leads and muzzles can also be incorporated into these detection roles, if appropriate for the search environment

General procedures

Dog sourcing

Detection dogs are generally selected based on temperament, not breed or sex. Many dog breeds and crossbreeds are working successfully as conservation detection dogs (e.g. Dahlgren *et al.* 2012). Candidate dogs will have (1) high toy or food motivation that persists in new environments and among distractions; (2) handler engagement; (3) good sociability; (4) confidence in novel environments; and (5) low motivation to chase or harm wildlife (Jamieson *et al.* 2017). Dogs should also be physically sound and agile, enabling them to work in often complex and challenging environments (Jamieson *et al.* 2017). Ideally, they should be of a size that allows them to be carried by handlers when necessary (e.g. if a severe injury is sustained).

Costs and benefits are associated with sourcing a dog from a breeder or rescue organisation. Dogs sourced from ethical breeders typically have a known history. Previous generations of dogs can be viewed to gauge working ability and puppies sourced from breeders can be socialised from a young age. However, typically < 50% of dogs purpose bred for working roles complete training (Jamieson *et al.* 2017). This outcome is both financially inefficient and an animal welfare concern (Cobb *et al.* 2015). Alternatively, rescued dogs can be sourced as adults, which can provide more-reliable behaviour indicators from aptitude evaluations than puppies. However, rescue dogs can have behavioural problems and an unknown learning history. Both purpose-bred and rescue dogs can develop behavioural problems throughout their working lives; these issues will need to be planned for and addressed by handlers.

Dog training

Currently, no standard training protocol is available for using detection dogs for wildlife detection work (Oldenburg *et al.* 2016). Training can typically be separated into three areas: (1) adaptations and responsiveness in the training/field environment; (2) imprinting to target odour; and (3) odour discrimination and problem-solving (Fischer-Tenhagen *et al.* 2011). Selected training methods should be science- and reward-based, and safeguard animal welfare. Current training methods often use associative learning theory through operant conditioning, where a stimulus (target odour) is immediately followed by the appearance of a reward. To maximise skill acquisition, training sessions should be brief and reward-based (Demant *et al.* 2011). Training should include both odour recognition and odour discrimination tasks in a variety of environments, and include trials where the target is absent. In addition, at a minimum for safety, operational detection dogs should be able to reliably perform immediate recalls and emergency stops (dog freezes in its position).

Testing

Assessments should resemble, as closely as possible, real-world working scenarios, with detection rates and field safety being assessed (ideally including behaviour around animals). Location and number of samples during testing should be unknown to the handler to ensure that they do not cue their dog and bias the results (Lit *et al.* 2011). Accuracy testing (i.e. proportion of targets found relative to the number of targets deployed (Cablk and Heaton 2006)) is often important for ecological surveys, particularly if detection dog-generated data are used to compare results (e.g. distribution or density between sites and years), or if missing the target odour would have dire consequences (e.g. environmental impact assessments). Odour discrimination can also be assessed (e.g. proportion of non-targets ignored relative to the number of non-targets deployed).

Search performance and field safety skills should be assessed in environments that mimic field conditions, including the search scale and environmental context (Rutter *et al.* 2021a), and designed to ensure they resemble survey requirements. Inappropriately designed assessments may introduce bias in the measure of accuracy and/or discrimination by the dog. Trial designs need to be statistically robust, including elements of randomness and replication. Dogs should be tested alongside the handler whom they will be working with in the field, as detection performance can vary between handlers (Jamieson *et al.* 2018). If appropriate, the handler should also be assessed to ensure they can identify target samples accurately.

Dog deployment

Like other survey methods, detectability performance when using detection dogs will be affected by environmental and other factors, which, if systematic, can create biases. Biases, when they cannot be avoided (e.g. by randomisation of search order between control and treatment sites), need to be measured, accounted for or, at a minimum, acknowledged (for a thorough review of dog-induced biases, see Gutzwiller 1990).

The search pattern when relying on olfactory rather than visual cues is of critical importance. Effective surveys require consideration of environmental factors, including wind, temperature, precipitation, humidity, terrain and vegetation structure (Reed *et al.* 2011). Environmental conditions affect survey time because of their influence on dogs' health, scent movement and concentration, and search effectiveness. High air temperatures affect dogs' abilities to detect scent as their panting rates increase to regulate their temperature (Goldblatt *et al.* 2009). Therefore, surveying during high temperatures can be inefficient and ineffective. Restricting detection dog survey times to early morning, or late afternoon, is commonly used to manage the dogs' welfare, but also for survey efficiency.

Continuous monitoring of individual dogs in the field is required to evaluate welfare, behaviour and survey efficiency. Field monitoring will include regular respiration, locomotion and alertness checks, and overall behaviour monitoring. If respiration is abnormal the dog should be rested and its mucous membrane colour checked. If monitored signs become abnormal and do not return to normal (specific to each dog) after a period of full rest, the dog should be deemed unfit to work for the rest of the day. Where recovery is slow, veterinary advice should be sought.

Consideration should also be given to biosecurity measures relevant to each survey site and/or detection targets, including preventing the movement of organic material to reduce the risk of spread of invasive seeds and fungi, including chytrid fungus (*Batrachochytrium dendrobatidis*) and cinnamon fungus or 'dieback' (*Phytophthora cinnamomi*).

Citizen scientist and detection dogs

Citizen science (see Chapter 10) plays an important part in many areas of conservation and has been suggested as a potential alternative way to access detection dogs for budget-restricted research programs (Dahlgren *et al.* 2012; Byosiere *et al.* 2019; Rutter *et al.* 2021a). Suitable citizen scientists and their pet dogs can be successfully trained by professionals to search natural environments for training odours (Rutter *et al.* 2021a) and conservation-related target odours (Rutter *et al.* 2021b). Volunteer teams need to be tested in field conditions they will be deployed in, and only deployed when they are safe, and their detection performance standards meet project requirements. Supervised volunteer teams can undertake cost-effective surveys and cover large areas by simultaneously deploying multiple teams.

Animal treatment, withdrawal and euthanasia

During their working life, detection dogs need to be checked regularly by their veterinarian, who needs to be aware of the working conditions, and by their handler for any injury or pain that should preclude work. As dogs age, their health, motivation and stamina need to be monitored to facilitate transition to light duties and retirement.

Equipment and maintenance

Housing and transport

Detection dogs must be provided with housing facilities year-round. Transportation vehicles should be safe, secure and ideally insulated. Housing must meet minimum standards set in relevant codes of practice for domestic dogs and working dogs in the appropriate state or territory. At a minimum, housing must ensure that dogs are secure, protected from weather conditions, and have their physical, social and mental needs met. To achieve optimal performance from a detection dog, housing and transport strategies which ensure positive welfare should be given appropriate consideration (Rooney *et al.* 2009). Preventing disease transmission and minimising stress by providing appropriate enrichment and stimulation are essential for welfare and working performance (Rooney *et al.* 2009).

Training and testing

Target and non-target odours can often be difficult to secure. Target and non-target odours should be sourced from captive populations, where species can be correctly identified (i.e. no risk of misclassified odours) and should be stored appropriately to avoid contaminating the target odour. New samples should be used for testing to ensure that the dogs have no prior exposure or learning history associated with specific samples.

Deployment

During deployment, general equipment items may include:

- identification jacket to make detection dogs more visible and identifiable to the public (Figure 5.4)
- lead and/or long line, if required
- GPS tracking collar to enable plotting of the area covered by the dog and to calculate survey effort
- muzzle, if needed when a low risk of 1080 poison baiting in the area is present (dogs are usually not deployed if the 1080 baiting risk is medium/high)
- protective boots in areas of rough terrain or vegetation
- water available at frequent intervals during deployments
- communication item for safety, such as two-way radio or emergency beacon
- first aid kits for the dog and handler.

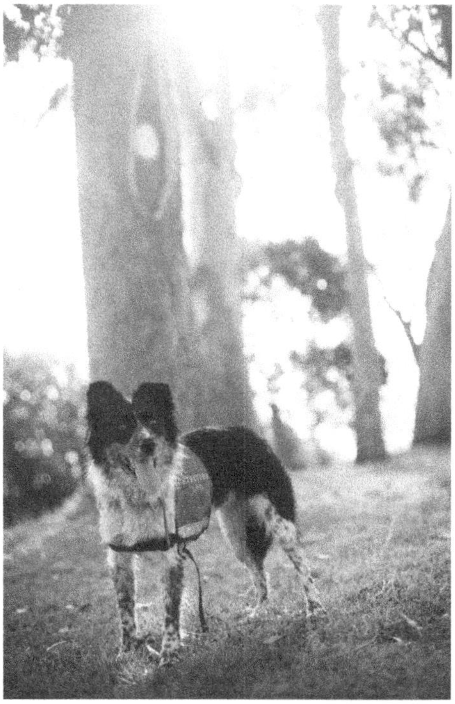

Figure 5.4: Maya the koala (*Phascolarctos cinereus*) scat detection dog, fitted with a reflective identification jacket. Photo © Marie Colibri.

Specific qualification, experience and training

No current government recognised certifications are available for dog-handler teams. However, dog handlers can be assessed for a fee, or detection dogs can be tested internally or by external funding bodies. Guidelines are available through the Australasian Conservation Dog Network (conservationdognetwork.com.au). It is recommended that once teams have successfully met internally developed criteria, where possible assessments are conducted by an independent third party. Minimum requirements are outlined in Table 5.2.

Workplace health and safety

Standard procedures relating to field work and working in remote areas should be addressed through organisational risk management processes. Dog safety also needs to be considered; specific risks to dog safety are considered below.

Heat

Dogs are prone to overheating. Handlers should be aware of physical and behavioural changes associated with overheating, such as excessive panting and lethargy. Adapting working to the coolest time of the day or year, providing frequent rest and water, and even cooling jackets, can be used for heat management.

Parasites and snake bites

Detection dogs need to be treated regularly for ticks (and other ectoparasites), especially in areas where paralysis ticks (*Ixodes holocyclus*) are present. Handlers should manage the risk of snake bite by avoiding long grass or

Table 5.2: Competency requirements for personnel using conservation detection dogs.

Competency category	Competency requirement
Dog responsive to handler cues	Handler has knowledge of dog behaviour and training principles, and a strong dog-handler bond. Dog is responsive to all cues provided by handler, including safety and search cues.
Team can search area efficiently	Handler has knowledge of scent theory and environmental influences. Dog can be directed through the environment and can problem-solve.
Identification of target odour/samples	Handler has target species training/knowledge (or is collaborating with species expert).
Odour accuracy/discrimination	Dog is able to accurately detect target species, whilst correctly discriminating against non-target species.
Safety of dog	Handler has knowledge of animal welfare and first aid. Dog behaves safely around wildlife.
Safety of wildlife	Handler has knowledge of wildlife and dog behaviour to ensure target and non-target wildlife are safe.
Fragile ecosystems	Handler has knowledge of the specific ecosystem and any special environmental considerations (e.g. significant plant species, relevant biosecurity protocols or culturally significant sites).

carrying dogs through high-risk areas. Handlers should have a list of the nearest emergency veterinary clinics with antivenom, when on deployment. Snake aversion training is possible, although its adoption varies with personal preference. Aversion training cannot prevent all snake encounters, such as accidental encounters, and should be considered with caution. Previous research on kiwi (*Apteryx* spp.) aversion training also highlighted the importance of completing aversion training on live animals, as when dogs are trained on training stimuli the dogs' aversion to the live animal is questionable (see Dale *et al.* 2017). Legislation surrounding the use of aversion training varies between Australian states and territories.

Poison baiting

In Australia, baiting with 1080 poison is widespread and presents a considerable risk to dogs (Goh *et al.* 2005). Risk assessments should be conducted for each deployment, as the risk will vary with the type of bait (e.g. manufactured, meat or grain) and the methods (e.g. aerial baiting, buried baits or injector-style baits) used. Buffers should be implemented in terms of space and time since baiting. Time is required so that the poison has time to degrade and become innocuous, which is dependent on environmental conditions. A spatial buffer accounts for wildlife moving baits outside the designated baiting area. Personal protective equipment (i.e. a muzzle) is insufficient to decrease the risk to dogs to an acceptable level, although it is a useful tool to use in conjunction with other mitigation methods. Handlers should discuss emergency treatment options with a veterinarian before deployment of their dog.

Alternative procedures

Detection dogs are a low-impact and minimally invasive monitoring method. For some target species and applications, detection dogs may be a successful stand-alone method for monitoring a variety of taxa. They can also be a complementary method to various monitoring methods, including camera traps (see 'Camera trapping' earlier in this chapter), live capture (Chapter 7), visual observations (Chapter 4) and thermography (Karp 2020). However, detection dogs are generally deployed when other methods are unsuccessful (low accuracy or low efficiency, for example) for detecting or monitoring target species.

REFERENCES

Adams MD, Law BS, Gibson MS (2010) Reliable automation of bat call identification for eastern New South Wales, Australia, using classification trees and AnaScheme software. *Acta Chiropterologica* **12**, 231–245. doi:10.3161/150811010X504725

Ballard AG, Meek PD, Doak S, Fleming P, Sparkes J (2014) Camera traps, sand plots and known events: what do camera traps miss? In *Camera Trapping: Wildlife Management and Research*. (Eds PD Meek, P Fleming, AG Ballard, PB Banks, A Claridge, J Sanderson and D Swann) pp. 189–202. CSIRO Publishing, Melbourne.

Barrott E (1999) Census techniques, habitat use and distribution of koalas in the Pilliga State Forests. BSc (Hons) thesis. The University of Sydney, Australia.

Berry O, Algar D, Angus J, Hamilton N, Hilmer S, Sutherland D (2012) Genetic tagging reveals a significant impact of poison baiting on an invasive species. *The Journal of Wildlife Management* **76**, 729–739. doi:10.1002/jwmg.295

Bleach IT, Beckmann C, Both C, Brown GP, Shine R (2015) Noisy neighbours at the frog pond: effects of invasive cane toads on the calling behaviour of native Australian frogs. *Behavioral Ecology and Sociobiology* **69**, 675–683. doi:10.1007/s00265-015-1879-z

Blumstein DT, Mennill DJ, Clemins P, Girod L, Yao K, Patricelli G, Deppe JL, Krakauer AH, Clark C, Cortopassi KA, Hanser SF, McCowan B, Ali AM, Kirschel NG (2011) Acoustic monitoring in terrestrial environments using microphone arrays: applications, technological considerations and prospectus. *Journal of Applied Ecology* **48**, 758–767. doi:10.1111/j.1365-2664.2011.01993.x

Brunner H, Coman BJ (1974) *The Identification of Mammalian Hair.* Inkata Press, Melbourne.

Burns PA, Parrott ML, Rowe KC, Phillips BL (2018) Identification of threatened rodent species using infrared and white-flash camera traps. *Australian Mammalogy* **40**, 188–197. doi:10.1071/AM17016

Byosiere S-E, Feng LC, Rutter NJ (2019) Factors that may affect the success of scent detection dogs: Exploring non-conventional models of preparation and deployment. *Comparative Cognition & Behavior Reviews* **14**, 81–86. doi:10.3819/CCBR.2019.140009

Cablk M, Heaton J (2006) Accuracy and reliability of dogs in surveying for desert tortoise (*Gopherus agassizii*). *Ecological Applications* **16**, 1926–1935. doi:10.1890/1051-0761(2006)016[1926:AARODI]2.0.CO;2

Chambers CL, Vojta CD, Mering ED, Davenport B (2015) Efficacy of scent-detection dogs for locating bat roosts in trees and snags. *Wildlife Society Bulletin* **39**, 780–787. doi:10.1002/wsb.598

Charlton BD, Whisson DA, Reby D (2013) Free-ranging male koalas use size-related variation in formant frequencies to assess rival males. *PLoS One* **8**, e70279. doi:10.1371/journal.pone.0070279

Claridge AW, Paull DJ (2014) How long is a piece of string? Camera trapping methodology is question dependent. In *Camera Trapping Wildlife Management and Research.* (Eds PD Meek, AG Ballard, PB Banks, AW Claridge, PJS Fleming, JG Sanderson and DE Swann) pp. 205–214. CSIRO Publishing, Melbourne.

Claridge AW, Paull DJ, Barry SC (2010) Detection of medium-sized ground-dwelling mammals using infrared digital cameras: an alternative way forward? *Australian Mammalogy* **32**, 165–171. doi:10.1071/AM09039

Cobb M, Branson N, McGreevy P, Lill A, Bennett P (2015) The advent of canine performance science: Offering a sustainable future for working dogs. *Behavioural Processes* **110**, 94–104. doi:10.1016/j.beproc.2014.10.012

Crisp H, Pedler R, Moseby K (2018) The use of hair tubes in detecting irruptive arid-zone rodents. *Australian Mammalogy* **40**, 230–233. doi:10.1071/AM15025

Cristescu RH, Foley E, Markula A, Jackson G, Jones D, Frère C (2015) Accuracy and efficiency of detection dogs: a powerful new tool for koala conservation and management. *Scientific Reports* **5**, 8349. doi:10.1038/srep08349

Cristescu RH, Miller RL, Frère CH (2020) Sniffing out solutions to enhance conservation: How detection dogs can maximise research and management outcomes, through the example of koalas. *Australian Zoologist* **40**, 416–432. doi:10.7882/AZ.2019.030

Crouch WB, Paton PW (2002) Assessing the use of call surveys to monitor breeding anurans in Rhode Island. *Journal of Herpetology* **36**, 185–192. doi:10.1670/0022-1511(2002)036[0185:ATUOCS]2.0.CO;2

Crump PS, Houlahan J (2017) Designing better frog call recognition models. *Ecology and Evolution* **7**, 3087–3099. doi:10.1002/ece3.2730

Cutler TL, Swann DE (1999) Using remote photography in wildlife ecology: a review. *Wildlife Society Bulletin* **27**, 571–581.

Dahlgren DK, Elmore RD, Smith DA, Hurt A, Arnett E, Connelly J (2012) Use of dogs in wildlife research and management. In *Wildlife Techniques Manual* 7th edn. (Ed NJ Silvy) pp. 140–153. The John Hopkins University Press, Baltimore.

Dale AR, Podlesnik AC, Elliffe D (2017) Evaluation of an aversion-based program designed to reduce predation of native birds by dogs: an analysis of training records for 1156 dogs. *Applied Animal Behaviour Science* **191**, 59–66. doi:10.1016/j.applanim.2017.03.003

De Bondi N, White JG, Stevens M, Cooke R (2010) A comparison of the effectiveness of camera trapping and live trapping for sampling terrestrial small-mammal communities. *Wildlife Research* **37**, 456–465. doi:10.1071/WR10046

Demant H, Ladewig J, Balsby TJS, Dabelsteen T (2011) The effect of frequency and duration of training sessions on acquisition and long-term memory in dogs. *Applied Animal Behaviour Science* **133**, 228–234. doi:10.1016/j.applanim.2011.05.010

DECC (2009) *Threatened Species Survey and Assessment Guidelines: Field Survey Methods for Fauna (Amphibians).* Department of Environment and Climate Change, Sydney.

DEWHA (2010) *Survey Guidelines for Australia's Threatened Frogs.* Commonwealth of Australia, Canberra.

Dema T, Towsey M, Sherub S, Sonam J, Kinley K, Truskinger A, Brereton M, Roe P (2020) Acoustic detection and acoustic habitat characterisation of the critically endangered white-bellied heron (*Ardea insignis*) in Bhutan. *Freshwater Biology* **65**, 153–164. doi:10.1111/fwb.13217

DSEWPC (2011) *Survey Guidelines For Australia's Threatened Mammals.* Department of Sustainability, Environment, Water, Population and Communities, Canberra.

Duffy AM, Lumsden LF, Caddle CR, Chick RR, Newell GR (2000) The efficacy of Anabat ultrasonic detectors and harp traps for surveying microchiropterans in south-eastern Australia. *Acta Chiropterologica* **2**, 127–144.

Duggan JM, Heske EJ, Schooley RL, Hurt A, Whitelaw A (2011) Comparing detection dog and livetrapping surveys for a cryptic rodent. *The Journal of Wildlife Management* **75**, 1209–1217. doi:10.1002/jwmg.150

Ellis W, Bercovitch F, FitzGibbon S, Roe P, Wimmer J, Melzer A, Wilson R (2011) Koala bellows and their association with the spatial dynamics of free-ranging koalas. *Behavioral Ecology* **22**, 372–377. doi:10.1093/beheco/arq216

Eyre TJ, Buck RG (2005) The regional distribution of large gliding possums in southern Queensland, Australia. I. The yellow-bellied glider (*Petaurus australis*). *Biological Conservation* **125**, 65–86. doi:10.1016/j.biocon.2005.03.012

Fiehler CM, Cypher BL, Bremner-Harrison S, Pounds D (2007) A theft-resistant adjustable security box for digital cameras. *The Journal of Wildlife Management* **71**, 2077–2080. doi:10.2193/2006-298

Fischer-Tenhagen C, Wetterholm L, Tenhagen B, Heuwieser W (2011) Training dogs on a scent platform for oestrus detection in cows. *Applied Animal Behaviour Science* **131**, 63–70. doi:10.1016/j.applanim.2011.01.006

Garden JG, McAlpine CA, Possingham HP, Jones DN (2007) Using multiple survey methods to detect terrestrial reptiles and mammals: what are the most successful and cost-efficient combinations? *Wildlife Research* **34**, 218–227. doi:10.1071/WR06111

Goh CSS, Hodgson DR, Fearnside SM, Heller J, Malikides N (2005) Sodium monofluoroacetate (Compound 1080) poisoning in dogs. *Australian Veterinary Journal* **83**, 474–479.

Goldblatt A, Gazit I, Terkel J (2009) Olfaction and explosives detector dogs. In *Canine Egonomics: The Science of Working Dogs.* (Ed WS Helton) pp. 135–174, CRC Press, Boca Raton, Florida.

Goldingay RL (1994) Loud calls of the yellow-bellied glider, *Petaurus australis*: territorial behavior by an arboreal marsupial. *Australian Journal of Zoology* **42**, 279–293. doi:10.1071/ZO9940279

Goldingay RL, Rohweder D, Taylor BD (2013) Will arboreal mammals use rope-bridges across a highway in eastern Australia? *Australian Mammalogy* **35**, 30–38. doi:10.1071/AM12006

Griffiths SR, Lumsden LF, Robert KA, Lentini PE (2020) Nest boxes do not cause a shift in bat community composition in an urbanised landscape. *Scientific Reports* **10**, 6210. doi:10.1038/s41598-020-63003-w

Gutzwiller KJ (1990) Minimizing dog-induced biases in game bird research. *Wildlife Society Bulletin* **18**, 351–356.

Halfwerk W, Lea AM, Guerra MA, Page RA, Ryan MJ (2016) Vocal responses to noise reveal the presence of the Lombard effect in a frog. *Behavioral Ecology* **27**, 669–676. doi:10.1093/beheco/arv204

Hanke PU, Dickman CR (2013) Sniffing out the stakes: hair-snares for wild cats in arid environments. *Wildlife Research* **40**, 45–51. doi:10.1071/WR12210

Harley D (2015) The use of call imitation to establish territory occupancy by Leadbeater's possum (*Gymnobelideus leadbeateri*). *Australian Mammalogy* **37**, 116–119. doi:10.1071/AM14014

Harley DKP, Holland GJ, Hradsky BAK, Antrobus JS (2014) The use of camera traps to detect arboreal mammals: lessons from targeted surveys for the cryptic Leadbeater's Possum *Gymnobelideus leadbeateri*. In *Camera Trapping in Wildlife Research and Management*. (Eds PD Meek, AG Ballard, PB Banks, AW Claridge, PJS Fleming, JG Sanderson and DE Swann) pp. 233–243. CSIRO Publishing, Melbourne.

Harris RL, Nicol SC (2010) The effectiveness of hair traps for surveying mammals: results of a study in sandstone caves in the Tasmanian southern midlands. *Australian Mammalogy* **32**, 62–66. doi:10.1071/AM09019

Heinlein BW, Urbanek RE, Olfenbuttel C, Dukes CG (2020) Effects of different attractants and human scent on mesocarnivore detection at camera traps. *Wildlife Research* **47**, 338–348. doi:10.1071/WR19117

Heaton JS, Cablk ME, Nussear KE, Esque TC, Medica PA, Sagebiel JC, Francis SS (2008) Comparison of effects of humans versus wildlife-detector dogs. *The Southwestern Naturalist* **53**, 472–479. doi:10.1894/PAS-03.1

James MS, Stockwell MP, Clulow J, Clulow S, Mahony MJ (2015) Investigating behaviour for conservation goals: Conspecific call playback can be used to alter amphibian distributions within ponds. *Biological Conservation* **192**, 287–293. doi:10.1016/j.biocon.2015.10.001

Jamieson LJ, Baxter GS, Murray PJ (2017) Identifying suitable detection dogs. *Applied Animal Behaviour Science* **195**, 1–7. doi:10.1016/j.applanim.2017.06.010

Jamieson LJ, Baxter GS, Murray PJ (2018) You are not my handler! Impact of changing handlers on dogs' behaviours and detection performance. *Animals (Basel)* **8**, 176–187. doi:10.3390/ani8100176

Jamieson LJ, Hancock AL, Baxter GS, Murray PJ (2021) How quollified are northern and spotted-tailed quoll detect dogs? *Wildlife Research* **48**, 376–384. doi:10.1071/WR19243

Karanth KU, Nichols JD, Kumar NS, Hines JE (2006) Assessing tiger population dynamics using photographic capture-recapture sampling. *Ecology* **87**, 2925–2937. doi:10.1890/0012-9658(2006)87[2925:ATPDUP]2.0.CO;2

Karp D (2020) Detecting small and cryptic animals by combining thermography and a wildlife detection dog. *Scientific Reports* **10**, doi:10.1038/s41598-020-61594-y

Kavanagh RP, Rohan-Jones WG (1982) Calling behaviour of the yellow-bellied glider, *Petaurus australis* Shaw (Marsupialia: Petauridae). *Australian Mammalogy* **5**, 95–111.

Kays R, Slauson K (2008) Remote cameras. In *Non-invasive Survey Methods for Carnivores*. (Eds RA Long, P MacKay, J Ray and W Zielinsk.) pp. 110–140. Island Press, Washington.

Law BS, Reinhold L, Pennay M (2002) Geographic variation in the echolocation calls of *Vespadelus* spp. (Vespertilionidae) from New South Wales and Queensland, Australia. *Acta Chiropterologica* **4**, 201–215. doi:10.3161/001.004.0208

Larrucea ES, Brussard PF, Jaeger MM, Barrett RH (2007) Cameras, coyotes, and the assumption of equal detectability. *The Journal of Wildlife Management* **71**, 1682–1689. doi:10.2193/2006-407

Lemckert F, Mahony M (2008) Core calling periods of the frogs of temperate New South Wales, Australia. *Herpetological Conservation and Biology* **3**, 71–76.

Lincoln A, Wirsing A, Quinn T (2020) Long-term use of non-invasive sampling methods: does successful sampling of brown bears by hair snares and camera traps change over time? *Wildlife Research* **47**, 499–508. doi:10.1071/WR19156

Lit L, Schweitzer JB, Oberbauer AM (2011) Handler beliefs affect scent detection dog outcomes. *Animal Cognition* **14**, 387–394. doi:10.1007/s10071-010-0373-2

Lumsden LF, Bennett AF (2005) Scattered trees in rural landscapes: foraging habitat for insectivorous bats in south-eastern Australia. *Biological Conservation* **122**, 205–222. doi:10.1016/j.biocon.2004.07.006

Lumsden LF, Nelson JL, Todd CR, Scroggie MP, McNabb EG, Raadik TA, Smith SJ, Acevedo S, Cheers G, Jemison ML, Nicol MD (2013) 'A new strategic approach to biodiversity management – research component'. Arthur Rylah Institute for Environmental Research, Unpublished Client Report for the Department of Environment and Primary Industries, Heidelberg, Victoria.

McNabb EG (1994) Predator calls and prey response. *Victorian Naturalist* **111**, 190–195.

Measey GJ, Stevenson BC, Scott T, Altwegg R, Borchers DL (2017) Counting chirps: acoustic monitoring of cryptic frogs. *Journal of Applied Ecology* **54**, 894–902. doi:10.1111/1365-2664.12810

Meek P, Ballard G, Fleming P, Falzon G (2016) Are we getting the full picture? Animal responses to camera traps and implications for predator studies. *Ecology and Evolution* **6**, 3216–3225. doi:10.1002/ece3.2111

Meek PD, Ballard AG, Fleming PJS (2012) *An Introduction to Camera Trapping for Wildlife Surveys in Australia*. Invasive Animals CRC, Canberra.

Meek PD, Ballard GA, Fleming PJS, Schaefer M, Williams W, Falzon G (2014) Camera traps can be heard and seen by animals. *PLoS One* **9**, e110832. doi:10.1371/journal.pone.0110832

Meek PD, Ballard GA, Vernes K, Fleming PJS (2015) The history of wildlife camera trapping as a survey tool in Australia. *Australian Mammalogy* **37**, 1–12. doi:10.1071/AM14021

Mills DJ, Harris B, Claridge AW, Barry SC (2002) Efficacy of hair-sampling techniques for the detection of medium-sized terrestrial mammals. I. A comparison between hair-funnels, hair-tubes and indirect signs. *Wildlife Research* **29**, 379–387. doi:10.1071/WR01031

Milne DJ, Armstrong M, Fisher A, Flores T, Pavey CR (2004) A comparison of three survey methods for collecting bat echolocation calls and species-accumulation rates from nightly Anabat recordings. *Wildlife Research* **31**, 57–63. doi:10.1071/WR03011

Morrant DS, Wurster CM, Johnson CN, Butler JR, Congdon BC (2017) Prey use by dingoes in a contested landscape: ecosystem service provider or biodiversity threat? *Ecology and Evolution* **7**, 8927–8935. doi:10.1002/ece3.3345

Murray AJ (2005) A new low-cost hairtube design for the detection of the spotted-tailed quoll, *Dasyurus maculatus*, in southeastern Australia. *Australian Mammalogy* **27**, 81–84. doi:10.1071/AM05081

Nelson JL (2006) A comparison of three hair-tube types for the detection of the spotted-tailed quoll *Dasyurus maculatus* in south-eastern

New South Wales. *Australian Mammalogy* **28**, 229–233. doi:10.1071/AM06031

Nelson JL, Durkin LK, Cripps JK, Scroggie MP, Bryant DB, Macak PV, Lumsden LF (2017) 'Targeted surveys to improve Leadbeater's possum conservation'. Arthur Rylah Institute for Environmental Research, Technical Report Series No. 278. Department of Environment, Land, Water and Planning, Heidelberg, Victoria.

O'Connell AF, Nichols JD, Karanth KU (Eds) (2014) *Camera Traps in Animal Ecology.* Springer, Tokyo.

Oldenburg C, Schoon A, Heitkönig IMA (2016) Wildlife detection dog training: A case study on achieving generalization between target odor variations while retaining specificity. *Journal of Veterinary Behavior* **13**, 34–38. doi:10.1016/j.jveb.2016.03.008

Pérez-Granados C, Bota G, Giralt D, Barrero A, Gómez-Catasús J, Bustillo-de la Rosa D, Traba J (2019) Vocal activity rate index: a useful method to infer terrestrial bird abundance with acoustic monitoring. *The Ibis* **161**, 901–907. doi:10.1111/ibi.12728

Reed S, Bidlack AL, Hurt A, Getz MG (2011) Detection distance and environmental factors in conservation detection dog surveys. *The Journal of Wildlife Management* **75**, 243–251. doi:10.1002/jwmg.8

Robertson HA, Fraser JR (2009) Use of trained dogs to determine the age structure and conservation status of kiwi *Apteryx* spp. populations. *Bird Conservation International* **19**, 121–129. doi:10.1017/S0959270908007673

Rolland RM, Hamilton PK, Kraus SD, Davenport B, Gillet RM, Wasser SM (2006) Faecal sampling using detection dogs to study reproduction and health in North Atlantic right whales (*Eubalaena glacialis*). *The Journal of Cetacean Research and Management* **8**, 121–125.

Rooney N, Gaines S, Hiby E (2009) A practitioner's guide to working dog welfare. *Journal of Veterinary Behavior* **4**, 127–134. doi:10.1016/j.jveb.2008.10.037

Rutter NJ, Howell TJ, Stukas AA, Pascoe JH, Bennett PC (2021*a*) Diving in nose first: the influence of unfamiliar search scale and environmental context on the search performance of volunteer conservation detection dog-handler teams. *Animals (Basel)* **11**, 1177–1197. doi:10.3390/ani11041177

Rutter NJ, Howell TJ, Stukas AA, Pascoe JH, Bennett PC (2021*b*) Buzzing with possibilities: training and olfactory generalization in conservation detection dogs for an endangered stonefly species. *Aquatic Conservation* **31**, 984–989. doi:10.1002/aqc.3531

Sanecki GM, Green K (2005) A technique for using hair tubes beneath the snowpack to detect winter-active small mammals in the subnivean space. *European Journal of Wildlife Research* **51**, 41–47. doi:10.1007/s10344-004-0069-5

Scotts DJ, Craig SA (1988) Improved hair-sampling tube for the detection of rare mammals. *Australian Wildlife Research* **15**, 469–472. doi:10.1071/WR9880469

Séquin ES, Jaeger MM, Brussard PF, Barrett RH (2003) Wariness of coyotes to camera traps relative to social status and territory boundaries. *Canadian Journal of Zoology* **81**, 2015–2025. doi:10.1139/z03-204

Sharpe DJ, Goldingay RL (2009) Vocal behaviour of the squirrel glider (*Petaurus norfolcensis*). *Australian Journal of Zoology* **57**, 55–64. doi:10.1071/ZO08075

Smallwood KS, Bell DA, Standish S (2020) Dogs detect larger wind energy effects on bats and birds. *The Journal of Wildlife Management* **84**, 852–864. doi:10.1002/jwmg.21863

Smith DA, Ralls K, Davenport B, Adams B, Maldonado JE (2001) Canine assistants for conservationists. *Science* **291**, 435.

Suckling GC (1978) A hair sampling tube for the detection of small mammals in trees. *Australian Wildlife Research* **5**, 249–252. doi:10.1071/WR9780249

Sugai LSM, Desjonquères C, Silva TSF, Llusia D (2020) A roadmap for survey designs in terrestrial acoustic monitoring. *Remote Sensing in Ecology and Conservation* **6**, 220–235. doi:10.1002/rse2.131

Sugai LSM, Silva TSF, Ribeiro JW, Jr, Llusia D (2019) Terrestrial passive acoustic monitoring: review and perspectives. *Bioscience* **69**, 15–25. doi:10.1093/biosci/biy147

Swann DE, Hass CC, Dalton DC, Wolf SA (2004) Infrared-triggered cameras for detecting wildlife: an evaluation and review. *Wildlife Society Bulletin* **32**, 357–365. doi:10.2193/0091-7648(2004)32[357:ICFDWA]2.0.CO;2

Taggart PL, Peacock DE, Fancourt BA (2020) Camera trap flash-type does not influence the behaviour of feral cats (*Felis catus*). *Australian Mammalogy* **42**, 220–222. doi:10.1071/AM18056

Teixeira D, Maron M, van Rensburg BJ (2019) Bioacoustic monitoring of animal vocal behavior for conservation. *Conservation Science and Practice* **1**, e72. doi:10.1111/csp2.72

Thompson SA, Thompson GG, Withers PC, Bennett EM (2020) Conservation detection dog is better than human searcher in finding bilby (*Macrotis lagotis*). *Australian Zoologist* **41**, 86–93. doi:10.7882/AZ.2020.012

Vine SJ, Crowther MS, Lapidge SJ, Dickman CR, Mooney N, Piggott MP, English AW (2009) Comparison of methods to detect rare and cryptic species: a case study using the red fox (*Vulpes vulpes*). *Wildlife Research* **36**, 436–446. doi:10.1071/WR08069

Vinson SG, Johnson AP, Mikac KM (2020) Thermal cameras as a survey method for Australian arboreal mammals: a focus on the greater glider. *Australian Mammalogy* **42**, 367–374. doi:10.1071/AM19051

Vynne C, Skalski JR, Machado RB, Groom J, Jácomo ATA, Marinho-Filho J, Neto MBR, Pomilla C, Silveira L, Smith H, Wasser SK (2011) Effectiveness of scat-detection dogs in determining species presence in a tropical savanna landscape. *Conservation Biology* **25**, 154–162.

Wegge P, Pokheral C, Inawali SR (2004) Effects of trapping effort and trap shyness on estimates of tiger abundance from camera trap studies. *Animal Conservation* **7**, 251–256. doi:10.1017/S1367943004001441

Whitehouse-Tedd K, Richards N, Parker M (2020) Dogs and conservation: emerging themes and considerations. *Journal of Vertebrate Biology* **69**, E2004.1–E2004.4. doi:10.25225/jvb.E2004

Wintle BA, Kavanagh RP, McCarthy MA, Burgman MA (2005) Estimating and dealing with detectability in occupancy surveys for forest owls and arboreal marsupials. *The Journal of Wildlife Management* **69**, 905–917. doi:10.2193/0022-541X(2005)069[0905:EADWDI]2.0.CO;2

Zimmerman F, Rovero F (2016) Field deployment of camera traps. In *Camera Trapping for Wildlife Research.* (Eds F Rovero and F Zimmerman.) pp. 23–32. Pelagic Press, Exeter.

6 Studying wildlife from the air

Debbie Saunders, Tony Pople and Steve McLeod

INTRODUCTION

Aerial surveys are integral to the research and management of many native and introduced wildlife species. Surveys employing human-piloted aircraft (including aeroplanes and helicopters) are often used to obtain abundance, distribution and time series information about populations of large animals that are visible from the air. They can cover large and inaccessible areas rapidly and can be used across both aquatic and terrestrial ecosystems. The expanding use of remotely piloted aircraft (RPA or drones) in wildlife research also provides new opportunities to gain unique perspectives and data on wildlife and their habitats. These opportunities include undertaking surveys at spatial and temporal scales suitable for studying populations, aggregations and individual animals. Drones are often used to survey smaller geographical areas, and can be deployed frequently in a flexible, yet targeted manner. This chapter provides general operating procedures (GOPs) and guidelines for aerial surveys undertaken with human-piloted and RPA.

HELICOPTERS AND FIXED-WING AIRCRAFT

Tony Pople and Steve McLeod

Target taxa

This GOP applies to all free-living large vertebrates that are sufficiently large to be seen from the air (either as individuals or aggregations) in terrestrial and aquatic environments, including terrestrial ungulates (Chapter 24), marine mammals (Chapter 25), crocodiles (Chapter 26), sharks (Chapter 31), aggregations of aquatic birds (Chapter 35) and large terrestrial birds (Chapter 36).

Context and scope

Fixed-wing aircraft and helicopters are used for determining the abundance and distribution of vertebrate wildlife. Surveys are flown with human observers, but remote airborne photography is increasingly being used as an alternative (Lethbridge *et al.* 2019). The target taxa, or their sign (e.g. nests and warrens), must be sufficiently large to be visible from the air. These aircraft are used in other areas of wildlife research, such as capture and transport, but such activities can have markedly different effects on wildlife, being more or less intrusive, respectively, and so must be treated separately. Both types of aircraft are also used to track wildlife with radio tags, akin to surveying small areas (also see Chapter 9). Aerial surveys are able to generate lengthy time series to help understand the population dynamics and distribution of terrestrial fauna, particularly introduced ungulate species, kangaroos (*Macropus* and *Osphranter* spp.) and emus (*Dromaius novaehollandiae*), and large marine and freshwater taxa in Australia (e.g. Preen *et al.* 1997; Kingsford *et al.* 1999; Pople *et al.* 2018).

Aerial surveys are integral to the management of many wildlife species for conservation, harvest and population reduction. Management may require accurate estimates of abundance to set harvest quotas as a proportion of population size, e.g. for kangaroos (Pople 2004). In conservation, a repeatable index of abundance may be sufficient to detect declines or recoveries of a threatened species. For invasive species control, aerial surveys can be used to monitor the effectiveness of management interventions, such as culling or poison baiting, by determining the extent of population reduction (Lethbridge *et al.* 2016).

Aerial surveys are usually the most cost-effective method for obtaining broad-scale (hundreds of square kilometres) estimates of abundance of wildlife. Fixed-wing aircraft have a long range, allowing good coverage of Australia's extensive rangelands where kangaroos are harvested (Caughley and Grigg 1981) and across swathes of coastal waters for monitoring aquatic animals, e.g. dugongs (*Dugong dugon*) (Preen *et al.* 1997). Helicopters are more expensive per flying hour and have a smaller range, but have advantages where vegetation cover is heavier and detection probability is lower, and in rugged terrain where constant height can be hard to maintain (Clancy *et al.* 1997). Ultralights and drones (see the next GOP in this chapter) provide alternative platforms for aerial survey, but are currently restricted to smaller survey areas; they also have smaller payloads (i.e. aircraft carrying capacity, including cargo and crew), limiting the survey methods that can be employed (i.e. multiple observers and bulky or heavy sensors).

Animal welfare considerations

Short-term responses to noise and animal disturbance

Aircraft, particularly helicopters, are noisy and animals respond with increased vigilance and movement over varying distances. This movement makes them more visible to observers, but they may also hide. Substantial movement can violate assumptions of the survey method and bias the resulting density estimates (Buckland *et al.* 2015). The reaction of target and non-target taxa to aircraft noise is the primary animal welfare concern associated with this type of survey, but in most cases the immediate effects are relatively minor. Nevertheless, instances of panic responses have led to mortalities in avian species (e.g. king penguins, *Aptenodytes patagonicus*) (Hughes *et al.* 2008)) and substantial responsive movements in some species (e.g. light geese (*Chen* and *Anser* spp.) (Gilbert *et al.* 2020)) so it is difficult to generalise.

The nature and duration of animals' responses to aircraft vary across taxa and environments. Mountain ungulates show marked responses to helicopters approaching within 500 m, leading to recommendations for minimum approach or overpass distances of < 1500 m (Côté *et al.* 2013; Brambilla and Brivio 2018). Similar recommendations have been given for hauled-out seals (Born *et al.* 1999). However, Tracey and Fleming (2007) found no detrimental short- or long-term effects from strong responses of introduced goats (*Capra hircus*) to helicopter surveys in eastern Australia. Antarctic seals and penguins in the pack ice showed only small movements in response to helicopter surveys (Southwell 2005). Gilbert *et al.* (2020) concluded that probability of disturbance was low for aerial surveys of waterbirds in central USA but, again, responses among species varied. Cetaceans commonly dive in response to low-flying aircraft (Luksenburg and Parsons 2009); this can negatively bias densities estimated by aerial survey. However, the effect sizes are often small, suggesting this potential bias is a greater problem for more-intensive activities, such as whale watching. All of these concerns are relevant to wildlife telemetry using light aircraft. However, with telemetry, any effect is often restricted to a smaller number of animals with radio-collars or tags, and their response and survival can be readily monitored.

Long-term effects of disturbance

The impact of an infrequent (e.g. annual) survey of a wildlife population must be distinguished from the effects of chronic disturbance. In the longer term, frequent noise from aircraft and other anthropogenic sources may alter animal behaviour, resulting in reduced time foraging, less time spent in preferred habitats and ultimately reduced body condition, survival and fecundity (Barber *et al.* 2010). Habituation may alleviate some of these effects, but does not always occur even with chronic disturbance (e.g. Côté *et al.* 2013) and is unlikely with infrequent surveys. In contrast, wildlife populations subjected to aerial shooting exhibit greater flight responses (Stankowich 2008) and animals readily seek refuge, reducing detection probability during aerial surveys (Tracey and Fleming 2007). Long-term effects of disturbance are difficult to measure. The long time series of abundance generated by aerial surveys could detect such an effect, but it would need to be separated from other factors driving population trends. Where sampling intensity is low (e.g. large study areas), population-level effects are unlikely.

General procedures

Survey bias

It is well recognised that counts of animals from the air in a survey plot or transect are incomplete, as animals are often missed. This visibility bias will be influenced by a range of factors, including the observers, features of the target species, aircraft height and speed, weather, time of day, sea state and vegetation. Considerable effort has gone into standardising or correcting for these effects to ensure density estimates are repeatable and, where necessary, accurate (see Marsh and Sinclair 1989 and Pople 2004). Investigators should consider these factors in the design phase of their study.

Survey height and timing

With human observers, survey height is generally < 150 m (e.g. kangaroos surveyed at 76 m by fixed-wing aircraft, Caughley and Grigg 1981; and 61 m by helicopter, Clancy *et al.* 1997). Ground speed ranges from 50 kn (helicopter) to 100 kn (fixed-wing). Detection probability declines with increasing height above ground level, as does noise level and disturbance. Species identification also becomes harder – this issue is an important consideration for surveys of mixed species, such as waterbirds and kangaroos. Consequently, it is hard to minimise disturbance without compromising accuracy. In Australia, surveys of ungulates and kangaroos are undertaken in winter 3 hours after dawn and before dusk when animals are more likely to be active and most visible.

Survey area and design

Aerial surveys generally sample the landscape along randomly or systematically placed transect lines. Alternative survey designs are possible depending on the dispersion of the study animal and size of the study area. Less than 2% of an extensive rangeland study area may be surveyed (Caughley and Grigg 1981). Alternatively, a survey may involve intensive counts in small blocks where a large percentage of a small population may be counted. Disturbance will be higher in small bocks where animals are deliberately flushed from cover than in larger areas. This principle also applies to radio tracking using light aircraft. Animals, particularly ungulates, can move considerable distances in response to aircraft. Thus, transects need to be spaced so as to avoid double counting.

Since its inception in Australia in the mid-1900s, aerial survey methodology has advanced from counts in strip transects to surveys along line transects (i.e. distance sampling), providing survey-specific correction for visibility bias (Buckland *et al.* 2015). Rather than counting all animals within a strip, a line transect involves recording perpendicular distances (or distance intervals) to clusters of one or more animals. With two observers surveying the same transect, a further adjustment can be made for animals missed on the line, in order to meet a critical assumption of the technique (mark–recapture distance sampling or MRDS; Burt *et al.* 2014). Where animals are hidden from observers (e.g. underwater or in a burrow), this availability bias (Marsh and Sinclair 1989) needs to be quantified (e.g. using telemetry) to estimate density of the entire population.

Aerial telemetry

For aerial radio tracking, procedures are well described (e.g. Seddon and Maloney 2004). Animals can be tracked using antennae attached to the aircraft, an antenna that is handheld from within a helicopter or a radio tracking system can be attached to a drone (see next section). For general considerations for radio tracking studies refer to Chapter 9.

Animal treatment, withdrawal and euthanasia

Surveys need to be designed to meet the assumptions of the sampling method. However, avoiding predetermined adverse responses from wildlife can be included as a survey requirement. For example, when flying over agricultural land, minimising disturbance to livestock (e.g. avoiding flying directly over mustered herds or naïve young animals, or bunching animals in fence corners) is often a requirement of landholders. Surveys should be modified or aborted if pre-conditions are not being met. Animal responses to disturbance may not be readily apparent from the air, requiring monitoring on the ground. Pilot studies may be needed to gauge wildlife responses to aircraft if insufficient guidance is available from the literature. Triggers need to be taxa-specific.

Equipment and maintenance

High-wing aircraft are used for fixed-wing surveys. Some states in Australia require government employees to use turbine- rather than piston-powered helicopters on safety grounds. MRDS requires observers in two seats on at least one side of the aircraft. Counts are usually made on both sides of the aircraft. Doing so can be important for line transect sampling of low-density populations where a sufficient number of sightings (> 60; Buckland *et al.* 2015) is needed to model detection probability. Adequate precision will generally require 10–20 transects.

For line transect sampling, sighting poles, booms, window markings or inclinometers are required to determine perpendicular distances from the transect line on the ground. If affixed to the aircraft, they will need certification by the Civil Aviation Safety Authority (CASA). For strip transect sampling, the strip width will need to be identified; this process is commonly done with streamers on the wing struts. Survey height is ideally maintained with the assistance of a radar altimeter.

Counts can be recorded on paper, voice recorders or data loggers. The latter have the advantage of being able to be linked to a global positioning system (GPS), so sightings can be georeferenced. Cameras are usually fixed to the aircraft with thermal or colour video (Lethbridge *et al.* 2019) or stills reviewed after the survey. Transect lines and survey blocks can be determined by GPS.

Specific qualifications, experience and training

Trainee observers require time counting wildlife from the air (e.g. > 40 h counting kangaroos from a fixed-wing aircraft; Beard 1999) before they routinely record similar numbers to an experienced observer. Not all people are suitable as observers (e.g. those who experience airsickness). Many organisations require observers in helicopters to undertake courses on flying safely in an aircraft, particularly on being aware of hazards, such as wires and towers. Australian governments usually set minimum standards for aircraft (see 'Equipment and maintenance') and pilots contracted for surveys. In Australia, pilots require a low-level endorsement to fly below 152 m (500 feet) above ground level.

Workplace health and safety

Aerial hazards

Hazards include power lines, towers, emergent vegetation and birds. Pilots and passengers must watch for these pieces of infrastructure and other light aircraft, particularly helicopters undertaking mustering, and be in communication with known local aircraft and sometimes landholders. Most surveys will be undertaken outside of controlled airspace.

Remote area aviation protocols

Many aerial surveys are undertaken in remote areas, requiring search and rescue protocols. Emergency equipment should be carried, such as satellite phone, satellite-based safety devices, spare GPS and survival kits.

Alternative procedures

Aerial surveys are often the only feasible method for monitoring abundance on a broad scale, especially for species inhabiting remote areas at low densities, such as introduced camels (*Camelus dromedarius*) (Lethbridge *et al.* 2016). Further, alternative methods, such as ground surveys (e.g. mark–recapture and vehicle surveys) may be more intrusive. Nevertheless, surveys can be timed to minimise disturbance and avoid susceptible periods, such as nesting or calving. Survey frequency can also be reduced if objectives are not compromised. Improvements in the resolution and analysis of aerial photography and videography will probably see human observers replaced in aerial surveys sometime in the future (e.g. Buckland *et al.* 2012), allowing surveys to be flown at higher altitudes to reduce disturbance. Imagery is already useful for counts of relatively static wildlife in open areas (e.g. cetaceans, seal haul-outs and waterbirds), but is not yet a suitable replacement in other situations (e.g. Gentle *et al.* 2018).

REMOTELY PILOTED AIRCRAFT (DRONES)

Debbie Saunders

Target taxa

This GOP relates to all free-living vertebrates.

Context and scope

Drones are used for a variety of applications relating to surveying vertebrate wildlife. A range of fixed-wing and multi-rotor drone platforms and sensors is available for aerial surveys of wildlife at different spatial and temporal scales. The types of drones and sensors used are largely determined by the environment they are being used in, the research question being addressed, and the characteristics of the taxa being studied. Drone technology has been used to study wildlife across diverse habitats, including wetlands, forests and grasslands, and marine and polar environments. Generally, the more difficult the landscape is to access or navigate on the ground, or the more challenging a species is to study (e.g. sensitive or aggressive species; Chabot and Bird 2015), the greater the applicability of drone technology. Importantly, drones can be a more-effective and lower-impact means of data collection compared to a range of traditional procedures (see Table 6.1 for examples).

Table 6.1: Examples of the benefits of drone use in wildlife research.

Activity	Procedure
Reduce survey times during breeding periods.	Conduct rapid aerial targeted surveys during breeding seasons to minimise disturbance compared to ground-based surveys.
Remotely track multiple animals simultaneously.	Radio track multiple animals simultaneously without needing to get close to them, or disturb natural behaviour or habitats.
Detect mortality radio signals remotely.	Rapidly detect and locate mortality signals remotely with drone radio-tracking system to enable targeted on-ground action.
Protect habitat.	Use aerial survey to reduce trampling of habitats in rookery/nesting areas, ground/understorey vegetation cover and sensitive habitats (e.g. alpine areas, bogs, burnt or flooded habitats).
Locate real-time positions of multiple animals.	Remotely locate multiple animals in real time to enable time critical on-ground actions, such as health inspections and management interventions.
Thermal and visual population monitoring.	Rapidly quantify population densities of large wildlife that are otherwise difficult to survey.
Remote GPS download.	Remotely download close proximity GPS with drone radio-tracking system without the need to get close to the animal; particularly useful for sensitive/wary species.
Remote acoustic recording.	Remotely and non-invasively record the acoustics of species in areas that are difficult to access on the ground.
Deter wildlife from danger.	Use deterrent drones (variable flight paths and noisy obtrusive drone platforms) to keep animals away from dangerous areas (e.g. airports) and crops to minimise culling of animals.
Capture dangerous animals safely.	E.g. crocodiles can be rapidly and ethically noosed using a drone, enabling safe and injury-free handling.
Collect biological/virological/morphological samples remotely.	Collect sample data unobtrusively for examining individual health, such as whale spout sampling and body condition data.

Drones are well-suited for collecting data at small to intermediate spatial scales that fill the niche between ground surveys and large-scale human piloted aircraft surveys. They provide a unique perspective on natural environments and wildlife habitat use. A recent survey of drone pilots across Australia (D. Saunders, unpublished data) revealed that a wider diversity of species had been observed or studied using drones than had been cited in published research, including aquatic species (such as whales, seals, crocodiles (*Crocodylus* spp.), turtles, sharks and dugongs) and invasive species (such as introduced pigs, *Sus scrofa*; deer; wild dogs/dingoes, *Canis* spp.; cats, *Felis catus*; and goats). Other mammals studied include flying-foxes, kangaroos and wombats (*Vombatus* and *Lasiorhinus* spp.), and a diversity of bird species ranging from water birds to parrots.

Animal welfare considerations

The use of drones for wildlife research has the potential to affect target and non-target species. However, with appropriate testing and protocols, drones can perform surveys with increased frequency, higher data resolution and less disturbance of wildlife than traditional methods that involve people being present on the ground (Hodgson *et al.* 2016), enabling more-robust programs for monitoring in some cases (McIntosh *et al.* 2018). Survey data collected by drones can also complement detailed ground-based observations (Callaghan *et al.* 2018). Before undertaking a drone-based study, investigators should consider potential effects on target and non-target species. Examples are outlined in Table 6.2. Given the diversity of responses between species, species' characteristics and the potential impacts on natural behaviour should be clearly documented and evaluated for each project (Ornithological Council 2018). This assessment should include consideration of the flight parameters and the types of drones and sensors used to collect data, since these factors influence the nature and extent of impacts.

Disturbance of natural behaviour

Responses of different species to the presence of drones vary depending on the type of animal, life-history stages and levels of aggregation (Mulero- Pázmány *et al.* 2017). For example, Bevan *et al.* (2018) found no obvious

Table 6.2: Procedures to minimise effects of drone use on wildlife.

Potential impact	Procedures for minimising effects on wildlife
Species-specific responses	Evaluate target and non-target species' characteristics in relation to potential impacts from drones before commencing study. Conduct trial flights before initiating the study to observe and document species-specific behaviour before, during and after the flights.
Low-altitude flights	Fly at a height that does not alter the species' behaviour; heights will vary depending on the drone used, species studied and habitat structure.
Proximity of flights	Use a zoom or longer focal length camera to provide an alternative to lower drone flights. Abort flights if the drone causes unavoidable large disturbance of animals.
Angle of approach	Identify the least disturbing angle of approach for the target species.
Loud drone noise	Use quieter battery-operated rather than fuel-powered drones.
Drone shape	Select a drone design fit for purpose and least likely to affect behaviour.
Threatening flight pattern	Targeted drones should not hover, chase or follow animals if natural behaviour is disturbed.
Seasonal sensitivity	Unless the study or survey pertains to some aspect of breeding, avoid flights near breeding/nesting sites during the breeding season. When monitoring nests, use wildlife spotters in addition to drone pilots to monitor the behaviour and alert pilot should flight changes be required to minimise impacts. Avoid flying close to nests when young are soon to fledge, so as to avoid provoking premature fledging. Non-breeding and aggregated animals may be more likely to have a strong behavioural response than breeding animals, so adjust flights accordingly.
Habituation flights	Reduce risk of bird strike by first doing a slow and low flight nearby to enable birds to habituate and for the pilot to gauge the birds' responses before proceeding with survey.
Blinding spotlight	Minimise the time the spotlight is shone directly on wildlife (2 min), using an appropriate light intensity spotlight (see Chapter 4).. Where possible use infrared sensors.
Launch/land disturbance	Launch/land drones at a distance or out of sight of the target species to minimise disturbance.
Physiological stress	Understand the physiological response of animals, but also evaluate impacts of implanted sensors versus short-term disturbance of drones.
Negative behavioural response	Allow animals to become habituated to drones to minimise collision risk and/or reduce responses to the drone's presence.
Animal strike	Where possible, maintain visual line of sight to enable evasive action to be taken if needed, such as flying directly upwards and/or moving away when birds of prey or swooping birds show an interest in the drone. Use a strobe light on top of the drone to deter raptors from approaching from above. Be aware of greater risk of interactions with raptors when operating in conditions that are windy or suitable for creating thermals. Where available and during high-risk flights, use protective guards around propellers so that direct contact with moving parts is minimised.

behavioural effects on nesting sea turtles even when they were in proximity to the drone, but crocodiles and crested terns displayed clear disturbance behaviours when a small drone was flown < 60 m altitude. Ramos *et al.* (2018) noted that bottlenose dolphins (*Tursiops truncatus*) were less sensitive to drones than Antillean manatees (*Trichechus manatus manatus*) when followed with a drone. Weimerskirch *et al.* (2018) found that adult king penguins (*Aptenodytes patagonicus*) breeding in large colonies showed little behavioural response even when the drone was close, whereas other species, such as giant petrels (*Macronectes* spp.), appeared highly sensitive to drone approaches.

In addition to flight altitude, the effects of proximity of take-off and landing locations also vary among species (Weston *et al.* 2020). Also, while adults with young in a nest or den often do not display obvious behavioural changes, they may have strong physiological responses, such as increased heart rate (Ditmer *et al.* 2015). Such responses can be reduced through habituation to drones (Ditmer *et al.* 2019). When using drones to track wildlife radio-transmitter signals, greater distances can be maintained from the target species compared to during terrestrial surveys. Consequently, using drones for radio tracking can actually reduce the effects of traditional handheld radio-tracking techniques on tagged animals (also see Chapter 9).

Risk of injury and fatality

Mid-air drone–wildlife collisions may result in injuries or fatalities (Davy *et al.* 2017). In the absence of published and established methods for the most effective ways to avert collisions and interactions, anecdotal evidence from drone pilots provides some ideas to reduce risks. Having spotters dedicated to monitoring responses of wildlife in the air, using strobe lights on top of the drone to deter approaches from birds flying above, flying upwards to move above approaching raptors and undertaking habituation flights may reduce the risk of collision and associated injuries.

The temporary effects of drones from infrequent surveys (e.g. annual, quarterly or monthly) must be distinguished from chronic disturbance (e.g. daily or weekly). However, where drones are used frequently, habituation may alleviate some of the effects (Ditmer *et al.* 2019). Potentially disproportional impacts may result from even short-term disturbances during the breeding season. For example, if cliff-nesting birds are flushed from their nests by drones and predators are nearby, the nests may be at greater risk of predation (Brisson-Curadeau *et al.* 2017). Investigators must remain vigilant in observing both target and non-target species, and be prepared to abort or change flight operations where such risks become evident.

Drone radio tracking enables tagged animals to be tracked from a distance, minimising disturbance of the target animals (Cliff *et al.* 2018) when compared to manual radio tracking. Conversely, where wildlife inhabits dangerous areas or human–wildlife conflict zones, such as near airports or in agricultural fields, intentional disturbance using drones with predator shape characteristics may prevent injuries or fatalities from other sources (Egan *et al.* 2020).

General procedures

Flight planning

In Australia, CASA airspace regulations require all standard drone operations to occur below 120 m (400 ft) above ground level; therefore, the bulk of wildlife research operations occur within this height range. Airspace regulations also require special permissions to be obtained within some restricted airspace (i.e. within 5.5 km of controlled airports) or when operating outside standard operating procedures.

Optimising the flying height of drones for visual aerial surveys of wildlife is a balance of minimising disturbance of natural behaviour, covering a large area and having a camera of sufficient resolution to be able to photograph and identify animals or habitat features accurately (Burke *et al.* 2019). Increasingly, evidence shows that negative effects are reduced when drones are flown at altitudes of ≥ 60 m, depending on the characteristics of the target species (McEvoy *et al.* 2016).

Nest surveys often require flights at much closer proximity (3–20 m) for finer resolution imagery and are more likely to cause disturbance than surveys at greater heights. However, these rapid surveys are often limited to 1–3 min and pose less risk of disturbance than traditional manual survey techniques, which take much longer (Junda *et al.* 2015). The distance of launch and landing sites from wildlife (Weston *et al.* 2020), and the angle of approach, can also be used to minimise disruptions of drone flights on natural behaviour while maximising data collection (Vas *et al.* 2015).

Drone platforms

The diversity of drone models makes generalisations on behavioural impacts difficult. However, most visual wildlife surveys use lightweight fixed-wing or multi-rotor drone platforms that are battery powered and have a small, high-resolution camera on board. Larger fuel-powered drones have also been used, but have evoked stronger reactions from wildlife than smaller drones (Mulero- Pázmány *et al.* 2017). The shape, size and wing profile of drones can also influence the response of some species, such as waterfowl. However, these impacts can be minimised by taking off and landing out of sight and flying at the correct altitude when approaching the survey animals (McEvoy *et al.* 2016).

Monitoring behaviour, survival and health of individual animals

The most common drone sensors used for wildlife surveys are high-resolution red green blue (RGB) visual cameras and thermal infrared (IR) cameras. Visual and thermal drone surveys tend to focus on species that are sufficiently large to be observed from the air, enabling density estimates of large aggregations (Sorrell *et al.* 2019) through to individual body condition assessments (Christiansen *et al.* 2016) and virological sampling (Geoghegan *et al.* 2018). It is also possible to conduct acoustic surveys (Fu *et al.* 2018) and to radio track animals using drones (Wildlife Drones 2020). The radio-tracking sensors can be used to rapidly survey multiple animals simultaneously, collect mortality signal data, and download GPS data for both large and small animals remotely (Wildlife Drones 2020). As a result, investigators have more time to determine the cause of mortality and to collect additional health, habitat or behavioural observation data.

Drone sensors – radio tracking

The collection of accurate data on individual animals can be challenging for many small, cryptic species, particularly those living in complex structural environments (Corcoran *et al.* 2019). However, radio-tracking sensors can detect and locate up to 40 tagged animals rapidly and simultaneously, enable increased detectability of tags, and access rugged and remote terrain (e.g. Wildlife Drones 2020). Unlike visual sensors, radio-tracking sensors minimise impacts on natural behaviour since individual animals can be located from a distance using triangulation techniques, removing the need to fly over or near them (Cliff *et al.* 2018). Also, radio-tracking data can be collected, processed and mapped in real time, enabling researchers to spend more time conducting research and less time searching for tag signals (Wildlife Drones 2020). When radio tracking, the drone can be flown at greater heights than when taking photographs, since the sensors are listening for signals rather than capturing images. Radio-tracking flights currently involve rotating the drone to sample signals from all directions, moving to another location and repeating the process to enable rapid triangulation of tagged animals (Cliff *et al.* 2018). Consequently, radio-tracking sensors can cover large areas rapidly, without needing to fly in grid patterns or to fly directly over target animals.

Drone sensors – visual cameras

Cameras can capture images of individuals or groups of animals when flown near or above them. By selecting cameras with optical zoom capabilities and image stabilisation, image data capture may be achieved from greater heights, minimising the risk of affecting the natural behaviours of the target species. Imagery from these sensors can include videos or photographs; data extraction is often conducted during post-processing.

Visual surveys typically involve pre-programmed flight paths with set flight speeds, heights and overlapping images based on the cameras used and the landscapes being surveyed. This process ensures overlap in the field of view to obtain a complete survey of an area using a systematic grid flight pattern. However, when searching for specific species manual flight modes may also be used.

The direction of flight approach can influence the level of disturbance to animals, with horizontal flight approaches being less threatening than vertical approaches for some birds, although different species have differing flight height tolerances (Vas *et al.* 2015). Lower flight heights generally cause more disturbance than higher ones (Weston *et al.* 2020). Imaging angle and sensor resolution are also important considerations when determining appropriate flight parameters (Horton *et al.* 2019). Challenges associated with collecting visual images over water also emphasise the importance of ground-truthing for maintaining data quality control (Joyce *et al.* 2019).

Drone sensors – thermal cameras

Thermal IR cameras can be used for evaluating population densities and identifying locations of cryptic or elusive species. Thermal data are often needed in real time so that activities, such as capturing and tagging or controlling the target species, can be conducted without delay on the ground. Artificial intelligence can also be used to post-process visual and thermal imagery data (Corcoran *et al.* 2021); however, enabling the ability to process results in real time using this technology is yet to be fully realised.

Thermal wildlife surveys typically include a combination of grid and manual flights conducted at night or in the early morning, and include different visual representations of the data, such as hot-spot object detection showing wildlife in contrast to the surrounding environment (Havens and Sharp 2015). To verify the species detected, the drone may need to be flown at different angles to get a better indication of the animal's shape, or visual drone surveys the following morning can be undertaken. Alternative verification techniques include the use of momentary flash photography, spotlighting or ground-truthing to enable further on-ground actions (Beranek *et al.* 2020).

The success of thermal surveys can be reduced where surveys are conducted during windy or wet conditions (Havens and Sharp 2015). Where vegetation cover is an issue, adjusting the camera angle may allow partial thermal signatures to be detected (Burke *et al.* 2019). Undertaking thermal surveys where thermal radiation emanates from objects can be challenging, particularly in landscapes that emit solar radiation that has been absorbed by rocks, bare soil and water bodies. Therefore, thermal surveys need to be undertaken at a time when the background environment is as thermally stable as possible, enabling radiation from wildlife to be differentiated more easily from that of the background environment (Havens and Sharp 2015).

Data collection and analysis

Radio-tracking data can be processed and analysed in real time, enabling immediate action on the ground where needed. These data can also be made available in a format for importing directly into statistical or mapping software, removing the need for post-processing of data. However, given the capacity of visual and thermal drone sensors to collect large quantities of data that often require post-processing, the collection, verification and extraction of data can prove challenging and time-consuming (Barnas *et al.* 2019). With increasing automation, artificial intelligence and machine-learning capabilities, including open-source software, such large-scale image processing is becoming more accessible and more precise over time (Lyons *et al.* 2019). However, training such algorithms with large quantities of verified data can be a limiting factor. Until such tools become more broadly applicable, robust and available to use in real time, ground-truthing of results while in the field will continue to play an important role in image data capture.

Animal treatment, withdrawal and euthanasia

Drone surveys are typically designed to collect data on wildlife remotely. Consequently, direct contact with animals is rare. However, if drones collide with wildlife, the operator must evaluate options for treatment or euthanasia. Where tracked animals appear stressed or panicked, or if the drone is being approached by a raptor, the operator should modify their flying technique or abandon the activity.

Equipment and maintenance

Equipment used will vary depending on the local environment, the study objectives and the species being studied. Having sufficient battery power to do the required work is critical for all drone-based studies. Depending on flight time, the distance needed to travel and weather conditions, it is advisable to purchase a large set of batteries and have them charged and ready, or have a smaller set of batteries and charge them regularly in the field. When deploying drones, it is important to bring enough equipment and spare parts to allow for contingencies and redundancies. Typical equipment for drone surveys is listed in Table 6.3.

Specific qualification, experience and training

The skills required to undertake drone-based surveys vary depending on the complexity of the environment being surveyed, the sensitivity of the study species and the study objectives. When proposing a project, pilots should state

Table 6.3: Suggested equipment and materials for drone-based fieldwork.

Drone platforms and permits	Sensors	Supporting equipment
• Multi-rotor, fixed-wing or vertical take-off and land (VTOL) drone • Remote controller • Multiple drone batteries • Multiple controller batteries • Relevant firmware/software installed on drone, batteries and controllers • CASA flight authorisations (RePL and/or ReOC) • Specialised authorisations (as required based on operations) for night flying or beyond visual line of sight (BVLOS) flights • Relevant flight planning software (if required) • Weather forecast software	• Radio-tracking receiver • RGB camera – still and/or video • Thermal camera • Sensor batteries • Base station – for real-time data feeds (radio tracking) and/or post processing of images (visual sensors) • USB drive for field data backup • GPS tag remote download system to attach to VHF antenna • Relevant sensor software	• Spare batteries • Battery chargers • Generator/charging system (if battery supply small) • Landing pad • Spare parts for drone (e.g. propellers, screws) • Spare parts for sensors • Waterproof and dustproof cover/case for equipment • Towel for wiping any moisture off equipment • 'Blower' for clearing fine dirt/grit out of electrical equipment (drone and sensors) • Base station booster power supply

clearly the nature of their previous experience, including flight hours and the drone platforms and sensors used. Australia's CASA currently requires drone operators to obtain a remote drone pilot licence (RePL) when flying a drone that weighs > 2 kg. Anyone operating outside of the standard safety rules, or flying the drone for paid work will also need a remote operator's certificate (ReOC). Regulations are regularly updated, so it is advised that investigators check the latest CASA information online for current requirements. Many modern drone platforms are easy to fly once basic training has been obtained, although the greatest challenges and risks are faced when unexpected events occur or appropriate flight precautions have not been adhered to. Suggested competency levels for drone pilot researchers are listed in Table 6.4.

Workplace health and safety

Aerial hazards

Drone pilots must constantly monitor potential hazards, including power lines, towers, emergent vegetation and flying wildlife (birds and bats). They also need to ensure that the drone does not pose a hazard to approaching aircraft.

Drone equipment safety

Standard drone operations must keep > 30 m from all people and property. This rule should generally apply to animals too unless closer flights are required for a specific purpose. Most lightweight drone systems used for wildlife research are powered by lithium polymer (LiPo) batteries, which are potentially hazardous and need to be handled with care to avoid damage and risk of fire.

Alternative procedures

Drones enable unique insights to be gained for wildlife research by collecting data at different spatial and temporal scales to traditional ground and human piloted aerial surveys, and often with lower-impact on target species. Drones surveys can be used as a lower-impact alternative to more invasive survey techniques. For example, large dangerous species, such as crocodiles, can be trapped rapidly and ethically using a drone to lure and noose the animal in < 15 min and without injury to the animal (Brien *et al.* 2020). Similarly, surveying raptor nests using drones can reduce the period of disturbance and risks to the researchers who would otherwise have to climb up to the nest (Junda *et al.* 2015) and be exposed to attacks from raptors. However, where welfare risks posed by drones are considered unacceptable, reverting to traditional or alternative low-impact methods on the ground may need to be considered (see Chapters 4 and 5).

Table 6.4: Suggested competency requirements for researchers using drones for wildlife studies.

Competency category	Competency requirement	Competency assessment
Experienced	Previous experience flying drones Licensed drone pilot (RePL) Operator's certificate authorisation (ReOC)	Licensed to fly the relevant category of drone, e.g. multi-rotor or fixed-wing of various weight classes (i.e. < 2 kg, < 7 kg, < 25 kg, > 25 kg). Experience using the flight techniques proposed. Experience flying in environments similar to those proposed for surveys. Flight hours should exceed the basic number of hours required to obtain a licence from CASA. Experience implementing evasive measures to minimise impacts on wildlife.
Limited	Limited experience flying drones No drone pilot licence or Drone pilot licence (RePL) but no operator's certificate	Some experience flying small drones (< 2 kg) using the flight techniques proposed. Experience flying in environments similar to those proposed for surveys. Flight hours should exceed the basic number of hours required to obtain a licence from CASA. Understand the features to check before take-off to ensure a safe flight (e.g. strong GPS signal, controller connected, drone operating as expected) Understand how to implement evasive measures and minimise impacts on wildlife.
Novice	No experience flying drones	Pilot should be trained or supervised by authorised person and practise their flying skills within relevant environments until they have at least limited competency before undertaking wildlife surveys.

ACKNOWLEDGEMENTS

Valuable information used in the remotely piloted aircraft (drones) GOP was obtained from many (anonymous) drone pilots and researchers who completed an online survey.

REFERENCES

Barber J, Crooks K, Fristrup K (2010) The costs of chronic noise exposure for terrestrial organisms. *Trends in Ecology & Evolution* **25**, 180–189. doi:10.1016/j.tree.2009.08.002

Barnas A, Darby B, Vandeberg G, Rockwell R, Ellis-Felege S (2019) A comparison of drone imagery and ground-based methods for estimating the extent of habitat destruction by lesser snow geese (*Anser caerulescens caerulescens*) in La Perouse Bay. *PLoS One* **14**, e0217049. doi:10.1371/journal.pone.0217049

Beard LA (1999) Training observers. *Australian Zoologist* **31**, 287–291. doi:10.7882/AZ.1999.029

Beranek C, Roff A, Denholm B, Howell L, Witt R (2020) Trialling a real-time drone detection and validation protocol for the koala (*Phascolarctos cinereus*). *Australian Mammalogy* **43**, 260–264. doi:10.1071/AM20043

Bevan E, Whiting S, Tucker T, Guinea M, Raith A, Douglas R (2018) Measuring behavioral responses of sea turtles, saltwater crocodiles, and crested terns to drone disturbance to define ethical operating thresholds. *PLoS One* **13**, e0194460. doi:10.1371/journal.pone.0194460

Born E, Riget F, Dietz R, Andriashek D (1999) Escape responses of hauled out ringed seals (*Phoca hispida*) to aircraft disturbance. *Polar Biology* **21**, 171–178. doi:10.1007/s003000050349

Brambilla A, Brivio F (2018) Assessing the effects of helicopter disturbance in a mountain ungulate on different time scales. *Mammalian Biology* **90**, 30–37. doi:10.1016/j.mambio.2018.02.001

Brien M, Booth S, Beri P, Coulson S, Frisby T, Perera D, Joyce M (2020) A novel method of using a drone to capture saltwater crocodiles (*Crocodylus porosus*). *Herpetological Review* **51**, 32–37.

Brisson-Curadeau E, Bird D, Burke C, Fifield D, Pace P, Sherley R, Elliott K (2017) Seabird species vary in behavioural response to drone census. *Scientific Reports* **7**, 17884. doi:10.1038/s41598-017-18202-3

Buckland S, Burt M, Rexstad E, Mellor M, Williams A, Woodward R (2012) Aerial surveys of seabirds: the advent of digital methods. *Journal of Applied Ecology* **49**, 960–967. doi:10.1111/j.1365-2664.2012.02150.x

Buckland S, Rexstad E, Marques T, Oedekoven C (2015) *Distance Sampling: Methods and Applications*. Springer, London.

Burke C, Rashman M, Wich S, Symons A, Theron C, Longmore S (2019) Optimizing observing strategies for monitoring animals using drone-mounted thermal infrared cameras. *International Journal of Remote Sensing* **40**, 439–467. doi:10.1080/01431161.2018.1558372

Burt M, Borchers D, Jenkins K, Marques T (2014) Using mark–recapture distance sampling methods on line transect surveys. *Methods in Ecology and Evolution* **5**, 1180–1191. doi:10.1111/2041-210X.12294

Callaghan C, Brandis K, Lyons M, Ryall S, Kingsford R (2018) A comment on the limitations of UAVS in wildlife research – the example of colonial nesting waterbirds. *Journal of Avian Biology* **49**, e01825. doi:10.1111/jav.01825

Caughley G, Grigg G (1981) Surveys of the distribution and density of kangaroos in the pastoral zone of South Australia and their bearing on the feasibility of aerial survey in large and remote areas. *Australian Wildlife Research* **8**, 1–11. doi:10.1071/WR9810001

Chabot D, Bird D (2015) Wildlife research and management methods in the 21st century: where do unmanned aircraft fit in? *Journal of Unmanned Vehicle Systems* **3**, 137–155. doi:10.1139/juvs-2015-0021

Christiansen F, Dujon A, Sprogis K, Arnould J, Bejder L (2016) Noninvasive unmanned aerial vehicle provides estimates of the energetic cost of reproduction in humpback whales. *Ecosphere* **7**, e01468. doi:10.1002/ecs2.1468

Clancy T, Pople A, Gibson L (1997) Comparison of helicopter line transects with walked line transects for estimating densities of kangaroos. *Wildlife Research* **24**, 397–409. doi:10.1071/WR96103

Cliff O, Saunders D, Fitch R (2018) Robotic ecology: tracking small dynamic animals with an autonomous aerial vehicle. *Science Robotics* **3**, eaat8409. doi:10.1126/scirobotics.aat8409

Corcoran E, Denman S, Hanger J, Wilson B, Hamilton G (2019) Automated detection of koalas using low-level aerial surveillance and machine learning. *Scientific Reports* **9**, 3208. doi:10.1038/s41598-019-39917-5

Corcoran E, Winsen M, Sudholz A, Hamilton G (2021) Automated detection of wildlife using drones: synthesis, opportunities and constraints. *Methods in Ecology and Evolution* **12**, 1103–1114. doi:10.1111/2041-210X.13581

Côté S, Hamel S, St-Louis A, Mainguy J (2013) Do mountain goats habituate to helicopter disturbance? *The Journal of Wildlife Management* **77**, 1244–1248. doi:10.1002/jwmg.565

Davy CM, Ford AT, Fraser KC (2017) Aeroconservation for the fragmented skies. *Conservation Letters* **10**, 773–780. doi:10.1111/conl.12347

Ditmer M, Vincent J, Werden L, Tanner J, Laske T, Iaisso P, Garshelis D, Fieberg J (2015) Bears show a physiological but limited behavioral response to unmanned aerial vehicles. *Current Biology* **25**, 2278–2283. doi:10.1016/j.cub.2015.07.024

Ditmer M, Werden L, Tanner J, Vincent J, Callahan P, Iaizzo P, Laske T, Garshelis D (2019) Bears habituate to the repeated exposure of a novel stimulus, unmanned aircraft systems. *Conservation Physiology* **7**, coy067. doi:10.1093/conphys/coy067

Egan C, Blackwell B, Fernandez-Juricic E, Klug PE (2020) Corrigendum: Testing a key assumption of using drones as frightening devices: do birds perceive drones as risky? *The Condor* **122**, duaa025. doi:10.1093/condor/duaa025

Fu Y, Kinniry M, Kloepper L (2018) The chirocopter: a UAV for recording sound and video of bats at altitude. *Methods in Ecology and Evolution* **9**, 1531–1535. doi:10.1111/2041-210X.12992

Gentle M, Finch N, Speed J, Pople A (2018) A comparison of unmanned aerial vehicles (drones) and manned helicopters for monitoring macropod populations. *Wildlife Research* **45**, 586–594. doi:10.1071/WR18034

Geoghegan J, Pirotta V, Harvey E, Smith A, Buchmann J, Ostrowski M, Eden J, Harcourt R, Holmes E (2018) Virological sampling of inaccessible wildlife with drones. *Viruses* **10**, 300. doi:10.3390/v10060300

Gilbert A, Jacques C, Lancaster J, Yetter A, Hagy H (2020) Disturbance caused by aerial waterfowl surveys during the nonbreeding season. *The Journal of Wildlife Management* **84**, 1063–1071. doi:10.1002/jwmg.21874

Havens K, Sharp E (2015) *Thermal Imaging Techniques to Survey and Monitor Animals in the Wild: a Methodology*. Academic Press, Sydney.

Hodgson J, Baylis S, Mott R, Herrod A, Clarke R (2016) Precision wildlife monitoring using unmanned aerial vehicles. *Scientific Reports* **6**, 22574. doi:10.1038/srep22574

Horton T, Hauser N, Cassel S, Klaus K, Fettermann T, Key N (2019) Doctor drone: non-invasive measurement of humpback whale vital signs using unoccupied aerial system infrared thermography. *Frontiers in Marine Science* **6**. doi:10.3389/fmars.2019.00466

Hughes K, Waluda C, Stone R, Ridout M, Shears J (2008) Short-term responses of king penguins *Aptenodytes patagonicus* to helicopter disturbance at South Georgia. *Polar Biology* **31**, 1521–1530. doi:10.1007/s00300-008-0492-2

Joyce K, Duce S, Leahy S, Leon J, Maier S (2019) Principles and practice of acquiring drone-based image data in marine environments. *Marine and Freshwater Research* **70**, 952–963. doi:10.1071/MF17380

Junda J, Greene E, Bird D (2015) Proper flight technique for using a small rotarywinged drone aircraft to safely, quickly, and accurately survey raptor nests. *Journal of Unmanned Vehicle Systems* **3**, 222–236. doi:10.1139/juvs-2015-0003

Kingsford R, Wong P, Braithwaite L, Maher M (1999) Waterbird abundance in eastern Australia, 1983–1992. *Wildlife Research* **26**, 351–366. doi:10.1071/WR96062

Lethbridge M, Saalfeld KW, Edwards GP (2016) Measured reductions in the density of camels under the Australian Feral Camel Management Project. *The Rangeland Journal* **38**, 173–179. doi:10.1071/RJ15106

Lethbridge M, Stead M, Wells C (2019) Estimating kangaroo density by aerial survey: a comparison of thermal cameras with human observers. *Wildlife Research* **46**, 639–648. doi:10.1071/WR18122

Luksenburg J, Parsons E (2009) The effects of aircraft on cetaceans: implications for aerial whale watching. In *Proceedings of the 61st Meeting of the International Whaling Commission.* May 2009, Madeira, Portugal.

Lyons M, Brandis K, Murray N, Wilshire J, McCann J, Kingsford R, Callaghan C (2019) Monitoring large and complex wildlife aggregations with drones. *Methods in Ecology and Evolution* **10**, 1024–1035. doi:10.1111/2041-210X.13194

Marsh H, Sinclair D (1989) Correcting for visibility bias in strip transect aerial surveys of aquatic fauna. *The Journal of Wildlife Management* **53**, 1017–1024. doi:10.2307/3809604

McEvoy J, Hall G, McDonald P (2016) Evaluation of unmanned aerial vehicle shape, flight path and camera type for waterfowl surveys: disturbance effects and species recognition. *PeerJ* **4**, e1831. doi:10.7717/peerj.1831

McIntosh R, Holmberg R, Dann P (2018) Looking without landing using remote piloted aircraft to monitor fur seal populations without disturbance. *Frontiers in Marine Science* **5**. doi:10.3389/fmars.2018.00202

Mulero- Pázmány M, Jenni-Eiermann S, Strebel N, Sattler T, Negr J, Tablado Z (2017) Unmanned aircraft systems as a new source of disturbance for wildlife: a systematic review. *PLoS One* **12**, e0178448. doi:10.1371/journal.pone.0178448

Ornithological Council (2018) *Guidelines to the use of wild birds in research. summary of literature reporting use of drones to study birds (2018 Supplement).* <https://birdnet.org/wp-content/uploads/2018/02/Drones-OCGuidelines.pdf>.

Pople A (2004) Population monitoring for kangaroo management. *Australian Mammalogy* **26**, 37–44. doi:10.1071/AM04037

Pople A, Gentle M, Brennan M (2018) Achieving pest control through sustainable wildlife use. In *Advances in Conservation through Sustainable Use of Wildlife.* (Eds G. Baxter, N. Finch, P. Murray) pp. 151–161. The University of Queensland, Brisbane.

Preen A, Marsh H, Lawler I, Prince R, Shepherd R (1997) Distribution and abundance of dugongs, turtles, dolphins and other megafauna in Shark Bay, Ningaloo Reef and Exmouth Gulf, Western Australia. *Wildlife Research* **24**, 185–208. doi:10.1071/WR95078

Ramos E, Maloney B, Magnasco M, Reiss D (2018) Bottlenose dolphins and Antillean manatees respond to small multi-rotor unmanned aerial systems. *Frontiers in Marine Science* **5**, 316. doi:10.3389/fmars.2018.00316

Seddon P, Maloney R (2004) *Tracking Wildlife Radio-tag Signals by Light Fixed-wing Aircraft.* Department of Conservation, Wellington.

Sorrell K, Clarke R, Holmberg R, McIntosh R (2019) Remotely piloted aircraft improve precision of capture-mark resight population estimates of Australian fur seals. *Ecosphere* **10**, e02812. doi:10.1002/ecs2.2812

Southwell C (2005) Response behaviour of seals and penguins to helicopter surveys over the pack ice off East Antarctica. *Antarctic Science* **17**, 328–334. doi:10.1017/S0954102005002798

Stankowich T (2008) Ungulate flight responses to human disturbance: a review and meta-analysis. *Biological Conservation* **141**, 2159–2173. doi:10.1016/j.biocon.2008.06.026

Tracey JP, Fleming PJ (2007) Behavioural responses of feral goats (*Capra hircus*) to helicopters. *Applied Animal Behaviour Science* **108**, 114–128. doi:10.1016/j.applanim.2006.10.009

Vas E, Lescroel A, Duriez O, Boguszewski G, Gremillet D (2015) Approaching birds with drones: first experiments and ethical guidelines. *Biology Letters* **11**, 20140754. doi:10.1098/rsbl.2014.0754

Weimerskirch H, Prudor A, Schull Q (2018) Flights of drones over sub-Antarctic seabirds show species- and status-specific behavioural and physiological responses. *Polar Biology* **41**, 259–266. doi:10.1007/s00300-017-2187-z

Weston M, O'Brien C, Kostoglou K, Symonds M (2020) Escape responses of terrestrial and aquatic birds to drones: towards a code of practice to minimize disturbance. *Journal of Applied Ecology* **57**, 777–785. doi:10.1111/1365-2664.13575

Wildlife Drones (2020) *Recent advances in drone radio-tracking technology.* Wildlife Drones, Canberra. <https://www.wildlifedrones.net>.

7 Wildlife capture methods

Helen P. Waudby, James M. Turner, Graeme Coulson, David A. Taggart, David Watson, Andrew J. Bengsen, Paul D. Meek, Deborah S. Bower, Scott Thompson, Lindy F. Lumsden, Jordan O. Hampton, Clare Death, Graham Thompson, Graeme Finlayson, David G. Hamilton, Sophie Petit, Judy Dunlop, Jocelyn Bentley, Eric Vanderduys, Guy A. Ballard and Damian S. Morrant

INTRODUCTION

Capturing animals enables the collection of data that cannot necessarily be collected with other methods. For example, information on morphology, abundance, population status, demographics, health and reproduction can be collected from trapped animals. Additionally, trapping is often required for collection of biological samples, including scats, tissue samples and voucher specimens. This chapter details general operating procedures (GOPs) for capturing terrestrial mammals, bats, reptiles and amphibians, and birds with mist nets. Capture methods for aquatic animals are covered elsewhere in this book (see Chapters 12–14), as are additional methods for the capture of birds (Chapter 15). Capture methods are diverse; this chapter is not intended to provide an exhaustive review of techniques, but focuses on those that are often the subject of research applications to animal ethics committees. The impacts of these methods on study and non-target animals can be mitigated through careful planning, proper resourcing, and ensuring that personnel have appropriate training and experience.

FUNNEL, CAGE, ALUMINIUM BOX, PITFALL AND PIPE TRAPS

Helen P. Waudby, Scott Thompson, Sophie Petit, James M. Turner, David A. Taggart, Graham Thompson, David G. Hamilton, Paul D. Meek, Clare Death, Jocelyn Bentley, Judy Dunlop and Deborah S. Bower

Target taxa

This GOP applies to dasyurids (Chapter 18), bandicoots, bilbies, possums, gliders and occasionally wombats (Chapter 19), small wallabies and potorids (Chapter 21), cats and red foxes (Chapter 22), rodents, European rabbits and hares (Chapter 24), snakes and lizards (Chapter 26), and amphibians (Chapter 27).

Context and scope

This GOP describes the capture of animals with funnel, cage, aluminium box (typically Elliott, Sherman or Longworth traps), dry pitfall (pitfalls), and arboreal and terrestrial pipe traps (Figure 7.1). A range of context-dependent animal welfare considerations is associated with these trap types, but most are manageable with careful planning by experienced personnel. The effectiveness of the proposed trap design relative to its expected financial and ethical costs should be evaluated before undertaking work (Waudby *et al.* 2019). Trapping programs that rely on static traps left *in situ* for a time must be designed so that sufficient resources are available for all traps to be checked in an appropriate time frame.

Funnel traps are used for capturing frogs and reptiles. Small mammals are occasionally caught, but rodents will often chew their way out of funnel traps. Sizes of animals caught in traps range from tiny juvenile geckoes up to snakes around 2 m in length. Davis *et al.* (2008) reported that tree-mounted funnel traps caught small arboreal geckoes and skinks effectively. Others noted that funnel traps rarely caught small ground-dwelling mammals (e.g. small rodents and dasyurids), but were effective for catching medium- and large-sized terrestrial snakes, widely foraging, medium-sized skinks and dragon lizards, and arboreal geckos that can climb out of pitfalls

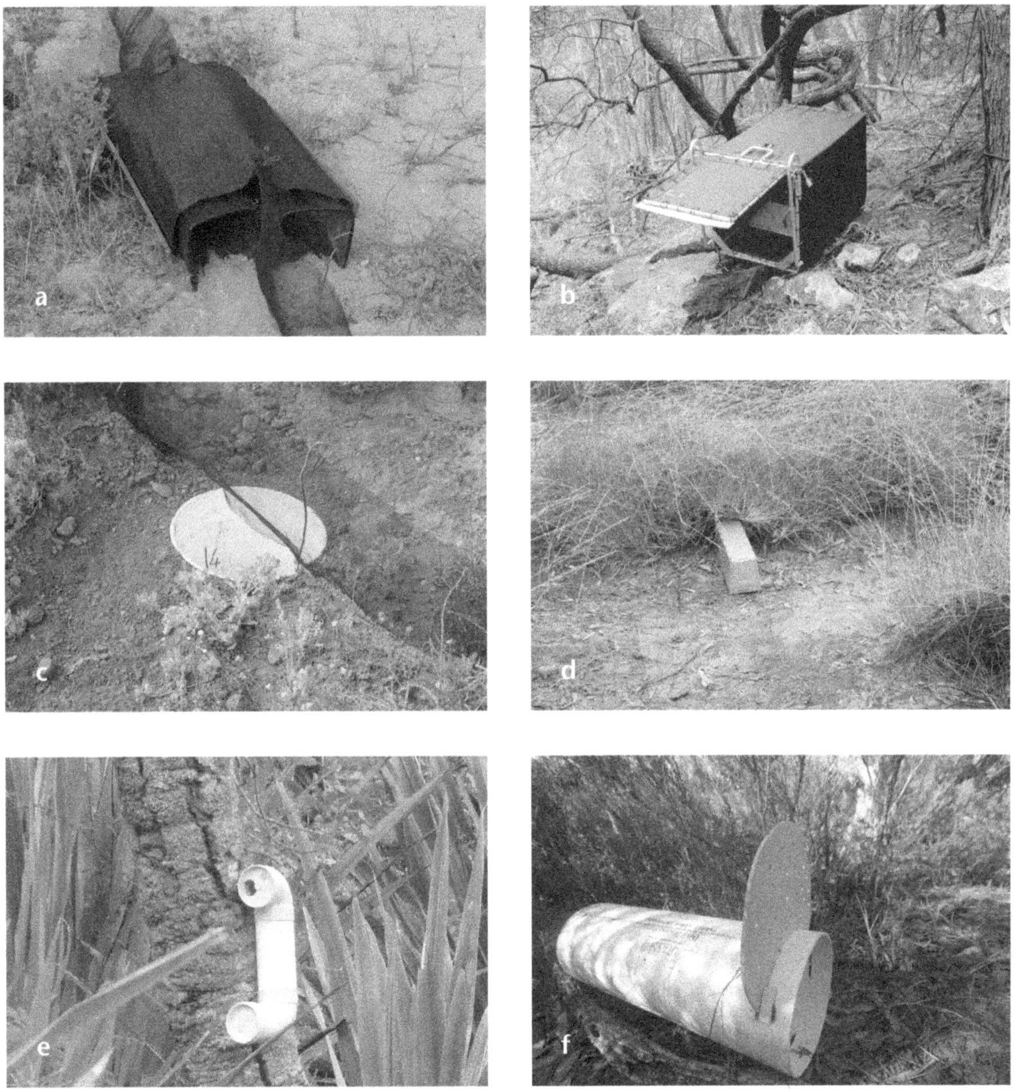

Figure 7.1: (a) Funnel traps with shade covers positioned alongside drift net fencing. Photo by Terrestrial Ecosystems. (b) Soft-sided cage trap often used for wallaby capture. Photo by David Taggart. (c) Pitfall trap for capturing ground-dwelling fauna. Photo by Helen P. Waudby. (d) Aluminium box trap placed near vegetative shelter. Photo by Helen P. Waudby. (e) Arboreal pipe trap. Photo by James M. Turner. (f) Ground-based pipe trap for catching large dasyurids. Photo by David Hamilton.

(Thompson and Thompson 2007). Funnel traps consist of shade cloth stretched over a foldable sprung frame, which can be single- or double-ended, although most have openings at both ends to increase likelihood of capture. A zippered opening allows removal of captured animals. Funnel traps vary in size, but their dimensions are typically ~750 × 180 × 180 mm with an internal funnel entrance diameter of around 40 mm. Funnel traps are usually set alongside drift net fencing when targeting ground-dwelling animals and may be installed with pitfall traps to capture species not targeted by pitfalls (Eyre *et al.* 2018).

Typically, cage traps are used for trapping larger dasyurids and rodents, possums, gliders, bandicoots, bilbies, bare-nosed wombats (*Vombatus ursinus*) in some instances (see Chapter 19 for specific considerations relating to wombats), small macropods, cats (*Felis catus*), red foxes (*Vulpes vulpes*), and medium- to large-sized reptiles and mammals, including *Tiliqua* spp. Cage traps can be used to capture terrestrial animals or mounted to a tree to target arboreal mammals. Wire cage traps have either an internal treadle mechanism or a hook for attaching the bait. When either is touched, a mechanism that closes the door is released. Traps should be covered with shadecloth or hessian to provide protection from the elements and to reduce stress in trapped animals. Trap sizes and construction material (e.g. steel, aluminium, or shade cloth) vary depending on the manufacturer and are target-species specific. Collapsible traps are available in various sizes, and in rigid wire or foldable form. The gauge of a cage trap's wire should be small enough that animals cannot push their noses through the wire, which can result in facial injuries. Cage traps can also have soft sides to reduce injuries, such as soft-sided traps for rock wallabies (Figure 7.1) and double-layer traps for swamp (*Wallabia bicolor*) (Di Stefano *et al.* 2005) and red-necked wallabies (*Notamacropus rufogriseus*) (Garnick and Coulson 2020). Doors can be external or enclosed within the trap. Internal closing spring-loaded doors are useful if traps are rolled over (cage traps with gravity-triggered doors may open if the trap is tipped upside down). For some species, such as quolls (*Dasyurus* spp.) and cats, the cage trap should be secured so that it cannot roll (i.e. pegged against a log or secured with other materials).

Dimensions of aluminium box traps vary among brands, but typical dimensions (i.e. for Elliott traps) are large (15 × 15 × 46 cm), medium (9 × 10 × 33 cm) and small (8 × 9 × 23 cm). Elliott and Sherman traps consist of aluminium sheets with an internal treadle that closes the door when an animal enters the trap and stands on it. Longworth traps are similar, but comprise a tunnel containing a hair-trigger that closes the trap when touched; a housing and bedding area is attached to the back of the tunnel. Care should be taken to file or bend sharp edges on new traps before use. Like cage traps, box traps are sometimes mounted in a tree to capture arboreal animals (e.g. Meek 2000). Johnson (1996) described a locking mechanism to minimise the risk of certain small mammal species, such as *Phascogale* spp., opening the door and escaping. Pitfalls typically consist of polyvinyl chloride (PVC) piping, rolled plastic sheets, plastic or metal buckets (Petit and Waudby 2012). The typical genera targeted by pitfalls are those of *Rattus* (mammals), *Ctenotus* (skinks), and snakes with body lengths less than the pitfall depth (Fitch 1987). Pitfalls are also used to target non-arboreal frogs (Willson and Gibbons 2009). In general, different pitfall designs are effective for targeting different taxa (e.g. Friend *et al.* 1989; Thompson *et al.* 2005; Waudby *et al.* 2019).

Arboreal pipe traps are mounted on tree trunks or limbs. They typically target small arboreal possums and gliders, but also scansorial species, such as *Antechinus* spp. and lizards. The trap comprises a vertical length of PVC pipe (9 cm diameter, around 50 cm in length) fitted with an 90° elbow at either end and a 10 cm piece with a screw cap attached to the lower elbow, which acts as the capture chamber (Winning and King 2007). A small hole is drilled in the floor of the chamber for drainage. A second cap, with a small entrance hole, can be fitted to the upper elbow to target small species, such as pygmy possums (*Cercartetus* spp.). The animal investigates the open upper elbow, falls inside and cannot climb up the smooth pipe surface.

Large terrestrial pipe traps (N. Mooney and D. Ralph, unpublished data) are designed specifically to capture Tasmanian devils (*Sarcophilus harrisii*), but can also target smaller dasyurids, including spotted-tailed (*Dasyurus maculatus*) and eastern (*D. viverrinus*) quolls. Traps are constructed of lengths of PVC pipe (length 875 mm, depth 315 mm) with a hinged door at one end. The door contains ventilation holes, one of which lines up with a pin mechanism attached to the body of the trap; this mechanism holds the door open. A length of degradable string is tied to a piece of bait (generally lamb or macropod) and threaded through a hole in the rear of the pipe so that the bait is flush against the roof of the trap. The exterior end of the string is tied to the pin holding the door open. When the bait is pulled, the pin is removed from the door, causing it to fall and close the trap. A second pin is triggered when the door falls, locking the door shut. Ventilation holes are also present in the closed end of the trap, and along the bottom of the body. These holes, combined with the PVC material, make the traps easy to sanitise after use (an important consideration when dealing with Tasmanian devils, which are affected by a highly transmissible form of cancer – see Chapter 18). Cage, aluminium box and pipe traps are baited; funnel traps and pitfalls are not. A mixture of honey and water is sometimes sprayed near arboreal pipe traps and aluminium box traps that are affixed to trees.

Animal welfare considerations

Stress, mortality or injuries from other animals caught in the same trap

One funnel or pitfall trap can catch multiple individuals and species (cage, box and pipe traps occasionally do, too), which can increase stress and the risk of fatal interactions between trapped animals. Predatory invertebrates, such as beetles, centipedes and ants, may also attack and kill other animals in the trap. The risk can be reduced by frequent trap checking and careful placement during installation. Pitfalls should be furnished with a shelter (or several) to provide some protection to animals from one another and the weather. Invertebrates should be removed from pitfalls each time they are checked and released at a reasonable distance from the trap to reduce the likelihood of recapture.

Ant-related stress or mortality

Attacks on trapped animals by ants can be an issue for all trap types, but particularly with baited traps that may attract them. Ant attack can cause rapid death of small vertebrates confined in a trap. Some ant species inflict painful bites and others appear to attract conspecifics when disturbed (S. Thompson, pers. obs.). Large numbers of ants can congregate in and around traps, biting captured animals, inflicting wounds, pain and stress. Before installation, researchers should scrutinise the site for the presence of large ant species, such as *Iridomyrmex*, *Camponotus* and *Myrmecia* species, although smaller species can be problematic if present in high numbers. Traps need to be located away from ant nests and obvious ant trails. Ideally, an alternative site is chosen if ant nests are nearby. Underground nest sites may not be visible, and *C. terebrans*, for example, is mostly active at night, so it is useful to check for ant activity after dark. Personnel may also 'stomp' the ground to check for jumping ants (*Myrmecia* spp.).

It can be difficult to avoid ants altogether through strategic trap placement. Insecticides should be avoided, but are used under certain conditions (DBCA 2018). Odourless pyrethrum-based sprays may be necessary in situations where ants are ubiquitous; the effects of short-term exposure of native animals to pyrethroids are not well understood. However, attacks by ants will almost certainly result in painful deaths for small trapped animals. Anecdotally, some researchers report seeing no impact on trapped frogs and reptiles if used in small amounts (cited in Petit and Waudby 2012). However, pyrethroids may be toxic to reptiles and frogs (DBCA 2018), bioaccumulate in bats, and are considered endocrine disrupters, altering testosterone production in rats (cited in Oliveiraa *et al.* 2020), so they are not without risk. Personnel should consider the implications of off-label use, including (for example) completing a risk assessment that considers the potential exposure dose of different species based on the planned strategy of application, the species' likely sensitivity to that dose and the potential effects on the environment. The chemical's safety data sheet must be read before use.

It can be impractical to place pyrethroid powder or spray around each trap if large numbers of traps are affected by ants, and it is possible (although apparently untested) that using chemicals around a trap will deter animals. If used, powders should be applied sparingly and mixed through the soil around the traps. Personnel can also spray (with a weed-spraying container or similar) the ground beneath the trap and then lay the trap on top of the soil, or spray the pyrethroid around a pit trap (but not in the trap). Doing so means that animals captured in the trap may have less contact with the insecticide - particularly important in a pitfall, where sand-swimming skinks would be exposed if the spray has been applied to soil inside a trap. If a particular trap line or trap is infested by ants, then it should be closed or moved. For pitfalls, placing a thin stem or blade of grass reaching from the base of the pitfall to its lip may allow ants and other non-target invertebrates to escape. For aluminium box traps, avoiding using certain bait mixtures (e.g. containing honey or tuna) may reduce ant activity near traps. Bait should be removed when the trap is not in use and disposed of appropriately (i.e. not discarded in the local environment).

Drowning

The risk of drowning in all of these trap types is relatively low as water from rain will flow through them, but drowning may occur if traps become inundated completely. Placing traps in ephemeral creek lines should be avoided when heavy rain is a possibility. Pitfalls and pipe traps should be designed with appropriate drainage capacity. For some pitfalls (e.g. pipes), the base can be fashioned from aluminium mesh or a similar material. For bucket-style pitfalls, holes that are sufficiently small to prevent trapped animals (e.g. small skinks) from escaping through them can be drilled into the base. Drilling should be done from inside the bucket to ensure that any lip created through drilling will not interfere with drainage. Some soil types (i.e. those rich in clay minerals) may impede drainage. Pitfalls can be furnished with objects or shelters that float and also provide shade or shelter, such as foam meat trays, stubby holders or cork disks, taking into consideration risks caused by ingestion. If rain is forecast, researchers should evaluate the risk that access to traps may be prevented, or that they may flood. If doubt exists, traps are to be closed and reopened when the weather has cleared.

Extreme temperatures

Trap placement should always consider the best site for protection of the target taxa during extreme conditions (e.g. avoid placing traps where they receive afternoon sun). Climatic conditions for the area should be monitored regularly. The combination of rain and cool temperature, or low humidity and high temperatures can produce poor welfare outcomes (or increase death rates), so decisions should be made based on expected conditions and the physiology of animals likely to be captured. Death from overheating or desiccation may occur in pitfalls when ambient temperatures reach 40°C (or less for some species) and if trapped small mammals are very active in the trap, thus raising their body temperature (e.g. Read and Kearney 2016). However, trap temperature can be much higher than ambient temperatures, particularly in aluminium box traps that are not completely in the shade. Heat radiating from the ground into traps should also be considered. If forecast temperatures exceed 40°C, researchers should consider closing their pitfalls (although capture rates of some species increase during hotter temperatures; Read and Kearney 2016) or increasing the number of daily checks and providing water if it does not attract undesirable species in a particular area.

If appropriate, funnel traps can be placed either under or on the southern and eastern edges of vegetation. If opened during the day in warmer weather, aluminium box traps and wire cage traps require a shade cover unless they are placed under vegetation where they receive constant shade. Moveable traps can be placed in or near vegetation or provided with additional shade. Shade is provided by vegetative material (branches, leaves) or artificial materials (shade cloth, hessian, air-cell glare shield). For funnel traps, using two shade cloth or jute/hessian bag covers may reduce temperatures and prolong the period before trap temperatures reach potentially lethal levels (Thompson and Thompson 2009). However, wrapping the entire funnel or cage trap might result in limited airflow, increasing the internal ambient temperature instead of allowing it to disperse. Shade should cover one end of the funnel, as animals tend to hide in a corner of the trap rather than in the middle, even if the shade is centred evenly across the trap.

Shade may be added to pitfall traps to reduce internal temperatures, but it may affect capture rates (Thompson and Thompson 2005). A layer of sand or soil in the bottom of pitfalls provides shelter for fossorial reptiles. A wet sponge or other moist substrate may increase survival, particularly of frogs. The sponge should be monitored to ensure that it does not attract ants (Read and Kearney 2016 and references therein) and may dry quickly, becoming ineffective. Pitfalls should always contain a shelter that will reduce solar radiation and buffer cool overnight temperatures (Petit and Waudby 2012), such as (for example) stubby holders, foam trays cut in half or PVC tubing stuffed with towelling or similar in one end. Bedding (e.g. coconut fibre, wool, a square of neoprene or polar fleece, sleeping bag filling) may be placed in aluminium box traps for small mammals, although in some cases investigators may avoid materials with loose fibres because animals may catch their feet on them. Closed-cell foam sheets can be placed underneath box traps to insulate them from the ground and traps can be placed inside a plastic bag to protect them from precipitation or dew, when condensation inside the bag is not an issue. If low overnight temperatures are likely to affect animals, researchers should consider closing traps earlier in the evening (Tasker and Dickman 2001; Waudby *et al.* 2019). Aluminium box traps heat quickly, and must be always shaded completely in warm weather (either by vegetation or with heavy jute bags).

Exposure to predators

Currawongs (*Strepera* spp.), Australian magpies (*Gymnorhina tibicens*), goannas (*Varanus* spp.), snakes, dingoes (*Canis dingo*), foxes and cats may be attracted to trap sites (Petit and Waudby 2012). Some carnivorous marsupials, such as *Dasycercus* spp., will enter pitfalls to eat trapped animals (C. Dickman, pers. comm. in Petit and Waudby 2012). Deep pitfalls (≥ 60 cm) may offer protection from large predators and reduce escapes, especially when combined with a funnel and jar capture point (see Doughty *et al.* 2011). However, ghost bats (*Macroderma gigas*) can enter 65-cm deep pitfalls to prey on trapped rodents, becoming caught themselves (Diete *et al.* 2016). All trap types may be tampered with by larger predators and some corvids may learn to remove pins from box traps. In these scenarios, traps may need to be secured to the ground in some way or trapping ceased if the problem continues. Shelters in pitfalls may provide some protection to trapped animals. Personnel should not discard food or other waste (including body waste and bait) in proximity to trap sites to avoid attracting predators, including ants. Similarly, animals that are being released may become easy targets for watching predators if disorientated or in a panic to escape. In an extreme case, one author observed a released fawn-footed melomys (*Melomys cervipes*) run directly into the mouth of a goanna that was following her down the trap line (J. Bentley, pers. obs.). Others have observed corvids at traps sites prey on bush rats (*Rattus fuscipes*) as they were released (P. Meek, pers. obs.). In these situations, predators may need to be chased away or the animal held until the predators have left. Ultimately, researchers should monitor and evaluate the situation and consider if a trapping site should be closed because of predation. Camera traps focused on trap arrays may help to detect trap interference.

Repeated recaptures

Trapping may increase stress in study animals, resulting in reduced body mass and increased corticosterone levels (e.g. Pearson *et al.* 2003; Bosson *et al.* 2012). Little research has been undertaken on the long-term impacts of repeated recaptures on individual animals' welfare. Researchers should mark animals (permanently or temporarily depending on their objectives) to clarify recapture rates, and remain alert to signs of stress (e.g. reduced body mass or hydration between sessions). Recaptured animals should be released immediately when their data are not required. In cases where overall recapture rates are high or the same individual is being caught repeatedly, researchers should consider if sufficient data have been collected, and close the site. Typically, trapping should be paused temporarily after 3 or 4 days and nights if recapture rates are high (Tasker and Dickman 2001; C. Pavey, pers. comm. in Petit and Waudby 2012) or ceased if personnel deem that sufficient data have been collected to meet the study objectives. Some researchers release recaptured animals on the opposite side of the pitfall drift fence to their initial release location in the hope that it may reduce the likelihood of recapture because they are not trying to return to a shelter, burrow or territory on the other side of the fence (Petit and Waudby 2012). Recapturing lactating females may affect dependent young. Avoiding trapping in the seasons where animals have large pouch young, dens or nests helps to minimise impact.

Disruptions to natural activities

Small mammals that are removed from traps with obvious signs of nursing (extended teats sometimes with dried milk visible or an open pouch) or with pouch young present should be processed immediately and released near cover, 20–40 m from the point of capture. Traps that recapture the same lactating female repeatedly within a session may be closed (DBCA 2018). Where females are caught in traps with young at foot, the individuals should be kept together, and released together. Some small mammal species with high energetic requirements (e.g. honey possums, *Tarsipes rostratus*) may need to be fed a sugar solution before release (DBCA 2018).

Capture of non-target species

All trap types catch non-target species. For pitfalls, choosing the most appropriate pitfall design for the target species reduces the likelihood of non-target capture. Non-target species should be released as soon as possible into habitat that provides some initial protection to give them time to adjust, and typically ~20–40 m from the trap. Providing shelters in traps (e.g. pieces of PVC pipe or similar) may help reduce impacts on non-target species, including injury from other animals caught in the same trap (Waudby *et al.* 2019).

Injury from falling into pitfalls or moving traps

Injury from falling into a pitfall appears to be rare (or at least difficult to determine), but it may be a greater risk with deep pitfalls (i.e. > 40 cm in depth). Providing a layer of sand or a soft substrate in the bottom of the pitfall trap may assist in reducing the risk. Cage and terrestrial pipe traps should be secured properly. In particular, tubular pipe traps can roll around if not secured, causing considerable stress to trapped animals. Similarly, Tasmanian devils are strong and may attempt to get into a closed trap with an animal in it, dislodging the trap in the process, unless it is well secured. These traps can be secured by placing them between trees, or securing them between rocks on both sides so that they do not roll.

Poor funnel trap clearance

Small reptiles and a range of invertebrates can hide under the funnels, so it is important that the zipper be opened, and the funnel traps properly searched for animals. Ideally, funnels should be picked up and looked through to search corners, to avoid small reptiles going undetected. Occasionally, large snakes will retreat under the shade cover, between the funnel and the drift fence or under the funnel trap.

General procedures

Planning

Personnel should identify their target species or taxa, an appropriate trap type and design, trapping array, and suitable sites that will deliver study objectives, but also where hazards (such as ants) appear low. They should evaluate the anticipated effectiveness of the proposed design relative to its financial and ethical costs beforehand (Waudby *et al.* 2019). Personnel should design their study in such a way to ensure that they can check all open multi-catch traps (e.g. pitfall traps) with appropriate frequency with the resources they will have available to them. Single-catch traps can be closed during the day following trap checks, and reopened late in the afternoon, although this requirement is context- and species-specific, and researchers may leave traps open if risks to animal welfare are low. For example, pipe and cage traps used for Tasmanian devils and some larger quoll species (i.e. spotted-tailed quolls) are typically left open for 24 h periods and only checked once, in the morning, because risks from overheating, hypothermia and starvation for these species are less than for smaller species (see Chapter 18 for further details), and traps are generally not targeted by devils or quolls at these times (D. Hamilton, unpublished data). Conversely, smaller northern quolls (*D. hallucatus*) are sometimes active during the day in winter and may enter open traps and overheat (J. Dunlop, pers. comm.). Capture myopathy may also be a risk for species that are prone to it if they are caught soon after trap checks and not removed until the next check. Personnel should evaluate the likelihood and degree of welfare impacts for target and non-target species versus the anticipated scientific benefits, if leaving traps open for 24 h periods. Generally, doing so is not recommended in warmer climates, including in arid or semi-arid zones and the tropics (see Chapter 18 for details on trapping large dasyurids), and especially when using traps that absorb heat, such as aluminium traps. Temperatures experienced by animals in traps may be higher than forecast temperatures because of reflective heat. If checking traps once per 24 h period, adequate bedding and food should be provided. Decisions should not be made based purely on logistical constraints.

Ideally, personnel should identify the anticipated location of trapping sites before commencing field work. The specific location of each trap can be determined in the field. Selecting an appropriate location based on vegetation cover and shade is important for all trap types, but particularly for aluminium box and wire cage traps. In warmer months, personnel should place traps where they will receive the least amount of direct sunlight (if left open at any point during the day).

Installing traps

Traps are usually deployed in a systematic manner (i.e. consecutive numbering), often in lines or grids, so that they can be easily located and checked. Personnel should mark and record the location of each individual trap (preferably with a GPS) and the general site location. Reflective tape on trees or long pieces of flagging tape (with trap site details written on them) assist with locating traps and sites at night. However, personnel should ensure that marking sites in this way will not interfere with (for example) land management activities (i.e. different combinations of coloured flagging tape can be used to demarcate logging coupes or similar on some tenures) and are unlikely to attract predators to trapping sites.

Funnel traps are typically placed in pairs on either side of a flywire drift fence and secured to the fence. Various configurations have been tested for drift fences and funnel traps (e.g. even trap spacing along a transect line; a 'T' or 'Y' formation); personnel should select one appropriate to their study objectives. Funnel traps are usually spaced along drift fences in pairs and secured to the drift fence with bulldog clips or similar. For funnel traps, a ramp of substrate is placed at the entrance to each funnel to provide a smooth transition from the substrate into the funnel for animals moving along the drift fence. Two shade cloth covers should be placed over funnel traps in warm to hot weather and a single shade cloth cover in cooler conditions.

When conducting ground-based trapping, personnel should set aluminium box and cage traps on firm flat bases to minimise movement of the trap, which will discourage animals from entering it. For trapping arboreal species, box traps are typically mounted on platforms fixed to trees or branches; pipe traps are attached to platforms with wire or metal brackets with the entrance facing the tree trunk. Once aluminium box and wire cage traps are set, personnel should check the mechanism operation to ensure that the door closes properly and is free from obstructions. For wire cage traps, substrate may be placed in the bottom of the cage, to minimise the animal walking on wire mesh and encourage it to enter the cage. Terrestrial pipe traps should be secured on flat ground with trees or rocks lining both sides of the trap. The entrance and rear of these traps must be flush with the ground so that the trap does not tip if an animal puts its weight on either end. Traps should be set along runways, near crevices, logs or tree roots, or under vegetation cover (Tasker and Dickman 2001).

Traps are baited with an attractant appropriate to the target animals. Bait should be fresh and not contain pathogenic organisms (i.e. honey is not used by some agencies because it may contain microorganisms as well as attracting ants). Peanut butter and oats are used for many species, but bait should be biologically suitable for the target species. Bait should not be discarded in the field or moved between sites (Eyre *et al.* 2018) and ingredients that may germinate should be rendered inert before use to avoid the risk of weed invasion. For some taxa, particularly those with high metabolic demands (e.g. small dasyurids and pygmy possums), providing sufficient and appropriate bait may reduce impacts on individuals substantially, particularly those that are recaptured repeatedly or in cold weather. Anecdotally, doing so may contribute to reduced mortality, particularly if trapping in years when animals are in poor condition (J. Bentley, pers. obs.).

Personnel should dig holes and insert pitfalls so that the edge is level with the ground, and the pitfall lip is not visible. Pitfall lines may be arranged in any manner that fulfils the study objectives, but personnel need to avoid placing curves or sharp angles in drift net fencing. Angles may direct animals away from the trap line and change the area that is being sampled, which is an issue if multiple sites are being compared. If used, drift net fencing should be placed over the centre of each pitfall in a continuous line and held in place by steel pegs. Drift net fencing may consist of fine aluminium mesh ('fly wire'), plastic sheeting (often black) or shade cloth, and should be maintained regularly. Drift nets increase capture rates for many species caught in pitfalls (Petit and Waudby 2012 and references therein). Funnels or cones, inserted into the top of the pitfall, may increase capture success for some mammal species (e.g. hopping mice, *Notomys* spp.); a board or other flat cover placed over the pitfall, but elevated just slightly, may be useful for targeting snakes (Fitch 1987). Numbers can be written inside the pitfalls to assist with recording data.

Traps must be provided with sufficient bedding and/or shelters, which may need to be increased during cold conditions. In these conditions, aluminium box traps should contain bedding that prevents the animal from coming into contact with the trap's cold metal floor, or the traps should be closed. See additional comments under 'Animal welfare considerations'.

Trapping times and duration

Trapping times depend on the study objectives and ecology of the target species. Similarly, trapping duration varies depending on the selected method, habitat, target species and objectives. Typically, three to five consecutive nights are recommended for threatened mammals (DSEWPC 2011a), although additional species may be detected if trapping operates for longer in some environments (Moseby and Read 2001), and monitoring of Tasmanian devils is typically conducted over seven to 10 nights (the point at which capture rates of new individuals start to diminish) (Lazenby *et al.* 2018; Cunningham *et al.* 2021).

All trap types can be left open for 24 h periods if required, providing that personnel plan for an appropriate checking regime, which should focus on animal welfare and integrity of data collection. Typically, traps should be checked at least twice if left open for 24 h (i.e. in the morning and in the late afternoon or early evening), although this requirement is context- and species-specific (see 'Planning'). If researchers propose one check per 24 h, then they must have a reasonable level of confidence that welfare of target and non-target species will not be compromised and that any potential risk is outweighed by the scientific benefits. Checking traps regularly allows personnel to replenish bait, which may be eaten by ants and non-target vertebrates, to release non-target species, and to reduce the time of captivity in the traps.

In very hot weather, traps should be checked more frequently to minimise heat stress and desiccation, or closed if doing so is not possible. Similarly, in cold weather, traps may be checked more frequently or during the night to minimise the time animals are contained in a trap, or closed earlier in the night. Checking time will vary depending on local conditions and study objectives. Ideally, personnel should check traps close to dawn (before sunrise) to remove and release nocturnal animals while light levels are still relatively low, although within 2–3 h of sunrise is generally acceptable depending on conditions. Checking traps early in the morning can result in crepuscular animals that are active early in the day being caught early in the morning and then remaining in the traps during the midday heat. Providing internal shelters and bedding material, and external shelters or shade, and increasing checks of traps during warmer weather minimise this risk. When surveying for all species present at a site (rather than targeted surveys for particular species), pit trapping should be undertaken for 8–10 nights to detect all species, especially rare or cryptic species (DSEWPAC 2011a).

Checking traps and removing animals

Personnel should record trap shut and open times consistently, so that trap effort can be calculated accurately. A designated person should ensure that all traps are accounted for during each check by maintaining a tally or check list (DBCA 2018). Personnel need to confirm what type of animal is in a trap before they attempt to remove it, especially if it is a venomous snake. They may be able to see scales or fur through the gaps in the sides of aluminium box traps without picking it up. Animals caught in box or pipe traps can be confirmed by lowering the door of the box trap slightly or tilting the screw cap on a pipe trap and looking through the gap, although care should be taken to ensure the animal does not attempt to leap through the gap. Often the trap's weight (or smell) will provide an indication of what might have been caught. Closed arboreal box traps may need to be detached from the platform or branch for checking. Personnel should check pitfalls carefully before reaching into a pitfall (a head torch may be necessary for deep pitfalls) and use long-handled tongs to examine shelters and under substrate. In general, personnel should check pitfall traps meticulously, including sifting through sand inside the pitfall, to ensure that small species like centipedes, scorpions and fossorial reptiles (e.g. *Lerista* spp.) are not missed. The latter are over-represented in mortalities (Read and Kearney 2016). Invertebrates should be removed from traps (an insect aspirator can be used if necessary).

Gloves may be worn to remove animals from traps and during handling, but some handlers believe that doing so reduces sensation and the ability to handle animals appropriately. Where disease transmission between target animals is a consideration (e.g. when working with Tasmanian devils or frogs), then gloves must be worn throughout the process and changed between animals (see Chapter 27 for a review of handling practices for frogs and tadpoles, including glove use). For box, cage and pipe traps, placing an appropriately sized catch bag over the trap entrance and encouraging the animal into the bag can be used to secure medium-sized captured animals. If animals are removed from a trap by hand, they should be grasped gently, but firmly, and placed immediately into a clean calico trap bag with the seams turned inside out to avoid claws or teeth snagging on them. Only one animal should be placed in each bag, and bags are preferably not reused for a new animal until they have been washed, to avoid parasite and disease transfer. It is important that animals cannot see through the bag into which they are being transferred for handling, and that the bag be placed securely in a cool, dark or shaded location before processing. Dark-coloured or opaque bags may assist in reducing stress for nocturnal animals. Animals typically remain very quiet once bagged and placed in a shaded and dark location.

Animals can be processed at the site or transported to a central processing area. If transported, animals should be kept in their tightly closed and labelled (masking tape can be used for labelling) calico bags, but placed inside a hard container, such as a plastic aquarium or large bucket, to avoid accidental squashing. Unless the animal is very small, it is generally easiest to measure, sex and assess an animal in a catch bag and probably less stressful for the animal than to hold it outside of the bag during processing. Keeping mammals' eyes covered as much as possible during processing will reduce animal and handler stress significantly. For appropriate handling techniques for each taxon, refer to the appropriate chapters in Section 3.

Animals must be released near their point of capture. Exact distances will depend on the species and environment, but small rodents, dasyurids and reptiles generally should be released 20–40 m from the trap site if the traps are left open. All trapped animals should be released near shelter and observed until they access it. Personnel should be aware of any potential predators. See the recommendations under 'Animal welfare considerations'.

Removing traps

Personnel should always count and record the number of box, cage and pipe traps deployed and retrieved. Each trap location should be recorded with a GPS. When checking traps, a simple checklist can be used to ensure that every trap has been checked. It is very easy to miss a trap, so this step should not be skipped. Pitfalls may be left closed *in situ* if they are to be used again. Pitfalls that are used regularly should be furnished with a stick that reaches from the bottom of the pitfall to its lip, but does not prevent the lid from being closed. The stick may help some animals escape if the lid becomes compromised. Lids must fit the trap properly, be fastened on securely, and be checked regularly to ensure that they are in good working order. Plastic lids will perish more quickly than PVC screw-on lids. A layer of soil placed over lids between sessions extends their integrity. Placing stones or dead branches over the trap may help locate it in the future and deter large animals from walking over it, damaging the lid in the process. Traps that are left for extended periods (e.g. > 6 months depending on the environment) must be filled with sandbags, soil (with care not to introduce animals into the traps), rocks, or another substrate and the lid replaced securely (clicked in or screwed on). Where hard-hoofed ungulates are present, pitfalls may need metal lids. All equipment moved between sites is to be cleaned and disinfected before reuse, including in areas affected by dieback (*Phytophthora cinnamomi*) (DBCA 2018), myrtle rust (*Austropuccinia psidii*), amphibian chytrid fungus (*Batrachochytrium dendrobatidis*) (DPIE 2020) and devil facial tumour disease. Researchers should articulate their plan for maintenance and/or removal.

Hygiene

Personnel should wash catch bags after every field trip. For species where disease transmission is a major concern (Tasmanian devils and amphibians), catch bags will need to be single use. Ideally, catch bags are used for one animal before being retired for washing, and allowed to dry completely in the sun before reuse. Ticks and mites will not necessarily die in a warm water wash, so where animals have ticks, catch bags will need to be checked and ticks removed and killed, although eggs and microscopic life stages will not be visible. Bags can be immersed in methylated spirits or 70% alcohol to kill parasites, but must be washed and dried before use. Single-use plastic bags can be used for amphibians. Aluminium box traps should be washed and disinfected after each trapping session. Funnel traps will need to be inspected to remove seeds, vegetation and dead insects before they are reused. Wire cage traps need to be checked to ensure all remnant bait and vegetation is removed and that traps are clean. Terrestrial pipe traps being used to target Tasmanian devils are cleaned thoroughly and sanitised with veterinary disinfectant (F10) after every animal capture, and again at the end of the trip. Personnel should consider the risk of transmission of anthropozoonoses to study animals and prepare accordingly; consulting with Wildlife Health Australia may assist with preparedness (e.g. Wildlife Health Australia 2018).

Animal treatment, withdrawal and euthanasia

Researchers should monitor the situation continually. Personnel make a decision to euthanase injured animals based on likelihood of survival, anticipated additional pain and stress if transportation is required to seek treatment from a veterinarian (i.e. if working in remote areas), and the skill set of personnel. Injured animals that are unlikely to survive if released should be euthanased by experienced personnel (or those under the supervision of experienced personnel) in line with accepted published procedures and protocols (see the relevant species chapters in Section 3). If capture numbers are high and traps cannot be checked in a timely manner (context-specific), then either all or some traps must be closed temporarily. Trapping may cease temporarily in very hot or cold weather, during rain, or if personnel anticipate that trap sites may become inaccessible (i.e. because of predicted flooding or bushfire). Unexpected changes in weather sometimes occur; these changes can be difficult to anticipate and may result in higher trap death rates (e.g. Lemckert *et al.* 2006; Waudby *et al.* 2019). Personnel should monitor local weather reports carefully and be ready to modify their trapping or trap-checking regime in response, where possible.

Equipment and maintenance

The equipment required will vary depending on the target species or taxon, local environment and study objectives. Typical items are listed in Table 7.1. All traps should be scrutinised before installation and again as they are packed away to ensure that they are clean and in good working order. Doing so is important to minimise the hazard that traps pose to animals, but also to ensure that they are working properly and collecting useable data. Aluminium box traps are susceptible to being bent out of shape and should be assessed regularly to ensure that the release mechanism remains sufficiently sensitive to trap target animals. Pitfall traps left *in situ* are assessed during each trapping session or every 12 months to ensure that they are not deteriorating and presenting a hazard to animals between trapping sessions. All traps and equipment used to install traps should be cleaned and disinfected before being used at sites and between each trapping session (in the case of removable traps), to minimise the risk of spreading pathogens such as amphibian chytrid fungus, *P. cinnamomi* and diseases such as Tasmanian devil facial tumour disease.

Table 7.1: Suggested equipment and materials required for the installation and operation of funnel, cage, aluminium box, pitfall, and arboreal and ground-based pipe traps.

Installing and opening traps	Checking traps	Processing animals	Maintenance and closing
• Traps • Shade covers for traps • Drift fences for attaching to funnel traps • Mattock or similar for creating drift-fence trenches • Flagging tape • Global positioning system • Permanent marker and grey lead pencil • Drift net fencing and pegs for pitfall traps • Digging implements • Crowbar • Shelters • Bedding material for box and pipe traps • Closed cell foam mats and plastic bags for box traps • Floating substrate • Moist substrate • Flagging or reflective tape • Poles or star pickets for marking sites and traps • Compass to position traps in lines or grids • Bait for box and cage traps	• Gloves • Insect aspirator • Long-handled tongs • Snake hook • Head torch • Identification books and reference material • Soup ladles or scoops	• Callipers • Clear plastic ruler • Scales • Calico bags (dark/opaque) • Clipboards and data sheets • Previously collected data • Animal identification guides • Animal marking implements • Solid container for animal transportation • Permanent marker/grey lead pencil • Masking tape • String • Vials for samples • 70–90% alcohol for disinfection of equipment Solution for sample preservation • Snap lock bags • Hand-lens or magnifying glass • Face mask • Hand wash • Disinfectant or sanitiser for hands or gloves	• Spare drift-fence and pegs for repairs • Equipment and ties for rolling up and securing drift fencing • Sandbags or similar • Shovels • Spare pitfall lids • Spare traps • Sticks that fit inside length of pitfalls • Equipment for trap maintenance • Cable ties

Specific qualifications, experience and training

The skills required to undertake trapping-based studies vary depending on sensitivity of the study species to the presence of humans and disturbance, and the nature of the study. Ideally, the primary investigator should be competent in the technique proposed, and in procedures for setting and clearing traps. They should be very familiar with the species or similar taxa, having undertaken similar work (including capture and handling). Preferably, at least someone in the team should have experience in removing animals (particularly venomous snakes) from traps and in handling the target or similar species, to teach and supervise others.

Workplace health and safety

Bites, scratches, and stings

Tucking pants into socks and checking clothes and body for ticks and mites is important following some field work. A dedicated first aid kit for bites and stings is kept close by, and personnel should carry sufficient snake-bite bandages. When checking pitfalls, the risk of being bitten, scratched or stung by trapped animals can be minimised by checking the base of traps carefully with a tool, such as long-handled tongs, before reaching in to remove animals. Tongs should be used to check the soil for animals, including venomous snakes and invertebrates. Shelters can be checked by holding them with a set of tongs. Ladles or scoops can be used to remove invertebrates such as spiders and scorpions. Personnel may use a head torch to see into the bottom of deep and narrow pitfalls. Personnel may wear gloves to avoid bites during handling, but doing so may reduce sensation and their capacity to handle animals effectively.

All traps will potentially catch large snakes. For funnel traps, leaving the zipper open for a brief period will often be sufficient for the snake to vacate the trap of its own accord, which is the safest strategy. Snakes that feel threatened will often search the funnel trap rapidly for an exit and may find one of the openings at the end of the funnel. In this case they often leave the funnel quickly and to the surprise of the researcher. Removing the wire pin that holds an Elliott trap together is the safest strategy for releasing snakes from these types of aluminium box traps. Propping the door of a wire cage trap open and allowing the snake to leave of its own accord is the safest strategy. The screw cap of arboreal pipe traps can be removed, and the capture chamber left open. Snakes should be removed from pitfalls by experienced personnel. If removal by hand is not possible, snakes can be removed with a snake hook or similar.

Manual handling (digging and leaning over)

Personnel should follow standard procedures for manual handling. Only personnel who are sufficiently fit and healthy should install and check traps. Installation of pitfalls can require considerable exertion, particularly if being installed manually.

Alternative procedures

The trapping methods described in this GOP are used to answer questions about the presence/absence, abundance, and/or population demographics of small and often cryptic animals. It can be difficult to answer such questions without capturing the species of interest. However, researchers should consider if study questions could be answered with remote monitoring equipment or indirect detection methods (see Chapters 4 and 5).

MIST NETS, HARP TRAPS AND TRIP LINING FOR BIRDS AND BATS

David Watson, Lindy F. Lumsden and Sophie Petit

Target taxa

This GOP applies to microbats and megabats (Chapter 23) and smaller bird species, including several passerine groups (Chapter 33).

Context and scope

This GOP describes the use of mist nets for the capture of birds and bats, and the use of harp traps and trip lining for the capture of bats. Most birds and all bats use active flight for locomotion, with the requisite energetic demands affecting most aspects of their anatomy, ecology and life history. Powered flight affords birds and bats access to locations and resources beyond the reach of other vertebrates, but also adds to the challenge of studying them. While many aspects of bird ecology and behaviour can be gleaned from observational work, it is more difficult to observe bats at night. Consequently, research involving bats often relies on their capture (although monitoring increasingly uses acoustic recorders: see Chapter 5). A variety of nets and traps are used to capture these animals, with mist nets the most widely used method for birds. In Australia, microbats are mostly caught using harp traps, although mist nets and trip lining are useful in some environments and for some species. Flying-foxes are caught using both mist nets and mega harp traps. These methods require considerable training to ensure they are deployed correctly and that trapped animals are freed, handled, processed and released in ways that minimise animal welfare impacts.

Animal welfare considerations

Entanglement and physical damage

Mist nets and harp traps are passive capture devices that intercept actively flying animals and hold them safely until they are removed by experienced handlers. Harp traps have been designed to capture and hold bats for extended periods (often deployed overnight), whereas mist nets require active checking to remove captured animals. A correctly set microbat harp trap should not entangle bats – rather, the 'harp' of taut monofilament fishing line intercepts bats in flight, and they then slide down into the canvas bag below and crawl beneath the overhanging plastic sheet (Tidemann and Woodside 1978). For megabat harp traps, individuals slide down the nylon-covered wire cables and are caught by hand at the base (Tidemann and Loughland 1993).

Mist nets catch animals in flight. Animals become suspended in the net, their weight supported by the netting and tensioned shelf strings. The longer an animal remains in the net, the more likely it is to struggle, becoming further entangled and attracting the attention of predators. When extracting animals from mist nets, particular care is needed with the wings of bats and the legs of birds, which have fine, delicate bones and can become snarled in the net. Also, many birds protrude their tongues while calling and panting – for honeyeaters and other birds with arrow-shaped tongues, netting can become caught around the base of the tongue. Such netting is best removed with an awl while the bird's body is supported.

Trip lining, which is often used in conjunction with mist netting, involves tautly stretching multiple strands of fine fishing line parallel to the surface of the water, several centimetres above it (Churchill 2008). As bats fly down to drink, they trip on the fishing line and fall into the water. Most species are unable to take flight from the water's surface and need to swim to shore, where they can be collected by hand. This technique should only be used where the water's edge is clear from vegetation so that the bats do not become entangled in vegetation and can be seen easily when they reach the shore. Care needs to be taken to ensure personnel do not stand on bats that are still on the ground.

Bats and birds can easily become tangled on loose threads on the inside of catch bags. Before using cloth bags for holding live animals, personnel ensure the seams are on the outside and any loose thread inside has been removed, or use bags with double seams.

Disruption to dependent young

When using harp traps to capture bats it is good practice to check the traps regularly throughout the night, so that bats can resume foraging. Doing so is especially important during the breeding season when females are lactating; harp traps should then be checked multiple times during the night and closed several hours before dawn to allow sufficient time for processing and release before it starts to get light so that females can return to their young. As roosts may be a considerable distance from the capture point (e.g. up to 12 km for lesser long-eared bats, *Nyctophilus geoffroyi*, and Gould's wattled bats, *Chalinolobus gouldii*; Lumsden *et al.* 2002), personnel should allow sufficient time for this return flight.

Exposure

Birds caught in mist nets are less able to regulate their temperature, with their feathers disrupted and their position relative to sun and shade, wind and rain constrained. For most applications, mist nets should be set in the shade and not be deployed in inclement or hot (> 30°C) weather. Harp traps provide greater protection for microbats from wind and rain, and bats' ability to enter torpor enables them to tolerate colder temperatures. Ideally, all bats should be released during the night of capture, before sunrise. However, if left in traps during the day they can be exposed to extremely hot temperatures (Ellis 2016), so traps left open all night should be checked early in the morning (within 2–3 h of sunrise if not earlier, depending on predicted temperatures) before temperatures rise. The fur of bats caught using trip lining will be wet and must be dried before release. As this technique is typically used on warm nights, drying usually occurs while they are held in cloth bags out of the wind, awaiting processing. Mist nets can be furled temporarily, which is advisable if a large number of animals are caught or if conditions become inclement (Keyes and Grue 1982). Harp traps can accommodate many individuals, so the only time that traps would need to be moved to reduce overcrowding is when set at a roost (e.g. cave entrance). Bats should not be released during the day because of the risk of predation by diurnal birds, so if any traps are checked after sunrise, trapped individuals must be kept secure until dusk (see Chapter 23 for details around transport and captivity).

Predators

Predators may be attracted to animals caught in mist nets or harp traps. In addition to harming or killing captured animals, predators can also become caught. When locating mist nets and harp traps, researchers should consider the local predator community. If predators seem to be attracted to captured animals, checking frequency should be increased. If the issue remains, the mist net or harp trap should be relocated. If an owl is observed targeting sites where bats are released, traps can be moved several hundred metres away, or the bat held for a time (e.g. 1 h) until the owl loses interest. Personnel should ensure that no potential runway is present, such as logs that lead up to the harp trap hips that would give terrestrial animals (e.g. rats) access to the bag (Lumsden 1989).

By-catch

While the likelihood of capturing target species can be increased by careful placement, mist nets can catch non-target species, including snakes and large insects, which can be difficult to extract unharmed. When targeting bats, mist nets should not be deployed until dusk to avoid catching diurnal birds. Harp traps will occasionally catch birds; however, non-target captures are usually very low (e.g. < 0.1% of captures; L. Lumsden, unpublished data). Large animals like kangaroos and cattle can stumble into nets or harp traps, rarely becoming captured for long, but invariably rendering the equipment unusable. By ensuring the lower shelf of the mist net is well clear of the ground or water and staying away from animal trackways, non-target captures can be minimised.

General procedures

Mist nets, trip lining and harp traps are used to catch free-flying animals, so the likelihood of the target species being captured is enhanced by observing their habits and noting those areas that are frequently used or consistently avoided. Nectarivorous and frugivorous species focus their foraging activities around food plants in full flower and full fruit, respectively. Many arid-zone species are attracted to standing water for drinking, bathing and foraging. When capturing bats, harp traps are regarded as less stressful (to both personnel and bats), but mist nets are preferred for some groups (e.g. bats with fluttering flight in the Hipposideridae and Rhinolophidae, and large-bodied bats in the Megadermatidae that chew through harp trap bags), contexts (over water or upper canopy deployment) or situations (remote fieldwork with space and weight restrictions for equipment; Francis 1989). Although these methods are non-selective, the likelihood of capturing particular target species (of both birds and bats) can be enhanced with judicious placement (next to known roosts, near favoured resources or in flight paths) or use of acoustic lures. The use of acoustic lures to increase trap success of microbats in harp traps is an emerging technique in Australia, and is showing promising results (Hill *et al.* 2015).

Mist nets

Personnel should spend time in target areas to decide where best to place nets (Figure 7.2). Animal trails and ant nests need to be avoided and fallen sticks and low branches cleared within ~1 m either side of the intended mist net location. Personnel should choose the most appropriate mesh size for the target species. For most work on small to medium-sized birds, 32-mm mesh size is ideal, while 24-mm mesh size is recommended if target species are very small birds, and 60-mm mesh size for larger songbirds (Pardieck and Waide 1992). Finer monofilament mist nets are typically used for catching microbats. Personnel should erect the net, ensuring that the bottom shelf remains clear of the ground, including when it contains a captured bird, unless targeting ground-active bird species. Nets are tensioned so that the shelf strings are tight – the fine nylon mesh will naturally billow to support captured animals. Personnel should

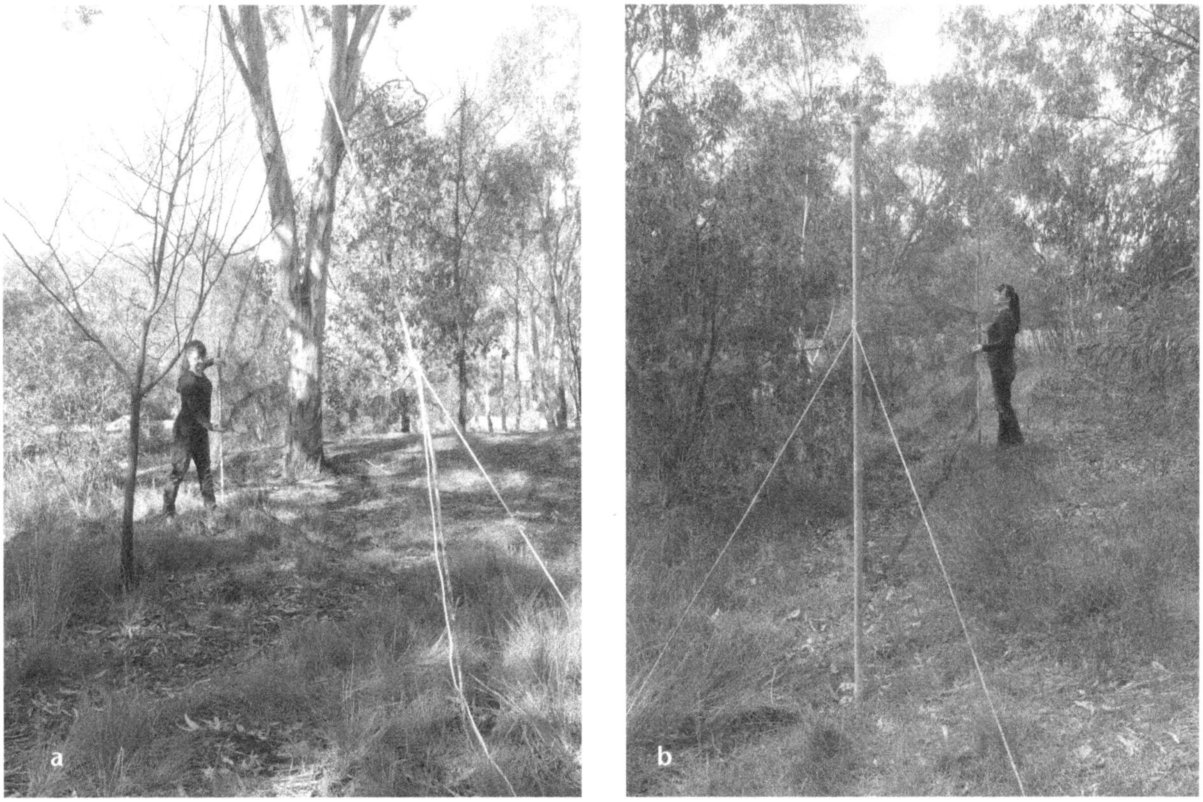

Figure 7.2: A mist net deployed for birds, set (a) poorly and (b) properly. Rather than position the net across an animal trail in direct sunlight, it should be located in the shade adjacent to a high visitation area – in this case, between two nectar-bearing plants. Instead of leaning into branches with the base touching the ground and catching on sticks, the net should be at least 300 mm clear of vegetation either side of the net and the bottom shelf. Rather than sagging from a flimsy cane and a bright single guy rope, the net should be tensioned from a sturdy pole secured with two dull-coloured guy ropes, shelf strings evenly spaced. Note the personnel wearing dark clothing without external fasteners – buttons readily catch on mist nets and are difficult to remove. Photos by David Watson.

check that the shelves of the net are spaced correctly by ensuring the cords at either end of the net (perpendicular to the shelf strings) are taut. When mist netting for birds, once nets are set, personnel should stay away from the nets to minimise disturbance. For birds, nets are checked every 20–30 min, or more frequently if conditions are damp or windy (Ralph *et al.* 1993). If check times take > 20 min, personnel should remove and process all trapped animals, and furl some nets immediately to reduce capture rates and removal times. To check nets, it is essential to know on what side of the net the animal was caught. Personnel should approach each net and examine the ground beneath it, then grasp the net mesh beneath the shelf string and enclose the body and wings of the animal to minimise risk of injury to the animal and handler. A seam ripper or fine scissors should always be available when checking nets. If an animal is visibly stressed and unable to be extracted quickly from the net, a strand or two should be cut to expedite removal, ensuring that no loose threads are left attached to the animal (Spotswood *et al.* 2012).

Bats can chew their way out of a monofilament mist net in less than 1 min, or become very tangled if left longer. When mist netting for microbats, nets should be checked every 1–5 min, so an appropriate number of nets and personnel, and the time to check nets should be considered during planning. A bat detector can alert personnel to a bat flying nearby and colliding with the nets and then a light shone along the length of each net to check for bats. Similarly to birds, individuals should be extracted from the side of the net on which they were caught, freeing the tail and feet first. When mist netting for flying-foxes, two people should be present: one to restrain the bat (one hand around neck, another holding the body) and the other to untangle it.

The size of the nets used in a trapping session should be recorded, as well as duration of use to determine the trapping effort (S. Petit and T. Reardon, pers. comm.). One mist net hour is equivalent to one 12 m net open for 1 h (Kalko and Handley 2001).

Trip lining

Trip lining is most effective at small bodies of water in dry or arid areas with little other water nearby, and in hot weather when bats are more likely to come down to drink. The banks of the water body should be free of vegetation and only gently sloping. Fishing line should be stretched across the water in parallel lines ~2 m apart and pulled tightly to prevent sagging. The fishing line can be held in place by wrapping it around tent pegs or sturdy sticks stuck into the ground at the edge of the water. Trip lines need to be monitored continually. A bat detector can alert personnel to a bat in the area. The sound of a bat plopping into the water is the signal to turn the light on to see where it has landed. At least two people are needed for this technique with one person on either side of the water body. One person shines a light at the bat, resulting in it swimming in the opposite direction, towards the second person who keeps their light off until the bat reaches the shore, where it can be quickly picked up. Having only one light shining on the bat reduces the risk of it swimming in circles, which occurs if a light is shone from both sides. Bats are surprisingly good swimmers; however, it is important to reduce the amount of time the bat is in the water. Personnel need to be prepared to wade into the water to rescue a bat on the rare occasion that one gets into difficulty.

Harp traps

Harp traps are best set up by two people in the late afternoon. When choosing trapping locations, positions are chosen that act as natural funnels such as along tracks, gaps between trees, creek lines or gullies (Figure 7.3). Optimal trapping locations have dense vegetation on either side of, and above the trap (Churchill 2008). As with mist nets, harp traps need to be tensioned correctly – too taut and flying bats will bounce off the fishing line; too loose and the bats will fly straight through. When tying the canvas bag, the sides should be pulled in firmly so that only a narrow gap is present between the plastic sheets through which the bats slide into the bag, to prevent bats escaping. For deployment over water, personnel should ensure that the bag is well clear of the surface, allowing for sudden changes in water depth. Guy ropes should be used to stabilise the trap to prevent it blowing over in the wind. If set at the entrances to mines and caves, harp traps should be monitored continually so that traps can be moved out of the flight path or individuals removed promptly to prevent overcrowding if large numbers are caught. Harp traps must be positioned well away from ant nests. When checking the harp trap, personnel need to ensure that all corners of the bag are checked thoroughly so that no bat is missed. When dismantling the trap, the bag should be taken off and thoroughly checked again, then inverted and any debris shaken out.

Harp traps used to catch flying-foxes work on the same principle as those used for microbats but are made

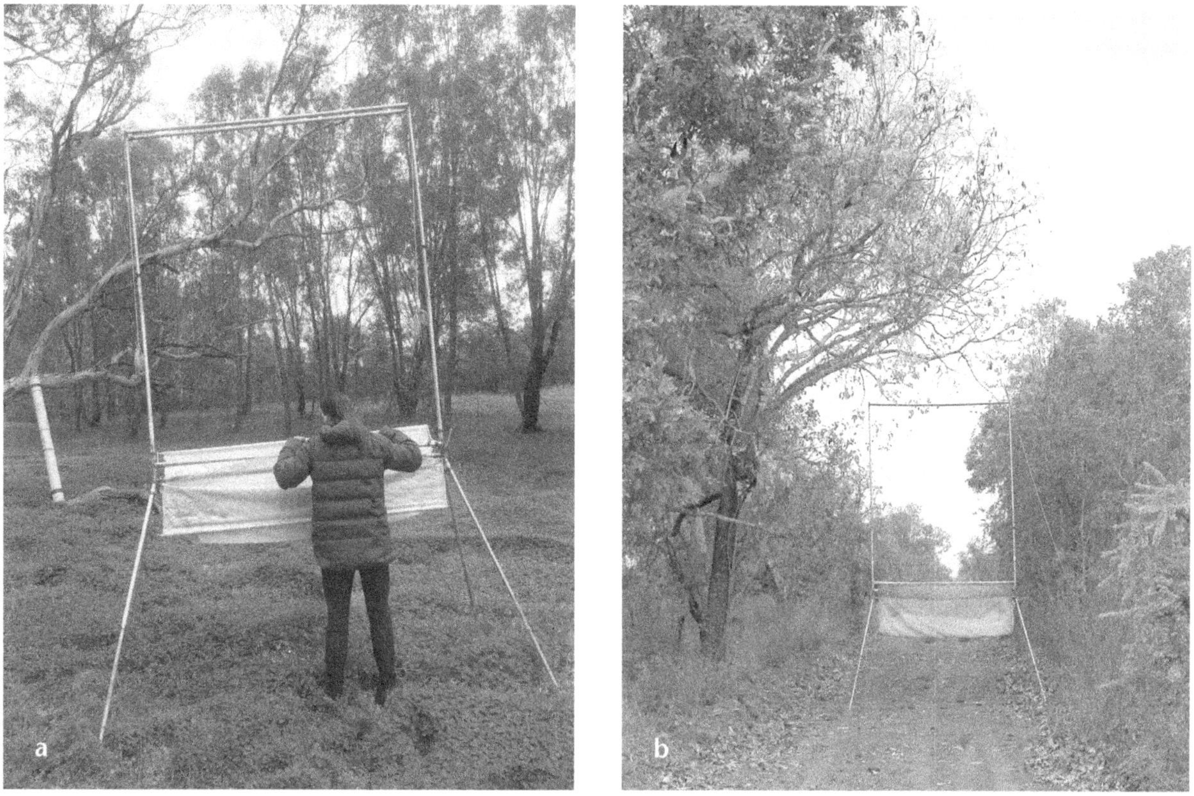

Figure 7.3: A harp trap deployed (a) less than optimally and (b) properly. More bats will be captured when the trap is placed in a fly way, such as along a track, and with vegetation on either side and above, than in the open as shown on the left. Adjust the legs to the height which maximises filling the gap in the vegetation. Guy ropes from the top corners of the trap should be tied to pegs or adjacent sturdy vegetation to ensure stability. When checking the bag, keep the bag ties done up and lower one side of the bag carrier as shown on the left. Doing so enables easy access to the bats while reducing the space within the bag from which bats could fly out. Photos by David Watson (a) and Lindy Lumsden (b).

of yacht masts with horizontal wire cables stretched between them attached at the top and bottom, from which two banks of vertical, nylon-covered wire cables are strung tightly. The trap stands 14 m high and 16 m long, with 120 vertical wires (Tidemann and Loughland 1993). A bag is not used with the megabat harp trap: personnel are stationed nearby ready to catch bats as they slide down to the ground. Trapping is usually undertaken adjacent to a flying-fox camp, on dusk or before dawn.

Animal treatment, withdrawal and euthanasia

Small-bodied and nectarivorous bird species should not be kept for longer than 1 h post-capture. If they are showing signs of stress (drooping eyelids, nodding and/or trembling) they should be placed in a calico bag somewhere dark and warm where they will often improve rapidly. Many birds undergo partial fright moult when caught or removed from mist nets, so some loss of contour or tail feathers can occur. It is important not to grasp the tail of any bird during handling (Lowe 1989). If a bird is in poor condition or obvious stress, personnel should try placing it in a safe, shaded area. Often, after several minutes, the bird's condition will improve, and it will fly away. If the animal is still there after 10 min or if signs of injury (blood, wings or tongue held strangely) are apparent, the bird should be treated by an experienced veterinarian. Bats captured in harp traps that are removed after dawn should be kept during the day to be released at the capture point that night on dusk. During the day they should be housed in small numbers in a cloth bag (no more than 10 individuals, if they were together in the trap, otherwise alone) and hung in a dark quiet room or shaded environment. Bats will often enter torpor during the day and so should be well warmed before being released. Euthanasia is rarely needed, and only if for major injuries (e.g. broken limb). If used correctly, injuries and trap deaths in harp traps are very rare.

Equipment and maintenance

Mist nets

Nets can only be purchased from specialist distributors, and in Australia are only available for researchers with a mist net endorsement from the Australian Bird and Bat Banding Scheme (ABBBS) or an appropriate state wildlife research permit. Nets should be stored in their own bag, with any sticks or other debris removed before packing. When erecting or packing up mist nets, they are best kept under tension and should never be allowed to touch the ground. Any broken strands (from branches, animals or personnel) can be readily mended, noting that animals can become badly tangled in nets with large holes. Badly damaged nets should be destroyed. It is usually not possible to repair the very fine monofilament nets used for microbats. Poles can be lengths of bamboo, or fashioned from readily available camping equipment, but very smooth poles are difficult to work with as shelf string loops can slip under tension. Other equipment needed for mist netting are guy ropes, pegs, clean catch bags, plus equipment for processing the animals (this equipment typically includes banding pliers if bird banding is to be undertaken, callipers and weighing scales). A steel 300-mm rule with a perpendicular lip added to one end (a bander's rule) is especially useful for measuring wing length in birds (Lowe 1989). Where ground pathogens such as phytophthora may be spread, mist nets and any equipment having been in contact with soil or animals should be cleaned and dipped in or sprayed with alcohol (70–90%) and dried before storing securely.

Trip lines

Trip lining simply requires fine fishing line (e.g. 3 kg breaking strength), tent pegs, lights and animal processing gear.

Harp traps

Harp traps are manufactured and sold by specialist distributors in Australia. Harp traps come packed inside a length of sturdy PVC pipe or flexible carry bag. Equipment needed for processing the animals includes callipers, scales and recording equipment. Correctly deployed harp traps that are packed away properly need little cleaning or maintenance, and remain serviceable even with several broken strings. Like mist nets, if ground pathogen such as phytophthora are a risk, then sections having been in contact with soil should be cleaned and dipped in or sprayed with alcohol (70–90%) and dried before storing. If multiple strings are broken (by a branch or wayward animal), they are best repaired indoors by experienced and patient personnel. Harp trap bags need to be completely dry before storage, otherwise they will go mouldy.

Specific qualifications, experience and training

It takes many hours to attain competency in setting mist nets and extracting, identifying, measuring and marking animals safely and efficiently. This competency is best gained under the close supervision of experienced personnel. Setting harp traps and extracting and processing bats are also highly skilled procedures, best learned by working closely with experienced personnel. If banding of trapped animals is planned, personnel will need to gain an appropriate ABBBS permit.

Workplace health and safety

General risks

Using harp traps or mist nets to capture birds and bats is a relatively low-risk activity, with best practice use involving the usual precautions for working outdoors (e.g. personal protective equipment and safe manual handling procedures; see Wildlife Health Australia 2020a). Other than low risk of disease exposure and injury (especially to the hands), personnel should be mindful of trips and falls when moving harp traps and mist net poles. Otherwise, any conditions where additional care is needed (exposure to extreme temperatures, floodwaters) or locations where additional caution is warranted (beside nests of stinging insects, curious livestock or water bodies containing crocodiles) should be avoided. When trip lining, care is needed to avoid tripping over obstacles when moving around in the dark.

Bites and scratches

Both bats and birds can bite and scratch people, but serious injuries are rare. Two groups of birds are noteworthy. Parrots have sharp and very powerful beaks, and bites from even small species routinely break the skin, so all parrots should be handled carefully, paying particular attention to the head, holding the head away from the hand with two fingers braced either side of the neck (see Chapters 15 and 33). Raptors use their sharp claws and strong feet to dispatch prey, so all owls and birds of prey should be handled with particular attention to their feet, safely held by grasping their legs (see Chapter 34). Although gloves can be useful to minimise injury while handling larger birds, extracting birds from nets relies on locating very fine nylon strands, and is best performed without gloves. Flying-foxes have large sharp teeth and claws on their feet and thumbs and should be handled using thick leather gloves. Although the teeth of microbats are much smaller, they can at times break the surface of the skin. The risk of contracting Australian bat lyssavirus (ABLV) is low, but all researchers should wear gloves, such as nitrile, or thin leather golfing gloves, and be vaccinated (see Chapter 23 for additional details).

Disease

Both bats and birds can transmit diseases to people. For birds this risk includes psittacosis (especially from pigeons and parrots), and various forms of influenza (Whitworth *et al.* 2007). In addition to biting or scratching, transmission of some of these diseases occurs via airborne particles. The coronavirus that causes COVID-19, while linked to bats overseas, has not been recorded in any Australian wildlife (Wildlife Health Australia 2020b). However, the virus could be transmitted by humans to bats (Botto Nuñez *et al.* 2020), and appropriate precautions should be taken (see Wildlife Health Australia 2020b). ABLV is the main disease of concern for bat researchers. The virus has been recorded in all Australian mainland species of flying-foxes and the yellow-bellied sheathtail bat (*Saccolaimus flaviventris*) (Field 2018). Antibodies for ABLV have also been recorded in a range of other microbat species (Field 2018; Prada *et al.* 2019), and so precautions should be taken when handling any species. Anyone handling bats should have a current rabies vaccination and wear puncture-proof gloves. To minimise cross-infection between captured animals, catch bags should only be used for single individuals, or for small groups of individuals if already clustered together such as in a harp trap. Bags should be washed before re-use, and both mist nets and harp traps should be cleaned of any animal traces (including droppings, feathers and fur) and soil (see 'General procedures') and sprayed with disinfectant such as methylated spirits, before being completely dried ahead of storage.

Alternative procedures

For those applications where birds or bats need to be captured to be measured, marked or tagged, the only other suitable alternatives are alternative capture methods, including cage traps, canon nets or other propelled nets (see Chapter 15 for birds), or the extraction of bats from nest boxes (Chapter 23). Observational identification and counts of birds and bat colonies, and the use of species-specific calls for identification purposes (either *in situ* or via passive acoustic recorders), usually suffice for most survey and monitoring objectives (Ralph *et al.* 1993); acoustic monitoring is becoming more widely used with bats as call libraries improve (Chapter 5). However, for poorly sampled regions or species, bats may still need to be caught to be definitively identified and to compile local call libraries. Capture may also be required for detailed ecological studies.

CAPTURING UNGULATES WITH CORRAL AND PEN TRAPS

Andrew J. Bengsen and Jordan O. Hampton

Target taxa

Corral and pen traps are used to capture large-bodied (> 20 kg), free-living, terrestrial mammals. In Australia, they are most commonly used to capture ungulates, such as pigs (*Sus scrofa*), goats (*Capra aegagrus hircus*), deer (Cervidae) and horses (*Equus caballus*) (Chapter 24).

Context and scope

Corral and pen traps include a diverse range of enclosures designed to capture multiple individuals of gregarious species at once. The materials and structure used vary depending on target species, but all comprise a rigid physical barrier around a lure (usually bait) or attractive landscape feature (usually a water point), with one or more entry points (Figure 7.4). They can be portable or semi-permanent. Corral (enclosure) traps typically range in area from 0.25 to 4 ha and aim to catch social groups of animals at once. Corral traps fitted with long fenced wings to guide driven animals towards the entrance have occasionally been used in Australia, but this technique is not recommended because animals enter the trap in an excited state, which can result in elevated injury and mortality rates (Hampton *et al.* 2019). Pen traps are smaller than corrals and hold fewer individuals. Specific types of pen traps are also known by other names, including panel, silo and figure 6 traps.

Smaller traps designed to capture single large-bodied animals include box, and Clover and Stephenson traps. Enclosures > 4 ha are generally referred to as paddock traps and are not usually used to capture animals for research. Large box and paddock traps are not covered in this GOP.

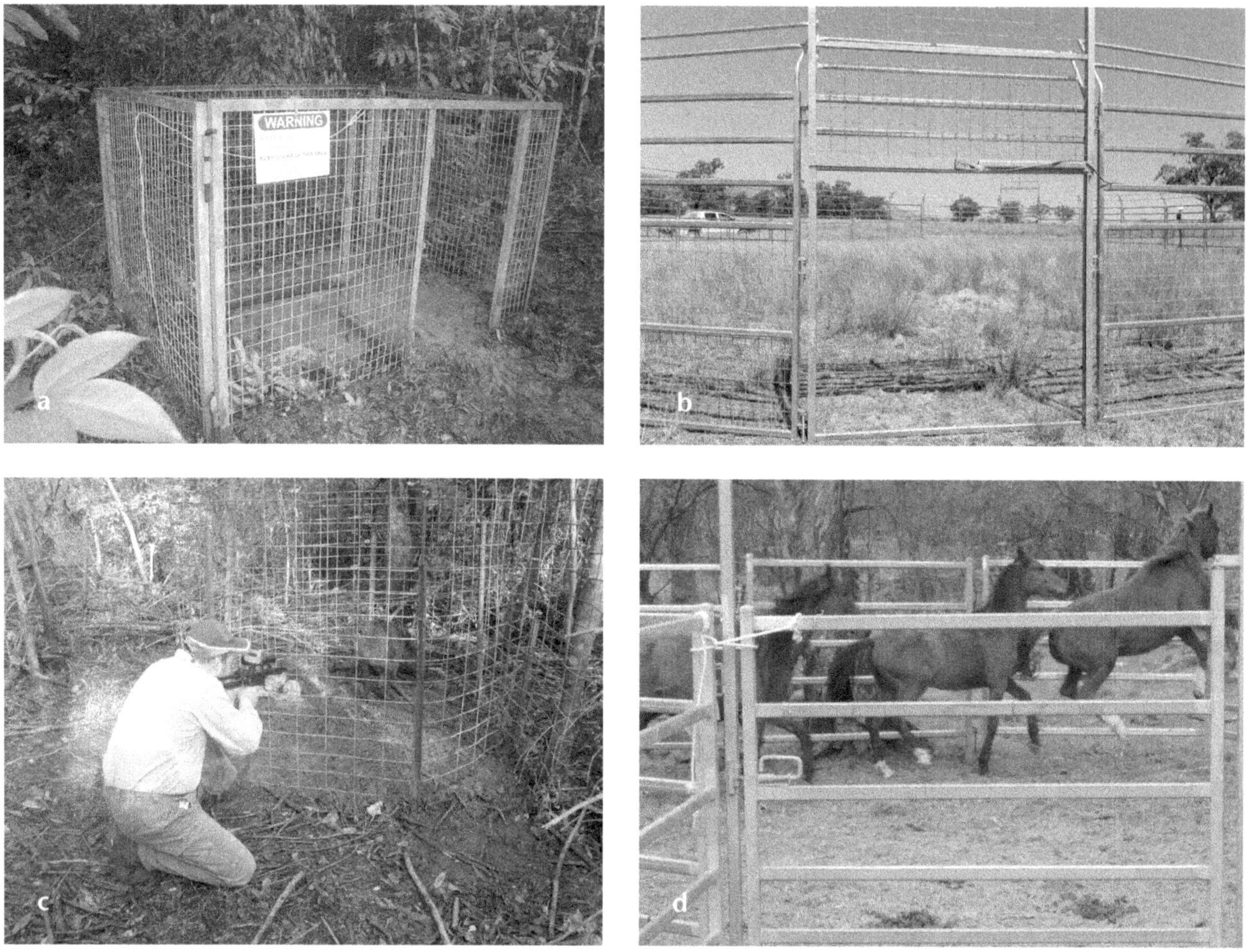

Figure 7.4: Examples of corral and pen trap construction. (a) Panel-style feral pig pen trap with a push-through side-swinging gate triggered by a rooting bar to reduce non-target captures. Photo by Andrew Bengsen. (b) Corral trap for fallow deer (*Dama dama*) made with cattle panels and mesh with multiple remotely triggered drop gates. Photo by Andrew Bengsen. (c) Feral pig pen trap with a push-through entry made from steel reinforcing mesh bent in on itself in a figure 6 shape. Photo by Peter Adams. (d) Horses in a corral trap showing the potential for self-trauma. Photo by Rob Gibbs, NSW NPWS.

Animal welfare considerations

Corral and pen traps can cause serious physical injury or death to trapped animals if they are not carefully constructed and operated. Reported frequencies of injury and mortality are variable for ungulates captured in corral or pen traps – for example, 2% mortality for feral horses (Scasta 2020) and 6% for feral pigs (Barasona *et al.* 2013). Causes of injury or death can be grouped into four main categories: (1) physical trauma from the trap (including self-trauma); (2) physiological distress from prolonged confinement and exposure to stressors; (3) thermal distress from prolonged exposure to heat or cold; and (4) isolation of dependent young.

Traps should be designed and situated to be as target-specific as possible, so that non-target animals are not unnecessarily exposed to these hazards. Gates, gate triggers and other entry points should reduce the risk of capturing non-target species. For example, deer traps can deploy high tripwires to avoid being triggered by macropods (Mitchell 2016) and pig traps can make use of rooting bars to reduce the risk of being triggered by many species (e.g. Figure 7.4a). Remotely triggered electronic latches (e.g. Figure 7.4b) allow precise control of gate closure timing and can be useful when combined with cameras that send imagery from the trap to a remote location, but they only provide a single capture event. One-way push-through gates (e.g. Figure 7.4c) allow continuous capture of multiple animals. Remotely triggered traps that use 4G technology to enable multiple captures are also now available (Lavelle *et al.* 2019).

Physical injury

Animals caught in traps sometimes charge and crash into the trap panels or gates during attempts to escape, when startled or when approached by humans, resulting in injuries, such as snout or muzzle lacerations, fractures and avulsed lips (Sweitzer *et al.* 1997). Animals can also be injured while attempting to jump out of the trap (e.g. broken necks in feral horses; Scasta 2020; Figure 7.4d). The potential for trap-related injury can be reduced through careful selection of trap location, trap construction materials and methods, and methods for approaching and handling trapped animals (see Chapter 24).

Physiological distress

Physiological distress includes a range of potentially harmful physiological responses to stressors, such as the perception of danger, confinement in unfamiliar environments and overcrowding in traps. Acute stress may result in hyperthermia and dehydration. Prolonged distress can cause capture myopathy. Trapping and handling procedures must aim to reduce fear, excitation and exertion in trapped animals.

Capture myopathy comprises a suite of syndromes that arise from prolonged distress and physical exertion associated with the pursuit, capture and restraint of wild animals (Spraker 1993). It is invariably fatal and characterised by severe muscle breakdown and hyperthermia leading to kidney failure (Breed *et al.* 2019). No reliable treatment is available, so prevention and minimisation are essential (Breed *et al.* 2019). A comparison of corral and pen traps found that biological indicators associated with capture myopathy were greatest in pigs captured in corral traps, probably because the larger area within the traps allowed greater physical exertion before handling than in smaller pen traps (Barasona *et al.* 2013). Other studies have also reported higher stress and injury rates in pigs captured in larger traps (Sweitzer *et al.* 1997). It is often easier to immobilise animals in pen traps than in large corrals (Figure 7.4c). Hence, although smaller pen traps may be less efficient than corrals for capturing large numbers of animals at once, they often produce lower rates of capture myopathy and higher rates of survival.

Animals targeted for capture in corral traps are gregarious species, but overcrowding or confinement with individuals from different social groups can cause prolonged distress and physical injury from fighting. Very young animals can also be crushed underfoot. If corral traps are to be used, they should be large enough to provide freedom of movement for large numbers of animals and to allow animals to avoid each other while accessing important resources within the corral, such as water and shade.

Exposure and dehydration

Animals captured in corral or pen traps have limited opportunity to shelter from extreme ambient temperatures. Prolonged exposure to very high or low ambient temperatures can cause dehydration, hyperthermia or hypothermia, all of which can be fatal. High temperatures also increase the risk and severity of capture myopathy (Breed *et al.* 2019; Spraker 1993). The best ways to reduce exposure are to avoid trapping at times and locations where exposure to extreme temperatures is likely, and to check traps and clear animals from them regularly. Building traps around or beneath trees provides both shade and transpiration cooling. It may be necessary to provide water in hot environments. Traps should be checked at least daily, and animals should not be held for > 24 h.

Separation of dependent young

Dependent young that do not enter traps with their mother may become separated and die from starvation. Traps should not be set during seasonal birth pulses in species with seasonal reproduction.

General procedures

Trap siting

Traps should be sited at locations with a high probability of being encountered and entered by the target species and low probability of being entered by non-target species. Large mammals often use regular trails ('pads') to commute between shelter and feeding areas. Areas on these trails will often satisfy this requirement. Traps should be sited in areas where they are unlikely to be encountered by other people. They should also be positioned in a location where they can be observed remotely and approached by personnel with minimal disturbance. Camera traps linked to communication networks can sometimes be used for remote observation. Trap locations should provide protection from extreme temperatures (i.e. shaded and not placed at a high altitude).

Trap construction

Construction materials, methods and design must be guided by the morphology and behaviour of target and likely non-target species, but certain features can reduce the risk of injury or mortality for all species. Traps are usually constructed using wire netting or panels of rigid wire mesh or metal rails, depending on the target species (Figure 7.4). Post and rail construction are common for horses. In all cases, trap construction must aim to prevent physical injury to target and non-target species, and to minimise exertion and physiological distress during capture and handling.

Pen traps are often preferable to corrals. Corrals and large pens should be round, rather than acutely angular, as corners can impede the natural flow of animals through the trap and form pressure points where animals can be crushed. Drafting and handling facilities may be necessary to enable safe restraint, handling and release of trapped animals (e.g. Moriarty 2004).

Panels and gates must be able to withstand repeated impact from trapped animals. Panels must be secured to the ground or sufficiently heavy to prevent them from being tipped over or lifted. They must be free of sharp surfaces, edges or projections that can cause injury and any wiring must be finished on the outside of the trap. Mesh size should be sufficiently small to reduce the risk of animals forcing their heads, or parts of their heads, through the mesh under pressure (e.g. ≤ 10 cm for feral pigs; Figure 7.4a, c) (Sharp 2012; Lavelle *et al.* 2019).

Entry points or gate triggers should be designed to reduce accessibility to non-target species. All gates must be checked to ensure that they work cleanly and close completely so that they do not pose a risk of animals getting stuck while attempting to escape. Gates should close quietly so that they do not induce a startle response.

Personnel should consider whether a shroud is appropriate. A hessian or shade cloth shroud around trap panels provides a physical and visual barrier that can help to reduce excitation and escape attempts in trapped animals (Lavelle *et al.* 2019). Shrouding the top section of fences or wire panels can also reduce the risk of macropods being caught by their hind legs when attempting to jump out of the trap (Sharp 2005). Low (0.9–1.2 m) panels or fences can allow macropods to escape from goat traps but will be too low for most other species. Pig traps, for example, should be at least 1.5 m high, or be covered, to prevent pigs from escaping.

Free-feeding

Free-feeding is the provision of food at the trap site to condition animals to use the area and enter the trap. Effective free-feeding maximises the number of animals available for capture, reduces the risk of non-target capture and may reduce stress in captured animals. Free-feeding should begin before the trap is constructed using a feed that is safe and attractive for the target species while minimising non-target species that would be susceptible to trapping. Camera traps can be used to identify species consuming feed. Concurrent feeding at several sites can help to identify sites where most effort should be invested. Once target animals have begun feeding regularly, trap materials can be introduced to the site and the trap constructed. The trap can be built in stages to reduce neophobic avoidance. Free-feeding should continue once the trap is built so that target animals become accustomed to entering and feeding within the trap. No feed should be provided outside the trap at this point. Goat traps with a jump-down entrance should have an open exit gate during free-feeding.

Setting the trap

The trap can be set once target animals are regularly feeding within it. Traps can be open at any time, but should not be armed and set to capture animals during periods of high ambient temperature or when target individuals are likely to be in late stages of pregnancy or have dependent young. To reduce the risk of hyperthermia in hot conditions, traps can be armed only at night and locked open or closed during the day. The inverse approach can be used for diurnal species during cold conditions that may predispose to hypothermia. This approach may also reduce the risk of capturing diurnal or nocturnal non-target species, respectively. The number of traps active at any one time should not exceed the number that can be checked and cleared within a reasonable time frame.

Approaching the trap

Prior to approaching the trap, it should be observed from a remote or concealed location to determine how many and what type of animals have been captured. If animals have been captured, the trap should only be approached once all required personnel and equipment are prepared for the necessary handling and release operation. The trap should be approached quietly, preferably from the main gate side to prevent animals putting pressure on this section of the trap.

Handling and releasing trapped animals

Specific handling procedures will depend on the target species and the tasks that need to be completed. Common tasks include tissue sampling, ear tagging and the fitting of tracking collars. These techniques are covered in Chapters 8 and 9, respectively. Handling and immobilisation of ungulates are covered in Chapter 24. All procedures should aim to minimise stress and excitation, both in animals and in handlers, and to complete all operations as efficiently as possible. Chemical immobilisation will often be required, depending on the nature of the tasks to be completed, although some simple tasks such as ear tagging can sometimes be achieved using physical restraint alone (Chapter 8). Handling and chemical immobilisation of ungulates are discussed in Chapters 16 and 24. If chemical immobilisation is required, trapped animals can be darted at close range using a dart gun (Figure 7.4c) or blow pipe, or an injection pole may be used. Mammals captured in corral or pen traps are susceptible to hyperthermia and capture myopathy. Water for dousing should be available to cool animals while they are being handled and before release (Sawicka *et al.* 2015).

Animal treatment, withdrawal and euthanasia

Corral and pen trapping can injure trapped animals severely, requiring euthanasia or treatment. Personnel must be able to deal with injured animals promptly and effectively. Procedures for managing possible adverse events must be documented and understood by the trapping team before the commencement of operations. Procedures should specify consumables, equipment and personnel that are required on-site to manage injured animals. Procedures for trapping operations must specify monitoring requirements to detect lacerations, fractures, hyperthermia and capture myopathy. Trapping teams must also be equipped to euthanase animals. Additional procedures will be required if animals are to be chemically immobilised. Procedures must also specify classes of animal to be excluded from specific treatments, such as excluding animals in poor condition from being burdened with tracking collars. Minor lacerations (if treated) can be managed by applying a topical antibiotic or antiseptic. Hyperthermia can be managed by dousing with cool water (Sawicka *et al.* 2015). Serious injury, illness or failure to fully recover from chemical immobilisation will usually require euthanasia *in situ* (see Chapter 24).

Equipment and maintenance

Equipment required for trapping will depend on the target species and context. Typical items may include:

- trap panels, gates, gate triggers, posts and wire
- fencing pliers, post drivers
- feed, water troughs
- consumables and equipment for minor first aid
- firearms and ammunition for euthanasia.

Specific qualifications, experience and training

Lead investigators or team leaders should have experience in building and operating traps for the target or similar species. At least one person on the trapping team should have experience, and preferably formal training, in euthanasia and chemical immobilisation of wild ungulates. If using firearms, personnel must have undertaken a firearms safety course and have appropriate certification. Ideally, they would have also undertaken a course in humane destruction of large ungulates. Personnel constructing and operating traps, and handling animals, should have demonstrated practical experience in those techniques, under the supervision of someone who has worked with those species or similar taxa.

Workplace health and safety

Trap construction and operation, and handling animals

Trap construction and operation present physical injury hazards relating to heavy lifting, crushes and minor cuts and abrasions. Trapping team members must practise safe lifting methods and should wear robust gloves. Eye protection should be considered. Trapped animals can injure handlers through kicking, biting, crushing or striking with antlers or horns. Handlers should have experience in handling trapped animals of the target or similar species or be under the supervision of somebody with appropriate experience. All handlers must follow prearranged procedures, have clear roles and understand other team members' roles. Handlers should practise appropriate hygiene and protective measures, such as wearing gloves, to reduce the risk of contracting zoonoses, such as brucellosis, leptospirosis and Q fever.

Alternative procedures

Single animals can be trapped in box traps or similar (e.g. Clover traps). They can also be captured using immobilisation drugs delivered by dart projectors, from ground- or helicopter-mounted shooters. Deer and pigs have been captured in drive nets and from net guns fired by helicopter-mounted shooters. Each of these methods has its own hazards and benefits (e.g. Hampton *et al.* 2019).

CAPTURING ARBOREAL MAMMALS BY HOOK AND NET

James M. Turner

Target taxa

This GOP applies to possums and gliders (Chapter 19).

Context and scope

The technique described in this GOP was born from a need to capture medium-sized arboreal mammals that do not enter standard cage or box traps readily and when tranquiliser-darting, branch-shooting or noose poles are inappropriate (W. Foley, K. Marsh and P. Beale, pers. comm.). Given that the target species are usually nocturnal, the method is conducted in combination with spotlighting (see Chapter 4). While few publications describe the hook and net method, it has been used to catch mountain and silky cuscuses, and coppery ringtail possums (*Phalanger carmelitae*, *P. sericeus* and *Pseudochirops cupreus*, respectively; Salas and Stephens 2004), rock ringtail possums (*Petropseudes dahli*; Runcie 2002) and Lumholtz's tree-kangaroos (*Dendrolagus lumholtzi*; Procter-Gray and Ganslosser 1986). It may also be used to encourage gliding behaviour in greater gliders, *Petauroides volans* (NHMRC 2014). Other authors describe shaking small trees to dislodge possums, but without the use of a hook and net (e.g. How *et al.* 1984; Pahl 1987; Munks 1991; Rawlins and Handasyde 2002). It is likely that the method is not often described explicitly in published research. Instead, the technique may simply be disguised as 'hand capture', which, while true, does not let the reader assess the technique's potential impacts on the animal and study results. Flagging methods for koalas are described in Chapter 20.

The hook and net technique is used when animal capture is necessary for investigation that cannot occur remotely, such as measurement of body mass or morphology, tissue sampling, collar attachment or transponder implantation. Animals are sought actively so baits or lures are not needed. This method typically requires a large sampling effort to catch a sufficient number of individuals, which can be time-consuming and physically demanding, depending on landscape and vegetation types. Capture itself is often rapid, but the duration varies with the position of the target individual on a tree and the density of surrounding vegetation, which can affect pole manoeuvrability.

Animal welfare considerations

Capturing an animal by shaking it out of a tree is stressful to the animal. The active process can last from seconds to minutes and ends in an animal's capture or its escape. While no impact of the technique has been reported in the literature, it can be assumed that it causes fear or distress, and at least a short-term stress response based on published knowledge of animal stress responses to capture (e.g. Buddle *et al.* 1992; Romero *et al.* 2008; Morellet *et al.* 2009; Breed *et al.* 2019). Other negative effects on welfare may include physical injury, disruption of normal behaviour or activities, and the alerting of predators to an individual's presence.

Physiological stress

Tree-shaking and capture are likely to induce a hormonal stress response in target animals; this response has the potential to reduce animal fitness in the long term, although the extent of long-term impact is difficult to predict. Ensuring that personnel are experienced and efficient in all procedures associated with the method will help minimise stress to study animals, because often a subjective judgment must be made in the field on the basis of animal behaviour. For example, if an animal has not been successfully captured after a few minutes of shaking, and it begins to look around and climb with rapid, 'panicked' movements, the capture attempt should be abandoned to avoid causing additional stress. Similarly, if after a few minutes it is apparent that an animal is in a position in the tree where it is unlikely to be dislodged with continued shaking, the attempt should be stopped.

Physical injury

The trajectory of a falling animal is difficult to predict, and an individual may not land in the net after shaking. An animal may strike a branch as it falls or land on the ground awkwardly, causing injury. All animals that miss the net immediately run for the closest tree or dense ground cover; observations of escape behaviour and physical examinations after capture have not revealed notable injury. To minimise the risk of injury from falling, it is important not to shake tree branches that are situated above rocky or debris-covered ground or hardened roads/paths.

Behaviour modification

Tree-shaking induces in animals a flight response, which could lead to home range displacement if they leave their current home ranges to escape capture. It may also increase hiding or vigilance behaviour in individuals, reducing the time spent accessing food resources, which could decrease body condition, or the ability to find mates, affecting reproductive success. In general, capture, or attempts at capture, interrupts the normal daily activities of target species, which may result in short- or long-term modifications in behaviour (Morellet *et al.* 2009). Studies on animal behaviour or spatial ecology should interpret data collected soon after capture with caution (Morellet *et al.* 2009). The impact of the hook and net technique on animal behaviour may be reduced by minimising site visitation duration or frequency.

Alerting predators

The location of an animal may be revealed to potential predators during or after shaking through illumination of an individual in a spotlight, noise from tree-shaking, defensive vocalisations of animals or olfactory cues from, for example, urination. Predation risk could be minimised by reducing the duration of capture attempts, reducing site visitation frequency, or avoiding an area if the presence of known predators, such as powerful owls (*Ninox strenua*), appears to increase.

General procedures

Locating study animals

Personnel search the study area on foot or from a vehicle if necessary (although vehicle noise may scare target animals), using a spotlight fitted with a red filter (Chapter 4) if the target species is nocturnal.

Tree-shaking

After an individual animal has been located, team members keep their distance to minimise disturbance. The pole is assembled as required, depending on animal height above ground, and lifted to the vertical position. Team members approach the tree and assume their roles, depending on team size; ideally, the team includes one pole operator, one or two catchers with nets, one or two people ready to intercept an animal if it runs towards a nearby tree, and one person to maintain a spotlight on the animal. Higher numbers of personnel may be less efficient or impractical in some situations, and capture is possible with fewer people (at least two are required). The pole operator slowly moves the hook towards the branch, taking care not to bump the trunk or other branches on the way, because doing so may motivate the animal to escape by climbing higher (out of reach of the pole) or jumping to a nearby tree. As soon as the hook is on the branch, between the trunk and animal if possible, the pole operator shakes it vigorously to dislodge the animal. If the animal runs towards and over the hook, shaking is ceased to avoid accidental injury. If possible, a branch or small tree can be bent towards the ground so that the animal can be captured by hand, avoiding any risk of injury from falling.

Catching

The net should be held loosely so that an animal does not bounce out of it upon impact. After an animal has fallen into the net, the two sides should be quickly brought together, and the net moved to the ground to increase entanglement and stop an escape. The animal can then be removed from the net carefully and placed in a cotton bag for processing.

Animal treatment, withdrawal and euthanasia

Despite the high-impact nature of the technique, injuries are infrequent (W. Foley, K. Marsh and P. Beale, pers. comm., pers. obs.). Withdrawal from a study may be considered if individuals are often recaptured and frequently exposed to the risk of stress or injury.

Equipment and maintenance

This technique requires custom-made equipment consisting of a pole with a hook for shaking the branch, similar to a traditional panking pole used to shake fruit from a tree, and a net for catching the animal. The pole may vary in design, but the one described below, adapted from a design developed by W. Foley (pers. comm.), has been used successfully by the author of this section to capture common ringtail possums.

The pole consists of three 2 m lengths of interlocking aluminium sections (Figure 7.5). The diameter of each section is 30 mm with a thickness of 3 mm. Two of the poles have a 26 cm length of steel tubing welded and riveted within their ends, with half protruding, to connect the sections. The base of one pole can then slide over the steel tube of a second pole. Whereas the poles consist of aluminium to reduce weight, these interlocking sections are made of steel for strength. These joins are a weak point of the pole. Aluminium joins tend to bend under

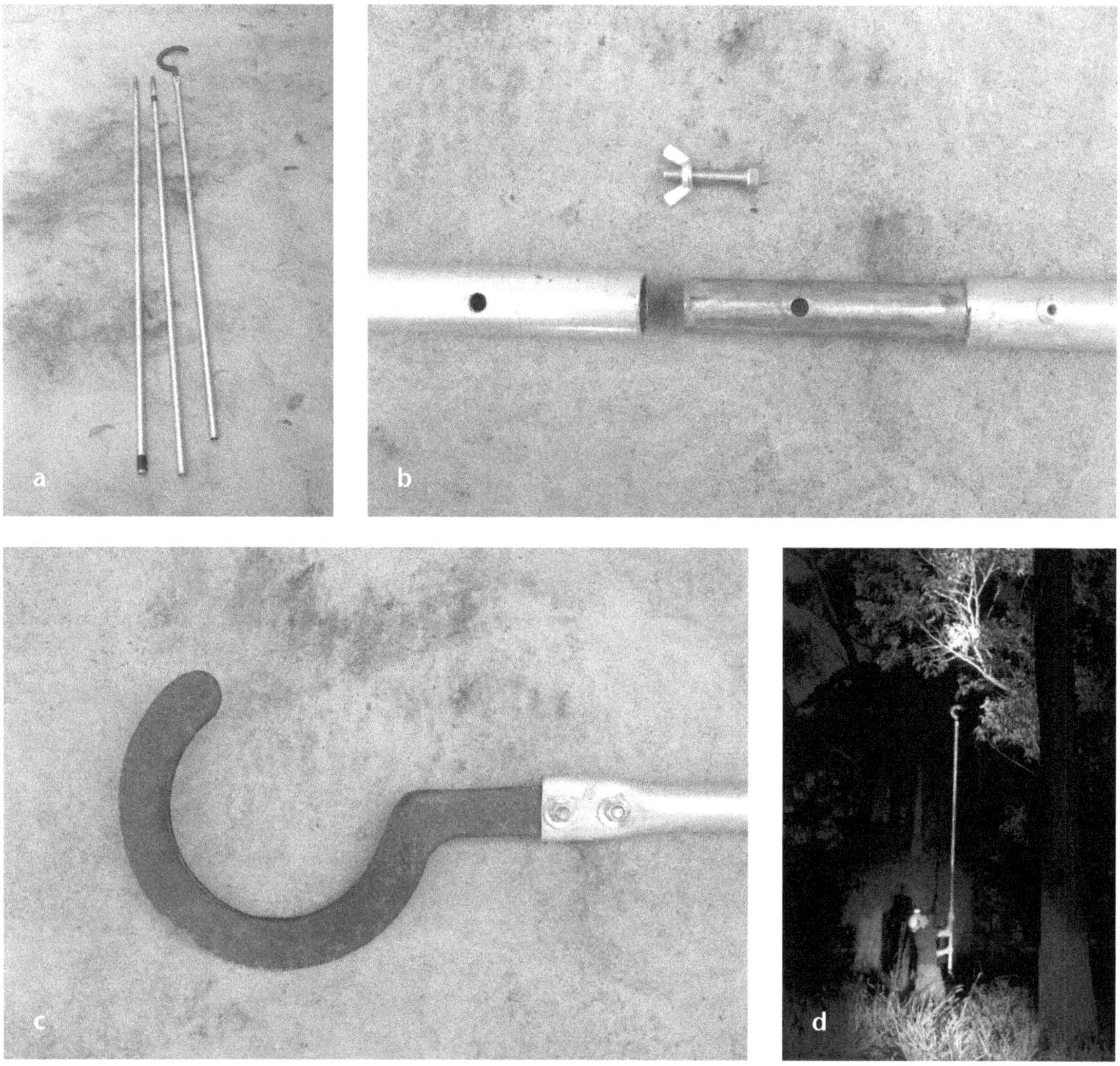

Figure 7.5: Pole with hook for the capture of arboreal mammals. The pole consists of (a) three aluminium sections, which are (c) interlocked with steel tubing and fastened with a wingnut and bolt. One section contains (c) a steel hook. Photograph (d) shows the pole, with two sections connected, being used to reach a tree branch. Photos by James M. Turner.

the pressure of the pole's weight when raising it from the ground and should be avoided. An 8 mm diameter hole is drilled halfway up the protruding steel tubing and at the corresponding point at the base of the next pole section. An 8 mm bolt can then be inserted through the poles to join them and a wingnut allows rapid fastening by hand. The third pole has a steel hook with a 210 mm diameter and 5 mm thickness, permanently fastened to its end with two bolts. A pole in three sections allows possums to be accessed at three different heights and simplifies transport.

The net should be sufficiently large to minimise catcher error. The net should contain loose folds to allow it to stretch when a possum falls inside, softening the landing, and of a mesh size that allows claws and fingers to pass easily through and become entangled. Typically, 5 mm anti-bird netting used to cover food plants works well. The net is strung along the lengths of two wooden poles (e.g. broom handles) using cable ties. When a possum falls in, this design allows the two sides of the net to be brought together quickly to prevent the animal from escaping. Other commercially sold nets may be available, but would probably need modification before their use as possum catchers; the use of camper's hammocks (Lemos de Sá and Glander 1993) and blankets (Salas and Stephens 2004) in catching falling animals has also been reported.

Other useful equipment items will depend on the study objective and the measurements to be made. Equipment may include that used for handling and processing an animal, such as gloves, a cotton handling bag, a spring balance and callipers. Maintenance includes regularly checking for cracks and bends in the pole and tightening the hook's bolts. The net is also checked for holes, entanglements and loose attachment points.

Specific qualifications, experience and training

The hook and net technique is not used broadly, so prior communication or training with an experienced person is essential. As a minimum, team leaders should have experience with field observations of mammal behaviour so that they can make apt, on-the-spot decisions on whether a capture attempt should be continued or stopped. It is useful for team personnel to have spotlighting and animal handling experience and skills, preferably with the target species.

Workplace health and safety

Falling branches and debris

Falling branches, twigs, leaves, bark, dust and other debris may fall onto personnel while shaking a tree. To minimise risk, only the shaker and the net-catcher stand directly under an animal. These personnel should wear protective equipment, including helmets and safety glasses. Other team members stand back from the tree, watch for falling objects and communicate any hazard to the shaker and catcher. All personnel wear personal protective equipment appropriate for working in the bush, such as sturdy footwear and long pants.

Injury from a captured animal

Possums may become defensive when captured and personnel may be scratched or bitten, which may result in infections, including from potential zoonoses. Appropriate personal protective equipment, such as leather gloves, should be worn when handling and processing animals. Any injuries should be treated immediately.

Alternative procedures

Alternative procedures may include tranquiliser darting (Chapter 16), but the appropriateness of this method will depend on the size of the target species. For example, darting of possums may be unsuccessful if darts bounce off individuals with relatively thin soft tissue layers (Webb 2018). Additionally, employing a sharpshooter to shoot the branch on which the possum is sitting may result in injury if the possum clings to the branch instead of bracing for impact. Use of a noose pole may be restricted by the height above ground of the target animal. These methods are not necessarily lower impact than the hook and method procedure and require specialist expertise. Baited cage traps (see other GOPs in this chapter) may be used depending on the target species but, again, are not necessarily lower-impact methods, particularly if an animal is caught within a trap for several hours. Additionally, while several studies have used cage traps to capture ringtail possums (e.g. Pahl 1987), success may be site-specific and depend on food availability, habitat type, wariness of traps and humans, familiarity with non-natural items and animal nesting behaviour.

TARGETED SEARCHES FOR REPTILES AND AMPHIBIANS

Deborah S. Bower, Eric Vanderduys and Helen P. Waudby

Target taxa

Procedures outlined in this GOP are appropriate for most small to medium-sized reptiles (Chapter 26) and amphibians (Chapter 27).

Context and scope

This GOP describes general techniques and considerations for targeted (active) searching of specific habitat features (e.g. underneath rocks, litter, timber or peeling bark) and the subsequent hand capture of reptiles and amphibians. These methods are sometimes referred to as visual encounter surveys when targeting frogs. Targeted surveys focus on habitat features that study taxa are expected to use for at least part of the day, night or season (DSEWPC 2011b). Subsequent hand capture, where necessary, permits data collection (e.g. checking sex, body measurements), allows handlers to perform techniques such as mark–recapture and radio tracking, and is required to collect animals (e.g. for use in experimental studies). Targeted searches may be once-off or repeated, depending on the research objectives.

Animal welfare considerations

These methods are likely to be low impact if completed quickly and with appropriate handling procedures for the species of interest. The main potential effects are changes in habitat use as a result of disturbance during active searching. Effects of hand capture on animals vary depending on the physiology of the species and personality of the individual (e.g. some monitor species respond defensively following capture and handling (Ward-Fear *et al.* 2018)). These effects will vary according to the length of time, conditions and procedure undertaken (Langkilde and Shine 2006).

Disruptions to daily activities and habitat use, and alerting of predators

Hand capture of reptiles and amphibians in the wild will disrupt their normal activities (e.g. feeding and foraging, reproduction, social interactions). Factors likely to influence the magnitude of this impact include the duration of handling following capture, the climate where handling occurs (temperature, moisture), seasonality (e.g. if handling occurs at a critical point in the breeding season, such as capture of frogs while calling), and territoriality or habitat use (e.g. if the animal follows the same route regularly). Investigators should also consider potential negative effects on animals associated with disturbing habitat to search for target individuals (e.g. turning over rocks or logs to search for animals). For example, rocks that were displaced in Sydney sandstone had larger and cooler crevices than did restored rocks, reducing their occupancy by reptiles, although the negative effects on habitat use were mitigated to some extent by replacing rocks precisely (Pike *et al.* 2010). Activities may lead to modifications in behaviour, such as increased refuge use, changes in habitat use and patterns of activity (Kerr *et al.* 2004) and reduced thermoregulatory time, which may impose physiological and behavioural costs (Martín and Lopéz 1999). Study animals may experience increased visibility at their point of release, which could increase the risk of predators targeting them. Animals should always be released in proximity to their shelter or cover and monitored to ensure that they move to cover successfully.

Physiological stress

Physiological stress occurs from prolonged or invasive procedures that may accompany hand capture (Langkilde and Shine 2006). Stress responses could include vomiting, defecating, everting reproductive organs, or laying eggs. Autotomy can occur during handling in lizards and will cause stress to individuals (Langkilde and Shine 2006). In the alpine she-oak skink (*Cyclodomorphus praealtus*), temperature, lizard length and observer experiences all influenced the probability of autotomy (Scroggie and Clemann 2009). Skinks also showed a characteristic tail wagging behaviour before autotomy. Cooling the lizard after capture, pausing activity if tail wagging is observed and training handlers on non-endangered species beforehand may reduce the risk of negatively impacting individuals (Scroggie and Clemann 2009). Causes and triggers of stress will vary among species so knowledge of the biology of the target species will enable researchers to reduce stress during handling.

Accidental mortality and disease transmission

Accidental mortality can result from animals overheating or being handled incorrectly (e.g. where breathing is inhibited). For fossorial and rainforest species (with a low critical thermal maximum), direct handling should be avoided where possible. For small skinks, a calico bag can be placed over the handler's hand and used to scoop individuals and move them between places to minimise heat transfer (Read and Kearney 2016); frogs can be kept cool and hydrated in a plastic container filled with water. Animals should be handled in a manner appropriate to their morphology (see Chapters 26 and 27). Investigators should also follow appropriate hygiene protocols when handling multiple individuals to minimise the risk of spreading diseases, such as the amphibian chytrid fungus, particularly when working with amphibians (see Chapter 27 for specific protocols).

General procedures

General considerations

Researchers select an appropriate survey method and sampling regime, which will depend on the study objectives and species. For evaluation of species persisting at low densities, or with limited or patchy distributions, surveys may need to be replicated across the study area, randomly or systematically (DSEWPC 2011b). Researchers should document the survey effort, including the number of personnel involved in searching for target taxa and the duration of surveys, and record details on environmental conditions and habitat. Active searching can be destructive to habitat and, once displaced, most habitat resources are unlikely to provide the same conditions for the target or non-target taxa. Wherever possible, displaced rocks, timber and other resources should be replaced as precisely as possible.

Consideration must be given to the species' requirements, such as moisture and temperature needs. Shade is required while handling animals in hot climates. Small, cold-adapted animals can perish rapidly in the heat of hands. Amphibians, particularly tadpoles, require constant hydration. Protocols to reduce the spread of pathogens must be adhered to, such as using single-use plastic bags for amphibians and disinfecting equipment between individuals or populations. The observer should have the appropriate safety equipment (e.g. gloves, bandages) to handle venomous species and species that can inflict damaging wounds (e.g. goannas, crocodiles). However, each study species will have different requirements, and these can change between age classes. For example, nitrile gloves are useful to handle frogs, but are toxic to some tadpole species (Cashins *et al.* 2008).

Locating the study animal

The researcher should identify appropriate methods for locating the animal (e.g. active search of specific substrates). Considerations that will determine how to locate the animal will include its movement patterns; diel behaviour patterns (nocturnal, diurnal, crepuscular) and seasonality; the level of risk that the animals pose to the observer if they become distressed; density of the population; and other research techniques being undertaken (e.g. radio-telemetry).

Diurnal active or hand searches are typically employed to target species that use particular habitat resources, such as underneath bark on tree trunks or fallen timber, crevices or weathering rocky outcrops, and under rocks, to name a few. Personnel can wear thick work gloves to turn substrate safely if required and may use a plastic rake or similar implements to check leaf litter for litter-dwelling reptiles. Substrates (timber, rocks) should be lifted carefully and away from the handler to minimise the risk of being bitten by a snake. Personnel should remain calm and avoid suddenly dropping substrates back onto animals (i.e. if startled suddenly). Rocks and timber or similar substrates should be replaced in the same position once the animal has been captured. Complete removal of bark from trees should be avoided where possible. Leaf litter should be raked firmly (i.e. so that the rake's prongs reach the soil layer) and with consistent movements and replaced afterwards.

Restraining the study animal

Once located, movements and noises that may alert, startle or alter the animal's behaviour should be avoided, unless they are required to assist capture. The handler should swiftly and safely restrain the animal using appropriate techniques. Care should be taken not to pin animals against spikes or other objects that could cause harm, which are particular hazards when capturing free-living reptiles and amphibians. The amount of handheld pressure and method of appropriate restraint will vary according to the animal's taxon. For example, gently holding the base of the tail while supporting the forebody will assist in restraint of an agamid lizard, but will often result in autotomy in skinks, legless lizards and geckos. Restraint should be achieved in a manner that avoids damage to vital organs. Restraint methods may change for different size classes of the same species (e.g. hatchling crocodiles compared to adult crocodiles – Chapter 26). An appropriately firm grip is required because animals may twist, jump or scratch suddenly if not restrained. Experience and careful training dictate the level of pressure required to maintain a firm grip. If animals are to be released, they should be replaced next to or, ideally, under their original substrate, without being squashed.

Animal treatment, withdrawal and euthanasia

The risk of injuring an animal directly through active searching and handling varies according to the species. Injuries may occur if the study animal becomes chronically stressed, exceeds its temperature limits, if the handler inflicts physical damage, or if predation increases. If treatment or euthanasia is required, suitably trained personnel should use a technique appropriate to their study species or seek veterinary advice. Factors that may result in a decision to withdraw from the study at any given point include obvious changes in the behaviour of the study species, such as changes in habitat use over time (i.e. where the same habitat is searched repeatedly over a period of time). During handling, animals should be monitored continuously for behavioural changes that may indicate signs of stress, such as postural change, sudden limpness, increased breathing rate, tail wagging in lizards, colour change, and a reduction in alertness. Monitoring should continue after release while the animal is in sight.

Equipment and maintenance

Equipment will vary depending on the species or taxon, and the nature of the study, but general items may include:

- containment suited to the study species (e.g. plastic bags for amphibians, plastic tubs or calico bags for small reptiles)
- pathogen protection (e.g. gloves, bags, disinfectant), including materials for disinfecting equipment

- first aid equipment (e.g. snake bandage, first aid kit, eye wash)
- note-taking equipment (e.g. notebook, laptop, tablet, voice recorder, clipboard)
- equipment for processing (e.g. callipers, camera, marking equipment) and animal handling (e.g. snake hooks)
- shade (e.g. gazebo, tree cover)
- water for amphibians.

Where ground-based pathogens, such as phytophthora, are a risk, all equipment that has come into contact with the soil should be cleaned thoroughly and disinfected before being moved to another site.

Specific qualifications, experience and training

The qualifications and experience required to perform the procedure vary depending on the sensitivity of the study species or taxon to handling and design of the study. In general, personnel should have been deemed competent in the technique by a more-experienced investigator, and have used the method on the target species or similar taxa. Personnel capturing and handling venomous snakes should have specific experience in doing so.

Workplace health and safety

Dangerous plants and animals

In some cases, personnel may wear or employ protective equipment (e.g. gloves for venomous snakes). For some species it will be important for personnel to complete hand capture in pairs (at least) to minimise the risk of injury to researchers (e.g. when handling dangerous species such as large goannas, venomous snakes and crocodiles). Additionally, personnel should pay attention to their surroundings as hand capture of harmless animals such as frogs has resulted in medical emergencies for handlers when snakes and spiders were in the process of preying on the target animal and envenomed the handler during the capture event (J. Clulow, pers. comm.). Handlers should also be aware of other dangerous plants and animals nearby during hand capture; centipedes can be mistaken for squamates and spiny plants can inflict damage to the handler and target animal.

Alternative procedures

Researchers should consider if study questions could be answered with, for example, remote monitoring equipment (e.g. acoustic recorders and wildlife monitoring cameras), or other technologies (e.g. long distance photography) that may be appropriate to answer study questions, and potentially lower in impact than active searching and hand capture.

CAPTURING MACROPODS WITH DRAW-STRING TRAPS

Graeme Coulson and Clare Death

Target taxa

Draw-string traps allow the capture and safe handling of medium- to large-bodied macropods, such as red-necked wallabies and eastern grey kangaroos (*Macropus giganteus*) (Coulson 1996; Coulson *et al.* 2003) (Chapter 21). The technique may also be applicable to other mammals, such as bare-nosed wombats that habitually move under fences (e.g. Coates 2013) (Chapter 19).

Context and scope

This GOP describes a method for capturing medium- to large-bodied macropods in situations where they routinely move through fences, often squeezing underneath or through narrow gaps. Chemical immobilisation, which is required immediately after initial capture and manual restraint, is covered elsewhere in the book (Chapters 16 and 21).

Animal welfare considerations

Several categories of potential animal welfare impacts are associated with draw-string traps: (1) stress and trauma from being pushed towards a trap before darting; (2) pain, stress and injury from confinement and restraint during capture; (c) stress when evading capture; (d) anaesthetic complications; and (e) capture myopathy. Of these, serious injury and myopathy are generally associated only with passive, unattended traps as used in New Zealand (Latham *et al.* 2020). The authors strongly advise against the use of such traps, which should never be left unattended. In contrast, draw-string traps that are operated actively have very few negative effects on welfare (Coulson *et al.* 2003).

Stress before and after capture

Exertion caused by driving animals towards a trap can increase the risk of hyperthermia and physical trauma from collisions with fencing and other solid objects. Confinement in netting and manual restraint induce immediate stress and involve some risk of physical trauma while struggling against restraint. Prolonged confinement before immobilisation is likely to exacerbate these effects and must be avoided. Large pouch young are at particular risk if ejected or escaped from the pouch; they must be quickly separated from the mother and placed in a cloth bag to avoid injury from kicks while the mother is restrained manually.

Failure to capture

Transient stress can occur when the trap is closed too soon, causing the animal to back away and flee, or closed too late, allowing the animal to force a passage through the draw-string and escape. This risk minimised by ensuring that personnel are experienced and/or trained by more experienced people.

Anaesthetic complications

Field anaesthesia is challenging, and immobilised animals can experience a range of complications, which are covered elsewhere in the book (Chapters 16 and 21).

Capture myopathy

Capture myopathy is possible if excessive 'pushing' occurs before capture, especially during warmer weather. Myopathy would be inevitable if confinement in the trap is prolonged, but that is not an element of the method, as all trapped animals are attended to immediately. This issue is discussed in detail elsewhere (Chapters 16 and 21).

General procedures

Installing traps

Draw-string traps should be installed in places where animals have already established a runway and are regularly pushing under or through the fence (Figure 7.6a). The fence can be further modified by enlarging the passage at the trap site to encourage its use, as well as

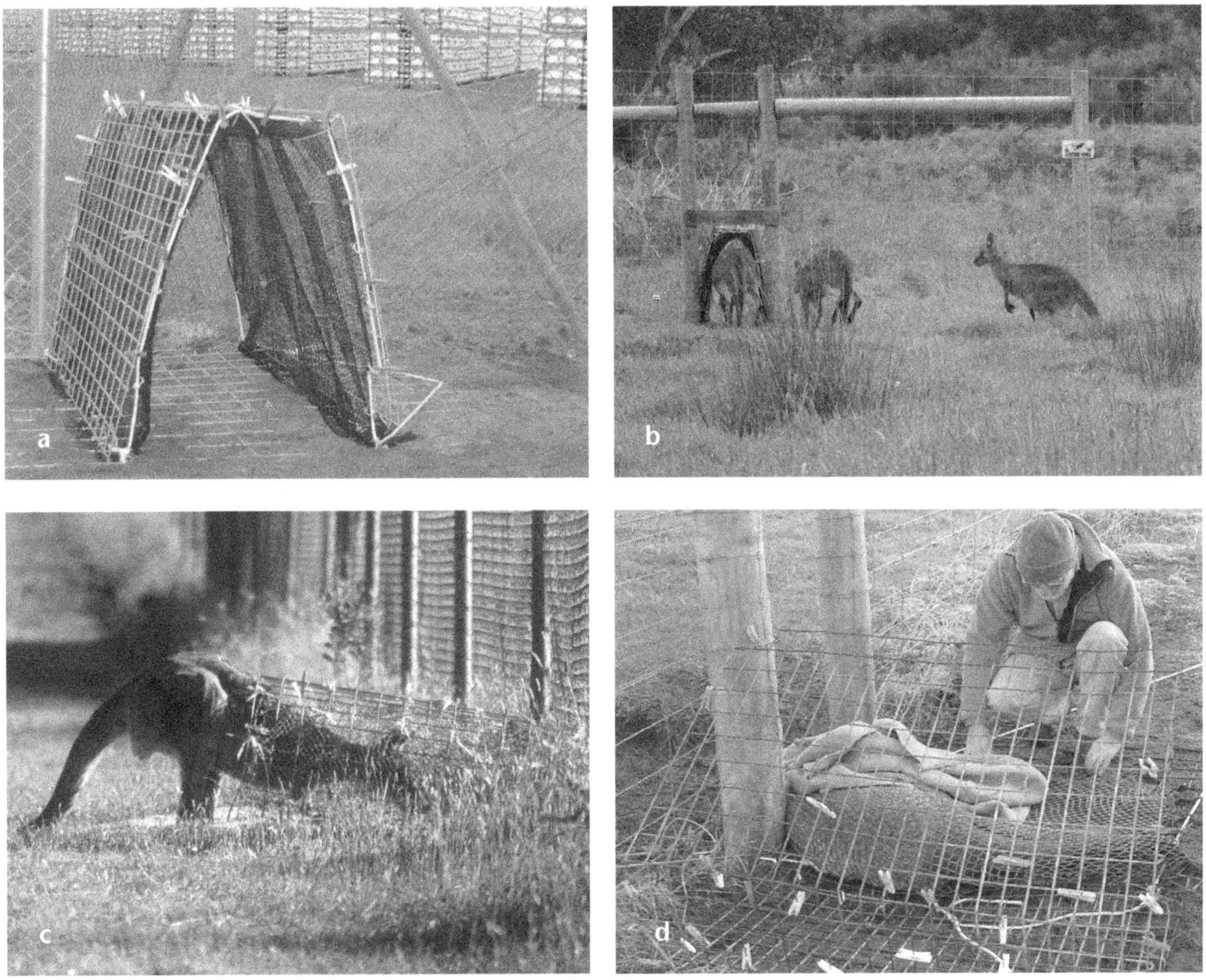

Figure 7.6: Use of the draw-string trap to capture eastern grey kangaroos (*Macropus giganteus*). (a) A trap set in a gap in a security fence. (b) One kangaroo enters a trap, as two others follow. (c) A kangaroo enters the trap, as viewed by the operator in the hide. (d) A recumbent kangaroo in the trap netting after chemical immobilisation. Photos by Graeme Coulson (a, b, c) and Sophie Petit (d).

eliminating alternative access points by reinforcing the fence and blocking holes beneath it. Traps are installed by placing a weld-mesh frame at right angles to the hole in the fence and securing a second weld-mesh floor to the ground. Care should be taken to ensure that all metal components are smooth and do not project into the runway. Once the trap site is being used consistently by the target species, the trap can be erected in stages to allow the animals to habituate to it. A section of netting is suspended within the weld-mesh frame and tied to the floor to create a tunnel. Draw-strings at each end of the tunnel are closed by an operator pulling the connected rope from a permanent hide, erected 10–20 m from the trap, on the same side of the fence. All ropes and other materials should be installed before a trapping session.

Trapping times and duration

Draw-string traps rely on natural movements of the target species, so trapping is normally conducted at dawn and dusk, when animals move between foraging areas and cover. Familiarity with the site, including the daily movement habits of the target species, is essential to the success of this trapping method. Trapping can be accelerated by encouraging target animals to approach the trap, which is best done by positioning one or two people in the open, at a non-threatening distance from the animals, to induce animals to seek refuge sooner in the morning; this approach usually cannot be used in reverse in the evening. Additional people should be coordinated by hand signals, mobile phones or two-way radios, but silence must be maintained as animals approach the trap. The active 'pushing' of animals is generally unproductive (Coulson 1996) and poses the risk of the animals colliding with fences and other objects or becoming stressed and/or hyperthermic. In hot weather, natural movements are likely to be restricted to cooler times of day, but trapping should be conducted only at safe temperatures (e.g. < 30°C). Trapping is also possible at night, under natural or artificial light aided by binoculars or night-vision devices (Coulson 1996), although identification of target animals is then more difficult. Trapping can be continued until no additional animal approaches the trap. However, each capture causes disturbance to target animals nearby, and resetting the trap will deter them, so the interval between sequential captures could be at least 30 min.

Operating traps and removing animals

A trap is operated from inside the hide. The method is highly selective; the operator can allow non-target animals to pass through the trap while waiting for a target animal to approach (Figure 7.6b, c). Once the target animal has entered the trap, the operator pulls the rope vigorously to close each end of the netting rapidly and secures the rope before leaving the hide and going to the trap. The operator then restrains the animal by squatting or kneeling on the netting on either side of the animal, injects the immobilising agent into the hind limb musculature, and maintains physical restraint during induction. Placing a fabric cover over the eyes of restrained animals is advisable while awaiting the onset of sedation (Figure 7.6d). Once the animal is immobilised, the operator releases the draw-strings and the animal can be removed from the trap.

Chemical selection and dosage calculation

The chemicals chosen for immobilisation and their recommended dosages are covered in more detail elsewhere in the book (Chapter 21). Zoletil® (tiletamine–zolazepam) has been used to immobilise animals in all draw-string trapping projects to date (e.g. Wilson *et al.* 2013; Death *et al.* 2019).

Securing traps between sessions

Animals are encouraged to continue to move through the trap between capture sessions by tying the netting securely to the outer frame, so that animals can pass through it. Failure to do so will result in the netting becoming dislodged over time so that it hangs down, partially blocking the route through the fence and creating an entanglement hazard.

Animal treatment, withdrawal and euthanasia

Manually operated draw-string traps pose few risks to target animals. Minor abrasions, from contact with the substrate or netting, can be treated by cleaning the area with a topical skin cleansing agent (e.g. dilute chlorhexidine or povidone–iodine) and/or application of a topical wound spray or powder if deemed appropriate by the advising veterinarian. Severe trap injuries will be avoided if no sharp edge is present in the trap construction. Veterinary opinion and treatment may be necessary for trapped animals that have incurred severe injuries or appear to be suffering from capture myopathy (as per Vogelnest and Woods 2008).

Equipment and maintenance

Equipment required for draw-string trapping includes:

- binoculars
- night-vision equipment (if required)
- mobile phone (for text messaging field assistants)
- syringes and needles of appropriate volumes and gauges (ensure you have more than you need)
- if appropriate, gloves and mask
- veterinary chemicals (ensure more than is needed is on hand)
- data sheets and veterinary chemical use logbooks
- spare batteries or power banks for electronic equipment
- materials for cleaning and disinfecting equipment before moving to next site
- spare clothes pegs, tent pegs, rope, etc. for trap repair.

Specific qualifications, experience and training

Personnel should have practical experience in capturing and handling large wild animals. Personnel administering veterinary chemicals will typically need to be working under the direct supervision of a veterinarian or possess accreditation to perform the method (requirements vary by jurisdiction). Ideally, personnel will have completed a chemical immobilisation training course.

Workplace health and safety

Draw-string trapping is a low-risk technique for field biologists. Safety risks include (1) self-injection with immobilisation chemicals; (2) being scratched or kicked by recumbent animals; and (3) zoonotic hazards, such as urine, faeces, blood- or saliva-borne pathogens (e.g. Q fever). All staff should be trained in appropriate responses to self-injection. Animal handlers should be vaccinated against Q fever, wash hands after captures, and avoid inhaling dust that may be contaminated by animal urine, faeces or birthing fluids.

Alternative procedures

Alternative capture methods that can be used in place of draw-string traps are cage traps for medium-sized macropods (e.g. Di Stefano *et al.* 2005), such as wallabies (see earlier GOPs in this chapter), and pole syringe (e.g. King *et al.* 2011) or darting (e.g. Roberts *et al.* 2010) for larger species (see Chapter 16).

CAPTURING WOMBATS AND MACROPODS BY STUNNING AND NETTING

David A. Taggart, Graeme Finlayson and Graeme Coulson

Target taxa

This GOP applies to wombats (Chapter 19) and macropods (Chapter 21), but may also apply to European rabbits (Chapter 24).

Context and scope

This GOP describes the capture of wombats and macropods via stunning followed by netting (or sometimes simply by manual restraint). The method is effective for capturing a range of species, including European rabbits (*Oryctolagus cuniculus*; Shepherd *et al.* 1978), red (*Osphranter rufus*), eastern grey (Jaremovic and Croft 1987) and western grey kangaroos (*M. fuliginosus*) (Robertson and Gepp 1982), and southern hairy-nosed wombats (*Lasiorhinus latifrons*) (Taggart *et al.* 2003). Detail is also provided for some of the specific capture and handling details associated with this method for key taxa. Other aspects of handling and immobilisation of these taxa are covered in Chapters 19 and 21.

Stunning was developed originally for capturing macropods (Robertson and Gepp 1982). Stunning relies on a combination of light and sound that interferes with the natural behaviour of the target animal, and improves the likelihood of capture considerably. Stunning occurs as a bullet travels at supersonic speed ~10–20 cm above an animal's head, or between its ears, with the sound wave created by the bullet temporarily deafening or confusing the animal. This sound or shock wave is the consequence of the bullet travelling faster than the sound waves it produces, causing the wave fronts to pile up on one another, and resulting in the constructive interference of many wave fronts (Halliday *et al.* 1993). This interference is believed to create the pressure that temporarily deafens the target animal. If successful for macropods, a targeted animal will drop its head and stand still for up to 30 s until disturbed. In other species, such as European rabbits, the resulting shock wave causes an apparent confusion, such that the rabbit does not flee, but runs around in proximity to where it was stunned, increasing the probability of capture. In all cases, the dazzling of the target animal with a spotlight at the same time allows the netter to approach undetected. Stunning is the most efficient method of capturing wombats, with one in every three or four wombats observed at night caught, and is superior to cage trapping, which should only be used if a particular animal needs to be caught from a known warren (e.g. for collar removal or a health check). For wombats, if the stunning is successful, the animal will remain motionless for 1–2 min (Taggart *et al.* 2003).

Animal welfare considerations

Several categories of potential animal welfare impacts are associated with the capture and handling of wombats and macropods by stunning: (1) stress, pain and trauma from restraint during capture; (2) stress when evading capture; (3) anaesthetic complications; (4) capture myopathy (mainly an issue for macropods); and (5) stress and trauma during transportation and handling.

When using firearms for stunning

Firing a bullet near a target animal presents a risk of death and stress to the animal. Firearms safety procedures must be adhered to during stunning. Only one trained and skilled shooter should be responsible for all firearms, ammunition and shooting components of this method, on any one field trip. The risk of animals being shot is negligible if the shooter remains constant, the rifle is fitted with a variable telescopic sight, the shot is taken from a resting position, and the shot placed no closer than 10–20 cm above the animal's head.

During netting

Confinement in netting and manual restraint induce immediate stress in target animals and involve some risk of physical trauma while they struggle against restraint. This risk is more pronounced in macropods than in wombats because macropods typically kick out with their hind legs or attempt to jump while netted. Prolonged confinement before immobilisation is likely to exacerbate these effects and must be avoided, particularly in macropods. Southern hairy-nosed wombats tend to settle quickly in a net if undisturbed, whereas bare-nosed wombats remain very active in the net following capture. For macropods, ejection or escape of medium to large pouch young is a real risk, so they must be separated quickly from the mother and placed in a cloth bag to avoid injury from kicks while the mother is restrained. Unlike macropods, wombats do not eject pouch young during capture or handling – possibly because of the tightness of the pouch during all pouch young stages, and the shorter limbs and lack of overall flexibility of wombats compared to that of macropods.

During failed capture attempts

Failed capture attempts result in only transient stress. Macropods that evade capture by netting or stunning simply hop away. Unsuccessful netting or stunning of a wombat results in the animal retreating underground for a period of time, but this response is a negligible issue in terms of welfare.

Risks associated with anaesthesia

Field anaesthesia can be challenging, and immobilised animals can experience a range of complications, which are covered elsewhere in the book (Chapters 16, 19 and 21).

Capture myopathy

Capture myopathy is not a risk for wombats. However, larger macropods are particularly prone to myopathy, as are some smaller macropod species (e.g. rock-wallabies), but not others (e.g. tammar wallaby, *N. eugenii*) (McMahon *et al.* 2013). Capture myopathy is possible if excessive 'pushing' occurs before capture, especially during warmer weather. Myopathy would be inevitable if confinement in a net was prolonged, but that is not an element of either method, as all captured animals are attended to rapidly. Treatment with injectable vitamin E and selenium has been advocated for prevention and therapy, but reports of efficacy are anecdotal (Vogelnest and Woods 2008).

General procedures

Netting and stunning

Wombats can be captured at night by spotlighting and netting, or by spotlighting, stunning and netting (Taggart *et al.* 2003; see Chapter 4 for more details relating to spotlighting). These activities are generally undertaken by personnel positioned on the back of a utility vehicle, which is driven slowly (< 10 km h^{-1}). The procedure requires a driver, one or two netters, a spotlighter, and a shooter. When a wombat is sighted (~30–80 m), the vehicle is stopped. The shooter then aims the rifle 10–20 cm above the wombat's head while the spotlighter trains the spotlight on the animal. Silence is essential. The shot is fired, and the netters then run along the edge of the spotlight beam until they reach and net the wombat. To secure animals following netting, personnel should stand on the handle or frame of the net until assistance arrives. Doing so is particularly important for wombats, which are very strong.

Macropods can be captured by stunning in much the same way as wombats, but a larger crew is required. Once a target animal has been located and is 'propped' in the beam of the spotlight, two pairs of 'runners' wait beside the vehicle until the shooter fires the shot. If the stun is successful, the animal will drop its head and remain motionless. Immediately after the shot, the 'runners' sprint along the edge of the beam and restrain the macropod manually, the first pair holding it by the tail or using a body tackle, and the second pair approaching to restrain the hind feet, tail and head. Additional personnel may be required to hold large animals. As soon as they are tackled, macropods regain consciousness and will struggle vigorously, so a high degree of handling skill and team coordination is required. A brief procedure, such as quickly fitting ear tags or a collar, can be completed by experienced personnel while the animal is restrained. Afterwards, it can be allowed to leave by first releasing the limbs and, once personnel are out of the way, releasing the tail. Longer procedures will require chemical immobilisation to avoid restraint-induced myopathy.

Transfer of captured animals from nets to bags

Once netted, animals are restrained within the net and generally transferred into a hessian sack or similar (see 'Equipment and maintenance') for processing. Wombats are powerful animals that are difficult to restrain. In order to transfer the wombat from the capture net to a bag, the wombat should be manoeuvred and blocked into a corner of the net. The loose netting around the wombat is then gathered in behind the animal's forearms, so that no loose netting is present around the animal's body from the forearms forward. The wombat, tightly secured within the net, and the net and handle, are picked up together and the wombat, rear end first, is dropped gently into the open bag. The bag is held wide open by two other personnel. These personnel are responsible for closing and securing the bag rapidly. Personnel should be aware that wombats can jump, although not very high. Bags should be double-tied as wombats can push the tie off the end of a bag if not secured properly. Once inside the dark bag or sack, wombats become calm very rapidly, and may fall asleep. Alternatively, some operators restrain common wombats in the net by standing on the frame and mesh, injecting them with Zoletil®, and then removing them from the net and placing them in the sack.

Small- to medium-sized macropods should be secured by the base of the tail, removed from the net and placed head first into an open sack held by other personnel (see Chapter 21). The sack should be pulled up over the animal rather than the handler trying to move the animal down into the sack. This procedure will prevent the animal grabbing hold of the sack rim as it is directed into the bag. The hind legs and toes must be facing away from all personnel as animals may kick out. Some medium-sized macropods may try and spin during bagging. To stop this movement, the animal should be allowed to put its forearms on the ground, and the procedure repeated rapidly. Animals will typically remain relatively quiet if a dark sack is placed over their heads and noise kept to a minimum.

Stunning and netting

This method only works at night when the spotlight hides the approach of the netters, but otherwise can occur at any time when the animals are active. Nights with little or no moonlight are best. Time from sighting to capture typically takes < 5 min. Stunning of wombats works best between 12–18°C, with few stuns achieved below 6°C and above 24°C, and also works best at higher humidity ≥ 50%.

Transport to a site for processing

If animals are being transported away from the capture site by vehicle for processing, they must be secured in their sacks to the vehicle tray or the sack placed in a pet crate to ensure that animals do not roll or bounce off the utility's tray once the vehicle is moving. Sedation for transporting small macropods or wombats is unnecessary. The authors of this GOP have transported over 100 small macropods in darkened pet crates or suspended sacks over hundreds of kilometres without incident. Wombats are always transported in secured sacks (clipped to the vehicle) so that they are not at risk of rolling or bouncing off a moving vehicle. Risks of myopathy in macropods are greatest at capture and on warm days, and not during transport. The authors' experience has been that once placed in the dark (e.g. individual darkened pet crates, or hanging suspended in sacks) with adequate ventilation, macropods remain calm and very quiet during transport. Additionally, some forms of sedation (e.g. diazepam) can be detrimental as sedated animals may lose the ability to regulate body heat and posture resulting in death. For example, the authors are aware of the death of multiple bridled nailtail (*Onychogalea fraenata*) and tammar wallabies following sedation and transport (D. Schultz, pers. comm).

Chemical selection and dosage calculation

The chemicals chosen for immobilisation of macropods and wombats and their recommended dosages are covered in more detail elsewhere (Chapters 16, 19 and 21). Zoletil® (tiletamine–zolazepam) has been used to immobilise large macropods and wombats in most trapping-based research projects to date (Taggart *et al.*1998; Finlayson *et al.* 2010; Wilson *et al.* 2013; Death *et al.* 2019).

Animal treatment, withdrawal and euthanasia

Generally, no specific animal injury that would warrant withdrawal or euthanasia is associated with stunning and netting wombats. Veterinary opinion should be sought and treatment may be necessary for trapped macropods that appear to be suffering from capture myopathy (as described in Vogelnest and Woods 2008) although, in mild cases, maintaining animals in a cool, dark, quiet location can alleviate distress markedly, and render animals fit for release.

Equipment and maintenance

Key equipment required for the capture of macropods and wombats includes:

- spotlight (100 W hand-held or car-mounted halogen, or equivalent).
- long-handled, heavy-duty, hand-held capture nets: wombat nets (made from tennis court netting) with a net area of 70 × 65 cm and 170 cm handle; macropod and rabbit nets with an 80 cm hoop diameter and 150 cm handle.
- 0.22 calibre magnum, bolt action rifle with telescopic sights (× 4 magnification minimum).
- sturdy utility vehicle with a flat tray back to allow for easy and rapid dismount, and a spotlighting and shooting frame mounted on its tray.
- roof-mounted gun rack
- catch bags or sacks – for large macropods and wombats, sacks can consist of hessian or green stripe bags (Colquhoun's Pty Ltd, South Australia)
- GPS to record location of animal captures.

Specific qualifications, experience and training

Personnel should have practical experience in capturing and handling large wild animals before attempting to capture animals on their own. Shooters will need to possess a firearms licence (Table 7.2) and must have demonstrated experience in this method before being deemed competent by a more-experienced supervisor. Importantly, the same shooter or shooters should be used for each field trip and each evening. Personnel administering veterinary chemicals will typically need to be working under the direct supervision of a veterinarian or possess accreditation to perform the method (requirements vary by jurisdiction). Ideally, personnel will have completed a chemical immobilisation training course.

Table 7.2: Relevant firearms legislation and codes.

Jurisdiction	Firearms legislation and regulations
Commonwealth	*National Firearms Safety Code 2002*
Victoria	*Victoria Firearms Act 1996* *Firearms Regulations 2018*
Tasmania	*Tasmania Firearms Act 1996* *Firearms Regulations 2016*
South Australia	*South Australia Firearms Act 2015* *Firearms Regulation 2017*
New South Wales	*New South Wales Firearms Act 1996* *Firearms Regulation 2017*
Queensland	*Queensland Weapons Act 1990* *Weapons Regulation 2016*
Western Australia	*Western Australia Firearms Act 1973* *Firearms Regulations 1974*
Australian Capital Territory	*Firearms Act 1996*
Northern Territory	*Firearms Act 1997*

Workplace health and safety

Safety risks include (1) self-injection with immobilisation chemicals; (2) being scratched, bitten or kicked by recumbent animals; and (3) zoonotic hazards, such as urine, faeces, blood- or saliva-borne pathogens (e.g. Q fever). All staff should be trained in appropriate responses to self-injection. Animal handlers should be vaccinated against Q fever, wash hands after captures, and avoid inhaling dust that may be contaminated by animal urine, faeces or birthing fluids. Stunning and netting are low to moderate risk techniques for field biologists. Apart from the risks mentioned above, additional safety risks include (1) tripping over while running in darkness to catch an animal; (2) not holding onto the safety bars and rails available on the vehicle and falling off the back of a very slow (< 10 km h^{-1}) moving or stationary vehicle; and (3) lifting injuries. Being shot is not a risk associated with stunning, as no person should leave the back of the vehicle until the stunning shot is fired.

Alternative procedures

For macropods, alternative procedures may include capture with drawstring or cage traps (see earlier GOPs in this chapter) and immobilisation by darting (Chapter 16). For southern hairy-nosed wombats, stunning provides a substantially increased rate of capture compared to just chasing an animal under spotlight with a net, and both methods have a far superior success rate than that associated with cage trapping wombats. Similarly for European rabbits and kangaroos, without using a shot fired above the animal, capture success with a hand-held net is greatly reduced or near impossible.

FOOTHOLD TRAPPING FOR EUTHERIAN CARNIVORES

Paul D. Meek, Damian S. Morrant and Guy A. Ballard

Target taxa

This GOP applies to eutherian carnivores (see Chapter 22).

Context and scope

Foothold trapping is widely used to capture dingoes, feral dogs, hybrid dogs/dingoes (*Canis* spp.), red foxes and cats in Australia (Meek *et al.* 1995; Meek *et al.* 2018), for control purposes and research. The method involves deploying rubber-lined, off-set jaw traps to capture target species by the front foot where they are tethered until released. Traps are placed in specific locations frequented by the target species (e.g. scent marking stations, resting locations, feeding areas or travel paths). Traps are commonly set along roads, but exact placement depends on species, habitat and season. Consequently, traps may also be set along water courses, fence lines, edges of ploughed fields and animal pads. Animals can be lured to trap-sets with olfactory (scent-based), auditory (sound) or visual lures. Alternatively, experienced investigators can set unlured traps successfully along tracks and pop-holes in fences (Fournier 2011). Foothold traps are generally the most efficacious means of capturing introduced mammalian carnivores for research purposes. These trap types pose a range of risks to captured animals. Recommendations for minimising risks have been described in detail in existing standard operating procedures (SOPs), codes of practice (COPs) and best practice guidelines (BPGs) (Sharp and Saunders 2008; also see Chapter 22), which personnel should familiarise themselves with.

Animal welfare considerations

Foothold trapping may cause high stress and injury to captured animals (Kreeger *et al.*1990; Lossa *et al.* 2007; Marks 2010). It should only be undertaken by experienced practitioners following detailed SOP, legislation and BPG, as noted above.

Physiological stress, exhaustion and dehydration

Capture and restraint by a trap will cause stress to animals (Kreeger *et al.* 1990; White *et al.* 1991; Marks 2010), although common behaviours of trapped animals also include extended periods of resting and sleeping (P. D. Meek, pers. obs.). Approaching trapped animals elevates anxiety and promotes attempts to escape. Risk of injury may be greatest at this time. Captured animals should be restrained and/or sedated promptly or euthanased swiftly where euthanasia is necessary. Where injuries are sustained, post-release myopathy can occur (Cattet *et al.* 2003). Animals caught in foothold traps typically expend energy attempting to escape. Effort varies between species, individuals and can be influenced by seasonal behaviours, such as breeding. Animals can display symptoms of exhaustion and dehydration (Powell 2005) depending on local conditions.

Direct injury

Injury during capture ranges from mild bruising and localised swelling to lacerations, damaged teeth, dislocations, broken bones and, rarely, death (Meek *et al.* 1995; Fleming *et al.* 1998; Marks 2010). Well-maintained traps with appropriate swivels and springs should be used, and traps should be checked as soon as possible after sunrise each day. Irrespective of treatment, released animals may experience post-release soreness, ischaemia and myopathy (Cattet *et al.* 2008), or show no effect (Bubela *et al.* 1998). While these techniques are associated with a low risk of indirect effects, such as exposure or predation, foothold trapping with rubber-lined, off-set jaw traps very rarely results in death (Fleming *et al.* 1998).

Abandonment of young and pack separation

Animals that travel in packs, with mates, siblings or young may be separated during capture, but risk of abandonment is low because most species leave young at dens while foraging. Dependent young could be disadvantaged if a parent is restrained for extended periods. This risk can be minimised by ensuring that traps are checked regularly, including during the breeding season.

Exposure to predation

Although predation of trapped animals (targets and non-targets) by other predators, including wedge-tailed eagles (*Aquila audax*), red foxes, and other canines does occur (Meek and Brown 2017), the occurrence and risk are generally low. Trapping of adults during whelping season might result in an increased risk of predation on juveniles.

General procedures

Preparation

Foothold trapping requires a good understanding of the target species' biology and ecology to ensure selection of appropriate traps sites and lures. Awareness of how animals use their landscape is valuable. Reconnaissance to locate spoor, with and without the aid of sniffer dogs (Chapter 5), and camera trapping can be informative. Detecting relevant animal signs, including that of non-targets, assists in making sound decisions about trap placement to maximise the likelihood of catching the target species, and minimising or removing the possibility of capturing non-target animals. Familiarity with COPs, SOPs and BPGs will ensure trapping programs are undertaken with due diligence. Appropriate trap type and trap fittings specific to capturing the target animal are necessary. Placement of traps must minimise risk of indirect injury to trapped animals during capture escape attempts. Trappers must be experienced and familiar with the safe removal of study animals from foothold traps and safe practices for euthanasia.

Assess exposure risk

Trappers must undertake a risk assessment to ensure all traps can be visited as soon as possible after the animal has been captured. Since this timing is difficult to predict in practice, it often means checking traps as soon as practicable after sunrise and before midday (depending on site weather). Checking traps at those times means that most animals spend few hours in traps because most predators are nocturnal or crepuscular. More frequent checks may be required depending on local conditions. Continually assessing weather conditions before and during trapping programs helps ensure trapped animals are not exposed to heavy rainfall, extreme heat or cold and other dangerous conditions. Trapper servicing of traps within 24 h of setting must be assured – this can mean checking water crossings and monitoring track conditions with respect to wet weather.

Trap choice and maintenance

A wide range of traps is used in Australia (Meek *et al.* 2018). Suggestions that bigger traps are faster and better than smaller traps are unfounded (Meek *et al.* 2019a). Trap type and size should be decided based on the target species and any risks posed by the preferred trap design. In research trapping programs, traps larger than size # 3 and those with four-coil springs are generally too large and over-engineered for safe use. Likewise, long drag chains (> 50 cm) and drags with sharp points tend to promote unacceptable injuries. Traps should be carefully checked and serviced (no sharp edge or burr, intact rubbers, free-moving swivels and operating springs) to ensure no additional risk is posed to animals by the device during capture or restraint in the trap.

Appropriate trap location selection

Traps should be placed to minimise any additional injury or duress from capture. Traps must not be set where risks to captured animals, including non-target species, are likely. Risks such as exposure, drowning, entanglement, puncture wounds, interference by members of the public, pets, guardian animals and insect attack need to be considered. Personnel should avoid setting traps in proximity to obvious ant nests and trails.

Trap devices and alerts

Lethal trap devices and trap alerts can be used in areas where visitation to traps is problematic. Lethal trap devices (Meek *et al.* 2019b) should only be used where animals are not required alive for the study. Trap alerts are intended to enable trap checking to be undertaken remotely (e.g. via satellite) and are triggered irrespective of target or non-target captures (Meek *et al.* 2020). Tranquiliser trap devices (Marks *et al.* 2004) are not used in Australia, but do offer a means of reducing capture stress.

Animal treatment, withdrawal and euthanasia

Deciding when not to trap, or to cease trapping, can be difficult, but is extremely important. When injuries are sustained by an animal during capture and handling, practitioners must decide whether to continue, treat, euthanase or release the animal. Treatment for swelling at the point of capture must be undertaken as soon as the trap is removed (see Chapter 22). Where injuries are severe, euthanasia must be undertaken. Researchers and trappers should be prepared for this eventuation.

Equipment and maintenance

Trapping equipment will vary with practitioners' preferences and study objectives, but would typically include the following:

- suitable traps for the target species and conditions (influenced by relevant jurisdictional legislation and approvals)
- chain assemblies, including heavy duty swivels, in-line springs and stakes or drags
- trap-setting tools
- gloves
- lures
- camera traps
- lethal trap devices or tranquiliser trap devices
- restraining and handling equipment
- rifle and ammunition or other legal means of euthanising animals
- consumables for treatment of captured animals, such as Hirudoid® cream for trapped feet, and chloramide or Cetrigen® sprays for treating minor wounds.
- hand cleaning and other hygiene consumables
- trapping signs
- GPS receiver or suitable phone app for relocating traps
- notebook or similar.

Specific qualifications, experience and training

Foothold trapping for research should not be undertaken without some level of training for the procedure or without direct supervision of a competent trapper. If euthanising animals with a rifle, personnel should hold an appropriate firearms licence (see Table 7.2). Additional competencies may be required to undertake chemical euthanasia, depending on legislation and the governing ethics committee's requirements.

Workplace health and safety

Trapping carnivores poses a range of workplace safety risks for the practitioner and the public, including vehicular accidents, injuries from trapping and animal-handling equipment, injuries from trapped animals and zoonotic diseases during handling, and from euthanasia procedures.

Access

Trapping can be undertaken on roads or off-trail, so road-associated danger exists especially in working forests, rubbish tips, farms or mine sites where machinery can be operating. Quad bikes and side-by-side vehicles are widely used by trapping practitioners; relevant safe work practices must be adhered to.

Trap setting

Trapping related injuries from padded foothold traps are less likely than with steel-jaw traps. Lacerations and bruising can occur to the operator during setting, such as when jaws are triggered accidently. Back injury can occur when attempting to remove trap stakes.

Animal handling

Procedures for removing trapped animals from traps are outlined in Chapter 22, including risks from bites and scratches.

Hygiene

Parasites carried by eutherian carnivores pose serious health risks to practitioners from direct contamination or secondary contamination from trap and equipment handling. Safe work practices must be adopted, disposable nitrile gloves should be used, and soap, water and hand sanitiser should be readily available for washing handling equipment and hands. Handling traps and trap paraphernalia (including lures) with bare hands should be avoided.

Firearms and lethal drugs

Firearms or approved chemicals for lethal injection must be carried with appropriate permissions and licences. Requirements should be discussed with land managers well ahead of trapping programs. Firearms and veterinary chemicals must be stored appropriately, consistently with legislation and protocols.

Alternative procedures

Foothold traps are the most effective means of catching eutherian carnivores for wildlife research that requires direct use of the animal. Alternative, less efficacious methods include cage trapping, snaring, netting and darting. However, these alternatives are not necessarily of lower impact than foothold trapping.

REFERENCES

Barasona JA, López-Olvera JR, Beltrán-Beck B, Gortázar C, Vicente J (2013) Trap-effectiveness and response to tiletamine-zolazepam and medetomidine anaesthesia in Eurasian wild boar captured with cage and corral traps. *BMC Veterinary Research* **9**, 107 http://www.biomedcentral.com/1746-6148/9/107. doi:10.1186/1746-6148-9-107

Bosson CO, Islam Z, Boonstra R (2012) The impact of live trapping and trap model on the stress profiles of North American red squirrels. *Journal of Zoology* **288**, 159–169. doi:10.1111/j.1469-7998.2012.00941.x

Botto Nuñez G, Cunningham A, Bakwo Fils EM, Frick W, Islam Md N, Jolliffe T, Kading R, Kepel A, Kingston T, Leopardi S, Medellín R, Mendenhall I, Parsons S, Racey P, Russo D, Shapiro JT, Vicente-Santos A, Víquez-R L, Vu Dinh T (2020) 'Recommended strategy for researchers to reduce the risk of transmission of SARS-CoV-2 from humans to bats'. IUCN SSC Bat Specialist Group. <https://www.iucnbsg.org/bsg-publications.html>.

Breed D, Meyer LCR, Stey JCA, Goddard A, Burroughs R, Kohn TA (2019) Conserving wildlife in a changing world: understanding capture myopathy – a malignant outcome of stress during capture and translocation. *Conservation Physiology* **7**, coz027. doi:10.1093/conphys/coz027

Bubela T, Bartell R, Muller W (1998) Factors affecting the trappability of red foxes in Kosciusko National Park. *Wildlife Research* **25**, 199–208. doi:10.1071/WR95046

Buddle BM, Aldwell FE, Jowett G, Thomson A, Jackson R, Paterson BM (1992) Influence of stress of capture on haematological values and cellular immune responses in the Australian brushtail possum (*Trichosurus vulpecula*). *New Zealand Veterinary Journal* **40**, 155–159. doi:10.1080/00480169.1992.35721

Cashins SD, Alford RA, Skerratt LF (2008) Lethal effect of latex, nitrile, and vinyl gloves on tadpoles. *Herpetological Review* **39**, 298–301.

Cattet M, Boulanger J, Stenhouse G, Powell RA, Reynolds-Hogland MJ (2008) An evaluation of long-term capture effects in ursids: implications for wildlife welfare and research. *Journal of Mammalogy* **89**, 973–990. doi:10.1644/08-MAMM-A-095.1

Cattet MRL, Christison K, Caulkett NA, Stenhouse GB (2003) Physiologic responses of grizzly bears to different methods of capture. *Journal of Wildlife Diseases* **39**, 649–654. doi:10.7589/0090-3558-39.3.649

Churchill S (2008) *Australian Bats.* 2nd edn. Allen and Unwin, Sydney.

Coates TD (2013) The performance of wombat gates in controlling wildlife movement through a predator fence. *Australian Mammalogy* **35**, 184–187. doi:10.1071/AM12030

Coulson G (1996) A safe and selective draw-string trap to capture kangaroos moving under fences. *Wildlife Research* **23**, 621–627. doi:10.1071/WR9960621

Coulson G, Poiani A, Nave CD (2003) A modified draw-string trap for capture of kangaroos at fences. *Australian Mammalogy* **25**, 177–182. doi:10.1071/AM03177

Cunningham CX, Comte S, McCallum H, Hamilton DG, Hamede R, Storfer A, Hollings T, Ruiz-Aravena M, Kerlin DH, Brook BW, Hocking G, Jones ME (2021) Quantifying 25 years of disease-caused declines in Tasmanian devil populations: host density drives spatial pathogen spread. *Ecology Letters* **24**, 958–969. doi:10.1111/ele.13703

Davis C, Fleming P, Craig MD, Grigg A, Hardy D (2008) A funnel trap for capture of small arboreal reptiles. *Amphibia-Reptilia* **29**, 413–423. doi:10.1163/156853808785112039

DBCA (2018) *Standard Operating Procedure: Dry Pitfall Trapping for Vertebrates and Invertebrates.* Department of Biodiversity, Conservation and Attractions, Perth.

Death CE, Coulson G, Hufschmid J, Morris WK, Gould J, Stevenson M (2019) When less is more: a comparison of models to predict fluoride accumulation in free-ranging kangaroos. *The Science of the Total Environment* **660**, 531–540. doi:10.1016/j.scitotenv.2018.12.203

Diete RL, Dixon KM, Barden PA (2016) Predation of pitfall-trapped rodents by the ghost bat, *Macroderma gigas*. *Australian Mammalogy* **38**, 249–252. doi:10.1071/AM15022

Di Stefano J, Moyle R, Coulson G (2005) A soft-walled, double-layered trap for capture of swamp wallabies *Wallabia bicolor*. *Australian Mammalogy* **27**, 235–238. doi:10.1071/AM05235

Doughty P, Rolfe JK, Burbidge AH, Pearson DJ, Kendrick PG (2011) Herpetological assemblages of the Pilbara biogeographic region, Western Australia: ecological associations, biogeographic patterns and conservation. *Records of the Western Australian Museum* **78**, 315–341. doi:10.18195/issn.0313-122x.78(2).2011.315-341

DPIE (2020) *Saving our Species Hygiene Guidelines: Protocols to Protect Priority Biodiversity Areas in NSW from* Phytophora cinnamomi, *Mmyrtle Rust, Amphibian Chytrid Fungus and Invasive Plants.* Department of Planning, Industry and Environment, Sydney.

DSEWPC (2011a) *Survey Guidelines for Australia's Threatened Mammals. Guidelines for Detecting Mammals Listed as Threatened under the* Environment Protection and Biodiversity Conservation Act 1999. Department of Sustainability, Environment, Water, Population and Communities, Canberra.

DSEWPC (2011b) *Survey Guidelines for Australia's Threatened Reptiles. Guidelines for Detecting Mammals Listed as Threatened under the* Environment Protection and Biodiversity Conservation Act 1999. Department of Sustainability, Environment, Water, Population and Communities, Canberra.

Ellis MV (2016) How hot does it get in a harp trap bag? *Australasian Bat Society Newsletter* **47**, 22–26.

Eyre TJ, Ferguson DJ, Hourigan CL, Smith GC, Mathieson MT, Kelly AL, Venz MF, Hogan LD, Rowland J (2018) *Terrestrial Vertebrate Fauna Survey Assessment Guidelines for Queensland.* Department of Environment and Science, Queensland Government, Brisbane.

Field HE (2018) Evidence of Australian bat lyssavirus infection in diverse Australian bat taxa. *Zoonoses and Public Health* **65**, 742–748. doi:10.1111/zph.12480

Finlayson G, White CR, Dibben RG, Shimmin C, Taggart DA (2010) Activity patterns of the southern hairy-nosed wombat (*Lasiorhinus latifrons*) (Marsupialia: Vombatidae) in the South Australian Murraylands. *Australian Mammalogy* **32**, 39–46. doi:10.1071/AM09024

Fitch HS (1987) Collecting and life-history techniques. In *Snakes: Ecology and Evolutionary Biology.* (Eds RA Seigel, JT Collins, and SS Novak) pp. 143–164. Macmillan Publishing Company, New York, NY.

Fleming PJS, Allen LR, Berghout MJ, Meek PD, Pavlov PM, Stevens P, Strong K, Thompson JA, Thomson PC (1998) The performance of wild-canid traps in Australia: efficiency, selectivity and trap-related injuries. *Wildlife Research* **25**, 327–338. doi:10.1071/WR95066

Fournier G (2011) *Training Guide Canid Trapping and Management.* Federation der Trappeurs Gestionnaires du Quebec, Quebec, Canada.

Francis CM (1989) A comparison of mist nets and two designs of harp traps for capturing bats. *Journal of Mammalogy* **70**, 865–870. doi:10.2307/1381730

Friend GR, Smith GT, Mitchell DS, Dickman CR (1989) Influence of pitfall and drift fence design on capture rates of small vertebrates in semi-arid habitats of Western Australia. *Australian Wildlife Research* **16**, 1–10. doi:10.1071/WR9890001

Garnick S, Coulson G (2020) Population persistence, breeding seasonality and sexual dimorphism in the red-necked wallaby. *Australian Mammalogy.* doi:10.1071/AM19059

Halliday D, Resnick R, Walker J (1993) *Fundamentals of Physics.* 4th edn. John Wiley and Sons Inc, New York, NY.

Hampton JO, Finch NA, Watter K, Amos M, Pople T, Moriarty A, Jacotine A, Panther D, McGhie C, Davies C, Mitchell J, Forsyth DM (2019) A review of methods used to capture and restrain introduced wild deer in Australia. *Australian Mammalogy* **41**, 1–11. doi:10.1071/AM17047

Hill DA, Armstrong KN, Barden PA (2015) Preliminary assessment suggests that acoustic lures can increase capture rates of Australian echolocating bats. *Australian Mammalogy* **37**, 104–106. doi:10.1071/AM14019

How RA, Barnett JL, Bradley AJ, Humphreys WF, Martin R (1984). The biology of *Pseudocheirus peregrinus* in a *Leptospermum laevigatum* thicket. In *Possums and Gliders*. (Eds AP Smith and ID Hume) pp. 261–268. Australian Mammal Society, Sydney.

Iossa G, Soulsbury CD, Harris S (2007) Mammal trapping: a review of animal welfare standards of killing and restraining traps. *Animal Welfare (South Mimms, England)* **16**, 335–352.

Jaremovic RV, Croft DB (1987) Comparison of techniques to determine eastern grey kangaroo home range. *The Journal of Wildlife Management* **51**, 921–930.

Johnson BW (1996) A locking mechanism for Elliott mammal traps to improve capture efficiency. *Wildlife Research* **23**, 119–120. doi:10.1071/WR9960119

Kalko EKV, Handley CO (2001) Neotropical bats in the canopy: diversity, community structure, and implications for conservation. *Plant Ecology* **153**, 319–333. doi:10.1023/A:1017590007861

Keyes BE, Grue CE (1982) Capturing birds with mist nets: a review. *North American Bird Bander* **7**, 2–14.

Kerr GD, Bull CM, Mackay D (2004) Human disturbance and stride frequency in the sleepy lizard (*Tiliqua rugosa*): implications for behavioural studies. *Journal of Herpetology* **38**, 519–526. doi:10.1670/13-04A

King WJ, Wilson ME, Allen T, Festa-Bianchet M, Coulson G (2011) A capture technique for free-ranging eastern grey kangaroos (*Macropus giganteus*) habituated to humans. *Australian Mammalogy* **33**, 47–51. doi:10.1071/AM10029

Kreeger TJ, White PJ, Seal US, Tester JR (1990) Pathological responses of red foxes to foothold traps. *The Journal of Wildlife Management* **54**, 147–160. doi:10.2307/3808915

Langkilde T, Shine R (2006) How much stress do researchers inflict on their study animals? A case study using a scincid lizard, *Eulamprus heatwolei*. *The Journal of Experimental Biology* **209**, 1035–1043. doi:10.1242/jeb.02112

Latham ADM, Davidson B, Warburton B, Yockney I, Hampton JO (2020) Efficacy and animal welfare impacts of novel capture methods for two species of invasive wild mammals in New Zealand. *Animals* **10**, 44. doi:10.3390/ani10010044

Lavelle MJ, Snow NP, Ellis CK, Halseth JM, Glow MP, VanNatta EH, Sanders HN, VerCauteren KC (2019) When pigs fly: reducing injury and flight response when capturing wild pigs. *Applied Animal Behaviour Science* **215**, 21–25. doi:10.1016/j.applanim.2019.03.014

Lazenby BT, Tobler MW, Brown WE, Hawkins CE, Hocking GJ, Hume F, Huxtable S, Iles P, Jones ME, Lawrence C, Thalmann S, Wise P, Williams H, Fox S, Pemberton D (2018) Density trends and demographic signals uncover the long-term impact of transmissible cancer in Tasmanian devils. *Journal of Applied Ecology* **55**, 1368–1379. doi:10.1111/1365-2664.13088

Lemckert F, Brassil T, Kavanagh R, Law B (2006) Trapping small mammals for research and management: how many die and why? *Australian Mammalogy* **28**, 201–207. doi:10.1071/AM06028

Lemos de Sá RM, Glander KE (1993) Capture techniques and morphometrics for the woolly spider monkey, or muriqui (*Brachyteles arachnoides*, E. Geoffroy 1806). *American Journal of Primatology* **29**, 145–153. doi:10.1002/ajp.1350290206

Lowe KW (1989) *The Australian Bird Bander's Manual*. Australian Bird and Bat Banding Schemes and Australian National Parks and Wildlife Service, Canberra.

Lossa G, Soulsbury CD, Harris S (2007) Mammal trapping: a review of animal welfare standards of killing and restraining traps. *Animal Welfare* **16**, 335–352.

Lumsden LF (1989) Predation by a bush rat (*Rattus fuscipes*) of bats captive in a harp trap. *Macroderma* **5**, 41–42.

Lumsden LF, Bennett AF, Silins JE (2002) Location of roosts of the lesser long-eared bat *Nyctophilus geoffroyi* and Gould's wattled bat *Chalinolobus gouldii* in a fragmented landscape in south-eastern Australia. *Biological Conservation* **106**, 237–249. doi:10.1016/S0006-3207(01)00250-6

Marks CA (2010) Haematological and biochemical responses of red foxes (*Vulpes vulpes*) to different capture methods and shooting. *Animal Welfare* **19**, 223–234.

Marks CA, Allen L, Gigliotti F, Busana F, Gonzalez T, Lindeman M, Fisher PM (2004) Evaluation of the trap tranquiliser device (TTD) for improving the humaneness of dingo trapping. *Animal Welfare* **13**, 393–399.

Martín J, Lopéz P (1999) An experimental test of the costs of antipredatory refuge use in the wall lizard, *Podarcis mularis*. *Oikos* **84**, 499–505. doi:10.2307/3546428

McMahon C.R, Wiggins NL, French V, McCallum HI, Bowman DMJS (2013) A report of capture myopathy in the Tasmanian pademelon (*Thylogale billardierii*). *Animal Welfare* **22**, 1–4. doi:10.7120/09627286.22.1.001

Meek PD (2000) The decline and current status of the Christmas Island shrew *Crocidura attentuata trichura* on Christmas Island, Indian Ocean. *Australian Mammalogy* **22**, 43–49. doi:10.1071/AM00043

Meek PD, Ballard GA, Fleming PJS (2018) Techniques and practices of Australian pest animal trappers. *Pacific Conservation Biology* **25**, 257–265. doi:10.1071/PC18044

Meek PD, Brown SC (2017) It's a dog eat dog world: observations of dingo (*Canis familiaris*) cannibalism. *Australian Mammalogy* **39**, 92–94. doi:10.1071/AM16018

Meek PD, Jenkins DJ, Morris B, Ardler AJ, Hawksby RJ (1995) Use of two humane leg-hold traps for catching pest species. *Wildlife Research* **22**, 733–739. doi:10.1071/WR9950733

Meek PD, Shorter K, Falzon G (2019a) Do lethal trap devices threaten foot-hold trap capture efficacy? *International Journal of Pest Management* **65**, 66–71. doi:10.1080/09670874.2018.1462538

Meek PD, Brown SC, Wishart J, Milne H, Aylett P, Humphrys S, Ballard G, Fleming P (2019b) Efficacy of lethal-trap devices to improve the welfare of trapped wild dogs. *Wildlife Research* **46**, 89–95. doi:10.1071/WR18129

Meek P, Ballard G, Milne H, Croft S, Lawson G, Fleming P (2020) Satellite and telecommunication alert system for foot-hold trapping. *Wildlife Research*. doi:10.1071/WR20043

Mitchell JL (2016) *'Corral Trapping Chital Deer (*Axis axis*)'*. FeralFix Services, Charters Towers.

Morellet N, Verheyden H, Angibault JM, Cargnelutti B, Lourtet B, Hewison MAJ (2009) The effect of capture on ranging behaviour and activity of the European roe deer *Capreolus*. *Wildlife Biology* **15**, 278–287. doi:10.2981/08-084

Moriarty AJ (2004) Ecology and environmental impact of Javan rusa deer (*Cervus timorensis russa*) in the Royal National Park. PhD thesis. The University of Western Sydney, Australia.

Moseby KE, Read JL (2001) Factors affecting pitfall capture rates of small ground vertebrates in arid South Australia. II. Optimum pitfall trapping effort. *Wildlife Research* **28**, 61–71. doi:10.1071/WR99058

Munks SA (1991) Ecological energetics and reproduction in the common ringtail possum, *Pseudocheirus peregrinus* (Marsupialia: Phalangeroidea). PhD thesis. The University of Tasmania, Australia.

NHMRC (2014) *A Guide to the Care and Use of Australian Native Mammals in Research and Teaching*. National Health and Medical Research Council, Canberra.

Oliveiraa JM, Destrob ALF, Freitasb MB, Oliveiraa LL (2020) How do pesticides affect bats? – A brief review of recent publications. *Brazilian Journal of Biology*. doi:10.1590/1519-6984.225330

Pahl LI (1987) Survival, age-determination and population age structure of the common ringtail possum, *Pseudocheirus peregrinus*, in a *Eucalyptus* woodland and a *Leptospermum* thicket in southern Victoria. *Australian Journal of Zoology* **35**, 625–639. doi:10.1071/ZO9870625

Pardieck K, Waide RB (1992) Mesh size as a factor in avian community studies using mist nets. *Journal of Field Ornithology* **63**, 250–255. www.jstor.org/stable/4513703.

Pearson DE, Ortega YK, Ruggiero LF (2003) Trap-induced mass declines in small mammals: mass as a population index. *The Journal of Wildlife Management* **67**, 684–691. doi:10.2307/3802675

Petit S, Waudby HP (2012) Standard operating procedures for aluminium box, wire cage, and pitfall trapping, handling, and temporary housing of small wild rodents and marsupials. *Australian Journal of Zoology* **60**, 392–401. doi:10.1071/ZO12102

Pike DA, Croak BM, Webb JK, Shine R (2010) Subtle – but easily reversible – anthropogenic disturbance seriously degrades habitat quality for rock-dwelling reptiles. *Animal Conservation* **13**, 411–418. doi:10.1111/j.1469-1795.2010.00356.x

Powell RA (2005) Evaluating welfare of American black bears (*Ursus americanus*) captured in foot snares and in winter dens. *Journal of Mammalogy* **86**, 1171–1177. doi:10.1644/05-MAMM-A-014R2.1

Prada D, Boyd V, Baker M, Jackson B, O'Dea M (2019) Insights into Australian bat lyssavirus in insectivorous bats of Western Australia. *Tropical Medicine and Infectious Disease* **4**, 46. doi:10.3390/tropicalmed4010046

Procter-Gray E, Ganslosser U (1986) The individual behaviors of Lumholtz's tree-kangaroo: repertoire and taxonomic implications. *Journal of Mammalogy* **67**, 343–352. doi:10.2307/1380888

Ralph CJ, Geupel GR, Pyle P, Martin TE, DeSante DF (1993) *Handbook of Field Methods for Monitoring Landbirds.* United States Department of Agriculture Forest Service, Albany, CA.

Rawlins DR, Handasyde KA (2002) The feeding ecology of the striped possum *Dactylopsila trivirgata* (Marsupialia: Petauridae) in far north Queensland, Australia. *Journal of Zoology* **257**, 195–206. doi:10.1017/S0952836902000808

Read JL, Kearney MR (2016) Too hot to handle? Balancing increased trappabilitiy with capture mortality in hot weather pitfall trapping. *Austral Ecology* **41**, 918–926. doi:10.1111/aec.12384

Roberts MW, Neaves LE, Claassens R, Herbert CA (2010) Darting eastern grey kangaroos: a protocol for free-ranging populations. In *Macropods: The Biology of Kangaroos, Wallabies and Rat-kangaroos.* (Eds G Coulson and MDB Eldridge) pp. 325–339. CSIRO Publishing, Melbourne.

Robertson GG, Gepp B (1982) Capture of kangaroos by 'stunning'. *Australian Wildlife Research* **9**, 393–396. doi:10.1071/WR9820393

Romero LM, Meister CJ, Cyr NE, Kenagy GJ, Wingfield JC (2008) Seasonal glucocorticoid responses to capture in wild free-living mammals. *American Journal of Physiology. Regulatory, Integrative and Comparative Physiology* **294**, R614–R622. doi:10.1152/ajpregu.00752.2007

Runcie MJ (2002) Behaviour and ecology of tropical rock-possums: the rock-haunting possum, *Petropseudes dahli* and the scaly-tailed possum, *Wyulda squamicaudata.* PhD thesis. Northern Territory University, Australia.

Salas LA, Stephens SA (2004) Capture and immobilisation of cuscuses and ringtail possums in Papua New Guinea. *Wildlife Research* **31**, 101–107. doi:10.1071/WR01078

Sawicka J, Fuller A, Fick LG, Hetem RS, Meyer LC (2015) Efficacy of different cooling methods for capture-induced hyperthermia in antelope. *African Journal of Wildlife Research* **45**, 100–110. doi:10.3957/056.045.0111

Scasta JD (2020) Mortality and operational attributes relative to feral horse and burro capture techniques based on publicly available data from 2010–2019. *Journal of Equine Veterinary Science* **86**, 102893. doi:10.1016/j.jevs.2019.102893

Scroggie M, Clemann N (2009) Handling-related tail loss in an endangered skink: incidence, correlates and a possible solution. *Journal of Zoology* **277**, 214–220. doi:10.1111/j.1469-7998.2008.00528.x

Sharp T (2005) *'GOA004: Trapping of Feral Goats'.* Invasive Animals Cooperative Research Centre, Canberra.

Sharp T (2012) *'PIG001: Trapping of Feral Pigs'.* Invasive Animals Cooperative Research Centre, Canberra.

Sharp T, Saunders G (2008) *A Model for Assessing the Relative Humaneness of Pest Animal Control Methods.* 2nd edn. Australian Government Department of Agriculture, Fisheries and Forestry, Canberra.

Shepherd RCH, Noland IF, Edmonds JW (1978) A review of methods to capture live wild rabbits in Victoria. *The Journal of Wildlife Management* **42**, 179–184. doi:10.2307/3800710

Spotswood EN, Goodman KR, Carlisle J, Cormier RL, Humple DL, Rousseau J, Guers SL, Barton GG (2012) How safe is mist netting? Evaluating the risk of injury and mortality to birds. *Methods in Ecology and Evolution* **3**, 29–38. doi:10.1111/j.2041-210X.2011.00123.x

Spraker TR (1993) Stress and capture myopathy in artiodactylids. In *Zoo and Wild Animal Medicine: Current Therapy 3.* (Ed ME Fowler) pp. 481–488. WB Saunders, Philadelphia, PA.

Sweitzer RA, Gonzales BJ, Gardner IA, Vuren D, Waithman JD, Boyce WM (1997) A modified panel trap and immobilization technique for capturing multiple wild pig. *Wildlife Society Bulletin* **25**, 699–705.

Taggart DA, Finlayson GR, Richings NM, Shimmin G, Dibben R, Adcock J, Temple-Smith PD (2003) Environmental factors affecting the capture of southern hairy-nosed wombats (*Lasiorhinus latifrons*) by stunning. *Wildlife Research* **30**, 539–546. doi:10.1071/WR01105

Taggart DA, Steele VR, Schultz D, Temple-Smith PD (1998) Semen collection and cryopreservation in the southern hairy-nosed wombat (*Lasiorhinus latifrons*): implications for the conservation of the northern hairy-nosed wombat (*Lasiorhinus krefftii*). In *Wombats in Australia.* (Ed R Wells) pp. 195–206, Surrey Beatty and Sons Ltd, Sydney.

Tasker EM, Dickman CR (2001) A review of Elliott trapping methods for small mammals in Australia. *Australian Mammalogy* **23**, 77–87. doi:10.1071/AM01077

Thompson GG, Thompson SA (2007) Usefulness of funnel traps in catching small reptiles and mammals, with comments on the effectiveness of the alternatives? *Wildlife Research* **34**, 491–497. doi:10.1071/WR06081

Thompson GG, Thompson SA (2009) Comparative temperature in funnel and pit traps. *Australian Journal of Zoology* **57**, 311–316. doi:10.1071/ZO09052

Thompson SA, Thompson GG (2005) Temporal variation in reptile assemblages in the Goldfields of Western Australia. *Journal of the Royal Society of Western Australia* **8**, 25–36.

Thompson SA, Thompson GG, Withers PC (2005) Influence of pit-trap type on the interpretation of fauna diversity. *Wildlife Research* **32**, 131–137. doi:10.1071/WR03117

Tidemann CR, Loughland RA (1993) A harp trap for large megachiropterans. *Wildlife Research* **20**, 607–611. doi:10.1071/WR9930607

Tidemann CR, Woodside DP (1978) A collapsible bat-trap and a comparison of results obtained with the trap and with mist-nets. *Australian Wildlife Research* **5**, 355–362. doi:10.1071/WR9780355

Vogelnest L, Woods R (2008) *Medicine of Australian Mammals.* CSIRO Publishing, Melbourne.

Ward-Fear G, Brown GP, Pearson DJ, West A, Rollins LA, Shine R (2018) The ecological and life history correlates of boldness in free-ranging lizards. *Ecosphere* **9**, e02125. doi:10.1002/ecs2.2125

Waudby HP, Petit S, Gill MJ (2019) The scientific, financial and ethical implications of three common wildlife-trapping designs. *Wildlife Research* **46**, 690–700. doi:10.1071/WR19084

Webb M (2018) *Wild rock-ringtail possums and my zenith moments.* <http://www.myfanwywebb.com/story-5-wild-rock-ringtail-possums-and-my-zenith-moments-7-min-read/>.

White PJ, Kreeger TJ, Seal US, Tester JR (1991) Pathological responses of red foxes to capture in box traps. *The Journal of Wildlife Management* **55**, 75–80. doi:10.2307/3809243

Whitworth D, Newman S, Mundkur T, Harris P (2007) *Wild Birds and Avian Influenza: An Introduction to Applied Field Research and Disease Sampling Techniques.* FAO Animal Production and Health, Food and Agriculture Organisation of the United Nations, Rome, Italy.

Wildlife Health Australia (2018) *National Wildlife Biosecurity Guidelines.* Wildlife Health Australia, Sydney.

Wildlife Health Australia (2020a) Personal protective equipment (PPE) information for bat handlers. <https://wildlifehealthaustralia.com.au/Portals/0/Documents/ProgramProjects/PPE_Info_for_Bat_Handlers.pdf>.

Wildlife Health Australia (2020b) *COVID-19 and Australian bats – information for bat carers, researchers and others interacting with bats.* Wildlife Health Australia. <https://www.wildlifehealthaustralia.com.au/Portals/0/Documents/ProgramProjects/COVID-19_Aust_bat_carers_researchers_Oct2020.pdf>.

Willson JD, Gibbons W (2009) Drift fences, coverboards, and other traps. In *Amphibian Ecology and Conservation: A Handbook of Techniques.* (Ed. CK Dodd Jr) pp. 229–245. Oxford University Press, Oxford, UK.

Wilson ME, Coulson G, Shaw G, Renfree MB (2013) Deslorelin implants in free-ranging female eastern grey kangaroos (*Macropus giganteus*): mechanism of action and contraceptive efficacy. *Wildlife Research* **40**, 403–412. doi:10.1071/WR13050

Winning G, King J (2007) A new trap design for capturing squirrel gliders and sugar gliders. *Australian Mammalogy* **29**, 245–249. doi:10.1071/AM07029

8 Wildlife marking methods

Helen P. Waudby, Phoebe A. Burns, Melissa A. Jensen, Jordan O. Hampton, David Hunter, Donald T. McKnight, Angela J. L. Pestell, Andrew J. Bengsen, Deborah Bower, Graeme Coulson, Geoffrey Heard, Alana de Laive, Chris J. Jolly, Susannah Hale, Bronwyn A. Fancourt, Shannon R. Kelleher, Sophie Petit, Linda Behrendorff, Lindy F. Lumsden and Mel McGregor

INTRODUCTION

This chapter details techniques to mark mammals, reptiles, and amphibians permanently or semi-permanently. All marking methods cause some level of stress and pain to animals. The benefit of one method over another is context and species-specific, and often the greatest effects on animal welfare are associated with the handling of animals for marking rather than the marking procedure itself. Contentious methods (e.g. toe or toe-bud clipping of small mammals) that are still used for some purposes (e.g. Fisher and Blomberg 2009) are not covered in this chapter. Their use for these taxa is likely to dwindle as less-invasive methods are developed and adopted (Jung *et al.* 2020). Bird and bat banding is subject to existing regulatory and best practice guidelines, and overseen by a national regulatory body (www.environment.gov.au/science/bird-and-bat-banding), so is not covered in this chapter (but see Chapter 15 for an overview of marking methods for birds and Chapter 23 for details on banding bats). Researchers should evaluate carefully the need for permanent marking, particularly if tissue collection is unnecessary. If recaptures are expected to be low between sessions (i.e. over time), then these techniques may not contribute sufficient data for some types of capture–mark–recapture (CMR) analyses, although some form of marking is advisable even if it is simply to identify and avoid reprocessing recaptured animals. In these cases, very low impact non-permanent techniques, including marking tails, ears or ventral surfaces with a permanent marker, painting claws with nail polish or correction fluid, or trimming a small amount of fur, may be appropriate instead. However, the potential toxicity of materials for small animals should be considered.

MICROCHIPPING MAMMALS, REPTILES AND AMPHIBIANS

Melissa A. Jensen, Alana de Laive, Chris J. Jolly, Deborah S. Bower and Lindy F. Lumsden

Target taxa

This general operating procedure (GOP) applies to monotremes (Chapter 17), dasyurids (Chapter 18), wombats, bandicoots, bilbies, possums and gliders (Chapter 19), eutherian carnivores (Chapter 22), bats (Chapter 23), rodents (Chapter 24), reptiles (Chapter 26) and amphibians (Chapter 27).

Context and scope

This GOP describes the permanent marking of a range of taxa with passive integrated transponder (PIT) tags or microchips via subcutaneous insertion (referred to as microchips or microchipping throughout). It applies to mammals, amphibians, and reptiles (refer to Chapters 12 and 13 for an overview of some marking methods for fishes and marine mammals). Typically, microchipping is not the preferred method for marking wild birds (except for some species, such as penguins) and is not covered here (see Chapter 15 for a review of bird marking methods). Microchipping is used for long-term population monitoring and CMR studies where individual identification of recaptured animals is required. Small microchips that transmit a unique number when scanned are implanted under the skin, using a hypodermic needle. Anaesthetisation of the animal is generally unnecessary, meaning that animals can be marked in the field. This technique allows for long-term individual identification of recaptured animals in the hand, or when an animal passes under or through mounted automatic scanning plates or rings deployed in the field (Mali and Forstner 2014). The application of microchips subcutaneously is generally appropriate for most wildlife species in Australia. The application of microchips intramuscularly or into the body cavity is not covered in this GOP.

PIT tags are electronic microchips encased in biocompatible glass or plastic. The casing protects the electronic components and prevents tissue irritation (Gibbons and Andrews 2004). Brands used routinely in Australia are available in two sizes (e.g. Trovan® produces a microchip measuring 11.5 mm long with a 2.12-mm diameter, and a smaller 'midi' microchip measuring 8 mm long with a 1.4-mm diameter) to suit animals of different sizes. Once inserted, microchips have little to no effect on the behaviour, appearance, growth rate, mating performance, predator susceptibility, or swimming speed of tagged individuals, and can operate for a long period and under a range of environmental conditions (Jemison *et al.* 1995; Gibbons and Andrews 2004; Mellor *et al.* 2004). However, microchips are not without their limitations, including their high purchase cost, which may render them impractical for marking large numbers of individuals, their low detection distance, incompatibility between some brands of tags and scanners, their ability to move around the body of large animals, and their potential to be lost altogether by falling out immediately following insertion or later expulsion (e.g. Roark and Dorcus 2000).

Microchipping is an effective long-term marking technique, and the preferred marking technique for platypus, bandicoots and bilbies, for which other marking techniques are generally unsuitable (Chapters 17 and 19, respectively DBCA 2017; Arid Recovery 2019). Microchipping is also a useful technique for long-term remote monitoring of microbats, via detection by readers set at roost entrances such as bat boxes (e.g. Godinho *et al.* 2015), or in caves (van Harten *et al.* 2019) (see Chapter 23). Microchipping is not always preferred for marking reptiles and amphibians, as other less expensive and equally effective means of identification (see other GOPs in this chapter) are available (Jemison *et al.* 1995; Ferner and Plummer 2016). Also, the ability of some reptile and possibly amphibian species to expel microchips (Roark and Dorcus 2000) may make microchipping unsuitable for these taxa. Nevertheless, this method can be an effective, long-lasting means of marking most reptile and amphibian species – in general, microchips should have a long residence time beneath the skin of most reptiles and amphibians when following taxon-specific tagging procedures (Brown 1997).

Animal welfare considerations

Risks and limitations

Microchipping, although generally safe and quick, is invasive, requiring penetration of the skin, and will cause some pain during the application process. Microchips can be inserted into both adult and juvenile animals (including furred marsupial pouch young), provided that the microchip-to-body-mass ratio does not exceed 10% in very small animals (Mellor *et al.* 2004; DBCA 2017). Microchips have a low risk of side effects, but they do occur occasionally. If subcutaneous blood vessels are accidentally struck with the applicator needle, haemorrhage is possible. While they appear to be rare, lethal outcomes are also possible, including fatal intravascular blood clot formation if microchips are accidentally injected into arteries, or neoplasia (cancers) of a certain type (sarcomas) that can occur because of an immune system response. One international study reports accidental arterial microchip insertion causing obstruction of the iliac artery in a Chilean flamingo (*Phoenicopterus chilensis*; Olds *et al.* 2016). Another described the development of an aggressive sarcoma associated with a microchip in an Egyptian fruit bat (*Rousettus aegyptiacus*; Siegal-Willott *et al.* 2007).

General procedures

Equipment preparation

Several types of microchips are produced by multiple manufacturers. For most types, a needle containing the microchip is removed from the sterile packaging and screwed into a non-sterile applicator, with personnel advised to keep the needle capped until ready for use. Personnel then scan the needle with the scanner to ensure the microchip works and record the microchip number.

Microchip packaging contains stickers labelled with the microchip number. These stickers can be applied to data sheets and sample tubes.

Microchipping procedure

Handling techniques differ depending on the species or taxon being microchipped. Once the animal has been restrained appropriately (see the relevant species chapters in Section 3), personnel should scan the animal to ensure that it does not already have a microchip. As microchips can move around the body, sometimes it is appropriate to scan the whole animal. The animal should be held securely in a cloth handling bag (or other taxon-specific restraint) with the target area exposed, preferably with the head and rest of the body covered. Except for amphibians, personnel should disinfect the target area with a povidone–iodine solution or alcohol swab. See below for specific methods for preparing amphibians. The animal should be held gently, but firmly so that it cannot move if startled. Depending on the species being microchipped, microchipping may be easier with two people: one to restrain the animal and another to insert the microchip.

Typically, the needle should be inserted towards the animal's head, but insertion methods may be taxon-specific (see the species chapters in Section 3 to confirm direction of insertion). For most species, personnel can lift the loose skin at the microchip insertion location until it resembles a tent (see Table 8.1 for general recommendations on insertion locations). For all species, the needle should be kept parallel to the animal's body to ensure that the microchip remains under the skin and does not enter the body cavity. Once the needle has passed through the skin and entered the subcutaneous space, personnel should depress the plunger on the applicator to insert the microchip. Some people choose to rotate the needle 180° before depressing the plunger (DBCA 2017). To ensure that the microchip does not come out as the needle is removed, personnel should feel for the microchip using the fingers and hold the skin around it while gently removing the needle (with the plunger still depressed). Needles should be disposed of in a sharps container. Tissue adhesive may be used to close the insertion point (Pyke 2005; DBCA 2017; Recio *et al.* 2019; van Harten *et al.* 2020). When microchipping mammals, personnel should inspect the fur around the insertion site to ensure that the microchip has not come out. The animal should be allowed to move freely about the handling bag and then scanned to ensure the microchip is transmitting correctly. Animals can usually be released immediately.

The reading range of microchips (i.e. how close the reader must be to the microchip to detect it) depends on several factors, including size and orientation of the tag, type and brand of the microchip and reader, and species' morphology and individual body condition, with a more-robust body condition increasing the required read distance (Davenport *et al.* 2011). In general, handheld readers have a reading range of ~5 cm. The small transmission distance of microchips means that this marking technique generally requires the animal to be recaptured to scan and identify it (unless automated systems are in place). Recent advances in the use of high-performance tags and a large (15 m long) loop antennae have resulted in the ability to detect

Table 8.1: General guide to appropriate taxon-specific implantation sites for microchips.

Taxa	Implantation site
Mammals	Subcutaneously between the scapula (shoulder blades)
Snakes	Subcutaneously between lateral scales, typically just anterior to the cloaca (i.e. in the side of the snake just in front of the cloaca)
Lizards	Subcutaneously between lateral scales, typically just anterior to the hind limb (i.e. in the side of the lizard just in front of the hind limb)
Freshwater turtles	Subcutaneously into the hind limb, parallel with the femur
Sea turtles	Subcutaneously into a flipper
Crocodiles	Subcutaneously under scutes, typically in the base of the tail or in the neck. The fore limb is another appropriate implantation site that may limit movement of tags (Manolis and Webb 2016)
Frogs	Subcutaneously, typically in the lateral region just anterior to the hind limb (i.e. in the side of the frog just in front of the hind limb)
Tadpoles	Tadpoles are typically not microchipped, but VIA tags can be inserted subcutaneously, usually in the lateral region just anterior to the tail base (i.e. in the side of the tadpole just anterior to the tail base)

bats flying 1 m either side of an 8 m^2 vertical detection plane within a cave, logging over 1.4 million unique detections over a three-year period (van Harten *et al.* 2019).

Microchipping mammals

Mammals can be microchipped in many ways. For large mammals, like dingoes (*Canis dingo*), some personnel will fold the dorsal shoulder skin over away from the head and insert the needle into the fold. As the skin comes back, the microchip is left where it was inserted. However, to microchip most mammal species, personnel can use one hand to lift the loose skin between the shoulder blades so that it resembles a tent, as per standard practice for general subcutaneous injections (Chapter 16). Using the other hand, the needle is uncapped and gently but firmly pushed through the skin at the base of the tent. Skin texture and thickness can vary among mammal species. For example, the skin of the greater bilby (*Macrotis lagotis*) is thin and can tear easily, while bandicoots tend to have relatively thick skin, which can be tough to puncture. Personnel must ensure that they do not push the needle too far, puncturing the skin on the other side of the tent (resulting in a double puncture). However, the needle must be inserted so that the microchip is inserted subcutaneously, rather than into the animal's skin (intradermal injection), which is associated with strong resistance when the plunger of the applicator is pushed. For specific advice on microchipping monotremes, see Chapter 17.

Microchipping reptiles (lizards, snakes, turtles and crocodiles)

Handling techniques for reptiles are often species-specific (e.g. tubes for venomous elapids, head and leg restraint for large varanids, *Varanus* spp.) and should only be attempted by experienced personnel or those under supervision of an experienced handler. Tagging of very large reptiles will almost certainly require two or more people. Inserting microchips subcutaneously is best practice for most reptile species. Doing so reduces the risk of injury, microchip loss via expulsion and microchips migrating beyond the detection distance of the reader within the body cavity. Personnel can use one hand to lift the skin away from the underlying muscle gently, and using the other hand insert the needle through the skin.

Microchipping amphibians

Generally, amphibians with a snout–vent length of ≥ 40 mm can be microchipped (Pyke 2005). Adult amphibians (frogs and toads) are usually restrained by holding the fully extended hind limbs together with one hand. Amphibian skin is often thin and can tear easily. The injection location for most adult amphibians is just anterior to where the hind limb meets the body, along the lateral body surface (Table 8.1). Personnel should dry and disinfect the target area by swabbing it with a benzalkonium–lidocaine solution such as Bactine®. Ideally, microchips in amphibians should be inserted subcutaneously. With forefinger and thumb, personnel can gently lift the skin away from the underlying muscle and insert the needle through the skin. Subcutaneous microchips can be moved below the surface of the skin with gentle pressure. Microchips should be encouraged to move away from the injection point, so they are not expelled via this opening. Tissue adhesive can be used to seal the wound, but great care should be taken when applying tissue glue to frogs, applying only a very small amount. Larval amphibians (i.e. tadpoles) tend to be too small to microchip. If tadpoles need to be individually identifiable, smaller visible implant alphanumeric (VIA) tags can be used (Courtois *et al.* 2013) as can visible implant elastomer. These marks are inserted subcutaneously into the lateral body of tadpoles, just anterior to the tail base, in much the same way microchips are inserted into amphibians (see later GOPs in this chapter).

Post-procedure monitoring (all species)

Following microchipping, personnel should monitor the animal for signs of distress. Momentary distress as the needle is inserted can be expected for most species, but continued distress is abnormal. Once the animal is moving normally it can be released.

Animal treatment, withdrawal, and euthanasia

Animals should be monitored continuously for signs of distress. If bleeding occurs, personnel should apply gentle pressure and monitor the animal until the bleeding stops, absorbing excess blood with a gauze before disinfection (if desired) and release. If excessive bleeding or injury occurs following microchipping, advice should be sought from a wildlife veterinarian. On very rare occasions, microchipping may cause serious injury or death, usually because of human error (Olds *et al.* 2016). Only experienced personnel, or those under direct supervision of experienced personnel, should undertake

Table 8.2: Suggested equipment and materials for marking mammals, reptiles and amphibians with microchips.

Marking equipment	Data collection	Post-marking
• Microchip in sterile packaging in appropriate size for target species • Microchip applicator • Microchip scanner (note: not all scanners can read all microchip brands) • Handling bags • Disinfectant for insertion site (alcohol swab, povidone–iodine solution or Bactine®)	• Clipboard and datasheets or electronic database	• Gauze • Tissue glue • Sharps container • Wound disinfectant appropriate for the taxon, if desired

this marking technique. Species prone to capture myopathy should be identified before microchipping and the time taken to restrain and microchip the animal considered.

Equipment and maintenance

Suggested equipment required for microchipping animals is listed in Table 8.2.

Specific qualifications, experience, or training

Researchers should be familiar with the species or similar taxa, comfortable with handling and restraining the species, and aware of signs of excessive agitation relevant to the species. Researchers should be trained in the use of the microchip applicator and supervised by an experienced researcher until deemed competent. Participation in a microchipping course may be advantageous, but is not a replacement for additional training in the field under the guidance of an experienced researcher.

Workplace health and safety

Microchipping is associated with the risk of needlestick injury. Needles are to remain capped when not in use. Appropriate first aid should be applied in the case of injury. All needles are single use and are disposed of in a sharps container immediately after use.

Alternative procedures

Alternative techniques will vary among taxa, but may include ear tagging, ear or scute notching or clipping, tattooing, ventral scale clipping, toe clipping (see other GOPs in this chapter) or photographic identification. If permanent marking is not required, less-invasive methods, such as marking with non-toxic marker pens or hair trimming, may suffice.

EAR TAGGING LARGE MAMMALS

Jordan O. Hampton, Andrew J. Bengsen, Graeme Coulson, Angela J.L. Pestell and Linda Behrendorff

Target taxa

This GOP applies to wombats (Chapter 19), koalas (Chapter 20), macropods (Chapter 21), eutherian carnivores (Chapter 22) and ungulates (Chapter 24).

Context and scope

This GOP describes the application of ear tags for marking large-bodied mammals, so that they can be identified during recapture or re-sighting activities. Ear tags provide a long-term marking method that can be useful for demographic, movement and behavioural studies. Tags are usually marked with unique alphanumeric codes that allow individuals to be identified visually. Combinations of tag colour, size and shape can be used to denote specific individuals, groups or cohorts of animals for easy identification from a distance. Adhesive reflective material in matching colours can also be affixed to tags to assist location and identification by spotlight at night. Sex recognition is often facilitated by applying tags on different ears for females and males. Tags can also carry radio transmitters that emit signals on a unique frequency for different individuals (typically VHF frequencies) or unique identification data via radio-frequency identification (RFID). Large tags can carry global positioning system (GPS) loggers that collect and store movement data. Some tag-mounted GPS loggers can transmit these data for collection via mobile data networks or radio transmitters.

Two-piece plastic livestock ear tags, or swivel tags, are most commonly used for large mammals. A two-piece tag comprises a tag or round button with a stud that pierces the outer ear (pinna) and locks into a hole in the main tag on the other side of the pinna (Figure 8.1). These tags are available in a range of sizes. In ungulates, the main tag,

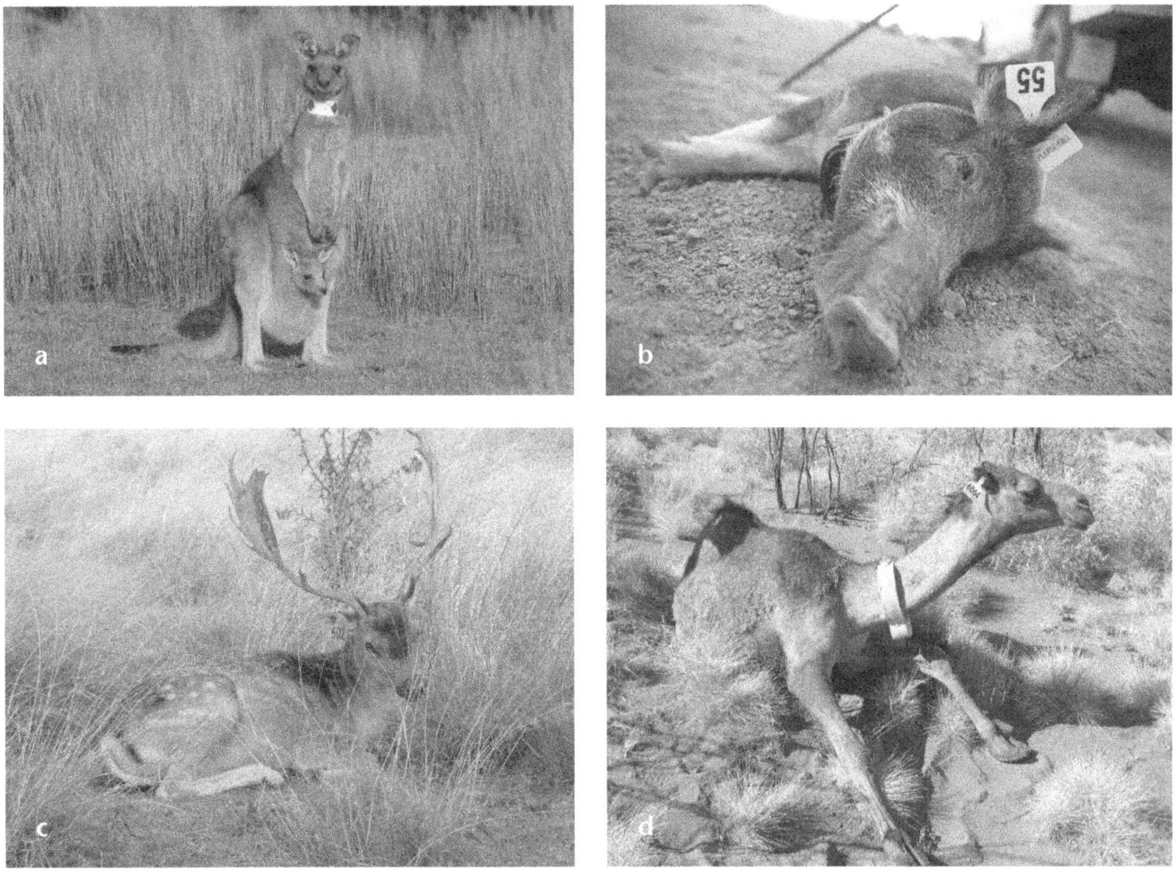

Figure 8.1: Individually marked ear tags applied to (a) an eastern grey kangaroo (*Macropus giganteus*) (photo by Graeme Coulson); (b) a wild pig (*Sus scrofa*) (photo by Andrew Hull); (c) a fallow deer (*Dama dama*) (photo by Michael Featherstone); and (d) a wild camel (*Camelus dromedarius*) (photo by Jordan Hampton).

which is the most visible part, is positioned on the anterior surface of the pinna. Macropod pinnae are carried higher and are more mobile, so the smaller tag is normally positioned on the anterior part of the pinna with the larger tag on the posterior side. For dingoes, tags sit on the anterior surface of the pinna. One or both tags are usually marked with an individual identification code and can also carry written information such as contact details (Figure 8.1b). Large plastic tags allow the identification code to be read from a distance, enabling animals to be identified without physical handling.

Folding one-piece tags are occasionally used to mark large mammals, but are used more commonly for small mammals (see 'Ear tagging small mammals' later in this chapter). These tags comprise a single piece of plastic or metal that forms a loop through the pinna. They are smaller than most two-piece tags and generally require the animal to be recaptured for the identification code to be read. They are not recommended for large mammals because they usually have lower retention rates and present a greater risk of injury to the ear than two-piece tags.

Animal welfare considerations

Ear tags are quick and simple to apply relative to other long-term marking procedures, such as telemetry collars, tattoos and brands. Ear tag application is an invasive procedure, but it does not usually cause prolonged distress and is rarely considered a major intervention. Ear tags are not known to affect the survival or behaviour of wild mammals after the initial period of discomfort. Nonetheless, poorly applied tags can affect animal welfare adversely and some types of tags are more likely to cause harm than others.

Tag application

In addition to the distress caused by capture and handling, piercing of the outer ear will cause short-term pain. Pain and stress may be increased if the interlocking parts of the tag are not properly aligned during application, resulting in longer handling time, or if large blood vessels or cartilage ridges are damaged from poor placement. The ear must be held securely to ensure that it does not fold during application. For eutherian carnivores, a biopsy hole, sometimes made while the animal is sedated (see Chapters 16 and 22) and before tag insertion, will reduce most issues involving misaligned tag application. Studies of animal welfare outcomes in domestic livestock have shown that two-piece tags are often easier to insert and produce fewer signs of distress at the time of application (e.g. Johnston and Edwards 1996; Edwards *et al.* 2001) than do folding one-piece tags.

Infection and sagging

The wound created when the pinna is pierced during tag application may become infected. This risk can be reduced by cleaning the pinna before piercing with topical antiseptic solution (e.g. povidone–iodine) and dipping the stud in antiseptic before application. Injectable antibiotics are rarely used in this instance and the efficacy of doing so is unknown. Tags that are too heavy for the animal's ear or misplaced may cause sagging of the ear, which may be aggravating for the animal; tag selection must consider the integrity of the ear and life-stage of the animal. For dingoes, puncturing the ear with a biopsy needle (while the animal is sedated) and treating the wound may reduce infection rate.

Long-term ear damage and tag loss

In the longer term, the tag can tear the pinna if the tagged animal tries to remove it (self-trauma) or a conspecific grips it (i.e. through aggressive interactions, such as biting behaviour in pigs; intraspecific fighting; or if it becomes snagged on a foreign object, such as vegetation or fencing). This risk may be exacerbated if the pinna becomes infected because of poor hygiene or processes during tag application. Similarly, if the tag does not swivel freely and skin remains snagged, it is more likely to become infected.

All ear tag types are prone to becoming snagged or otherwise lost, but simple two-piece tags usually have high (> 90%) retention rates in ungulates. An evaluation of ear tag retention in a large sample (n = 3844) of free-ranging white-tailed deer (*Odocoileus virginianus*) reported a 96% annual retention rate for large two-piece plastic ear tags, whereas one-piece folding metal tags had a 91% retention rate (Belser *et al.* 2017). Tags burdened with bulky transmitters often have comparatively low retention rates (e.g. 62% in feral horses, *Equus cabbalus*; Kluever *et al.* 2012). Tag loss also has implications for the experimental design of studies because it violates the assumptions of demographic models, producing biased parameter estimates. One-piece tags should not be applied to animals whose pinnae are not fully developed because they will hinder growth if they are applied tightly, or pose a high risk of becoming snagged if they are applied loosely to allow for future growth.

General procedures

Equipment selection

The tags and tag applicator should be suitable for the task required. Larger tags provide greater visibility and readability, but may be more prone to snagging or loss in some situations. Larger tags are also more likely to cause ears to droop or collapse, particularly in smaller species (e.g. wallabies) and younger animals. Tags can be trimmed to suit smaller animals, such as pouch young, or sit on the anterior surface of the pinna without hindering most animals. Brightly coloured or high-contrast tags are more visible to researchers and wildlife managers, but may also make animals more visible to hunters or predators. All parts of the tagging system must be compatible. Anterior and posterior sections of two-piece tags must match, and the applicator must be suitable for the type of tag. Investigators must read the instructions for the system selected and test the equipment before capturing animals.

Tag application

Correct tag application will reduce the severity of harm to tagged animals while maximising tag retention and readability. Broadly, the tagging process is as follows:

- The tag is loaded into the applicator following the instructions for the system being used; personnel check the alignment by lightly squeezing the applicator together.
- The tag stud is disinfected by spraying or dipping the applicator and tag stud into a disinfectant solution (e.g. povidone–iodine; chlorhexidine). The applicator or tag is kept clean and does not touch soil or potentially contaminated material.
- The animal is restrained or sedated (see Chapter 16) and its head secured to prevent unnecessary movement, following appropriate restraint procedures.
- The application site is identified; it should be close to the base of the pinna and located away from large blood

vessels and cartilage ridges (these should be visible and palpable). The site is cleaned of debris before being wiped with disinfectant solution. It may be necessary to part the fur of species with furry ears, such as koalas (*Phascolarctos cinereus*). A small torch, held against the outer part of the ear, can be used to highlight large blood vessels.

- Most ear tags are self-piercing. However, if a tissue sample is desired (e.g. for DNA analysis), a biopsy punch or tissue collection system (e.g. Allflex® Tissue Sampling Unit) can first be used to pierce the pinna before the tag is applied through the resulting hole. Bare-nosed wombats (*Vombatus ursinus*) and dingoes have particularly thick pinnae, so a biopsy tool must be used first to allow a tag to penetrate the ear.
- The loaded applicator is positioned over the application site. For ungulates, the stud is placed behind the ear and the main tag at the front, with the identification code facing forward (anteriorly). The position of the stud and main tag is reversed for macropods.
- The applicator is squeezed until the tag snaps together, then released and removed. The tagging process usually displaces some tissue, which can be collected as a simple alternative to tissue sampling.
- The tag is checked to ensure that it has snapped together properly, and the site inspected for any unexpected damage. The tag should also be checked so that it swivels freely by removing any fur caught in the tag before releasing the animal or moving on to the next procedure. Sedated animals should be placed with their tagged ear towards the ground to prevent pooling of fluid or blood (if any is present).

Animal treatment, withdrawal and euthanasia

Ear tag application is unlikely to cause harm that would require major treatment or euthanasia. Excessive bleeding from ear tag application should be treated by applying pressure to the site with clean, absorbent material. Sedated animals are laid with the tagged ear down after the procedure. Tags are not applied to ears that are compromised by existing injuries, such as large tears or haematomas. Animals should not be burdened with excessively large tags that may cause the ear to collapse or sag.

Equipment and maintenance

Equipment required for ear tag application includes ear tags (ensure that more than are required are kept on hand), an applicator (including a spare), gloves, antiseptic and disinfectant. A biopsy punch, fine forceps and sample tubes, or a self-contained tissue sampling unit, will be required if tissue is to be collected for DNA analysis, as well as up-to-date paperwork pertaining to the specific project that details tags and numbers already administered. Depending on the study objectives, it may be most efficient to have separate tags and applicators ready to apply to males and females.

Specific qualifications, experience and training

Personnel performing the procedure unsupervised should have demonstrated experience handling the target or similar species, and experience in applying ear tags to them. Inexperienced personnel should be supervised closely until deemed competent and should practise the method on a carcass or other non-living substrate before attempting it on live animals.

Workplace health and safety

Ear tag application requires handlers to place their hands on an animal's head; doing so increases the risk of being bitten or scratched or suffering crush injuries to hands from sudden violent movements of animals with large heads (e.g. horses). It can also expose handlers to zoonotic hazards, such as blood- or saliva-borne pathogens (e.g. Q fever). Handlers should follow appropriate sanitisation protocols. For some species, such as koalas and wombats, personnel may wear leather gauntlets that cover their forearms up to the elbows to reduce the risk of being scratched by the species' sharp claws. Restraining boards may be used for non-sedated dingoes (see Chapter 22). Other hazards arising from capture, restraint and handling of wild animals (e.g. kick injuries) also apply and should be assessed for risk during the study's planning phase.

Alternative procedures

Ear tags provide a well-established, reliable method for long-term marking of animals, but less-invasive alternatives are sometimes appropriate. Paints, dyes and fur trimming can be used if short-lived markings are sufficient. Naturally occurring marks, such as coat patterns or prominent scarring can sometimes be used as long-term marks, but these marks must be obvious and consistent over time. Broad neck bands or collars marked with individual patterns or identification codes have also been used to identify eastern grey kangaroos (*Macropus giganteus*) (e.g. Mulder *et al.* 2010; Figure 8.1a).

EAR TAGGING SMALL MAMMALS

Phoebe A. Burns, Melissa A. Jensen and Susannah Hale

Target taxa

This GOP applies to some dasyurid species (Chapter 18), larger bandicoots, possums and gliders (Chapter 19), small potoroids (Chapter 21) and rodents (Chapter 24).

Context and scope

This GOP describes the marking of small- to medium-sized mammals by ear tagging. It applies to mammals ranging from the smallest marsupials and rodents to medium-sized species such as brushtail possums (*Trichosurus* spp.) (tagging of larger species is covered earlier in this chapter). Ear tags are generally used for long-term population monitoring and CMR studies where individual identification is required. Small metal ear tags stamped with unique numbers allow for individual identification of recaptured animals in-hand. Placement of ear tags in particular ears (e.g. left for male and right for female) can facilitate identification of sexes from a distance or on camera trap images. Reflective tape adhered to fingerling ear tags has been successfully used to perform CMR on yellow-bellied gliders (*Petaurus australis*) (Goldingay and Kavanagh 1990).

Ear tagging is an inexpensive method of marking mammals, but is not an effective long-term marking technique for many species as tags may be lost during grooming, combat with conspecifics, or through entanglement with vegetation. While medium-sized mammals (e.g. quolls, *Dasyurus* spp.; bettongs, *Bettongia* spp.; and possums) tend to retain ear tags well, tagging is not suitable for mammals with thin, delicate pinnae, such as bilbies, pygmy possums and small rodents, as they are highly susceptible to tag loss and ear damage (DBCA 2017; Arid Recovery 2019). Ear tagging is also discouraged for smaller bandicoots (individuals of *Isoodon and Perameles* spp.), phascogales (*Phascogale* spp.), dunnarts (*Sminthopsis* spp.) and antechinus (*Antechinus* spp.) because of the risk of tags tearing out during fights or excessive clawing at tags causing damage to the ear (DBCA 2017; Arid Recovery 2019).

Failure to retain ear tags is an issue both for loss of data if individuals are not identifiable, and as an ethical concern when tags are torn out, causing injury to the animal. If the risk of ear tag loss is high, consider applying an ear tag in each ear or using a second or alternative marking method (Silvy *et al.* 2005) such as ear notching with a unique numbering system, microtattooing, or microchipping (see other GOPs in this chapter). Ear tagging may be appropriate in situations where the risk of loss is low, microchipping is too expensive, ears are too small or dark for tattooing, or where natural wear and tear and minor ear damage make ear notching impractical.

Animal welfare considerations

Ear tagging requires injury to the ear and carries the risk of pain and infection during the application process and following release if tags are partially or fully torn out during the course of the animal's normal activities (grooming, fighting and movement through vegetation). Infection or inflammation of the insertion site may occur in some species with fleshier ears (e.g. brushtail possums and potoroos, *Potorous* spp.). Ear tags are generally only applied to the ears of adult animals; application of ear tags to juveniles may affect ear development and is not recommended (DBCA 2017). Tagging will cause temporary pain, which may be reduced by applying a topical anaesthetic to the mark site before marking (left in place for ≥ 5 min before marking), although the efficacy of this method in reducing pain is contentious (see the discussion in 'Tattooing mammals and lizards' later in this chapter) and it is not recommended if doing so is likely to increase handling time appreciably.

General procedures

Ear tag selection

Self-piercing metal 'fingerling' tags are commonly used to tag small- to medium-sized mammals and are available from laboratory supply companies. The smallest tags commonly available are 6 mm in internal length and are suitable for medium-large rodents and quolls. Tags with an internal length of 11 mm are suitable for medium-sized mammals, such as brushtail possums and bettongs.

Positioning of the tag

The tag should be positioned low on the front edge of the ear, close to the head, to prevent the weight of the tag folding the ear over. For species with thin pinnae that may be weighed down by the tag even in this position, the tag can be placed along the lower edge of the ear, close to the head, or an alternative marking technique can be considered. Tags should be placed sufficiently far inside the ear to minimise the amount of tag protruding from the ear, thus reducing the likelihood of the tag being torn out (e.g. when moving through vegetation). This placement can be achieved by ensuring the folded edge of the tag is flush with the outside edge of the ear before closure of the applicator. Care must be taken to avoid cartilage and blood vessels during the application process.

Tag application

Personnel should select an appropriately sized tag for the species and record the number. The animal can be held securely in a cloth handling bag with the target ear exposed, preferably with the eyes, nose and body covered. Personnel should disinfect the ear, the tag and the tag applicator with ≥ 70% alcohol, and place the tag in the applicator, ensuring the hole in the tag is against the indentation in the applicator. The applicator is positioned over the ear in the desired location as described above, ensuring that the ear tag number is on the outside of the ear. The applicator is operated in a decisive motion while personnel maintain a secure hold on the animal. The tag must fully puncture the ear and personnel should check that it has closed itself as designed. The applicator should be disengaged carefully, but swiftly to minimise the risk of tearing the ear if the animal suddenly moves or pulls away. Personnel should then check that the tag has closed properly, disinfect the ear again with a povidone–iodine solution, if desired, and double-check the tag number. The animal should then be allowed to move freely in the handling bag. Personnel must monitor the animal for signs of distress – momentary distress as the ear is punctured can be expected for most species, but continued distress is abnormal. Once the animal is seen to be moving normally and any bleeding has stopped, it may be released. The tag applicator should be disinfected. If an ear tag has been incorrectly fitted it may be necessary to remove it with pliers or metal snips. However, the risk of causing further trauma to the animal should be evaluated against the benefit of repositioning the tag (DBCA 2017).

Animal treatment, withdrawal and euthanasia

Animals should be monitored continuously for signs of distress. If bleeding occurs, personnel should apply pressure to the site with clean, absorbent material and monitor the animal until any bleeding stops. Excess blood can be cleaned away using gauze; some personnel may choose to apply a povidone–iodine solution or ≥ 70% alcohol to the wound, although this may sting the animal. Upon recapture of a tagged animal, the tag site should be inspected for signs of infection (i.e. inflammation, weeping or bleeding). If excessive bleeding occurs following tagging, or a recaptured animal shows signs of severe infection, personnel should seek advice from a wildlife veterinarian and consider removing the tag. Injuries from ear tagging rarely lead to euthanasia. Species prone to capture myopathy should be identified before ear tagging, and the time taken to restrain and ear tag the animal taken into consideration (i.e. reduced as much as possible).

Equipment and maintenance

Equipment should be kept meticulously clean and free from rust or oxidisation. Typical equipment items required may include:

- individually numbered ear tags of an appropriate size for target species
- ear tag applicator
- handling bags
- disinfectant for ear and equipment (≥ 70% alcohol or povidone–iodine solution)
- gauze for swabbing ears and equipment
- clipboard and data sheets or an electronic database
- needle-nosed pliers or metal snips for emergency ear tag removal.

Specific qualifications, experience and training

Researchers should be familiar with the species or similar taxa, comfortable with handling and restraining the species, and aware of signs of excessive agitation for the species. Researchers should be trained or supervised by people who are experienced in the use of the chosen marking technique until deemed competent. Prior to use on a live animal, the technique should be practised on paper or cloth until the researcher is comfortable and confident with operating the applicator.

Workplace health and safety

Few specific safety risks are associated with this technique. Personnel should consider the potential for bites, scratches, or transmission of zoonoses or parasites from their study species.

Alternative procedures

Ear tagging small mammals has a higher risk of data loss than most other common individual marking methods (P. Burns, pers. obs.). Investigators should consider whether the following alternative techniques would be better suited to their study species before employing ear tagging: ear notching, ear or tail tattooing, microchipping (see other GOPs in this chapter). If permanent marking is not required, investigators should consider low-impact methods, such as non-toxic marker pens or hair trimming.

EAR NOTCHING FOR MARKING AND COLLECTION OF TISSUE SAMPLES

Helen P. Waudby, Angela J.L. Pestell, Phoebe A. Burns, Melissa A. Jensen and Bronwyn A. Fancourt

Target taxa

This GOP applies to dasyurids (Chapter 18), bandicoots, pygmy possums and gliders (Chapter 19) and rodents (Chapter 24).

Context and scope

This GOP describes the permanent marking of small to medium-sized mammals by ear notching. It applies to mammals ranging from around the size of the smallest planigale (*Planigale* spp.) up to around the size of quolls. It should not be used on microbats (see Chapter 23). Typically, ear notching is used to collect genetic samples and/or mark mammals permanently for long-term studies or management activities. When used in conjunction with a numbering system, the method allows for identification of recaptured individuals. Permanent marking to identify individuals is typically used for long-term studies that employ CMR methods (repeated capture of individuals over time) as the retention and readability of marks to identify individuals is important for these types of analyses. CMR approaches are used widely to estimate abundance, density and demography of target species (Jung *et al.* 2020). Studies that involve ear notching, puncturing or other permanent marking methods should demonstrate clearly that no other alternative is available (Petit and Waudby 2012). Where long-term studies have used these methods for many years, researchers may be reluctant to introduce new methods that could result in error or misreading of marks (affecting study results and potentially, animal welfare outcomes). In these cases, new methods should be tested to ensure that study objectives can still be achieved (D. Lunney, pers. comm. in Petit and Waudby 2012).

Animal welfare considerations

Infection and bleeding

Notching requires making an open wound to the ear, which on rare occasions may cause infection if the equipment and/or wound site are not disinfected properly. Equipment should be disinfected immediately before and after undertaking notching, and the mark site disinfected before creating the notch. Solutions of ≥ 70% alcohol should be used for disinfection of equipment, but alcohol should be allowed to evaporate or be flamed before being used, to avoid stinging open wounds. Personnel should release animals only once bleeding has stopped. Recaptured animals are checked for signs of infection at the wound site (i.e. obvious swelling, unusual redness or weeping or bleeding). Depending on the severity of the infection or bleeding and the remoteness of the study location, the animal can be treated by experienced personnel or transported to a veterinary facility. Euthanasia is unlikely to be required as a result of ear notching.

Pain during mark application

Ear notching may cause temporary mild to moderate pain and distress in marked animals, depending on the species and how the procedure is applied. The efficacy of topical anaesthetics is debated, but probably does reduce the pain of invasive marking methods to some extent (see Kasanen *et al.* 2011; Keating *et al.* 2012). If used, a lignocaine-based local anaesthetic gel or cream (typically available from pharmacies or medical suppliers) is applied to the intended wound site and left for ≥ 5 min before notching. Doing so is not recommended if application is likely to increase handling time appreciably. Personnel should remain calm and speak quietly while completing the procedure. Scissors or punches must be maintained in a sharp and clean condition (equipment should be checked regularly). Pain and stress are reduced by ensuring that inexperienced personnel are trained by more-experienced personnel and have practised the method on other substrates (e.g. paper or aluminium foil) beforehand.

Changed interactions among conspecifics and visibility to predators

No evidence is available to suggest that interactions change among marked animals because of notching, although it is possible. The wound site should be cleaned of blood and personnel should ensure that bleeding has ceased before the animal is released. For many species bleeding is likely to be minimal when the procedure has been performed properly, if it occurs at all.

General procedures

Planning

If permanent marking or tissue collection is unnecessary to meet the study objectives, personnel should

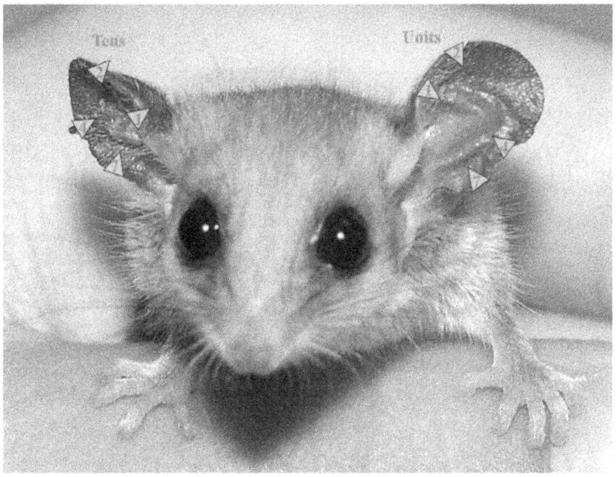

Figure 8.2: Potential ear notching numbering system demonstrated on a western pygmy possum (*Cercartetus concinnus*). The marks are positions 1, 2, 4, and 7; the left ear displays units and the right displays tens. For example, to mark an animal as number 22, personnel notch position 2 on the right ear (20) and position 2 on the left ear (2). Image adapted from Pestell and Petit (2007).

consider alternatives, including non-permanent or less invasive forms of marking instead. Typically, some form of marking is advisable, even if doing so is required to avoid reprocessing recaptured animals rather than for analytical purposes. If ear notching is selected, an appropriate numbering system is required that will allow investigators to identify individuals with relative ease (e.g. Figure 8.2).

Disinfecting and anaesthetising the site

An appropriate location on the ear should be identified. Personnel should avoid notching on scar tissue, or visible blood vessels (unless, e.g., the procedure is also being used for blood collection) where possible as these areas are more prone to bleeding and are likely to be more painful. The notch site should be disinfected with a ≥ 70% alcohol solution, which should be allowed to dry before notching. If desired, numbing agent (e.g. lignocaine gel) can be applied to the site by putting it on two gloved fingers and grasping the ear gently between these fingers, and left for at least 5 min. Personnel may process the animal while the numbing agent is working. All equipment should be disinfected immediately before use, including trays, scissors, biopsy punches and tweezers, with ≥ 70% alcohol. Personnel may wear non-powdered nitrile disposable gloves to protect themselves from potential zoonoses, and the animal from potential zooanthroponoses.

Notching

Personnel should hold the animal securely in a calico bag or similar. Ideally, the animal's eyes and the rest of its body are covered by part of the bag while notching takes place. Personnel may wear a head torch to make the wound site and any blood vessels more obvious. Personnel can use small sharp embroidery or medical scissors to cut a triangular notch at the edge of the ear, or a biopsy punch (which should typically only be used once as they become blunt quickly when used multiple times) or reusable mouse ear punch to punch a partial rounded notch at the edge of the ear. Punching an enclosed circle is not advised as the hole may be prone to snagging and tearing. Notches created with scissors are typically triangular in shape; care should be taken not to make the notch too deep. Notches should be sufficiently large to be visible on later inspection and less likely to be mistaken for a tear or bite (see Figure 8.2 for examples of good marks). Small, pointed tweezers can be used to help remove excised tissue and place it in a storage solution (e.g. a 50:50 saline and 100% alcohol solution, or ≥ 70% alcohol), if necessary. Any blood should be removed from the wound site with cotton wool or gauze. Some personnel treat wounds with a povidone-iodine solution, although doing so may sting the animal. The animal can be released once it is clearly active and moving normally and any bleeding has stopped. All equipment should be disinfected.

Animal treatment, withdrawal and euthanasia

Personnel should monitor animals throughout the process. Signs of stress will depend on the study species. Pressure can be applied to bleeding wound sites, which may occur if a notch has been cut too far into the ear. The animal should be monitored to ensure that the bleeding stops completely before release. If an animal struggles excessively during handling and restraint, and/or appears to go limp, it should be released immediately into the bag and allowed to recover. Some rodent species may be particularly susceptible to stress induced by handling in general (Petit *et al.* 2012) and should be observed carefully. If an animal flinches obviously during the procedure, then personnel should reassess the situation and apply numbing agents for a longer period before applying notches.

Equipment and maintenance

Typical items required for ear notching are listed in Table 8.3. All equipment should be kept as clean as possible. A dedicated field toolkit for storing the equipment is highly recommended as it will assist with overall organisation as well as cleanliness. Reusable mouse ear punches can be sharpened by using the tool to puncture aluminium foil.

Specific qualifications, experience and training

Personnel should be supervised closely by other experienced personnel until they are deemed competent and should have practised the method on pieces of paper or another substrate. They should already be confident in handling their target species or similar taxa, and able to use appropriate restraint methods, before using the procedure.

Workplace health and safety

Specific safety concerns associated with this method are few. However, personnel should take care to avoid cutting injuries when using scissors or biopsy punches and have access to appropriate first aid. They should consider the potential for transmission of zoonoses or parasites from the species they are handling. Personnel should take care not to burn themselves if sterilising notching equipment by flame.

Alternative procedures

If applied appropriately, ear notching causes minimal obvious distress to study animals (i.e. a lack of obvious flinching or other retraction movements in small animals). Other methods of permanent marking, such as tattooing with ultraviolet ink, may be more appropriate for some species, including sensitive rodents (e.g. Petit *et al.* 2012), although they are not necessarily quicker, and are less obvious than ear notches. Microchipping (see 'Microchipping mammals, reptiles and amphibians' earlier in this chapter) may also be a suitable alternative, although this method requires access to additional equipment (i.e. microchip readers).

MARKING REPTILES AND AMPHIBIANS WITH VISIBLE IMPLANT ELASTOMER AND VISIBLE IMPLANT ALPHANUMERIC TAGS

Helen P. Waudby, Geoffrey Heard and Sophie Petit

Target taxa

This GOP applies to reptiles (Chapter 26) and amphibians (Chapter 27).

Context and scope

This GOP describes the marking of juvenile and adult stages of reptiles and amphibians with visible implant elastomer and visible implant alphanumeric tags (VIE and VIA, respectively). These tags are biocompatible and silicone-based, and often used for marking reptiles and amphibians (e.g. Heard *et al.* 2008; Waudby and Petit 2011), including tadpoles and metamorph frogs (Courtois *et al.* 2013; Bainbridge *et al.* 2015), fishes (Sandford *et al.* 2020), and amphibian egg masses in the case of VIE (Regester and Woosley 2005). Visible implant elastomer has also been used to mark earthworms, crustaceans and cephalopods (e.g. Butt and Lowe 2007; Davis *et al.* 2005; Replinger and Wood 2007), and possibly has applications for marking small mammals (Jung *et al.* 2020).

Table 8.3: Suggested equipment and materials required for ear notching small to medium-sized mammals.

Marking	Data collection	Post-marking
• Small sharp embroidery or medical scissors, biopsy punch or small-sized livestock or laboratory mouse ear-notching equipment • Pointed tweezers • Diagram of notch locations and numbers • ≥ 70% alcohol (for disinfection of equipment and marking site prior to marking) • Butane torch or lighter to flame reusable notching equipment • Cotton cosmetic wipes (for swabbing equipment) • Gauze • Gloves • Face mask • Topical anaesthetic if desired • Container to hold equipment	• Clipboard and data sheets • List of available notch numbers • Vials of solution for tissue preservation • Transportable fridge or cool box (for some types of tissue collection) • Hard surface (e.g. a tray or table) on which to place animals while notching	• Povidone–iodine solution for wound disinfection, if desired • Plastic aquaria or similar for monitoring marked animals if required • Container to hold used swabs or gauze

Procedures for marking mammals, egg and larval stages of amphibians, and fish are not covered by this GOP.

Marking with VIE is useful for very small animals that would otherwise be difficult to mark. For example, Waudby and Petit (2011) marked skinks as small as < 1.0 g with VIE. The substance is created by mixing a coloured elastomer with a curing agent that is injected under the animal's epidermis. Over time, the material solidifies (the rate of curing depends on ambient temperature). Visible implant alphanumeric tags comprise the same biocompatible elastomer as VIE but are available in two sizes as pre-made coloured rectangles displaying an alphanumeric code printed in black (Northwest Marine Technology Inc. 2017). Both tag types are available in various colours. Some VIE colours fluoresce under UV light, as do all VIA tags. Typically, VIE marks are applied with a needle and VIA with a specialised injector. By using a combination of colours and body locations, animals can be allocated individual marks. For example, Jung *et al.* (2000) used three colours and four body locations to create 255 individual codes in a study of salamanders. For VIA tags, 2500 unique marks are possible per colour (fluorescent orange, yellow, green or red), but multiple tags can be used to create greater numbers of marks (www.nmt.us/vi-alpha).

Animal welfare considerations

Animal welfare considerations for these marking methods primarily relate to tag retention and readability (which affects data collection and effectiveness of animal use) and the potential for pain, distress, and changes to survival and detectability as a result of marking. Marking with VIE and VIA is sometimes cited as an alternative to toe clipping (e.g. Heard *et al.* 2008; Waudby and Petit 2011).

Infection

Marking with VIE and VIA requires the subject's epidermis to be punctured. Infection may occur if the equipment and wound site are not disinfected properly, although reports of infection in amphibians and reptiles are limited. Penney *et al.* (2001) marked threatened sand skinks (*Neoseps reynoldsi*) without any observable infection. Heard *et al.* (2008) observed no infection in extensive tagging of metamorph growling grass frogs (*Litoria raniformis*), both in laboratory and field settings. It is unclear if marking methods that puncture the epidermis increase the susceptibility of amphibians to infectious diseases, such as chytridiomycosis, by disrupting the symbiotic bacterial communities in their skin or depleting their peptide stores (Antwis *et al.* 2014). Following appropriate disinfection procedures will minimise the risk of infection.

Pain during mark application

Mark application may cause temporary pain and distress. For reptiles, a lignocaine-based numbing gel or cream can be applied to the intended mark site (left in place for ≥ 5 min before marking), although the efficacy of this method in reducing pain is contentious (see the discussion around tattooing elsewhere in this chapter). Pain and stress are reduced by ensuring that inexperienced personnel are trained by more experienced personnel and have practised the method on preserved specimens, road-killed individuals or proxies (e.g. a sausage, potato or faux skin) beforehand. Needles and other injecting equipment should be sharp and changed or maintained regularly. Using the manual injector (Northwest Marine Technology Inc. 2017) supplied with the kit may improve the speed with which VIE can be applied, particularly if marking large numbers of animals. When marking certain lizard taxa with VIE, inserting the needle against the direction of the scales will make it easier to puncture the skin and avoid inadvertent scale removal. Visible implant elastomer is particularly effective for marking geckoes because of their translucent skin, but their epidermis can be difficult to puncture as it sometimes 'bags' under the needle, which must be sharp to avoid this issue (Waudby and Petit 2011).

For VIA tags, Heard *et al.* (2008) reported that it was preferable for their focal frog species to create an incision in the skin rather than puncturing it using the specialised injector, before inserting tags because of difficulties in keeping the injector suitably sharp, and the risk of damaging the underlying muscle tissue or puncturing the peritoneal cavity. Anaesthesia may be used on target animals, but doing so creates additional welfare issues and is probably unnecessary if handling techniques are appropriate and personnel are experienced.

Stress, and health and fitness costs

Studies of reptile and amphibian physiological stress responses to marking with VIE and VIA are few. Assessment of urinary corticosterone metabolites in wild-caught Asian toads (*Duttaphrynus melanostictus*) demonstrated that acute stress responses to marking with

VIE were not worse than those experienced during handling, capture or marking with a sham material (saline solution) (Narayan and Gramapurohit 2019). Red-eyed tree frogs (*Agalychnis callidryas*) showed no adrenal response (represented by faecal glucocorticoid metabolite concentrations) or peptide production as a result of marking with VIE, although microbial abundance was slightly higher on the skin of marked frogs 2 weeks after tagging (Antwis *et al.* 2014).

No study is available to indicate if marking with VIE or VIA has a long-term negative effect on the health and fitness of study animals. Schmidt and Schwarzkopf (2010) found that immediately after marking with VIE, locomotor performance (jump distance) of striped rocket frogs (*L. nasuta*) was reduced, but that the effect was greater for toe clipping than for VIE. After 2 weeks, locomotor performance was lower than at the start of the experiment for all marking methods. Immediately after marking, VIE reduced endurance of open-litter rainbow skinks (*Carlia pectoralis*), although toe clipping had a stronger negative effect on running speed than did VIE. After 2 weeks, endurance and running speed increased to above the initial measurement irrespective of marking method. Sapsford *et al.* (2014) found no effect of VIE marking on movement or survival rates on tree frogs in the 3 weeks post-marking. Regester and Woosley (2005) marked spotted salamander (*Ambystoma maculatum*) eggs with VIE with no effect on embryo hatching, body size, or hatchling developmental size. Heard *et al.* (2008) examined the effect of VIA tagging on survival and growth of 52 juvenile growling grass frogs under laboratory conditions over 12 weeks and found that neither was adversely affected (all frogs survived, and growth rates of marked individuals were slightly higher than controls). Field studies reported by Heard *et al.* (2008) suggest that long-term effects are minimal, with animals being recaptured up to 18 months after marking.

Tag retention and visibility

Visibility of VIE marks depends, in part, on the extent of pigmentation and scale thickness (Northwest Marine Technology Inc. 2017). Typically, the ventral surface is less pigmented than the dorsum, so choosing locations on the abdomen may improve mark visibility (Waudby and Petit 2011). Penney *et al.* (2001) noted that mark migration may be most likely to occur in young individuals as they grow and in individuals that have been marked for some time (e.g. > 2 years), although marks of 12 of 13 sand skinks recaptured after 2 years were still readable. Spacing marks widely might help reduce misidentification resulting from mark migration (Penney *et al.* 2001).

Reported retention of VIE is typically high for reptiles (at least over study durations), but conflicting information is available on VIE tag retention for amphibians. For example, 50% of VIE tags moved (resulting in potential misidentification of ~71% of individuals) in an 8-week study comparing VIE beads and PIT tag marking of 53 captive leopard frogs (*Lithobates pipiens*) and Kihansi spray toads (*Nectophrynoides asperginis*) (Brannelly *et al.* 2013). Similarly, in a comparison of four marking methods, VIE was the least-effective method for identifying alpine tree frogs (*Litoria verreauxii alpina*) with tags correctly identified only ~19% of the time (Brannelly *et al.* 2014).

In species with thick or heavily pigmented skin, VIA numbers may be obscured. Clemas *et al.* (2009) found that the pigmented skin of growling grass frogs obscured numbers, but that VIA tags were reliable for tagging adult brown tree frogs. However, Heard *et al.* (2008) marked juvenile growling grass frogs with VIA tags and found they remained highly readable. Using a UV light likely improves detection and readability of VIA tags. Retention of VIA marks by amphibians may be affected by mark location. Heard *et al.* (2008) noted that tags implanted on the dorso-lateral area of growling grass frogs (below the dorso-lateral fold) were less likely to be lost than those implanted into the thigh (7% loss rate for tags implanted dorso-laterally versus 59% loss rate for tags implanted on the thigh). Tags were rarely misidentified (3% of 208 trials), although accuracy varied among observers. Caballero-Gini *et al.* (2019) evaluated marking of adult and juvenile neotropical treefrogs with VIA and toe clipping. Of 196 marked individuals, 57 were recaptured in the 7-month study period. Only one VIA mark was unreadable because it was located deep under the skin; these authors also noted one case of tag expulsion and two inverted tags. If wounds take some time to heal, tags may be expelled in the meantime, but using a wound sealant may reduce that risk (Heard *et al.* 2008). Lunghi and Veith (2017) recommend avoiding inserting tags into the tails of salamanders that can autotomise them.

General procedures

Planning

Personnel should determine an appropriate numbering or coding system before embarking on the study (e.g. Figure 8.3 for VIE), including colour combinations

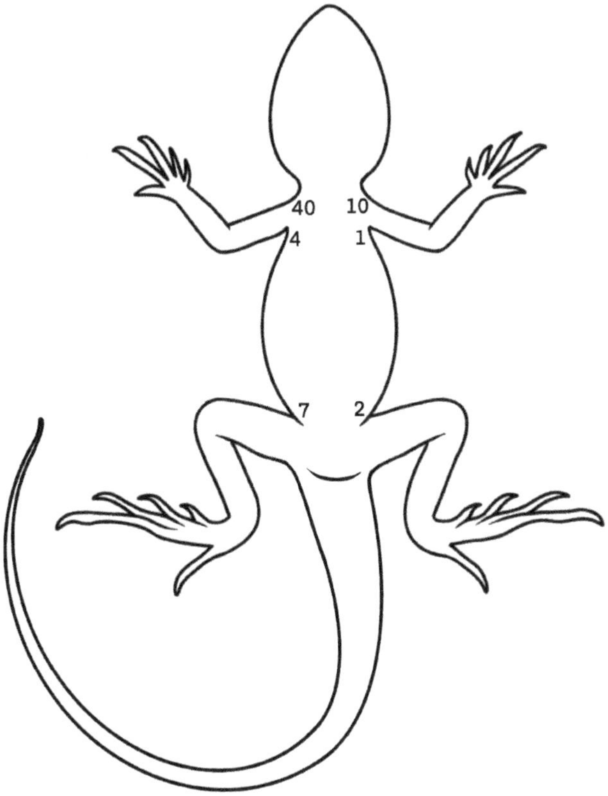

Figure 8.3: Potential numbering system when using VIE demonstrated on a reptile's ventral surface. The mark are positions 1, 2, 4, 7, 40 and 10. For example, to mark an animal as number 12, personnel mark position 10 near the front left leg and position 2 near the left leg (2). Illustration by Alana de Laive.

and mark locations (e.g. Figure 8.4 for VIA). Fluorescent colours are useful for species with pigmented skin; their visibility is increased at night or in dark areas by illuminating them with an ultraviolet (UV) light. The manufacturers recommend that fluorescing colours of VIE are favoured first (Northwest Marine Technology Inc. 2017).

Mark locations may become crowded on small lizards, so choosing a system requiring the least number of marks is sensible for those taxa when using VIE (Waudby and Petit 2011). Reptiles can be tagged successfully with VIE on their ventral side, in the upper legs and in the tail (Waudby and Petit 2011). Turtles, including hatchlings, have been tagged by injecting VIE into their limbs (Davy *et al.* 2010) or into the plastron to create individual tag numbers (Anderson *et al.* 2015).

For frogs, potential VIE tagging sites include between the toes (Naulerwaerts 2000), on the upper hind leg of frogs. Ideally, personnel choose a tagging location that is not heavily pigmented. For very small lizards, or species with absent or reduced limbs, locations on the abdomen are most appropriate (Waudby and Petit 2011). Typical VIA tagging locations for amphibians include the inner thigh (Caballero-Gini *et al.* 2019), and the side of the thorax or body (Heard *et al.* 2008; Figure 8.4), and the limbs of salamanders that can autotomise their tails (Lunghi and Veith 2017).

Disinfecting and anaesthetising the site

An appropriate location on the animal's body should be identified. For reptiles, the mark location should be disinfected with ≥ 70% alcohol and allowed to dry before the needle is inserted or insertion made. If desired, for reptiles, a lignocaine-based gel can be applied to the mark site with a cotton ear bud and left for ≥ 5 min. For amphibians, the implantation site may be disinfected with Bactine®, which is a disinfectant recommended for use with amphibians that also contains a weak anaesthetic (lignocaine). All equipment should be disinfected immediately before use, including trays and needles, with a ≥ 70% alcohol. When handling amphibians, personnel wear disposable gloves, or use a lightweight plastic bag, both changed between individuals (see Chapter 27). All glove types may affect amphibians, but nitrile gloves may be particularly toxic to tadpoles; vinyl appears to be the best choice (Cashins *et al.* 2008). General anaesthesia is unnecessary for marking with VIE or VIA tags. However, in some cases with VIA researchers do so to improve ease of handling and reduce stress on the animal (i.e. Nauwelaerts and Coeck 2000). Personnel should follow appropriate procedures for anaesthetising reptiles and amphibians (Chapters 16, 26 and 27) if they choose to do so.

Applying the mark

Reptiles or amphibians should be captured and handled using appropriate methods (Chapters 26 and 27). Personnel should mix VIE following the manufacturer's instructions and load the mixture into a 0.3 cm^3 insulin syringe with a 29 G needle. Animals should be restrained and turned so that the area to be marked faces the researcher. The needle should be inserted under the skin of the animal (against the direction of the scales for reptiles), with the bevel facing upwards, and the syringe depressed slightly. The needle only needs to be inserted to the depth of the needle's bevel at an angle of 5–10°. Personnel should stop depressing the needle before it is removed to reduce the chance of VIE being extruded back through the puncture site (i.e. where it may solidify and be pulled from the

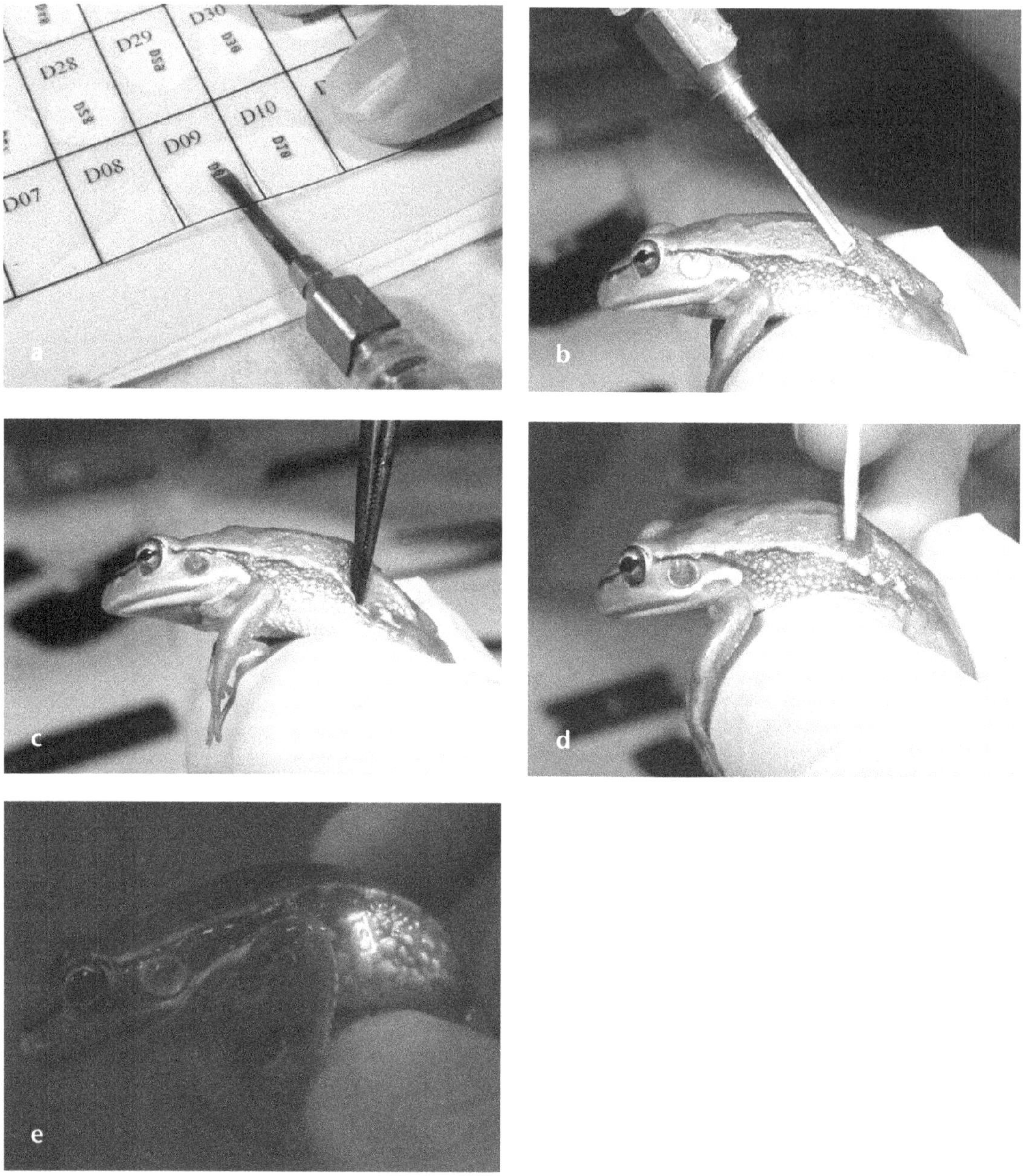

Figure 8.4: Example of VIA tag placement in a growling grass frog (*Litoria raniformis*). (a) Selection of VIA tag and placement in applicator. (b) Insertion of tag with the applicator. (c) Manipulation of the tag with tweezers. (d) Sealing of the wound with tissue adhesive. (e) Confirmation of the tag's location and readability. Photos by Geoffrey Heard.

animal's body). A small amount of topical tissue adhesive can be applied to the puncture wound, if necessary, to reduce the risk of solidified VIE extruding from the animal's body before it heals.

Alpha tags (Figure 8.4a) can be implanted either using the injector that can be purchased from the supplier or through an incision. Making a small incision first may be more efficient than using the injector to do so (as above) (Heard *et al.* 2008), with the injector then used solely to insert the tag through the incision. If doing so, personnel can make a small incision in the epidermis (i.e. around 3 mm) with small surgical scissors or nail clippers over the underlying muscle. The tag should be inserted under the epidermis and through this incision using the injector supplied with the tags (Figure 8.4b). External manipulation of the tag with blunt forceps may be required to ensure that the tag is inserted properly, or to move it to the desired location (Figure 8.4c). The wound should be sealed with a topical tissue adhesive (Figure 8.4d) (Heard *et al.* 2008). Additional detailed instructions and advice for applying the mark are available from the supplier (Northwest Marine Technology Inc. 2019). Personnel can treat the puncture with a povidone–iodine solution (for reptiles) or Bactine® (for amphibians), if desired, and then release animals.

Animal treatment, withdrawal and euthanasia

Personnel should monitor animals throughout the process. Signs of stress are difficult to assess in reptiles and amphibians and will depend on the study species (Chapters 26 and 27). Typically, animals can be released immediately after marking, but may be observed for a period if doing so does not create additional unnecessary stress.

Equipment and maintenance

Suggested equipment required for marking animals with VIE and VIA is listed in Table 8.4. Kits containing the materials for mixing VIE and applying marks can be obtained from the supplier.

Specific qualifications, experience or training

Personnel should be supervised closely by other experienced personnel until they are deemed confident and should have practised the method on dead specimens or another substrate. Experience handling and restraining the target species is vital, as errors and injuries to either the marker or the animal often result from the animal 'breaking free' of the restraining hold. Personnel should receive training by others experienced in handling and restraining the focal species, or similar species, and should be able to demonstrate the capacity to secure and restrain quickly the animals to be marked. Doing so is particularly important because most issues that arise during marking are related to poor handling.

Workplace health and safety

Personnel may inadvertently injure themselves with needles or scalpels, either while marking or if used needles are not secured, with a risk of infection and transmission of blood-borne zoonoses. Personnel should consider wearing gloves to reduce the risk of injury during marking, although doing so may reduce sensation, increasing the risk of injury. Used needles must be disposed of in a sharps container immediately after use. Needles should never be left unsecured (i.e. in equipment kits). Personnel must follow appropriate first aid procedures if a needlestick injury occurs. A material safety data sheet is available from the supplier's instruction manual (Northwest Marine Technology Inc. 2017).

Alternative procedures

If applied appropriately, these procedures should cause minimal distress to study animals. The methods are often cited as alternatives to toe clipping, although their use should be evaluated against the likely retention and readability rates over the duration of the study. Long-term studies may require an additional or alternative permanent marking method. Other methods of permanent or semi-permanent marking, such as tattooing, toe clipping, and microchipping (see other GOPs in this chapter) can be used, although they are not necessarily lower impact than VIE or VIA and are associated with their own suite of considerations.

Table 8.4: Suggested equipment and materials for marking reptiles and amphibians with VIE and VIA.

Marking equipment	Data collection	Post-marking
• 0.3 cm^3 insulin syringe with a 29 G needle • VIE constituents • VIA tags and injector • Scalpels • Diagram of mark locations and numbers • ≥ 70% alcohol (for disinfection of equipment and marking site) • Cotton cosmetic wipes (for swabbing equipment) • Hard surface (e.g. a portable tray, table or lid) on which to place animals while marking • Means of keeping mixed VIE cool (e.g. portable cool box or refrigerator) • Topical anaesthetic, if desired	• Clipboard and data sheets • List of available mark numbers	• Povidone–iodine solution or Bactine® for disinfecting wound, if desired • Plastic aquaria or similar for monitoring of marked animals if required • Container to hold used swabs/gauze • Sharps container • UV light (for viewing fluorescing colours) • Tissue adhesive for sealing wounds

TATTOOING MAMMALS AND LIZARDS

Helen P. Waudby, Sophie Petit and Mel McGregor

Target taxa

This method has applications for a range of taxa, but particularly dasyurids (Chapter 18), possums and gliders (Chapter 19), rodents and lagomorphs (Chapter 24) and lizards (Chapter 26).

Context and scope

This GOP describes permanent marking of terrestrial mammals (e.g. Lindner and Fuelling 2002; Petit *et al.* 2012; McGregor and Jones 2016) and lizards (Petit *et al.* 2012) by tattooing. Tattooing is a relatively simple and cost-effective method for permanently marking animals. When undertaken by experienced personnel the method is quick (e.g. can be completed in ≤ 2–5 min) and can be completed in the field (Lindner and Fuelling 2002; McGregor and Jones 2016). Typically, tattoos are made by injecting ink under the epidermis with a needle (Soderquist and Dickman 1988; Petit *et al.* 2012), battery-operated tattoo pens (McGregor and Jones 2016), or tattoo pliers (Lindner and Fuelling 2002). The method is potentially useful for small mammal species that are prone to stress associated with other marking methods, such as ear notching, and has been used to mark very small reptiles (e.g. dwarf skinks; Petit *et al.* 2012). The method has also been used for amphibians (Perret and Joly 2002), but may be less suitable for these taxa (Halliday 1996). Typically, snakes are no longer marked by tattooing as other methods (such as scale clipping – see later in this chapter), are more successful for long-term identification (Plummer and Ferner 2012). The method has also been used for marking bats (Bumrungsri *et al.* 2007); refer to Chapter 23 for additional details about marking microbats with tattoos.

Animal welfare considerations

Animal welfare issues associated with tattooing primarily relate to legibility of marks (which affects data collection and effectiveness of animal use), and short-term pain and physiological stress associated with marking. Special consideration should be given to applying tattoos to undeveloped pouch young of some smaller marsupial species and the use of fluorescing ink where predators that use ultraviolet (UV) cues may be present (see below).

Physiological stress and pain

Relatively few studies have examined physiological effects of tattooing on wild animals or evaluated pain responses to the technique. A laboratory-based study of eight white rabbits examined the effectiveness of a topical lidocaine- and prilocaine-based anaesthetic for reducing pain during ear tattooing. Tattooing without the anaesthetic produced significantly higher pain-related behaviours than when it was used, including higher peak heart rate, systolic and mean arterial blood pressure. However, behavioural changes 1 h post-treatment were not identifiable in any treatment group, and serum corticosterone responses did not differ between sham and tattoo treatments. The authors concluded that ear tattooing caused temporary and potentially severe pain in rabbits, which is preventable by the prior application of a topical local anaesthetic (Keating *et al.* 2012). Similarly, tattooing without anaesthetic or analgesia caused significant cardiovascular changes in rats, which may be indicative of pain and physiological stress (Kasanen *et al.* 2011). A study of the usefulness of fluorescing tattoo marks in small wild mammals and reptiles noted occasional retraction movements in western pygmy possums (*Cercartetus concinnus*) and some rodent species, even after application of a lignocaine-based topical anaesthetic, but these movements also occurred when tail hairs were simply touched (Petit *et al.* 2012). Automated tattoo pens make a buzzing noise when in use (akin to a battery-operated personal hair trimmer), which may bother target species a little. Turning on the pen before using it around an animal's head helps to prevent sudden startling.

While general anaesthesia is sometimes recommended to prevent the pain associated with tattooing in laboratory animals, doing so creates additional risks to the animal, particularly for smaller mammals (Keating *et al.* 2012), and is not necessarily practical in field situations. However, applying a topical anaesthetic may reduce pain. Pain and stress are also minimised by ensuring that inexperienced personnel are trained properly and have practiced the method on other substrates beforehand (e.g. a sausage, potato, orange or faux skin). Needles and other tattooing equipment should be sharp.

Health and fitness costs

A study examining the effects of marking with fluorescent tattoo ink in small lizards and mammals found that all recaptured animals (92 of 657) appeared to be in good health, with no evidence of infection in any individual and no significant difference in the body mass of recaptured male western pygmy possums (Petit *et al.* 2012). Lindner and Fuelling (2002) noted that tattooing with pliers did appear to affect body mass of recaptured grey-sided voles (*Myodes rufocanus*). McGregor and Jones (2016) did not observe signs of infection or other negative effects when marking northern brown bandicoots (*Isoodon macrourus*) and common brushtail possums with tattoo pens – many individuals displayed trap-happy behaviours after marking. While evaluations are relatively few, it seems unlikely that the method has greater long-term health or fitness effects on individuals than any other similar permanent marking method. However, it should be noted that scant information is available on the toxicological risks of tattoo inks for humans, let alone non-human animals, including their potential for phototoxicity, migration of inks and conversion of ink ingredients into toxic substances (Grant *et al.* 2015; Laux *et al.* 2016; Schreiver *et al.* 2017).

Suitability for marking pouch young

Soderquist and Dickman (1988) marked the pinnae of house mouse (*Mus musculus*) pinkies, and pouch young of western quolls (*Dasyurus geoffroii*) and southern brown bandicoots (*Isoodon obesulus*) with fluorescent tattoos, without obvious effects on marked individuals. However, the method may not be suitable for species that bear very small undeveloped pouch young (e.g. around 4 mm long in *Antechinus* sp.) and have moist skin that absorbs oxygen (Fisher and Blomberg 2009). Fisher and Blomberg (2009) suggest that tattooing (or other marking methods) of the skin of young of these species may affect their ability to absorb oxygen. Also, *Antechinus* spp. mothers will clean young attached to their teats constantly, which may harm young if they are trying to remove a mark (A. Cockburn, pers. comm. in Fisher and Blomberg 2009). Tattoo pliers may not be suitable for smaller mammals because ear size can be limiting, for example, Lindner and Fuelling (2002) recommended avoiding tattooing ears of small grey-sided voles with tattoo pliers, because personnel would often run out of room to complete marks on the small ears, possibly an issue for several smaller Australian rodent and dasyurid species.

Infection and risk of disease transfer

Tattooing requires the subject's epidermis to be punctured, so it is possible that infection may occur if the equipment and wound site are not disinfected properly. However, reports of infection appear negligible in studies of wild animals (e.g. Lindner and Fuelling 2002). Following appropriate disinfection procedures will minimise the risk.

Susceptibility to predators and changed interactions

Some raptor species use UV cues in their prey's urine to hunt them. Vision of many diurnal bird and reptile species, and some mammal and amphibian species, is often in or near the UV spectrum (Honkavaara *et al.* 2002; Jones *et al.* 2007), which may present an increased predation risk to individuals marked with fluorescent tattoo ink. Similarly, it is possible (although apparently untested) that fluorescing marks may be detected by the invertebrate prey of marked individuals, potentially reducing hunting success. Social interactions of some small vertebrate species could be affected by fluorescent marks since UV signals are used in social interactions of some bird and reptile species (e.g. Honkavaara *et al.* 2002), although this effect is also untested. Placing marks in less-visible locations, including ventral locations, will likely help minimise these potential risks. Ultimately, if the risk is considered a realistic one, personnel should avoid using fluorescing ink.

Tag retention and visibility

In a study of grey-sided voles, ~90% of recaptured individuals retained individually identifiable marks over 15 days. The actual rate was probably higher, but recently marked individuals still had too much ink smeared over their marked ear for marks to be readable (Lindner and Fuelling 2002). Tattooing may not be suitable for species with heavily pigmented skin. For example, Petit *et al.* (2012) avoided marking the tails of dunnarts, although they suggest that other locations (e.g. ears) could have been used instead. Tattoo marks may degrade over time. For example, black-ink tattoos on the tails of eastern pygmy possums lost definition over time, but the alternative method (ear notching) was unreliable because animals sometimes had torn ears (Bladon *et al.* 2002). Petit *et al.* (2012) reported that the longest time between marking and recapture for a western pygmy possum was 252 days, with fluorescent marks on the tail still clearly visible. Brushtail possums and northern brown bandicoots recaptured over ~2.5 years retained legible marks after marking with tattoo pens (McGregor and Jones 2016).

General procedures

Planning and choosing mark locations

Personnel should determine an appropriate numbering or coding system before embarking on the study (Figure 8.3 demonstrates potential reptile marking locations), including colour combinations, mark locations, and digits or symbols to be used. Lizards can be marked on their ventral side, in the upper legs, and in the tail (Waudby and Petit 2011). Typically, suitable tattooing locations for mammals include their tail (Petit *et al.* 2012), ears (Lindner and Fuelling 2002), and potentially their feet (Leclercq and Rozenfeld 2001). Tattooing ears of juvenile mammals may be difficult if they are very thin, undeveloped or wrinkled (Lindner and Fuelling 2002), although Soderquist and Dickman (1988) successfully marked the pinnae of 5 day old house mice, and pouch young of western quolls and southern brown bandicoots with fluorescent tattoos. Tattooing very thin ears (e.g. of some rodent and *Antechnius* spp.) can be difficult with a tattoo pen; marking lower on the ear (towards the head) is an alternative for these species (M. McGregor, pers. obs.).

Disinfecting and anaesthetising the site

Personnel should disinfect the mark location with ≥ 70% alcohol or a povidone–iodine solution and allow it to dry before tattooing starts. All equipment must be disinfected immediately before use with the alcohol solution. General anaesthesia is unnecessary for this marking method. However, if desired, a topical anaesthetic (i.e. lignocaine-, or lidocaine- and prilocaine-based) can be applied to the mark site with a cotton ear bud and left for ≥ 5 min before being wiped away.

Applying the mark

Animals should be captured and handled using taxon-appropriate methods (refer to Section 3). After cleaning and disinfecting the mark site, personnel can use a pre-filled needle (0.5 cc syringes with 30 G needles have been used for small mammals and reptiles; Petit *et al.* 2012), tattoo pen (McGregor and Jones 2016), or pliers (Lindner and Fuelling 2002) to inject or apply tattoo ink to the skin of animals. Needles are changed between every animal. Pliers should be immersed completely in alcohol before use. Tattoo ink designed specifically for use in animals is available, but some authors have used ink designed for use in humans without obvious issues (Petit *et al.* 2012).

Tattoo pliers can be used to mark the ears of mammals and are typically available as devices with revolving heads and fixed digits (letters or numbers) or with moveable digits that are changed as required to make new marks. Spring-loaded pliers are often preferred because they remove the ear from the device as the pliers are released (West 2016). For pliers with moveable digits, personnel should select and place the digits in the pliers before restraining the animal, and test the planned mark on a piece of paper first. Typically, marks are placed inside the ear; the side of the pliers containing the digits is placed inside the ear. Personnel should place the ear between the digits and the rubber backing of the device (ensuring that the ear is not wrinkled) and squeeze so that the ear is punctured, and the pliers closed completely. Caution must be taken when releasing the pliers to ensure that the ear fully detaches from the device and is not torn. Personnel can work ink into the punctures; the ink becomes fixed as the wounds heal. Alternatively, a cotton swab or fingers can be used to work ink into the holes. Personnel should use a thin ink rather than a paste because it is easier to rub into the punctures. Excess ink is not removed. Personnel can apply a thin film of petroleum jelly over the tattoo if desired, which seals the punctures temporarily while they heal. It is preferable to puncture the ear completely rather than apply too little pressure and produce an illegible mark (West 2016).

Tattoo pens are automated devices used as an alternative to traditional tattooing methods, to mark ears of mammals (e.g. McGregor and Jones 2016). A weighted ink well is filled with ink, the needle is placed inside, and the ink coats the needle. Ink wells should be kept full to avoid the needle touching the bottom. Holding the ear taut is important. If desired, personnel may draw the mark on the ear first using non-toxic marker or ones supplied for use in tattooing, although the mark must be cleaned away once the tattoo has been made to ensure that the tattoo is legible. Personnel should turn on the device and use it in a pen-like fashion, making contact with the skin and tracing over the pre-drawn mark if one was made. If desired, a small amount of petroleum jelly can be smeared on to the mark to assist with healing and protect the wound. Petroleum jelly can be applied before the tattoo begins to minimise running. Personnel should replace the protective cap once the pen has been cleaned.

Animal treatment, withdrawal and euthanasia

Personnel should monitor animals throughout the handling and tattooing process. Signs of stress will depend on the study species. If animals appear stressed, personnel should review the marking process and handling methods. Excessive stress may be related to the nature and duration of handling rather than the marking method as such. Having two people (one to hold the animal securely in a bag with its eyes covered and one to perform the tattooing) may help calm highly stressed animals. Tattooing has been used successfully for sensitive rodents that appear prone to death during the handling associated with other marking techniques, such as ear notching (Petit *et al.* 2012). Animals can be released immediately after tattooing, but may be observed for a period of time providing that doing so does not create additional unnecessary stress.

Equipment and maintenance

Specific equipment needs will depend on the tattooing method selected. Suggested equipment required for performing the procedure is listed in Table 8.5.

Specific qualifications, experience and training

Personnel should be supervised closely by other experienced personnel until they are deemed confident and should have practised the method on another substrate, such as sausage, potato, orange or false skin (available from tattoo suppliers) before attempting it on an animal.

Workplace health and safety

Personnel should refer to considerations detailed for marking reptiles and amphibians with VIE and VIA. A material safety data sheet for the specific brand of tattoo ink should be reviewed and kept on hand.

Alternative procedures

If applied appropriately, the procedures probably cause minimal distress to study animals. Other methods of permanent or semi-permanent marking, such the use of visible implant elastomer or alphanumeric tags, toe or scale clipping, and microchipping (see other GOPs in this chapter) may be appropriate, although they are not necessarily quicker or lower impact than tattooing and are associated with their own suite of potential animal welfare impacts.

MARKING REPTILES AND AMPHIBIANS BY TOE, SCALE AND TAIL-TIP CLIPPING

David Hunter, Shannon R. Kelleher and Deborah S. Bower

Target taxa

This GOP applies to lizards, snakes (Chapter 26) and amphibians (Chapter 27).

Context and scope

This GOP details procedures for permanently marking or obtaining a tissue sample from reptiles and amphibians using toe clipping, scale clipping, or by removing a small section of the tail tip (tail clipping). Toe clipping is also used for marking small mammals, although its use for these taxa is expected to decline in favour of other methods (Jung *et al.* 2020). Procedures for marking mammals are not included in this GOP. The partial removal of toes, scales and tails have been standard research procedures for reptile and amphibian studies for some time (Dunham *et al.* 1988; Perry *et al.* 2011). These procedures are particularly useful for marking individuals and cohorts (a group of animals from the same species and generation). These techniques often serve a dual purpose of obtaining tissue samples for genetic and histological analysis, or whole toes for studies of skeletochronology. Their application is often critical for answering questions about taxonomy, genetic diversity, and population demography.

As with any marking method, the application of these methods requires careful consideration of potential impacts on study species. Toe clipping has received considerable attention following the study of McCarthy and Parris (2004), who documented decreasing return rates (apparent survival) for several frog species with increasing numbers of toes removed. The ethics and value of toe clipping frogs was questioned by McCarthy and Parris (2004), whose work was echoed in a

Table 8.5: Suggested equipment and materials for tattooing mammals and herpetofauna.

Marking equipment	Data collection	Post-marking
• Appropriately sized syringes and needles, pens or pliers • Tattoo ink • ≥ 70% alcohol (for disinfection of equipment and marking site) • Cotton wipes or swabs (for disinfecting equipment) • Hard surface (e.g. a portable tray, table or lid) on which to place animals while marking • Topical anaesthetic if desired • Petroleum jelly • Gloves and face mask if required	• Clipboard and data sheets • List of available mark numbers and marking diagram	• Plastic aquaria or similar for monitoring of marked animals if required • Container to hold used swabs/gauze • Sharps container • UV light (for viewing fluorescing colours)

subsequent opinion article by May (2004). Funk *et al.* (2005) pointed out that toe clipping does not always reduce apparent survival, and that in many cases the benefits of toe clipping for conservation management may be argued to outweigh possible negatives (depending on how values are prioritised and what system of ethics is applied). In a detailed review, Perry *et al.* (2011) concluded that toe clipping reptiles and amphibians can be argued to impose acceptable animal welfare impacts where it meets study needs.

Animal welfare considerations

Since the potential impact of these methods varies among species, and possibly also different environments, the decision to use these techniques is context-specific. As with all marking methods, clear justification for the work and consideration of alternatives are important. Personnel should ask themselves: are suitable alternatives available; do the anticipated research outcomes balance the possible stress or negative effects on the target species; and is tissue removal required to answer the research question?

Reduced apparent survival

Following issues raised by McCarthy and Parris (2004), numerous studies have examined the effects of toe clipping on apparent survival (the probability that an individual is still alive and in the population during subsequent censuses) in different frog species. While some level of reduced apparent survival has been observed for some species (Grafe *et al.* 2011), most studies have found no effect of toe clipping (Phillott *et al.* 2008; Grafe *et al.* 2011; Ginnan *et al.* 2014; Olivera-Tlahuel *et al.* 2017). Similarly, earlier studies found no effect of toe clipping on survivorship of salamander and newt species (Arntzen *et al.* 1999; Ott and Scott 1999), or various lizard species (Paulissen and Meyer 2000; Jones and Bell 2007). More recently, reduced apparent survival with increasing numbers of toes removed has been documented for some lizard species (Olivera-Tlahuel *et al.* 2017). Considered together, these studies indicate that the effects of toe clipping are highly species- and context-specific. Studies should be designed so that potential negative effects are reduced and can be quantified. Effects on individual survival from the removal of a single toe are likely to be low. No evidence is available to suggest that scale or tail-tip clipping affects short- or long-term survival (e.g. for larval salamanders, Polich *et al.* 2013).

Infection

Infection is a risk for all procedures that cause an open wound, and may explain reduced apparent survival in studies using toe clipping for individual identification (McCarthy and Parris 2004). Infection and necrosis associated with removing amphibian toes have been observed in many species (Golay and Durrer 1994; Lemckert 1996; Brannelly *et al.* 2014). Since tail loss is a normal aspect of the biology of many lizards, and scale clipping causes a relatively superficial wound, these techniques carry less risk of serious infection. Regardless of the technique, it is important to maintain good hygiene practices when undertaking these methods, as detailed in 'general procedures'.

Disruptions to normal behaviour and fitness

Toe clipping may impair the normal behaviour and fitness of amphibians and reptiles, although reported effects vary. Slower body mass gain was observed in a toe-clipped salamander species (Davis and Ovaska 2001). Locomotor performance was initially reduced in a skink species (Schmidt and Schwarzkopf 2010) and clinging ability in an anolis lizard species (Bloch and Irschick 2005). Other studies have shown no effect of toe clipping on locomotor performance for amphibians (Hudson *et al.* 2017; Zamora-Camacho 2018) or lizards (Borges-Landáez and Shine 2003), or ability to climb walls in an arboreal gecko species (Paulissen and Meyer 2000). Toe clipping did not affect growth rate or body condition in cane toads (Hudson *et al.* 2017). Risks associated with toe clipping can be reduced by not removing toes with specific functions, such as toes with nuptial pads or the longest toes, which can facilitate sexual selection, successful amplexus, efficient locomotion and foraging (Wells 2007).

General procedures

Key principles

Aseptic techniques are difficult to maintain in the field. However, the area to be clipped should at least be kept free of obvious dirt or debris by spraying clean, filtered water over the area and gently wiping it with a delicate task wipe (e.g. Kimwipes™). Personnel should use sharp stainless-steel surgical scissors or scalpel of an appropriate size. Equipment must be clean and sterile, and sterilised between each individual by flaming after soaking in ≥ 70% alcohol, and then rinsed with sterile water. Doing so is also necessary to avoid cross-contamination of tissue collected for genetic analyses, and to reduce the potential spread of bacteria and infectious disease.

Tail-tipping procedures

Personnel should not remove tail tips from species where the tail tip may be important for function (e.g. caudal luring). The minimum amount of tail necessary should be removed, although the exact amount will depend on the size of the species (e.g. ranging from a few mm for small skinks to around 1 cm for larger agamids) and on whether a tissue sample is required. Where possible, personnel should remove the tip of the tail by physically pulling the tail so that it breaks along the natural fracture lines. Where tail tip removal along fracture lines is not appropriate, personnel quickly cut the tail tip using small sharp surgical scissors.

Toe clipping

When toe clipping for individual identification, personnel should aim to use a system that minimises the number of toes clipped (see Donnelly *et al.* 1994), but toes can regrow in some species. Where possible, personnel only clip one toe per foot, particularly for arboreal species. Otherwise, no more than two adjacent toes should be removed on one foot. Personnel should also avoid removing toes that are essential for specific functions (e.g. some frog toes have nuptial pads; the longest toe on the hind limbs may be important for removing shed skin; elongated toes on lizards may be important for sprint speed). For removal of whole toes, the clip should be made at the interphalangeal joint. For studies where only a small amount of tissue needs to be removed, personnel should snip just the very tip of the toe with sharp scissors (i.e. the toe pad). Similarly, for short-term studies (i.e. within a season) personnel should consider removing only the most distal toe. Personnel may apply an antiseptic to the open wound (e.g. Bactine®), if desired.

Scale clipping

Scale clipping typically requires two people: one to restrain the animal, and the other to undertake the procedure. The coding system should focus on ventral and lateral scales for snakes (see Brown and Parker 1976 for detailed methods). Personnel should ensure that the head is restrained before clipping the animal. Scales are cleaned from debris or dirt before incising. Personnel should not cut the first complete scale above the vent. They can remove the scale to the white connective tissue using either surgical scissors or a scalpel (multiple cuts may be required to remove an entire scale). Personnel should remove the minimum number of scales necessary.

Animal treatment, withdrawal and euthanasia

Personnel should monitor the animals continually. Signs of stress are difficult to assess in reptiles and amphibians and will depend on the study species (see Chapters 26 and 27), but may include behaviours such as flinching, body flattening, and continued struggling associated with undertaking the procedure. Typically, animals can be released immediately after marking, but may be observed for a period providing that doing so does not create additional unnecessary stress.

Equipment and maintenance

Specific equipment will vary depending on the context of the study and the study species. Suggested equipment is detailed in Table 8.6.

Specific qualifications, experience and training

Only personnel with appropriate experience (i.e. they have used the method at least two or three times and were deemed competent by a more-experienced person) should be undertaking these methods unsupervised. Personnel may consider gaining experience and confidence by practising the methods on preserved animals first, if available.

Table 8.6: Suggested equipment and materials for marking herpetofauna by toe, tail or scale clipping.

Marking equipment	Data collection	Post-marking
• Surgical scissors • Scalpels • Cotton cosmetic wipes (for swabbing equipment) • Delicate task wipes and filtered water (for cleaning the area before clipping) • Alcohol, lighter and sterile water (for disinfecting and cleaning equipment between individuals) • Disposable gloves appropriate for the taxon	• Clipboard and data sheets • List of available mark numbers or locations	• Bactine® or similar for disinfecting the wound, if desired • Plastic bags for holding amphibians if necessary • Eppendorf tubes or appropriate containers to hold tissue samples • Sharps container • Tissue adhesive for sealing wounds, if desired

Workplace health and safety

Personnel should consider the risk of cutting injuries (see details in earlier GOPs in this chapter) and be aware of potential risks associated with their specific study taxa.

Alternative procedures

One study found PIT tagging and marking with VIE less accurate than toe clipping for identifying animals (Brannelly *et al.* 2014). It is also difficult to assess the level of stress caused by different techniques. For example, the assumption that stress associated with toe clipping will exceed that caused by handling may not be valid (Fisher *et al.* 2013). Other techniques often proposed as suitable alternatives, such as PIT tagging (Langkilde and Shine 2006; see earlier in this chapter) and buccal swabs for collecting genetic material (Pidancier *et al.* 2003) are associated with their own suite of ethical and animal welfare considerations. However, handling time should be an important consideration when comparing potential alternative techniques (Phillott *et al.* 2008).

The decision to use alternative techniques should take into account the trade-off between efficiency and accuracy versus perceived stress and effects on fitness. The methods detailed in this GOP are efficient and require minimal handling time, which arguably may be more stressful to an animal than the procedure itself. These methods also provide a readable and long-term mark and can be used to collect genetic samples. Consideration of these trade-offs led Phillott *et al.* (2008) to conclude that toe clipping is often a viable technique for individual identification of frogs. The most desirable alternative for individual identification may be pattern recognition (e.g. Bradfield 2004), which in some cases can be undertaken without handling (Patel and Das 2020). However, detailed studies of the target species are typically required before using these methods and they often require parallel marking systems (e.g. toe clipping or microchipping) because individual patterns may change over time. Other alternative marking methods may include tattooing, VIA and VIE (see earlier GOPs in this chapter).

ACKNOWLEDGEMENTS

Thank you to Jodi Rowley for her review of and comments on this GOP.

MARKING FRESHWATER TURTLES BY SHELL NOTCHING

Donald T. McKnight

Target taxa

This GOP applies to freshwater turtles (Chapter 26).

Context and scope

This GOP describes the marking of freshwater turtles by filing or drilling notches or holes into their marginal scutes (Cagle 1939). Considerations and methods vary by species and size, but notches are effective and permanent for most species and size classes of turtle, and they are associated with relatively few animal welfare issues.

Animal welfare considerations

Animal handling

Handling and shell notching may cause short-term stress to target animals. Turtles should be handled by experienced researchers and processed in a cool area out of direct sunlight.

Number of marks

Notching is a minimally invasive marking technique. However, animals may experience stress and discomfort during the procedure. Therefore, coding systems that minimise the number of marks per animal are preferred.

Vascularized scutes and damage to tissues

Most scutes can be notched without bleeding. However, the scutes along the bridge (always the 5th and 6th scute, and sometimes the 7th and 8th) are vascularised and should be avoided (Cagle 1939). Similarly, care should be taken to avoid deep notches (> half the scute) and, on some individuals, scutes may need to be avoided if they are unusually small, close to the tissue, or damaged. Care should be taken to avoid injuring any soft tissues while marking turtles, particularly when using a drill or rotary tool. Risks can be minimised by restraining turtles' limbs appropriately, avoiding scutes that are narrow and close to the skin, and not making marks that are more than half the depth of the scute.

Young individuals

Very young individuals have soft shells that are not fully calcified. They must be notched carefully, and methods that result in a lot of strain on the shell (e.g., when using a file) should be avoided to prevent damage. Notches on very young turtles may become difficult to read as they grow, and other marking methods such as VIE should be considered.

General procedures

Notching systems

Most turtle species have 11 or 12 marginal scutes on each side of the shell. Within species, the number can vary slightly among individuals; therefore, counting should always start from the anterior part of the turtle. Individuals can easily be given unique identifying marks by notching or drilling a unique set of these scutes. Numerous systems are available for assigning unique marks (Plummer and Ferner 2012). Many common systems involve assigning a number to each scute, then assigning an identification number to each individual by taking the sum of the numbers for the marked scutes. However, these systems often require more than four marks (often up to eight) for an individual, even if only a few turtles are involved in a study, which makes the coding more time consuming and invasive. Additionally, notches can become difficult to read if an animal is captured many years after being marked (particularly if it was young when it was initially marked), and systems that require many notches increase the probability that a code will be difficult to accurately read in the future.

A simpler method that is faster to implement and requires fewer marks per individual involves simply recording what scutes were marked, with each side of the turtle being recorded as 'L' (left) and 'R' (right) and counting starting at the first anterior scute on each side (Figure 8.5). Thus, the first turtle captured in a study would receive marks on the first two scutes on the right side and would be recorded as 'R1,R2' (or simply 'R1,2'). The next turtle would be 'R1,R3', followed by 'R1,R4', followed by 'R1,R7' (scutes 5 and 6 are skipped), etc. Following 'R1,R12' the counting would move to the left side, and the next turtle would be 'R1,L1'. After 'R1,L12', the marking would resume on the right side with 'R2,R3'. Once all two-mark codes have been exhausted, a three-mark system can be used starting with 'R1,R2,R3', then 'R1,R2,R4', etc. Using this system, for a species with 12 marginal scutes on each side, it is possible to mark 190 individuals with two notches, 1140 with three notches, and 4845 with four notches (skipping the 5th and 6th scute). An alternate labelling system that results in the same number of marks per turtle involves describing each scute with a letter (A–L on the right, and N–Y on the left) (Nagle *et al.* 2017). Thus, 'R1,R2' is recorded as 'AB', 'R1,L1' is recorded as 'AN', etc. This notation minimises the length of records and reduces the chance of errors.

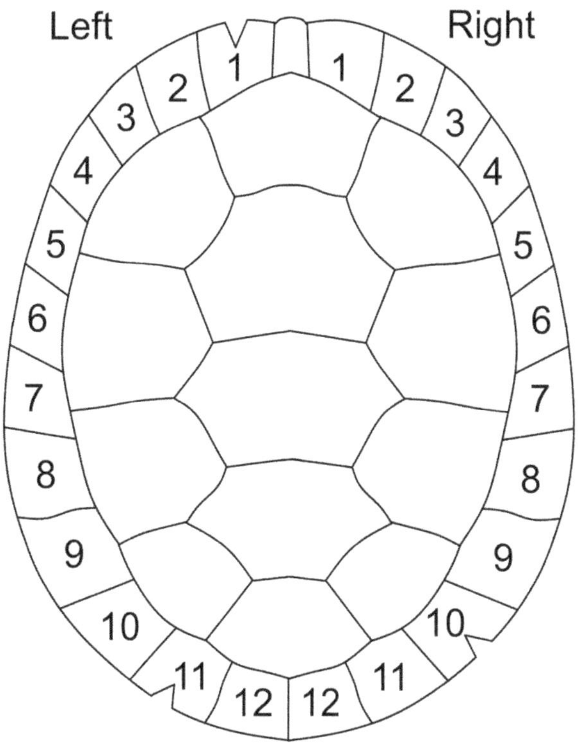

Figure 8.5: Diagram of a turtle shell showing the notch code R10, L1, L11 (or JNX using the Nagle *et al.* 2017 notation). Illustration by Donald T. McKnight.

Handling turtles

Turtles should be held by experienced researchers. For small individuals, it is usually possible for a single researcher to hold an animal with one hand and notch it with the other; however, for large individuals, it may be necessary for one researcher to hold the animal while another makes the marks (holding a turtle from below by gripping both sides of the posterior plastron lobe is also useful). Limbs should be pressed in and held tightly against an individual's body to avoid contact with the drill's bit, rotary tool's blade, file, or hacksaw. Similarly, when marking anterior scutes, the head should either be held out of the way or restrained inside the shell using a small wooden stick (e.g., pencil) or, for some species, a finger.

Making marks

Marks should be made in the centre of a given scute and should be less than half the depth of the scute, where depth is defined as the distance from the outer edge of the scute to the inner edge. Marks can be made either by using a drill to make a hole in the centre of a scute (or using a syringe needle for hatchlings) or by using a triangular file, rotary tool, or hacksaw to cut a notch into the scute from the outer edge (for hatchlings, surgical scissors or nail clippers can be used). Battery-operated rotary tools with reinforced cutting blades are generally the fastest method and provide the greatest user control and least strain on turtles' shells.

Animal treatment, withdrawal and euthanasia

Notches should be checked for bleeding (uncommon) and, if it occurs, antiseptic and surgical or veterinary glue should be applied to stop the bleeding. If an injury to a limb or the head occurs, the animal should be treated by a veterinarian.

Equipment and maintenance

Equipment varies by turtle size and researcher preference, but may include the following:

- Surgical scissors or toenail clippers are cheap and work well for hatchlings but cannot be used for larger turtles.
- Syringe needles can be used for hatchlings to make a small hole in the scute through which a piece of fishing line is passed (tied at each end). The fishing line falls out over time, but the hole remains.
- Triangular files and hacksaws are inexpensive, do not require electricity/batteries (making them good for remote field work), and can be used on all size classes except hatchlings, but they can be slow, particularly when working with large individuals or large numbers of individuals.
- Rotary tools (e.g., Dremel®) with reinforced cutting blades provide good user control and allow rapid notching of all size classes with minimal strain to turtles' shells. However, they are more expensive than files and require electricity/batteries.
- Drills allow the rapid marking of most size classes (except very small turtles) but provide less user control than rotary tools. They are more expensive than files and require electricity/batteries.
- Protective equipment, such as goggles, gloves, suitable clothing, and, in some cases, masks (to avoid inhaling dust from rotary tools) covers health and safety requirements.

Specific qualifications, experience and training

Researchers should be trained by individuals with experience notching turtles before attempting the method. Researchers can be trained on dead animals first.

Workplace health and safety

Using drills and rotary tools often results in small particles of shell flying into the air. Eye protection and a mask should be worn to prevent particles from entering the eyes and respiratory system. Rotary tool blades may also occasionally break (particularly if using blades that are not reinforced) and can injure a researcher's eyes if eye protection is not worn. Researchers should be careful to avoid cutting or stabbing themselves when working with drills, rotary tools, hacksaws, and syringes. Abrasions can also occur from triangular files.

Alternative procedures

Notching turtles is one of the most effective, inexpensive, and non-invasive marking techniques. Alternatives include photo identification (which is time consuming and unreliable for many species), microchipping (requires specialised equipment to identify an animal and injecting a tag into an animal), and VIE (the elastomer has to be refrigerated and is most effective on hatchlings). Procedures for marking with VIE and microchipping are detailed in earlier GOPs in this chapter. Notches are generally permanent, but for some species and small individuals, it may be advisable to use two marking methods (e.g. notches and microchipping) to ensure reliable future identification.

REFERENCES

Anderson KP, Byer NW, McGhee RJ, Richards-Dimitrie T (2015) A new system for marking hatchling turtles using visible implant elastomer. *Herpetological Review* **46**, 25–27. doi:10.13140/2.1.3643.1361

Antwis RE, Purcell R, Walker SL, Fidgett AL, Preziosi RF (2014) Effects of visible implant elastomer marking on physiological traits of frogs. *Conservation Physiology* **2**, cou042. doi:10.1093/conphys/cou042

Arid Recovery (2019) *Processing Reintroduced Mammals Procedure.* Arid Recovery, Roxby Downs.

Arntzen JW, Smithson A, Oldham RS (1999) Marking and tissue sampling effects on body condition and survival in the newt *Triturus cristatus*. *Journal of Herpetology* **33**, 567–576. doi:10.2307/1565573

Bainbridge L, Stockwell M, Valdez J, Klop-Toker K, Clulow S, Clulow J, Mahony M (2015) Tagging tadpoles: retention rates and impacts of visible implant elastomer (VIE) tags from the larval to adult amphibian stages. *The Herpetological Journal* **25**, 133–140.

Belser EH, Hewitt DG, Reitz RL, Gann KR, Lewis JS, Hellickson MW (2017) Ear tag and PIT tag retention by white-tailed deer. *Wildlife Society Bulletin* **41**, 752–757. doi:10.1002/wsb.831

Bladon RV, Dickman CR, Hume ID (2002) Effects of habitat fragmentation on the demography, movements and social organisation of the eastern pygmy-possum (*Cercartetus nanus*) in northern New South Wales. *Wildlife Research* **29**, 105–116. doi:10.1071/WR01024

Bloch NI, Irschick DJ (2005) Toe-clipping dramatically reduces clinging performance in a pad-bearing lizard (*Anolis carolinensis*). *Journal of Herpetology* **39**, 288–293. doi:10.1670/97-04N

Borges-Landáez PA, Shine R (2003) Influence of toe-clipping on running speed in *Eulamprus quoyii*, an Australian scincid lizard. *Journal of Herpetology* **37**, 592–595. doi:10.1670/26-02N

Bradfield KS (2004) *Photographic Identification of Individual Archey's Frogs,* Leiopelma archeyi, *from Natural Markings'.* Department of Conservation, Wellington, New Zealand.

Brannelly LA, Berger L, Skerrat LF (2014) Comparison of three widely used marking techniques for adult anuran species *Litoria verreauxii alpina. Herpetological Conservation and Biology* **9**, 428–435.

Brannelly LA, Chatfield MWH, Richards-Zawacki CL (2013) Visible implant elastomer (VIE) tags are an unreliable method of identification in adult anurans. *The Herpetological Journal* **23**, 125–129.

Brown LJ (1997) An evaluation of some marking and trapping techniques currently used in the study of anuran population dynamics. *Journal of Herpetology* **31**, 410–419. doi:10.2307/1565670

Brown WS, Parker WS (1976) A ventral scale clipping system for permanently marking snakes (Reptilia, Serpentes). *Journal of Herpetology* **10**, 247–249. doi:10.2307/1562986

Bumrungsri S, Leelapaibul W, Racey PA (2007) Resource partitioning in sympatric *Cynopterus* bats in lowland tropical rainforest, Thailand. *Biotropica* **39**, 241–248. doi:10.1111/j.1744-7429.2006.00245.x

Butt KR, Lowe CN (2007) A viable technique for tagging earthworms using visible implant elastomer. *Applied Soil Ecology* **35**, 454–457. doi:10.1016/j.apsoil.2006.06.004

Caballero-Gini A, Villafane DB, Romero L, Ferreira M, Cañete L, Laino R, Musalem K (2019) Visible implant alphanumeric (VIA) as a marking method in the lesser snouted treefrog *Scinax nasicus. Acta Herpetologica* **14**, 129–133. doi:10.13128/a_h-7751

Cagle FR (1939) A system of marking turtles for future identification. *Copeia* **1939**, 170–173. doi:10.2307/1436818

Cashins SD, Alford RA, Skerratt LF (2008) Lethal effect of latex, nitrile, and vinyl gloves on tadpoles. *Herpetological Review* **39**, 298–301.

Clemas RJ, Germano JM, Speare R, Bishop PJ (2009) Use of three individual marking methods in Australian frogs (Genus: *Litoria*) with notes on the placement of visible implant alphanumeric tags. *New Zealand Natural Sciences* **34**, 1–7.

Courtois EA, Lelong C, Calvez O, Loyau A, Schmeller DS (2013) The use of visible implant elastomer tags for anuran tadpoles. *Herpetological Review* **44**, 428–435.

Davenport J, Plot V, Georges JY, Doyle TK, James MC (2011) Pleated turtle escapes the box-shape changes in *Dermochelys coriacea. The Journal of Experimental Biology* **214**, 3474–3479. doi:10.1242/jeb.057182

Davis JLD, Young-Williams AC, Hines AH, Zohar Y (2005) Assessing the potential for stock enhancement in the case of the Chesapeake Bay blue crab (*Callinectes sapidus*). *Canadian Journal of Fisheries and Aquatic Sciences* **62**, 109–122. doi:10.1139/f04-150

Davis TM, Ovaska K (2001) Individual recognition of amphibians: effects of toe clipping and fluorescent tagging on the salamander *Plethodon vehiculum. Journal of Herpetology* **35**, 217–225. doi:10.2307/1566111

Davy CM, Coombes SM, Whitear AK, MacKenzie AS (2010) Visible implant elastomer: a simple, non-harmful method for marking hatchling turtles. *Herpetological Review* **41**, 442–445.

DBCA (2017) *Standard Operating Procedure: Semi-permanent Marking of Mammals using Ear Tags.* Department of Biodiversity, Conservation and Attractions, Perth.

Donnelly MA, Guyer C, Juterbock JE, Alford RA (1994) Techniques for marking amphibians. In *Measuring and Monitoring Biological Diversity: Standard Methods for Amphibians.* (Eds WR Heyer, MA Donnelly, RW McDiarmid, LC Hayek and MS Foster) pp. 277–284. Smithsonian Institution Press, Washington, DC.

Dunham AE, Morin PJ, Wilbur HM (1988) Methods for the study of reptile populations. In: *Biology of the Reptilia*, Volume 16. (Eds C Gans and RB Huey) pp. 330–386. Alan R Liss, New York, NY.

Edwards D, Johnston A, Pfeiffer D (2001) A comparison of commonly used ear tags on the ear damage of sheep. *Animal Welfare (South Mimms, England)* **10**, 141–151.

Ferner JW, Plummer MV (2016) Marking and measuring reptiles. In *Reptile Ecology and Conservation: A Handbook of Techniques.* (Ed. CK Dodd) pp. 45–59. Oxford University Press, Oxford, UK.

Fisher DO, Blomberg SP (2009) Toe-bud clipping of juvenile small marsupials for ecological field research: No detectable negative effects on growth or survival. *Austral Ecology* **34**, 858–865. doi:10.1111/j.1442-9993.2009.01991.x

Fisher KJ, Guilfoyle KJ, Hatch KA (2013) Stress induced by toe-clipping in cane toads (*Rhinella marina*). *Copeia* **2013**, 539–542. doi:10.1643/CP-12-149

Funk WC, Donnelly MA, Lips KR (2005) Alternative views of amphibian toe-clipping. *Nature* **433**, 193. doi:10.1038/433193c

Godino LN, Lumsden LF, Coulson F, Griffiths SR (2015) Network analysis reveals cryptic seasonal patterns of association in Gould's wattled bat (*Chalinolobus gouldii*) roosting in bat-boxes. *Behaviour* **152**, 2079–2105.

Golay N, Durrer H (1994) Inflammation due to toe-clipping in Natterjack toads (*Bufo calamita*). *Amphibia-Reptilia* **15**, 81–83. doi:10.1163/156853894X00560

Goldingay R, Kavanagh R (1990) Socioecology of the Yellow-bellied Glider, *Petaurus australis*, at Waratah Creek, NSW. *Australian Journal of Zoology* **38**, 327–341. doi:10.1071/ZO9900327

Gibbons WJ, Andrews KM (2004) Microchipping: simple technology at its best. *Bioscience* **54**, 447–454. doi:10.1641/0006-3568(2004)054[0447:PTSTAI]2.0.CO;2

Ginnan NA, Lawrence JR, Russell ME, Eggett DL, Hatch KA (2014) Toe clipping does not affect the survival of leopard frogs (*Rana pipiens*). *Copeia* **2014**, 650–653. doi:10.1643/CH-14-064

Grafe TU, Stewart MM, Lampert KP, Rödel MO (2011) Putting toe clipping into perspective: a viable method for marking anurans. *Journal of Herpetology* **45**, 28–35. doi:10.1670/10-016.1

Grant CA, Twigg PC, Baker R, Tobin DJ (2015) Tattoo ink nanoparticles in skin tissue and fibroblasts. *Journal of Nanotechnology* **6**, 1183–1191. doi:10.3762/bjnano.6.120

Halliday T (1996) Amphibians. In *Ecological Census Techniques, A Handbook.* (Ed WJ Sutherland) pp. 205–217. Cambridge University Press, Cambridge.

Heard GW, Scroggie MP, Malone BS (2008) Visible Implant Alphanumeric tags as an alternative to toe-clipping for marking amphibians – a case study. *Wildlife Research* **35**, 747–759. doi:10.1071/WR08060

Honkavaara J, Koivula M, Korpimäki E, Siitari H, Viitala J (2002) Ultraviolet vision and foraging in terrestrial vertebrates. *Oikos* **98**, 505–511. doi:10.1034/j.1600-0706.2002.980315.x

Hudson CM, Brown GP, Shine R (2017) Effects of toe-clipping on growth, body condition, and locomotion of cane toads (*Rhinella marina*). *Copeia* **105**, 257–260. doi:10.1643/CE-16-564

Jemison SC, Bishop LA, May PG, Farrel TM (1995) The impact of PIT-tags on growth and movement of the rattlesnake, *Sistrurus miliarius. Journal of Herpetology* **29**, 129–132. doi:10.2307/1565098

Johnston AM, Edwards DS (1996) Welfare implications of identification of cattle by ear tags. *The Veterinary Record* **138**, 612–614. doi:10.1136/vr.138.25.612

Jones C, Bell T (2007) Does toe clipping reduce recapture rates of McCann's skinks? *New Zealand Journal of Zoology* **34**, 265.

Jones MP, Pierce KE, Ward D (2007) Avian vision: a review of form and function with special consideration to birds of prey. *Journal of Exotic Pet Medicine* **16**, 69–87. doi:10.1053/j.jepm.2007.03.012

Jung RE, Droege S, Sauer JR, Landy RB (2000) Evaluation of terrestrial and streamside salamander monitoring techniques at Shenandoah National Park. *Environmental Monitoring and Assessment* **63**, 65–79. doi:10.1023/A:1006413603057

Jung TS, Boonstra R, Krebs CJ (2020) Mark my words: expert's choice of marking methods used in capture-mark-recapture studies of small mammals. *Journal of Mammalogy* **101**, 307–317. doi:10.1093/jmammal/gyz188

Kasanen IHE, Voipio H-M, Leskinen H, Luodonpää M, Nevalainen TO (2011) Comparison of ear tattoo, ear notching and microtattoo in rats undergoing cardiovascular telemetry. *Laboratory Animals* **45**, 154–159. doi:10.1258/la.2011.010113

Keating SCJ, Thomas AA, Flecknell PA, Leach MC (2012) Evaluation of EMLA cream for preventing pain during tattooing of rabbits: changes in physiological, behavioural and facial expression responses. *PLoS One* **7**, e44437. doi:10.1371/journal.pone.0044437

Kluever BM, Lagos L, Breck SW, Howery LD, Sanmartín ML, Bergman DL, Bárcena F (2012) Integrity and retention of ear-tag radiotransmitters in domestic cattle and feral horses. *Wildlife Society Bulletin* **36**, 189–193. doi:10.1002/wsb.95

Langkilde T, Shine R (2006) How much stress do researchers inflict on their study animals? A case study using a scincid lizard, *Eulamprus heatwolei*. *The Journal of Experimental Biology* **209**, 1035–1043. doi:10.1242/jeb.02112

Laux P, Tralau T, Tentschert J, Blume A, Al Dahouk S, Bäumler W, *et al.* (2016) A medical-toxicological view of tattooing. *Lancet* **387**, 395–402. doi:10.1016/S0140-6736(15)60215-X

Leclercq GG, Rozenfeld FM (2001) A permanent marking method to identify individual small rodents from birth to sexual maturity. *Journal of Zoology* **254**, 203–206. doi:10.1017/S0952836901000711

Lemckert F (1996) Effects of toe-clipping on the survival and behaviour of the Australian frog *Crinia signifera*. *Amphibia-Reptilia* **17**, 287–290. doi:10.1163/156853896X00450

Lindner E, Fuelling O (2002) Marking methods in small mammals: ear-tattoo as an alternative toe-clipping. *Journal of Zoology* **256**, 159–163. doi:10.1017/S0952836902000195

Lunghi E, Veith M (2017) Are visual implant alpha tags adequate for individually marking European cave salamanders (genus *Hydromantes*)? *Salamandra (Frankfurt)* **53**, 541–544.

Mali I, Forstner MRJ (2014) Use of stationary microchip reader for monitoring interpond movement of freshwater turtles. *Herpetological Review* **45**, 22–25.

Manolis SC, Webb GJW (2016) *Best Management Practices for Crocodilian Farming*. Version 1. IUCN-SSC Crocodile Specialist Group, Darwin.

May RM (2004) Ecology: ethics and amphibians. *Nature* **431**, 403. doi:10.1038/431403a

McCarthy MA, Parris KM (2004) Clarifying the effect of toe clipping on frogs with Bayesian statistics. *Journal of Applied Ecology* **41**, 780–786. doi:10.1111/j.0021-8901.2004.00919.x

McGregor M, Jones D (2016) Tattoo pens as a low-cost approach to in-field permanent identification of medium-sized mammals. *Wildlife Society Bulletin* **40**, 169–173. doi:10.1002/wsb.631

Mellor DJ, Beausoleil NJ, Stafford KJ (2004) *Marking Amphibians, Reptiles and Marine Mammals: Animal Welfare, Practicalities and Public Perceptions in New Zealand*. New Zealand Department of Conservation, Wellington, New Zealand.

Mulder RA, Guay P-J, Wilson M, Coulson G (2010) Citizen science: recruiting residents for studies of tagged urban wildlife. *Wildlife Research* **37**, 440–446. doi:10.1071/WR10007

Nagle RD, Kinney OM, Gibbons JW, Congdon JD (2017) A simple and reliable system for marking hard-shelled turtles: the North American code. *Herpetological Review* **48**, 327–330.

Narayan J, Gramapurohit NP (2019) Urinary corticosterone metabolite response to capture and visible elastomer tagging in the Asian toad (*Duttaphrynus melanostictus*). *The Herpetological Journal* **30**, 179–183. doi:10.33256/hj29.3.179183

Nauwelaerts S, Coeck J (2000) Visible implant elastomer as a method for marking adult anurans. *Herpetological Review* **31**, 154–155.

Northwest Marine Technology Inc (2017) *Visible Implant Elastomer Tag Project Manual: Guidelines on Planning and Conducting Projects using VIE*. Northwest Marine Technology Inc., Washington, DC.

Northwest Marine Technology Inc (2019) *Instructions for Visible Implant Alpha Tags*. Northwest Marine Technology Inc., Washington, DC.

Olds JE, Ewing J, Arruda P, Kuyper J, Riedesel E, Miles KM (2016) Iatrogenic microchip arterial embolism in a Chilean flamingo (*Phoenicopterus chilensis*). *Journal of Zoo and Wildlife Medicine* **47**, 686–690. doi:10.1638/2015-0168.1

Olivera-Tlahuel C, Pérez-Mendoza H, Zúñiga-Vega J, Rubio-Rocha L, Bock BC, Rojas-González RI *et al.* (compilers) (2017) *Best Management Practices for Crocodilian Farming*. IUCN-SSC Crocodile Specialist Group, Darwin.

Ott JA, Scott DE (1999) Effects of toe-clipping and PIT-tagging on growth and survival in metamorphic *Ambystoma opacum*. *Journal of Herpetology* **33**, 344–348. doi:10.2307/1565740

Patel NG, Das A (2020) Shot the spots: a reliable field method for individual identification of *Amolops formosus* (Anura, Ranidae). *Herpetozoa (Wien)* **33**, 7–15. doi:10.3897/herpetozoa.33.e47279

Paulissen MA, Meyer HA (2000) The effect of toe-clipping on the gecko *Hemidactylus turcicus*. *Journal of Herpetology* **34**, 282–285. doi:10.2307/1565425

Penney KM, Gianopulos KD, McCoy ED (2001) The visible implant elastomer marking technique in use for small reptiles. *Herpetological Review* **32**, 236–241.

Perret N, Joly P (2002) Impacts of tattooing and pit-tagging on survival and fecundity in the alpine newt (*Triturus alpestris*). *Herpetologica* **58**, 131–138. doi:10.1655/0018-0831(2002)058[0131:IOTAPO]2.0.CO;2

Perry G, Wallace MC, Perry D, Curzer H, Muhlberger P (2011) Toe clipping of amphibians and reptiles: science, ethics, and the law. *Journal of Herpetology* **45**, 547–555. doi:10.1670/11-037.1

Pestell AJL, Petit S (2007) Methods and ethical considerations of pitfall trapping for the western pygmy possum (*Cercartetus concinnus* Gould) (Marsupialia: Burramyidae), with observations on capture patterns and nest sites. *Wildlife Research* **34**, 296–305. doi:10.1071/WR06090

Petit S, Waudby HP, Walker AT, Zanker R, Rau G (2012) A non-mutilating method for marking small wild mammals and reptiles. *Australian Journal of Zoology* **60**, 64–71. doi:10.1071/ZO11088

Petit S, Waudby HP (2012) Standard operating procedures for aluminium box, wire cage, and pitfall trapping, handling, and temporary housing of small wild rodents and marsupials. *Australian Journal of Zoology* **60**, 392–401. doi:10.1071/ZO12102

Phillott AD, Skerratt LF, McDonald KR, Lemckert FL, Hines HB, Clarke JM, Alford RA, Speare R (2008) Toe clipping of anurans for mark-recapture studies: acceptable if justified. That's what we said! *Herpetological Review* **39**, 149–150.

Pidancier N, Miquel C, Miaud C (2003) Buccal swabs as a non-destructive tissue sampling method for DNA analysis in amphibians. *The Herpetological Journal* **13**, 175–178.

Plummer MV, Ferner JW (2012) Marking reptiles. In *Reptile Biodiversity: Standard Methods for Inventory and Monitoring.* (Eds RW McDiarmid, S Mercedes, S Foster, G Guyer, JW Gibbons and N Chernoff) pp. 143–150. University of California Press.

Polich RL, Searcy CA, Shaffer HB (2013) Effects of tail-clipping on survivorship and growth of larval salamanders. *The Journal of Wildlife Management* **77**, 1420–1425. doi:10.1002/jwmg.596

Pyke GH (2005) The use of PIT tags in capture-recapture studies of frogs: a field evaluation. *Herpetological Review* **36**, 281–285.

Regester KJ, Woosley LB (2005) Marking salamander egg masses with visible fluorescent elastomer: retention time and effect on embryonic development. *American Midland Naturalist* **153**, 52–60. doi:10.1674/0003-0031(2005)153[0052:MSEMWV]2.0.CO;2

Replinger SE, Wood JB (2007) A preliminary investigation of the use of subcutaneous tagging in Caribbean reef squid *Sepioteuthis sepioidea* (Cephalopoda: Loliginidae). *Fisheries Research* **84**, 308–313. doi:10.1016/j.fishres.2006.11.028

Roark AW, Dorcus ME (2000) Regional body temperature variation in corn snakes measured using temperature-sensitive passive integrated transponders. *Journal of Herpetology* **34**, 481–485. doi:10.2307/1565378

Recio P, Rodríguez-Ruiz G, Ortega J, Martín J (2019) PIT-Tags as a technique for marking fossorial reptiles: insights from a long-term field study of the amphisbaenian *Trogonophis wiegmanni*. *Acta Herpetologica* **14**, 101–107.

Sandford M, Castillo G, Hung T-C (2020) A review of fish identification methods applied on small fish. *Reviews in Aquaculture* **12**, 542–554. doi:10.1111/raq.12339

Sapsford SJ, Roznik EA, Alford RA, Schwarzkopf L (2014) Visible implant elastomer marking does not affect short-term movements or survival rates of the treefrog *Litoria rheocola*. *Herpetologica* **70**, 23–33. doi:10.1655/HERPETOLOGICA-D-13-0004

Schmidt K, Schwarzkopf L (2010) Visible implant elastomer tagging and toe-clipping: effects of marking on locomotor performance of frogs and skinks. *The Herpetological Journal* **20**, 99–105.

Schreiver I, Hesse B, Seim C, Castillo-Michel H, Villanova J, Laux P, *et al.* (2017) Synchrotron-based ν-XRF mapping and μ-FTIR microscopy enable to look into the fate and effects of tattoo pigments in human skin. *Scientific Reports* **7**, 11395. doi:10.1038/s41598-017-11721-z

Siegal-Willott J, Heard D, Sliess N, Naydan D, Roberts J (2007) Microchip-associated leiomyosarcoma in an Egyptian fruit bat (*Rousettus aegypticacus*). *Journal of Zoo and Wildlife Medicine* **38**, 352–356. doi:10.1638/1042-7260(2007)038[0352:MLIAEF]2.0.CO;2

Silvy NJ, Lopez RR, Peterson MJ (2005). Wildlife marking techniques. In *Techniques for Wildlife Investigations and Management 6th Edn* (Ed CE Braun) pp. 339-376. The Wildlife Society, Maryland, USA.

Soderquist TR, Dickman CR (1988) A technique for marking marsupial pouch young with fluorescent pigment tattoos. *Australian Wildlife Research* **15**, 561–563. doi:10.1071/WR9880561

van Harten E, Reardon T, Lumsden LF, Meyers N, Prowse TAA, Weyland J, Lawrence R (2019) High detectability with low impact: optimising large PIT tracking systems for cave-dwelling bats. *Ecology and Evolution* **9**, 10916–10928. doi:10.1002/ece3.5482

van Harten E, Reardon T, Holz PH, Lawrence R, Prowse TAA, Lumsden LF (2020) Recovery of southern bent-winged bats (*Miniopterus orianae bassanii*) after PIT-tagging and the use of surgical adhesive. *Australian Mammalogy* **42**, 216–219. doi:10.1071/AM19024

Waudby HP, Petit S (2011) Comments on the efficacy and use of Visible Implant Elastomer (VIE) for marking lizards. *South Australian Naturalist* **85**, 7–13.

Wells K (2007) *The Ecology and Behaviour of Amphibians.* University of Chicago Press, London, UK.

West T (2016) *Instructions for Tattooing Rabbits.* Ohio State University, College of Food, Agricultural and Environmental Sciences, Columbus, OH.

Zamora-Camacho FJ (2018) Toe-clipping does not affect toad's short-term locomotor performance. *Annales Zoologici Fennici* **55**, 237–246. doi:10.5735/086.055.0606

9 Wildlife tracking methods

Damian S. Morrant, James M. Turner, Melissa A. Jensen, Nicole A. Hansen, Deborah S. Bower, Gerhard Körtner, Paul D. Meek, Angela J.L. Pestell, Peggy D. Rismiller, Helen P. Waudby and Carmen Amos

INTRODUCTION

Scientists and wildlife managers track animals by fitting them with telemetry collars, tags, harnesses, adhesive transmitters, implants or other devices to help them understand how animals use the landscape, study their behaviour, or to locate animals for management purposes. The first published wildlife telemetry research used implanted transmitters for three woodchucks (a.k.a. groundhogs, *Marmota monax*; LeMunyan *et al.* 1959). Cochran and Lord (1963) attached transmitters to eastern cottontail rabbits (*Sylvilagus floridanus*) and striped skunks (*Mephitis mephitis*) with harnesses (but did not find them satisfactory), and then trialled collars for the same animals in addition to raccoons (*Procyon lotor*). Very high frequency (VHF) radio tracking revolutionised the study of wild-animal movements. By March 1979, one of the leading commercial suppliers of radio-tracking equipment had sold > 17 500 radio collars (Mech 1980). Since then, researchers have developed a plethora of devices to study and understand animal movements, including global positioning system (GPS) loggers, passive integrated transponder (PIT) tags (Chapter 8), sensors (e.g. activity and proximity; temperature, humidity and light; video and still cameras), and data-sharing devices (e.g. that can share data among collars in an animal group) (Latham *et al.* 2015).

Ever smaller and efficient batteries, transmitters and circuitry have improved signal strength, detection range, and the computing power and precision of tracking devices. For some taxa, researchers are already able to monitor movements and behaviour of individual animals throughout their life cycle, providing data of immense value for biodiversity conservation. Wildlife telemetry provides insights into the ways that animals interact with each other, their food or prey, humans, climate and the landscape in general. Tracking affords researchers the opportunity to analyse animal movement data using sophisticated statistical methods, and in some instances also allows researchers to visualise and follow the same paths as their study animals, viewing the landscape from a similar perspective. Despite the benefits to species' conservation, telemetry (and associated) devices can pose several risks to the wellbeing of individual study animals (Hennig *et al.* 2020), and must be evaluated before undertaking any study. The general operating procedures (GOPs) detailed in this chapter discuss some of these risks and propose ways to mitigate them.

SURGICAL IMPLANTATION OF RADIO TRANSMITTERS

James M. Turner, Gerhard Körtner and Peggy D. Rismiller

Target taxa

These methods apply to tetrapod vertebrates, including terrestrial mammals (Chapters 17–24), reptiles (Chapter 26), amphibians (Chapter 27) and birds (Chapters 33–36).

Context and scope

This GOP outlines general procedures for surgically implanting small electronic radio transmitters into animals for research. Surgery is moderately complex and describing the many nuanced variables that change with species is beyond the scope of this GOP. Instead, it provides an overview of best practice methods based on the authors' experiences. Where practicable, these methods should be performed by a veterinarian, and thorough training in surgical procedures is imperative for the methods described here. While the methods *per se* apply to animals in captive or laboratory settings, and can be used for data loggers, transponders or other devices designed to measure a broad range of physiological variables, this GOP focuses on transmitters implanted into wildlife for the purpose of radio-tracking studies.

Implanted radio transmitters were initially developed in the late 1950s and used to relay physiological information such as body temperature, respiration rate or electrocardiograms to a receiver (Adams 1965). Technological miniaturisation in the decades since have reduced this 122.5 g, 7.5 × 4.0 × 1.4 cm prototype into pea-sized transmitters that weigh < 1 g. Importantly, this advancement has reduced the impact of surgery on study subjects.

An advantage of internally located transmitters compared to externally attached devices (see other GOPs in this chapter for examples) is the capability to measure physiological variables and provide the animal's location simultaneously. This capability has allowed ecophysiological research to expand. Biologists now have a better understanding of how animals function in the wild and can confidently describe physiological mechanisms underlying observed behavioural traits and ecological patterns. Additionally, external transmitters can affect locomotion, thermoregulation, energy expenditure, visibility, predation risk, risk of entanglement, an animal's profile (important for flying, swimming or burrowing), parasite load and various behaviours, and may cause skin, hair or feather damage (reviewed in Casper 2009; Horning *et al.* 2017). Implanted transmitters may be less likely to cause behavioural changes in mammals than devices attached with collars (Koehler *et al.* 1987). External transmitters are also vulnerable to damage during the study animal's normal activities and need to be more rugged than an implanted unit. However, implantation can cause severe impacts on some species (e.g. Meyers *et al.* 1998) and the transmission range of internal transmitters with small loop antennas can be considerably reduced in comparison to similarly sized external transmitters with a whip antenna. Finally, GPS transmitters cannot be implanted as the weak radio waves transmitted by satellites do not penetrate body tissue.

Animal welfare considerations

Surgery is an invasive technique that will cause at least some pain and distress to study animals (Chapter 16). Animals need to be caught, removed temporarily from their natural habitat, and are sometimes transported to an operating theatre, which may be at a field station. However, surgery may be performed *in situ* (Fiorello *et al.* 2016), especially for large species that are difficult to transport, e.g. moose, *Alces alces* (Græsli *et al.* 2020). Implanted animals then need to be held in captivity for a recovery period before release. It is in the researchers' best interests that surgery is minimally invasive and animals recover quickly and completely because compromised data collected from impaired animals will not reflect natural activity nor meet study objectives (Casper 2009).

Physical injury

Most internal transmitters are implanted intraperitoneally, but on occasions subcutaneous implantation is appropriate. Implantation requires a surgical incision through skin, muscle, serous membranes (thin membranes that lines the internal body cavities and organs), to open a body cavity. While the techniques used are designed to minimise injury and a full recovery of the animal is always the intended outcome, surgery is unavoidably invasive. Animals will feel pain and distress after the procedure and although the surgical wound is likely to heal, the resulting scar will not have the same integrity as surrounding tissue (Anderson 1996). The long-term effects of the incision can be minimised through good hygiene practices, and careful and accurate surgical technique during implantation and subsequent suturing of the wound.

Physiological stress

A stress response is likely to be induced in a study animal during capture, transportation to the operating theatre, anaesthetic induction, recovery and time in captivity (Casper 2009). Stress can be minimised by performing surgery as soon as possible after capture. For small species, stress can be reduced by keeping the animal in a darkened bag or box in a quiet place (Fiorello *et al.* 2016). After surgery, analgesic and anti-inflammatory drugs (Chapter 16) can reduce discomfort and stress and enable animals to be released at their point of capture promptly. Stress following implantation has the potential to cause a long-term reduction in fitness, but the extent of the impact varies among species (Sexson *et al.* 2014).

Bearing a load

A valid concern of equipping an animal with any type of device is that of instantly increasing the load it carries and whether this load may affect behaviour, fitness, survival or other physiological or ecological factors. Researchers often quote a 3%, 5% or 10% 'rule' – marking the upper limit of an animal's body mass that a transmitter should weigh. However, the load that an animal can bear varies greatly with body shape and mass, life-history stage and method of locomotion (Aldridge and Brigham 1988; Casper 2009; Rojas *et al.* 2010). Also, the mass of young carried by a female *in utero*, in eggs, in a pouch or on the back can greatly exceed 10% of her body mass, and mass gain caused by seasonal fattening of many hibernating mammals is often 100% of summer weight. Indeed, if a transmitter is implanted close to an animal's centre of gravity, any effect is likely to be smaller than that imposed by applying the same mass to, for example, a collar located close to one end of the body (Casper 2009). Therefore, while the mass and size of a transmitter is an important consideration, the authors recommend first scrutinising a species' biology instead of following an arbitrary rule. Ultimately, lighter and smaller transmitters are likely to minimise negative impacts on an animal, but researchers must be careful not to jeopardise data quality and the outcomes of the study.

General procedures

Common anaesthetics and analgesics are described in Chapter 16.

Know the study species

Researchers must be familiar with the physiology and anatomy of their study species. This information will influence the type and dosage of drugs to be administered, the location of the surgical wound and transmitter positioning, the equipment needed to perform surgery, including suture materials and methods, and the required level of post-surgical care, among other factors. For example, a midline incision can minimise muscle damage and is advisable for many small mammals and birds. In contrast, in many reptiles a major central blood vessel prohibits such an approach. Furthermore, the effect of surgery can differ seasonally. For example, the body temperature of an animal is important for the healing process, and surgery during the cooler months of the year should be avoided in ectothermic animals (reptiles, amphibians and fish). Similar problems can occur in animals that undergo daily torpor or hibernation.

Anaesthesia induction and maintenance

The anaesthetic chosen must be suitable for the species and the individual's age and developmental stage. Researchers should refer to Chapter 16 for more detailed procedures..

Pre-operative considerations

Before implantation, transmitters can be coated in an inert resin or wax to add a waterproof layer and prevent any tissue reactions. They then need to be sterilised in, for example, ethanol or formaldehyde. Standard veterinary surgical procedures (Fiorello *et al.* 2016) should be followed to ensure aseptic technique. Ideally, surgery should be conducted on a cleaned surface in a quiet room, but doing so is not always practical, especially if it needs to be done in the field (Fiorello *et al.* 2016). Where possible, personnel conducting the procedure should wear gloves, a mask, a head covering and a robe. The animal needs to be kept warm, which is particularly important for ectotherms (reptiles and amphibians) whose metabolism is directly related to ambient temperature. The same applies to small endotherms (mammals and birds) as thermoregulation is impaired during anaesthesia. A warm room, heat pad, circulating warm-water blanket, forced warm-air blanket, parenteral administration of warm fluids or a warm bath can be used to maintain animal warmth.

The surgical site must be prepared and the skin exposed. Mammal hair can be shaved using clippers and/or a razor blade or removed using a depilatory cream. Bird feathers can be wetted and pushed aside so that only a few require plucking. Reptile scales need only be cleaned. The site can be sterilised with chlorhexidine gluconate or povidone–iodine concentrate. However, soaps, detergents, isopropyl alcohol or povidone–iodine products are not recommended for amphibians (Gentz 2007).

Implantation procedure

Here the procedure for implanting a transmitter into the peritoneal cavity (birds and mammals) or coelom (amphibians and reptiles) of a study animal is described. Larger animals may only need subcutaneous implantation, depending on the physiological variable to be examined.

A longitudinal midline incision can be made with dissecting scissors or a reversed scalpel blade, depending on skin thickness. The cut should be made in the skin between the scales of reptiles, or on the interfacing side between belly and dorsal scales in snakes, and inferior to the keel in birds. Tissues can be held using tissue forceps. Taking care to avoid the abdominal vein in reptiles and amphibians, the muscle layer and underlying peritoneum are then cut. Retractors may be needed to hold the wound open in larger animals. The incision should be kept as small as possible to minimise wound size but large enough to allow the transmitter to be inserted without further damaging tissue. The transmitter may be tethered to the abdominal wall in larger animals to avoid migration or sutured to a rib in pythons to prevent encapsulation into the gut and subsequent expulsion with faeces (Pearson and Shine 2002). After the transmitter is inserted and in a satisfactory position, the wound can be closed. The peritoneum and muscle layer can be sutured together with absorbable swaged sutures with a curved needle (e.g. chromic gut or Vicryl®); low-profile swaged needles are particularly important for reptiles with inelastic skin. The skin is sutured separately; continuous sutures should be avoided if the animal can easily reach the wound and remove the suture. Surgical glue and staples are alternatives for wound closure. Surgical glue is especially useful for thin-skinned species, such as amphibians and some reptiles, and can be used by itself or in addition to sutures; for example, individual sutures between reptile scales in combination with glue is an effective technique. Staples are regularly used in laboratory mice and rats and could be used if the study species (rodents and diprotodont marsupials, for example) is able to pull out stitches with its incisors.

Post-operative considerations

After wound closure, precautions must be made to prevent damage to the surgical site, avoid infection and minimise pain. Typically, a combination of a species-appropriate broad-spectrum antibiotic (which can also be applied to the wound before closure), analgesic (injected, topical or oral), topical antiseptic, non-steroidal anti-inflammatory and parasiticide are administered. Non-adherent bandages can be used to protect the wounds of species that are unlikely to remove them. These can be glued in place on reptiles such as snakes and goannas; the wound is often healed by the time they have worn off. In other cases, a waterproof spray bandage can be used. Topical anaesthetics can reduce itchiness caused by inflammation and have an unpleasant taste that may deter grooming of the wound.

Individuals should be monitored after surgery to look for any adverse effects, including shock, external bleeding or bruising. Indicators of post-operative pain may include restlessness, lethargy, reduced activity, panting or shallow breathing and lameness (Price *et al.* 2003). The time it takes for wounds to heal is highly variable, but collagen and scar tissue can maintain wound integrity as soon as 7 days post-surgery in mammals (Anderson 1996). Healing times in reptiles and amphibians are greatly protracted owing to their low rates of metabolism and dependence on ambient temperature for normal physiological processes; reptiles can take seven times as long to heal as a similarly sized mammal (Alworth *et al.* 2011). The duration of time that a study animal is held in captivity before release varies widely in the literature from hours to months. Animals may even be released immediately after surgery without decreased survival (Fiorello *et al.* 2016). In fact, in our experience, short-beaked echidnas (*Tachyglossus aculeatus*) and goannas (*Varanus* spp.) released into the wild as soon as possible are less likely to become stressed and show improved healing and recovery than animals maintained in captivity (P. Rismiller, pers. obs.). Ultimately, researchers need to be confident that animals have recovered from surgery enough to display normal behaviours in the wild, thereby not adversely affecting their welfare or negatively influencing the objectives or outcomes of the study.

Explantation procedure

Implanted transmitters are often left inside study animals to avoid a second surgery. However, if a device needs to be retrieved, for instance to avoid impeding egg-laying in reptiles, explantation procedures are usually identical to those used for implantation. Care needs to be taken if the transmitter has become encapsulated by tissue and attached to the abdominal wall. During explantation, any sequelae (conditions that are the consequence of a previous injury) should be recorded, treated and potentially used to improve future surgical techniques with the aim of avoiding their occurrence.

Animal treatment, withdrawal and euthanasia

Generally, problems are more likely to be associated with anaesthesia than with the surgical procedure itself. Modern inhalation anaesthetics such as isoflurane have a high safety margin (Chapter 16), but species specificity, stress, body condition and perhaps health issues that are sometimes difficult to anticipate may still affect surgery outcomes. These factors are particularly relevant for wildlife studies where the history, age and health of the individual is unknown and previous experience with a particular species is limited or non-existent. In contrast, the risk of a trained surgeon causing accidental irreparable injury during implantation is likely to be low. If an accident occurs, the surgeon should be sufficiently skilled to repair the injury and minimise any additional impact on the animal, or if the injury is severe enough to preclude recovery, euthanase the animal. If unpredicted complications or acute pain are identified after surgery while an animal is recovering and cannot be quickly remedied, informed judgment must be used when deciding if a second surgery, which has the potential to prolong recovery and cause additional stress, is needed or whether euthanasia is appropriate.

Equipment and maintenance

Given that, in most cases, the mechanical procedure will be simple incision, minimal equipment is required. However, particular species may require specialised equipment. For instance, an oscillating sagittal saw is needed to remove a section of a turtle plastron (shell underside) and its reinstalment requires an acrylic glue and epoxy resin (Alworth *et al.* 2011).

Specific qualifications, experience and training

In some states, animal surgery is considered an 'act of veterinary science' and can only legally be performed by a veterinarian (Australian Veterinary Association 2017). The level of training that the surgeon requires also varies with organisational animal ethics committees (AECs). AECs may require veterinary qualifications for surgical procedures; some committees accept certification gained from short experimental surgical techniques training courses or informal training received from an experienced or qualified senior researcher. Veterinary support may also be appropriate where specialised equipment is required or restricted drugs will be used. If fieldwork is to be conducted in a remote area, animal capture success is low and/or animal transport is difficult, it may be impractical to rely on the involvement of a professional veterinarian and researchers should undergo appropriate training from qualified personnel. Personnel should be familiar with the study species and all drugs required for surgery, and should be competent in all aspects of the required surgical technique, including maintenance of anaesthesia and pre- and post-operative care. They should either hold a formal qualification in veterinary medicine or have undergone sufficient training with an expert mentor.

Workplace health and safety

Surgery precautions

Personal protective equipment (PPE) to prevent infection with zoonoses is needed (see Chapter 16). Adequate ventilation of room air is required to minimise inhalation of fumes from anaesthetics and other chemicals. Care must be taken when using sharp surgical instruments and syringe needles. Typical equipment and materials for surgically implanted transmitters includes:

- surgical PPE (gloves, face mask, hair covering, robe, protective eyewear)
- surgical drapes and adhesive tape/clips to hold them in place
- equipment to hold animals in place such as rope or adhesive tape
- equipment to keep an animal warm such as a heat mat, warm air blanket or water bath
- anaesthetic machine
- veterinary drugs – anaesthetics, analgesics and other post-operative drugs
- needles and syringes
- razor blade/clippers/depilatory cream to remove hair
- skin sterilisers
- magnifying glasses or lamp for very small species
- autoclaved surgery kit, including a minimum of: scalpel, forceps, dissecting scissors, needle-drivers and haemostats; in the field, chemical sterilisation of equipment is acceptable using, for instance, 100% ethanol
- sutures with low-profile swaged needles
- sterile gauze, bandages and/or spray bandage
- animal housing for recovery.

Alternative procedures

The decision to use implants is usually related to a species' anatomy or behaviour; see later GOPs in this chapter for alternative device attachment options for telemetry studies. If the measurement of a physiological variable is desired, implanted transmitters are often the most viable option. However, alternatives may include external temperature-sensitive transmitters located on collars or glued to an animal's skin, which are sometimes used to record skin temperature as a proxy for core body temperature, and studies doing so often cite animal welfare considerations as justification. In larger ungulates, an ingested transmitter lodged in the rumen is also a viable option (Signer *et al.* 2010) and ingested transmitters are regularly used in snakes (Shine 1987). These methods can be successful for some species but depend on the study objectives, animal morphology and behaviour, ambient temperature and transmitter placement (Willis and Brigham 2003; Dausmann 2005). Also, in recent years collar-mounted devices that measure dynamic body acceleration (accelerometers) have gained traction as a robust alternative to implanted heart rate transmitters in studies of free-ranging animal metabolism (Wilson *et al.* 2020).

TELEMETRY DEVICES ATTACHED WITH COLLARS

Damian S. Morrant, Paul D. Meek and Melissa A. Jensen

Target taxa

This GOP applies to dasyurids (Chapter 18), wombats, possums and gliders (Chapter 19), koalas (Chapter 20), macropods (Chapter 21), eutherian carnivores (Chapter 22), bats (Chapter 23), and rodents, lagomorphs and terrestrial ungulates (Chapter 24).

Context and scope

This GOP describes key considerations for studies that track animal movements using collars. The methods described in this GOP are only suitable for animals with clearly defined necks. Consequently, devices attached with collars are generally deployed on mammals and rarely on other taxa. Collars may support a range of sensors and transmitters, including very high frequency (VHF) beacons, GPS, satellite or short message service (SMS) communication devices, accelerometers, ultra-high frequency (UHF) communication devices, digital cameras, and sensors for temperature and humidity. General considerations are similar for all devices.

VHF tracking involves using a directional antenna and receiver to follow the signal given off by a transmitter that is attached to a collar to determine the exact location of the collared animal. The operator programs the receiver with the transmitter frequency and rotates the antenna until the loudest signal is heard. This signal is followed, with the operator regularly checking the direction of the signal and fine-tuning the receiver, until the animal is located. VHF signals may be reflected, or 'bounce', from hard, smooth surfaces such as rocks and trees, sometimes making it difficult to locate the precise location of the animal. Signals may also be emitted by a range of electronic sources. For example, mobile phones and electric fences emit a pulse that may be received like a weak and/or flat 'ping' from the animal's collar. The effects of radio-frequency interference are usually greatest in peri-urban areas. GPS devices in collars use precise time and location data, from satellite broadcasts, to determine their location (Latham *et al.* 2015). They can be programmed to record data at desired time intervals and location data are stored in a memory chip within the collar. In many cases data can also be uploaded remotely or downloaded either manually or automatically via SMS, VHF, UHF or satellite. Most GPS collars used in Australia have a VHF capability so they can be located and monitored in the field.

Animal welfare considerations

Animal welfare issues associated with collaring animals are influenced by the means of capture, duration of handling, type of collar, the tightness with which the collar is fitted, operator experience, the age class, body mass and breeding status of the animal, species, local environmental conditions and the reliability of the equipment. Collars may cause animals to increase their energy consumption and compromise fundamental life-history traits, such as survival and breeding success (McMahon *et al.* 2011). Devices may also influence an animal's hunting, navigation and use of natural structures, and ability to groom. In extreme cases, collared animals may asphyxiate or experience rubbing wounds if the collar is too tight, or the collar may become entangled (e.g. on a fence or foliage, or entrapment of a leg) if too loose (Jones et al. 2012). Care should be taken to remove any knobs or crimps from the end of whip collars, as they may become lodged in cracks in logs/trunks and entrap animals. Careful consideration is needed when designing a tracking study, and choosing collar materials and design.

Capture methods

Animals may experience stress during capture and handling. Researchers must be experienced in the capture, handling and collar fitting processes suitable for the target species, or be trained and supervised by people who are. Options for mitigating stress or injury in captured animals include anaesthesia, restraining boards (Chapter 7), restraints, and head or eye covers (i.e. hood or blindfold). However, for most small- to medium-sized animals, restraining the animal in a soft, dark bag with their head and eyes covered, is usually sufficient. As with all procedures involving animal handling, stress can be minimised via competent handling by experienced operators, undertaken in a calm and competent manner.

A well-designed study will mitigate many of the potential impacts on study animals, by ensuring that appropriate equipment, sample size and study duration are chosen, and that the researcher has the necessary skills and equipment to respond to issues that may arise. Thus, researchers should begin their telemetry study by defining their research questions (White and Garrott 1990; Fieberg and Börger 2012; Latham *et al.* 2015), and then choose the appropriate technology, study design and data analysis strategy to answer them (Fieberg and Börger 2012).

Collar dimensions

It is vital that collars are acquired and fitted to animals only after careful consideration of the study species' ecology, behaviour, reproductive cycle, anatomy and physiology. Collars should allow the animal natural mobility and not impair activities such as hunting and foraging, grooming/preening, sleeping or provisioning young. The potential effects on pelage integrity and insulation should be considered, particularly in extremely hot or cold climates (McMahon *et al.* 2011). Collars can cause pelage damage even when fitted correctly. If they are too tight, they may impede movement, swallowing and breathing, rub or break the skin around the animal's neck or, in extreme cases, cause skin necrosis. If they are too loose, they may fall off (e.g. during grooming, playing or fighting), move around and cause chafing, become entangled in foliage, or the animal may slip a foot through the collar and be unable to remove it (Jones *et al.* 2012).

Neck circumferences tend to vary as animals mature, during lactation, and as they store fat across seasons. Therefore, it is important to consider not only the neck circumference when fitting the collar, but also potential changes in girth during the study. Collars on juvenile animals may be fitted slightly looser than on adults, to allow for growth. Collar fit can be species-specific, but generally researchers should be able to fit two to four fingers under the collar on medium- to large-sized mammals (Kenward 2000; Matthews *et al.* 2013) and one or two fingers under the collar of smaller mammals. Collar dimensions and tightness should be modified according to the shape of the collar and girth of the animals' temporomandibular joints. For some species without well-developed necks, such as feral pigs (*Sus scrofa*), collars need to be fitted more tightly to avoid them being shed (Quy *et al.* 2014), whereas collars fitted to numbats (*Myrmecobius fasciatus*), for example, should be fitted as loosely as possible, but tight enough that the collar cannot be pulled off over the numbat's head (see Chapter 18). Collars should be rotated around the neck once they have been fitted to ensure that pelage is not caught in the locking mechanism(s).

Collar mass

Refer to 'Surgical implantation of radio transmitters' for general considerations in relation to device mass as a percentage of animal body mass. Battery, GPS and VHF components are usually housed under the animal's ventral neck in a 'box' (Figure 9.1a), which may act as a counterweight to the GPS antenna at the top, if fitted. Information about appropriate collar dimensions and materials should be sought from a range of sources, including previous studies and the collar manufacturer. Where possible, the collar should be customised for the study species and the load of the electronic components should be distributed evenly (Matthews *et al.* 2013). Strong belting material and internal antennae can be used for predators and large herbivores, as weak belting and external components can be damaged or chewed during play, hunting and agonistic interactions.

Timing and duration of the study

Careful planning and design are required to identify appropriate methods, sample sizes, and study durations, noting that extra animals may need to be collared in case some data are not recovered (Latham *et al.* 2015). For example, Matthews *et al.* (2013) recommended deploying 20% extra collars to account for animal deaths, collar shedding and failure. If too few animals are tracked, or they are not tracked for long enough, the ability to detect the effect(s) of interest is reduced and the study animals undergo distress for a less-productive outcome. Similarly, unnecessary impacts may occur if too many animals are tracked or if they are tracked for longer than necessary to achieve the study aims.

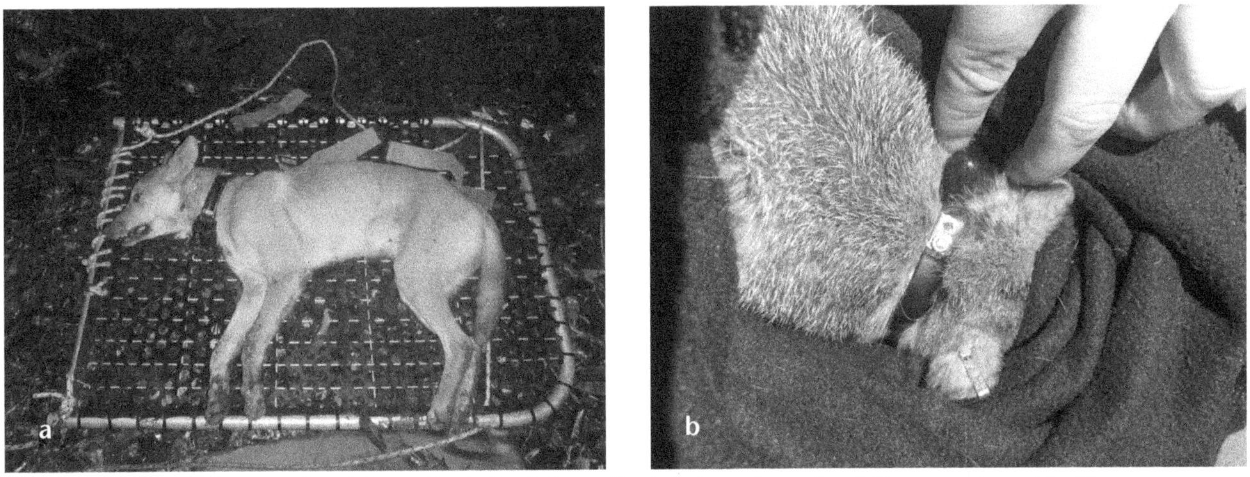

Figure 9.1: (a) Sedated, GPS-collared dingo (*Canis dingo*), immediately before release. A sedative reversal agent had been administered shortly before the photograph was taken. Photo by Damian S. Morrant. (b) Non-sedated burrowing bettong (*Bettongia lesueur*) fitted with a radio-tracking collar. Photo by Melissa A. Jensen.

Monitoring study animal welfare

GPS and satellite tracking devices allow researchers to gather telemetry data remotely, reducing labour costs, impacts on animal behaviour, and environmental disturbances. However, this technology can reduce monitoring of animal welfare following release, and accidents and wounds in study animals, or equipment failures, may go unnoticed (Cowan *et al.* 2020). Routine monitoring should be undertaken to enable researchers to respond to problems in a timely manner and improve animal welfare.

VHF transmitters on collars can often be programmed to change their signal rate depending on the animal's activity. Common options include signals for moving, stationary, and after a predefined period of inactivity (i.e. mortality) (Hampton *et al.* 2021). The mortality period should be chosen based on the best available knowledge of the animal's behaviour and activity patterns. Animal locations that do not change as expected, or mortality signals, may indicate that intervention is required (Matthews *et al.* 2013). Camera traps (Chapter 5) can be deployed in activity hotspots derived from telemetry data, where it is necessary to monitor study animals more intensively. Imagery can enable the researcher to assess the study animal's condition and concurrently collect information about activity patterns and behaviour. Obvious signs of weight loss or injury may indicate that intervention is required. Reflective tape may be added to collars to facilitate identification of individual animals (Meek and Saunders 2000). Periodic recapture of collared animals, where practical, may also facilitate the early detection of any issues caused by the collar (e.g. rubbing wounds) and allow for collars to be readjusted following weight gain or loss. However, the stress imposed by additional capture events would have to be balanced against any potential benefit from regular monitoring.

Collar cannot be located

Signal transmission from collars can fail; this situation has financial and research implications, but also poses animal welfare concerns. If the collar is not transmitting, study animals cannot be located or monitored, and it may not be possible to remove their collars. If battery failure is the cause of signal loss, other components may have also failed, including the timed-release mechanism (if fitted). All reasonable attempts should be made to relocate and recapture animals to remove collars from which no signal can be obtained, noting that some animals may roam and disperse over large distances. Available options to increase detection likelihood include extensive searches on foot, from a vehicle with or without a mounted antenna, from an elevated platform such as a tall building or fire tower, or from an aircraft. VHF signals are strongest where an unobstructed path is located between the transmitter and the receiver, enabling line-of-sight communication.

Collar removal

Animals should be freed from collars as soon as possible after sufficient data have been collected to answer research questions or if rubbing wounds caused by the collar are detected. In the past, researchers have recaptured animals, or added biodegradable weak links to collars (e.g. metal wire prone to corrosion or cotton/embroidery thread) that fall off after the link breaks. More recently, timed-release mechanisms have enabled researchers to retrieve collars at a predetermined time or on command via a remote signal (e.g. a drained battery or compromised animal welfare). Weak links may be incorporated in addition to timed-release devices; however, a premature break could cost valuable data (Matthews *et al.* 2013) and this mechanism is not always reliable (Rayner *et al.* 2021). Timed-release mechanisms increase collar mass, and so are often not appropriate for studies of smaller mammals. They may also be dispensed with for study animals that are easily recaptured.

General procedures

Planning

It can be easy to become overwhelmed by the myriad of options for collecting and analysing telemetry data. In addition to the text below, the reference section of this chapter is a good place to start for a broad oversight of the subject. For example, Matthews *et al.* (2013) provide an overview of logistics and discuss the strengths and weaknesses of GPS telemetry, gained from numerous studies involving 13 Australian mammal species.

Fitting collars

Once the animal has been captured, and physically and/or chemically restrained, the collar can be fitted (Figure 9.1). Once the desired fit has been determined (discussed in 'Collar dimensions'), new holes can be drilled for the attachment bolts and excess collar belting may be cut off, if required. For small mammals, embroidery thread or cable ties threaded through plastic tubing may be used. These attachments should also be trimmed to the required length. Researchers should ensure that cutting or drilling the belting will not damage the transmitter or internal electronics. The animal should be inspected for injuries, deformities or other ailments that could be exacerbated by collaring and should not be collared if these are found. Wounds and swelling should be treated before release. Prior to fitting the collar, or at minimum before releasing the animal, the collar should be checked to ensure that it is correctly programmed, batteries are activated, and VHF beacon, and other options such as remote download, are functional. Once the collar has been secured, Loctite® glue can be applied to bolts to prolong attachment, if required. Heat shrink tubing may also be applied to collars to reduce the risk of rubbing. Important data such as collar number, VHF frequency, and remote communication codes should be recorded. The animal can be released after the collar has been fitted. Animals should be monitored after release, until they have moved away from the capture site and out of sight.

Tracking

Routine field tracking enables researchers to monitor animal wellbeing and retrieve movement data, while making observations about the study scenario that may inform future analyses. Where expediency is required, it may be possible to locate animals by affixing an antenna to a vehicle and programming the VHF receiver to cycle through collar frequencies while driving through parts of the study area that are accessible. Animal behaviour can also be monitored via data sent by satellite or SMS. Regardless of the method of collection, data should be checked for unusual behaviour or inactivity that might indicate that intervention is required.

Collar retrieval

Efforts to remove collars must be undertaken on completion of the study, which ideally should occur via a timed-release mechanism where available. Timed release may not always be feasible or practical. For example, the collar may be too small or light to house the additional components, or the animals may be easily recaptured. It may be necessary to release the collar before the planned end date, for example for animal welfare concerns or low battery. If the collar does not release, and no degradable link has been incorporated, the researcher will need to consider other means of collar removal, such as recapturing the animal. Killing (e.g. by rifle shot) may be an option, but this practice should only be considered when working with invasive species or where vital to the project aims (e.g. an epidemiologist may need to collect tissue or blood samples).

Animal treatment, withdrawal and euthanasia

Researchers should act immediately if an animal's wellbeing appears to be compromised. Ideally the animal would be recaptured and assessed, the collar removed, and the animal taken to a veterinarian if warranted. Not all personnel will be able to transport animals to a veterinarian and doing so may result in additional stress and trauma to the animal. The principal researcher should plan for this scenario. Where an animal cannot be recaptured, information to support decisions about treatment, withdrawal and euthanasia can be obtained via a range of other sources, including targeted camera trap deployments (Chapter 5) or observation from hides (both with or without sound/odour/food lures – Chapter 4), visits to hotspots, and discussions with landholders who may encounter the animals. Mortally injured animals must be euthanased by experienced personnel, although these types of injuries are rare using these methods.

Equipment and maintenance

Equipment requirements will vary depending on the target species or taxon, local environment and study objectives. All equipment should be inspected before deployment and again as it is packed away to ensure good working order. Magnets or other means of activation and deactivation should be checked to ensure they are configured correctly. Software, collars and other equipment should be prepared and checked before deploying so that there are no delays when handling animals. Suggested equipment and materials for telemetry studies using collars, including collaring and tracking, are presented in Table 9.1.

Specific qualifications, experience and training

The skills required to undertake telemetry research vary according to the behaviour of the animal and its response to capture, and the nature of the study. The primary investigator should be competent in the techniques proposed, procedures for capture, handling and restraint of the study species, and should have undertaken similar work. Personnel should detail their previous experience applying the proposed methods. Design, conduct, analysis and interpretation of telemetry studies can be overwhelming and prone to errors. An experienced mentor should be engaged to advise on unfamiliar procedures, particularly involving handling and administering restricted medicines to animals (Chapter 16).

Workplace health and safety

Personnel may be exposed to a risk of zoonotic disease and/or bites and scratches during animal handling and associated activities (e.g. handling faeces, blood and raw or rotten meat bait). Considerations and risk minimisation practices for catching and handling particular taxa are identified in their relevant chapters in Section 3. Personnel should have procedures in place for remote area work where appropriate.

Table 9.1: Suggested equipment items for telemetry studies using collars.

Collar preparation and deployment	Tracking
• Trapping and restraint equipment • Tracking equipment (e.g. receiver) to test collar functionality before releasing animal • Tools (e.g. pliers, screwdrivers or spanners) or similar (to fasten bolts), drill (to create holes in collar belting for improved fit) and shears or scissors (to cut belting, tubing, thread or cable ties) • Collar materials (e.g. belting, plastic tubing, embroidery thread or cable ties) • Microchips and tools • Ear tags and tools (e.g. DNA collection kit) • Note-taking equipment (e.g. notebook, laptop, tablet, voice recorder, clipboard and datasheets) • Personal protective equipment • Spare batteries for electronic equipment • First aid kit • Loctite® glue • Heat shrink tubing, heat pen and leather to protect animal while using the heat pen • Magnet to turn the transmitter on	• VHF frequencies of collars* • Remote access codes for collars* • Field computer with collar-manufacturer supplied software installed* • GPS • Manufacturer supplied electronic cables and UHF download device* • VHF receiver* • Antennae and cables (e.g. Yagi, roof-mounted)* • Remote download equipment to download GPS data from animals tracked in the field* • Extension pole to increase antenna range • First aid kit • Note-taking equipment • Navigation equipment, including cadastral boundaries if likely to traverse multiple properties • Landholder contact information where access must be requested • Emergency response equipment and communications • Personal protective equipment • Site-marking and recording equipment (e.g. flagging tape, permanent markers or GPS)

* These items should be tested for functionality before deployment or release of the animal.

Alternative procedures

The use of transmitters attached with collars is ideal for long-term monitoring of individuals. However, if long-term monitoring is not required or collars are not a suitable option for the study species, alternative tracking methods may include the use of glue-on transmitters, surgically implanted transmitters or fluorescent powers (see other GOPs in this chapter). Some questions about animal movement and land use can also be investigated using alternative procedures (Latham *et al.* 2015). For example, habitat use can be investigated via stable isotope analysis (e.g. carbon ratios are markedly different between grassland and woodland; this 'signature' passes and can be detected throughout the food chain; e.g. Morrant *et al.* 2017). Migratory or nomadic movements can be investigated by collecting DNA samples (e.g. from feathers or hair) at locations of interest (Chapter 5), from which individual or species movements among locations can be identified from matching or related genetic sequences. Observations of conspicuously patterned or artificially marked animals at different locations provides insights into their movements (e.g. ear tags on mammals or bands on birds; Chapters 8 and 15, respectively). Animal movement and density estimates can be derived via pattern recognition from camera trap images (Chapter 5), although this method is not broadly applicable to many species.

TELEMETRY DEVICES ATTACHED WITH BELTS AND HARNESSES

Deborah S. Bower

Target taxa

This section outlines procedures required to fit telemetry devices to lizards (Chapter 26) and frogs (Chapter 27) with belts or harnesses.

Context and scope

Belts and harnesses are an effective means of securing tracking devices to many Australian frog and lizard species. Devices may include radiotelemetry, GPS transmitters or harmonic diodes for smaller species that cannot be tracked using radiotelemetry because of mass restrictions (e.g. the common mist frog, *Litoria rheocola*) (Gourret et al. 2011).

Animal welfare considerations

Effects on energy expenditure and activity

The shape, mass and location of the tracking device are important considerations and should be designed to minimise their encumbrance on the target animal (Hawkins 2004). Heavier attachments require the target animal to expend more energy when active (Wilson and McMahon 2006). Generally, it is accepted that devices should not exceed 5–10% of the target animal's mass (Heyer *et al.* 1994; Blomquist and Hunter 2007; Kingsbury and Robinson 2016). However, researchers need to consider the context and requirements of their specific target animals. For example, heavily gravid animals will have heavier body masses, but they may already be nearing the limit of their energetic resources. Additionally, reductions in vagility and escape behaviour have resulted from belt attachments in frogs (Blomquist and Hunter 2007). Therefore, researchers should consider the habitat, behavioural needs and condition of the target animal during the experimental design stage and consider the potential effect of attachments carefully when drawing inferences from these data. See the additional discussion under 'Surgical implantation of radio transmitters' earlier in this chapter.

External injury

Belts and harnesses must be fitted firmly to amphibians or lizards to prevent individuals from slipping out of them or becoming entangled. The attachment must not be so tight that it causes abrasion, although abrasions can also occur if attachments are fitted too loosely. Most risks can be minimised through undertaking short pilot studies before release and by locating the released target animal frequently. Some species (e.g. green and golden bell frogs, *L. aurea*) are susceptible to skin damage from the belt abrasion on the skin and this risk increases when individuals are more active. In the worst case, individuals may become tangled in vegetation and die. This risk is minimised by fitting the attachment properly and locating the target animal frequently to confirm its status. The specific means of attachment used needs to balance comfort, flexibility and durability and will depend on the specific behaviour and morphology of the target species. Determining and trialling the attachment before release is recommended where feasible.

General procedures

Handling

A single-use glove (e.g. latex-free or vinyl) may be used when handling amphibians to reduce transmission of pathogens (Murray *et al.* 2011; Chapter 27).

Fitting belts or harnesses

For frogs, a silicon tube or strip of elastic forms a band around the target animal's waist. Glass beads around the elastic are sometimes added to the belt (Blomquist and Hunter 2007). Cotton stitching is used to attach two ends of the elastic, or a knot to join cotton inside the silicon tube ensures that if animals are not recovered, the string will rot and fall off. Leuser's frog (*L. lesueuri)* fitted with harmonic diodes attached using a waistband were more active than frogs in the control group; researchers should be aware that behavioural differences can result from attachments in the first 24 h of a tracking study (Langkilde and Alford 2002; Rowley and Alford 2007). Direct attachments to frogs (e.g. glue) will be shed within hours and are not recommended for amphibians.

For larger skinks and dragons, vests can be made from nylon mesh with superglue used to secure the harness and the transmitter (e.g. used for jacky dragons, *Amphibolurus muricatus*, and Australian water dragons, *Physignathus lesueurii*; Warner *et al.* 2006; Doody *et al.* 2009). For heavier equipment (e.g. GPS packs), back-packs can be crafted from super-grip fabric and nylon meshes, or denim material to attach and hold GPS transmitters either in a vest or directly to the animal's scales with contact cement (Flesch *et al.* 2009; Price-Rees and Shine 2011). For aquatic animals, nylon mesh is advisable because it does not become waterlogged or break down (Doody *et al.* 2009).

Geckos can be tracked using belts (made from dialysis tubing that consists of cellulose acetate, a semi-permeable membrane) (Nordberg and Schwarzkopf 2019). Careful consideration of the harness material is necessary (e.g. rubber is not recommended) and monitoring is required because the soft skin of geckoes is susceptible to damage from abrasion (Van Winkel and Ji 2014).

Animal treatment, withdrawal and euthanasia

Belts or harnesses may cause abrasions on the skin of tracked individuals or interfere with sloughing of scales. Regular monitoring will help detect issues early and belts or harnesses may need to be readjusted or removed. Where target animals are suffering from severe wounds, the belt or harness should be removed, and the animals evaluated and treated, or euthanased, according to the study protocols.

Equipment and maintenance

Specific equipment requirements will vary depending on the target species and method of tracking. Note-taking and tracking equipment will be similar to telemetry devices attached with collars. Basic equipment requirements include the chosen attachment materials (belt or harness), materials to secure the transmitter device to the attachment (e.g. adhesive or sewing materials) and material to secure the attachment to the animal (e.g. cotton threat, adhesive, cable ties).

Specific qualifications, experience and training

Formal training is not required to fit an animal with a belt or harness. The target animal's behaviour and habitat use (e.g. aquatic, arboreal or fossorial), and potential for materials to impede their movement or cause injury, should inform the design and materials chosen for attachment. Personnel should be familiar with suitable handling methods for their target species.

Workplace health and safety

Infection by pathogens may occur during animal handling and associated activities. The considerations and risk minimisation practices for handling reptiles and frogs are identified in Chapters 26 and 27, respectively.

Alternative procedures

Alternatives to telemetry should be considered where research questions can be answered without the risks to animal health and wellbeing that telemetry studies can impose. The use of tracking techniques that avoid belt and harnesses (including dye tracking, surgical implants, or direct attachment onto the skin with adhesive) may be optimal or necessary for species that cannot be fitted with harnesses or belts (e.g. monitors, legless lizards) see 'Small transmitters and chemi-tags secured with adhesives' next in this chapter.

SMALL TRANSMITTERS AND CHEMI-TAGS SECURED WITH ADHESIVES

Melissa A. Jensen, Angela J.L. Pestell, Damian S. Morrant and Helen P. Waudby

Target taxa

This GOP applies to monotremes (Chapter 17), dasyurids (Chapter 18), bandicoots, wombats, possums and gliders (Chapter 19), microbats (Chapter 23), rodents (Chapter 24), and lizards, turtles and crocodiles (Chapter 26).

Context and scope

This GOP describes the tagging of a range of taxa with small transmitters and fluorescent chemi-tags (also known as cyalume capsules, glow sticks or light tags) secured with adhesives. It applies to small- to medium-sized mammals and reptiles. The use of transmitters secured with adhesives for tagging marine mammals and birds is covered in Chapters 12 and 15, respectively. The use of tail-mounted transmitters for bilbies and some bandicoot species is discussed in Chapter 19. Transmitters may also be attached to turtles by drilling small holes in the carapace and bolting the transmitter to it; attachment to marine turtles via carapace drilling is covered in Chapter 12.

Transmitters secured with adhesives, also known as glue-on transmitters, are generally used for short-term monitoring of individuals. Small transmitters (usually VHF) that transmit a unique frequency, and that can be programmed and monitored via a receiver, are glued onto the animal using an adhesive, such as medical latex glue (e.g. SAUER Skin Adhesive®), Vetbond®, Uro-Bond IV®, or other cyanoacrylate-based glue (e.g. superglue) or epoxy. Chemi-tags are typically used for the short-term tracking of individuals where the objective of the study is to follow the animal visually immediately after release to gather data on habitat use, to track it back to its shelter, or to identify individual microbats for echolocation call recording. Typically, these tags are also attached to the animal using a cyanoacrylate-based glue. Anaesthetising the animal is generally unnecessary, so animals can be tagged in the field and released as soon as the adhesive has dried.

Glue-on transmitters can be particularly useful for species for which traditional transmitter attachment methods are unfavourable, including species that are too small to carry transmitters attached by other means (e.g. microbats and pygmy possums), species that have a body shape that makes it difficult to fit radio collars (e.g. bandicoots; Coetsee *et al.* 2016), and species for which other transmitter attachment methods cause irritation. Additionally, as the transmitters generally fall off the animal unassisted, this technique can be effective for species that are difficult to capture, eliminating the need to recapture the animal to remove the transmitter.

Glue-on transmitters appear to have minimal and relatively short-lived effects on the pelage of mammals. For example, Morrant and Petit (2012) recaptured two western pygmy possums (*Cercartetus concinnus*), 2–3 months after they were tracked and found that their hair had almost completely regrown at the attachment site. Similarly, Shark Bay bandicoots (*Perameles bougainville*) have been recaptured only weeks after the loss of a transmitter with fur completely regrown at the attachment site (M. Jensen, unpublished data). Glue-on transmitters and chemi-tags are useful for gathering data that are otherwise difficult to capture, such as habitat use, feeding behaviour, bat echolocation, and nest or shelter use (Bullen and McKenzie 2001; Jensen 2012; Pestell and Petit 2007; Morrant and Petit 2012). However, the varying and often short retention times of glue-on transmitters and chemi-tags mean that this technique is generally only suitable for studies during which the species is only required to be monitored for a short period of time.

Animal welfare considerations

Pain and infection

The application of transmitters and chemi-tags secured with adhesives is generally painless and has a low risk of infection when conducted correctly. However, before use researchers must consider the setting time of the chosen adhesive (which influences the duration required to hold the animal), and the likelihood of any associated injuries to the animal resulting from the transmitter being torn off the animal, before using this technique. Some adhesives (e.g. Vetbond®) are designed to break down quickly, reducing retention time.

Mass consideration

Transmitters and chemi-tags attached with adhesives can be used on adult and juvenile animals. Typically, transmitter and chemi-tag weights should not exceed 4–5% of the animal's body mass (Cochran 1980; White and Garrot 1990), although these values are context- and species-specific, and greater masses may be justified in some situations (refer to 'Surgical implantation of radio transmitters'). Care must also be taken to ensure that the positioning of the transmitter does not impede the animal's full range of movement (including foraging, grooming, mating, flying, access to the pouch and predator evasion). The positioning of the transmitter may also affect the transmitter's signal strength and retention time.

General procedures

Equipment preparation

Personnel should weigh the animal to ensure that the transmitter or chemi-tag does not exceed the predetermined carrying weight for that individual. The transmitter should be turned on and checked to confirm that it is transmitting. Personnel should record the transmitter frequency and program the transmitter frequency into the receiver. The frequency may be adjusted up or down slightly to improve the signal strength. Antennae may need to be trimmed if personnel consider that a foraging or nesting animal is at risk of becoming snagged. Personnel should seek advice from the manufacturer regarding appropriate length and the effect of shortening the antenna on signal strength. Chemi-tags need to be activated (cracked and shaken until fluorescing) before being attached to the animal. All other animal processing must be completed before tagging the animal.

General tagging procedures

Handling techniques differ depending on the species or taxon being tagged. Once the animal has been processed it should be appropriately restrained (see taxa-specific chapters for restraint methods). In general, the animal should be held securely in a cloth handling bag (or other taxa-specific restraint) with the target area exposed, preferably with the head and rest of the body covered. Depending on the species being tagged, tagging may be easier with two people: one to restrain the animal and another to attach the transmitter.

Attaching devices

Glue-on transmitters and chemi-tags are typically positioned between or just below the shoulder blades, or on the rump of small mammals. Generally, transmitters or chemi-tags should be adhered to the fur of the animal, not to the skin. However, transmitters are applied directly to the skin of microbats (Chapter 23) and the scales of lizards (Chapter 26) – see Figure 9.2. Personnel should select the target location and trim hairs (if required) using small clippers or scissors. Transmitters can be attached using a medical latex glue or cyanoacrylate-based glue (e.g. superglue; most common for mammals) or epoxy (more common for lizards). Glue should be applied to the underside of the transmitter or chemi-tag, which is immediately placed onto the target location and held in place until the glue has set. For

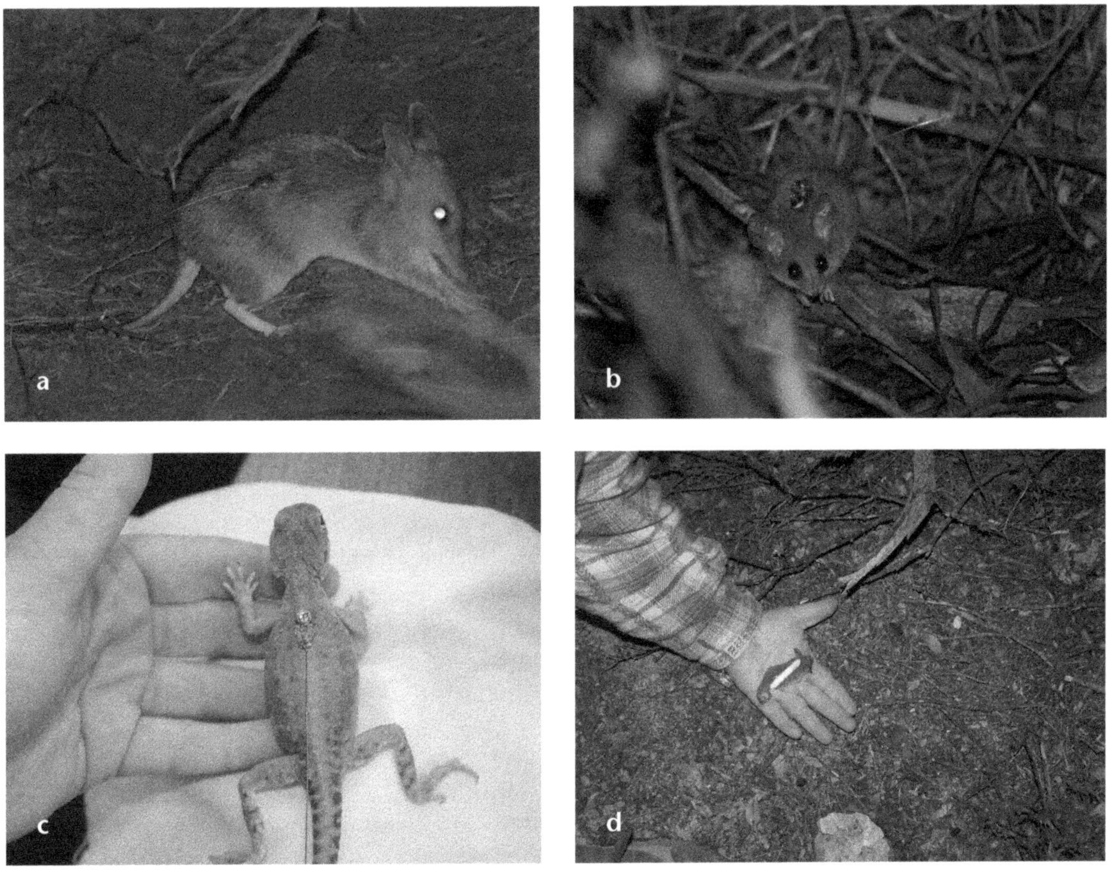

Figure 9.2: (a) Shark Bay bandicoot (*Perameles bougainville*) fitted with a glue-on transmitter. Photo by Melissa A. Jensen. (b) Western pygmy possum (*Cercartetus concinnus*) fitted with a glue-on transmitter. Photo by Damian S. Morrant. (c) Transmitter attached to a gibber dragon (*Ctenophorus gibba*) with epoxy. Photo by Helen. P. Waudby. (d) Western pygmy possum about to be released with a chemi-tag attached. Photo by Angela J.L. Pestell.

some species with easily shed guard hairs (e.g. some bandicoot species), trimming a few guard hairs and adhering the transmitter to the under-hairs may improve retention times and reduce the risk of skin lesions (Jensen 2012; M. Jensen, unpublished data; Coetsee *et al.* 2016). Similarly, to improve retention time in species with long fur, personnel may lift some of the hair at the target location and apply glue to both the top and sides of the transmitter, and adhere the surrounding fur to the transmitter.

To increase the surface area and improve retention times, researchers may also glue a piece of cotton gauze to the animal and adhere the transmitter to the gauze. For lizards, covering the transmitter with a small piece of flesh-coloured paper tape may reduce the risk of the transmitter reflecting light and attracting predators (H. P. Waudby, pers. obs.). Once the glue has set and the transmitter or chemi-tag is in place, the animal is allowed to move freely in the handling bag. Personnel should check that the transmitter is still transmitting correctly or that the chemi-tag has not dislodged. Animals can usually be released immediately. Specific methods for attaching transmitters to monotremes and microbats are covered in Chapters 17 and 23, respectively.

Animal treatment, withdrawal, and euthanasia

Animals should be monitored continuously for signs of distress during the handling and transmitter attachment process. The application of transmitters or chemi-tags secured with adhesive is unlikely to cause harm that would require major treatment or euthanasia. However, transmitters may be torn off the animal after application, the glue may inhibit the water resistance of the pelage, and antennae may become snagged (e.g. one of the authors has seen a pygmy possum snagged on a *Eucalyptus* sp. infructescence). Personnel should seek advice from a wildlife veterinarian if any recaptured animals show signs of injury or infection. Species prone to capture myopathy (Breed *et al.* 2019) should be identified before tagging and the time taken to restrain and tag the animal considered.

Equipment and maintenance

Suggested equipment and materials required for securing transmitters and chemi-tags using adhesives include:

- transmitter or chemi-tag
- clipboard and datasheets or electronic database (to record transmitter frequency)
- receiver (to ensure transmitter is transmitting before use)
- adhesive
- handling bags
- scissors or clippers (for trimming hair)
- gauze (for removing any excess adhesive)
- acetone or other solvent to remove spilled and excess adhesive
- soldering iron and solder for connecting circuits in small transmitters
- magnet (if required to turn transmitter on)
- tweezers/forceps
- gloves (if required)
- scales.

Specific qualifications, experience or training

Researchers should be familiar with the species or similar taxa, comfortable with handling and restraining the species, and aware of signs of excessive agitation for the species. Researchers should be trained or supervised by an experienced researcher who is experienced in the use of the chosen marking technique until deemed competent.

Workplace health and safety

Adhesive injury

Care must be taken when working with adhesives. They should remain capped when not in use and spills cleaned immediately. Appropriate first aid should be applied in the case of injury. Consult the material safety data sheet for the chosen adhesive for further advice.

Alternative procedures

The use of small transmitters and chemi-tags secured with adhesives is generally not suitable for long-term monitoring of individuals. Should long-term monitoring be required, alternative transmitter application techniques may include radio collars, harnesses or belts, tail-mounted transmitters, or surgically implanted transmitters (see other GOPs in this chapter). If long-term monitoring is not required, less-invasive methods, such as tracking with fluorescent powder may suffice (see other GOPs in this chapter).

TRACKING WITH FLUORESCENT POWDER

Nicole A. Hansen and Carmen Amos

Target taxa

This method is applicable to a range of nocturnal small- and medium-sized mammals (Chapters 18, 19 and 24), reptiles (Chapter 26) and amphibians (Chapter 27).

Context and scope

This GOP describes the use of fluorescent powder for tracking nocturnal terrestrial mammals, reptiles and amphibians and considerations for animal welfare when using this technique. This method has been shown to be generally safe for small rodents (Stapp *et al.* 1994), some snake species (Furman *et al.* 2011), small reptiles (Dodd 1992; Hansen *et al.* 2020), frogs (Rittenhouse *et al.* 2006; Okamiya and Kusano 2018) and salamanders (Williams *et al.* 2014). However, harmful effects have been recorded for some amphibian (Gourevitch and Downie 2018) and rodent (Stapp *et al.* 1994) species. This technique is non-invasive (Stapp *et al.* 1994; Rittenhouse *et al.* 2006) and low-cost, and can be performed successfully with little training (Furman *et al.* 2011). By following appropriate safeguards, powders can be applied with minimal animal handling time compared to other tracking techniques (e.g. can be completed in < 1 min; Ramírez *et al.* (2017)). Moreover, no anaesthetic, tracking device or attachment (or retrieval of attachment) is required.

Animals are dusted with a fluorescent powder that then leaves a trail or is deposited on other individuals, leaving a traceable record of the individuals' movements, habitat use, social interactions or foraging behaviour (Furman *et al.* 2011; Okamiya and Kusano 2018). The trail is typically short lived (lasting < 4 days), generally carries low physiological cost (e.g. < 0.5 g in mass) and can be used on juveniles or species too small for tracking devices (Hansen *et al.* 2020). When used on frogs, the powder will mostly wash off if the tracked frog enters the water, so the trail will be shorter-lived for purely aquatic amphibians. Adverse effects of powder tracking on behaviour, reproduction and survivorship are little reported, but the authors recommend that researchers consider animal welfare, physiological stress, increased predation risk and the potential for toxicity of powders and inadvertent spread of pathogens.

Animal welfare considerations

Animal welfare issues associated with fluorescent powder are minimal. However, increased predation risk (bright powders may make animals more conspicuous to predators, prey and/or conspecifics that detect fluorescence), risk of ingestion, and physiological stress through handling and application may occur. The method applies to a wide range of taxa and environments, so negative effects may not be consistent or predictable across species. In the absence of species-specific information, powder should be tested experimentally to understand its limits and effectiveness. While these impacts are specifically associated with the technique of fluorescent powder, an animal may also experience other impacts from associated procedures such as trapping and capture. Consideration should be given to selecting appropriate non-toxic powders and avoid applying powders to animals that are active during the day (or releasing animals covered in powder in daylight) to minimise predation risk. Where possible, powders should be applied to the ventral and lateral parts of the animal to minimise effects on heat absorption and reduce visibility.

Physiological stress of handling and application

Relatively few studies have evaluated the physiological impacts of applying fluorescent powders on wild animals or if the application has lasting effects over subsequent nights (e.g. possible effects of prolonged exposure, or if powder remains on the animal for longer than planned; see Ramírez *et al.* 2017). Several authors observed unnatural movement patterns, quick retreats to cover sites or the extended use of retreat sites, which may indicate stress associated with handling during application of powder (Dodd 1992; Furman *et al.* 2011; Sozio *et al.* 2013; Ramírez *et al.* 2017). Ramírez *et al.* (2017) noted that the use of fluorescent powder did not appear to influence the movements of Maud Island frogs (*Leiopelma pakeka*) negatively, with distances travelled by powdered and unpowdered frogs similar and no overall ill effects observed (e.g. death or attempts to remove powder). Orlofske *et al.* (2009) found that fluorescent powder did not affect respiration of lungless red-backed salamanders (*Plethodon cinereus*) or lunged terrestrial red-spotted newts (*Notophthalmus viridescens*). Similarly, Rittenhouse *et al.* (2006) did not observe short-term or long-term effects of fluorescent powder on the growth, survival or rate of water loss for wood frogs (*Rana sylvatica*) or spotted salamanders (*Ambystoma maculatum*) during a 6 week study.

Sozio *et al.* (2013) did not observe any negative effects (on health or behaviour) when marking three species of mice, but could not exclude species-specific effects of handling or marking on subsequent behaviour. Fluorescent powder may influence thermoregulation in reptiles (Fellers and Drost 1989). However, applying powder to ventral and lateral surfaces would minimise this risk. While evaluations are few, given the temporary nature of the marking method (e.g. typically < 4 days), it seems unlikely that individuals are affected by stress impacts in the long term, compared to other conventional tracking methods.

Increased predation risk and changed interactions

Many fluorescent powders show up as brightly coloured under ambient light or alter cryptic coloration of animals, potentially making diurnal species more conspicuous during the day, as well as being seen at night by predators, conspecifics or prey that can detect fluorescence (Rittenhouse *et al.* 2006) (also see 'Tattooing mammals and lizards' in Chapter 8). Restricting powder to the ventral or lateral areas of the animal, selecting colours that correspond with surrounding vegetation and avoiding highly contrasting colours will help reduce visibility of marked animals to predators. Powder in an animal's eyes may also interfere with the ability to avoid predators. Application of fluorescent powder could affect intraspecific social signalling of marked animals, particularly reptile species that respond to colour-based visual cues and those outside the spectrum visible to humans (Whiting and Noble 2018).

Toxicity of powders

Fluorescent powders are generally considered to be non-toxic. However, chemicals used in commercial powders can vary, powders may not be suitable for all species. Some powders have been found to have toxic, sublethal effects and, if absorbed through the skin during application or ingested in large amounts during subsequent self-grooming, can have acute and chronic systemic effects, including death (Stapp *et al.* 1994). For amphibians, the direct application of powder may interfere with cutaneous respiration and water exchange. Stressed amphibians may exhibit water-holding behaviour that could change activity levels or microhabitat use (Wisely and Golightly 2003). Of the few studies testing for ill effects, one study discontinued use of fluorescent powder, with no further description of effects, and pursued alternative tracking methods (Gourevitch and Downie 2018).

Repeated application of powder may affect respiration over time; however, important characteristics like growth rate appear to be unaffected (Rittenhouse *et al.* 2006). The physical presence or taste of the powder may trigger excessive grooming and incidental consumption of toxic levels of powder, particularly for small mammals. Stapp *et al.* (1994) examined impacts of powdered fluorescent pigments on wild deer mice (*Peromyscus maniculatus*), finding that mice ingested particles that typically passed through the gastrointestinal tract with no adverse reaction. Mild to moderate histiocytic pneumonia was detected in some mice and presumably associated with inhalation of powder. Stapp *et al.* (1994) recommended minimising the exposure of study animals to large quantities of powder to reduce pathological effects. The authors noted that fluorescent powder is a generally safe technique for tracking amphibians, reptiles and frogs. However, given the potentially harmful effects, caution must be used when selecting powders to consider the toxicity and product composition.

Spread of disease

Personnel must be aware of the possibility of pathogens or parasite transfer between individuals and locations if handling animals at multiple sites. Good hygiene practices should be maintained, with equipment cleaned and disinfected between animals. Ensure gloves are changed between individuals, avoid reusing powder that may be contaminated by another animal and ensure fluorescent powder containers are sealed after each use to reduce the risk of spreading pathogens between animals and sites. For specific hygiene protocols related to handling frogs refer to Chapter 27.

General procedures

Applying the powder and release

Captured animals should be handled in a manner that minimises stress, and for as long as required to coat and process them (usually ≤ 5 min), and released at the point of capture. Minimising injury and stress are best done with firm and quiet handling, using sufficiently competent personnel to restrain the animal and using techniques that are appropriate to the species. Applying powder strategically (e.g. to the ventral side, abdomen, hind limbs or feet; Figure 9.3) to minimise predation risk and inhalation may be difficult as the powder is easily dispersed. Researchers may choose to use differently coloured powders if tracking multiple animals or species. Some colours (e.g. pink and orange) may appear similar under UV light, so colours should be selected carefully if it is important to differentiate between individuals or species. Powdering technique used will depend on the species. For example, for frogs and reptiles, powder may be applied by placing the animal on top of the powder to cover the ventral surface, legs and feet (Ramírez *et al.* 2017; Hansen *et al.* 2020) or brush against an applicator (Okamiya and Kusano 2018). Furman *et al.* (2011) applied powder to snakes by placing their

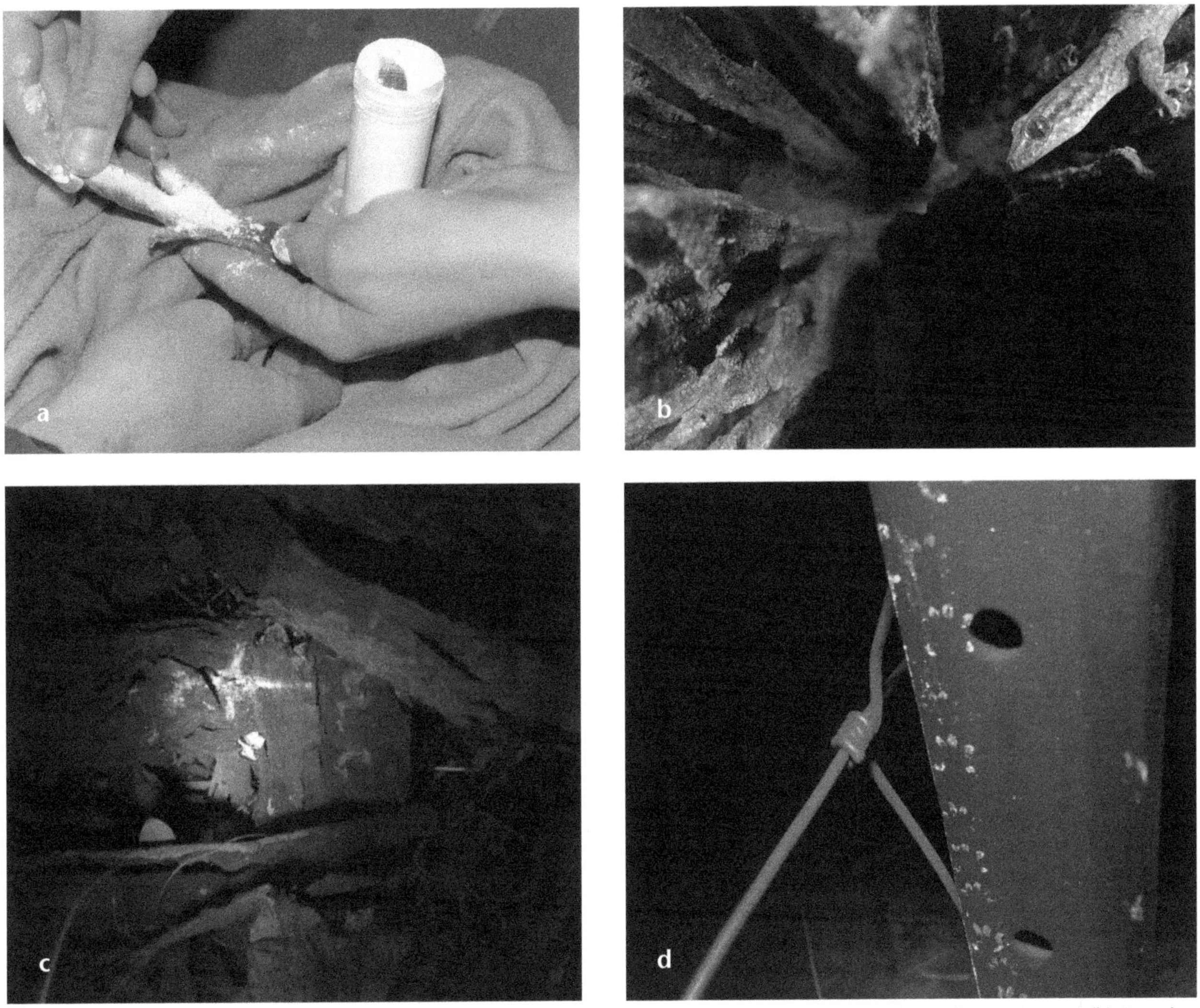

Figure 9.3: (a) Applying powder to the hind foot of a burrowing bettong (*Bettongia lesueur*). Photo by Melissa A. Jensen. (b) A gecko with powder applied to its underbody. (c) A 'splat' pattern made by a gecko that had leapt off a perch. (d) Fluorescing gecko tracks on a fence post. Photos b, c and d by Nicole Hansen.

bodies in a plastic bag with 2.5 cm of powder and gently tipping the bag back and forth to coat all sides of the snake. During powdering, the snake's head should be kept out of the bag, ensuring powder is not applied to the eyes or mouth. Ideally, handling should be undertaken during the cooler periods of the day (dawn/dusk) and animals released at a time when they are normally active. When releasing the animal, the researcher should check for any predators in the area (e.g. raptors, snakes and goannas) and delay release until they have moved on.

Animal treatment, withdrawal and euthanasia

Personnel must monitor animals continually throughout application. Signs of stress will vary among species. If animals appear excessively stressed, personnel should review the marking process and handling methods. Excessive stress may be related to the nature of the handling rather than the marking method. Typically, animals can be released immediately after powder application at point of capture, but may be observed for a short time providing this does not create additional unnecessary stress.

Equipment and maintenance

Equipment requirements are few depending on the objectives of the study. Typical items may include:

- appropriate non-toxic powder (ensure application, specific considerations and storage instructions are followed)

- species-appropriate applicator, container or bag to facilitate application
- plastic clip lock bag to hold used material
- gloves
- ultraviolet light for viewing fluorescing colours and monitoring marked animals.

Specific qualifications, experience and training

Fluorescent powder application requires very little training; however, experience and knowledge in animal handling for the relevant species are required to apply the powder quickly, efficiently and appropriately (e.g. to avoid excessively covering the animal and to recognise signs of excessive stress). Similarly, personnel should understand the types of movements likely to be made by their species when evaluating tracks (e.g. frogs tracks can be difficult to follow if they have jumped a far distance). Personnel should be trained or supervised by those experienced in using the method until they are deemed competent. Personnel must be able to correctly identify the species they're likely to encounter and confidently handle mammals.

Workplace health and safety

Personnel may develop contact allergies to powder. Personnel with allergies should wear appropriate PPE, and personnel with respiratory conditions should consider wearing a mask. A material safety data sheet for the powder should be obtained and reviewed.

Alternative procedures

If fluorescent powder is applied as recommended, the method should cause minimal distress to study animals following the procedures described in this GOP. Other methods of permanent or semi-permanent marking of animals to understand fine-scale movements include trapping (Chapter 7), visible implant elastomer (Chapter 8), radio or GPS tracking (see earlier GOPs in this chapter), or light emitting diodes or coloured bands. However, these techniques are associated with their own suite of potential animal welfare impacts and are not necessarily lower impact than tracking with fluorescent powder.

REFERENCES

Adams L (1965) Progress in ecological biotelemetry. *Bioscience* **15**, 83–86. doi:10.2307/1293341

Aldridge HDJN, Brigham RM (1988) Load carrying and manoeuvrability in an insectivorous bat: a test of the 5% 'rule' of radio-telemetry. *Journal of Mammalogy* **69**, 379–382. doi:10.2307/1381393

Alworth LC, Hernandez SM, Divers SJ (2011) Laboratory reptile surgery: principles and techniques. *Journal of the American Association for Laboratory Animal Science; JAALAS* **50**, 11–26.

Anderson D (1996) Wound management in small animal practice. *In Practice* **18**, 115–128. doi:10.1136/inpract.18.3.115

Australian Veterinary Association (2017) *Restricted Acts of Veterinary Science*. Australian Veterinary Association, Melbourne.

Blomquist SM, Hunter ML (2007) Externally attached radio-transmitters have limited effects on the antipredator behavior and vagility of *Rana pipiens* and *Rana sylvatica*. *Journal of Herpetology* **41**, 430–438. doi:10.1670/0022-1511(2007)41[430:EARHLE]2.0.CO;2

Breed D, Meyer LC, Steyl JC, Goddard A, Burroughs R, Kohn TA (2019) Conserving wildlife in a changing world: Understanding capture myopathy – a malignant outcome of stress during capture and translocation. *Conservation Physiology* **7**, coz027. doi:10.1093/conphys/coz027

Bullen RD, McKenzie NL (2001) Differentiating Western Australian *Nyctophilus* (Chiroptera: Vespertilionidae) echolocation calls. *Australian Mammalogy* **23**, 89–93. doi:10.1071/AM01089

Casper RM (2009) Guidelines for the instrumentation of wild birds and mammals. *Animal Behaviour* **78**, 1477–1483. doi:10.1016/j.anbehav.2009.09.023

Cochran WW, Lord RD, Jr (1963) A radio-tracking system for wild animals. *The Journal of Wildlife Management* **27**, 9–24. doi:10.2307/3797775

Cochran WW (1980) Wildlife telemetry. In *Wildlife Management Techniques Manual*. (Ed. SD Schemnitz). The Wildlife Society, Washington, DC.

Coetsee A, Harley D, Lynch M, Coulson G, de Milliano J, Cooper M, Groenewegen R (2016) Radio-transmitter attachment methods for monitoring the endangered eastern barred bandicoot (*Perameles gunnii*). *Australian Mammalogy* **38**, 221–231. doi:10.1071/AM15029

Cowan M, Blythman M, Angus J, Gibson L (2020) Post-release monitoring of western grey kangaroos (*Macropus fuliginosus*) relocated from an urban development site. *Animals (Basel)* **10**, 1914. doi:10.3390/ani10101914

Dausmann KH (2005) Measuring body temperature in the field – evaluation of external vs. implanted transmitters in a small mammal. *Journal of Thermal Biology* **30**, 195–202. doi:10.1016/j.jtherbio.2004.11.003

Dodd CK (1992) Fluorescent powder is only partially successful in tracking movements of the six-lined racerunner. *Florida Field Naturalist* **20**, 8–14.

Doody JS, Roe J, Mayes P, Ishiyama L (2009) Telemetry tagging methods for some freshwater reptiles. *Marine and Freshwater Research* **60**, 293–298. doi:10.1071/MF08158

Fellers GM, Drost CA (1989) Fluorescent powder – a method for tracking reptiles. *Herpetological Review* **20**, 91–92.

Fieberg J, Börger L (2012) Could you please phrase 'home range' as a question? *Journal of Mammalogy* **93**, 890–902. doi:10.1644/11-MAMM-S-172.1

Fiorello CV, Harms CA, Chinnadurai SK, Strahl-Heldreth D (2016) Best-practice guidelines for field-based surgery and anesthesia on free-ranging wildlife. II. Surgery. *Journal of Wildlife Diseases* **52**, S28–S39. doi:10.7589/52.2S.S28

Flesch JS, Duncan MG, Pascoe JH, Mulley RC (2009) A simple method of attaching GPS tracking devices to free-ranging lace monitors (*Varanus varius*). *Herpetological Conservation and Biology* **4**, 411–414.

Furman BLS, Scheffers BR, Paszkowski CA (2011) The use of fluorescent powdered pigments as a tracking technique for snakes. *Herpetological Conservation and Biology* **6**, 473–478.

Gentz EJ (2007) Medicine and surgery of amphibians. *ILAR Journal* **48**, 255–259. doi:10.1093/ilar.48.3.255

Gourevitch EHZ, Downie JR (2018) Evaluation of tree frog tracking methods using *Phyllomedusa trinitatis* (Anura: Phyllomedusidae). *Journal of Herpetology* **17**, 233–246. doi:10.11606/issn.2316-9079.v17i2p233-246

Gourret A, Alford R, Schwarzkopf L (2011) Very small, light dipole harmonic tags for tracking small animals. *Herpetological Review* **42**, 522–525.

Græsli AR, Thiel A, Fuchs B, Singh NJ, Stenbacka F, Ericsson G, Neumann W, Arnemo JM, Evans AL (2020) Seasonal hypometabolism in female moose. *Frontiers in Ecology and Evolution* **8**, 107.

Hampton JO, Amos M, Pople A, Brennan M, Forsyth DM (2011) Minimising mortalities in capturing wildlife: refinement of helicopter darting of chital deer (*Axis axis*) in Australia. *Wildlife Research* **48**, 304–313. doi:10.1071/WR20106

Hansen NA, Driscoll DA, Michael DR, Lindenmayer DB (2020) Movement patterns of an arboreal gecko in fragmented agricultural landscapes reveal matrix avoidance. *Animal Conservation* **23**, 48–59. doi:10.1111/acv.12505

Hawkins P (2004) Bio-logging and animal welfare: practical refinements. *Memoirs of the National Institute of Polar Research* **58**, 58–68.

Hennig JD, Scasta JD, Beck JL, Schoenecker KA, King SR (2020) Systematic review of equids and telemetry collars: implications for deployment and reporting. *Wildlife Research* **47**, 61–71. doi:10.1071/WR19229

Hetem RS, Strauss WM, Fick LG, Maloney SK, Meyer LC, Shobrak M, Fuller A, Mitchell D (2012) Activity re-assignment and microclimate selection of free-living Arabian oryx: responses that could minimise the effects of climate change on homeostasis? *Zoology (Jena, Germany)* **115**, 411–416. doi:10.1016/j.zool.2012.04.005

Heyer WR, Donnelly MA, McDiarmid RW, Hayek L-AC, Foster MS (1994) Supplemental approaches to studying amphibian biodiversity. In *Measuring and Monitoring Biological Diversity: Standard Methods for Amphibians.* (Ed. WR Heyer) pp. 143–182. Smithsonian Institution Press, Washington.

Horning M, Andrews RD, Bishop AM, Boveng PL, Costa DP, Crocker DE, *et al.* (2017) Best practice recommendations for the use of fully implanted telemetry devices in pinnipeds. *Animal Biotelemetry* **5**, 13. doi:10.1186/s40317-017-0128-9

Jensen M (2012) Habitat use of the western barred bandicoot (*Perameles bougainville*) within the Arid Recovery Reserve. Honours thesis. The University of Adelaide, Adelaide.

Jones M, Hamede R, McCallum H, Banks P, Lunney D, Dickman C (2012) The devil is in the detail: conservation biology, animal philosophies and the role of animal ethics committees. In *Science under Siege: Zoology under Threat* (Eds P Banks, D Lunney and C Dickman.) pp. 79–88. Royal Zoological Society of New South Wales, Mosman.

Kenward RE (2000) *A Manual for Wildlife Radio Tagging.* Academic Press, London.

Kingsbury B, Robinson NJ (2016) Movement patterns and telemetry. In *Reptile Ecology and Conservation: A Handbook of Techniques.* (Ed DJC Kenneth) pp. 11–120. Oxford University Press, Oxford, UK.

Koehler DK, Reynolds TD, Anderson SH (1987) Radio-transmitter implants in four species of small mammals. *The Journal of Wildlife Management* **51**, 105–108. doi:10.2307/3801638

Langkilde T, Alford RA (2002) The tail wags the frog: harmonic radar transponders affect movement behavior in *Litoria lesueuri*. *Journal of Herpetology* **36**, 711–715. doi:10.1670/0022-1511(2002)036[0711:TTWTFH]2.0.CO;2

Latham AD, Latham MC, Anderson DP, Cruz J, Herries D, Hebblewhite M (2015) The GPS craze: six questions to address before deciding to deploy GPS technology on wildlife. *New Zealand Journal of Ecology* **39**, 143–152.

LeMunyan CD, White W, Nyberg E, Christian JJ (1959) Design of a miniature radio transmitter for use in animal studies. *The Journal of Wildlife Management* **23**, 107–110. doi:10.2307/3797755

Matthews A, Ruykys L, Ellis B, FitzGibbon S, Lunney D, Crowther MS, *et al.* (2013) The success of GPS collar deployments on mammals in Australia. *Australian Mammalogy* **35**, 65–83. doi:10.1071/AM12021

McMahon CR, Collier N, Northfield JK, Glen F (2011) Taking the time to assess the effects of remote sensing and tracking devices on animals. *Animal Welfare (South Mimms, England)* **20**, 515–521.

Mech LD (1980) Making the most of radio tracking – a summary of wolf studies in northeastern Minnesota. In *A Handbook on Biotelemetry and Radio Tracking (Proceedings of an International Conference on Telemetry and Radio Tracking in Biology and Medicine, Oxford).* (Eds CJ Jr Amlaner and DW Macdonald) pp. 85–95. Pergamon Press, New York.

Meek PD, Saunders G (2000) Home range and movement of foxes (*Vulpes vulpes*) in coastal New South Wales, Australia. Wildlife Research **27**, 663–668. doi:10.1071/WR98030

Meyers PM, Hatch SA, Mulcahy DM (1998) Effect of implanted satellite transmitters on the nesting behavior of murres. *The Condor* **100**, 172–174. doi:10.2307/1369912

Morrant DS, Petit S (2012) Strategies of a small nectarivorous marsupial, the western pygmy-possum, in response to seasonal variation in food availability. *Journal of Mammalogy* **93**, 1525–1535. doi:10.1644/12-MAMM-A-031.1

Morrant DS, Wurster CM, Johnson CN, Butler JRA, Congdon BC (2017) Prey use by dingoes in a contested landscape: ecosystem service provider or biodiversity threat? *Ecology and Evolution* **7**, 8927–8935. doi:10.1002/ece3.3345

Murray K, Skerratt L, Marantelli G, Berger L, Hunter D, Mahony M, Hines H (2011) *Hygiene Protocols for the Control of Diseases in Australian Frogs. A Report for the Australian Government Department of Sustainability, Environment, Water, Population and Communities.* Department of Sustainability, Environment, Water, Population and Communities, Canberra.

Nordberg EJ, Schwarzkopf L (2019) Heat seekers: a tropical nocturnal lizard uses behavioral thermoregulation to exploit rare microclimates at night. *Journal of Thermal Biology* **82**, 107–114. doi:10.1016/j.jtherbio.2019.03.018

Okamiya H, Kusano T (2018) Evaluating movement patterns and microhabitat selection of the Japanese common toad (*Bufo japonicus formosus*) using fluorescent powder tracking. *Zoological Science* **35**, 153–160. doi:10.2108/zs170101

Orlofske SA, Grayson KL, Hopkins WA (2009) The effects of fluorescent tracking powder on oxygen consumption in salamanders using either cutaneous or bimodal respiration. *Copeia* **2009**, 623–627. doi:10.1643/CP-08-155

Pearson DJ, Shine RT (2002) Expulsion of intraperitoneally-implanted radiotransmitters by Australian pythons. *Herpetological Review* **33**, 261–262.

Pestell AJL, Petit S (2007) Methods and ethical considerations of pitfall trapping for the western pygmy possum (*Cercartetus concinnus* Gould) (Marsupialia: Burramyidae), with observations on capture patterns and nest sites. *Wildlife Research* **34**, 296–305. doi:10.1071/WR06090

Price J, Catriona S, Welsh EM, Waran NK (2003) Preliminary evaluation of a behaviour-based system for assessment of post-operative pain in horses following arthroscopic surgery. *Veterinary Anaesthesia and Analgesia* **30**, 124–137. doi:10.1046/j.1467-2995.2003.00139.x

Price-Rees SJ, Shine R (2011) A backpack method for attaching GPS transmitters to bluetongue lizards (*Tiliqua*, Scincidae). *Herpetological Conservation and Biology* **6**, 155–161.

Quy RJ, Massei G, Lambert MS, Coats J, Miller LA, Cowan DP (2014) Effects of a GnRH vaccine on the movement and activity of free-living wild boar (*Sus scrofa*). *Wildlife Research* **41**, 185–193. doi:10.1071/WR14035

Ramírez PA, Bell BD, Germano JM, Bishop PJ, Nelson NJ (2017) Tracking a small cryptic amphibian with fluorescent powders. *New Zealand Journal of Ecology* **41**, 134–138. doi:10.20417/nzjecol.41.2

Rayner K, Sullivan M, Sims C, Cowen S (2021) A pain in the neck: weak links are not a reliable release mechanism for radio-collars. *Australian Mammalogy*. Online early. doi:10.1071/AM20065

Rittenhouse TAG, Altnether TT, Semlitsch RD (2006) Fluorescent powder pigments as a harmless tracking method for ambystomatids and ranids. *Herpetological Review* **37**, 188–191.

Rojas AD, Körtner G, Geiser F (2010) Do implanted transmitters affect maximum running speed of two small marsupials? *Journal of Mammalogy* **91**, 1360–1364. doi:10.1644/10-MAMM-A-052.1

Rowley J, Alford R (2007) Techniques for tracking amphibians: the effects of tag attachment, and harmonic direction finding versus radio telemetry. *Amphibia-Reptilia* **28**, 367–376. doi:10.1163/156853807781374755

Sexson MG, Mulcahy DM, Spriggs M, Myers GE (2014) Factors influencing immediate post-release survival of spectacled eiders following surgical implantation of transmitters with percutaneous antennae. *The Journal of Wildlife Management* **78**, 550–560. doi:10.1002/jwmg.690

Shine R (1987) Intraspecific variation in thermoregulation, movements and habitat use by Australian blacksnakes, *Pseudechis porphyriacus* (Elapidae). *Journal of Herpetology* **21**, 165–177. doi:10.2307/1564479

Signer C, Ruf T, Schober F, Fluch G, Paumann T, Arnold W (2010) A versatile telemetry system for continuous measurement of heart rate, body temperature and locomotor activity in free-ranging ruminants. *Methods in Ecology and Evolution* **1**, 75–85. doi:10.1111/j.2041-210X.2009.00010.x

Sozio G, Mortelliti A, Boitani L (2013) Mice on the move: wheat rows as a means to increase permeability in agricultural landscapes. *Biological Conservation* **165**, 198–202. doi:10.1016/j.biocon.2013.05.022

Stapp P, Young JK, VandeWoude S, VanHorne B (1994) An evaluation of the pathological effects of fluorescent powder on deer mice (*Peromyscus maniculatus*). *Journal of Mammalogy* **75**, 704–709. doi:10.2307/1382519

Van Winkel D, Ji W (2014) Attaching radio-transmitters to geckos: trials and tribulations. *Herpetological Review* **45**, 13–17.

Warner D, Thomas J, Shine R (2006) A simple and reliable method for attaching radio-transmitters to lizards. *Herpetological Conservation and Biology* **1**, 129–131.

Whiting MJ, Noble DWA (2018) Lizards – measuring cognition: practical challenges and the influence of ecology and social behaviour. In *Field and Laboratory Methods in Animal Cognition*. (Eds N Bueno-Guerra and F Amici) pp. 266–285. Cambridge University Press, Cambridge, UK.

White GC, Garrot RA (1990) *Analysis of Wildlife Radio-tracking Data*. Academic Press, San Diego, CA.

Williams ST, Powell SD, Gorman TA, Haas CA (2014) Pioneering the utility of a mineral oil mixture for fluorescent powder tracking of salamanders. *Herpetological Review* **45**, 20–22.

Willis CKR, Brigham RM (2003) Defining torpor in free-ranging bats: experimental evaluation of external temperature-sensitive radiotransmitters and the concept of active temperature. *Journal of Comparative Physiology. B, Biochemical, Systemic, and Environmental Physiology* **173**, 379–389. doi:10.1007/s00360-003-0343-y

Wilson RP, Börger L, Holton MD, Scantlebury DM, Gómez-Laich A, Quintana F, *et al.* (2020) Estimates for energy expenditure in free-living animals using acceleration proxies: a reappraisal. *Journal of Animal Ecology* **89**, 161–172. doi:10.1111/1365-2656.13040

Wilson RP, McMahon CR (2006) Measuring devices on wild animals: what constitutes acceptable practice? *Frontiers in Ecology and the Environment* **4**, 147–154. doi:10.1890/1540-9295(2006)004[0147:MDOWAW]2.0.CO;2

Wisely SM, Golightly RT (2003) Behavioral and ecological adaptations to water economy in two plethodontid salamanders, *Ensatina eschscholtzii* and *Batrachoseps attenuatus*. *Journal of Herpetology* **37**, 659–665. doi:10.1670/5-03A

10 Citizen science and education

Helen P. Waudby, Gregory D. Kerr, Erin Roger, Matthew J. Gill, Sophie Petit and Tegan K. Douglas

INTRODUCTION

Connection to nature (Whitburn *et al.* 2020; Keith *et al.* 2021) and nature-based environmental education (Otto and Pensini 2017) are drivers of pro-environmental behaviours. However, opportunities to establish connections with nature are probably declining, with much of the world's population living in urban areas, influencing the ways in which people interact with the natural world (Keith *et al.* 2021). These opportunities can be facilitated, at least in part, by incorporating studies of natural history and wildlife into education, and engaging people in citizen science programs. The study of large-scale patterns in the natural world requires data to be collected over extensive spatial and temporal scales. Such programs can be difficult to resource, particularly in view of limited funding for wildlife research. The growth of citizen science over the past 20 years has provided an opportunity to collect extensive data on species occurrences and distributions, boost science literacy, and foster environmental and ecological awareness. Similarly, collaborating with the education sector on citizen scientist projects can provide a means of engaging students on conservation issues and introducing them to the scientific method. Accordingly, many citizen science–focused activities are now geared towards the education sector. For example, school-based citizen science projects have investigated the presence of insects in urban environments (Saunders *et al.* 2018), the impacts of urban bird feeding (Soanes *et al.* 2020, and the effects of vegetation cover on nest predation (Gracanin *et al.* 2020). Teaching with wildlife educates people about the environment in a meaningful and practical way. Similarly, direct interactions with animals are an important component of many tertiary courses that aim to provide students with comprehensive wildlife management and research skills. This chapter highlights general principles for managing animal welfare outcomes in citizen science and education sectors.

WILDLIFE-FOCUSED CITIZEN SCIENCE

Helen P. Waudby, Gregory D. Kerr, Erin Roger, Matthew J. Gill, Sophie Petit and Tegan Douglas

Target taxa

Citizen science is applicable to all species and taxa depending on the study objectives and expertise of participants.

Context and scope

This general operating procedure (GOP) details considerations and principles for the use of wildlife in citizen science projects. It assumes that investigators have determined that animal ethics approval is required for their research (see Chapter 3 for further discussion on animal ethics approval processes and citizen science). Definitions of citizen science are diverse and often include community engagement and education goals in addition to scientific ones. Citizen science approaches have evolved over the past 20 years to include (among other components) the integration of explicit and tested protocols for collecting data, vetting of data by professional scientists, and incorporation of specific and measurable goals for public education (Roger *et al.* 2020). Importantly, programs should seek to answer a clear research question or objective. A review of threatened species–focused citizen science projects in Australia found that only 2% of projects stated clear research questions (Steven *et al.* 2019).

Citizen science is becoming an increasingly popular and effective means of collecting scientific data. Its rise has been facilitated, at least in part, by the advent of accessible and user-friendly data collection tools, such as smartphone applications and web-based resources (Saunders *et al.* 2018). Citizen science-based projects are being used to answer diverse questions about wildlife (Table 10.1). Effective training and data management are critical to achieving research objectives and ensuring acceptable animal welfare outcomes. The involvement of 'non-trained' participants can lead to a decline in scientific rigour (and potentially animal welfare) if inappropriate or inconsistent data collection methods are employed.

While wildlife-focused citizen science projects often employ low-impact methods, some level of impact on study species is likely in many cases, and it can be difficult for primary investigators to maintain close

Table 10.1: Examples of wildlife-focused citizen science projects.

Focus	Species examples	Mode of data collection
Assessing population trends of target species	Humpback whales (Pirotta *et al.* 2020); green sea turtles (Hof *et al.* 2017); koalas (Predavec *et al.* 2017); Carnaby's black-cockatoo (Williams *et al.* 2016).	Long-term dataset of shore-based observations (Pirotta *et al.* 2020); capture–mark–recapture program implemented by citizen scientists (Hof *et al.* 2017); postal and web-based surveys of community members in target areas (Predavec *et al.* 2017); annual synchronised surveys (the Great Cocky Count) of known roosting locations (Williams *et al.* 2016).
Tracking dispersal or seasonal movements of target species	Australian fairy tern; sulphur-crested cockatoo; Australian brush turkey; Australian white ibis; Pacific gull; migratory shorebird species.	Participants submit photos or reports of locations of marked animals via a smartphone application (e.g. Cockatoo Wingtags), on dedicated social media pages (South-west Fairy-tern Network; shorebird leg-flag sightings in the East Asian–Australasian Flyway).
Patterns of road mortality	Eastern long-necked turtles (Santori *et al.* 2018).	Purpose-built website (Turtle SAT) to which citizens upload turtle sightings (Santori *et al.* 2018).
Invasive species surveillance	Red squirrels (Goldstein *et al.* 2014). Broad-scale surveillance of invasive species (Centre for Invasive Species Solutions 2020).	Supported by a media campaign; participants reported sightings through a dedicated website, by mail or over the phone (Goldstein *et al.* 2014). FeralScan program supported by a dedicated website and smartphone application (Centre for Invasive Species Solutions 2020).
Broad-scale assessments of specific taxa (abundance, biodiversity, distribution)	Frogs (Rowley *et al.* 2019) and birds (Callaghan *et al.* 2021). Common bottlenose dolphin (Bartram and Bartram 2011).	Participants submit data through smartphone applications (e.g. Birdata e-Bird, FrogID, iNaturalist Atlas of Living Australia, DolphinWatch), or online portals (e.g. EP Birds Online Portal).
Evaluation of human–wildlife interactions and community education and engagement	Bluetongue lizards, possums, Australian magpies and spiders (Roetman and Daniels 2011). Multiple species evaluations through BioBlitzes (Hepburn *et al.* 2015).	Intensive promotion through local radio and social media; participants contributed data through an online survey during a 13-week period (Roetman and Daniels 2011). BioBlitzes are at the interface between citizen science and education and are typically an intensive survey of an area for all biodiversity present over a set period of time (Hepburn *et al.* 2015).
Mapping ecosystem recovery using citizen science wildlife observational data as indicators	Large-scale evaluation of the effects of wildfire on biodiversity (Kirchhoff *et al.* 2020).	Rapid response project launched in response to the 2019–20 south-eastern Australian bushfires; data collected by participants via a smartphone application (iNaturalist) and supported by a media campaign.

supervision over citizen scientists, particularly when projects are undertaken over large geographical and spatial scales. We suggest the following principles for designing wildlife-based citizen science projects:

- Research questions are clearly defined and articulated to participants.
- The project design minimises interactions between citizen scientists and target animals (e.g. participants record animal calls rather than photograph them at close range), particularly for self-directed programs.
- If citizen scientists are involved in collection of data from animals (which may include close observation or even handling in some cases), participants are under the direct supervision of a principal or other experienced investigator. Alternatively, for observation-only work, maximum approach distances are defined depending on the sensitivity of the target species. Participants are trained according to strict criteria defined by the investigators.
- Some activities (e.g. observation of nesting or breeding animals) are only undertaken by experienced citizen scientists with specialised training.

Animal welfare considerations

Few studies have examined the actual or potential effects of citizen science programs on animal welfare. In general, impacts are context-specific, depending on the research objectives, sensitivity of the study taxa, data collection methods, experience of participants and local environment. Investigators should remember that even simple observation can affect wildlife, for example through disruption of an animal's activity patterns or increased stress levels, or indirectly via changes in habitat (Liddle 1997; Green and Higginbottom 2000). Extent of impact will also be influenced by the attitudes and behaviours of participants who are not necessarily under the direct control of principal investigators. For example, a program that encourages the recording of animal calls through a smartphone application should, intuitively, be low impact. However, if participants choose to search for a calling animal, perhaps to photograph it or collect a better recording, then impacts may be heightened. Ultimately, some risks associated with citizen scientist-type projects are difficult to control. Table 10.2 details a range of generic impacts that investigators may consider during planning stages.

Table 10.2: Potential impacts of citizen science programs on animal welfare.

Potential impact	Examples	Mitigation options
Direct and indirect disturbance	Disturbance to habitat, such as turning of rocks or fallen timber. Repeated participant visits to a site creating trails for predators. Attempts to observe animals at breeding sites at close range.	Data collection methods require negligible or minimal disturbance. Unambiguous instructions provided to participants about appropriate interactions. Project open to selected participants (i.e. not a broad call for participation).
Revealing locations of rare, sensitive and threatened species	Sensitive species may be particularly prone to disturbance. Risk of collection or additional disturbance of species by other members of the public attempting to access sites and species if locations are revealed.	Sensitive location data should be protected. For example, some national programs and databases buffer the locations of threatened or rare species. Participants made aware of the issues around revealing the location of sensitive species. Minimal permanent markers and tags, such as tree tags, left in the field outside of monitoring sessions.
Cumulative impacts	Distress because of repeated visits to a site by the same or different participants. Distress from repeated deliberate disturbance (e.g. frequent unnecessary checking of nest boxes; frequent use of drones for monitoring purposes).	Investigators consider potential impacts in view of the sensitivity of study species. Participants trained in appropriate data collection techniques and provided with unambiguous instructions. Participants have allocated sites to monitor.
Spread of pathogens	Spread of pathogens, such as chytrid fungus (*Batrachochytrium dendrobatidis*), which may affect individuals and populations of amphibians directly. Spread of pathogens, such as *Phytophthora cinnamomi*, which will affect habitat.	Participants may be supervised by experienced investigators where the risk of pathogen spread is high. Avoid actions that may increase risk of disease in habitat.

General procedures

Broadly, the process for planning and implementing field-based citizen science projects led by professional scientists, involves:

1. defining a research question (ideally in collaboration with the intended participants)
2. forming a scientist/educator/technical expert/evaluator team
3. developing, testing and refining protocols, data forms and educational support materials
4. recruiting and training participants, and clarifying expectations around ownership of data (which should belong to the project)
5. recording, editing, and displaying data
6. providing community members with access to data
7. analysing and interpreting data
8. disseminating results
9. measuring and reporting on outcomes, including educational ones.

Pre-planning

Investigators should plan their project in accordance with principles for citizen science projects (Australian Citizen Science Association 2018), and in view of their target demographic or audience (e.g. school children; Soanes *et al.* 2020). In their protocols, investigators should clearly state the research questions or objectives being addressed, the experimental design used to test them and the target audience, including their anticipated experience and knowledge levels – for example, a group of field naturalists with extensive knowledge of a specific area or species versus community members of a broad geographical area.

Investigators should define the type of data being collected from animal subjects by citizen science participants. Ideally, the data should be simple to collect with minimal disturbance to study animals. For example, the recording and submission of animal vocalisations, such as those of calling male frogs during their breeding season, or bird surveys using binoculars or telescopes, would be considered low impact. However, bird surveys using call playback would need to articulate clearly the procedures to minimise negative impacts on birds. Investigators should consider any animal welfare-related laws or policies relating to their study species and incorporate them into the program (e.g. rules around interactions with cetaceans or raptors).

Data collection methods

Investigators should define how data will be collected, recorded and submitted by participants (see examples in Table 10.1). Data may be recorded on data sheets, notebooks, by uploading records to websites or be collated and uploaded through smartphone applications. Smartphone applications are increasingly popular and offer many advantages (e.g. ease of use; *in situ* error and completion checks; can be supported by online reference material) over traditional paper-based methods, but will not necessarily cater to all demographics. Paper-based collection methods are typically easy to prepare and accessible by most participants, but may become lost, damaged, incomplete, illegible or remain unsubmitted. Investigators should be mindful of applications that employ a gamification or competition strategy of wildlife record collection. Gamification (see Chapter 3 for further discussion) is useful for incentivising participation, but could have increased negative effects on wildlife, particularly through cumulative impacts.

Launch of programs and participant training

Investigators should provide training (e.g. in data collection methods, life-history characteristics of the target species, and hygiene and animal welfare protocols). Doing so creates an opportunity to reinforce sound methodological practices and engage participants in the project.

Dissemination of results

Study results must be articulated to participants (Silvertown 2009; Van der Wal *et al.* 2016; Zhou *et al.* 2020). Ideally, participants are provided with an opportunity to ask questions and comment on the study. Depending on the nature of the project, feedback may be provided at regular intervals through the program or at its culmination. Investigators should choose a mode of communicating results (e.g. via newsletters or websites, follow-up workshops, presentations and social media) appropriate to their target demographic. Providing access to the dataset for citizen scientists is an important part of building buy-in to the work. However, careful consideration about what data can be disclosed is necessary (Table 10.2); investigators should remain mindful about sharing data relating to the locations of threatened and culturally important species (Roger *et al.* 2020), including being aware of the sensitive data species policies of some platforms. Limitations on data sharing should be made clear to participants early on in the study.

Animal treatment, withdrawal and euthanasia

Knowing when to revise or withdraw a program relies on knowledge of (often unreported) effects of the study on animals, and is difficult to gauge for programs where participants are not under direct supervision of primary investigators. Citizen scientists can be asked to report signs of stress in animals if they are observing or interacting with them directly. Investigators can consider tracking how often participants visit certain sites and when, as an indication of potential cumulative impacts in any given area.

Equipment and maintenance

Equipment requirements depend on the type of research being conducted. For some studies, participants may simply require access to a smartphone and the ability to download an application. For other projects, participants may require specialised equipment. For example, access to high-quality binoculars or spotting scopes may markedly improve the quality of data collected in bird surveys.

Specific qualifications, experience and training

Required qualifications or training will depend entirely on the nature of the study. Investigators must be satisfied that their participants, or likely participants, will have an appropriate level of skills and expertise to participate in the study effectively. In some cases, cultivating local 'champions' who help with motivating and training other participants may be helpful. Critically, investigators must regularly reiterate the requirements of the study to participants, including expectations around animal treatment (Hepburn *et al.* 2015).

Workplace health and safety

Investigators should consider the health and safety of citizen scientists involved in their projects and provide them with appropriate advice. Potential risks and advice are context- and project-specific, but may include:

- considerations around site access on private and public land, including seeking landholder permission and specific risks relating to certain sites (e.g. contaminated land, livestock, barbed wire fences, fire risk with cars, and presence of phytophthora)
- suitable clothing, including personal protective equipment
- specific equipment (e.g. head torches, waders)
- protocols for appropriate, community-minded use of optical and audio recording equipment in public spaces (e.g. using binoculars near private homes and schools)
- the need for insect repellent and sunscreen
- protocols for inclement weather and for working in remote areas (e.g. maps, compasses, GPS, emergency beacons, safety itineraries and contacts, fire danger)
- potential for harm of participants by animals (including transmission of zoonoses if they are in to be close contact with wildlife or habitat)
- habitat- or geography-specific risks, including for remote areas (e.g. areas known to have a high prevalence of ticks or mites, water bodies, or survey in isolated locations outside phone reception).

Alternative procedures

Typically, citizen science projects use low-impact methods that involve little to no direct interaction with animals, particularly where the skill levels of participants are variable. Often, citizen science approaches complement other methods as part of the same study. Those running projects that rely on more-direct interaction with animals should consider if other less-interactive methods are more suitable, for example assessment of signs and traces (Chapter 4) and camera trapping without lures (Chapter 5).

TEACHING WITH WILDLIFE

Gregory D. Kerr, Helen P. Waudby, Erin Roger, Matthew J. Gill, Sophie Petit and Tegan K. Douglas

Target taxa

Potentially, all species and taxa may be used for educational purposes depending on the ages and experience levels of students, and the program objectives. The sensitivity of target taxa to the proposed activities and the risk that working with the species presents to students should be assessed before embarking on the program.

Context and scope

This general operating procedure (GOP) details principles for the use of wildlife to facilitate teaching programs at primary, secondary and tertiary levels. It assumes that educators have determined that animal ethics is required for their proposed teaching activity (Table 10.3 details relevant state policies, guidelines and other resources). This GOP does not discuss the pedagogy of using animals for invasive procedures.

Table 10.3: Animal welfare policy, guidelines and resources for schools.

Jurisdiction	Guidelines and resources
National	Australian Code for the Care and Use of Animals for Scientific Purposes The Australian Guide to Running a BioBlitz (Hepburn *et al.* 2015)
Australian Capital Territory	Care and Use of Animals in ACT Schools Policy
New South Wales	Animals in Schools: Animal Welfare Guidelines for Teachers
Northern Territory	Animals in Schools Policy and the Animals in Schools Risk Management Plan
Queensland	Use of Animals in Education Procedure: Animals in Queensland State Schools
South Australia	Standard Operating Procedures for the use of Animals in Schools, Preschools and Child Care Centres Animal Welfare Codes of Practice
Tasmania	Infection Prevention and Control Guidelines
Victoria	Policy, Guidelines and Resources for Teaching with Animals Victorian Codes of Practice for Animal Welfare Wildlife in Schools (school authorisation permits)
Western Australia	Use of Animals in Public Schools Policy and Procedures

The benefits to student social function, performance, and educational outcomes, from using living animals in classrooms (Gee *et al.* 2015) are well documented. In general, contact with nature is linked to improved health and wellbeing (Kaplan 1995; Martin *et al.* 2020). Simply explaining ecological interactions or conservation issues to students is unlikely to instil a long-term sense of respect or appreciation for the environment (Hungerford and Peyton 1994). Contact with the natural world, particularly during childhood, is important for forming meaningful bonds to nature (Kellert 2002). Additionally, working with wildlife is a facet of many science- and land management-based occupations that are the focus of tertiary courses. The practical animal handling, identification and assessment skills needed by students to obtain these positions often can only be gained effectively through working with animals directly (McCleery *et al.* 2005). Developing these skills in a controlled educational setting will improve animal welfare outcomes when students enter wildlife-based professions.

Animal welfare considerations

Teachers have a duty to show a caring and humane approach in their work with animals, and education institutions must follow the relevant codes of practice for the welfare of animals when using animals for teaching purposes (Table 10.3). As with research-focused activities, educators must demonstrate that animal use in teaching is essential in view of the 'three Rs' (Chapter 1). Potential impacts on animal welfare are context-specific. For example, impacts on amphibians that have been bred and kept in a classroom, so that primary school students can observe metamorphosis, are likely to be different from those on wild small mammals being trapped by tertiary students to learn capture and handling techniques.

Observation versus interactive activities

Typically, teaching with animals can be classed as purely observational or interactive (e.g. physical manipulation of an animal or its habitat). Observation-based activities are often lower impact than interactive ones, but the duration and intensity of the impact will depend on whether or not the animal is captive-bred, habituated, or being dealt with in the wild. Educators should refer to the relevant chapters in Section 3 of this book and other GOPs dealing with their planned capture, handling or marking technique to assess specific potential impacts on their target taxa.

Inexperienced students

Stress to animals may be exacerbated by interactions with inexperienced students. Educators must articulate clearly to their students the potential impacts of their behaviour on animals and acceptable standards for interacting with animals. Key principles should be reiterated consistently and regularly to students. Students should be taught that animals are individuals and not all will behave in the same way. Students should be supervised closely. Importantly, students who handle animals should be trained to remain calm during these interactions as the demeanour of the handler directly affects the stress of the animal subject.

Educators taking students to interact with animals in the wild must consider the impact of observation on wild animals and balance it against the anticipated educational outcomes (Higginbottom *et al.* 2001). An observer's presence can result in behavioural changes even when animals appear habituated to humans (Caine 1990), although the degree of behavioural change can vary with the level of habituation (Labra and Leonard 1999), or with observer proximity and visibility. For example, in reptiles, observer presence may lead to increased refuge use, changes in habitat use and patterns of activity (Kerr *et al.* 2004) and reduced basking time, which may impose physiological and behavioural costs (Martín and Lopéz 1999).

General procedures

Articulation of educational outcomes

Educators articulate the objective of animal use within their teaching and learning plans, and reiterate these objectives to students. It should be clear that animal use is not 'recreational' and is being undertaken for a specific purpose. At all times, educators should demonstrate respect for study animals and require the same of students. Poor treatment of, or attitude towards, animals should not be tolerated.

Animal husbandry and collection of animals

Educators should determine if activities will focus on captive animals or free-living wild animals. Captive animals should be monitored daily, providing that doing so does not cause them additional unnecessary stress. Teachers must be practised in the handling and husbandry requirements of species in their care, and know when to seek veterinary advice. Animals cannot be taken from the wild without permits. For example, it is illegal to collect frog spawn and tadpoles.

Student supervision and training

Where students are working directly with animals, they must remain under close supervision by an experienced educator at all times. Students must also be trained and practised in proper handling techniques. Ideally, students practise the procedure or movements on a 'dummy' animal (e.g. a plush toy) before attempting on a live animal. In tertiary settings where students will handle and interact directly with animals, educators can consider requiring students to complete simple theory-based sessions to improve their knowledge of animal behaviour before having direct contact (e.g. Old and Spencer 2011).

Group numbers should be maintained at appropriate levels for the animals and program objectives. In general, teachers should aim to mitigate the negative impacts of a disturbance, such as high numbers of students, by designing measures to manage their numbers, spatial distribution, and location (in relation to the animals) or temporal distribution. Consideration may also need to be given to the effects of individual student behaviour on animal welfare; if detrimental impacts are possible, measures to modify student behaviour – either directly or through modifying their expectations and attitudes – should be taken. For example, students surveying waterbirds might share a class set of binoculars and observe the birds from a bird hide rather than setting off individually.

End of the activity or project

For animals that are kept in captivity, educators should plan for the management or appropriate disposal of that animal once teaching has finished. Discussion with the students and reflection on interactions with the animals emphasise learning outcomes and respect for wildlife.

Animal treatment, withdrawal and euthanasia

Where an incident compromising the welfare of any animal occurs, the immediate needs of the animal must be assessed and attended to by the lead educator or other appropriately trained person (such as a veterinarian). Educators should take the opportunity to review with students the events that may have contributed to the animal's injury or death and discuss how procedures could be improved to prevent or minimise such events in the future. Similarly, if animal euthanasia is required, educators should consider demonstrating appropriate methods. Students' needs for counselling are also assessed.

Equipment and maintenance

Equipment needs depend entirely on the nature of the educational activity.

Specific qualifications, experience and training

The lead educator or handler should be appropriately qualified and experienced to undertake all planned activities, and ideally should have worked with the target taxa beforehand. Some activities will require lead personnel to have formal accreditations (Figure 10.1).

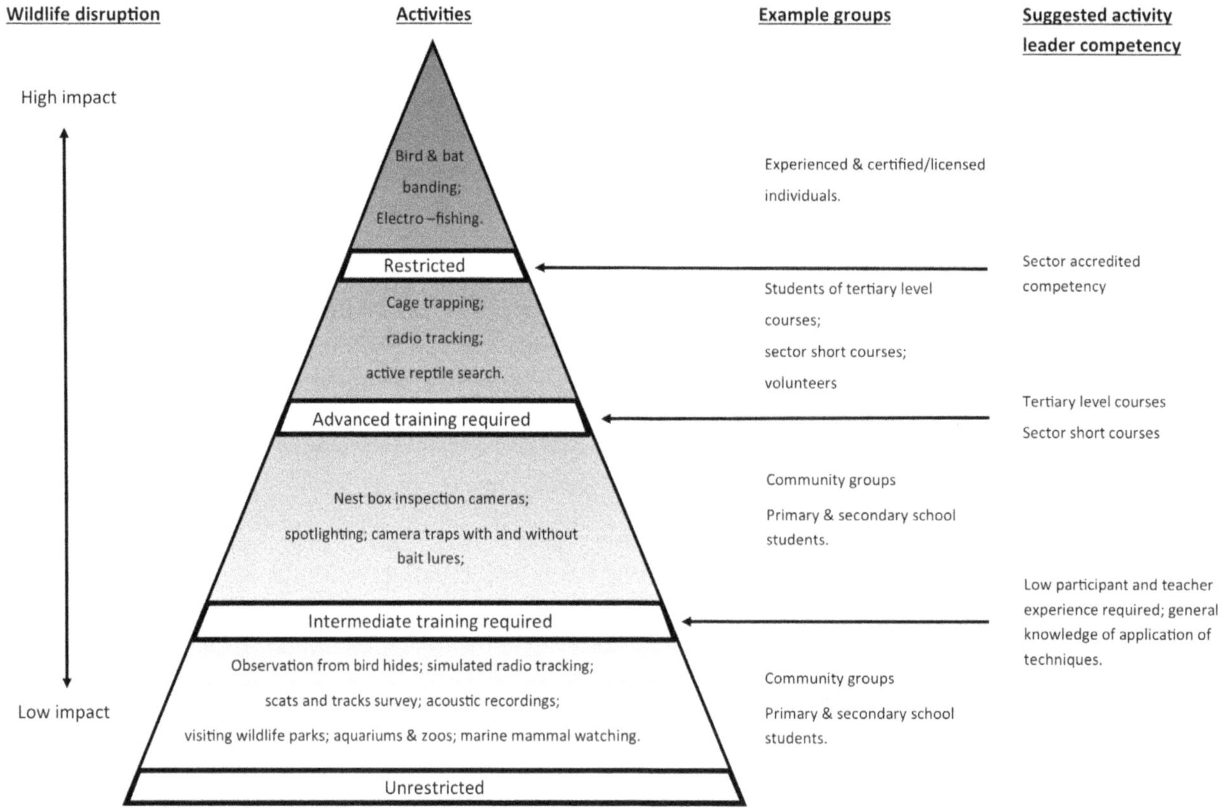

Figure 10.1: Recommended target audiences and competency levels for educators for wildlife-related activities with varying levels of potential impact. Illustration by Matthew J. Gill.

Workplace health and safety

Potential disease hazards and other occupational health and safety issues are associated with the presence, care and use of animals in schools. Risk management of animal activities ensures the health, safety and wellbeing of students, staff and others involved. If animals are kept on site, schools should develop a biosecurity plan to identify potential issues around animals and their water, bedding material and food being brought into the school, animal health management, treatment of pests and diseases, animal and student hygiene, equipment hygiene, removal and treatment of wastes, fencing or caging design and maintenance, and staff and student training. Doing so provides an opportunity to educate students about biosecurity and help protect the school from the entry and spread of pests and diseases.

Alternative procedures

Direct use of animals may be unnecessary, particularly for primary and secondary students. For example, learning experiences might include classroom-linked field trips to zoos and aquariums or nature programs involving experiential learning outside of the classroom, and in nature parks or wildlife reserves rather than specific use of animals (Figure 10.1).

REFERENCES

Australian Citizen Science Association (2018) *10 principles of citizen science.* Australian Citizen Science Association, Sydney. <https://citizenscience.org.au/10-principles-of-citizen-science/>.

Bartram P, Bartram T (2011) Walking with dolphins Kangaroo Island Dolphin Watch. *Wildlife Australia* **48**, 12–15.

Caine NG (1990) Unrecognised anti-predator behaviour can bias observational data. *Animal Behaviour* **39**, 195–197. doi:10.1016/S0003-3472(05)80741-9

Callaghan CT, Nakagawa S, Cornwell WK (2021) Global abundance estimates for 9,700 bird species. *Proceedings of the National Academy of Sciences of the United States of America* **118**, e2023170118. doi:10.1073/pnas.2023170118

Centre for Invasive Species Solutions (2020) *FeralScan.* Centre for Invasive Species Solutions, Canberra. <https://www.feralscan.org.au/>.

Gee NR, Fine AH, Schuck S (2015) Animals in educational settings: research and practice. In *Handbook on Animal-assisted Therapy: Foundations and Guidelines for Animal-Assisted Interventions.* 4th edn. (Ed. A Fine) pp. 195–210. Elsevier Academic Press, Amsterdam, The Netherlands.

Goldstein EA, Lawton C, Sheehy E, Butler F (2014) Locating species range frontiers: a cost efficiency comparison of citizen science and hair-tube survey methods for use in tracking an invasive squirrel. *Wildlife Research* **41**, 64–75. doi:10.1071/WR13197

Gracanin A, Roger E, Katsis AC, O'Loughlin LS, Emery NJ, O'Cock JF, O'Hanlon JC (2020) An artificial bird nest experiment in urban environments: lessons from a school-based citizen science program. *Austral Ecology* **45**, 523–528. doi:10.1111/aec.12859

Green RJ, Higginbottom K (2000) The effects of non-consumptive wildlife tourism on free-ranging wildlife: a review. *Pacific Conservation Biology* **6**, 183–197. doi:10.1071/PC000183

Hepburn L, Tegart P, Roetman P, von Gavel S, Niedra S, Roger E, Miller S, Fyffe T, Brenton P, Lambkin C (2015) *The Australian Guide to Running a BioBlitz*. Atlas of Life, Atlas of Living Australia, Great Barrier Reef Foundation, Office of Environment and Heritage, Queensland Museum, Australian Government, Inspiring Australia. doi:10.13140/RG.2.1.2294.1289

Higginbottom K, Northrope C, Green R (2001) *Positive Effects of Wildlife Tourism on Wildlife*. Wildlife Tourism Research Report No. 6. Cooperative Research Centre for Sustainable Tourism, Gold Coast.

Hof CAM, Smallwood E, Meager J, Bell IP (2017) First citizen-science population abundance and growth rate estimates for green sea turtles *Chelonia mydas* foraging in the northern Great Barrier Reef, Australia. *Marine Ecology Progress Series* **574**, 181–191. doi:10.3354/meps12173

Hungerford HR, Peyton RB (1994) *Procedures for Developing an Environmental Education Curriculum: A Discussion Guide For UNESCO Training Seminars on Environmental Education (Revised)*. UNESCO-UNEP International Environmental Education Programme Environmental Education Series 22, Paris, France.

Kaplan S (1995) The restorative benefits of nature: towards an integrative framework. *Journal of Environmental Psychology* **15**, 169–182. doi:10.1016/0272-4944(95)90001-2

Keith RJ, Given LM, Martin JM, Hochuli DF (2021) Urban children's connections to nature and environmental behaviors differ with age and gender. *PLoS One*. doi:10.1371/journal.pone.0255421.

Kellert SR (2002) Experiencing nature: affective, cognitive and evaluative development in children. In *Children and Nature: Psychological, Sociological and Evolutionary Investigations*. (Eds PH Kahn Jr and SR Kellert) pp. 117–151. MIT Press, Cambridge, MA.

Kerr GD, Bull CM, Mackay D (2004) Human disturbance and stride frequency in the sleepy lizard (*Tiliqua rugosa*): implications for behavioural studies. *Journal of Herpetology* **38**, 519–526. doi:10.1670/13-04A

Kirchhoff C, Callaghan C, Keith DA, Indiarto D, Taseski G, Ooi MKJ, Le Breton TD, Mesaglio T, Kingsford TR, Cornwell W (2020) Rapidly mapping fire effects on biodiversity at a large scale using citizen science. *EcoEvoRxiv Preprints*. doi:10.32942/osf.io/vc6ry

Labra A, Leonard R (1999) Intraspecific variation in antipredator responses of three species of lizard (Liolaemus): possible effects of human presence. *Journal of Herpetology* **33**, 441–448. doi:10.2307/1565641

Liddle MJ (1997) *Recreation Ecology: The Ecological Impact of Outdoor Recreation and Ecotourism*. Chapman and Hall, London, UK.

Martín J, Lopéz P (1999) An experimental test of the costs of antipredatory refuge use in the wall lizard, *Podarcis mularis*. *Oikos* **84**, 499–505. doi:10.2307/3546428

Martin L, White MP, Hunt A, Richardson M, Pahl S, Burt J (2020) Nature contact, nature connectedness and associations with health, wellbeing and pro-environmental behaviours. *Journal of Environmental Psychology* **68**, 101389. doi:10.1016/j.jenvp.2020.101389

McCleery RA, Lopez RR, Harveson LA, Silvy NJ, Slack RD (2005) Integrating on-campus wildlife research projects into the wildlife curriculum. *Wildlife Society Bulletin* **33**, 802–809. doi:10.2193/0091-7648(2005)33[802:IOWRPI]2.0.CO;2

Old JM, Spencer RJ (2011) Development of online learning activities to enhance student knowledge of animal behaviour prior to engaging in live animal handling practical sessions. *Open Journal of Animal Sciences* **1**, 65–74. doi:10.4236/ojas.2011.12009

Otto S, Pensini P (2017) Nature-based environmental education of children: environmental knowledge and connectedness to nature, together, are related to ecological behaviour. *Global Environmental Change* **47**, 88–94. doi:10.1016/j.gloenvcha.2017.09.009

Pirotta V, Reynolds W, Ross G, Jonsen I, Grech A, Slip D, Harcourt R (2020) A citizen science approach to long-term monitoring of humpback whales (*Megaptera novaeangliae*) off Sydney, Australia. *Marine Mammal Science* **36**, 472–485. doi:10.1111/mms.12651

Predavec M, Lunney D, Shannon I, Lemon J, Sonawane I, Crowther M (2017) Using repeat citizen science surveys of koalas to assess their population trend in the north-west of New South Wales: scale matters. *Australian Mammalogy* **40**, 47–57. doi:10.1071/AM16059

Roetman PEJ, Daniels CB (2011) The benefits of citizen science in research, education and community engagement. In *Creating Sustainable Communities in a Changing World*. (Eds PEJ Roetman and CB Daniels) pp. 249–260. Crawford House Publishing, Adelaide.

Roger E, Tegart P, Dowsett R, Kinsela MA, Harley MD, Ortac G (2020) Maximising the potential for citizen science in NSW. *Australian Zoologist* **40**, 449–461. doi:10.7882/AZ.2019.023

Rowley JJL, Callaghan CT, Cutajar T, Portway C, Potter K, Mahony St, Trembath DF, Flemons P, Woods A (2019) FrogID: citizen scientists provide validated biodiversity data on frogs of Australia. *Herpetological Conservation and Biodiversity* **14**, 155–170.

Santori C, Spencer R-J, Van Dyke JU, Thompson MB (2018) Road mortality of the eastern long-necked turtle (*Chelodina longicollis*) along the Murray River, Australia: an assessment using citizen science. *Australian Journal of Zoology* **66**, 41–49. doi:10.1071/ZO17065

Saunders ME, Roger E, Geary WL, Meredith F, Welbourne DJ, Bako A, *et al.* (2018) Citizen science in schools: engaging students in research on urban habitat for pollinators. *Austral Ecology* **43**, 635–642. doi:10.1111/aec.12608

Silvertown J (2009) A new dawn for citizen science. *Trends in Ecology & Evolution* **24**, 467–471. doi:10.1016/j.tree.2009.03.017

Soanes K, Cranney K, Dade MC, Edwards AM, Palavalli-Nettimi R, Doherty TS (2020) How to work with children and animals: a guide for school-based citizen science in wildlife research. *Austral Ecology* **45**, 3–14. doi:10.1111/aec.12836

Steven R, Barnes M, Garnett ST, Garrard G, O'Connor J, Oliver JL, Robinson C, Tulloch A, Fuller RA (2019) Aligning citizen science with best practice: threatened species conservation in Australia. *Conservation Science and Practice* **1**, e100. doi:10.1111/csp2.100

Van der Wal R, Sharma N, Mellish C, Robinson A, Siddharthan A (2016) The role of automated feedback in training and retaining biological recorders for citizen science. *Conservation Biology* **30**, 550–561. doi:10.1111/cobi.12705

Whitburn J, Linklater W, Abrahamse W (2020) Meta-analysis of human connection to nature and proenviromental behaviour. *Conservation Biology* **34**, 180–193. doi:10.1111/cobi.13381

Williams MR, Yates CJ, Stock WD, Barrett GW, Finn HC (2016) Citizen science monitoring reveals a significant ongoing decline of the endangered Carnaby's black-cockatoo *Calyptorhynchus latirostris*. *Oryx* **50**, 626–635. doi:10.1017/S0030605315000320

Zhou X, Tang J, Zhao YC, Wang T (2020) Effects of feedback design and dispositional goal orientations on volunteer performance in citizen science projects. *Computers in Human Behavior* **107**, 106266. doi:10.1016/j.chb.2020.106266

11 Deterring and repelling wildlife

Bradley P. Smith, Lysanne Snijders, Jorge Tobajas, Katherine Whitehouse-Tedd, Linda van Bommel, Benjamin J. Pitcher, Colleen Cassady St. Clair, Robert G. Appleby, Neil R. Jordan and Alison L. Greggor

INTRODUCTION

This chapter provides general operating procedures (GOPs) and guidelines for a variety of non-lethal techniques, which seek to interrupt, reduce or modify the behaviour of wildlife to decrease the occurrence of 'unwanted' or 'undesirable' behaviours. In Australia such methods are mostly employed for threatened species protection as part of introduced predator management, and for protecting agricultural interests from wildlife (e.g. to keep carnivores from attacking livestock, or kangaroos from accessing grazing land). However, non-lethal techniques as described in this chapter can be applied to a multitude of management and research contexts (e.g. to protect humans from shark attack). Methods covered include guardian animals, disruptive stimuli (frightening devices, lights, sounds), conditioned taste aversion (odours and chemicals) and electric deterrents (fences, shields, collars). These guidelines are written to be complementary to each other given the overlap in many themes that exist across the techniques. A great deal of the literature referred to is drawn from international sources where many of the problems, solutions and ethical implications are similar.

Disruptive stimuli are intentional anthropogenic efforts to exclude or perturb wild animals. They can be defined as 'undesirable stimuli that prevent or alter particular behaviors of animals', while aversive stimuli are 'any stimuli that cause discomfort, pain, or an otherwise negative experience and are paired with specific behaviors to achieve conditioning against these behaviors' (Shivik and Martin 2000, p. 112). Accordingly, the use of aversive stimuli allows the animal to learn by 'punishment' (i.e. consequences that reduce the likelihood of a behaviour occurring) and so develop an association between a behaviour undesired by humans and the animal-aversive stimulus (Snijders *et al.* 2019). Strategic application of these techniques can result in the ceasing or modification of behaviour, with the strength and duration of the association (retention) depending on the treatment procedure (Smith *et al.* 2000).

Any disruptive technique or aversive conditioning procedure has the potential to negatively affect the welfare of animals. Indeed, the very intention of these methods is to change behaviour via exposure to discomforting stimuli. As such, the process involves the deliberate cause of short-term pain or discomfort to induce fear, escape and avoidance. The effectiveness of the method relies on the animal being conditioned to avoid the situation in the future. However, learning from transient aversive situations is not unnatural or uncommon for wildlife (Appleby *et al.* 2017a). In fact, such associative learning is evolutionarily programmed into animals (including humans) as it enables individuals to increase their probability of survival by learning about temporary unfavourable experiences (e.g. fear; Gaynor *et al.* 2021), and avoiding more severe and permanent unfavourable situations (e.g. injury or death) in the future (Domjan 2018).

The effectiveness of disruptive and aversive management techniques rely on behavioural responses from animals. One of the potential advantages of these techniques over lethal methods is that individuals have the opportunity to learn and persist in the environment where they can maintain ecological functions, compete with conspecifics, and in some cases pass on knowledge of cues to other individuals (Thorogood *et al.* 2018). For these reasons, understanding the cognitive processes that underlie the desired response, including perception, learning and decision-making, makes it possible to design interventions where only a few unpleasant exposures are needed, which minimises harm to realise long-term behavioural change (Greggor *et al.* 2014).

Human–wildlife conflicts are diverse and no single technique will be effective across all situations. Whenever possible, one should first attempt to alter the human practice that is causing the conflict (Dubois *et al.* 2017). The greatest chance of reducing conflict successfully involves applying an approach strategically in conjunction with other critical management approaches (Appleby *et al.* 2017a). In particular, management of the 'human' dimension of wildlife–human interactions is critical for changing the occurrence and perception of conflict (IUCN 2020). Then, effective disruptive or aversive stimuli become complementary tools in the toolbox of human–wildlife conflict management.

USING GUARDIAN ANIMALS TO MANAGE WILDLIFE

Linda van Bommel and Katherine Whitehouse-Tedd

Target taxa

Guardian animals have been used to manage a variety of Australian wildlife, but are most typically targeted to wombats (Chapter 19), macropods (Chapter 21), eutherian carnivores (Chapter 22) and ungulates (Chapter 24).

Context and scope

This GOP reviews factors and considerations for the use of guardian animals to deter wildlife (i.e. the target taxa listed above) under field conditions. These strategies are intended to cause a behavioural change in the targeted individuals or groups, by altering or modifying behaviour, presenting a barrier or deterrent, or causing animals to move away from the guarded area temporarily (van Bommel and Johnson 2014). Guardian animals include livestock guardian dogs (LGDs; *Canis familiaris*), llamas (*Lama glama*), alpacas (*Vicugna pacos*), donkeys (*Equus asinus*) and mules (*Equus mulus*) that are used to protect livestock and wildlife from predation (Figure 11.1). Guardian animals are employed in multiple contexts and environments. Often regarded as a form of responsible livestock management they are considered largely effective in reducing livestock depredation where they have been evaluated (e.g. Eklund *et al.* 2017; van Eeden *et al.* 2018).

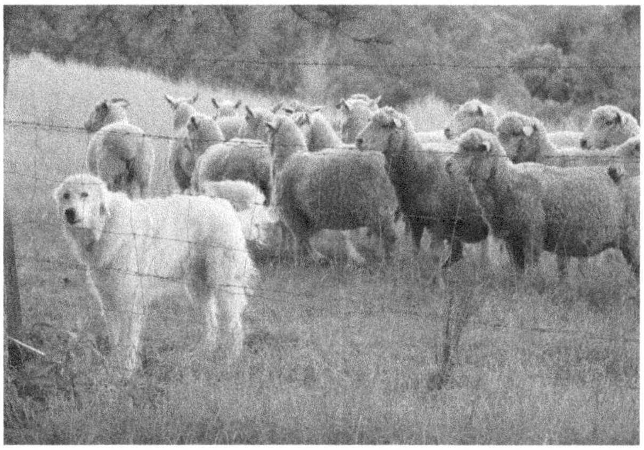

Figure 11.1: A livestock guarding dog protecting a flock of domestic sheep. The dog forms a strong bond with the flock and defends them against predators. Photo by Andy Fitzsimon, CC BY-SA 2.0.

Animal welfare considerations

When using guardian animals, the welfare of several groups of animals that may be intentionally or unintentionally affected should be considered: the guardian animals themselves, the species being guarded, the target wildlife (that the guardian animals are guarding against), and non-target wildlife that guardian animals may interact with (Smith *et al.* 2020d). Monitoring protocols should include consideration of the frequency, severity and characteristics of guardian animal interactions with wildlife (Chestley and Whiting 2015). For the purposes of this GOP, only those activities occurring during the animals' lives (i.e. before death) are considered.

Welfare considerations for the guardian animal

Negative effects on guardian animals can include injury or stress from confrontations with wildlife, and irregular access to water or food, and can be exacerbated by duration and type of daily activity (Lorenz *et al.* 1986).

Environmental risks include interactions with dangerous animals, challenging terrain, weather extremes, variable access to shelter, and hoof or paw wear. Vehicle collisions, other dogs and neighbouring farmers can also create risks (i.e. of being chased, attacked or shot/poisoned). The decision to use solitary or groups of guardians will depend on the species' natural social structure and the nature of the conflict (van Bommel 2010). Transfer of infectious diseases and parasites between dogs, livestock and wildlife is a possibility and should be monitored (Smith *et al.* 2020d). Positive effects include the forming of bonds between the guardian animal and the guarded species, providing constant access to social interaction and companionship for the guardians. The guardian animals should also be free to engage in natural behaviours without limitation.

Welfare considerations for species guarded

Appropriately trained and managed guardian animals should be trustworthy with and protective of the animals they are guarding (Coppinger and Coppinger 2001). Negative effects for guarded species can include increased stress (e.g. if unfamiliar with LGDs, guarded species can initially consider them to be predators); injuries from the guarder (undesirable behaviours); disease or parasite transmission; and competition for resources. However, these risks can be prevented or rectified by following standardised LGD training protocols. Positive effects can include reduced stress (i.e. reduced vigilance, improved feed conversion and wider dispersal/foraging); bond with guarder (social interaction and affiliative behaviours); and protection during periods of vulnerability (e.g. LGDs staying with lame or birthing animals).

Welfare considerations for wildlife (target and non-target)

Interactions between wildlife and guardian animals should (1) be targeted towards damage-causing individuals of a species; (2) function predominantly as a deterrent without physical interaction; and (3) be as rare as possible (relative to the incidence of threats and population size of threatening wildlife). Negative effects can include lethal and non-lethal injuries, stress or fear from confrontations; reduced fitness as a result of confrontation or habitat exclusion; competition for resources; and disease/parasite transmission (Smith *et al.* 2020d). Most literature relating to the effect on wildlife is specific to guardian dogs, with a lack of equivalent research relating to the impact of using other guardian species. Positive effects can include reduced or mitigated persecution of wildlife by humans because of a reduction in negative human–wildlife interactions (Johnson *et al.* 2019; Smith *et al.* 2020d).

General procedures

If guardian animals are to be included in a project, several important considerations must be made. First, the suitability of the guardian species to the context must be considered. Second, the suitability of the age, sex and behaviour of the guardian animals must be ensured, as well as de-sexing (neutering) where appropriate. Third, regular monitoring must be part of the research design, and especially in the initial introduction stage, as well as ensuring the project has the capacity to detect undesirable behaviour and provide appropriate intervention. Lastly, guardian animal retirement needs to be considered. Criteria for this decision (e.g. age, health status, guardian effectiveness, behavioural, owner non-compliance) and options for the animal after retirement (e.g. rehoming, rescue organisation) should be confirmed before engaging a guardian animal.

Guardian dogs

van Bommel (2010) published guidelines for the management and training of LGDs in Australia. When choosing breeds for guardian dogs, some consideration should be given to the breed of dog most suitable for the situation. A range of different breeds exist worldwide, although only a limited number are available in Australia (van Bommel 2010). Each breed has specific temperament and physical characteristics which should be considered. Key points to consider when implementing guardian dogs are as follows:

- Early bonding with the species they need to guard is crucial, and correct management and raising of pups will prevent many undesirable behaviours.
- If undesirable behaviours do occur, they need to be corrected. Most guardian dogs go through a juvenile or subadult phase where undesirable behaviour is more likely and will need close supervision and management during this time.
- Dogs may take up to 2 years to mature and before this should not be considered effective working dogs.
- Appropriate feeding and healthcare are required.
- Whether solitary dogs will be required, or pairs or groups of dogs, is context-specific.
- The sex of the dog and species to be guarded does not appear to influence guardian effectiveness; however,

reproductively intact and fertile animals may be more prone to roaming and show undesirable behaviours associated with sexual activity.

Guardian llamas, alpacas and donkeys

Although these species have demonstrated efficacy in guarding livestock because of their protective characteristics, physical strength and capacity to confront predators, they are themselves prey species. As such, they may be more likely to fall prey to predators than guardian dogs. It is unclear if they can be effective in managing non-predator species of wildlife, unless the animals under their protection are threatened directly. Guidelines for the use of these species have been published by Dohner (2007); and the Canadian Ministry of Agriculture have published guidelines for the use of donkeys (www.omafra.gov.on.ca). Key points to consider when using these species include the following:

- They need time to bond to the species to be guarded.
- If starting with a young guardian animal, they take time to mature.
- Individuals need to be selected carefully – not all individuals will make good guardians.
- Sex – entire males can try to mate the females of the species they are meant to guard.
- Group composition – single or in pairs works best, as larger numbers tend to prefer the company of their own species over that of the species they are guarding. This situation has consequences for the number of individuals and size of the area that can be protected.
- Management is essential, including shearing for llamas/alpacas, hoof care for donkeys/mules and adequate fencing.
- Appropriate feeding and healthcare are required.

Animal treatment or withdrawal

Removal or intervention (e.g. veterinary attention, change in management, corrective training or replacement) should be implemented if the parameters outlined in Table 11.1 are observed.

Equipment and maintenance

Resources required for guardian animal implementation include:

- guardian animals, including:
  - appropriate selection and sourcing of the animal from proven working lines and reputable breeders
  - care, nutrition, veterinary care (preventative and responsive), sterilisation, maintenance (shearing/foot/hoof care, coat maintenance, etc)
  - bonding/training programs
  - appropriate housing/fencing
  - transport (placement and monitoring)
- caretakers/managers, and their training if required
- monitoring officers whose role is to monitor animal welfare, training/bonding, problem resolution, animal replacement, and program management.

Resources required for researching the impacts of guardian animals will relate to the context, species and environment. Control sites should be monitored concurrently, where possible. Types of research questions (which will dictate the type of equipment or tools required) might relate to determining the following:

- *Effectiveness against predators.* Empirical measures of losses and injuries of the guarded species prior to and following placement of guardian animals; could include spatiotemporal monitoring of the guardian and guarded animals, and stakeholder-reported records of losses/injuries or other measures of predator impacts.

Table 11.1: Events, related to guardian animals, the guarded species and wildlife, which will require intervention by owners, managers or researchers.

Guardian animal	Guarded species	Wildlife
• Abuse or neglect, or poor guardian animal management • Poor physical health that is unresponsive to treatment • Injury • Inappropriate behaviour towards wildlife (e.g. any non-defensive interaction), guarded animals (e.g. biting, chasing and mounting), or humans (e.g. aggression, inability to catch/handle)	• Injuries or death caused by guardian animal (must rule out scavenging) • Behavioural, health or production changes associated with stress or fear linked to the guardian animal	• Unacceptable incidence of morbidity or mortality inflicted on wildlife • Guardian animal–induced disease • Non-target species interactions or damaging interactions with endangered species of wildlife • Competition for resources with non-target wildlife • Change in non-target wildlife behaviour, resource/habitat use, or population status which is a proven consequence of the guardian animal placement

- *Effectiveness against non-predator wildlife.* Population estimates and grazing impact estimates before and after the implementation of guardian animals; could also include spatiotemporal monitoring of the species.
- *Socio-economic impacts.* Stakeholder surveys (qualitative and quantitative approaches), market/economic surveys or legal surveys.
- *Guarded species impacts.* Techniques to measure productivity and animal welfare parameters.
- *Ecological impacts.* Telemetry, camera trapping, transect surveys, population parameter surveys, dietary analyses and spatiotemporal analyses.

Specific qualifications, experience and training

Guardian animal training, conditioning and placements should only be implemented by experienced practitioners. Inappropriate training or interventions can result in ineffective guardians at best, or compromised animal welfare (for guardians, livestock or wildlife) at worst. If experienced practitioners are not available, training should be undertaken by a suitable candidate before the start of the project. Guardian animals require regular monitoring for physical and behavioural suitability to the role, and oversight of health and animal welfare, by an experienced practitioner. In cases where guardian animals are placed as part of a research project, but anticipated to remain *in situ* beyond the duration of the research project, researchers must ensure appropriate monitoring of guardian animals for the duration of the animals' lives.

Workplace health and safety

Working with animals comes with a risk, including for example direct physical harm to the handler (i.e. bite, kick or being trodden on), as well as property damage, transferral of disease or parasites, and third-party liability. Most situations can be avoided with proper selection, training and management (of both guardian animals and handlers). It should be clear where responsibility lies should an incident occur and what action should be triggered following an incident.

Guardian animal handling

Handling guardian animals for transport, veterinary care or other husbandry practice increases the risk of incidents occurring. To reduce the risks, do the following:

- Use low-stress handling methods (e.g. calm interactions with the guardian and guarded animals).
- Desensitise the guardian to different situations from a young age.
- Use appropriate restraints (leads, head collars etc); where necessary, use a sedative (under veterinary supervision/approval), or a muzzle on dogs.
- Ensure the handler is experienced.
- Monitor the guardian animal for signs of stress, adjust its management accordingly.
- Create a handling protocol for specific situations, which includes proper hygiene to prevent disease/parasite transmission.

To reduce the risk when handling a guardian animal for research, do the following:

- Ensure proper placement of research units (e.g. GPS collar) and monitor animal welfare with units on, intervene if it negatively affects animal welfare – ill-fitting units can make the animal uncomfortable, increasing the risk of incidents.
- For some breeds of dogs, the researcher may require an introduction to the guardian before entering the area they are working in.
- Do not surprise the guardian animal – let it know you are there.
- Do not threaten the animals its guarding or the guardian animal itself – ignore both where possible.
- If threatened, leave the area, and come back later.

Guardian animal escape

Escapes can be prevented via training, fences, and/or specially modified collars (e.g. triangles) for dogs (van Bommel 2010), and ensuring that guardian animals have proper identifiers (e.g. collar tags, microchipping, brands that are species dependent and appropriate). Researchers or caretakers should always inform neighbours of animal presence prior to or at the commencement of the project, and request notification if the animal strays onto their property. In the event of an escape, the caretaker should inform the researchers as soon as possible. If an animal is missing it could be located using tracking technology, if available. Neighbours can be asked for assistance and relevant local rangers or authorities informed. Repeat offenders need better containment systems or retraining.

Guardian animal aggression towards humans

The risk of aggression and attacks can be minimised via protocols for proper training and socialisation of the guardian animals relevant to their deployment situation.

Ensuring proper approach and management of the guardian animals by humans (e.g. regular handlers or researchers/general public if on public lands) is important. On public land, information signs should be installed to instruct the public about guardian animal presence, proper behaviour and contacts in case of problems.

In the event that a person is threatened or attacked by the animal, the person should stay calm and non-threatening (i.e. do not scream, run away or hit the animal – doing so is likely to escalate the problem) and retreat from the area as soon as possible. Vulnerable body parts should be shielded and an attempt made to place a physical barrier between the person and the animal. A call for help should be made. It is never appropriate to retaliate physically. Lastly, the incident should be reported to the relevant organisation or person. After the incident, the responsible organisation or person should analyse the cause of attack, looking at, for example, illness or injury, lack of socialisation, location (e.g. incursion by public), and human behaviour (triggers). If reasons for the attack cannot be determined or managed and aggressive behaviour continues, the animal should be relocated or replaced.

Alternative procedures

Until the adverse impacts of guardian animals are more robustly defined, their use appears justified on the basis of the targeted and discriminatory nature of their desirable interactions with target wildlife and the rare incidence of undesirable interactions towards target and non-target species (Whitehouse-Tedd *et al.* 2020). Nevertheless, both animal welfare and conservation-relevant issues need to be considered (as debated between Allen *et al.* 2019 and Johnson *et al.* 2019). Alternative procedures as discussed in other sections of this chapter (and book) could be considered in areas where the use of guardian animals is not feasible.

DISRUPTIVE STIMULI (FRIGHTENING DEVICES, SOUND AND LIGHT)

Benjamin J. Pitcher, Bradley P. Smith, Alison L. Greggor, Lysanne Snijders, Colleen Cassady St. Clair, Rob G. Appleby and Neil R. Jordan

Target taxa

The procedures covered in this section can be applied to almost all free-living taxa, and have previously been used on terrestrial carnivores (Chapters 18 and 22), terrestrial herbivores (Chapters 19–21), bats (Chapter 23), rodents (Chapter 24), marine mammals (Chapter 25), birds (Chapters 33–36) and snakes (Chapter 26).

Context and scope

For almost all wildlife, certain stimuli will provoke fear, pain or irritation. Such 'undesirable' stimuli can be used as a disruptive stimuli to interrupt undesirable behaviour in the act (a repellent), or reduce the desire to enter or stay in a particular area (a deterrent) (Shivik and Martin 2000; Smith *et al.* 2000). These strategies are most often used in the resolution of human–wildlife conflict. Fear-evoking stimuli can include visual, auditory and olfactory stimuli; for a list of examples see Table 11.2. The most promising perhaps are those that take inspiration from nature, using biologically relevant scents and sounds (sometimes referred to as 'bioboundaries'). In many cases, multiple devices, or devices that target multiple modalities (e.g. light and sound), are used.

These disruptive strategies have the advantage of (often) being low in cost and simplistic in design, and many have shown some promise in both captive and field conditions. For example, Ausband *et al.* (2013) showed that territorial scent marks reduce wolf attacks on domestic sheep. However, many of the benefits or impacts of disruptive devices are often limited because of the effects of habituation. Habituation effects are particularly rapid for predators who have flexible behaviours and can quickly determine whether a stimulus is harmful or not. That is, the perception of the animal towards the stimulus changes as it is exposed to the device, with habituation occurring when no negative reinforcement is associated with it. In elk (*Cervus canadensis*), bolder individuals were quicker to increase flight responses when subjected to aversive conditioning, but they were also quicker to revert when conditioning ceased (Found and St. Clair 2018). Not all individuals respond to the stimuli in the same way, and indeed some disruptive stimuli may attract (e.g. predator inspection) rather than repel the target species.

Although only a relatively small repository of experimental studies is available in the Australian context, a large collection of international literature exists (see Table 11.2 and Appleby *et al.* 2017a for examples) that can be used to inform and guide decision-making processes. The evaluation and reporting of experiments are encouraged, as is the seeking of innovative non-lethal solutions.

Table 11.2: A selective summary of disruptive and fear evoking stimuli that have been used.

Many of these disruptive stimuli are often used in combination with one another.

Disruptive stimuli	Examples of application
Sound	Whip crack and foot stomp sounds have been used to protect western grey kangaroos (*Macropus fulignosus*) from roads (vehicle strike) and crop protection (Biedenweg *et al.* 2011). Acoustic deterrent or harassment devices have limited predation of fish farm stock by pinnipeds (seals and sealions) (Götz and Janik 2013). Acoustic cannons and electronic sounds have been used to deter birds at agricultural and industrial sites associated with airports, agriculture, aquaculture (Conover 2002).
Ultrasound	Ultrasound has been used to deter eastern grey kangaroos (*Macropus giganteus*) from grazing land (Bender 2003) and keep rodents off roads (Sousa-Guedes *et al.* 2020).
Lights	Flashing lights, strobe lights, lights that mimic flashlights have been used to deter carnivores (e.g. lions (*Pantera leo*) from attacking livestock (Lesilau *et al.* 2018) and African elephants (*Loxodonta africana*) from entering crop fields (Adams *et al.* 2020). Lasers have been used to deter birds from sites of conflict (Blackwell *et al.* 2002).
Firecrackers and noisemakers	Large firecracker-style explosives that may emit both a loud sound and a flash of light have been used to deter pinnipeds and cetaceans from fishing equipment (Jefferson and Curry 1996). Propane exploders have been used to deter white-tailed deer (*Odocoileus virginianus*) from crops (Belant *et al.*1996).
Chases by people, herding by dogs	Elk (*Cervus elaphus*) have been chased by people and herded by dogs (Kloppers *et al.* 2005), black bears (*Ursus americanus*) have been deterred from human-use areas by trained dogs (Beckmann *et al.* 2004). Handheld devices such as an air horn, water pistol, and whistle have been tested for their ability to deter approaching dingoes (*Canis dingo*) from humans (Appleby *et al.* 2017b).
Flagging/fladry	Fladry (colourful flags on a fence) has been used to prevent wolves (*Canis lupus*) from livestock enclosures (Musiani *et al.* 2003).
Effigies (human figures)	Effigies have been used to protect livestock from jaguar (*Panthera onca*) and pumas (*Puma concolor*) (Zarco-González and Monroy-Vilchis 2014), and deter captive dingoes from accessing food (Smith *et al.* 2020a). They have been effectively used to prevent birds from consuming farmed catfish (*Ictalurus punetatus*) (Stickley *et al.* 1995).
Predator models	Agricultural sites and airports have sought to deter pest birds with falconry (using kestrels, *Falco sparverius*) and hawk-shaped kites (Steensma *et al.* 2016), and turkey vultures (*Cathartes aura*) have been deterred from roost sites by hanging an upside-down taxidermied conspecific specimen (Blackwell and Fernandez-Juricic 2013).
Other	Artificial eye spots on livestock deter lion attacks (Radford *et al.* 2020). Beehive fences have been used to deter African elephants from crops (King *et al.* 2017).

Animal welfare considerations

Physiological stress, injury or death

Deployment of predator scent and sound is sometimes done under the landscape of fear paradigm (Miller and Schmitz 2019) and, as such, is expected to induce a fear response by design. Aversive devices used in a potentially dangerous situation may need to be piloted in more-benign circumstances before *in situ* tests. For example, where fleeing may result in response to devices, placement along roadways could increase mortality. Where protection of livestock or crops is intended, unintended responses, such as attraction, may be costly. Potential failure should be considered during planning, and potentially include the scope to compensate trial participants for losses.

Devices that employ explosions may cause physical injury to animals if they are used at unsafe close ranges. For example, marine mammals such as dolphins, have been reported suffering broken bones and other injuries from explosive devices (see Jefferson and Curry 1996).

Exposure to loud sounds has also been suggested to cause hearing impairment in some situations. Acoustic deterrent devices that use high source level sounds are designed to work on the principle that they cause physical discomfort or even pain, thereby prompting the target animal to move away from the sound source. Sounds at or near the pain threshold risk causing immediate hearing damage, while long-term exposure to moderate-to-high sound pressure levels can also lead to hearing loss (Götz and Janik 2013).

In relation to behavioural modification and the assessment of frequency and consequence of pain and distress, some aversive stimuli and experiments cause repeated experience of pain and distress, but most, by design, only cause temporary pain, minor discomfort or distress, and are alleviated quickly. Any experiments involving pain should be conducted as quickly and efficiently as possible so that a clear result is achieved in a short as possible time frame, and that the animals involved should be monitored and assessed to ensure their wellbeing is not disproportionately affected. Monitoring may entail direct observation and behavioural assessment, and the use of animal-borne devices to monitor activity and facilitate direct observations (Appleby *et al.* 2017a).

Factors relating to frequency and intensity of conditioning events have implications for successful interventions. For example, higher-intensity stimuli are more likely to generate a sensitisation response so that less conditioning may be needed in the future. Lower-intensity stimuli may seem less invasive, but may be counterproductive because they do not sufficiently mitigate habituation responses, in turn imposing a need for longer-term treatment and, if conflict remains unresolved, the possibility of lethal management (Groves and Thompson 1970).

Non-target species

Non-target species (including humans) may also be affected by deterrent devices, and it is possible that impacts on non-targets may be greater than on the intended target. Deterrent devices may not be effective against target species in a situation where the benefit of the protected resources outweighs the costs imposed by the deterrent. Conversely, if a non-target species does not gain a similar benefit from the resource they may not tolerate the cost of the deterrent and be unintentially impacted. Further, non-target species may have different perceptual ranges that make them more susceptible to devices. For example, non-target porpoises are likely to detect acoustic deterrents over longer distances than target pinnipeds, and may not readily habituate, resulting in them abandoning areas of their habitat (Götz and Janik 2013). Ideally, any impact monitoring should extend beyond the target species and include other species that may also be affected by the intervention. In this way the true cost of the intervention can be weighed against any benefits it delivers.

Environmental noise and signal masking

The introduction of additional noise (in any modality) into the environment is likely to affect both target and non-target species. These impacts may be both acute and chronic (Doherty *et al.* 2021). Acoustic stimuli that occur in the same bandwidth as other signals have the potential to mask their perception. For example, a loud noise from a deterrent device may make it difficult or impossible for animals in the environment to detect another animal's call or other acoustic cues they use in the environment. Similar masking can happen in other modalities such as olfactory and visual signals, and may disrupt communication networks, making signals harder to detect, or forcing animals to shift their signal frequency or intensity. Changes in behaviour may also be observed as animals compensate for masking in one sensory modality by or with, for example, increased vigilance where acoustic noise limits the ability to hear approaching predators, resulting in less time being available for other behaviours such as foraging. While some of these effects may be desirable and contribute to the effectiveness of deterrents, others may be unintended and must be considered when evaluating the animal welfare impacts of stimuli on both target and non-target animals (Hampton *et al.* 2021).

Consequences of removing lethal control and testing non-lethal techniques

Removing lethal control to test the impact of the non-lethal technique (using a randomly controlled trial for instance) is problematic both practically and ethically. For example, if seeking to reduce attacks on livestock, stakeholders who depend on livestock production for their livelihoods are unlikely to be willing to be in the 'no treatment' (control) condition. In these circumstances, the case is strong for compensation of losses through the experiment. In some cases, crossover trials also present a solution, so that a particular group or individual is not a permanent control. While control group participants may be expected to have greater losses, it should be acknowledged that attempted interventions can also result in losses, and appropriate planning and provisioning for such outcomes are essential. Where disruptive stimuli are effective, problems may simply shift to neighbouring properties or other areas; this should be considered at the outset and monitored throughout the trials.

The loss of livestock if the intervention does not work is also an important consideration.

When conducting pilot or preliminary trials of a new technique or device, it is important to ensure that only as many animals are used as are needed to reach statistical significance. This means, for instance, that if five trials are required to demonstrate a target effect size, and the first two trials did not appear to work, the experiment is not abandoned prematurely. Doing so would mean that any animal welfare impact incurred to that point is wasted without establishing whether the intervention worked or not. Power analyses can help determine how many trials or subjects may be needed in order to detect a given size of effect.

General procedures

Selecting the appropriate disruptive stimuli

Any technique employed should ideally be one that has been used previously on the same or similar problem (either species or problem), and has been shown to be satisfactory. Evidence for the effectiveness of any given intervention ideally should contain relevant control conditions and have been replicated in multiple contexts or conditions. While some reviews have examined the theory behind and case studies of deterrents (e.g. Schakner and Blumstein 2013; Appleby *et al.* 2017a), reviews of the diversity of aversion techniques are lacking. However, support and evidence repositories, such as (www.conservationevidence.com) can serve as useful sources. Whenever possible, relying on single studies to determine large policy changes should still be avoided because conflicting evidence often arises as more studies are conducted. If satisfactory evidence is unavailable for support of a given technique, then any attempts to use it should be considered exploratory and aim to collect data to help evaluate its effectiveness relative to other techniques (e.g. employing proof-of-concept and pilot studies that might use small numbers of animals). When developing novel techniques (i.e. where a sound evidence base does not yet exist), predicted responses and efficacy should be made on a sound theoretical basis, and ideally tested before implementation in the field.

Administering the disruptive stimuli

Aversion techniques should be designed such that the delivery is matched to the behaviour or problem of interest. The need to ensure appropriate learning is paramount across all disruptive interventions, and it is key to closely match the stimulus with the behaviour or context that it is meant to deter or exclude them from. For example, the use of projectiles to haze individuals, if not done correctly, will be ineffective because the target will not learn what behaviour is being conditioned.

Observation, monitoring and displacement events

When conducting trials of aversive and disruptive stimuli, wildlife should be monitored immediately before and after full implementation, and periodically thereafter. Monitoring should include the intended and unintended impacts on target and non-target species. For example, some stimuli could actually work as attractants, or the effective aversion could push the problem elsewhere (such that the animals have been moved from an area adopting non-lethal management to one where lethal methods are employed).

Reducing the risk of habituation

It is important to ensure the effectiveness of the approach for as long as possible, or at least during the periods when it is most needed. As such, some techniques should not be continuously implemented, particularly those that are not immutably aversive, as doing so is likely to lead to habituation and desensitisation of the tool (Shivik and Martin 2000). Effectiveness is generally achieved by (Smith, Appleby and Jordan 2020):

- restricting deployments to specific time periods or events (which also aids learning) or deploying deterrents in direct response to animal's approaching
- rotating or varying the use of each stimulus (device) sufficiently both in terms of the timing and other patterns of production (e.g. pulse rates, colours, frequencies), and the specific locations of disruptive devices at the problem site
- using multiple stimuli (modalities such as hearing and vision) simultaneously to counter individual variation and response
- employing methods that incorporate the biology of the species that relate to behaviour (e.g. territoriality, fear of novelty), physiology (e.g. sensitivity of hearing and sight) and cognition (e.g. intelligence and speed of learning or processing).

Beyond habituation, disruptive stimuli may ultimately have a 'dinner bell effect', where the originally aversive signal becomes a conditioned reinforcer of the unwanted behaviour. This effect has been observed in pinnipeds where trials of acoustic deterrent devices lead to an increase in predation (see Götz and Janik 2013). Similarly, a commercially available light device marketed to deter red foxes (*Vulpes vulpes*) led to an increase in fox activity and fewer piglet births when trialled in a free-range piggery (Hall and Fleming 2021).

Evaluating and determining 'success'

All aversive and disruptive stimuli should be evaluated properly, particularly before large-scale implementation. To begin, all studies need to establish what constitutes a success or failure, if this definition is realistic, and how success or failure will ultimately be measured. For example, it is unrealistic to expect 100% effectiveness in reducing livestock depredations, or area exclusion (lethal control methods cannot achieve this either). When comparing lethal and non-lethal methods, 'success' may differ according to the values or criteria (e.g. financial or animal-welfare related).

Smith *et al.* (2020b) propose the following steps for evaluating the success of non-lethal tools, including disruptive stimuli:

- Establish baseline information about the problem such that the intervention can be compared against (e.g. number of livestock losses, population).
- Develop a clear understanding of the concepts involved in trying to change the behaviour (e.g. principles of learning, habituation, reflecting the target species biology and behaviour).
- Determine the measure of success, ensuring it is realistic.
- Ensure that a sound experimental method is used to evaluate success (see Treves *et al.* 2019).

Evaluations of non-lethal tools may also need to consider longer-term monitoring, since habituation and learning will only become apparent when animals have had multiple opportunities to interact with the tool over time.

Animal treatment, withdrawal and euthanasia

The experiment should be ceased or suspended pending review if the device causes significant injury to target individuals, has been shown not to be effective, or if complaints are received from the public. Identification of adverse impacts on non-target species may also require premature termination of the study. Although unexpected impacts on non-target species are challenging to predict and set acceptable thresholds for, when they do occur they should fall into the same assessment framework as for the target species. Researchers have a responsibility to monitor and remain vigilant for adverse events beyond the target species and to consult their animal ethics committee (AEC) if impacts become apparent. For devices that have a high probability of causing injury to target and non-target species, a veterinarian should be present or on call to assist.

Equipment and maintenance

Typical items for experiments of aversive repellents and deterrents may include:

- the disruptive stimuli, which should incorporate:
  - a backup to be used in the event of malfunction or tampering by wildlife or humans
  - tamper-proof controls and material to avoid destruction and interference
  - weather-proofing
  - a power source (battery, solar, mains power) as required, including backup power in the event of malfunction
- monitoring equipment, such as:
  - video surveillance camera or sensor camera to observe interactions between wildlife and the device
  - animal-borne tracking devices (e.g. GPS) to monitor the effectiveness of the device in altering behaviour
- personal protective equipment as appropriate (e.g. gloves, goggles, face masks, safety earmuffs, and appropriate clothing)
- public signage.

Qualification, experience and training

Before the device is used in the field, all personnel should be trained in its operation. Ideally, training will take place while the device is being tested (i.e. does what it is designed to do consistently), and then in captive or field conditions to test the efficacy of the device on the target species. A standard operating procedure (SOP) for the use of the device should be developed to ensure safe handling and operation.

The use of certain disruptive stimuli might require a permit for its use, so it is important to check local and state government guidelines. For example, undertaking scaring activities (such as loud noises and gas guns) to manage kangaroos and wallabies in the state of Victoria often require a permit from the relevant state government's environmental agency. The need for ethical permission from an AEC should be investigated.

Workplace health and safety

Care must be taken when handling the devices, particularly those that can be dangerous to the operator or adjacent persons if unintentionally triggered (e.g. odours, loud sounds, explosives and projectiles). All commercially acquired devices should be used in-line with the provided operational instructions. Operators should use personal protective equipment appropriate to the device.

Residents (permanent or visiting) should be notified about activity in the area that may cause disruption (e.g. the use of explosives and loud noises) and the possibility of encountering aggressive or panicked animals in the area after exposure. Where possible, public ability to interfere with the devices should be mitigated to limit the risk of altering the equipment calibration (which may result in injury to target and non-target wildlife) or injury to the person. This risk may be reduced by preventing access to device controls, secure placement of the device, and appropriate signage in the area and adjacent to the device.

Alternative procedures

While management approaches that use aversive elements to achieve conflict resolution are almost always non-lethal (or meant to be), they can and do cause harm. From an animal welfare and ethical perspective, the least harmful but most consistently successful approach is likely to be the best choice. However, experimentation, particularly involving wildlife, often requires at least some flexibility when it comes to procedures and rightly, AECs often ask what procedures or alternatives will be available under certain circumstances, particularly if experiments do not go to plan. Careful consideration is required in determining how best to minimise any intentional or unintentional harms animals may experience as a result of experimental procedures, including during capture and handling, exposure to treatment conditions that involve pain or suffering, responses from conspecifics, unwanted changes in behaviour or condition, or reduction in survival and reproductive success.

AVERSIVE ODOURS AND CHEMICALS

Jorge Tobajas, Lysanne Snijders and Neil R. Jordan

Target taxa

The procedures covered in this section can be applied to almost all free-living taxa. They are most often applied to dasyurids (Chapter 18) and eutherian carnivores (Chapter 22), but also to macropods (Chapter 21), and certain marine mammal and shark species (Chapters 25 and 31, respectively).

Context and scope

This GOP provides advice on the use of aversive odours and chemicals under field conditions, including for strategies intended to cause a behavioural change in the targeted individuals or groups, by either altering or modifying behaviour, causing a barrier/threshold, or causing animals to relocate. Examples covered by this GOP include odours (e.g. predator odours) and chemicals (e.g. repellents and conditioned taste aversion (CTA)) that have been used for non-lethal management of wildlife (see Table 11.3). Repellents have a direct disruptive or aversive effect (e.g. deploying predator urine or faeces repels kangaroos,) without learning necessarily occurring. CTA involves an animal learning that a particular taste, or the ingestion of a particular substance, often in concert with another salient odour or visual cues, is associated with a feeling of illness (e.g. nausea). This response tends to cause avoidance of consumption of that substance in the future. CTA is especially relevant to minimising harm to animals since even a single experience with eating an item laced with nausea-inducing chemicals may encourage long-term avoidance of that food type (Garcia *et al.* 1974). The use of CTA should be restricted to conflicts involving particular food/prey consumption, while repellents can also be used to reduce site visitation.

Such approaches have been used in reducing conflict between humans and carnivores (Smith *et al.* 2000), pest management and agricultural crop protection (DeLiberto and Werner 2016), and threatened species management (O'Donnell *et al.* 2010). The methods employed vary, and relate to the species and context. Habituation is a major risk with the use of repellents. Additionally, in some instances odours that should promote avoidance, such as predator odours, encouraged approaches (Apfelbach *et al.* 2015; Parsons *et al.* 2018). In the case of CTA, in some species, such as coyotes and wolves, the ability to produce consistent avoidance responses has been mixed.

Animal welfare considerations

Repellents produce a short-term immediate effect and must always be present to generate the aversion. In contrast, CTA aims to induce one intense effect so that animals will avoid the target food without the ongoing presence of the substance. Thus, repellents cause repeated minor discomfort while CTA, in its most effective form,

Table 11.3: A selective summary of studies utilising aversive odours and conditioned taste aversion (CTA).

Odour	Examples of application
Conspecific urine and faeces	To influence the movement of carnivores- particularly from entering livestock production areas such as wolves (Ausband *et al.* 2013), as well as African wild dogs (*Lycaon pictus*), leopards (*Pathera pardus*) and cheetahs (*Acinonyx jubatus*)
Dead and decaying conspecifics	Some species of shark show avoidance behaviours when exposed to chemicals released by dead and decaying conspecifics. Many other shark specific chemical repellents have been trialled (see Hart and Collin 2015)
Predator urine, faeces, and fur	Used to prevent southern flying squirrels (*Glaucomys volans*) from interfering with roosting of red-cockaded woodpeckers (*Leuconotopicus borealis*) (Borgo *et al.* 2006)
Various chemical sprays (e.g. pepper; capsaicin)	Used for human protection against brown (*Ursus arctos*), polar (*Ursus maritimus*) and black bears (e.g. Mazur 2010)
Chemical	**Examples of applications in CTA studies**
Levamisole	Used in combination with an odour cue as a tool for reducing post-release predation during animal translocations (Tobajas *et al.* 2021).
Cinnamamide and ziram	Used to protect crops from European badgers (*Meles meles*) (Baker *et al.* 2005).
Lithium chloride or LiCl	Has been used with coyotes (*Canis latrans*) to condition them against livestock predation, such as domestic chickens (Conover *et al.* 1977).
Pulegone	To protect eggs of various species from predators (Conover and Lyons 2003).
Thiabendazole	To prevent livestock attack by dingoes (Gustavson *et al.* 1983). When combined with dead toads (*Rhinella marina*), northern quolls (*Dasyurus hallucatus*) could be conditioned not to consume cane toads (O'Donnell *et al.* 2010)
Sodium carbonate	To prevent predation of hooded plover eggs from red foxes (Maguire *et al.* 2009)

causes a single stronger discomfort followed by avoidance. Effectiveness of both methods varies with species and situation. A prediction should be made for the probable number of exposures necessary and the discomfort associated with each of these exposures so as to select the method that minimises the impact on individual animal welfare.

Physiological stress, and/or injury or death

Odours and chemical repellents produce different effects depending on the animal species and the chemical compound characteristics. When using odours from predators as repellents, responses of subjects were varied depending on if the odour was from a familiar predator, the threat the predator poses, and the size and defensive abilities of the (prey) subjects (Apfelbach *et al.* 2015). Responses included defensive and fear reactions, site avoidance, immobility and flight, and were always accompanied by a physiological stress reaction.

Contact with odour and taste repellents causes a short transient period of disgust, pain, fear and discomfort, generally resulting in brief and minor stress levels. However, with some repellents, such as anthraquinone, repellency is caused by post-ingestional distress through irritation of the gut (DeLiberto and Werner 2016), and the effect may be severe and long lasting.

Chemicals used to create CTA need a rigorous evaluation of the toxicological effects before their use, including an estimate of the effectiveness, level of discomfort, potential damage or other sublethal effects and the possibility of bioaccumulation. Doses should be set with a wide margin of toxicological safety to avoid intoxication, which otherwise can cause irreversible effects on an animal's health. Additionally, during the period of discomfort, animals may be especially vulnerable to predators and conspecifics. Consequently, it is also important to consider the presence of additional stressors and the availability of refuges.

Before work commences and to minimise the risk of poisoning, a review should be undertaken to assess the possible negative effects and the lowest possible doses expected to produce the desired aversive effect (Tobajas *et al.* 2019). In the absence of previous toxicological studies, these tests should be completed on captive animals to evaluate the effective doses, toxicological effects and (unexpected) behavioural changes. The doses and toxicological effects of the same substance can vary considerably between species (DeLiberto and Werner 2016; Tobajas *et al.* 2020). Consequently, the species-specific effects of potentially affected species must be considered, including potentially affected non-target species.

Non-target species

Repellents and aversive odours could have toxicological or repellent effects on non-target species should be considered, potentially inducing fear, site avoidance, reduced food intake or an increase in vigilance behaviours. Consequently, the potential effects on non-target species are a major consideration in the application of these often non-discriminatory methods. Also, doses that have been selected for the target species may be substantially higher than those considered safe for smaller non-target species. The potential effects of specific substances and exposure methods on non-target species should be reviewed in literature and evaluated in field experiments (Tobajas *et al.* 2019, 2020, 2021).

General procedures

Selecting the appropriate aversion

Methods using odours and chemicals have to be targeted because of their context- and species-specific effects (Apfelbach *et al.* 2015; DeLiberto and Werner 2016). Equally, doses of chemicals in CTA should be selected for a specific species (Tobajas *et al.* 2019). Thus, the best option is to first try methods that have been previously used on the same or similar species and proved to be satisfactory. In general, odour and chemical repellents are used to reduce predation, consumption or promote exclusion, and create avoidance *in situ*, but need to be in use constantly. Conversely, in effective CTA the long-lasting induced aversion is generalised to the particular food item with or without the noxious chemical, so it can be effective in protecting 'food items' in any location (e.g. ground-nests or released animals). Care should be taken when the conflict food item resembles important natural food resources of the target animal (Appleby *et al.* 2017a). During foraging, mammals may use smell as well as taste (e.g. Baker *et al.* 2008; Tobajas *et al.* 2021) and birds use visual cues. Consequently, aversions methods are associated with a risk of the target animal associating and consequently avoiding smells or colours that are shared with natural foods.

Observation and monitoring

The type of monitoring will depend on the nature of the research question and methods selected. If methods are being implemented to enact behaviour change, then the focus of monitoring should be the change in predation, consumption or activity. However, while the method may be deemed successful in changing the target behaviour, it could also have unintended effects on other behaviours or animal welfare parameters. Ideally, likely relevant behaviours and animal welfare parameters should be identified *a priori*, monitored and reported. See also 'Animal treatment, withdrawal and euthanasia'.

Habituation and extinction effects

Habituation from repeated exposures is a major risk of the use of chemical and odour repellents. However, in natural environments the loss of response over time can also be caused by chemical degradation of the signal (Walter *et al.* 2010; Apfelbach *et al.* 2015). Therefore, methods and repellents should be selected that minimise the likelihood of habituation occurring, including using alternative repellents or combing complementary methods to improve the efficiency (Walter *et al.* 2010; see also 'Disruptive stimuli (frightening devices, sound and light)'.

In CTA, the reduction of an aversive effect does not occur through habituation, but by extinction of the aversion. The rate of extinction will depend on several factors such as the dose used (i.e. the illness effect) and the number ingestions of referent food before and mainly after conditioning, leading the animal to associate the food as safe. The CTA can be reinitiated by reinforcement with a new exposure to the aversive chemical and the specific food item.

Animal treatment, withdrawal and euthanasia

Users of chemical and odour repellents should investigate and formulate species-specific and context-specific criteria for any anticipated impacts. These criteria should include the duration of the intended or observed impact (e.g. low grade, but chronic impact may equate to high grade but acute impact), and if the ends justify the means. When using chemicals, odours or CTA, the critical moment to monitor is when the animals come into contact with the chemical or odour and the degree of nausea induced. At this time, it is important to observe the effects on individuals as well as their general effectiveness. Trials should cease if disproportionate effects are observed or when the research question has been answered. Pilot testing of dose and impacts may assist with limiting harm. Monitoring should include identification of all species that interact with the chemicals or odours, and a quantification of its effects on them. For CTA, the treated species should be monitored after conditioning to observe possible detrimental effects of the treatment. Working with tagged individuals helps ensure adequate monitoring of individuals (Tobajas *et al.* 2020; see Figure 11.2).

Equipment and maintenance

Selected odours and chemical repellents application should:

- induce slight discomfort, fear or avoidance at the exposure or just after ingestion
- have low toxicological effects on target, non-target species and to the ecosystem
- not affect the viability and characteristics of the food in which it is applied (i.e. seeds)
- be stable for a long time in environmental conditions, maintaining its repellent capacity and intensity.

Resources required for CTA implementation (also detailed in Tobajas *et al.* 2019) include an averse compound that should:

- induce slight gastrointestinal adverse effects such as vomiting or diarrhoea
- have a wide acute toxicological margin of safety (acute margin of safety = toxic dose (median lethal dose (LD50))/effective dose (to produce vomiting)), which is required to avoid intoxication in the event that an individual consumes numerous doses
- be odourless and tasteless to avoid detection in the food item
- have a short period of latency (30 min to 2 h) to assure the correct learning of conditioned taste aversion

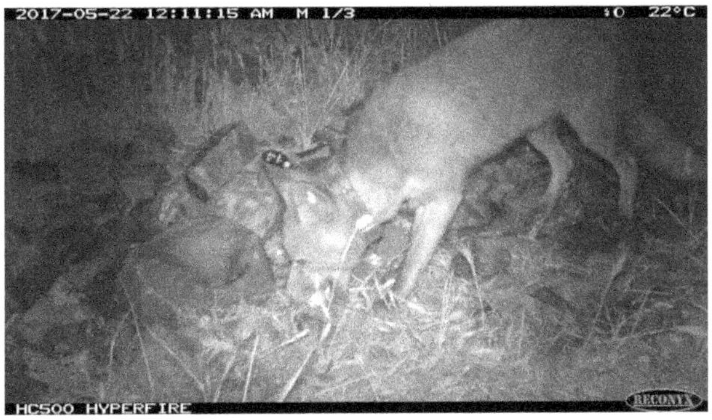

Figure 11.2: Remote sensor camera image showing a free-ranging red fox (*Vulpes vulpes*) tagged with GPS and ear tags, and eating an egg treated with thiram. Image taken from a study by Tobajas *et al.* (2020). Photo by Jorge Tobajas.

- be stable along time in environmental conditions
- be added to the conflict food item or a substitute that closely mimics the food item (e.g. in the case of endangered prey species).

Resources useful for implementing and monitoring outcomes and animal welfare (as shown in Figure 11.2), include:

- methods for tracking consumption by various animal species and potential effects on animal welfare (e.g. direct observations, Chapter 4; camera traps, Chapter 5)
- animal tracking devices (see Chapter 9)
- animal identification tags (Chapter 8)
- information signs or public notices (see advice on research in peri-urban and urban areas in Chapter 3).

Qualification, experience and training

The qualifications and experience required to perform the procedure will vary depending on the species, the nature of the chemical, and the context in which it is being applied. Many odour and chemical repellents are commercially available and can be applied by users who simply follow the instructions, so no special preparation is necessary for their application. However, with CTA, since chemicals are placed in nature with high associated risks of being misapplied, it must be carried out (or supervised) by those with solid training and capabilities of using CTA in the field.

Workplace health and safety

Any substances used should be handled with care and in compliance with all safety measures, material safety data sheets and protocols because of the possible adverse effects that may occur in the event of ingestion, inhaling or contact with the eyes or skin. These procedures are especially important for substances used as repellents, since the desired effect is commonly discomfort by exposure.

Chemical repellents can also be irritating or painful to humans, so care and practice are required for their safe use. In Australia, capsaicin-based and related sprays are restricted and illegal to carry in many Australian states and territories (Western Australia is an exception). Prolonged discomfort of animals could be considered unacceptable to members of the public, and place animals in jeopardising situations that they might otherwise not be in (e.g. they could be vulnerable to injury from people or other animals). If subjects are potentially dangerous animals, people being able to closely approach them, when normally this would not be possible, might also put such people at risk, particularly if the animals are irritable or feel threatened (see Appleby *et al.* 2017a).

Alternative procedures

In many cases, odour and CTA may be preferred over alternative methods, such as physical punishments and electric fences. Conditioned taste aversion has been used to reduce nest predation by red foxes (Tobajas *et al.* 2020; Figure 11.2) without lethal control. However, other novel methodologies, such as chemical camouflage, could offer alternatives with fewer impacts on animal welfare (Price and Banks 2012). In relation to livestock predation by large carnivores, alternative lower-impact non-lethal methods could be implemented, including guardian dogs and electric fences (both covered in this chapter). No methods are without potential effects on the welfare of target and non-target species, so an evaluation of alternatives must be undertaken before their implementation to ensure the selection of the most effective solution is adopted.

ELECTRIC STIMULI (FENCES, COLLARS AND SHIELDS)

Bradley P. Smith, Benjamin J. Pitcher, Rob A. Appleby and Lysanne Snijders

Target taxa

Devices utilising electric shocks have been used across a variety of taxa. Electric fences and netting are regularly used for terrestrial, arboreal and aquatic native fauna. Animal-borne collars have most often been used with eutherian carnivores (Chapter 22), but can be widely applied. Electric shields and repellents are typically used with sharks (Chapter 31).

Context and scope

Aversive techniques that utilise electric stimuli typically deliver a pulse of electricity at relatively high voltage and low amperages. Many variations of such devices are available, including permanency, materials, and energisers used to create the electrical stimulus. Electric shock is a powerful aversive stimulus because it is precise and contiguous; presentation of the shock stimulus is possible in relation to the target behaviour; and adjustment of stimulus characteristics, such as intensity and duration, is achievable. Electric stimuli are short lived, less prone to habituation than other methods (Appleby *et al.* 2017a), and are effective in various settings and applications. Electric stimuli can be employed in three main ways to deter wildlife.

Electric fencing and netting

Electric fences usually consist of one or several wires capable of carrying electric current produced by an 'energiser', such that if an animal touches a wire (and the ground) it receives a shock. When installed and operating correctly, these fences create a largely impenetrable physical barrier, and are among the most widely used and effective non-lethal methods for excluding or containing wildlife. For example, electric fences have been used to keep coyotes from livestock (Acorn and Dorrance 1994), to prevent pinnipeds (seals and sea lions) gaining access to fish farms in New Zealand (Kemper *et al.* 2003), as well as to keep bears in the USA from entering camp sites (Smith *et al.* 2018) and apiaries (Otto and Roloff 2015). Yet, mixed results have been reported for wild ungulates (Karhu and Anderson 2006). Although applied as a physical barrier, electric fencing is likely to also result in aversive conditioning of the animal.

Animal-borne shock collars

A brief electric shock can be delivered via wearable devices such as collars, often via metal probes that are in contact with the skin. The devices are triggered when the bearer enters an exclusion area, or when exhibiting a particular behaviour, and can be preceded by 'warning' stimuli such as tones or vibrations. Shock collars are logistically challenging to implement in field settings (Smith *et al.* 2020b), but can drastically and rapidly alter behaviour. Their application includes the potential to condition site-specific or behaviour-specific aversion – for example, preventing to approach or interaction with children, adults and human-related objects (Appleby 2015) or to thwart livestock/threatened species predation (coyotes: Andelt *et al.* 1999; wolves: Hawley *et al.* 2009; foxes: Cooper *et al.* 2005). For social animals such as gray wolves (*Canis lupus*), not all individuals may need to wear a collar for avoidance to develop within a pack (e.g. Rossler *et al.* 2012). In general, experiments utilising shock and other aversive collars are few, and often involve pilot-level trials on predators with varying methodology and low replication. The effectiveness of aversive collars in depredation management research has been largely positive (Shivik *et al.* 2002 being a notable exception), but ultimately the approach is likely to only be used in highly specific cases because of logistical and animal welfare considerations (Smith *et al.* 2020b). Nonetheless, these methods represent a valuable option for chronic problem situations and for populations of high conservation value (Rossler *et al.* 2012), particularly as collar technology improves.

Electric and magnetic repellents

Electric and magnet repellents are primarily used by divers, swimmers and surfers for preventing shark attacks (Hart and Collin 2015). These repellents can be divided into three broad categories: active electrical repellents, passive electrical repellents using electropositive metals, and passive electrical repellents using magnets (Hart and Collin 2015). These repellents exploit the highly sensitive electroreceptive system of sharks (Hart and Collin 2015), and are likely to have little impact on other species that lack electroreceptive capabilities (Broad *et al.* 2010). The repellents are designed to work by overstimulating the sensory system and could result in the aversive conditioning of the animal. Active devices are typically worn by divers and use a power supply to generate pulses at particular voltages, frequencies and waveforms. Their effectiveness appears to vary between manufacturers and shark species, but at least one model successfully deterred white sharks (*Carcharodon carcharias*) under test conditions (e.g. Kempster *et al.* 2016). Electropositive metals react with water and generate electrical potentials. Their smaller size makes them more suitable for use on fishing equipment, but they have a limited effective range, making them unsuitable for protecting people. Tests of their effectiveness have been mixed, and their cost and short life span are limitations to their uptake in commercial fisheries (Hart and Collin 2015). Permanent magnets are thought to act on shark sensory systems through electromagnetic induction (O'Connell *et al.* 2014). Like other passive repellents, their effectiveness has been mixed and their effective range is limited. However, recent work has incorporated magnets into visual barriers resembling strands of kelp (O'Connell *et al.* 2018) that may be suitable for beach bather protection. These barriers appear to be successful in excluding white sharks from areas while not restricting movements of teleosts and other small elasmobranch species (O'Connell *et al.* 2018).

Animal welfare considerations

Researchers should undertake an *a priori* risk assessment of the expected frequency and consequences of pain and distress in animals, avoiding any scenario where an animal will be exposed to severe pain or distress for prolonged periods of time. Monitoring of animals and their welfare should occur throughout. See Appleby *et al.* (2017a) for a detailed discussion of some of the animal welfare aspects of shock collars. Exposures to shock should be brief, and consist of a maximum of ~10, 0.5–3 s high-intensity shock events per individual in a given application. While this range is relatively arbitrary, in most circumstances (e.g. during training and maintenance shocks events) a higher rate of exposure could suggest that the shock is not adequately moderating behaviour.

The number of shock events required per individual will vary with species and context. Linhart *et al.* (1976) only required three to five shocks events, at 0.5–1 s per shock event, per individual to condition four out of five coyotes to avoid killing black rabbits (*Oryctolagus* sp.). Dale *et al.* (2017) delivered 0.5–1.5 s shocks in one or two behavioural evaluation events per dog per trial, and achieved 100% avoidance of kiwi (*Apteryx* spp.) related stimuli in conditioned dogs within five trials. One of the most serious animal welfare concerns relates to repeated shocks (e.g. being caught in an electric fence or being stuck in the exclusion zone). The former is prevented by good fence design and the latter by mechanisms in the device that prevent the delivery of repeated shocks. Indeed, most collars have in-built shut-offs after a certain period (e.g. 30 s).

The addition of warning cues (visual or auditory) is the primary means through which aversive conditioning using electric fences and shock collars can be facilitated, thereby making the devices effective without the need to always deliver electric shocks. Pairing with warning cues also improves animal welfare by increasing predictability and controllability of the shock for the animal (Destrez *et al.* 2013) through the development of escape through to avoidance responses. Animal welfare outcomes can be improved further by making the learning period that is needed for the animal to associate the cue with the shock as short as possible. This result is largely achieved by making the desired association as unambiguous as possible.

In the marine environment, electric and magnetic repellent devices act on electroreceptive species (Hart and Collin 2015), and are likely to have little effect on other species (Broad *et al.* 2010). Some studies (e.g. O'Connell *et al.* 2018) have noted that teleosts appear unaffected by magnetic repellents, while others have found that electric repellents are species-specific among sharks (see Hart and Collin 2015). Because the repellents act by overstimulating the sensory system and inducing an escape response, it is likely that prolonged constant exposure could have animal welfare impacts. However, given that repellent fields are only active over relatively small distances, and in a typical use the animal is free to move away from the repellent device, any impacts, based on current knowledge, are expected to be minimal and transient.

General procedures

General principles for electric fences and netting

Energised wires can be added to existing fencing, installed temporarily (e.g. as night pens or to protect bee hives), or erected permanently in a stand-alone fashion. Electrified netting can be used to avert animals from certain spatially fixed objects, such as fruit trees. Electric fences are effective and long lasting if well-constructed, and designed with the target species in mind. Construction faults are responsible for more failures than are maintenance issues and wear and tear (Frank and Eklund 2017). If conditioned avoidance is achieved, animals will likely exhibit this response to any similar looking fence, particularly if salient warning cues (e.g. fladry) are added (Lance *et al.* 2010). Solar-powered energisers can make use of electric fences in remote areas practical and affordable. However, electric fences are more effective, easier to erect and maintain, and have fewer unwanted costs when they are applied to small areas, pastures or herds (Durant *et al.* 2015; Smith *et al.* 2020c).

Many detailed guides are available for building and using electric fences for wildlife management, including Acorn and Dorrance (1994), Sowka (2013) and White and Hirons (2019). Broadly, key considerations relate to (1) the power supply (ensuring species-appropriate level of shocking power; stable grounding); (2) fence construction (avoid near-contact with other services (electricity, telephone, water) and vegetation; ensuring fence is the appropriate height, depth and wire spacing for target and non-target species; increasing practicality and safety with gateways, warning signs and visibility aids); and (3) maintenance (set up an appropriate monitoring schedule; be aware of relevant legislation). Long and Robley (2004) provide a comprehensive guide for using electric fencing to exclude several species of introduced animals found in Australia, including behavioural reactions, optimal fence heights, electrification, and spacing between electric wires.

General principles for animal-borne shock collars

The shock component of the collar is triggered when the collar or device comes in to proximity to either a radio-transmission device (such as buried transmission wire); via GPS, such that if a collared animal enters a zone predetermined by GPS points shock may occur; or is manually triggered via a handheld remote control when the animal is doing a specific behaviour (this requires someone monitoring the animal). Prior to a shock being delivered, usually a warning tone (or vibration) is initially emitted for 1 or 2 s. If the collared animal immediately moves away or changes behaviour when only the warning has occurred the shock will not be delivered. However, if it remains in an area or does not change behaviour, the shock will be delivered, and the process is repeated as necessary up to a predetermined maximum. Maximal effectiveness and minimal welfare impact is achieved when the target animals form an association between the shock event and either the 'problem' behaviour or the salient warning cues (Figure 11.3). While shock may still cause a temporary cessation of 'problem' behaviour, in the absence of such an association, no long-term (conditioned) avoidance is likely to occur.

Current iterations of shock collars are largely drawn from devices used in domestic dog applications. In turn, they have several immediate limitations in relation to wildlife application. The most important limitations relate to being able to regularly remove collars (i.e. to prevent pressure sores developing where probes meet the

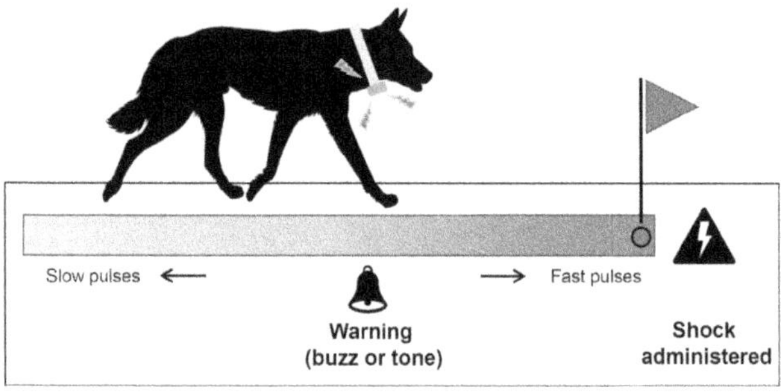

Figure 11.3: As the collared animal approaches the exclusion (shock) zone boundary, it receives a series of warning cues (typically a vibration or tone) that intensify as it approaches the boundary. The shock is paired with the warning, and the latter thus becomes the stimulus it conditions to (e.g. respond to with avoidance). Illustration by Bradley Smith.

skin) or recharging and replacing batteries. They may also not be robust enough for the rigors of the wild. As such, collars for domestic use usually require modifications and augmentation before deployment on wild animals.

Electronic collars are only ever likely to be deployed on a relatively small number of individuals, and current collars only have a limited operational life. It also requires the need to physically capture and handle animals, which itself requires specialist skills, raises welfare concerns of its own, and can be expensive. Cost, unit longevity and reduced weight may become less prohibitive as technology improves.

General principles for electric and magnetic repellents

Electric and magnetic repellents are designed for use with sharks to protect humans, but none is completely effective for deterring all species or individuals (Hart and Collin 2015). The effectiveness of the repellent depends on the strength and frequency of the electrical pulse, and the configuration of electrodes. Several brands/models of shark repellents, which may have different settings and efficacy depending on species and context, are available.

Animal treatment, withdrawal and euthanasia

Monitoring and observation

Upon release, and during all subsequent observations, the welfare of the collared animals should be monitored, both in relation to any potentially deleterious effects arising from collar burden, and those potentially arising from the experimental protocol. Examples include the animal becoming trapped, repeatedly receiving shocks, or getting injured following shock, such as running away and colliding with a nearby obstacle, getting entangled in a fence, or even running onto a road and risking a collision with a vehicle. Monitoring equipment can be placed on animals fitted with devices (e.g. which log the number of triggers), or at test sites (e.g. through motion detection cameras or direct observation). A collar system may be programmed to send a signal to researchers or even trigger a release should it detect that the animal is entangled and immobile, or should it not be operating as intended.

Impact on target and non-target species

Fences must be designed so that they are visible to wildlife and allow non-target herbivores to jump over them without tripping and getting caught. Other major implications of large-scale fencing projects include trapping species inside the fence, restricting access to critical resources and disrupting connectivity of wildlife, particularly for migratory and nomadic species (Durant *et al.* 2015; Smith, King and Allen 2020). In such cases especially, the use of collars and taxon-specific 'metaphorical' fences, rather than physical and electric fences, should be seriously considered (Hayward and Kerley 2009).

Injuries from animal-borne shock collars

Shock collar probes may cause lesions where they contact the skin (Hawley *et al.* 2009). Alternatively, the collars/devices may cause minor rubbing on the neck of the animals. Strategies to avoid such injuries include using a shock collar with rounded probes and placing the electric probes at the back of the neck instead of the front or underside (see Hawley *et al.* 2013). At any sign of skin irritation, the collar should be removed and treatment applied if possible. Collars should not be left on animals for extended periods of time, unless probes are retractable, and a reliable, automatic collar detachment mechanism should be used so that collared animals do not require recapture. Ideally, collars should include a remotely activated detachment capability.

Equipment and maintenance

Equipment must be checked to ensure that it is functioning as intended (ideally tested in controlled and field conditions), and be monitored throughout the study. A cautious approach is required when using devices that are commercially sourced, particularly if they are modified or used outside of the manufacturer's instructions, as well as those that are custom built. Most devices incorporate a mode for testing operation (e.g. aversive collars have lights that can be attached to the probes to show that they are activated). However, these mechanisms do not convey information about the shock intensity. All devices should include a mechanism to allow the devices to be turned off or otherwise made benign should issues arise. For all methods, information signs or public notices are useful for managing public concern.

Electric fencing and netting

Equipment required for studies involving electric fences and nets depends on the nature of the fence being constructed, but is likely to include:

- an energiser (with sufficient power to deliver species specific shock)
- a power supply (e.g. mains power 240 V, or 12 V battery, or solar)

- wire or netting (ideally at least 2 mm diameter for improved conductivity)
- a grounding system (i.e. at least one grounding rod, and wire from the ground rod to the ground terminal of the energiser)
- posts (made of nonconductive material)
- insulators (to place between the wire strands and the posts) if wood or metal is used
- a fence tester (voltmeter) to determine whether the energiser and grounding system is working – this is not to be confused with a voltage reader which only indicates if electric current is passing through the wire
- traditional fencing tools, such as wire splicers, cutters and tensioners
- equipment necessary for fence line preparation (including to control vegetation)
- visibility aids to ensure that wildlife can see the fence (e.g. white flags, reflective tape or reflective wire)
- warning signage for the public that adhere to legislation requirements.

Animal-borne shock collars

Typical items and considerations for studies involving animal-borne shock collars include:

- items necessary for capture (Chapter 7) and collaring (see Chapter 8 and species-specific chapters in this book)
- the aversive device:
  - total collar weighs less than 5% of the animal's body mass (but even then, animal welfare impacts should be evaluated), and fitted in a way that does not inhibit species specific behaviours (see Chapter 9 for considerations when using telemetry devices attached with collars)
  - the intensity of the shock is relative to the animal body mass
  - there is an automatic shutoff mechanism to prevent delivery of repeated shocks
  - there is the ability to manually disable the shock device (either via transmitter or collar)
  - there is a drop off mechanism for removing the collar, and a material back-up option if the mechanism fails (e.g. using fabric or cotton that will degrade quickly)
  - battery life is sufficient for the length of the trial
- scissors or hair clippers to trim hair or fur where prongs make contact with skin
- ability to track (e.g. GPS and VHF) and monitor (e.g. animal identification tags, and motion detection camera) the collared animal for potential effects on animal welfare.

Unfortunately, the literature examining aversive collars is sparse and mostly outdated. Equipment and methods that have been used previously quickly become obsolete. Researchers must ensure they remain up to date with recent advances in technology and methodology used in the design of aversive devices that utilise electric stimulation. No wildlife-specific shock collar designs appear to be available beyond prototype development stages.

Electric and magnetic repellents

Several brands and models of devices using electric and magnetic repellents, which may have different settings and efficacy, are available.

Qualification, experience and training

None of these methods currently requires formal qualifications or training. However, previous experience with the target species' behaviour, public engagement and conducting aversive experiments is likely to result in fewer problems while implementing the study, and provide better animal welfare outcomes. Intimate knowledge of learning theory and applied behaviour analysis are particularly relevant to studies involving aversion and aversive conditioning via electric stimuli. If the animals are required to be trapped and telemetry collars fitted, investigators should refer to Chapters 7 and 9 respectively.

Workplace health and safety

Care should be taken when working with electrical devices, although most do not contain electrical characteristics that are dangerous to humans or non-human animals. Accidental triggers should be largely avoided by keeping the device off until being used or tested, and following the manufacturer's instructions. Any devices that are observed to activate accidentally under normal operating parameters should not be used.

Electric fences may be encountered by members of the public, so ample warning (e.g. signage that meets regulations) and possibly an intermediate barrier may be required to minimise exposure. If built surrounding entire human-use areas, entry/exit points for people and vehicles will usually have to be included. The installation and maintenance of electric fencing must be done in accordance with Australian standards. Electric fences may present a fire risk, so care must be taken in areas of high bushfire risk (Long and Robley 2004).

Animals may become aggressive after stimulation via shock collars and attack nearby humans. Polsky (2000) commented on five cases where domestic dogs wearing aversive stimulus collars as part of pet containment systems exhibited aggressive behaviour towards people, correlating with shock events. However, this observation has not been described in any studies with wildlife, and has not occurred during experiments with dingoes (R. Appleby, pers. obs.). At least some such cases of redirected aggression may be related to the ambiguity of shock events from the animals' perspective; this could be eliminated by better experimental design and protocols (Appleby *et al.* 2017a).

Alternative procedures

In wildlife applications, conditioning animals to avoid specific areas or undertaking natural behaviours (e.g. hunting) is challenging. Electric fences are a widely used and highly successful example of influencing the behaviour of wildlife. Conversely, despite many similarities in potential animal welfare impacts and expectations in terms of potential success, the uptake of shock collars has been low – perhaps because of logistical issues, animal welfare concerns and associated controversy. Less-controversial forms of aversive or defensive stimuli (e.g. biofences and other techniques mentioned in this chapter) might be more suitable for testing in all but the most intractable cases.

ACKNOWLEDGEMENTS

Valuable feedback on the use of livestock guarding animals was provided by Deon Cilliers and Cyril Stannard from the Cheetah Outreach Trust.

REFERENCES

Acorn RC, Dorrance MJ (1994) An evaluation of anti-coyote electric fences. *Proceedings of the Vertebrate Pest Conference* **16**, 45–50.

Adams TS, Mwezi I, Jordan NR (2020) Panic at the disco: solar-powered strobe light barriers reduce field incursion by African elephants *Loxodonta africana* in Chobe District, Botswana. *Oryx*, 1–8 [Online early]. doi:10.1017/S0030605319001182

Allen BL, Allen LR, Ballard G, Drouilly M, Fleming PJS, Hampton JO, *et al.* (2019) Animal welfare considerations for using large carnivores and guardian dogs as vertebrate biocontrol tools against other animals. *Biological Conservation* **232**, 258–270. doi:10.1016/j.biocon.2019.02.019

Andelt WF, Phillips RL, Gruver KS, Guthrie JW (1999) Coyote predation on domestic sheep deterred with electronic dog-training collar. *Wildlife Society Bulletin* **27**, 12–18.

Apfelbach R, Parsons MH, Soini HA, Novotny MV (2015) Are single odourous components of a predator sufficient to elicit defensive behaviours in prey species? *Frontiers in Neuroscience* **9**, 263. doi:10.3389/fnins.2015.00263

Appleby R (2015) Dingo–human conflict: attacks on humans. In *The Dingo Debate: Origins, Behaviour and Conservation.* (Ed. B Smith) pp. 123–150. CSIRO Publishing, Melbourne.

Appleby R, Smith B, Bernede L, Jones D (2017*a*) Utlising aversive conditioning to manage the behaviour of Fraser Island dingoes (*Canis dingo*). *Pacific Conservation Biology* **23**, 335–358. doi:10.1071/PC17017

Appleby R, Smith B, Mackie J, Bernede L, Jones D (2017*b*) Preliminary observations of dingo responses to assumed aversive stimuli. *Pacific Conservation Biology* **23**, 295–301. doi:10.1071/PC17005

Ausband DE, Mitchell MS, Bassing SB, White C (2013) No trespassing: using a biofence to manipulate wolf movements. *Wildlife Research* **40**, 207–216. doi:10.1071/WR12176

Baker SE, Ellwood SA, Watkins R, MacDonald DW (2005) Non-lethal control of wildlife: using chemical repellents as feeding deterrents for the European badger *Meles meles*. *Journal of Applied Ecology* **42**, 921–931. doi:10.1111/j.1365-2664.2005.01069.x

Baker SE, Ellwood SA, Slater D, Watkins RW, Macdonald DW (2008) Food aversion plus odor cue protects crop from wild mammals. *The Journal of Wildlife Management* **72**, 785–791. doi:10.2193/2005-389

Beckmann JP, Lackey CW, Berger J (2004) Evaluation of deterrent techniques and dogs to alter behavior of 'nuisance' black bears. *Wildlife Society Bulletin* **32**, 1141–1146. doi:10.2193/0091-7648(2004)032[1141:EODTAD]2.0.CO;2

Bender H (2003) Deterrence of kangaroos from agricultural areas using ultrasonic frequencies: efficacy of a commercial device. *Wildlife Society Bulletin* **31**, 1037–1046. https://www.jstor.org/stable/3784449

Belant JL, Seamans TW, Dwyer CP (1996) Evaluation of propane exploders as white-tailed deer deterrents. *Crop Protection* **15**, 575–578. doi:10.1016/0261-2194(96)00027-0

Biedenweg TA, Parsons MH, Flemming PA, Blumstein DT (2011) Sounds scary? Lack of habituation following the presentation of novel sounds. *PLoS One* **6**, e14549. doi:10.1371/journal.pone.0014549

Blackwell B, Bernhardt G, Dolbeer R (2002) Lasers as nonlethal avian repellents. *The Journal of Wildlife Management* **66**, 250–258. doi:10.2307/3802891

Blackwell BF, Fernandez-Juricic E (2013) Behavior and physiology in the development and application of visual deterrents at airports. In *Wildlife in Airport Environments: Preventing Animal–aircraft Collisions through Science-based Management.* (Eds TL DeVault, BF Blackwell and JL Belant) pp. 11–22. Johns Hopkins University Press, Baltimore, MD.

Borgo JS, Conner LM, Conover MR (2006) Role of predator odor in roost site selection of southern flying squirrels. *Wildlife Society Bulletin* **34**, 144–149. doi:10.2193/0091-7648(2006)34[144:ROPOIR]2.0.CO;2

Broad A, Knott N, Turon X, Davis AR (2010) Effects of a shark repulsion device on rocky reef fishes: no shocking outcomes. *Marine Ecology Progress Series* **408**, 295–298. doi:10.3354/meps08591

Chestley ST, Whiting TL (2015) Conceptualising the ethical questions in the use of livestock protection dogs. *The Canadian Veterinary Journal. La Revue Veterinaire Canadienne* **56**, 625–628.

Conover MR, Francik JG, Miller DE (1977) An experimental evaluation of aversive conditioning for controlling coyote predation. *The Journal of Wildlife Management* **41**, 775–779. doi:10.2307/3800006

Conover MR, Lyons KS (2003) Reducing or delaying egg depredation by punishing free-ranging predators for opening eggs. *Applied Animal Behaviour Science* **83**, 177–185. doi:10.1016/S0168-1591(03)00132-1

Conover MR (2002) *Resolving Human–wildlife Conflicts: The Science of Wildlife Damage Management.* CRC Press, Boca Raton, FL.

Cooper DM, Kershner EL, Garcelon DK (2005) *The Use of Shock Collars to Prevent Island Fox (*Urocyon littoralis*) Predation on the Endangered San Clemente Loggerhead Shrike* (Lanius ludovicianus mearnsi*).* Institute for Wildlife Studies, Arcata, CA.

Coppinger R, Coppinger L (2001) *Dogs: A Startling New Understanding of Canine Origin, Behaviour & Evolution.* Scribner, New York, NY.

Dale AR, Podlesnik CA, Elliffe D (2017) Evaluation of an aversion-based program designed to reduce predation of native birds by dogs: an analysis of training records for 1156 dogs. *Applied Animal Behaviour Science* **191**, 59–66. doi:10.1016/j.applanim.2017.03.003

DeLiberto ST, Werner SJ (2016) Review of anthraquinone applications for pest management and agricultural crop protection. *Pest Management Science* **72**, 1813–1825. doi:10.1002/ps.4330

Destrez A, Deiss V, Leterrier C, Boivin X, Boissy A (2013) Long-term exposure to unpredictable and uncontrollable aversive events alters fearfulness in sheep. *Animal* **7**, 476–484. doi:10.1017/S1751731112001796

Doherty TS, Hays GC, Driscoll DA (2021) Human disturbance causes widespread disruption of animal movement. *Nature Ecology & Evolution* **5**, 513–519.

Dohner JV (2007) *Livestock Guardians: Using Dogs, Donkeys and Llamas to Protect Your Herd.* Storey Publishing, North Adams, MA.

Domjan M (2018) *The Essentials of Conditioning and Learning.* 4th edn. American Psychological Association, Washington, DC.

Dubois S, Fenwick N, Ryan EA, Baker L, Baker SE, Beausoleil NJ, *et al.* (2017) International consensus principles for ethical wildlife control. *Conservation Biology* **31**, 753–760. doi:10.1111/cobi.12896

Durant SM, Becker MS, Creel S, Bashir S, Dickman AJ, Beudels-Jamar RC, *et al.* (2015) Developing fencing policies for dryland ecosystems. *Journal of Applied Ecology* **52**, 544–551. doi:10.1111/1365-2664.12415

Eklund A, López-Bao J, Tourani M, Chapron G, Frank J (2017) Limited evidence on the effectiveness of interventions to reduce livestock predation by large carnivores. *Scientific Reports* **7**, 2097. doi:10.1038/s41598-017-02323-w

Found R, St. Clair CC (2018) Personality influences wildlife responses to aversive conditioning. *The Journal of Wildlife Management* **82**, 747–755. doi:10.1002/jwmg.21449

Frank J, Eklund A (2017) Poor construction, not time, takes its toll on subsidised fences designed to deter large carnivores. *PLoS One* **12**, e0175211. doi:10.1371/journal.pone.0175211

Garcia J, Hankins WG, Rusiniak KW (1974) Behavioural regulation of the milieu interne in man and rat. *Science* **185**, 824–831. doi:10.1126/science.185.4154.824

Gaynor KM, Cherry MJ, Gilbert SL, Kohl MT, Larson CL, Newsome TM, *et al.* (2021) An applied ecology of fear framework: linking theory to conservation practice. *Animal Conservation* **24**, 308–321. doi:10.1111/acv.12629

Götz T, Janik VM (2013) Acoustic deterrent devices to prevent pinniped depredation: efficiency, conservation concerns and possible solutions. *Marine Ecology Progress Series* **492**, 285–302. doi:10.3354/meps10482

Greggor AL, Clayton NS, Phalan B, Thornton A (2014) Comparative cognition for conservationists. *Trends in Ecology & Evolution* **29**, 489–495. doi:10.1016/j.tree.2014.06.004

Groves PM, Thompson RF (1970) Habituation: a dual-process theory. *Psychological Review* **77**, 419–450. doi:10.1037/h0029810

Gustavson CR, Gustavson JC, Holzer GA (1983) Thiabendazole-based taste aversions in dingoes (*Canis familiaris dingo*) and New Guinea wild dogs (*Canis familiaris hallstromi*). *Applied Animal Ethology* **10**, 385–388. doi:10.1016/0304-3762(83)90187-6

Hall KJ, Fleming PA (2021) In the spotlight: can lights be used to mitigate fox predation on a free-range piggery? *Applied Animal Behaviour Science* **242**, 105420. doi:10.1016/j.applanim.2021.105420

Hampton JO, Hyndman TH, Allen BL, Fischer B (2021) Animal harms and food production: informing ethical choices. *Animals* **11**, 1225.

Hart NS, Collin SP (2015) Sharks senses and shark repellents. *Integrative Zoology* **10**, 38–64. doi:10.1111/1749-4877.12095

Hawley JE, Gehring TM, Schultz RN, Rossler ST, Wydeven AP (2009) Assessment of shock collars as nonlethal management for wolves in Wisconsin. *The Journal of Wildlife Management* **73**, 518–525. doi:10.2193/2007-066

Hawley JE, Rossler ST, Gehring TM, Schultz RN, Callahan PA, Clark R, *et al.* (2013) Developing a new shock-collar design for safe and efficient use on wild wolves. *Wildlife Society Bulletin* **37**, 416–422. doi:10.1002/wsb.234

Hayward MW, Kerley GI (2009) Fencing for conservation: restriction of evolutionary potential or a riposte to threatening processes? *Biological Conservation* **142**, 1–13. doi:10.1016/j.biocon.2008.09.022

IUCN (2020) IUCN SSC Position Statement on the Management of Human-Wildlife Conflict. IUCN Species Survival Commission (SSC) Human-Wildlife Conflict Task Force. <www.iucn.org/theme/species/publications/policies-and-position-statements>.

Jefferson TA, Curry BE (1996) Acoustic methods of reducing or eliminating marine mammal-fishery interactions: do they work? *Ocean and Coastal Management* **31**, 41–70. doi:10.1016/0964-5691(95)00049-6

Johnson CN, van Bommel L, Williams D (2019) Livestock guardian dogs and animal welfare: comment on Allen et al. (2019) Animal welfare considerations for using large carnivores and guardian dogs as vertebrate biocontrol tools against other animals. *Biological Conservation* **236**, 580–581. doi:10.1016/j.biocon.2019.04.017

Karhu RR, Anderson SH (2006) The effect of high-tensile electric fence designs on big-game and livestock movements. *Wildlife Society Bulletin* **34**, 293–299. doi:10.2193/0091-7648(2006)34[293:TEOHEF]2.0.CO;2

Kemper CM, Pemberton D, Cawthorn M, Heinrich S, Mann J, Würsig B, Shaughnessy P, Gales R (2003) Aquaculture and marine mammals: co-existence or conflict. In *Marine Mammals: Fisheries, Tourism and Management Issues.* (Eds N Gales, M Hindell and R Kirkwood) pp. 208–225. CSIRO Publishing, Melbourne.

Kempster RM, Egeberg CA, Hart NS, Ryan L, Chapuis L, Kerr CC, *et al.* (2016) How close is too close? The effect of a non-lethal electric shark deterrent on white shark behaviour. *PLoS One* **11**, e0157717. doi:10.1371/journal.pone.0157717

King LE, Lala F, Nzumu H, Mwambingu E, Douglas-Hamilton I (2017) Beehive fences as a multidimensional conflict-mitigation tool for farmers coexisting with elephants. *Conservation Biology* **31**, 743–752. doi:10.1111/cobi.12898

Kloppers EL, St. Clair CC, Hurd TE (2005) Predator-resembling aversive conditioning for managing habituated wildlife. *Ecology and Society* **10**, 31. doi:10.5751/ES-01293-100131

Lance NJ, Breck SW, Sime C, Callahan P, Shivik JA (2010) Biological, technical, and social aspects of applying electrified fladry for livestock protection from wolves (*Canis lupus*). *Wildlife Research* **37**, 708–714. doi:10.1071/WR10022

Lesilau F, Fonck M, Gatta M, Musyoki C, van 't Zelfde M, Persoon GA, *et al.* (2018) Effectiveness of a LED flashlight technique in reducing livestock depredation by lions (*Panthera leo*) around Nairobi

National Park, Kenya. *PLoS One* **13**, e0190898. doi:10.1371/journal.pone.0190898
Linhart SB, Roberts JD, Shumake SA, Johnson R (1976) Avoidance of prey by captive coyotes punished with electric shock. *Proceedings of the Vertebrate Pest Conference* 7, 302–306.
Long K, Robley A (2004) *Cost Effective Feral Animal Exclusion Fencing for Areas of High Conservation Value in Australia.* Department of the Environment and Heritage, Canberra.
Lorenz JR, Coppinger RP, Sutherland MR (1986) Causes and economic effects of mortality in livestock guarding dogs. *Journal of Range Management* **39**, 293–295.
Maguire GS, Stojanovic D, Weston MA (2009) Conditioned taste aversion reduces fox depredation on model eggs on beaches. *Wildlife Research* **36**, 702–708. doi:10.1071/WR09123
Mazur RL (2010) Does aversive conditioning reduce human-black bear conflict? *The Journal of Wildlife Management* **74**, 48–54. doi:10.2193/2008-163
Miller JR, Schmitz OJ (2019) Landscape of fear and human-predator coexistence: applying spatial predator-prey interaction theory to understand and reduce carnivore-livestock conflict. *Biological Conservation* **236**, 464–473. doi:10.1016/j.biocon.2019.06.009
Musiani M, Mamo C, Boitani L, Callaghan C, Gates CC, Mattei L, *et al.* (2003) Wolf depredation trends and the use of fladry barriers to protect livestock in western North America. *Conservation Biology* **17**, 1538–1547. doi:10.1111/j.1523-1739.2003.00063.x
O'Connell CP, Andreotti S, Rutzen M, Matthee CA, Meÿer M, He P (2014) Effects of the Sharksafe barrier on white shark (*Carcharodon carcharias*) behavior and its implications for future conservation technologies. *Journal of Experimental Marine Biology and Ecology* **460**, 37–46. doi:10.1016/j.jembe.2014.06.004
O'Connell CP, Andreotti S, Rutzen M, Meÿer M, Matthee CA (2018) Testing the exclusion capabilities and durability of the Sharksafe Barrier to determine its viability as an eco-friendly alternative to current shark culling methodologies. *Aquatic Conservation* **28**, 252–258. doi:10.1002/aqc.2803
O'Donnell S, Webb JK, Shine R (2010) Conditioned taste aversion enhances the survival of an endangered predator imperilled by a toxic invader. *Journal of Applied Ecology* **47**, 558–565. doi:10.1111/j.1365-2664.2010.01802.x
Otto TE, Roloff GJ (2015) Black bear exclusion fences to protect mobile apiaries. *Human-Wildlife Interactions* **9**, 8. doi:10.26077/dn8a-3941
Parsons MH, Apfelbach R, Banks PB, Cameron EZ, Dickman CR, Frank AS, *et al.* (2018) Biologically meaningful scents: a framework for understanding predator–prey research across disciplines. *Biological Reviews of the Cambridge Philosophical Society* **93**, 98–114. doi:10.1111/brv.12334
Polsky R (2000) Can aggression in dogs be elicited through the use of electronic pet containment systems? *Journal of Applied Animal Welfare Science* **3**, 345–357. doi:10.1207/S15327604JAWS0304_6
Price CJ, Banks PB (2012) Exploiting olfactory learning in alien rats to protect birds' eggs. *Proceedings of the National Academy of Sciences of the United States of America* **109**, 19304–19309. doi:10.1073/pnas.1210981109
Radford C, McNutt JW, Rogers T, Maslen B, Jordan N (2020) Artificial eyespots on cattle reduce predation by large carnivores. *Communications Biology* **3**, 430. doi:10.1038/s42003-020-01156-0
Rossler ST, Gehring TM, Schultz RN, Rossler MT, Wydeven AP, Hawley JE (2012) Shock collars as a site-aversive conditioning tool for wolves. *Wildlife Society Bulletin* **36**, 176–184. doi:10.1002/wsb.93
Schakner ZA, Blumstein DT (2013) Behavioral biology of marine mammal deterrents: a review and prospectus. *Biological Conservation* **167**, 380–389. doi:10.1016/j.biocon.2013.08.024
Shivik JA, Asher V, Bradley L, Kunkel K, Phillips M, Breck S, Bangs E (2002) Electronic aversive conditioning for managing wolf predation. In *Proceedings of the Vertebrate Pest Conference* **20**, pp. 227–231.
Shivik JA, Martin DJ (2000) Aversive and disruptive stimulus applications for managing predation. *Wildlife Damage Management Conferences- Proceedings* **20**. <https://digitalcommons.unl.edu/icwdm_wdmconfproc/20>.
Smith B, Jaques N, Appleby R, Morris S, Jordan N (2020a) Automated shepherds: responses of captive dingoes to sound and an inflatable, moving effigy. *Pacific Conservation Biology* **27**, 195–201. doi:10.1071/PC20022
Smith B, Appleby R, Jordan N (2020b) Co-existing with dingoes: challenges and solutions to implementing non-lethal management. *Australian Zoologist.* doi:10.7882/AZ.2020.024[Online early]
Smith D, King R, Allen BL (2020c) Impacts of exclusion fencing on target and non-target fauna: a global review. *Biological Reviews of the Cambridge Philosophical Society.* doi:10.1111/brv.12631[Online early]
Smith BR, Yarnell RW, Uzal A, Whitehouse-Tedd K (2020d) The ecological effects of livestock guarding dogs (LSDs) on target and non-target wildlife. *Journal of Vertebrate Biology* **69**, 20103.1-17. doi:10.25225/jvb.20103
Smith ME, Linnell JD, Odden J, Swenson JE (2000) Review of methods to reduce livestock depredation II. Aversive conditioning, deterrents and repellents. *Acta Agriculturae Scandinavica* **50**, 304–315. doi:10.1080/090647000750069502
Smith TS, Hopkins B, Gookin J, Thompson S (2018) Portable electric fencing for bear deterrence and conservation. *Human-Wildlife Interactions* **12**, 3. doi:10.26077/h9sw-qg28
Snijders L, Greggor AL, Hilderink F (2019) Effectiveness of animal conditioning interventions in reducing human–wildlife conflict: a systematic map protocol. *Environmental Evidence* **8**, 10. doi:10.1186/s13750-019-0153-7
Sowka P (2013) *Living with Predators Resource Guide Series – Practical Electric Fencing Resource Guide: Controlling Predators.* The Living with Wildlife Foundation and the Montana Fish, Wildlife & Parks, Arlee, MT.
Steensma K, Lindell C, Leigh D, Burrows C, Wieferich S, Zwamborn E (2016) Bird damage to fruit crops: a comparison of several deterrent techniques. In *Proceedings of the Vertebrate Pest Conference* **27**. doi:10.5070/V427110693
Stickley A, Mott D, King J (1995) Short-term effects of an inflatable effigy on cormorants at catfish farms. *Wildlife Society Bulletin* **23**, 73–77. https://www.jstor.org/stable/3783197.
Sousa-Guedes D, Ribeiro H, Vaz-Freire MT, Mira A, Sillero N (2020) Ultrasonic device effectiveness in keeping rodents off the road. *European Journal of Wildlife Research* **66**, 23. doi:10.1007/s10344-020-1361-8
Thorogood R, Kokko H, Mappes J (2018) Social transmission of avoidance among predators facilitates the spread of novel prey. *Nature Ecology & Evolution* **2**, 254–261. doi:10.1038/s41559-017-0418-x
Tobajas J, Descalzo E, Jiménez J, Villafuerte R, Mateo R, Ferreras P (2021) Conditioned odor aversion as a tool for reducing post-release predation during animal translocations. *Animal Conservation* **24**, 373–385. doi:10.1111/acv.12643
Tobajas J, Descalzo E, Mateo R, Ferreras P (2020) Reducing nest predation of ground-nesting birds through conditioned food aversion. *Biological Conservation* **242**, 108405. doi:10.1016/j.biocon.2020.108405
Tobajas J, Gómez-Ramírez P, María-Mojica P, Navas I, García-Fernández AJ, Ferreras P, Mateo R (2019) Selection of new chemicals to be used in conditioned aversion for non-lethal predation control. *Behavioural Processes* **166**, 103905. doi:10.1016/j.beproc.2019.103905

Treves A, Krofel M, Ohrens O, van Eeden LM (2019) Predator control needs a standard of unbiased randomized experiments with cross-over design. *Frontiers in Ecology and Evolution* **7**, 462. doi:10.3389/fevo.2019.00462

van Bommel L (2010) *Guardian Dogs: Best Practice Manual for the Use of Livestock Guardian Dogs.* Invasive Animals CRC, Canberra.

van Bommel L, Johnson CN (2014) Protecting livestock while conserving ecosystem function: non-lethal management of wild predators. In *Carnivores of Australia: Past, Present and Future.* (Eds AS Glen and CR Dickman) pp. 323–354. CSIRO Publishing, Melbourne.

van Eeden LM, Crowther MS, Dickman CR, Macdonald DW, Ripple WJ, Ritchie EG, Newsome TM (2018) Managing conflict between large carnivores and livestock. *Conservation Biology* **32**, 26–34. doi:10.1111/cobi.12959

Walter WD, Lavelle MJ, Fischer JW, Johnson TL, Hygnstrom SE, VerCauteren KC (2010) Management of damage by elk (*Cervus elaphus*) in North America: a review. *Wildlife Research* **37**, 630–646. doi:10.1071/WR10021

White G, Hirons G (2019) *The Predator Exclusion Fence Manual: Guidance on the Use of Predator Exclusion Fences to reduce Mammallan Predation on Ground-Nesting Birds on RSPB Reserves.* Version 3. Royal Society for the Protection of Birds, London, UK.

Whitehouse-Tedd K, Wilkes R, Stannard C, Wettlaufer D, Cilliers D (2020) Reported livestock guarding dog-wildlife interactions: implications for conservation and animal welfare. *Biological Conservation* **241**, 108249. doi:10.1016/j.biocon.2019.108249

Zarco-González MM, Monroy-Vilchis O (2014) Decreasing predation with low-cost deterrents. *Animal Conservation* **17**, 371–378. doi:10.1111/acv.12104

12 Research methods for marine mammals and reptiles

Janet M. Lanyon, Roger J. Kirkwood and Ian P. Bell

INTRODUCTION

While some common themes exist, techniques for capture, restraint and sampling of marine mammals and reptiles are often species-specific. Accordingly, methods appropriate to these taxa are covered in this chapter. Marine mammals and reptiles are subject to high levels of legislative protection compared with marine invertebrates or fishes. Capture and handling require judicious planning to comply with these regulations and to ensure that the welfare of every individual is maintained. This chapter provides general operating procedures (GOPs) for common research methods for marine mammals and reptiles in Australia. These techniques are not necessarily transferable to other species. For example, among the pinnipeds, only otariids (fur seals and sea lions) occur in large numbers in Australia, so this chapter focuses on these taxa while realising that techniques for handling phocids (true seals) can differ. Target taxa in this chapter include cetaceans that occur regularly in Australian waters, pinnipeds, dugongs (*Dugong dugon*), marine turtles and sea snakes.

OBSERVATIONAL STUDIES

Target taxa

This GOP applies to cetaceans (dolphins, whales), pinnipeds (seals, sea lions), dugongs (Chapter 25), sea snakes and marine turtles (Chapter 26).

Context and scope

This GOP describes techniques for observational studies of wild marine mammals and reptiles, ranging from population surveys conducted from vessels, air-borne platforms or shore vantage points, to specific focal follows of individuals. Observational studies are often combined with targeted sampling. Real-time observations of fully aquatic species are usually restricted to animals at or close to the water surface, depending on water clarity. Seal and turtle rookeries can be surveyed from land-based vantage points or during colony walk-throughs. For observational studies, including population surveys, of fully aquatic marine mammals (cetaceans and dugongs) in Australian waters, observation platforms have consisted of ships or small boats (e.g. Parker 1978; Ansmann *et al.* 2015), manned aircraft or unmanned aerial vehicles (UAVs) (e.g. Hodgson *et al.* 2013), underwater passive acoustic stations or arrays (e.g. McCauley *et al.* 2018), coastal lookouts (e.g. Charlton *et al.* 2019) or some combination of these methods (e.g. Corkeron *et al.* 1994; Hedley *et al.* 2011). Demographic, behavioural and physiological aspects of marine turtle populations are also being monitored increasingly by UAVs such as quadcopters, balloons, blimps (Schofield *et al.* 2017) and drones (Chapter 6). It is rare to be able to document protracted underwater observations of marine mammals and reptiles via snorkel or SCUBA (but see Burns and Heatwole 1998; Arnold *et al.* 2005).

Animal welfare considerations

Disturbance or obstruction to normal behaviours

Observers' proximity, activities and noise must not obstruct natural behaviours of target and non-target species, including travel along migration paths and nursing. Monitoring to assess degree of behavioural response to disturbance is recommended, with subsequent pause or withdrawal of operations as necessary. For pinnipeds and sea turtles, observational studies or surveys may be conducted during their terrestrial phases – for example, in rookeries when observer presence may coincide with critical reproductive or moulting periods. Care should also be taken to minimise disturbance of non-target species, such as nesting seabirds, when undertaking terrestrial observations.

Disturbance of marine mammals is not usually an issue with fixed wing aircraft because flight altitude is generally at least 100–150 m (see Chapter 6). Helicopter noise is problematic, but may be alleviated by increasing altitude and positioning downwind. In contrast, fixed-wing and rotored UAVs are increasingly being used for survey (Hodgson *et al.* 2013; Bryson and Williams 2015), behavioural studies (Nielsen *et al.* 2019) and photogrammetry with flights at altitudes as low as 10–50 m (Sorrell *et al.* 2019; Christiansen *et al.* 2020). Noise levels underwater are below ambient noise levels when flying a UAV above 10 m altitude, so that the risk of marine mammals hearing the drone is probably low. No behavioural response was observed in southern right whale (*Eubalaena australis*) mother–calf pairs to controlled approaches with a UAV (Christiansen *et al.* 2020). Tethered blimps (e.g. Hodgson and Marsh 2007) and balloons equipped with cameras are relatively quiet, but limit the range of observation.

Injury and collision

Adhering to permitted approach distances and remaining aware of the positions of nearby target and non-target animals should reduce the likelihood of collisions at sea (i.e. between observer boats and animals).

General procedures

Key considerations

Observations of marine mammals at sea must be conducted in accordance with guidelines regarding approach distances for protected species, both on the water and from the air (DAWE 2020). Australian Commonwealth waters extend from 3–200 nm off the coast and include the Australian Whale Sanctuary within which federal standards apply to minimum approach distances for marine mammals. Within 3 nm of the Australian coast, state or territory regulations apply, and researchers are advised to check guidelines specific to their study area and species. Specific approach distances may apply where special management declarations are made (e.g. in marine parks). All observational studies require research permits and animal ethics committee (AEC) clearance; exceptions to approach distance regulations require special exemptions.

Boat-based observations of marine mammals and reptiles at sea

During boat-based work, in addition to maintaining legal allowable distance from focal animals, approach protocols should aim for minimal disturbance. For example, for cetaceans, vessels should approach animals parallel to and slightly to their rear, rather than head-on or directly from the rear of the animal. Researchers should remain quiet, avoiding disturbance of individuals and groups and separation of mothers and offspring, and move around the animals at no-wake speed. Approaching foraging dugongs from the shallow side risks scaring the entire herd towards deep water. During focal follows, researchers must not disturb, chase or block the path of target or non-target animals, and must avoid driving a vessel in such a way that pods or herds are divided into smaller groups, or are forced to veer off their migration path. Since some observational studies (e.g. photo identification, health assessment of cetaceans) require proximity to view identifiable markings on individuals (Figure 12.1), long-range binoculars (e.g. 7 × 50) and/or a camera with a zoom lens (e.g. 90–300 mm) are required. If offspring are in focal groups, a dedicated observer should monitor their positions, although young are often difficult to see. Non-motorised vessels (sailboat, kayak) are useful for close behavioural observations including acoustic studies (Corkeron *et al.* 1994). If marine mammals show signs of disturbance (including onset of rapid diving, changing direction erratically, separation of mother and offspring), observers must withdraw beyond the caution zone.

Aircraft-based observations of marine mammals and reptiles at sea

Observations can also be conducted using various aircraft depending on the research question (survey or

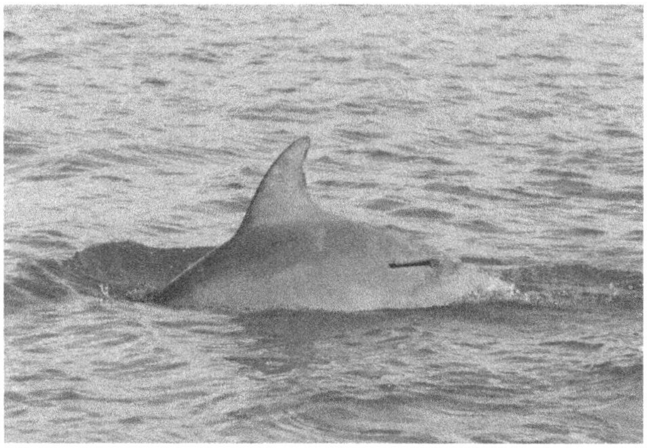

Figure 12.1: Photo of inshore bottlenose dolphin (*Tursiops aduncus*) in Moreton Bay Queensland, taken using a long-range zoom lens to identify the individual based on dorsal fin shape and body markings. A biopsy dart from Paxarms™ biopsy system is striking the dorsum. Photo by Ina Ansmann.

behaviour), extent of area to be covered and distribution of the target species (see Chapter 6 for general considerations). Fixed-wing aircraft have been used in line transect surveys for cetaceans offshore, at points along their migration paths and also within breeding and resting grounds (Bryden 1985; Bannister and Hedley 2001). Pinniped populations have also been monitored by aerial survey (Green *et al.* 1995; Shaughnessy *et al.* 2005). In Antarctica, helicopters have been important for surveys and censuses of pack-ice seals (Southwell *et al.* 2008). Dugongs have traditionally been surveyed via fixed-wing aircraft in their major foraging grounds using a modified strip transect method (Marsh and Sinclair 1989). Design of aerial survey needs to consider biological parameters including size, swim speed and diving behaviour of animals and their spatial and temporal patterns of distribution, and also factors that may affect detectability (e.g. glare, sea state, turbidity) (Bryson and Williams 2015).

Underwater observations

It is rare to be able to conduct direct underwater observations of marine mammals and turtles for periods long enough to be useful, and at proximity that allows collection of robust data without disturbance. However, underwater video stations have been used to monitor Weddell seals (*Leptonychotes weddellii*) under ice (Rouget *et al.* 2007). Sea snakes are generally easier to observe underwater than on the surface, once located. Boat surveys to spot sea snakes at the water surface, followed by underwater observations on SCUBA or snorkel, and underwater focal follows have been conducted for some common species in clear waters (Burns and Heatwole 1998). Underwater visual census (UVC) has been used to assess the distribution and abundance of sea snakes around coral reefs (Lukoschek *et al.* 2007). However, short survey times and depth constraints restrict the amount of habitat that can be surveyed. Sea snake species assemblages have also been surveyed remotely by baited remote underwater video stations (BRUVS) in the Great Barrier Reef region (Udyawer *et al.* 2014). In this case, mesh canisters of prey items (e.g. oily sardines) have been used to attract the snakes to within video range.

Observations of pinnipeds on land

In Australia, seals haul out mostly on offshore islands and remote mainland coasts. Access can require larger transit vessels and a small landing dingy, or a helicopter. Stepping ashore in a pinniped colony can be disruptive to seals, especially during breeding periods. Once ashore and overlooking a site, observations of seal numbers and terrestrial behaviours are possible by eye or binoculars and spotting scopes, or through camera equipment (e.g. Back *et al.* 2018). Alternatively, observations may be made from a vessel stationed offshore (e.g. Cowling *et al.* 2015), with drones (McIntosh *et al.* 2018; Allan *et al.* 2019) or remotely operated cameras (Garlepp *et al.* 2014).

Otariids can be distributed along sections of coast (e.g. caves, cliffs and boulders) that are difficult to access, in which case the best method for counting or approaching individuals to sample is to walk along the coast (i.e. effectively through the colony). Doing so can be highly disruptive to the seals and may be dangerous to the researcher; seals may bite if cornered. Accordingly, researchers must endeavour to not get between seals and their escape route to the water. Such walk-through procedures should be well planned to minimise the duration of disturbance to the seals. On sub-Antarctic islands and in Antarctica, phocid seals haul out on beaches or on sea ice. Southern elephant seals (*Mirounga leonina*) may tolerate people moving near them, so that their population status and on-land behaviour can be observed readily (e.g. Hindell and Burton 1987), but most pack-ice seals are flighty and require careful approach. Observations of Weddell seal behaviours have been conducted from hides established on the ice near tide-cracks, where the seals haul out (van Polanen Petel *et al.* 2007).

Observations of sea turtles on land

Nesting turtles approaching shore after dark are easily disturbed. It is important to minimise movement and artificial lights in their vicinity (Lutcavage *et al.* 1997). The first indication that a female turtle has left the ocean to attempt nesting may be a 'beach crawl' track, which will also allow identification of the species. Her crawl ashore and up the beach to locate a nesting site above the high tide mark can take up to an hour. Turtles are easily disturbed by lights and movement during this time, and may respond by returning to the ocean without laying a clutch of eggs. For this reason, nesting turtles should be approached only after they have completed oviposition and have commenced filling of the egg chamber using their hind flippers. At this stage, sampling may be conducted.

Animal treatment, withdrawal and euthanasia

Observational studies, if conducted appropriately, are unlikely to have detrimental effects on target animals. If the act of observing a wild animal results in a detectable behavioural change, the researcher(s) must pause or withdraw operations as appropriate. All reportable incidents (unexpected or adverse events) must be reported to the appropriate AEC and governmental marine conservation agency as soon as possible, as set out in the permit conditions.

Equipment and maintenance

Equipment needs will vary depending on the observational methods selected but may include equipment associated with safe operation of the survey platform (e.g. aircraft or vessel, SCUBA, associated safety gear), survey technique (e.g. camera, binoculars, theodolites, acoustic stations) and appropriate protective gear for researchers (wetsuits, robust footwear, sun protection, first aid gear). General paperwork will include navigational charts, datasheets, permits. All equipment should be kept in safe working order.

Specific qualifications, experience and training

If using a motorised boat or drone, the driver must hold the relevant licences and permits required for the activity by current legislation and be skilled in their operation. While no specific qualifications may be required for some observational studies, all techniques in this GOP should only be undertaken by experienced personnel who have worked with the target or similar taxa (ideally several times), or under the supervision of more experienced researchers.

Workplace health and safety

Boating and aircraft accidents

Researchers must hold appropriate licences or certificates and take all precautions to operate and deploy vessels and/or aircraft in a safe manner around target taxa.

Injury from bites and stings

Researchers should be aware of potential injury from non-target species (e.g. cryptic benthic animals, including razor clams (e.g. *Pinna bicolor*) and stonefish (*Synanceia* spp.) when standing in the shallows). In inshore tropical waters, box jellyfish and estuarine crocodiles may be a concern; location and season should be considered when planning fieldwork and appropriate protective measures should be taken. At some sites, the risk posed by these taxa may preclude safe in-water research.

Drowning risk and exposure

All in-water operators should be fit, competent and able to swim. Self-awareness and alertness regarding the positions and activities of other crew members are critical. Long periods of outdoor work are inherent in this field of study. Protection against the elements requires appropriate personal protective equipment (e.g. wetsuits, long sleeves, hat) and behaviour (e.g. seeking shade, frequent hydration).

Alternative procedures

The methods detailed in this GOP are relatively low impact, compared to, for example, capture and sampling techniques. Investigators should consider if techniques, such as RUV (remote underwater video), which do not require the regular presence of human observers, may be suitable for meeting study objectives.

CAPTURE METHODS

Target taxa

This GOP applies to cetaceans (dolphins, whales), pinnipeds (seals, sea lions), dugongs (Chapter 25), sea snakes and marine turtles (Chapter 26).

Context and scope

This section describes the capture of wild marine mammals and reptiles in Australia for research purposes, including to mark individuals, sample tissues (including parasites), or attach devices (e.g. dive recorders and tracking instruments). Alternatively, animals may be captured to provide animal welfare assistance to individuals harmed through anthropogenic processes – for example, to remove entangling marine debris (Groom and Coughran 2012), or to remove them from a dangerous situation (e.g. stranded on a public beach). Choice of capture and restraint techniques depends on multiple factors including species, location of the animal, ambient temperature when capturing or sampling animals on land, operator experience level and expected length of restraint required. Broadly, possible techniques are physical restraint alone, a combination of physical and chemical restraint, or chemical restraint alone.

For fully aquatic taxa, such as dugongs and dolphins, capture is conducted at sea. Capture of the semi-aquatic pinnipeds (seals and sea lions) usually occurs during their terrestrial resting periods, although at-sea captures are possible. Sea turtles can be captured at sea by crew deployed from a fast-moving boat or sampled on land at a rookery, while fully aquatic sea snakes are captured by a variety of techniques including by hand with snorkel or SCUBA, or by dip net from a boat. Equipment and techniques for capture may or may not include nets such as modified seine and hoop nets, which all target smaller marine mammals (< 4 m). Coastal dolphins, including bottlenose dolphins (*Tursiops* spp.) and Australian humpback dolphins (*Sousa sahulensis*) have been captured at sea in Australia for rescue and rehabilitation, for captive display historically, and more rarely for research purposes. Australian research programs that have captured dolphins to attach transmitters have used a breakaway hoop net to capture bow-riding bottlenose dolphins (Corkeron and Martin 2004) or a seine netting technique (Chilvers *et al.* 2001) following protocols largely developed overseas (e.g. Wells *et al.* 2004). Protocols for capturing dolphins at sea using seine nets are covered in this GOP. However, as netting is unlikely to be the best way to capture dugongs because of their propensity to roll and entangle, this method is not applied to dugongs in this GOP. Sampling of larger marine mammals (whales) is usually conducted without capture; any restraint may be for rescue only (Groom and Coughran 2012).

Animal welfare considerations

Drowning, injury, collision and entanglement

Marine mammals and reptiles must surface to breathe. In-water capture techniques must allow unfettered access to the water's surface at all times during the capture procedure. Use of nets or other equipment (if used) must not hinder passage to the water surface or form an obstacle or entanglement hazard that prevents an animal from surfacing freely. When using nets, mesh size that reduces the chances of entanglement of limbs or fins should be selected. In case of accidental entanglement, net knives must be carried in order to effect rapid release. If using sharp implements (e.g. net knives, tagging devices), care must be taken to sheath these when in proximity to the animal.

If operating in a marine protected area, special permits to exceed vessel speed limits or to access zoned areas may be required. For dugongs and sea turtles, which are both captured using an open water method, care must be taken to avoid collisions between the vessel and target animal, and also with other marine animals that may be encountered during pursuit. If an animal swims under the boat or towards the boat's outboard motors, the engine must be put into neutral immediately to avoid injuring the animal or damaging the propeller. If available, a 'forward' rather than a 'tiller' steered vessel should be used to avoid interaction with non-target animals. Once the animal is captured and held at the water's surface, handlers must not use it as a flotation device.

Exposure to gravity on land

For fully aquatic vertebrates, time out-of-water presents physical challenges. For any animal that relies on movement of its chest to breath and is normally buoyed in water, the thorax must not become so compressed that proper chest movement is impeded. Similarly, pregnant marine mammals may require body support in order to reduce weight on their ventrum.

Extreme temperatures and weather conditions

Capturing marine mammals and reptiles at sea in fair weather conditions will reduce risks associated with chaotic surface conditions. Visibility of animals is facilitated when skies are clear (low cloud cover, no glare) and sea state is low (Beaufort sea state < 2). In the case of dugongs with short surface intervals (< 10 s), in particularly murky inshore waters, the optimal time for sighting and visual tracking is usually around noon when light penetrance into the water is greatest. When pursuit of an animal or deployment of a net is involved, smooth seas permit a more controlled approach.

Timing of capture and sampling activities should avoid exposure to air temperatures that may chill or heat the animal's body beyond normal ambient temperature, when possible. Other factors to consider are wind (chill factor) and precipitation (rain, snow). Animals out-of-water may require full shade over the body, wet cotton placed over the body and/or periodic dousing to avoid rapid overheating. Body temperature may be monitored via rectal temperature (Little 1995) or in the case of the hindgut-fermenting dugong, through a proxy to body temperature (e.g. oral temperature; Lanyon *et al.* 2010b).

General procedures

Preparation

All personnel must have clearly defined roles, and a defined leader must be selected. The leader ensures that the capture team comprises sufficient experienced personnel to fill key positions required to capture and restrain a marine mammal or reptile safely. Check lists are handy to ensure that all required equipment is working and packed, and tasks completed in an efficient and timely manner. All personnel should be familiar with possible variations in the catch scenario so that they can be prepared to adapt the catch protocol according to environmental conditions, if necessary. Immediately before each capture event, a run-down on procedures or rehearsal should be conducted; this review should cover weather and sea state, boating plan, animals to be caught, crocodile or shark safety (if appropriate), the plan for moving animals once they are caught, individual staff roles, and what to do if staff feel unsafe or animals are injured. Immediately after each capture event, a debriefing should be conducted to review potential improvements in capture and animal welfare outcomes.

Open water capture of dugongs

Open water capture of dugongs involves a short boat pursuit before a person leaps from the boat and grasps the dugong (Lanyon *et al.* 2006). This process is known as the 'rodeo' method. The vessel must have capacity to hold the team, sufficient power to maintain contact with a rapidly swimming dugong capable of reaching burst speeds of > 20 kn, and sufficient manoeuvrability to follow a weaving dugong. A rigid hull inflatable vessel with low sides to facilitate entry and egress of the team from the water is an effective catch boat. Catcher(s) must be sufficiently physically strong and competent in water to restrain a 600 kg dugong.

Solitary dugongs and those on the periphery of herds, which may be coaxed away without disruption to the herds, are targeted preferentially. Cows with dependent calves ≥ 2 years have been captured, but cow–neonate pairs can be biopsied without capture (see below). Capture is best conducted in clear shallow waters (1.5–4 m) because dugongs spend little time at the surface, so must be tracked visually underwater during pursuit. Since dugongs tend to flee towards the closest deep-water refuge, shallow areas distant from deep water are preferred. Fair weather conditions (sunny, wind speed ≤ 10 kn) facilitate initial sighting and efficient tracking. During pursuit, the skipper attempts to remain in relatively close contact with the dugong and prevent its egress into deeper waters. A dugong is pursued until it is fatigued only to the extent that risk of injury to animal or catcher is reduced. Under Queensland protocols, a dugong can be pursued for a maximum of 10 min or until just after the third breath, whichever comes first (Lanyon *et al.* 2006, 2010b). Throughout pursuit, respiratory function of the dugong should be monitored closely to detect any respiratory abnormalities or other signs that capture should be aborted. The dugong is captured just after it has surfaced within reach of the bow, taken a breath unhampered, and before it dives away; failure to allow this breath may be fatal.

Capture involves a catcher leaping from the bow and grasping the dugong firmly around its peduncle (tail stock) so that the upper surface of the flukes is held firmly against the catcher's body, to prevent the dugong effecting a power stroke; the catcher can arch their back to reduce the downward power stroke further (Lanyon *et al.* 2006). An alternative approach is to have two catchers grasp the dugong's peduncle region to bring the dugong to a full stop. When the catchers exit the boat, the boat's engine(s) should be turned off. Personnel may assist in restraining the dugong at the surface by holding the base of each of the dugong's pectoral fins (Lanyon *et al.* 2006), may use an inflatable stretcher (Marsh and Rathbun 1990), or may secure the dugong to the side of the catch vessel (Holley 2006); pool noodles are useful in providing extra flotation. The aim of restraint is to prevent the dugong from escaping and to keep the dugong's head at the surface to facilitate regular breathing while processing occurs. A calm and quiet environment should be maintained.

If a dugong is to be removed from the water for health assessment or to collect biological samples (e.g. blood, urine) uncontaminated by seawater, a customised stretcher slung between two vessels has been used to transport the dugong to a mother ship, and a crane used to lift the dugong onto deck (Lanyon *et al.* 2010b). Dugongs can be held out of water on a closed-cell mattress with shade and seawater provided for temperature regulation. The highest priority for researchers removing a dugong from water is to establish regular and strong breathing by dousing of the head, since some dugongs have a propensity to stop breathing. Temperature pulse respiration (TPR) should be monitored throughout the out-of-water period (Lanyon *et al.* 2010b) and the dugong returned to the water at the onset of abnormal vital signs or behaviour. Dugongs are normally docile and still when out of water and do not need additional restraint.

Netting of coastal dolphins

Most captures of dolphins have been conducted by encircling animals with large-mesh seine nets that are run around them in shallow water. Once encircled, several experienced dolphin handlers positioned around the net restrain and disentangle the dolphin. Few Australian studies have attempted dolphin capture because this netting procedure is complex and requires a large team (eight or more people), several vessels including a special net boat, and a customised capture net. Furthermore, some dolphins may be prone to acute stress from capture and handling (Fair *et al.* 2014; Hart *et al.* 2015). If seine netting of dolphins is to be conducted, the capture procedure should be rehearsed for the local conditions, geography and target species. A seine net suitable for dolphin capture may be of variable length (400–500 m) but with a drop to match water depth, and a lead line on the bottom of the net and a float line along the top. Appropriate mesh size is large enough to reduce fouling organisms but small enough to prevent entanglement of fins; an example mesh size is 130–180 mm slack and 150–200 mm stretched (diamond to diamond).

Solitary dolphins are targeted preferentially for capture. However, the social nature of dolphins means that it is common to net more than one dolphin per capture event. Suitable locations in which to catch dolphins by seine net include shallow open water areas with sandy and muddy substrates; rocky/rubble reefs are usually avoided so as to reduce net obstruction and snagging. Dolphins can also be captured along a beach with the net run out in a semi-circle to prevent escape to deeper water. A suitable net boat is essential: this vessel must be large enough to hold a net folded into pleats, ideally has a removable transom so that the net can be deployed linearly from the stern as the boat encircles the target dolphin and must be capable of sufficient acceleration so as to close off the net securely either against itself, or against the shore before the dolphin can escape. As the net is deployed, one or more attendant boats, each with dolphin handlers on board, move into position along but just off the net perimeter. The number of attendant boats and handlers will depend on the length of net to be monitored and the number of dolphins to be captured and/or released. From these vessels, the crew can monitor the net in case of dolphin entanglement. An alternative approach places personnel at intervals around the net in standing-depth water.

It is critically important that the dolphins' positions within the net be monitored continuously. If any dolphin hits the net, the skippers must bring their attendant boats to the animal's aid, with staff lifting the animal in the net to allow it to breath at the surface. In the event of entanglement, the priority is to ensure that no staff become entangled in the net. The dolphin can then be supported to ensure that its blowhole is above the water surface so it can breathe freely. If at any time a dolphin becomes securely entangled so that its ability to breathe is compromised, the net must be cut immediately to free it; net knives should be held at the ready on each attendant boat. Once deployed, the size of the net can be lessened by either drawing it inwards towards the net boat in the case of a circular net, or by drawing the net towards the beach until the water is shallow enough for staff to stand. Once the dolphin is captured safely by hand, it can be lifted onto a suitable platform (e.g. stand-up paddleboard, stretcher or boat) for veterinary or other procedures. It is recommended that a minimum of four people should be involved in carrying a dolphin and should abide by safe work practices for heavy lifting. If a dolphin is contained by the net in shallow water near a beach, staff may approach the dolphin from the shore and apprehend it by grasping the animal's pectoral flippers from above and holding them in close against the animal's body. Other staff can assist by embracing the dolphin in their arms in front of the dorsal fin. Since the tail stock is very strong, it is a potentially harmful body part by which to restrain a dolphin. If a dolphin is to be sampled out of water, it is held in a recumbent position on a closed-cell mattress with full shade and doused frequently to assist in temperature regulation. Wild dolphins rarely have to be physically restrained while out of water, but proximity to the flukes is to be avoided.

Capture of pinnipeds

Techniques for capture and handling of pinnipeds are dependent on coastal geography, seal species (body size, nature and habits) and reason for capture (see Chapter 25). Site geography will influence each of approach time, working space, and safety considerations. For example, Australian fur seals (*Arctocephalus pusillus doriferus*) may occur in large numbers on open rocky coasts and will stampede *en masse* to the water if they detect humans. Consequently, capture can require lengthy approach times, including crawling into position so as not to scare them into the water too soon. New Zealand (or long-nosed) fur seals (*Arctocephalus forsteri*) can also occur in large numbers; they can haul out on sharp boulders along highly active coasts, and generally flee if they detect humans. In contrast, Australian sea lions (*Neophoca cinerea*) usually occur in small groups on open rocky or sand beach coasts and appear to be relatively nonchalant about human approaches. Itinerant Antarctic pinnipeds are sometimes encountered on Australian coasts and these include leopard seals (*Hydrurga leptonyx*), elephant seals (*Mirounga leonina*) and sub-Antarctic fur seals (*Arctocephalus tropicalis*). These species are usually single visitors, and often in poor body condition. Generally, they are left alone unless they have injuries judged to make their long-term survival unlikely. Captures may be performed to shift individuals to beaches less visited by humans, or to bring them into captivity for rehabilitation. Elephant seals on sub-Antarctic islands occupy sand and gravel beaches where windy, wet and cold conditions prevail. They are large (> 150 kg unless a pup), and while generally slow-moving, they can move suddenly and rapidly over short distances. In Antarctica, crabeater (*Lobodon carcinophagus*), leopard and Weddell seals are usually present in low densities, solitary or in low numbers, and rest on ice beside escape points that they can access in seconds. These differences in habits and habitats mean that approaches to capture vary greatly but most require judicious planning.

Capture technique is also dependent on required handling times, which can range from seconds (e.g. entanglement removal, marking), through minutes (e.g. device deployment, serological sampling) to hours (e.g. relocation). For brief periods, smaller seals may be restrained by hand or in a net. For periods longer than ~5 min or involving invasive procedures like tooth extraction, sedation or anaesthesia should be utilised to minimise stress.

Capture techniques for pinnipeds include 'run and grab' (pups), 'run and net' (Figure 12.2) or 'swim in and net' (for individuals ≤ 100 kg), or tranquilise (if > 100 kg or for individuals that would be difficult to net before they could enter the water) (Kirkwood and Goldsworthy 2013). A typical capture net comprises a pole with net at the end in the classic 'butterfly net' design. The hoop diameter is sufficiently large to allow entry of the animal and sufficiently deep to contain most of the animal's body within the net. Ideally, the seal's own momentum is harnessed to capture it quickly by placing the net opening in the seal's path of movement. Once in the net, seals will need to be restrained, for example, by placing bodyweight around the net (Figure 12.2) or tying off/twisting the hoop end so that the seal remains in the net. Doing so is especially important for otariids as they can use their powerful fore flippers to push off the ground; if possible, the fore flippers should be restrained along the side of the seal. For smaller seals, once restrained in a net, they may be carried or stretchered to spots that are more suitable for seal and researcher safety during processing (i.e. flatter and further from cliffs or wave action). 'Sausage nets' (wide-mouthed long nets with a flexible hoop, but no handle) and head bags can be used on larger phocid seals that are less mobile on land. Land captures of large individuals (> 100 kg) will usually require a chemical agent as part of their immobilisation. In large pinnipeds, immobilisation drugs are most often delivered remotely, by dart rifles, or a pole syringe (see Chapters 16 and 25).

Pinnipeds may also be captured in the water. A novel technique that proved successful in an offshore situation was to crane a large (6 × 4 m) dip net over the side of a fishing vessel to ~2 m depth, then bait the surface over the

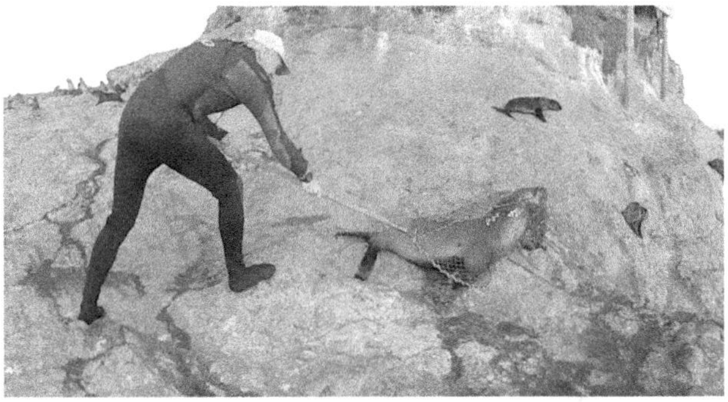

Figure 12.2: One of the authors (RJK) capturing a juvenile Australian fur seal (*Arctocephalus pusillus doriferus*) to recover tracking and dive recording devices previously attached to the back of the seal. The seal was restrained for < 2 min while the devices were removed by trimming the seal's fur underneath them. Photo by Marcus Salton.

net with fish. The net was hoisted when a seal passed over it and the seal was subsequently transferred to the deck of the ship (Tilzey *et al.* 2006).

Open water capture of marine turtles

The standard capture method for all marine turtles in Australian waters, except leatherbacks *Dermochelys coriacea*, is also via the rodeo method: by jumping on them from a small boat (Limpus and Walter 1980). As with dugongs, this method presents several challenges. Sea turtles are well camouflaged with a dark brown speckled patterned carapace making them inconspicuous within reefal or intertidal habitats. They maintain a cryptic lifestyle, only using shallow feeding flats during periods of high tide and leaving for deeper water at low tide. Since turtles move up onto the foraging flats and travel towards shore as the tide rises, it may take considerable time (1–2 h) for them to be 75–150 m inshore from deep water (> 2 m) and thus in a location where they can be pursued and caught. Upon disturbance, a turtle will generally swim rapidly towards and descend into deep water, allowing only seconds to manoeuvre a vessel into a position suitable for somebody to dive in and catch the turtle.

Vessels used to catch turtles are typically 4–5 m, rigid hulled, outboard motor-powered dinghies and are crewed by an experienced driver and several trained turtle spotters and catchers. The vessel layout should be such that all crew can maintain a watch for turtles and other nearby animals from the vessel's bow. Typically, a several hundred metre-wide strip of reef or tidal flat is searched in a zigzag pattern while working downwind and with the sun behind the boat to minimise glare and maximise chances of sighting movement through the water. Upon sighting a turtle, the skipper rapidly manoeuvres the vessel so that a catcher can enter the water from the bow of the boat directly onto the turtle. The catcher grasps the turtle by front and back edges of the carapace and, by tilting the turtle upwards, moves the turtle (even the largest ones) to the water surface. Once restrained at the surface, the vessel is brought alongside, and the turtle can be loaded into the boat (Limpus and Reed 1985).

Alternative methods of capture are sometimes used. Beach jumping is a modification of the open water method where a person catches turtles while walking over shallow foraging areas, jumping onto turtles as encountered (Miller 1994). Slow-swimming sea turtles can be captured by hand while snorkelling or SCUBA diving (Limpus and Reed 1985). Turtles can also be captured by dragging a seine net through a shallow water area or by block-netting (i.e. a blocking net is held across a gutter or channel draining a seagrass or reef flat). On a falling tide, the water flow will trap turtles within and against the net, allowing for hand capture (Miller 1994). In a few foraging grounds (e.g. Shoalwater Bay and Great Sandy Straits), some green turtles (*Chelonia mydas*) may remain stranded on the intertidal flats at low tide after foraging on mangroves, or basking (Read *et al.* 1996); these animals can be hand collected and brought to the water's edge for collection by boat or transported via wheeled transport (modified wheelbarrow) to a processing site nearby. Some basking turtles may be sampled on site and left *in situ*.

During sampling, turtles are monitored to ensure that they do not overheat, moving them to the shade if necessary or cooling with water. Turtles are typically placed on their plastrons with their eyes covered with a damp cloth or placed in a position within a vessel that restricts movement to prevent them wandering and abrading themselves unnecessarily. After sampling, turtles are usually returned to the water within a few hours of capture.

Capture of sea snakes

Capture of live sea snakes may be conducted opportunistically as they are brought up as by-catch in prawn trawlers (Courtney *et al.* 2010). In coastal habitats when targeted capture is required, sea snakes can be located by spotlighting the water's surface in early evening or at night from boats cruising at low speeds in shallow (< 10 m) waters (e.g. over seagrass beds) (Ukuwela *et al.* 2012; Gillett *et al.* 2015; Udyawer *et al.* 2017). In reef waters, during daylight hours and when conditions are fair (sunny, Beaufort sea state < 2), some sea snakes (e.g. olive sea snake, *Aipysurus laevis*) may be spotted at the surface by the sun reflecting off their bodies (Kerford 2005). Snakes may then be collected into a handheld, wide-mouth (45 cm square) dip net (Kerford 2005) or landing net (Gillett *et al.* 2015). Reefal species of sea snakes are also typically captured by researchers on SCUBA or snorkel by hand or directly into fish catch bags (Burns and Heatwole 1998; Lukoschek *et al.* 2007). When underwater, it is recommended that researchers take care, wear gloves and approach the snake using slow fluid movements before grasping it. If removing a sea snake from a trawler net, snake tongs may secure the animal behind its head (Redfield *et al.* 1978). Once captured, sea snakes require further care. Live snakes have been retained in floating cages (Shine *et al.* 2020), water-filled drums (Courtney *et al.* 2010) or open weave hessian sacks (Wassenberg *et al.* 1994) until sampled. It is important that snakes be kept out of temperature extremes and in a secure and ventilated receptacle (see Chapter 26).

Animal treatment, withdrawal and euthanasia

Unexpected or adverse events must be reported to the appropriate AEC and governmental marine conservation agency as soon as possible, as defined in the permit conditions. If a severely injured or diseased animal with poor potential to rehabilitate is captured, the decision may be made to euthanase the animal, usually by a veterinarian.

Equipment and maintenance

Equipment needs will vary depending on the capture methods selected but may include gear associated with safe operation of a vessel, snorkelling or SCUBA gear, gear to capture and handle animals (e.g. nets, net knives, snake tongs, spotlights), protective gear for animal handlers (e.g. wetsuits, helmets, gloves) and equipment for restraint of animal (e.g. platform, mattress, straps, shade). General paperwork will include navigational charts, maps, datasheets and permits. All equipment should be kept in safe working order.

Specific qualifications, experience and training

All techniques in this GOP should only be undertaken by experienced personnel who have worked with the target or similar taxa and the proposed methods, or under the supervision of more-experienced researchers. Personnel may require licences for operating boats or undertaking diving. Inexperienced personnel should start off by participating as observers or spotters before receiving training in direct capture methods.

Workplace health and safety

Injury from bites and crushing

Capture of large marine mammals and reptiles is associated with various risks to personnel, including bites. Bites from pinnipeds, dolphins, sea turtles and sea snakes can all cause serious injuries. Investigators should remain vigilant when working around the heads of carnivorous marine mammals and wear protective clothing (wet suits and dive booties are advised). Injuries may also be sustained from crushing or collisions, which may lead to concussion or worse in serious cases. The risk is minimised through planning and training of all personnel (see 'General procedures').

Sea snakes in Australian waters are elapids, so most species are dangerously venomous (except for the egg-eaters with vestigial fangs), delivering fast-acting immobilising neurotoxins and myotoxins; some are lethal to humans (Heatwole and Cogger 1994). How sea snakes are handled depends on the species and size of the snake but, in general, all sea snakes should be considered as potentially lethal. Only personnel familiar with handling venomous snakes should handle live sea snakes. Thick gloves, snake tongs, pressure bandages and first aid information form the basic safety kit for the sea snake researcher. Live snakes may have their heads secured within clear open-ended plastic or Perspex® tubing to reduce the risk of snakebite (Murphy 1971). Handling of dead or moribund sea snakes also poses a risk to the handler because the venom glands retain venom; a dead snake's head should be wrapped, or the jaws taped together securely, to avoid contact with the fangs.

Injury from nets, ropes

Nets and ropes should be kept coiled to avoid trip and entanglement hazards. Deployment and attendance of seine nets (dolphin capture) require operators to walk through the water and care must be taken, since entanglement is also a risk. Steel cables and winches on cranes used to hoist animals from the water present entanglement hazards. Refer to details under 'Observational studies'.

Alternative procedures

Capture is often necessary to collect biological information or attach devices. Investigators should consider if observation-only techniques may be suitable for meeting study objectives.

COLLECTING BIOLOGICAL SAMPLES AND MARKING ANIMALS

Target taxa

This GOP applies to cetaceans (dolphins, whales), pinnipeds (seals, sea lions), dugongs (Chapter 25), sea snakes and marine turtles (Chapter 26).

Context and scope

This GOP describes sampling methods including simple tissue biopsy through to more complex health assessment of wild marine mammals and reptiles, and also marking methods. Tissue biopsies yield information on genetics, reproductive condition, diet, health status and contaminants. Biological samples include skin, faeces, blood, urine, saliva and exhaled breath. Sampling techniques vary depending on the taxon and sample type and may range from distance sampling with little to no disturbance to the animal (i.e. without capture), to more-invasive biopsies and procedures after capture. Sampling of some more-tractable fully aquatic species may also be conducted out of water when samples other than skin and basic biological data are required. The value of carcasses as sources of biological materials cannot be overestimated. Several marine mammals (e.g. family Ziphidae, beaked whales) are known mostly or only from stranded carcasses (e.g. MacLeod *et al.* 2005) and necropsy of dead marine vertebrates has yielded biological information for populations and species (Beasley *et al.* 2019; Dalle Luche *et al.* 2019). For example, information on reproductive biology and diet of sea snakes has been compiled based largely on retrieval of by-catch from prawn trawlers in northern Australia (e.g. Fry *et al.* 2001; Marcos and Lanyon 2004). This GOP does not apply to large or oceanic whales, for which no routine method of capture is available.

Animal welfare considerations

Stress from handling

Only experienced practitioners should handle marine mammals and reptiles. Handling duration should be minimised to reduce the likelihood of acute stress. For fully aquatic animals sampled out of water, minimising duration of exposure and associate stress is essential. Monitoring vital signs (temperature, heart rate, respiration) and behaviour during processing is critical; abnormal signs may advise early release of the animals.

Injuries during sampling and marking

Confining marine animals out of water in small, unprotected spaces with hard substrates increases the risk of knocks, abrasion and associated infections. Marine turtles are usually immobilised by placing them on non-abrasive material (rubber matting) in a cool, shaded location. Marine mammals are usually held recumbent on smooth non-abrasive surfaces (e.g. fabric stretcher, closed-cell foam mattress, paddleboard) with physical restraint devices (e.g. foam mattresses, straps) if required.

Procedures such as tagging and biopsy may cause pain and/or infection. For turtles, a flipper tag can cause necrosis if it compresses tissue to the point of blocking vascular circulation (Balazs 1982). Improperly applied flipper tags, typically those with an excessively long piece of tag extending from the flipper, can be torn out if snagged. Tag longevity must be assessed against the risk of injury; wounds caused by abrasion can occur if tags remain attached to marine mammals for too long. In the past, hot-iron brands applied to southern elephant seals proved useful for conservation-based research, but attracted controversy (Green and Bradshaw 2004); the general consensus is that in Australia this method is ethically unacceptable for marking marine mammals.

Pain produced by the collection of a tissue biopsy sample, both at the time of collection and afterwards, is an important animal welfare consideration. The site and size of biopsy provide a rough guide as to what magnitude of pain might be expected. Using local anaesthesia to control pain at the biopsy site should be considered if practical. Capture provides the opportunity to collect tissue biopsy samples in a manner that minimises pain to an animal because local or general anaesthetics can be applied.

Exposure

Marine mammals and reptiles are susceptible to heat stress while being restrained on a boat or beach, especially during summer. Cooling may include provision of shade, wet cotton fabric placed across the body or regular dousing of the body with water. In cold extremes, space blankets (made of heat-reflective thin plastic sheeting) have been deployed to protect animals thermally. Whilst the eyes of sea turtles are protected by keratinised and mobile lids, personnel should reduce stress and avoid possible corneal sun damage by covering the animal's head while it is on land, without impeding respiration.

General procedures

Non-invasive biopsy collection from marine mammals

Common non-invasive biopsy samples collected from live marine mammals include faeces and sloughed skin from the water's surface, or scats from pinniped colonies (e.g. Kirkwood *et al.* 2008; Deagle *et al.* 2009). Faecal analysis is a powerful tool, but it is uncommon to collect freshly voided intact faecal samples from fully marine mammals and reptiles. Exceptions are dugongs in known foraging areas where faeces may float or sit on the benthos. Since many large whales feed around Antarctica and travel into Australian waters during their fasting period, it is rare to collect their faeces. Nevertheless, faeces from some large cetaceans have been collected opportunistically (Gill 2002; Stamation *et al.* 2007). Targeted collections of fresh faeces from individual cetaceans have also been achieved by trawling a fine-mesh net (0.5 mm) through slicks of defaecated material (Jarman *et al.* 2002; Nicol *et al.* 2010) or by leaning off the bow with a handheld net whilst following an animal. Odour detection dogs (see Chapter 5) that have been used to detect cetacean faeces elsewhere in the world (Rolland *et al.* 2007) have not yet been used in Australia. Sloughed skin shed from live whales can also be collected opportunistically and used for genetic characterisation (e.g. Gill 2002). Collection of environmental DNA (eDNA) in water is probably the least invasive method of all (see Chapter 4). Use of eDNA has provided insights into the distribution (presence/absence) of specific marine mammals, including in difficult-to-survey areas or where they are rare (e.g. Hunter *et al.* 2018). Although eDNA use is still in its infancy, with rigorous marker development and experimental validation it promises to expand the range of non-invasive survey techniques for marine wildlife. A novel non-invasive means of collecting excreted urine from phocid seals (e.g. Weddell seals) has been through sampling of ice (Constable *et al.* 2006).

Invasive biopsy collection from marine mammals without capture

Obtaining a biopsy of epidermis (skin) and/or blubber from a targeted marine mammal can provide information about individual identity and population assignment via genetics, sex and reproductive status through endocrinology, diet through stable isotope and fatty acid analysis, and health status through collection of samples allowing inference regarding exposure to infectious organisms, immunological function and toxicology. For large or fast marine mammals that may be difficult or impossible to capture, or for neonates whose capture presents some risk, methods of biopsy sampling require specialised sampling devices, which may comprise a firing, scraping or jabbing device that removes and retains a skin or underlying blubber sample. Each of these methods requires approaching the animal to within a distance from which a device can be deployed effectively.

Crossbows have been deployed to collect biopsy samples (Patenaude and White 1995) and to attach telemetry devices to free-swimming cetaceans, including humpback (*Megaptera novaeangliae*) and pygmy blue whales (*Balaenoptera musculus brevicauda*) in Australian waters (Gales *et al.* 2010) and from pinnipeds (Worthington Wilmer *et al.* 1999). Determining the appropriate combinations of biopsy tip lengths and diameters, and crossbow draw weights and distances, is important for obtaining a sample and reducing the wound severity respectively; prior testing on similar fresh carcasses is recommended (as per Patenaude and White, 1995). Crossbows have been largely unsuccessful on dugongs, perhaps because of their tough epidermis (R.W. Slade, pers. comm.). Crossbows are used less commonly in contemporary studies because of the need for large projectile size (the bolt), and accompanying limitations of relatively low accuracy and high impact energy, when compared to recently developed systems that use darts fired from a rifle.

Any dart rifle with a 13 mm diameter can be used to fire a biopsy dart. A commonly used dart rifle has been the Paxarms™ biopsy system (New Zealand), originally designed for small cetaceans (Krützen *et al.* 2002; Ansmann *et al.* 2015), but also used to sample whales (Gales *et al.* 2009; Attard *et al.* 2018). A more recently developed biopsy dart system has been developed by Pneu-Dart®. These systems typically fire floating (or tethered) plastic biopsy darts with a stainless-steel cutting head. The biopsy core may vary from a standard depth (2 cm, and 0.7 cm diameter) to sample epidermis, to deeper cores with dart depths of 3–20 cm and 0.8–9 mm diameter for sampling blubber. Sampling via biopsy dart relies on the dart striking then bouncing off the body (Figure 12.1). It causes mild short-term behavioural responses, and biopsy wounds that heal quickly and apparently without complications (Krützen *et al.* 2002). However, all forms of darting can create adverse animal welfare events (Hampton *et al.* 2021), and at least one mortality has been reported from a biopsy dart striking a small cetacean close to the spine with high kinetic energy (Bearzi 2000). When using such a firing device, experience and good aim to target particular body regions (e.g. dorsum), while avoiding the head region, are required. The animal also needs to be within firing range and remain at the surface for long enough for the sampler to take aim.

Handheld devices can be used to collect epidermal biopsies from marine mammals if they can be approached to within a few metres. These include biopsy syringe poles with biopsy corer ends (e.g. bow-riding dolphins, Bilgmann *et al.* 2007), skin scraping devices on the ends of poles, or even small hand-sized scrapers if the animal is within arm's reach (e.g. dugongs; Lanyon *et al.* 2010a) (Figure 12.3). This approach may be applied to mothers with neonates without the need for capture or risk of separating these individuals (e.g. dugong cows and calves; Lanyon *et al.* 2010a). Overseas, direct measurements of blubber thickness of southern right whales and North Atlantic right whales (*Eubalaena glacialis*) have been achieved using a pole-mounted ultrasound (Miller *et al.* 2011). Urine samples can be collected directly into a plastic bag attached to a long pole, such as when Weddell seals urinate during haul-out (Constable *et al.* 2006).

Over recent years, sampling in the air stream of the exhaled blow of marine mammals has allowed collection of mucosal cells from the respiratory tract for endocrine (Hogg *et al.* 2009) or genetic analysis (Frère *et al.* 2010), or samples of the respiratory tract microbiome and disease pathogens (Pirotta *et al.* 2017). A commonly used device is a collecting plate or tube (often coated with nylon tulle) on the end of a long (6–15 m) carbon fibre pole that is positioned over the animal's blowhole(s) (Hogg *et al.* 2009; Mingramm *et al.* 2019) (Figure 12.4). Biopsy collection through such close approaches of individuals is labour intensive and it may take years to collect enough samples for a robust population analysis (Seddon *et al.* 2014; Parra *et al.* 2018). Alternatively, drones can be used to collect samples. Drones equipped with sampling tubes have been directed into the exhaled airstream of large cetaceans (Pirotta *et al.* 2017; Domínguez-Sánchez *et al.* 2018) and particularly elusive dolphin species (Raudino *et al.* 2019). Photogrammetry of body size and shape to determine body condition and health status of marine mammals via drone has also become increasingly useful (Christiansen *et al.* 2018; van Aswegen *et al.* 2019).

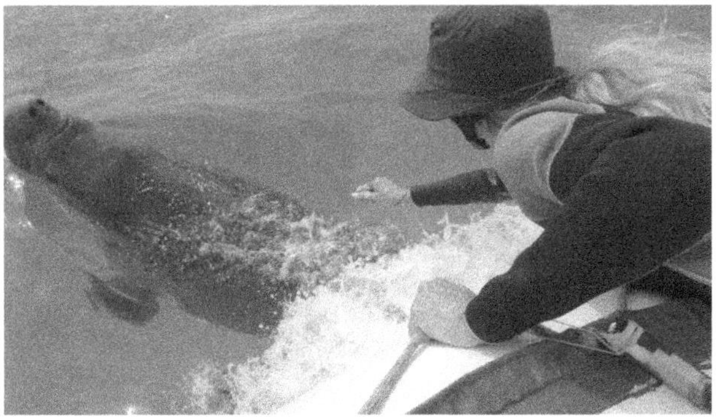

Figure 12.3: A handheld scrape device being used to collect a small skin sample from the dorsum of a surfacing dugong (*Dugong dugon*). Source: Janet Lanyon.

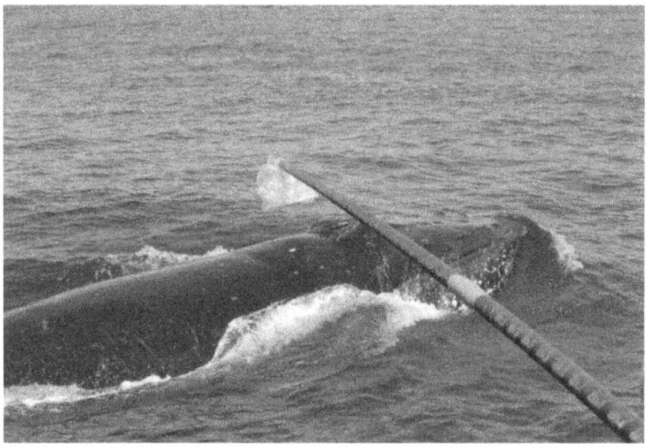

Figure 12.4: Collecting a sample of respiratory vapour (blow) from a migrating humpback whale (*Megaptera novaeangliae*) using a collecting dish on the end of a 6 m carbon fibre pole. Photo by Fletcher Mingramm.

Body morphometrics and condition

An animal's body condition (weight and muscle mass relative to body size) is a useful indicator of its overall health status. Body measurements, including standard body lengths, girths at intervals along the body or metrics of particular body parts can be measured directly for mammals < 4 m body length that are relatively docile or immobile at capture. For tractable fully marine mammals (dolphins, dugongs), it is easier to measure mid-body girths in water rather than out of water; precision and accuracy of in-water measures can then be validated through comparison with out-of-water measures (e.g. Lanyon *et al.* 2010b). Standard measures for turtles include carapace length, head length and width, plastron length, and tail length to carapace/plastron, tail length to carapace, plastron and tip to vent. Standard body measurements for sea snakes are as for most snake species (Chapter 26). Body weight determination is possible in certain situations. A gantry with weighing scale may be erected on land for pinnipeds and sea turtles, while dolphins and dugongs are hoisted in stretchers attached to a weighing device aboard a vessel.

Full body photography permits photogrammetry (interpreting measurements from photography) which is a useful tool for documenting and scaling body parts and for allometric size-weight relationships (e.g. Hodgson *et al.* 2020). Captured marine mammals can be sexed visually through examination of the anal-urinogenital region and through presence/absence of secondary sex characteristics. Animals should be visually examined for wounds, injuries and abnormal discharges from eyes, nares and body openings. The appearance of the animal's integument compared to its expected appearance is also useful as a health indicator. Beyond these superficial assessments, health is assessed by targeted sampling of blood, tissues and mucosal surfaces to survey for a range of pathogens and measure physiological parameters.

Marking animals post-capture

Recognising individual animals is essential for some behavioural and life history studies. An appropriate marking method is one that is permanent, unambiguous, and discriminates individuals effectively (Chapter 8). However, apart from some cetaceans that may be individually distinguished (e.g. humpback whales identified through unique pigmentation patterns, markings, scars or injury), for most species of marine mammal, all mostly look alike. Identity tags applied to marine mammals are diverse, often taxon-specific and include any of highly visible coloured and/or numerically coded tags that can be attached and allow for immediate identification of individuals. Other marking methods include subcutaneous implantation of tags, application of epidermal marks, or molecular tags.

Tags for pinnipeds include temporary marks, such as paint, glued material, glued devices (tracking and dive recorders), hair trimming and hair bleach (Kirkwood *et al.* 2010). Devices are typically glued to the fur of seals on the dorsal midline just posterior to the scapula, using marine-stable, two-part epoxy. Since most seals moult annually, these attachments will not last more than around 12 months. For longer-term identification, flipper tags (individually numbered) are attached to the proximal trailing edge of the fore or rear flipper (Wilkinson and Bester 1997).

Large cetaceans in Australian waters, including humpback whales (Forestell *et al.* 2011), pygmy blue whales (Jenner *et al.* 2008) and southern right whales (Charlton *et al.* 2019), are primarily identified through photo-identification. In most studies of free-ranging dolphins, photo-identification has been used to discriminate individuals (e.g. Ansmann *et al.* 2015). Despite some limitations to this approach (i.e. natural markings may change over time and some (especially young) individuals may not have recognisable marks), generally more than half of a cetacean population can usually be identified reliably (bottlenose dolphins; Markowitz *et al.* 2003). In a few studies, live free-ranging and stranded dolphins have been individually physically marked by freeze-branding the dorsal fin using iron numerals cooled in liquid nitrogen, then applied directly to the dorsal fin for between 10 and 30 s (Gales 1992; Gales and Waples 1993; Chilvers *et al.* 2001). Temporary paint tags have also been used for short-term marking. More recently, photo-identification has been combined with molecular tagging for population studies of cetacean populations (Ansmann *et al.* 2015; Parra *et al.* 2018).

In contrast, the most effective tags used for marking dugongs are always permanent gene tags based on a suite of microsatellite markers (Broderick *et al.* 2007). Combined with species-specific molecular sex markers, individual dugongs can be identified and sexed based on a skin fragment (Seddon *et al.* 2014). Dugongs have also been marked using numerically coded turtle tags applied to the trailing edge of the tail flukes, passive integrated transponder (PIT) tags that contain microchips implanted subcutaneously in the shoulder region, and a biopsy notch in the trailing fluke (Lanyon *et al.* 2006). Turtle tags have a 5 year retention rate of 80% and an 8 year retention rate of 50% on dugongs; retention rate of PIT tags is lower. Photo-identification is not appropriate for dugongs (*cf.* Anderson 1995) unless the animal has highly distinctive scarring or disfigurement. For short-term (1–5 days) marking, thick oil-based crayons (paint sticks) have been applied to the dugong's dorsum (Lanyon *et al.* 2006).

Coastal aggregations of feeding marine turtles (principally green, loggerhead and hawksbill) provide an opportunistic window of observation into otherwise widely dispersed populations (Stokes *et al.* 2014). Sea turtles in Australian foraging grounds have been studied since the 1980s and one of the keys to the success of such population level studies is identification of individuals, which leads to robust data on growth and reproductive rates. Sea turtles are individually marked with self-locking titanium tags, typically applied in the axillary position on a front flipper (Limpus and Reed 1985) (Figure 12.5). The axillary tagging position is through or immediately adjacent to the enlarged scale closest to the body on the trailing edge of either the left or right front flippers. Since all sea snakes look superficially similar, marking of individuals can be important in some studies; typical methods include microchipping (see Chapter 8) and occasionally freeze-branding (Burns and Heatwole 1998).

Collecting biopsies post-capture

In marine mammals, epidermis (skin and/or hair) can be sampled via a biopsy core (dolphins) (Bilgmann *et al.*

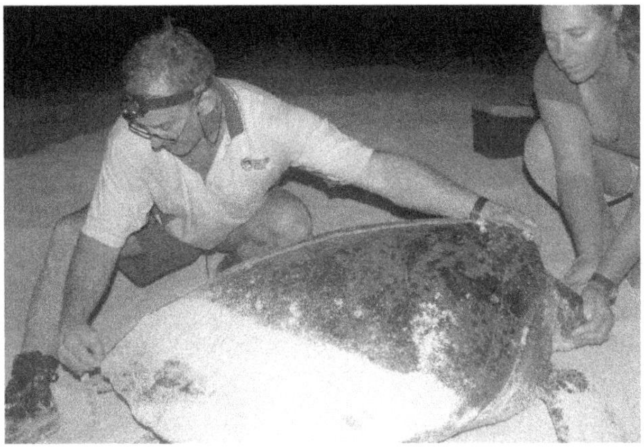

Figure 12.5: Measuring body size (carapace length) of an adult female green turtle (*Chelonia mydas*), after oviposition. Source: Ian Bell.

2007), whisker clip (otariids), hair trim (from the flank, otariids) (Lynch *et al.* 2012), skin clip from the trailing edge of the flippers (phocids, otariids) (Lancaster *et al.* 2010), skin clip from the trailing edge of the flukes (dugongs), or superficial skin scrape of the dorsum (dugongs), the final method replicating routine injury caused by tusks of conspecifics (Lanyon *et al.* 2006). In many cases, an epidermal scrub with antiseptic (e.g. povidine-iodine and/or 70% alcohol) is conducted before skin sampling, to reduce likelihood of infection of the biopsy site. Biopsy of epidermal lesions for pathology may include biopsy core, skin scrape or clip (as above) of normal and abnormal epidermis for comparison, and /or syringed aspiration of lumps. Most or all of these techniques can be conducted both in water and out of water. External parasites including barnacles on dugongs and mites on pinnipeds can be collected by hand, directly from the epidermis. Tissue samples can be stored frozen; for routine genetic analysis, samples are generally stored in 70–100% ethanol or in salt-saturated DMSO.

Skin biopsy from marine turtles usually consists of marginal carapace scute fragments sampled from the trailing edge of three posterior marginal bridging scales on each side of the carapace–plastron interface and the two supracaudal scutes. This area of carapace is scrubbed with a stiff bristled nylon brush and rinsed with seawater and 70% ethanol, before collecting ~1 g of scutes using sterilised handheld side cutters. Alternatively, for larger samples, the surgical site (typically the trailing edge of a flipper) is prepared by scrubbing with 70% alcohol before incision. Approximately 3 min after injection of lignocaine (local anaesthesia), a ~2 mm^2 piece of tissue is collected using a sterile scalpel blade. Methods for collecting tissues from snakes via tail clips are covered in Chapter 8

Blood sampling

General principles for blood collection from wildlife are detailed in Chapter 16. Blood has been successfully collected from each of pinnipeds, dolphins and dugongs out of water: phlebotomy collection sites and equipment vary among taxa, size class of the animal and researchers. Draw-in techniques vary between programs but may be via vacutainers or standard syringe. Degree of difficulty in blood collection differs between taxa. Researchers should aim to collect blood as soon as possible after capture to reduce acute stress effects on blood analytes.

For otariid pinnipeds, blood can be collected from several sites including the brachial vein, interdigitally from the hind flippers, from the extradural intravertebral vein (between vertebrae in the cervical region) or from the extramedullary vertebral sinus in the lumbar region of the spinal column (Lynch *et al.* 2012). Blood is usually collected using 18 G needles (> 38 mm in length) or butterfly needles.

For live wild dolphins, blood is typically collected by venipuncture of the plexus of superficial vessels in the dorsal surface of the tail fluke (Gales 1992) using 20–21 G needles. Blood has also been collected from the central fluke vein in a live immature Bryde's whale (*Balaenoptera edeni*) that was entrapped in a river in New South Wales (Priddel and Wheeler 1998).

In dugongs, vessels are situated more deeply and the only guaranteed site at this time is the brachial arterio-venous plexus between the ulna and radius with usual entry from the palmar surface of pectoral fin, although lateral entry is also effective. Since fusion of the ulna and radius occurs with age, the size of the collecting window is small in older dugongs. Phlebotomists should note that shifting the animal's bodyweight towards the sampled pectoral fin will assist with blood flow. Needles used are 19–21 G, and lengths vary from a standard 38 mm to larger needles for large dugongs.

Blood is collected from sea turtles from the cervical sinus (Owens and Ruiz 1980). Prior to collection, the turtle is orientated so that the head is lower than the tail, with the front flippers restrained. This may be achieved by placing the turtle on a sturdy box or digging a hole under the head if on the beach. The head is pulled forward gently until the neck is fully outstretched. The dermis of the neck is cleaned with 70% alcohol and any encrusting barnacles removed. A 21 G needle is inserted perpendicularly, approximately one cm to the side of the dorsocervical midline, in an attempt to locate the cervical sinus. After insertion, a small amount of suction is applied to the syringe and depending on turtle size, the needle may be inserted to a depth of 1–3 cm, before blood begins to flow. Blood can be drawn from sea snakes via the caudal (coccygeal) tail vein; phlebotomy is more challenging from snakes < 40 cm snout-to-vent length (Gillett *et al.* 2015).

Other body tissues

A range of body fluids/excreta can be sampled from marine mammals held out of water. Saliva can be swabbed from the oral cavities of all marine mammals via cotton swabs. After a freshwater rinse, tears can be sampled using absorbent eye spears or swabs. Exhaled breath can be collected by introducing sample tubes or plates directly into the exhaled airstream (Hogg *et al.* 2009). Faeces may be collected opportunistically from the water at capture, or from under a recumbent mammal on the sampling platform; placing shallow Frisbees™ under the anal and/or urinary orifices facilitates uncontaminated collection of faecal and urine samples (Lanyon *et al.* 2002). Alternatively, soft tubing (e.g. a latex equine yearling oesophageal tube) can be introduced into the distal rectum for an uncontaminated faecal sample for dugongs (Lanyon *et al.* 2002). Milk may be expressed from lactating dugong cows through gentle downwards squeezing of the axillary teat. In seals, administering 5–10 UI ml^{-1} oxytocin intramuscularly several minutes beforehand assists milk flow in studies of milk composition (Arnould and Hindell 1999). Pinniped scent has been collected for studies of individual chemical recognition by sea lions by rubbing clean cotton swabs against their fur (Wierucka *et al.* 2019).

To determine the recent diet of a dugong, mouth contents can be collected by hand. For a foraging turtle, an oesophageal lavage sample may be collected (Forbes and Limpus 1993). Turtles are placed plastron-down on a ~500 mm high stand. The head is gently extended posteriorly, and a 19 mm diameter PVC tube is inserted into the mouth to restrict the crushing effect exerted through the jaws. An 8 mm diameter soft plastic water-delivery tube is then inserted down through the PVC tube, along the oesophagus and into the anterior section of the crop, being careful to avoid entering the glottis. Clean seawater is introduced through the central smaller tube using a low-volume foot or hand operated pump to control flow rate. Discharged ingesta, along with waste water, is collected in a 1 mm mesh net held under the turtle's mouth. Sampling is conducted for a maximum of 2 min after tube insertion and water delivery, and turtles are then kept under observation before release.

Collection of data on nesting turtles and eggs

Typically, nesting females are released at the nest site within ~10 min of capture following tagging and measuring. Disturbance is kept within the level that the turtles are normally exposed to at that breeding site so that seasonal egg production of individual turtles is not altered. The main principles governing management of the research team's activities include not approaching turtles as they leave the sea or search for nest sites, and minimising use of lights visible to, and in close proximity of, a nesting turtle before her commencement of oviposition (egg laying). Turtles do not always lay eggs on each visit to a nesting beach. Turtles that have aborted a nesting attempt may be sampled before their return to the sea. Sampling a nesting turtle may include measurements of curved carapace (body) length and checking for flipper tags on the trailing edge of left and right front flippers and/or application of a tag (Eckert *et al.* 1999). Any visible injury to the turtle should be recorded.

If appropriate, the collection of morphometric data for eggs should be completed within 2 h of being laid. During the opening of the nest, lifting eggs from the nest, counting of the eggs, and returning eggs to the nest, there should be no vertical rotation of the eggs, and horizontal rotation of the eggs should be kept to a minimum. Eggs being relocated during the heat of the day should be kept shaded (Miller 1997). Except in specifically defined experiments, marine turtle hatchlings are kept at a temperature not exceeding the nest temperature for their beach (usually 25–32°C) and are kept dry until they are released at or adjacent to the nest site within 2 h of hatchling emergence. Because hatchlings do not drink or feed while digging from the nest, nor while crossing the beach, hatchlings are not offered food or water during the above period (Miller 1997). Magnetic imprinting occurs when the hatchlings are leaving the nest and crossing the beach (Lohmann *et al.* 2004), so hatchlings should not be retained in metal containers or wire cages – plastic mesh cages, cloth bags and plastic buckets are the preferred containers. Because there is a strong possibility that hatchlings undergo chemosensory imprinting when they first contact water, hatchlings should not be held in containers of water but instead released into natural seawater. Marine turtle hatchlings should be released on the beach to ensure that they are correctly oriented as they enter the sea and to allow natural imprinting processes that may occur whilst they cross the beach.

Animal treatment, withdrawal and euthanasia

Refer to 'Capture methods' earlier in this chapter.

Equipment and maintenance

Equipment needs will vary depending on the sampling methods selected. All equipment should be kept meticulously clean and in good working order. Non-disposable sampling equipment that is to be used for more than one animal should be cleaned and sterilised between uses (e.g. with 70% alcohol).

Specific qualifications, experience and training

Sampling wild marine mammals and reptiles requires specialist knowledge of where and when to locate them, their behavioural responses to approach, capture and handling, and experience in using sampling equipment. Each of the described programs is overseen by senior researchers. There may be no formal training requirement in general. However, most research programs in these fields will specifically train their staff and expect some close involvement in the program before being assigned pivotal roles. All key operators should be confident and competent and with sufficient background knowledge and experience to perform the tasks efficiently. New operators must be accompanied and trained by an experienced supervisor to ensure competency as determined by the organisation; this is usually a requirement of AECs. If using a motorised boat or drone, the driver must hold the relevant licences and permits required for the activity by current legislation and be skilled in their operation.

For some procedures, specialist veterinary experience /qualifications may be required, such as for advanced surgical procedures, management of challenging anaesthetic procedures (see Chapter 16), ultrasonography or other advanced diagnostic procedures in the case of necessary euthanasia.

Workplace health and safety

Refer to 'Capture methods' earlier in this chapter.

Alternative procedures

There may be value to sampling of marine wildlife by non-invasive means exclusively (e.g. through opportunistic collection of sloughed skin, faeces and shed hair), as long as the researcher is aware of problems that might arise because of the small amounts of material collected, degradation of samples (and DNA) exposed to the elements and uncertainty regarding identity of the individual.

ATTACHMENT OF DEVICES

Target taxa

This GOP applies to cetaceans (dolphins, whales), pinnipeds (seals, sea lions), and dugongs (Chapter 25), and sea snakes and marine turtles (Chapter 26).

Context and scope

This GOP describes methods and considerations for attaching external devices to marine mammals and reptiles to monitor movements, migrations and behaviour. Telemetric devices include global positioning system (GPS), satellite, VHF radio and acoustic tags. Behavioural trackers include time-depth recorders (TDRs), digital recording tags (DTAGs) and animal-mounted cameras. Choice of attachment method depends on the taxa, size and approachability of the animal, size of the device and required deployment period. Telemetric (tracking) tags may be attached to the animal subcutaneously (penetrating devices), with an external attachment to the epidermis or body part, or with a harness. Device configuration and design are specific to the research question and are not covered here, except for factors that affect animal welfare.

Animal welfare considerations

Key animal welfare considerations include changes to normal behaviour, and risk of injury and infection. Devices are intended to monitor 'normal' behaviour, so they must be designed to avoid impeding movement through increased drag, and avoid detectable energetic costs. The device must be sufficiently secure to maintain position and orientation on the animal's body without causing abrasion, and discrete so that it does not repel conspecifics or attract predators. In marine environments, corrosion of metallic components, and biofouling of devices by barnacles and algae, may occur over time; these may affect device function, increase drag or present injury risks.

Impediment to normal behaviours

Behavioural responses of an animal to the presence of an attached device should be considered. Some bottlenose dolphins undertake long-distance movements immediately after release with an attached device (Irvine *et al.* 1982; Mate *et al.* 1995) while others do not change behaviour appreciably (Chilvers *et al.* 2001). Similarly, some dugongs fitted with towed satellite transmitters immediately moved large distances (across embayments or between feeding grounds) (C. Limpus, pers. comm.); these behaviours do not normally occur after routine capture and health sampling. Size, positioning and drag of the device are all considerations when evaluating an animal's behavioural response to tagging.

Injury and infection

Attaching devices to marine mammals and reptiles comes with a risk of device migration (for implanted tags), injury (e.g. abrasion, tears/rips, pressure marks) or secondary infection over time. Deeper penetration to the underlying body musculature should be avoided when using penetrating tags because doing so may prolong attachment and create scarring. Prior knowledge of the target animal's anatomy and dermal composition is required. Devices attached via an external harness must comprise robust and resilient materials (UV and seawater-proof) and parts that contact the animal's skin directly must be uniformly smooth, non-abrasive and relatively non-corrodible; swivel attachments may reduce the risk of entanglement if protruding parts are involved. Deployment period must be considered so that fouling or deterioration of the device does not introduce risk to the animal or study objectives over time. A detachment or release method, or plan for retrieval, must be configured into the original device design and planning.

General procedures

Key considerations

The marine environment presents physical challenges to resilience and longevity of devices, and to detection of tracking signals and data retrieval. Seawater attenuates radio signals, so that placement of a tracking device high on an animal's body (e.g. high on dorsum, carapace or head) is critical to maximising the time that the signal or saltwater transmission switch is at or above the water's surface. Habits of the taxon or individual (e.g. time at surface and out of water) also influence the devices' efficacy and attachment methods.

Subcutaneous and carapace tags

Subcutaneous penetrant tags (e.g. e-tag, satellite tags) have been deployed on large cetaceans (e.g. humpback and pygmy blue whales) *sans* capture as projectiles fired from a compound crossbow or compressed air gun (Gales *et al.* 2009; Garcia-Rojas *et al.* 2018). In these cases, whales must be approached to within a safe and workable distance (e.g. within 5 m). When closer proximity is possible, syringe poles deployed from the bowsprit of a boat can be used to attach penetrating devices to cetaceans (Mate *et al.* 2000; Heide-Jørgensen *et al.* 2001). Penetrant tags must have sharp cutting edges for clean entry, must be applied with sufficient force to penetrate well within the blubber layer, and have recurved barbs to ensure retention.

For marine turtles, acoustic tags can be secured to the ventral surface of one (usually the left) supracaudal scute by drilling a 6 mm diameter hole, using a rechargeable electric drill, then passing a 6 × 50 mm stainless steel bolt through the tag and carapace, and securing the tag with a Nyloc™ self-locking nut. A second hole is drilled ~50 mm posterior to the initial attachment point and also fitted with a 6 × 50 mm stainless steel bolt and nut (Bell and Parmenter 2008).

Fin and suction-cup attachments

Only a few Australian studies have attached devices to dolphins, but all have used the dorsal fin as an anchor point. Transmitter packages have been attached directly to the dorsal fin using a snugly fitting belt with neoprene lining (Corkeron and Martin 2004), plastic Delrin® bolts (Gales and Waples 1993) or monofilament fishing line treaded through the fin and held by a corrodible steel washer so that the entire instrument would be shed after a time (Chilvers *et al.* 2001). Such attachments are associated with the risk of epidermal discolouration or necrosis, and migration of the fasteners out of the dorsal fin may cause disfigured or scarred fins. Less-invasive short-term device attachment methods include suction cups applied directly onto a whale's dorsum (Noad *et al.* 2004). A series of suction cups with DTAGs have been attached to the dorsum of humpback whales by making a slapping action with a 12 m long pole attached to a pivot on the bow of the boat; these attachments detach after ~4 h (Cato *et al.* 2012). Suction cups have been trialled on captive dugongs, but the animals' propensity to rub their dorsum along the benthos quickly dislodged the device.

Glued attachments following capture

For smaller, more-tractable marine mammals, or following anaesthesia, devices can be attached after capture. In pinnipeds, small devices (e.g. geolocators) may be glued to flipper tags, but generally devices are glued to the hair or fur. As with all marine animals, devices should be as hydrodynamic as possible to minimise drag; chiton-shaped devices are ideal. The weight and cross-sectional surface area of the device should be as small as possible and the placement location on the body chosen carefully to minimise drag (Kay *et al.* 2019). Tag placement must also take into consideration non-impedance of normal body movements (e.g. flipper motion) and ability to operate properly, for example, for tracking devices to transmit data to satellites while at sea. For example, for phocid seals, satellite tracking devices need to be placed on the head or just behind the neck, because when surfacing to breath (and collect or transmit location data) these seals often lift only their heads clear of the water. Accelerometers, that can measure movement in all directions and often aim to record feeding events, are also best placed on the head. As they are attached to the fur and most pinnipeds moult annually, the longest periods of attachment are obtained by attaching the devices as soon as possible after the animal has moulted. Often devices need to be recovered to retrieve their data, or to be reused. Recovery may involve trimming the fur under the instrument or cutting through a neoprene strip specifically used between the instrument and the integument to facilitate removal. Devices attached to seals in Australia, listed approximately by increasing size, include geolocators, VHF transmitters, accelerometers, heart-rate recorders, TDRs, satellite and GPS trackers, and crittercams (Hindell *et al.* 1991; Kirkwood *et al.* 2006; Volpov *et al.* 2015).

Satellite tags can be glued directly onto the carapace of hard-shelled turtles. The best location, to reduce hydrodynamic drag, is centrally on the carapace near the head. The attachment footprint should be only marginally larger than the tag base. The combined weight of the tag and glue should not exceed 3% of the turtle's body mass (NMFS 2008). Devices should only be attached to healthy individuals. Barnacles that may interfere with attachment are removed and the carapace cleaned with seawater and a scouring pad, then dried thoroughly. The section of carapace identified for the tag should be sanded to remove any encrusting algae or biofilm, using 180 grit sandpaper and cleaned with ≥ 70% alcohol. The tag should then be bedded in an epoxy adhesive and allowed to dry.

Belt and harness attachments

For dugongs, tracking devices (GPS, satellite tag, acoustic tag, TDR) are usually attached via a peduncle belt, modelled on a system designed for Florida manatees (*Trichechus manatus latirostris*) (Marsh and Rathbun 1990). The belt consists of a padded and adjustable peduncle loop attached to a semi-rigid tether (e.g. 2 m polypropylene rod) ending in a buoyant floating canister containing the transmitter (Marsh and Rathbun 1990). This design maximises the time that the transmitter is at the surface, while the dugong is foraging in shallow water (< 3 m). The peduncle belt must include a detachment device (e.g. corrodible link made of brass, steel or zinc bolts, and/or a pop-up device), to avoid excessively long deployment and wounding by the belt. Some issues do arise for dugongs using this device attachment method: the belt and transmitter housing are prone to biofouling, the belt covering (usually latex rubber) may deteriorate causing chafing over protracted deployments, and the towed transmitter housing may bump along the benthos even when dugongs are feeding in shallow (< 2 m) water. Towing a transmitter may cause behavioural irregularities, at least in the short term, but possibly over days, resulting in unusual long-range movements. Researchers are urged to review this design in future studies, considering the faster, more-pelagic nature of dugongs compared to Florida manatees.

For soft-shelled turtles, such as leatherbacks, two attachment methods can be used: a custom-fitted harness system (structured like a backpack) to hold a satellite tag in place above the carapace, or a direct attachment method, requiring drilling of the turtle's highly vascularised cartilaginous carapace. The direct attachment method requires channels to be drilled through the longitudinal carapacial ridges, and then wire, ties or other foreign materials are laced through the drill channels to secure the instruments. This method effectively precludes complete healing for as long as these materials are in place. Devices can only be attached to flatback turtles (*Natator depressus*), with the harness method.

Surgical implantation and ingestible devices

Small acoustic transmitters have been surgically implanted into the peritoneal cavity of sea snakes after administration of local anaesthetic (lignocaine) (Udyawer *et al.* 2017). The small ventrolateral incision (~2 cm) was closed using monofilament surgical sutures and the snakes allowed to recover in individual holding tanks for 4 or 5 days post-surgery before tracking experiments. Small acoustic transmitters have also been introduced into sea snakes via the digestive tract (Burns and Heatwole 1998). In this case, live foraging sea snakes were hand-fed small, fresh fish containing concealed transmitters. As the meal digested, the transmitter lodged in the snake's stomach. At the end of a 9 day period (as the battery signal weakened), the snakes were recaptured and regurgitation was induced to retrieve the transmitter, with no apparent adverse effects on the snakes (Burns and Heatwole 1998).

Animal treatment, withdrawal and euthanasia

Refer to 'Capture methods' earlier in this chapter.

Equipment and maintenance

Refer to 'Collecting biological samples and marking animals' earlier in this chapter.

Specific qualifications, experience and training

Techniques for attaching devices described in this GOP should only be undertaken by experienced personnel or under the direct supervision of more-experienced researchers. For some advanced technical procedures (e.g. anaesthesia) and under some permit regulations, veterinarians may need to participate.

Workplace health and safety

Refer to 'Capture methods' earlier in this chapter.

Alternative procedures

Attachment of devices is typically necessary to collect specific biological and life-history information, which is difficult with other techniques. Investigators should consider if observation-only techniques may be suitable for meeting study objectives.

REFERENCES

Allan BM, Ierodiaconou D, Hoskins AJ, Arnould JP (2019) A rapid UAV method for assessing body condition in fur seals. *Drones* **3**, 24. doi:10.3390/drones3010024

Anderson PK (1995) Scarring and photoidentification of dugongs (*Dugong dugong*) in Shark Bay, Western Australia. *Aquatic Mammals* **21**, 205–212.

Ansmann IC, Lanyon JM, Seddon JM, Parra GJ (2015) Habitat and resource partitioning among Indo-Pacific bottlenose dolphins in Moreton Bay, Australia. *Marine Mammal Science* **31**, 211–230. doi:10.1111/mms.12153

Arnold PW, Birtles RA, Sobtzick S, Matthews M, Dunstan A (2005) Gulping behaviour in rorqual whales: underwater observations and functional interpretation. *Memoirs of the Queensland Museum* **51**, 309–332.

Arnould JPY, Hindell MA (1999) The composition of Australian fur seal (*Arctocephalus pusillus doriferus*) milk throughout lactation. *Physiological and Biochemical Zoology* **72**, 605–612. doi:10.1086/316702

Attard CR, Beheregaray LB, Sandoval-Castillo J, Jenner KCS, Gill PC, Jenner MNM, *et al.* (2018) From conservation genetics to conservation genomics: a genome-wide assessment of blue whales (*Balaenoptera musculus*) in Australian feeding aggregations. *Royal Society Open Science* **5**, 170925. doi:10.1098/rsos.170925

Back J, Hoskins AJ, Kirkwood RJ, Arnould JPY (2018) Behavioral responses of Australian fur seals to boat approaches at a breeding colony. *Nature Conservation* **31**, 35–52. doi:10.3897/natureconservation.31.26263

Balazs GH (1982) Factors affecting the retention of metal tags on sea turtles. *Marine Turtle Newsletter* **20**, 11–14.

Bannister JL, Hedley SL (2001) Southern Hemisphere Group IV humpback whales: their status from recent aerial surveys. *Memoirs of the Queensland Museum* **47**, 587–598.

Bearzi GI (2000) First report of a common dolphin (*Delphinus delphis*) death following penetration of a biopsy dart. *The Journal of Cetacean Research and Management* **2**, 217–222.

Beasley I, Cherel Y, Robinson S, Betty E, Hagihara R, Gales R (2019) Stomach contents of long-finned pilot whales, *Globicephala melas* mass-stranded in Tasmania. *PLoS One* **14**, e0206747. doi:10.1371/journal.pone.0206747

Bell IP, Parmenter CJ (2008) The diving behavior of inter-nesting hawksbill turtles, *Eretmochelys imbricata* (Linnaeus 1766), on Milman Island reef, Queensland, Australia. *Herpetological Conservation and Biology* **3**, 254–263.

Bilgmann K, Griffiths OJ, Allen SJ, Möller LM (2007) A biopsy pole system for bow-riding dolphins: sampling success, behavioral responses, and test for sampling bias. *Marine Mammal Science* **23**, 218–225. doi:10.1111/j.1748-7692.2006.00099.x

Broderick D, Ovenden J, Slade R, Lanyon JM (2007) Characterisation of 26 new microsatellite loci in the dugong (*Dugong dugon*). *Molecular Ecology Notes* **7**, 1275–1277. doi:10.1111/j.1471-8286.2007.01853.x

Bryden MM (1985) Studies of humpback whales (*Megaptera novaeangliae*), Area V. In *Studies of Sea Mammals in South Latitudes* (Eds JK Ling and MM Bryden) pp. 115–23. South Australian Museum, Adelaide.

Bryson M, Williams S (2015) *Review of Unmanned Aerial Systems (UAS) for Marine Surveys*. Australian Centre for Field Robotics, University of Sydney.

Burns G, Heatwole H (1998) Home range and habitat use of the olive sea snake, *Aipysurus laevis*, on the Great Barrier Reef, Australia. *Journal of Herpetology* **32**, 350–358. doi:10.2307/1565449

Cato D, Noad M, Dunlop R, McCauley R, Gales N, Salgado-Kent C, Kniest H, Paton D, Jenner C, Noad J, Maggi A (2012) Project BRAHSS: behavioural response of Australian humpback whales to seismic surveys. In *Proceedings of the Acoustical Society of Australia*, 2012.

Charlton C, Ward R, McCauley RD, Brownell Jr RL, Salgado Kent C, Burnell S (2019) Southern right whale (*Eubalaena australis*), seasonal abundance and distribution at Head of Bight, South Australia. *Aquatic Conservation* **29**, 576–588. doi:10.1002/aqc.3032

Chilvers BL, Corkeron PJ, Blanshard WH, Long TR, Martin AR (2001) A new VHF tag and attachment technique for small cetaceans. *Aquatic Mammals* **27**, 11–15.

Christiansen F, Nielsen ML, Charlton C, Bejder L, Madsen PT (2020) Southern right whales show no behavioral response to low noise levels from a nearby unmanned aerial vehicle. *Marine Mammal Science* **36**, 953–963. doi:10.1111/mms.12699

Christiansen F, Vivier F, Charlton C, Ward R, Amerson A, Burnell S, Bejder L (2018) Maternal body size and condition determine calf growth rates in southern right whales. *Marine Ecology Progress Series* **592**, 267–281. doi:10.3354/meps12522

Constable S, Parslow A, Dutton G, Rogers T, Hogg C (2006) Urinary cortisol sampling: a non-invasive technique for examining cortisol concentrations in the Weddell seal, *Leptonychotes weddellii. Zoo Biology* **25**, 137–144. doi:10.1002/zoo.20088

Corkeron PJ, Brown M, Slade RW, Bryden MM (1994) Humpback whales, *Megaptera novaeangliae* (Cetaceaa: Balaenopteridae), in Hervey Bay, Queensland. *Wildlife Research* **21**, 293–305. doi:10.1071/WR9940293

Corkeron PJ, Martin AR (2004) Ranging and diving behaviour of two 'offshore' bottlenose dolphins, *Tursiops* sp., off eastern Australia. *Journal of the Marine Biological Association of the United Kingdom* **84**, 465. doi:10.1017/S0025315404009464h

Courtney AJ, Schemel BL, Wallace R, Campbell MJ, Mayer DG, Young B (2010) Reducing the impact of Queensland's trawl fisheries on protected sea snakes. FRDC Report Project No. 2005/053.

Cowling M, Kirkwood R, Boren L, Scarpaci C (2015) The effects of vessel approaches on the New Zealand fur seal (*Arctocephalus forsteri*) in the Bay of Plenty, New Zealand. *Marine Mammal Science* **31**, 501–519. doi:10.1111/mms.12171

Dalle Luche G, Bengtson Nash S, Kucklick J, Mingramm FM, Boggs S (2019) Liquid chromatography tandem mass spectrometry for the quantification of steroid hormone profiles in blubber from stranded humpback whales (*Megaptera novaeangliae*). *Conservation Physiology* **7**, coz030. doi:10.1093/conphys/coz030

DAWE (2020) Whale and dolphin watching. <http://www.environment.gov.au/marine/marine-species/cetaceans/whale-and-dolphin-watching>.

Deagle B, Kirkwood R, Jarman S (2009) Analysis of Australian fur seal diet by pyrosequencing prey DNA in faeces. *Molecular Ecology* **18**, 2022–2038. doi:10.1111/j.1365-294X.2009.04158.x

Domínguez-Sánchez CA, Acevedo-Whitehouse KA, Gendron D (2018) Effect of drone-based blow sampling on blue whale (*Balaenoptera musculus*) behavior. *Marine Mammal Science* **34**, 841–850. doi:10.1111/mms.12482

Eckert KL, Bjorndal KA, Abreu-Grobois FA, Donnelly M (1999) *Research and Management Techniques for the Conservation Of Sea Turtles.* IUCN/SSC Marine Turtle Specialist Group, Washington, DC.

Fair PA, Schaefer AM, Romano TA, Bossart GD, Lamb SV, Reif JS (2014) Stress response of wild bottlenose dolphins (*Tursiops truncatus*) during capture–release health assessment studies. *General and Comparative Endocrinology* **206**, 203–212. doi:10.1016/j.ygcen.2014.07.002

Forbes G, Limpus C (1993) A non-lethal method for retrieving stomach contents from sea turtles. *Wildlife Research* **20**, 339–343. doi:10.1071/WR9930339

Forestell PH, Kaufman GD, Chaloupka M (2011) Long term trends in abundance of humpback whales in Hervey Bay, Australia. *The Journal of Cetacean Research and Management* **3**, 237–241.

Frère CH, Krzyszczy E, Patterson EM, Hunter S, Ginsburg A (2010) Thar she blows! A novel method for DNA collection from cetacean blow. *PLoS One* **5**, e12299. doi:10.1371/journal.pone.0012299

Fry GC, Milton DA, Wassenberg TJ (2001) The reproductive biology and diet of sea snake bycatch of prawn trawling in northern Australia: characteristics important for assessing the impacts on populations. *Pacific Conservation Biology* **7**, 55–73. doi:10.1071/PC010055

Gales NJ (1992) Mass stranding of striped dolphin, *Stenella coeruleoalba*, at Augusta, Western Australia: notes on clinical pathology and general observations. *Journal of Wildlife Diseases* **28**, 651–655. doi:10.7589/0090-3558-28.4.651

Gales N, Waples K (1993) The rehabilitation and release of bottlenose dolphins from Atlantis Marine Park, Western Australia. *Aquatic Mammals* **19**, 49–59.

Gales NJ, Double MC, Robinson SA, Jenner CU, Jenner MI, King ER, Gedamke JA, Paton DA, Raymond B (2009) Satellite tracking of southbound East Australian humpback whales (*Megaptera novaeangliae*): challenging the feast or famine model for migrating whales. *International Whaling Commission*: SC61/SH17.

Gales N, Double MC, Robinson SA, Jenner CU, Jenner MI, King ER, Gedamke JA, Childerhouse SI, Paton DA (2010) Satellite tracking of Australian humpback (*Megaptera novaeangliae*) and pygmy blue whales (*Balaenoptera musculus brevicauda*). White paper presented to the Scientific Committee of the International Whaling Commission.

Garcia-Rojas MI, Jenner KCS, Gill PC, Jenner MNM, Sutton AL, McCauley RD (2018) Environmental evidence for a pygmy blue whale aggregation area in the Subtropical Convergence Zone south of Australia. *Marine Mammal Science* **34**, 901–923. doi:10.1111/mms.12494

Garlepp L, Logan M, Kirkwood R (2014) Climatic correlates of haul-out behaviour in Australian fur seals (*Arctocephalus pusillus doriferus*). *Marine Mammal Science* **30**, 978–993. doi:10.1111/mms.12094

Gill PC (2002) A blue whale (Balaenoptera musculus) feeding ground in a southern Australian coastal upwelling zone. *The Journal of Cetacean Research and Management* **4**, 179–184.

Gillett AK, Flint M, Hulse L, Hanger J, Mills PC (2015) Haematological and biochemical reference intervals for three species of hydrophiine sea snakes (*Hydrophis curtus, H. elegans and H. peronii*). *Australian Veterinary Journal* **204**, 275–281. doi:10.1016/j.tvjl.2015.04.008

Green JJ, Bradshaw CJ (2004) The 'capacity to reason' in conservation biology and policy: the southern elephant seal branding controversy. *Journal for Nature Conservation* **12**, 25–39. doi:10.1016/j.jnc.2004.04.001

Green K, Burton HR, Wong V, McFarlane RA, Flaherty AA, Pahl BC, Haigh SA (1995) Difficulties in assessing population status of ice seals. *Wildlife Research* **22**, 193–199. doi:10.1071/WR9950193

Groom CJ, Coughran DK (2012) Entanglements of baleen whales off the coast of Western Australia between 1982 and 2010: patterns of occurrence, outcomes and management responses. *Pacific Conservation Biology* **18**, 203–214.

Hampton JO, Arnemo JM, Barnsley R, Cattet M, Daoust PY, DeNicola AJ, Eccles G, Fletcher D, Hinds LA, Hunt R, Portas T (2021) Animal welfare testing for shooting and darting free-ranging wildlife: a review and recommendations. *Wildlife Research.* Online early. doi:10.1071/WR20107

Hart LB, Wells RS, Kellar N, Balmer BC, Hohn AA, Lamb SV, *et al.* (2015) Adrenal hormones in common bottlenose dolphins (*Tursiops truncatus*): Influential factors and reference intervals. *PLoS One* **10**, e0127432. doi:10.1371/journal.pone.0127432

Heatwole H, Cogger HG (1994) Sea snake toxinology. In *Sea snakes of Australia* (Eds H Heatwole and HG Cogger) pp. 167–205. Singapore University Press, Singapore.

Hedley SL, Bannister JL, Dunlop RA (2011) Abundance estimates of Southern Hemisphere breeding stock 'D' humpback whales from aerial and land-based surveys off Shark Bay, Western Australia 2008. *The Journal of Cetacean Research and Management* **3**, 209–221.

Heide-Jørgensen MP, Kleivane L, Ølen N, Laidre KL, Jensen MV (2001) A new technique for deploying satellite transmitters on baleen whales: Tracking a blue whale (*Balaenoptera musculus*) in the North Atlantic. *Marine Mammal Science* **17**, 949–954. doi:10.1111/j.1748-7692.2001.tb01309.x

Hindell MA, Burton HR (1987) Past and present status of the southern elephant seal (*Mirounga leonina*) at Macquarie Island. *Journal of Zoology* **213**, 365–380. doi:10.1111/j.1469-7998.1987.tb03712.x

Hindell MA, Slip DJ, Burton HR (1991) The diving behavior of adult male and female southern elephant seals, *Mirounga leonina* (Pinnipedia, Phocidae). *Australian Journal of Zoology* **39**, 595–619. doi:10.1071/ZO9910595

Hodgson A, Kelly N, Peel D (2013) Unmanned aerial vehicles (UAVs) for surveying marine fauna: a dugong case study. *PLoS One* **8**, e79556. doi:10.1371/journal.pone.0079556

Hodgson AJ, Marsh H (2007) Response of dugongs to boat traffic: the risk of disturbance and displacement. *Journal of Experimental Marine Biology and Ecology* **340**, 50–61. doi:10.1016/j.jembe.2006.08.006

Hodgson JC, Holman D, Terauds A, Koh LP, Goldsworthy SD (2020) Rapid condition monitoring of an endangered marine vertebrate using precise, non-invasive morphometrics. *Biological Conservation* **242**. doi:10.1016/j.biocon.2019.108402

Hogg CJ, Rogers TL, Shorter A, Barton K, Miller PJO, Nowacek D (2009) Determination of steroid hormones in whale blow: it is possible. *Marine Mammal Science* **25**, 605–618. doi:10.1111/j.1748-7692.2008.00277.x

Holley DK (2006) Movement patterns and habitat usage of Shark Bay dugongs. MSc thesis. Edith Cowan University, Australia.

Hunter ME, Meigs-Friend G, Ferrante JA, Takoukam AK, D'orazio RM, Keith-Diagne L, Luna F, Lanyon JM, Reid JP (2018) Surveys of environmental DNA (eDNA): a new approach to estimate occurrence in vulnerable manatee populations. *Endangered Species Research* **35**, 101–111. doi:10.3354/esr00880

Irvine AB, Wells RS, Scott MD (1982) An evaluation of techniques for tagging small odontocete cetaceans. *Fishery Bulletin* **80**, 135–143.

Jarman SN, Gales NJ, Tierney M, Gill PC, Elliott NG (2002) A DNA-based method for identification of krill species and its application to analysing the diet of marine vertebrate predators. *Molecular Ecology* **11**, 2679–2690. doi:10.1046/j.1365-294X.2002.01641.x

Jenner C, Jenner M, Burton C, Sturrock V, Salgado Kent C, Morrice M, Attard C, Möller L, Double M (2008) Mark recapture analysis of pygmy blue whales from the Perth Canyon, Western Australia 2000–2005. *Scientific Committee of the International Whaling Commission*, SC/60/SH16.

Kay WP, Naumann DS, Bowen HJ, Withers SJ, Evans BJ, Wilson RP, Stringell TB, Bull JC, Hopkins PW, Börger L (2019) Minimizing the impact of biologging devices: using computational fluid dynamics for optimizing tag design and positioning. *Methods in Ecology and Evolution* **10**, 1222–1233. doi:10.1111/2041-210X.13216

Kerford M (2005). The ecology of the bar bellied sea snake (*Hydrophis elegans*) in Shark Bay, Western Australia. PhD thesis. Simon Fraser University, Canada.

Kirkwood R, Goldsworthy SD (2013) *Fur Seals and Sea Lions*. Australian Natural History Series. CSIRO Publishing, Melbourne.

Kirkwood R, Hume F, Hindell M (2008) Sea temperature variations mediate annual changes in the diet of Australian fur seals in Bass Strait. *Marine Ecology Progress Series* **369**, 297–309. doi:10.3354/meps07633

Kirkwood R, Lynch M, Gales N, Dann P, Sumner M (2006) At sea movements and habitat use of adult male Australian fur seals (*Arctocephalus pusillus doriferus*). *Canadian Journal of Zoology* **84**, 1781–1788. doi:10.1139/z06-164

Kirkwood R, Pemberton D, Gales R, Hoskins AJ, Mitchell T, Shaughnessy PD, Arnould JPY (2010) Continued population recovery by Australian fur seals. *Marine and Freshwater Research* **61**, 695–701. doi:10.1071/MF09213

Krützen M, Barré LM, Möller LM, Heithaus MR, Simms C, Sherwin WB (2002) A biopsy system for small cetaceans: darting success and wound healing in *Tursiops* spp. *Marine Mammal Science* **18**, 863–878. doi:10.1111/j.1748-7692.2002.tb01078.x

Lancaster ML, Arnould JPY, Kirkwood R (2010) Genetic status of an endemic marine mammal, the Australian fur seal, following historical harvesting. *Animal Conservation* **13**, 247–255. doi:10.1111/j.1469-1795.2009.00325.x

Lanyon JM, Slade RW, Sneath HL, Broderick D, Kirkwood JM, Limpus D, Limpus CJ, Jessop T (2006) A method for capturing dugongs (*Dugong dugon*) in open water. *Aquatic Mammals* **32**, 196–201. doi:10.1578/AM.32.2.2006.196

Lanyon JM, Sneath HL, Kirkwood JM, Slade RW (2002) Establishing a mark-recapture program for dugongs in Moreton Bay, south-east Queensland. *Australian Mammalogy* **24**, 51–56. doi:10.1071/AM02051

Lanyon JM, Sneath HL, Long T (2010*a*) Three skin sampling methods for molecular characterisation of free-ranging dugong (*Dugong dugon*) populations. *Aquatic Mammals* **36**, 298–306. doi:10.1578/AM.36.3.2010.298

Lanyon JM, Sneath HL, Long T, Bonde RK (2010*b*) Physiological response of wild dugongs (*Dugong dugon*) to out-of-water sampling for health assessment. *Aquatic Mammals* **36**, 46–58. doi:10.1578/AM.36.1.2010.46

Limpus CJ, Reed PC (1985) The green turtle, *Chelonia mydas*, in Queensland: a preliminary description of the population structure in a coral reef feeding ground. In *Biology of Australasian frogs and reptiles*. (Eds G Grigg, R Shine and H Ehmann) pp. 47–52. Surrey Beatty and Sons, Sydney.

Limpus CJ, Walter DG (1980) The growth of immature green turtles (*Chelonia mydas*) under natural conditions. *Herpetologica* **1**, 162–165.

Little GJ (1995) Body temperature in the newborn southern elephant seal, *Mirounga leonina*, at Macquarie Island. *Marine Mammal Science* **11**, 480–490. doi:10.1111/j.1748-7692.1995.tb00671.x

Lohmann KJ, Lohmann CMF, Ehrhart LM, Bagley DA, Swing T (2004) Geomagnetic map used in sea-turtle navigation. *Nature* **428**, 909–910. doi:10.1038/428909a

Lukoschek V, Heatwole H, Grech A, Burns G, Marsh H (2007) Distribution of two species of sea snakes, Aipysurus laevis and Emydocephalus annulatus, in the southern Great Barrier Reef: metapopulation dynamics, marine protected areas and conservation. *Coral Reefs* **26**, 291–307. doi:10.1007/s00338-006-0192-8

Lutcavage ME, Plotkin P, Witherington BE, Lutz PL (1997) Human impacts on sea turtle survival. In *The Biology of Sea Turtles*. (Eds PL Lutz and JA Musick) pp. 387–409. CRC Press, Boca Raton, FL.

Lynch M, Kirkwood R, Gray R, Robson D, Burton G, Jones L, Sinclair R, Arnould JPY (2012) Characterization and causality investigations of an alopecia syndrome in Australian fur seals (Arctocephalus pusillus doriferus). *Journal of Mammalogy* **93**, 504–513. doi:10.1644/11-MAMM-A-279.1

MacLeod CD, Perrin WF, Pitman R, Barlow J, Ballance LD, Amico AA, *et al.* (2005) Known and inferred distributions of beaked whale species (Cetacea: Ziphiidae). *The Journal of Cetacean Research and Management* **7**, 271.

Marcos LA, Lanyon JM (2004) Dietary and morphometric analysis of three sea snake species caught as a single trawl by-catch assemblage around the Swain's Reefs, southern Great Barrier Reef, Queensland. *Proceedings of the Royal Society of Queensland* **111**, 63–71.

Markowitz TM, Harlin A, Würsig B (2003) Digital photography improves efficiency of individual dolphin identification. *Marine Mammal Science* **19**, 217–223. doi:10.1111/j.1748-7692.2003.tb01103.x

Marsh H, Rathbun GB (1990) Development and application of conventional and satellite radio tracking techniques for studying dugong movements and habitat use. *Wildlife Research* **17**, 83–100. doi:10.1071/WR9900083

Marsh H, Sinclair DF (1989) Correcting for visibility bias in strip transect aerial surveys of aquatic fauna. *The Journal of Wildlife Management* **53**, 1017–1024. doi:10.2307/3809604

Mate BR, Krutzikowsky GK, Winsor MH (2000) Satellite-monitored movements of radio-tagged bowhead whales in the Beaufort and Chukchi seas during the late-summer feeding season and fall migration. *Canadian Journal of Zoology* **78**, 1168–1181. doi:10.1139/z00-045

Mate BR, Rossbach KA, Nieukirk SL, Wells RS, Blair Irvine A, Scott MD, Read AJ (1995) Satellite-monitored movements and dive behavior of a bottlenose dolphin (*Tursiops truncatus*) in Tampa Bay, Florida. *Marine Mammal Science* **11**, 452–463. doi:10.1111/j.1748-7692.1995.tb00669.x

McCauley RD, Gavrilov AN, Jolliffe CD, Ward R, Gill PC (2018) Pygmy blue and Antarctic blue whale presence, distribution and population parameters in southern Australia based on passive acoustics. *Deep-sea Research. Part II, Topical Studies in Oceanography* **157–158**, 154–168. doi:10.1016/j.dsr2.2018.09.006

McIntosh R, Holmberg R, Dann P (2018) Looking without landing: using remote piloted aircraft to monitor fur seal populations without disturbance. *Frontiers in Marine Science* **5**, 202. doi:10.3389/fmars.2018.00202

Miller CA, Reeb D, Best PB, Knowlton AR, Brown MW, Moore MJ (2011) Blubber thickness in right whales *Eubalaena glacialis* and *Eubalaena australis* related with reproduction, life history status and prey abundance. *Marine Ecology Progress Series* **438**, 267–283. doi:10.3354/meps09174

Miller JD (1994) Describing sea turtle population structure in foraging areas: a review of current methods. In *Proceedings of the Australian Marine Turtle Conservation Workshop*. 14–17 November 1990, Gold Coast. (Ed R James) pp. 118–125. Australian Nature Conservation Agency, Canberra, Australia.

Miller JD (1997) Reproduction in sea turtles. In *Biology of Sea Turtles*. (Eds PL Lutz and JA Musick) pp. 51–81. CRC Press, Boca Raton, FL.

Mingramm FM, Keeley T, Whitworth DJ, Dunlop RA (2019) Relationships between blubber and respiratory vapour steroid hormone concentrations in humpback whales (*Megaptera novaeangliae*). *Aquatic Mammals* **45**, 465–477. doi:10.1578/AM.45.5.2019.465

Murphy JB (1971) A method for immobilising venomous snakes at Dallas Zoo. *International Zoo Yearbook* **11**, 233. doi:10.1111/j.1748-1090.1971.tb01915.x

National Marine Fisheries Service (NMFS) (2008) Sea Turtle Research Techniques Manual. *NOAA Technical Memorandum* NMFS-SEFSC-597, National Marine Fisheries Service Southwest Fisheries Science Centre. p. 92.

Nielsen ML, Sprogis KR, Bejder L, Madsen PT, Christiansen F (2019) Behavioural development in southern right whale calves. *Marine Ecology Progress Series* **629**, 219–234. doi:10.3354/meps13125

Noad MJ, Cato DH, Stokes MD (2004) Acoustic tracking of humpback whales: measuring interactions with the acoustic environment. *Proceedings of Acoustics 2004*. 3–5 November, Gold Coast, Australia, pp. 353–358.

Nicol S, Bowie A, Jarman S, Lannuzel D, Meiners KM, Van Der Merwe P (2010) Southern Ocean iron fertilization by baleen whales and Antarctic krill. *Fish and Fisheries* **11**, 203–209.

Owens DW, Ruiz GW (1980) New methods of obtaining blood and cerebrospinal fluid from marine turtles. *Herpetologica* **36**, 17–20.

Parker DAA (1978) Observations of whales on ANARE voyages between Australia and Antarctica. *Wildlife Research* **5**, 25–39. doi:10.1071/WR9780025

Parra GJ, Cagnazzi D, Jedensjo M, Ackermann C, Frere C, Seddon JM, Nikolic N, Krutzen M (2018) Low genetic diversity, limited gene flow and widespread genetic bottleneck effects in a threatened dolphin species, the Australian humpback dolphin. *Biological Conservation* **220**, 192–200. doi:10.1016/j.biocon.2017.12.028

Patenaude NJ, White BN (1995) Skin biopsy sampling of beluga whale carcasses: assessment of biopsy darting factors for minimal wounding and effective sample retrieval. *Marine Mammal Science* **11**, 163–171. doi:10.1111/j.1748-7692.1995.tb00515.x

Pirotta V, Smith A, Ostrowski M, Russell D, Jonsen ID, Grech A, Harcourt R (2017) An economical custom-built drone for assessing whale health. *Frontiers in Marine Science* **4**, 425. doi:10.3389/fmars.2017.00425

Priddel D, Wheeler R (1998) Hematology and blood chemistry of a Bryde's whale, *Balaenoptera edeni*, entrapped in the Manning River, New South Wales, Australia. *Marine Mammal Science* **14**, 72–81. doi:10.1111/j.1748-7692.1998.tb00691.x

Raudino HC, Tyne JA, Smith A, Ottewell K, McArthur S, Kopps AM, Chabanne D, Harcourt RG, Pirotta V, Waples K (2019) Challenges of collecting blow from small cetaceans. *Ecosphere* **10**, e02901. doi:10.1002/ecs2.2901

Read MA, Grigg GC, Limpus CJ (1996) Body temperature and winter feeding in immature green turtles, *Chelonia mydas*, in Moreton Bay, southeastern Queensland. *Journal of Herpetology* **30**, 262–265. doi:10.2307/1565520

Redfield JA, Holmes JC, Holmes RD (1978) Sea snakes of the eastern Gulf of Carpentaria. *Marine and Freshwater Research* **29**, 325–334. doi:10.1071/MF9780325

Rolland RM, Hamilton PK, Kraus SD, Davenport B, Gillett RM, Wasser SK (2007) Faecal sampling using detection dogs to study reproduction and health in North Atlantic right whales (*Eubalaena glacialis*). *The Journal of Cetacean Research and Management* **8**, 121–125.

Rouget PA, Terhune JM, Burton HR (2007) Weddell seal underwater calling rates during the winter and spring near Mawson Station, Antarctica. *Marine Mammal Science* **23**, 508–523. doi:10.1111/j.1748-7692.2007.00129.x

Schofield G, Katselidis KA, Lilley MKS, Reina RD, Hays GC (2017) Detecting elusive aspects of wildlife ecology using drones: new insights on the mating dynamics and operational sex ratios of sea turtles. *Functional Ecology* **31**, 2310–2319. doi:10.1111/1365-2435.12930

Seddon JM, Ovenden JR, Sneath HL, Broderick D, Dudgeon CL, Lanyon JM (2014) Fine scale population structure of dugongs (*Dugong dugon*) implies low gene flow along the southern Queensland coastline. *Biological Conservation* **15**, 1381–1392.

Shaughnessy PD, Dennis TE, Seager PG (2005) Status of Australian sea lions, *Neophoca cinerea*, and New Zealand fur seals, *Arctocephalus forsteri*, on Eyre Peninsula and the far west coast of South Australia. *Wildlife Research* **32**, 85–101. doi:10.1071/WR03068

Shine R, Shine TG, Brown GP, Goiran C (2020) Life history traits of the sea snake Emydocephalus annulatus, based on a 17 yr study. *Coral Reefs* **39**, 1407–1414. doi:10.1007/s00338-020-01974-y

Sorrell KJ, Clarke RH, Holmberg R, McIntosh RR (2019) Remotely piloted aircraft improve precision of capture–mark–resight population estimates of Australian fur seals. *Ecosphere* **10**, e02812. doi:10.1002/ecs2.2812

Southwell C, Paxton CGM, Borchers D, Boveng P, De La Mare W (2008) Taking account of dependent species in management of the Southern Ocean krill fishery: estimating crabeater seal abundance off east Antarctica. *Journal of Applied Ecology* **45**, 622–631. doi:10.1111/j.1365-2664.2007.01399.x

Stamation KA, Croft DB, Shaughnessy PD, Waples KA (2007) Observations of humpback whales (*Megaptera novaeangliae*) feeding during their southward migration along the coast of southeastern New South Wales, Australia: identification of a possible supplemental feeding ground. *Aquatic Mammals* **33**, 165. doi:10.1578/AM.33.2.2007.165

Stokes KL, Fuller WJ, Glen F, Godley BJ, Hodgson DJ, Rhodes KA, Snape RTE, Broderick CA (2014) Detecting green shoots of recovery: the importance of long-term individual-based monitoring of marine turtles. *Animal Conservation* **17**, 593–602. doi:10.1111/acv.12128

Tilzey R, Goldsworthy S, Cawthorn M, Calvert N, Hamer D, Russell S, Shaughnessy P, Wise B, Stewardson C (2006) Assessment of seal–fishery interactions in the winter blue grenadier fishery off west Tasmania and the development of fishing practices and Seal Exclusion Devices to mitigate seal bycatch by factory trawlers. *Fisheries Research and Development Corporation Project 2001/008, Final Report*. Bureau of Rural Sciences, Canberra, Australia.

Udyawer V, Cappo M, Simpfendorfer CA, Heupel MR, Lukoschek V (2014) Distribution of sea snakes in the Great Barrier Reef Marine Park: observations from 10 yrs of baited remote underwater video station (BRUVS) sampling. *Coral Reefs* **33**, 777–791. doi:10.1007/s00338-014-1152-3

Udyawer V, Simpfendorfer CA, Heupel MR, Clark TD (2017) Temporal and spatial activity-associated energy partitioning in free-swimming sea snakes. *Functional Ecology* **31**, 1739–1749. doi:10.1111/1365-2435.12882

Ukuwela KD, Sanders KL, Fry BG (2012) *Hydrophis donaldi* (Elapidae, Hydrophiinae), a highly distinctive new species of sea snake from northern Australia. *Zootaxa* **3201**, 45–57. doi:10.11646/zootaxa.3201.1.3

van Aswegen M, Christiansen F, Symons J, Mann J, Nicholson K, Sprogis K, Bejder L (2019) Morphological differences between coastal bottlenose dolphin (*Tursiops aduncus*) populations identified using non-invasive stereo-laser photogrammetry. *Scientific Reports* **9**, 12235. doi:10.1038/s41598-019-48419-3

van Polanen Petel T, Giese MA, Wotherspoon S, Hindell MA (2007) The behavioural response of lactating Weddell seals (*Leptonychotes weddellii*) to over-snow vehicles: a case study. *Canadian Journal of Zoology* **85**, 488–496. doi:10.1139/Z07-029

Volpov BL, Hoskins AJ, Battaile B, Viviant M, Wheatley KE, Marshall GJ, Abernathy K, Arnould JPY (2015) Identification of prey captures in Australian fur seals (*Arctocephalus pusillus doriferus*) using head-mounted accelerometers: field validation with animal-borne video cameras. *PLoS One* **10**, e0128789. doi:10.1371/journal.pone.0128789

Wassenberg TJ, Salini JP, Heatwole H, Kerr JD (1994) Incidental capture of sea-snakes (Hydrophiidae) by prawn trawlers in the Gulf of Carpentaria, Australia. *Marine and Freshwater Research* **45**, 429–443. doi:10.1071/MF9940429

Weinrich MT (1991) Behavioural response of humpback whales (*Megaptera novaeangliae*) in the southern Gulf of Maine to biopsy sampling. *Report of the International Whaling Commission* **13**, 91–97.

Wells RS, Rhinehart HL, Hansen LJ, Sweeney JC, Townsend FI, Stone R, *et al.* (2004) Bottlenose dolphins as marine ecosystem sentinels: developing a health monitoring system. *EcoHealth* **1**, 246–254. doi:10.1007/s10393-004-0094-6

Wierucka K, Barthes N, Harcourt RG, Schaal B, Charrier I, Pitcher BJ (2019) Chemical fingerprints suggest direct familiarisation rather than phenotype matching during olfactory recognition in Australian sea lions (*Neophoca cinerea*). *Journal of Experimental Marine Biology and Ecology* **517**, 49–53. doi:10.1016/j.jembe.2019.06.001

Wilkinson IS, Bester MN (1997) Tag-loss in southern elephant seals, *Mirounga leonina*, at Marion Island. *Antarctic Science* **9**, 162–167. doi:10.1017/S0954102097000217

Worthington Wilmer J, Allen PJ, Pomeroy PP, Twiss SD, Amos W (1999) Where have all the fathers gone? An extensive microsatellite analysis of paternity in the grey seal (*Halichoerus grypus*). *Molecular Ecology* **8**, 1417–1429. doi:10.1046/j.1365-294x.1999.00705.x

13 Research methods for marine and estuarine fishes

Bonnie J. Holmes, Samuel M. Williams, Adam Barnett, Cynthia A. Awruch, Leanne M. Currey-Randall, Luciana C. Ferreira, Charlie Huveneers, Rob L. Jones, Samantha J. Nowland, Andrea Taylor, Sean R. Tracey and Daniela Waltrick

INTRODUCTION

Teleosts (fishes) and chondrichthyans (sharks, rays and chimaeras) comprise multiple and diverse taxonomic groups, which occur in freshwater, estuarine and marine ecosystems. These taxa can occupy three-dimensional space within a habitat, with some species inhabiting the deepest oceans. Therefore, undertaking research on these taxa often requires nuanced ethical and practical considerations, including specialised methods for capture or observation, and lethal research. This chapter reviews contemporary best practice methods for field-based research involving teleosts and chondrichthyans. The general operating procedures (GOPs) detailed in this chapter provide guidance around animal welfare considerations when undertaking research on these taxa, and are complementary to Chapters 30 (teleosts) and 31 (chondrichthyans). Researchers should use this chapter as a guide while drawing on their own knowledge and experience, and those of other experienced researchers to select the most appropriate methods for their study. This chapter is focused primarily on marine and estuarine species, but the sections on biological sampling, tagging, transport and housing may also apply to freshwater fishes (Chapter 32), or species that use freshwater environments for part of their life cycle. Marine and estuarine researchers may find that other GOPs within this book (including Chapter 14, which describes capturing, observing and handling freshwater animals, including fish) will also be relevant to their work, particularly if conducting research across freshwater and terrestrial landscapes.

CAPTURE AND RELEASE METHODS

Charlie Huveneers and Leanne M. Currey-Randall

Context and scope

This GOP describes methods and guidelines for the capture, handling, and release of teleosts and chondrichthyans. It is not intended to replace detailed or step-by-step protocols. These wild animals are caught for scientific purposes for a variety of reasons, including lethal and non-lethal biological sampling, tagging (see other GOPs in this chapter), and sometimes require transport and housing for laboratory or aquaria research (see Chapters 30 and 31). Here, the diverse methods used to capture, handle and release teleosts and chondrichthyans at sea are summarised, and key methods used for these taxa highlighted.

Animal welfare considerations

Physiological stress

Capture and handling can cause physical trauma and physiological disruption (Barton 2002; Dapp *et al.* 2016a; Ellis *et al.* 2017), resulting in three levels of stress response. The primary response is typically shown as an immediate neuroendocrine response with rapid increases in circulatory levels of stress hormones, predominantly catecholamines and corticosteroids. Secondary responses comprise a suite of physiological and biochemical changes that are typically measured by changes in blood and muscle biochemistry (e.g. lactate, glucose, potassium, chloride, calcium and pH). Extreme physiological changes can lead to mortality, with sensitivity to capture and handling, and likelihood of severity varying between species (Dapp *et al.* 2016b). For example, Port Jackson (*Heterodontus portusjacksoni*) and wobbegong (*Orectolobus* spp.) sharks have high post-capture survival, while hammerheads (*Sphyrna* spp.) are more vulnerable to capture stress (Gallagher *et al.* 2014; Dapp *et al.* 2016a). Likewise, post-release survival varies among teleost species, from 98% for shallow-caught reef fishes (e.g. stripey snapper, *Lutjanus carponotatus*, and longfin rockcod, *Epinephelus quoyanus*) to 14% for demersal West Australian dhufish (*Glaucosoma hebraicum*) caught from 45 m depth (Ayvazian *et al.* 2002; St John and Syers 2005). Even in situations when an animal recovers physiologically from a stressful situation, sublethal tertiary effects on feeding, growth, reproduction and immune system function can ensue, with consequences possible at the population level (Wendelaar Bonga 1997; Skomal and Bernal 2010).

Physical trauma and injury

Physical trauma or injuries can also occur during capture and handling. These risks are minimised by ensuring that personnel are properly trained, and handling times are minimal. Elasmobranchs (sharks, rays and skates) comprise all chondrichthyans minus chimaeras. This group tend to heal quickly (Towner *et al.* 2012; Chin *et al.* 2015; Kessel *et al.* 2017) and can survive more severe injuries than those that typically occur during standard capture and handling processes. Similarly, some injuries to teleosts, such as swim bladder ruptures, can heal within as little as 24 h (Campbell *et al.* 2014).

Physical trauma and physiological stress can vary with equipment used (Veldhuizen *et al.* 2018), and environmental conditions (e.g. water temperature) at the time of capture. For example, organisms caught in gill nets are more likely to suffer from asphyxiation than those caught on hooks because fish can continue moving while caught on a hook (allowing oxygenated water to flow over their gills). Species that perform buccal pumping (when fish are able to pump water through their mouth and over their gills) while stationary (e.g. benthic or bottom dwelling species) are less likely to be affected by oxygen depletion from constrained movement (Dapp *et al.* 2016b). Researchers need to consider several issues when developing sampling procedures, accounting for the target species, possible by-catch (non-target species capture), safety considerations, and logistical constraints (e.g. size of research vessels, predominant weather condition) (Table 13.1). One capture or handling method will not be suitable across all species or for one species across all situations.

General procedures

Specific considerations for minimising the potential impacts of a range of capture, handling and release methods are detailed in Table 13.2. This table is not exhaustive. Other techniques may include lesser-used capture methods, such as fence or tunnel netting (where a diver/wader herds fish into a net), clove oil collections (popular for catching small reef fish species), cast netting (usually for bait or small fish collection), and hand and dip netting. Other types of nets (i.e. fyke) that may be used in estuarine waters, are covered in the freshwater section of this book (Chapter 14).

Capture

Teleosts and chondrichthyans can be captured via diverse methods (Table 13.2) with the most suitable methods depending on the species targeted, whether the animals are collected for lethal or non-lethal sampling, environmental conditions (e.g. weather), and field logistics (e.g. boat size, number of people present). The following recommendations should be considered by researchers when using the methods described in Table 13.2:

- Reduce capture duration as much as practicable. Gear should be checked frequently enough to reduce stress and avoid mortality, but not so often as to affect catch efficiency. Soak times will vary depending on gear used. For example, drumlines facilitate active swimming (and oxygenation) of animals, while gill nets require more regular checks.
- If possible, target teleosts in shallow water to reduce retrieval time to landing and potential barotrauma.
- Retrieve traps and deep-water bottom-set longlines slowly to reduce barotrauma.
- For all hook-based methods, use hooks that are least likely to be swallowed (typically circle hooks), are easy to remove, and that corrode if they cannot be removed.

Handling

Animal handling must maintain safety to the researcher and minimise stress to the animal. When handling teleosts, an Environet™ can reduce scale loss, and gloves

Table 13.1: Animal welfare considerations for selecting suitable capture, handling, and release methods for teleosts and chondrichthyans.

Concern	Consideration
Elevated hormonal and physiological stress	Selection of capture methods to reduce time caught before handling or processing; use handling methods minimising air exposure and handling duration.
Hooking injuries	Possible injuries when using line and reel, setlines, or longlines; ensure adequate hook size and type; use corrodible hooks; use capture methods that prevents foul and gut hooking; have appropriate training to safely remove hooks when possible.
Movement restriction	Occurs in gill nets, trawls, and setlines/drumlines via entanglements. If sampling species sensitive to asphyxiation, e.g. obligate ram ventilating, consider methods least likely to restrain movements.
Crushing injury	Occurs in trawls. Reduce trawl duration to avoid overcrowding in the cod end; ensure that by-catch reduction devices are used where appropriate.
Predation	Can occur when animals that have reduced ability to move and escape predation are caught. Reduce capture duration as much as possible; ensure that animals are released in good condition.
Injuries from sudden movements	Can occur during handling. Ensure that adequate restraints are used when handling animals and enough support is provided.
Released animals prone to infection via scale loss and removal of mucus	Can occur during capture and handling. Ensuring minimal removal of scales and fish mucus, which assists in healing and healthy immune response.
Barotrauma	While most likely to occur in teleosts, differences in pressure can also lead to elevated stress in deep-sea elasmobranchs. Ensure bringing animals up slowly if capturing from deep water or if species is known to be sensitive to barotrauma; venting of the swim bladder can be done on teleosts; release at depth can also be used when needed.

or wet towels can provide grip during de-hooking or removal from fishing apparatus, reducing the chance of injury to the fish and to the handler from spines or teeth. Researchers should wear sufficient coverage when handling elasmobranchs to avoid 'shark burn' caused by abrasion of elasmobranch denticles. Handling fish or elasmobranchs by their gills or spiracles (when present) should also be avoided. When de-hooking, animals should be supported in a horizontal position to avoid spinal and muscular injuries and not held vertically from the hook for an extended period, as some species are susceptible to injury (e.g. barramundi, *Lates calcarifer*; Gould and Grace 2009). Where removal of the hook is likely to cause injury (e.g. if the hook is swallowed and caught on internal organs) or is dangerous to remove (e.g. large sharks), researchers can cut the hook or the trace/line as close to the hook as possible. Hook selection should take into account target species' mouth morphology, feeding mode and the fishing style to reduce the likelihood of injury (Cooke and Suski 2004).

Selecting the best method to restrain the animal after capture depends on the size of the vessel and the procedure that will follow capture. Elasmobranchs and large teleosts (e.g. billfish) are often measured and tagged alongside vessels because of their large size, which enables water flow over gills and minimises physical handling. Sharks must be restrained securely to avoid injury to the animal and researcher, usually involving securing the hooked trace to one end of the vessel and a tail rope around the caudal peduncle to hold the shark outstretched, with the animal's ventral side facing up to facilitate tonic immobility (Kessel *et al.* 2015). Teleosts and smaller elasmobranchs can be brought on board, but require adequate restraints.

Holding and restraining fish

Holding and restraining fish are undertaken routinely to conduct various research procedures at sea. For small teleosts and chondrichthyans, some procedures may be done by transporting the animal on board the boat or the shoreline. This process can involve placing the fish in a water-filled trough (often using a cradle to support the fish) with its ventral side facing up, so that the ventral surface is above the water line, but the gills remain submerged. Handling should be completed quickly to reduce physiological stress or longer-term impairment caused by air exposure. Gills should remain submerged, have a continuous flow of pumped fresh sea/estuarine

Table 13.2: Some standard methods of capture for teleosts and chondrichthyans, including their main advantages and disadvantages.

Method	Description	Target	Advantages	Disadvantages
Trawl	Bottom-set or pelagic trawl with nets. Animals are typically released on deck into sorting trays.	Multi-species teleosts and elasmobranchs varying sizes.	Samples the community, efficient method to sample in deep water.	Potential for crushing injuries in the cod end and lengthy air exposure during sorting. High by-catch if only targeting specific species.
Seine netting	Vertically hanging net with bottom edge held down by weights and top edge buoyed by floats. Operated in shallow inshore areas. Individuals are circled by a net which is dragged onto shore.	Multi-species small to medium teleosts and rays.	Samples the community. Low stress and injuries.	Only usable in shallow environment. Can be done without boat but leads to safety concern (e.g. from dangerous animals). Limited sampling spatially with potentially low catch rate. High by-catch if only targeting specific species.
Gill netting	Vertically hanging net with bottom edge held down by weights and top edge buoyed by floats. Can be surface or bottom set. Entangles animals attempting to swim through the net.	Multi-species small to medium teleosts and elasmobranchs.	Efficient method to capture less-abundant teleosts and elasmobranchs. Can be size selective.	Animals caught via monofilament around gills and restrains movement. May lead to injury and low post-release survival. High by-catch if only targeting specific species but lower than trawl or seine netting.
Trap	Frame of steel wire with hole tapering inside the trap allowing fish to swim in, but not out.	Small to medium species.	Little to no injuries. By-catch species can be released (if not affected by barotrauma)	Potential for teleost barotrauma if brought to the surface too quickly or used in deep water; within-trap predation.
Hook and line (rod and reel/ handline)	Standard recreational fishing equipment.	Small to medium species.	Gear selection can enable high species- and size-selectivity. Minimal injuries and capture duration	Captures single or small number of individuals, therefore time-consuming.
Longline Setline	Long line with baited hooks attached at intervals by snoods/ gangions. Can be bottom or surface set. Length of line and number of hooks is variable.	Medium to large species.	Gear selection can enable high species- and size-selectivity. Animals can keep swimming, assisting post-release survival.	Animals can become entangled leading to asphyxiation if not monitored regularly. Some possible by-catch; possible human safety concerns due to large number of hooks.
Drumline Dropline	Float with a snood/trace and hook(s). Can either be drifting or bottom set with another line attached to an anchor.	Medium to large species.	Gear selection can enable high species- and size-selectivity. Animals can keep swimming, assisting post-release survival.	Captures one individual at a time. Animals can become entangled leading to asphyxiation if not monitored regularly. Some possible by-catch.
Hand spear Speargun	Long shaft with point at one end powered by rubber bands.	All trophic groups, small to medium animals.	Highly selective.	Labour intensive; restricted to breath-hold or diving depths; human safety concerns.

water, or be kept wet with a wet towel. Keeping teleosts wet ensures retention of their mucous layer, which assists in avoiding infection (Ángeles Esteban 2012); the use of a wet towel to cover eyes also reduces stress.

In-water tagging typically requires restraining the animal either by holding it (by pectoral and tail regions), or by securing the animal to the side of the vessel using a soft rope or a harness/cradle. Whichever method is used, the fish's gills must be kept underwater with water passing over the gills. The holding method will depend on the size of the fish, the size and configuration of the boat, and the fieldwork conditions. The use of anaesthetic to reduce stress during handling and procedures (e.g. internal tagging) is discussed later in this chapter, but the effect on recovery time of anaesthetised animals at sea should be considered.

Release

Barotrauma is a key issue affecting post-release survival of teleosts and typically occurs from capture at increased depths, with some species more sensitive than others (e.g. black jewfish, *Protonibea diacanthus*), which can suffer irreversible tissue damage when caught in as little as 10 m depth (Phelan *et al.* 2008). Efficacy of strategies to return fish to depth and reduce barotrauma are varied and species-specific (Cooke and Suski 2004; Sumpton *et al.* 2010). Venting is common and is achieved by inserting a needle into the swim bladder behind the pectoral fin to release gas. Release weights (shot-line) involve hooking the lip to weighted non-barbed hooks and sending the animal back to depth via swim bladder recompression (Butcher *et al.* 2012). Similarly, release cages can be used to lower animals to depth and small hyperbaric chambers have also indicated success for some species (Hughes *et al.* 2019). These techniques enable teleosts to seek shelter on the seabed, rather than remain at the surface waiting for the gas to release naturally, causing additional struggle-related stress and an increased risk of predation and death.

Predation of released animals can be reduced by releasing them at shallow depths to enable them to reach the safety of complex substrate quickly, however compromised individuals are more likely to be preyed on (Raby *et al.* 2014). Consequently, ensuring teleosts and chondrichthyans are in the best condition possible (e.g. recovered from procedures, vented, non-lethargic) will ensure high post-release survival. Monitoring of the animal before release is essential to ascertain normal movement or return of full equilibrium; the animal should be held in the water and should swim off with vigour. Elasmobranchs and large fish post-sedation (tonic immobility or chemical sedation) are often 'swum' by researchers, which involves moving the caudal fin to reorient the individual to the swimming motion or holding the vessel in gear to assist water flow over the gills (Kessel *et al.* 2015). Holding time post-procedure can be beneficial to an individual's recovery (e.g. to regain equilibrium after internal tagging), but the duration should not allow animal to become agitated. Some researchers hold teleosts on board or in a holding cage on the side of the vessel, but this technique should only be used if animals remain calm (Williams *et al.* 2015). Data collected should include handling time and release condition.

Animal treatment, withdrawal and euthanasia

Key triggers for animal welfare interventions are detailed in Table 13.3. Euthanasia should be considered if no body, eye or gill movement can be detected, if rigor mortis is setting in, or if the animal's condition is deteriorating. See other GOPs in this chapter for information on appropriate euthanasia techniques.

Table 13.3: Triggers that can be used to monitor animals throughout capture and handling and before release.

Trigger	Description
Injuries or bleeding	Consider whether healing can be helped with antiseptics or via suturing.
General movement	Vigorous movement, sluggish or no movement.
Gill movement	Regular gill movement, irregular gill movement, no movement or gill flaring in teleosts.
Rigidity	Stiffening of the body (rigor mortis).
Eye movement and colour	Eye movement is reduced and eyes become cloudy in teleosts as condition deteriorates.
Barotrauma	Exophthalmia (bulging eyes), swim bladder hyperextension or perforation, prolapse of intestine via vent or stomach out through mouth, and haemorrhaging of the gills, cornea and viscera.

Equipment and maintenance

Equipment requirements will depend on the chosen capture method, procedure to be conducted (e.g. lethal sampling, tagging), and if the animal will be released. Key equipment required for capture is detailed in Table 13.2. For handling and restraint, investigators may require:

- gloves and covered clothes for personal protection
- fresh seawater (plus aerators if feasible), or water tube and circulation of water flow over gills (e.g. via a bilge pump)
- holding container/tanks/tubs for teleosts on board
- hard or soft slings have been used for sharks, but tail and body ropes are now more common to restrain large sharks alongside vessels
- wet towels to restrain teleosts, and keep teleosts and elasmobranchs wet and calm
- foam mattress for support during on-board procedures.

For release procedures, investigators may require:

- needle-nosed pliers (for teleosts) or de-hooker to remove hook from mouth
- bolt cutters (for elasmobranchs) to cut hook shank if hook cannot be removed
- wire cutters (for elasmobranchs) to cut wire trace if hook shank cannot be cut
- venting needles, weighted hooks, or release cage to assist barotrauma-sensitive species.

All equipment should be in working order, sprayed with anti-rust or water-displacing spray (e.g. WD40), or replaced if showing signs of wear (e.g. frayed ropes or trace, seized cutters).

Specific qualifications, experience and training

No formal training is required for the capture, handling and release of teleosts and chondrichthyans. However, an experienced staff member should be present during work, and have trained or demonstrated methods to all crew. A level of competency in the capture and handling techniques specific to each field trip and project is required to avoid injury to the researchers and animals. While not essential, fishing experience (recreational or commercial) is beneficial.

Workplace health and safety

A project-specific risk assessment should be undertaken for each field trip and reviewed by all personnel. A safe environment is achieved through supervision by experienced staff members, and knowledge of the fishing method, handling procedures, release processes and potential risks. The variety of fishing gears used for capture (Table 13.2) have specific safety issues, which should be addressed and mitigated in the risk assessment. Crew and researcher safety are paramount, and several general risks should be considered, including gear maintenance, correct deployment of gear, and knowledge of local venomous or dangerous species and the relevant first aid.

Alternative procedures

Researchers must assess which capture and handling methods are the most effective while accounting for logistical constraints, the need to reduce animal stress and injuries, and maximising post-release survival (if released). Methods of capture, handling and release should be refined and replaced with alternatives if more adequate techniques can be achieved.

LETHAL BIOLOGICAL SAMPLING

Bonnie J. Holmes, Daniela Waltrick and Rob L. Jones

Context and scope

This GOP provides guidelines to assist researchers in developing detailed operating procedures for lethally sampling teleosts and chondrichthyans. Approval to conduct research on teleosts and chondrichthyans requires consideration of methods to euthanase these species. Lethal sampling of wild-caught teleosts and chondrichthyans for biological studies is common in Australia, and often includes research into critical life-history parameters that are required for stock (population) assessments (Heupel and Simpfendorfer 2010). These methods are undertaken for collection of internal tissues that currently cannot be non-lethally sampled. These investigations incorporate a wide variety of research disciplines, some of which are outlined in Table 13.4.

The authors recognise that different bioregions, jurisdictions, institutions and animal ethics committees (AECs) across Australia have different requirements in relation to lethal sampling of teleosts and chondrichthyans, and that a single guideline may not be suitable for all situations. Researchers are invited to use this GOP as a guide, but to draw on their own knowledge and experience in consultation with their respective AEC. Improvements to non-lethal sampling technologies and methodologies to undertake the same tasks are

Table 13.4: Overview of routine teleost and chondrichthyan research areas that require lethal sampling.

Research area	Collection required	Research importance
Reproduction	Reproductive organs, eggs, semen, amniotic fluids, *in utero* pups (chondrichthyans).	To undertake research on fecundity, reproductive seasonality, cycle and spawning, litter/clutch size, pup characteristics (chondrichthyans), egg development, sperm storage, size at maturity.
Age and growth	Otoliths in teleosts (located in head); vertebrae in chondrichthyans (usually 7–8 from the cervical region). Sometimes fin spines also used.	To determine longevity, size at birth, growth rates, growth band deposition and periodicity, differences in population growth, size at maturity.
Brain function, homeostasis, and sensory biology	Brains, eyes, ampullae of Lorenzini, olfactory lobes, lateral lines, muscle.	To understand brain morphology, activity and function, nervous systems and pain studies, lateralization and learning capabilities, cognition.
Diet, digestion, stable isotopes	Stomach content, tissue (muscle, liver, fin), intestinal chyme.	To determine prey preferences, ontogenetic shift, trophic niche, movements, ingestion/digestion, gastric function.
Biochemistry	Vertebrae, liver, blood and blood products, muscle, swim bladders.	To undertake research on liver oil composition, buoyancy, hormones and stress responses, biochemical constitutions, metabolic capacity.
Biomechanics	Teeth, jaws, tails, vertebrae and other skeletal parts, fins, scales/denticles.	To understand functional anatomy, feeding sequences, bite characteristics, filter feeding, muscle activity, acceleration and turning (swimming/hunting), predation avoidance.
Taxonomy	Whole animal.	To understand taxonomic classification, identify and describe new species, obtain voucher specimens for museums and other collections.
Parasites	Internal and external parasites. May be in gut, tissue, brain or other organs of the animal.	To determine parasitic load, species composition and life cycle, species specificity and range, impact on host and lethality.

continually being developed. These operating procedures broadly describe chemical and physical techniques that may be applied in the euthanasia of teleosts or chondrichthyans caught from the wild for scientific purposes. It covers the take of species that are sourced from freshwater, estuarine and marine environments. Anaesthesia for captive teleosts and chondrichthyans is covered in 'Internal tagging methods' later in this chapter. General considerations for use of sedatives and anaesthetics in wildlife are detailed in Chapter 16.

Animal welfare considerations

Teleosts and chondrichthyans are captured using a range of fishing apparatus selected for the purpose of the research (see Table 13.2). Currently, many research questions on these animals cannot be answered using non-lethal methods. Consequently, researchers often need to dispatch animals at sea rapidly and humanely. Euthanasia of teleosts and chondrichthyans is undertaken in a range of ways, depending on the size of the animal and whether handling occurs in the water or on board the vessel. Recommended practices may vary between jurisdictions.

General procedures

Key examples of chemical and physical methods that may be employed to reduce stress and undertake rapid euthanasia of teleosts and chondrichthyans for scientific purposes are detailed below. Methods relating to tissue and gut collection are covered in 'Non-lethal biological sampling' within this chapter.

Euthanasia of teleosts at sea with chemical methods

Immersion anaesthetic is added to the aqueous environment of the fishes' holding tank, forming a lethal solution that passes over the fish's gills to induce death. Application of this method in teleosts is analogous to gaseous inhalant anaesthesia in terrestrial animals (Chapter 16). When teleosts ventilate, the treated water enters their bloodstream through the gills and/or the skin, passing rapidly to the central nervous system (Neiffer and Stamper 2009). An overdose of anaesthetic is the method most recommended by scientific authorities in Australia and overseas for fish euthanasia (e.g. Barker *et al.* 2002; Leary *et al.* 2013; Jones and Daly 2014). Several chemical agents are suitable, but in Australia, many are only available by veterinary prescription. A commercial preparation that contains purified and standardised concentrations of the active constituent of clove oil (~50% iso-eugenol) is available (AQUI-S®). It was originally developed for harvesting of Atlantic salmon (*Salmo salar*) in New Zealand (Jones and Daly 2014).

Immersion methods for small teleosts that can be held in buckets or large plastic bins on vessels can involve an overdose of an anaesthetic agent, such as AQUI-S®. While AQUI-S® is readily available over the counter, it may cause skin, eye and organ damage (through prolonged use) to humans, and should only be used in calm seas where the appropriate workplace health and safety measures can be met. If conditions are not appropriate to the use of chemicals, physical methods for euthanasia should be employed (see below). AQUI-S® is appropriate for euthanasia of all tropical and temperate species (from small < 5 cm, to medium > 15 cm total length), providing that the fishes' own *in situ* water, in a volume of water appropriate to the fish size, is used (Jones and Daly 2014). Large or potentially dangerous teleosts (i.e. those > 1 m that require ram ventilation or are difficult to handle) that cannot be transported onto research vessels are not suitable for chemical euthanasia, and should be dispatched using the physical methods described below.

Euthanasia of chondrichthyans at sea with chemical methods

Like teleosts, small chondrichthyans that can be safely handled and placed in appropriately sized containers on board may be euthanased in a field situation in calm seas using AQUI-S®. Additionally, during initial handling of captured sharks, turning them over so that the ventral side is facing upward induces (in most elasmobranchs, but not all) a state referred to as 'tonic immobility' (Kessel *et al.* 2015). This process immediately reduces stress on the animal and allows for safer handling and application of the relevant euthanasia technique, noting that an animal will need to be turned back over to apply any physical method of euthanasia. Large elasmobranchs can only be safely handled while still in the water at the side of the vessel, so chemical methods for euthanasia are not able to be used.

Euthanasia using physical methods (at sea)

The adoption of physical methods of euthanasia requires consideration of specific circumstances, such as specimen body size and where handling occurs (in water or on board a vessel). With correctly applied physical methods of euthanasia, some post-mortem cadaveric spasms will probably be observed. These movements occur as the nerve cells continue to be triggered by electrical pulses, and the animal continues twitching, despite its deceased state. If physical methods have been correctly applied, the spasms should cease within a few minutes.

Large elasmobranchs should always be appropriately restrained by securing the head (or hooked trace if captured using drumline or longline gear for example) to the bow of the vessel, and using a soft rope to restrain the tail to the aft, facilitating safe handling by researchers. Secondarily, the use of a supporting strap (e.g. soft rope, or wide diameter snatch strap) can be placed around the midsection of the animal, posterior to the pectoral fins. Inducing them into tonic immobility before applying one of the physical procedures described below is advised where safe, should the operators have experience in this procedure.

Physical euthanasia of teleosts and small chondrichthyans

A range of methods suitable for euthanasia of teleosts and small chondrichthyans can be conducted on board a vessel or on shore. Pithing is also known as brain spiking or *ikejime*, and consists of inserting a sharp tool (e.g. pointed knife or screwdriver) into the animal's skull to cause brain destruction. Considering the small brain size of sharks and their relatives, this procedure should be carried out by a trained staff member with knowledge of the species' morphology to ensure a quick death (Diggles 2006).

Decapitation, or spinal transection, is the process of separating the brain from the spinal cord by inserting a sharp knife or scalpel blade to remove, or partly remove, the head. Fish are tolerant of hypoxia, so this method should always be followed immediately by pithing to stop brain activity. Cervical dislocation is similar in method to decapitation; however, it involves breaking the cervical bones near the head by inserting a thumb or a rod into the fish's mouth, holding the fish with the opposite hand and displacing the head dorsally (Close *et al.* 1997). This method is suitable for small teleosts only and is not acceptable for larger fish (Reilly 2001) or chondrichthyans. Percussive stunning, or cranial concussion, involves a blow to the head region with sufficient force to induce unconsciousness immediately. This method should immediately be followed by pithing (Reilly 2001) or decapitation (Close *et al.* 1997) to ensure death. This method can be used in both fish (except small specimens) and chondrichthyans. Rapid chilling, the rapid chilling by placing on an ice slurry (2–4°C), causing death by hypothermal shock, is only acceptable for small (< 5 cm) tropical fish. This method is not acceptable for teleosts larger than 5 cm, cold water teleosts and chondrichthyans (Leary *et al.* 2013; Jones and Daly 2014).

Physical euthanasia of large chondrichthyans

Depending on the operation, investigators should consider jurisdictional variations on the preferred methods for euthanasia of large sharks. Generally, a cervical transection method using a sharp instrument inserted caudal to the skull to sever the spinal cord (neural arch), the cervical vertebrae and the blood supply (haemal arch) is used as death is quick. This process should be followed by pithing. In jurisdictions with shark control programs in place, large sharks that are already being euthanased as part of those programs can often be obtained from the contractors to assist with biological research, negating the need for independent lethal sampling.

Animal treatment, withdrawal and euthanasia

See 'General procedures' in this GOP.

Equipment and maintenance

Equipment varies depending on the specific method chosen and the species, but typical items may include:

- ropes, slings, poles to secure animals safely
- anaesthetic if required for euthanasia (and appropriate material safety data sheets)
- latex gloves for handling anaesthetics or other chemicals
- sturdy cotton or cut-resistant gloves (wet) for handling fish
- appropriate type and size knives and spares in case of damage or loss overboard
- whetstone or other resharpening tool
- appropriate sharp tool or screwdriver for pithing
- hammer, mallet or a solid piece of wood for percussive stunning
- small and large holding containers, to apply chemical euthanasia to small animals
- field identification guide(s)
- copies of permits and approvals
- information signs with permit details
- data sheets, pencils, pens, waterproof marker
- data collection equipment (e.g. scales, rulers, fish measuring boards)
- containers or bags to store deceased animals for return to laboratory
- plastic sealable bags, containers or vials required for other samples
- for night sampling: torches, headlamps, spare batteries
- general personal protective equipment (e.g. personal floatation devices, long-sleeved shirts, hat, sunscreen, insect repellent)
- first aid kit
- hook remover
- bolt cutters.

Specific qualifications, experience and training

No formal training is required for most chemical and physical methods of euthanasia in teleosts and chondrichthyans. However, staff should have specific knowledge of the methods employed and always have an experienced staff member present during operations. Veterinary chemicals are registered under different 'schedules' according to the perceived risk they pose to the community in Australia (see Chapter 16). Using a Schedule 6 commercial preparation, such as AQUI-S®, negates the need to use more restricted (Schedule 4 or 8) veterinary drugs. However, researchers should be familiar with its use, and have undertaken similar activities on land (i.e. on aquaria specimens) before attempting its use at sea. It is also recommended that researchers be familiar with the various stages of anaesthesia in fish (Table 13.5).

Workplace health and safety

Bites and stings

Handling fish can pose a risk of injury to the crew that can be minimised by training and experience. As with any wild species, teleosts and chondrichthyans may be unpredictable when under stress and on board a vessel. Potential injuries include being struck or bitten (sharks), and stung and cut (rays and teleosts). An injury caused by stingray barbs (generally venomous) and teleost spines (generally not venomous) range from unpleasant to serious, and even life threatening, and require medical attention. The severity of a shark bite will obviously vary with species' size and location of the bite, but could be life threatening. Therefore, prior knowledge of the target

Table 13.5: Stages of anaesthesia in teleosts (adapted from Jones and Daly 2014).

Level	Level of anaesthesia	Signs associated with this level
0	Normal	Normal swimming behaviour and reaction to external stimuli
1	Light sedation	Still swimming but reduced reaction to external stimuli; equilibrium normal; normal opercular rate
2	Deep sedation/light anaesthesia	No swimming; loss of equilibrium (rolls over or belly up) but may still try to right itself; normal to slightly decreased opercular rate; still maintains a tail reaction*
3	Surgical anaesthesia	Complete loss of equilibrium; complete loss of reactivity (negative tail reaction); very slow opercular rate; slow heart rate
4	Medullary collapse	Total loss of opercular movement followed by cardiac arrest. Euthanasia achieved

* Tail reaction involves pinching the tail fin to see if a response occurs.

species, potential by-catch and best handling practices is crucial to guarantee safety on board.

Sharp implements

Sharp objects, such as knives and piths, should be kept handy, but secured in a sheath or inside a container or compartment that stops them from moving around the boat. Accidental injuries from such items may vary in degree of severity. Training and the use of cut-proof gloves is recommended to minimise potential accidents. Needles should be capped and used only by trained staff in appropriate conditions.

Chemicals

Using chemicals on board vessels should only be undertaken if deemed required for euthanasing the target species, and only in suitable at-sea conditions to minimise the risk of the safety of researchers. In most cases, physical methods for euthanasia may be used as an alternative method in these situations. Material safety data sheets for all chemicals (e.g. used for euthanasia) should be maintained and read by all investigators and personnel.

Alternative procedures

Sustainable use of teleosts and chondrichthyans often requires biological and ecological data that are needed for the development of effective regional conservation and management strategies (Cortés 2007). Demographic information on reproduction, age, growth, and mortality estimates are critical for understanding stock status and the susceptibility of populations to exploitation. Lethally sampling teleosts and chondrichthyans remains the most effective means of gathering these types of data for most species (Heupel and Simpfendorfer 2010). However, multi-disciplinary approaches are still being explored to develop alternatives to lethal techniques for generating necessary data, particularly for threatened species (Hammerschlag and Sulikowski 2011).

Given that many species of interest are often target species in commercial or recreational fisheries, fishery-derived specimens can sometimes be obtained in sufficient numbers to conduct the relevant biological research both temporally and seasonally. However, often researchers are interested in the fishery-independent aspect of the collections, as these data discriminate the spatial locations where a species is present or absent (rather than being biased by the 'targeting' nature of fishing operations), and can be conducted at specific time frames to ensure representative sampling is achieved. For chondrichthyans, taking advantage of existing shark control programs means that large specimens being 'culled' (or already deceased) as part of that program may be able to be further utilised for scientific research.

NON-LETHAL BIOLOGICAL SAMPLING

Samuel M. Williams and Cynthia A. Awruch

Context and scope

This GOP provides guidelines to assist researchers in developing detailed operating procedures for non-lethally sampling teleosts and chondrichthyans. It describes techniques and practices for non-lethal biological sampling of fishes and chondrichthyans. Where possible, non-lethal sampling is the preferred method for collecting biological information. A range of non-lethal approaches is commonly used for research purposes in Australia and elsewhere (Table 13.6). Several biological applications cannot be resolved through non-lethal approaches and, for those research purposes, the methods defined in lethal biological sampling section above are most appropriate. The approaches for capture and handling are

Table 13.6: Overview of non-lethal sampling techniques and their associated field of research, and invasiveness on the target species.

Sampling technique	Research type	Invasiveness/impact
Mucus swabs (epidermal)	Molecular analysis (e.g. genetics and stable isotope)	Negligible
Fin clipping (intramuscular)	Molecular analysis (e.g. genetics, genomics, stable isotope and fatty acid)	Low/medium
Biopsies (intramuscular)	Molecular analysis (e.g. genetics, genomics, stable isotope and fatty acid)	Low/medium
Vertebral staining (calcein injection) – intramuscular or intraperitoneally	Age and growth studies	Low/medium
Stomach flushing (intragastinal)	Stomach content and composition analysis	Low/medium
Blood samples (intravascular)	Physiology/endocrinology	Low/medium
Ultrasound and endoscopy (epidermal/ inter-renal)	Reproductive examination (e.g. embryos/egg capsules)	Low/medium

outlined in 'Capture and release methods' earlier in this chapter. They are complementary to the contents of this chapter and should be considered in addition to the procedures outlined herein.

Animal welfare considerations

Non-lethal sampling minimises the risk of injuries or mortality to fishes and chondrichthyans. However, specific considerations for reducing injuries or mortality may include minimising soak and holding times, correct training for appropriate handling and sample collection (e.g. for blood sampling), and an understanding of the target species (or a surrogate one). These approaches will aid in preventing high-stress situations, which could lead to increased physiological impairment or mortality. As non-lethal methods include the release of study animals, depredation (post-release predation by natural predators, such as large fishes, sharks or birds) represents a risk to released animals. Releasing physically injured or impaired animals can greatly increase the risk of post-release predation. Therefore, analgesics or anaesthesia are generally not recommended during non-invasive procedures.

General procedures

Procedure for fin clips and biopsies

Fin clipping and biopsies aim to collect tissue samples, often for molecular analysis. These approaches are considered minimally invasive. The short time period (often < 5 s) and low level of impacts required to conduct biopsy or fin clip sampling mean that analgesics or anaesthetics typically are not applied, with animals returned to the water as quickly as possible following the procedure. Holding animals for longer periods (i.e. for recovery) from minor procedures will often result in prolonged stress on the animal, and increase the likelihood of impairing fish behaviour and influence survival after release (i.e. predation; Cooke *et al.* 2016). Biopsy samples or fin clips can either be undertaken on restrained animals boat side, on board vessels or underwater (Williams *et al.* 2015; Bradford *et al.* 2016). Samples should be a sufficient size for the analytical technique, and small enough that they do not cause long-term injury to the fish. Biopsy and fin clip procedures should avoid areas adjacent to vital organs (e.g. lateral to the body cavity). Equipment should be pre-sterilised or immersed in antiseptic solutions, such as diluted povidone–iodine before use. Once the sample has been collected it should be placed into a dry sterile vial or 100% ethanol.

Procedure for epidermal mucus (swabs) sampling

Epidermal mucus is used increasingly for molecular analysis. Mucus sampling techniques are minimally invasive; however, researchers should consider whether sufficient quality samples can be collected for the intended analysis (e.g. where high-quality genomic DNA may be required in downstream processing). These approaches are in their infancy, and several recent techniques have emerged that include the use of different collection mediums (e.g. FTA® Elute Cards, buccal swabs, cotton cloths and toothbrushes). Techniques vary based on whether samples are collected on-water or in-water. On-water sampling occurs via a surface vessel and can be used on most species for which fin clipping and biopsy sampling are used (Lieber *et al.* 2013). Most in-water sampling is undertaken via SCUBA and focuses on large species that may be difficult or sensitive to capture (Kashiwagi *et al.* 2015; Balázs *et al.* 2020). Once the samples have been collected, they are stored in a freezer/on ice or transferred to an FTA® Elute Card to reduce degradation.

Procedure for stomach content collection

This procedure is mainly used on chondrichthyan species to facilitate regurgitation of stomach contents. Stomach flushing can be undertaken by inserting a plastic hose (the diameter will depend on the species size) through the mouth into the stomach. The hose is attached to an electric pump propelling water into the species' stomach. Once the stomach is filled with water, personnel remove the hose, and apply gentle pressure to the abdominal region until all contents have been regurgitated (Barnett *et al.* 2010). Personnel collect the regurgitated material in a sieve for storage in plastic containers/bags in the freezer or 70% ethanol.

Procedure for blood sampling

Non-lethal blood sampling is becoming a standard procedure to obtain biological information from fishes and chondrichthyans (e.g. reproductive parameters; health condition). Animals should be weighed before blood collection. No more than 1% of the animal's body mass should be removed during blood collection; personnel should assume that 1 mL of blood weighs ~1 g. For teleosts, fish may be anaesthetised prior collection. However, anaesthesia is not a common procedure for chondrichthyans. Suitable needles and syringes should be chosen with the needle gauge (the needle diameter) and length adjusted depending on the size of the animal. For example, for animals that are 1 m in length, a 22 G needle would be appropriate, while for large sharks, an 18–14 G needle should be used. Needle length can be up to 110 mm. Syringe size will vary according to the quantity of blood to be taken. Vacutainers® are also used for blood extraction. To avoid blood clotting, needles and syringes or collection vials must be coated with an anticoagulant (e.g. heparin, EDTA). However, it is important to ensure that the anticoagulant does not interfere with the blood properties being examined (see Campbell (2015) for more information on preferred anticoagulants). Blood samples in teleosts and chondrichthyans can be taken from several locations on the body, depending on the species and the sizes (Table 13.7). Once blood collection is finished, and if not using a vacutainer, blood should be transferred into storage vials. The needle must be removed from the syringe before expelling the blood through the syringe hub into the tube (to avoid haemolysis).

Ultrasound and endoscopy

Ultrasound can provide a precise diagnostic and minimise handling. Several types of ultrasounds equipment are available. Precise methods depend on the field/laboratory conditions and the ultrasound machine specifications (i.e. linear versus curve transducers, depth range and ultrasound frequency). Typically, linear transducers are used. However, for large teleosts and chondrichthyans, a curve transducer with deeper scan range is preferred. While some species remain under water during the procedure, others are kept out of water. While some transducers are applied ventrally, others may be applied either laterally or dorsally depending on the diagnostic (Whittamore *et al.* 2010; Guitreau *et al.* 2012; Novelo and Tiersch 2012; Anderson *et al.* 2018).

Endoscopy has the potential to be a valuable non-lethal tool, mainly when examining the reproductive tract or observing the presence/absence of embryos/egg capsules. However, it is important to reduce the risk of abortion. When considering an endoscopic procedure in fish, the anatomy of the species, how the species will be immobilised and the performance of the procedure should all be considered. In chondrichthyan species the endoscope is generally inserted through the cloaca, while in teleost species incisions are generally made above the base of the pelvic fin on the side of the fishes for insertion of the endoscope into the body cavity. It is highly recommended that an anaesthetic is applied (either general or local) for these invasive procedures on teleosts. For more information on chondrichthyans see Murray (2010), or for teleosts see Swenson *et al.* (2007).

Animal treatment, withdrawal and euthanasia

Animals often have good survival outcomes with all non-lethal procedures, if capture and handling practices are undertaken effectively. However, additional considerations apply when releasing animals in deep

Table 13.7: Common procedures for sampling blood from teleosts and chondrichthyans.

Adapted from Campbell (2015).

Method	Species target	Procedure	Comments
Caudal puncture	Teleosts and chondrichthyans (Figure 13.1)	Gently insert the needle perpendicular to the body along the ventral midline, guiding the needle towards the vertebral body into the caudal vein that lies just below the vertebrae. A slight suction from the syringe will create enough pressure to get the blood flowing. To identify if the vein was reached, the needle will touch the vertebrae (feels like a 'click'), then back ~1 mm to position the needle right into the vein and slowly suction the syringe to extract the blood. The suction pressure on the syringe should be gentle, as the vein may collapse and stop blood flow.	Chondrichthyan denticles provide a toughened barrier for the needle to go through, so areas closer to the fins (either ventral or anal) or just at the beginning of the cloaca may be more appropriate. If possible, animals should be restrained ventral side up on a stable surface. This type of procedure can also be done laterally.
Caudal sinus and dorsal sinus puncture	Large size elasmobranchs (Figure 13.2)	Gently insert the needle perpendicular or slightly inclined to the body into the dorsal or caudal sinus.	In whale sharks, blood can also be obtained from the dorsal side of the pelvic fin, or on the dorsal side of the pectoral fin.
Cardiac puncture	Many teleosts and batoid species. Cardiac puncture is used to obtain blood samples where it is difficult to do caudal puncture (Figure 13.3)	Gently insert the needle perpendicular to the ventral surface of the animal, in general the heart can be localised in the centre of an imaginary line between the anterior end of the pectoral fins. In some teleost species, the needle is inserted into the caudal margin of the operculum.	In many teleost species, blood can be drawn from the dorsal aorta, either by reaching the aorta through the animal's mouth or along the body axis and posterior to the anus. In many batoid species, blood can be drawn from the radial wing vessels. The mesopterygial vein provides quick vascular access located immediately ventrolateral to the metapterygium cartilage (Westmoreland *et al.* 2019).

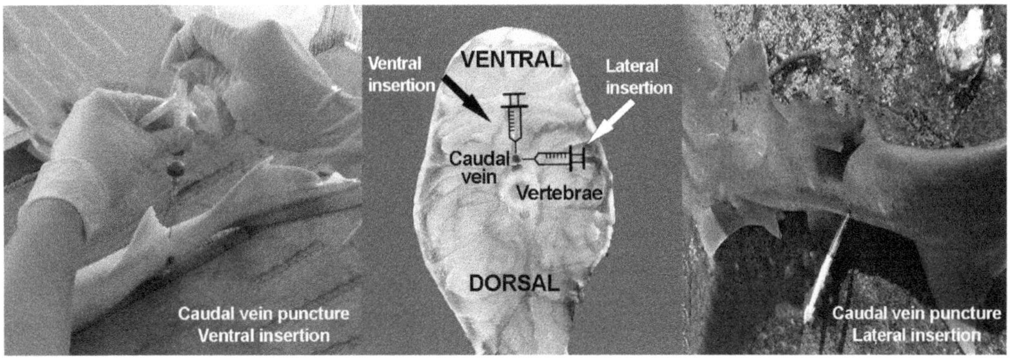

Figure 13.1: Caudal puncture blood sampling of fusiform elasmobranchs. Image by Cynthia Awruch.

water. If required, fish can be gently 'swum' manually through the water to wash oxygenated water over the gills until they regain equilibrium and swim off independently. The presence of possible predators should be checked. Animals with life-threatening injuries (e.g. severe barotrauma or badly torn gills) may need to be euthanased.

Equipment and maintenance

Specific equipment depends on the method selected, but general equipment may include:

- data collection equipment (e.g. wet gloves, scales, rulers and fish measuring boards)
- appropriate research vessel to allow effective handling of animals (e.g. low sides to provide easy

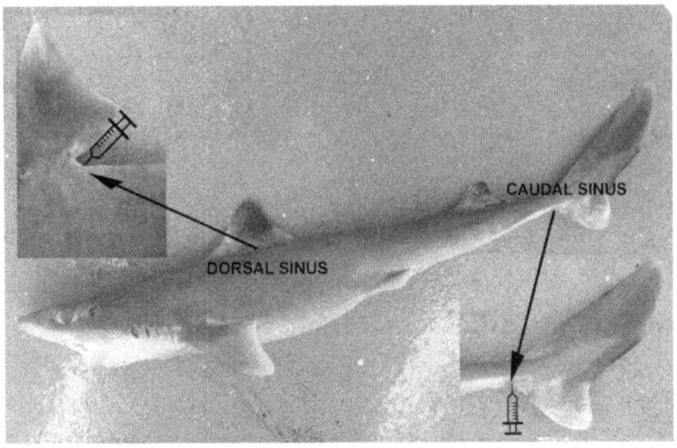

Figure 13.2: Dorsal and caudal sinus blood sampling of fusiform elasmobranchs. Image by Cynthia Awruch.

access to water or platforms for work on the boasts deck)

- data sheets, pencils, pens, waterproof marker
- field identification guide(s)
- fishing/sampling permits
- ice, esky or freezer.

More-specific items may include:

- sharp scissors, sheers or knife (tissue sampling)
- ethanol or diluted povidone-iodine for sterilising (tissue and biopsy sampling)
- sample vials with preservative such as DMSO or ethanol (tissue and biopsy sampling)
- plastic sealable bags, containers or vials required for samples (tissue and biopsy sampling)
- buccal swabs and zip lock bags/storage containers (mucus sampling)
- needle, syringes, tubes to place the blood and anticoagulants (blood sampling)
- large holding container, portable or plumbed aerator, spare batteries
- anaesthetic (if required)
- equipment for euthanasia
- latex gloves.

Specific qualifications, experience and training

Capturing wild fishes for research requires knowledge of where and when to find animals for capture, and of the equipment to be used. Non-lethal sampling approaches are generally considered low risk, and there is no formal training requirement for non-lethal sampling techniques on fishes, but researchers should first gain experience on the techniques with an experienced supervisor to ensure competency.

Workplace health and safety

Most health and safety considerations apply to capture and handling techniques associated with sampling techniques. Therefore, researchers working on these species must be properly trained in safe capture and handling techniques. Health and safety concerns associated with capture and handling techniques will vary considerably based on the target species, method, equipment, personnel experience level and location. Additional health and safety concerns that apply directly to non-lethal sampling methods include potential injury from sharp knives, sheers, needles or chemicals, which should be considered under workplace health and safety assessments.

Alternative procedures

Non-lethal sampling approaches are generally considered among the lowest-impact methods for answering biological questions about teleosts and chondrichthyans. Alternative non-lethal procedures include observational methods, such as baited remote underwater video

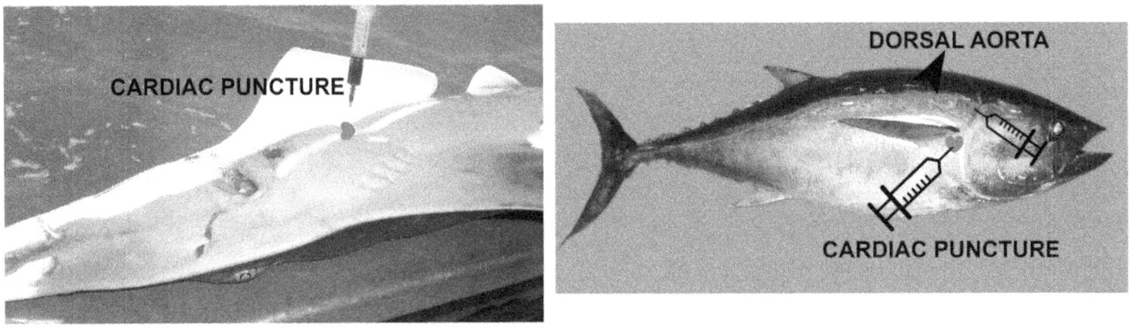

Figure 13.3: Cardiac puncture on ventral side of flat chondrichthyans and location of cardiac puncture and dorsal aorta on teleosts. Image by Cynthia Awruch.

stations (BRUVS) and the photo capture–recapture method (for species with distinct patterning, such as manta rays, *Mobula* spp., and whale sharks, *Rhincodon typus*), are often used to evaluate ecological research questions.

INTERNAL TAGGING METHODS

Adam Barnett

Context and scope

This GOP describes internal tagging methods for teleosts and chondrichthyans. Given the diversity in size, morphology, behaviour, life history and physiological tolerances of fish species and the highly variable environmental conditions between field work locations, no single standard procedure fits all species. Variations in method between species are discussed. In many cases, chosen method is a trade-off between best practice in a laboratory environment and what is practical in field locations where conditions can vary considerably – for example, from working from the bank of a lake, in small confined boats in coastal waters, to boats in the rough seas of the open ocean.

Animal welfare considerations

Anaesthesia

Most of the internal tagging techniques are invasive and some require minor medical procedures. Therefore, the potential for pain and distress needs consideration. Whether teleosts feel pain remains a contentious issue unable to be reached by scientific consensus (see Key 2016, and related commentaries in *Animal Sentience* Volume 1 2016). Notwithstanding, the ethical standpoint adopted here is a precautionary approach that would recommend anaesthesia be used in minor procedures such as internal tagging. However, before routinely using anaesthesia several considerations need to be addressed. In general, anaesthesia is not recommended when the risks from anaesthesia outweigh the benefits (Wargo Rub *et al.* 2014). Consideration must be given to the morphology and behaviour of each species and decisions made on a species-specific basis (Readman *et al.* 2017). The effects of anaesthetics are largely unknown for most teleosts and chondrichthyans (Neiffer and Stamper 2009; Cooke *et al.* 2016). Even between closely related taxa, the effects of anaesthesia may be vastly different and caution is required when using on a species for the first time (Readman *et al.* 2017). The effects of anaesthesia can also differ between life-history stages and environmental conditions (e.g. Cooke *et al.* 2016). Field work settings also need consideration (e.g. the ability to provide appropriate post-operative care). If used, the lightest plane of anaesthesia is recommended (Wargo Rub *et al.* 2014).

Tagging studies aim to minimise handling and surgery time and release tagged fish as fast as possible. Anaesthesia extends the handling time of the fish considerably and can impair fish behaviour and influence survival after release – for example, increase mortality from predation (Cooke *et al.* 2016). General anaesthesia on fish is typically administrated by immersing a fish in a container with diluted anaesthetic. This limits the size of the fish that can be anaesthetised in the field. For fast swimming obligate ram ventilators, anaesthesia is not recommended due to problems such as fish jumping out of the anaesthetising tub, anaesthesia killing fish due to unmet oxygen demands, or difficult recovery through impaired oxygen uptake. The hypnosis method, where an immobility reflex is induced by a strong flow of water through the branchial chamber (Wells *et al.* 2005), is more appropriate for these species. In this method, fish are turned upside down and a vigorous water flow is provided to stimulate the branchial chamber, inducing an immobility reflex referred to as the atonic immobility reflex (Wells *et al.* 2005). Normal behaviour returns immediately upon returning the fish to an upright position.

For chondrichthyans, many species are too large, too active and/or need to swim to breathe, preventing the use of a general anaesthetic and restraint for long periods. Little information is available on the effects of general anaesthesia on this group, including on their ability to breathe. Research to date suggests chondrichthyans do not have the physiological ability to feel pain like mammals do (Rose *et al.* 2014; Sneddon 2018). Historically, researchers have secured large sharks for procedures using tonic immobility, an innate reversible paralysis through dorso-ventral inversion which facilitates fast recovery (Kessel *et al.* 2015; Williamson *et al.* 2018). The local anaesthesia method described above for teleosts should also be considered here for the chondrichthyans as a precautionary measure when undertaking internal tagging procedures.

Size and weight of transmitter/tag

A central consideration for selecting a transmitter is the size and mass of the transmitter in relation to the body size or mass of the fish. The conservative 2% rule (Smircich and Kelly 2014), where the transmitter is ≤ 2% of the animal's body mass is commonly applied. However, in some instances, tags of up to 5–10% of body mass may be appropriate (Smircich and Kelly 2014; Sloman *et al.* 2019). Body cavity size in relation to organs and digestive track, dimensions of tag, and effects on buoyancy should also be considered (Cooke *et al.* 2011; Sloman *et al.* 2019). Therefore, the 2% rule is flexible (taxa-specific), but a useful guideline if no experimental evidence is available for specific taxa.

General procedures

Holding and restraining fish

Holding fish for tagging is either done with the fish removed from the water (on board the boat or the shoreline) or in-water, with the fish secured to the side of the boat or held in shallow water. For out of water tagging, fish should be kept wet and it is important to ensure that water is covering the gills to allow oxygen uptake. This process can involve placing the fish in a water-filled trough (with a high dissolved oxygen content) using a cradle (to support the fish) ventral side up, so that the ventral surface (i.e. area of implantation) is above the water line but the gills remain submerged, or by using a bilge pump and tube to continually pass water over the gills. A valve controlling water pressure should ideally be used so adjustments to the water flow can be made for differently sized fish.

In-water tagging typically requires restraining the animal by either holding it (by pectoral and tail regions), or by securing the animal to the side of the vessel using soft rope or a harness/cradle. It is important that whichever method is used, the fish's gills are underwater, and water is passing over the gills. The holding method will depend on the size of the fish, the size and configuration of the boat, and fieldwork conditions. Common procedures for internal tagging and marking are summarised in Table 13.8. These procedures are not exhaustive and technological advances are occurring rapidly. New applications (e.g. elasmobranch birthing tags, currently in prototype phase) should be considered as they arise.

Aseptic techniques

In field conditions, it is impossible to attain the level of aseptic standards in laboratory settings. Nevertheless, procedures should strive to be as sterile as possible (Wagner *et al.* 2011). Soaking transmitters and tools in chemicals is the most feasible aseptic technique in the field, but care must be taken as many sterilising chemicals are toxic to fish (Wargo Rub *et al.* 2014). Soaking transmitters and tools in antiseptic baths (e.g. chlorhexidine diacetate or povidone-iodine) before planned procedures in solutions of decreasing concentration can prevent chemicals irritating fish tissues. Sterile sutures should be used. The use of disposable gloves is desirable but can be impractical and/or not feasible in some conditions. Also, if gloved hands touch potentially contaminated surfaces (e.g. the fish's exterior, the boat or even seawater), they can be just as contaminated as bare hands. Washing fingers in an antiseptic bath (with or without gloves) before touching tools, the incision site and the transmitter is an option. Tools should be disinfected and rinsed between procedures and/or several sets of instruments used in rotation. Use a new scalpel blade for each animal.

Table 13.8: Common procedures for internal tagging and marking of fishes.

Method	Procedure	Comments
Acoustic transmitters	Internal tag implantation or external fitting	Transmitters send data to a receiver. Tag sizes allow use on a vast range of species and sizes.
Archival loggers/transmitters	Internal tag implantation or external fitting	Data stored in the tag. Mainly for species that will be recaptured.
Radio transmitters	Internal tag implantation or external fitting	Transmitters send data to a receiver. Only used in freshwater systems.
Passive integrated transponder (PIT tag)	Tag injected into fish or manually implanted	Recaptured fish is scanned by a PIT tag reader for identification.
Intra-gastric tagging(e.g. pH loggers)	Fish swallows tag, normally hidden in food	Tag is either regurgitated or passed days to weeks later.

An example of an aseptic process in field locations follows:

1. Soak tools and transmitters in 100% povidone–iodine well before surgery.
2. Prior to tag implantation, move the tools and transmitters into 50% povidone–iodine to 50% distilled/filtered water solution.
3. Immediately before implantation, dip transmitter in distilled/filtered water.

Other considerations for asepsis include the following:

1. Coating transmitters in paraffin or beeswax may increase tag retention in species that are prone to expelling transmitters (see Cooke *et al.* 2011), as coatings provide a layer of natural material that may encourage tissue encapsulation.
2. In some teleosts, the removal of some scales is needed to access the dermis. If scale removal is required, a minimal number should be removed using forceps by applying constant retraction in a caudal direction at a 45° angle (Wargo Rub *et al.* 2014).
3. The fish mucous layer is a physical barrier that inhibits infections and supports immune response. Therefore, applying chemical disinfectants to the incision site can be counterproductive (preventing the effectiveness of the mucous layer and delaying healing) or even harmful (e.g. irritate or damage the integument) (Wagner *et al.* 2011; Wargo Rub *et al.* 2014).

Procedure for surgically implanting transmitters, including anaesthesia

Preparation for internal tagging at sea should include consideration of the proposed field settings and target species, and researchers need to ensure that all necessary equipment and anaesthesia are prepared, organised and easily accessible, so that the tagging process is completed in a timely manner. As part of the animal ethical approvals, an assessment of whether general or local anaesthesia be used (decided on a species-by-species basis) would have been made. For assistance on this process, see Figure 13.4. Details on the capture, handling, monitoring and release procedures should also be planned well ahead of fieldwork commencing (see earlier GOPs in this chapter). Local anaesthesia through injections for internal tagging procedures is recommended for teleosts. By injecting a short-acting anaesthetic at the site of the tag insertion location, veterinarian advice is that tagging can proceed immediately with the anaesthesia taking full effect by the end of the procedure and providing pain relief for up to 24 h. Correct dosages for the chosen anaesthetic should be calculated at the start of the project during the project preparation and training stages, with a veterinarian. Anaesthesia is generally not recommended for chondrichthyans (see 'Animal welfare').

Transmitters are most often implanted through the ventral surface midway between the pelvic fin and cloaca into the peritoneal cavity. For teleosts, incision can also be done on lateral and parallel to the midline (for pros and cons of each incision positioning see Wagner *et al.* 2011). Body shape can also influence incision location – for example, in flat fish the peritoneal cavity may be accessed dorsally (Wargo Rub *et al.* 2014). A scalpel or sharp knife is used to make a small incision through the muscle layer until reaching the peritoneum. Care must be taken when the peritoneum is reached as a deep cut risks damage to internal organs. A finger or the blunt end of a scalpel handle can be used to gently penetrate the peritoneum. For smaller individuals, gently lifting the skin with forceps when making the incision can help avoid a cut passing through the peritoneum and nicking an organ. The incision should be only just large enough for the tag to tightly slide into the body cavity, normally ~1–4 cm long, depending on the size of the tag and fish (e.g. large sharks with thick muscle layers may need longer incisions on the outer muscle wall). Insert the tag into the body cavity either forwards or sideways (ventral for lateral incisions), so that the tag lies in line with the length of the fish but is sitting off the incision site.

The incision should be sutured with medical grade absorbable sutures. Suture size will vary depending on size of the fish, and where possible suturing both the muscle layer and then the skin layer is advised if conditions permit. In general, to minimise introduction of foreign material, the smallest suture material that will effectively hold tissues in apposition without tearing through skin at incision site should be used (Figure 13.5). Half-circle reverse cutting needles with coloured suture material are recommended. Archival transmitters and radio transmitters have trailing antennas and light stalks protruding outside of the body cavity. Suturing the incision should include placing sutures immediately posterior to the tag stalk to keep it from slipping back (CSIRO 2015).

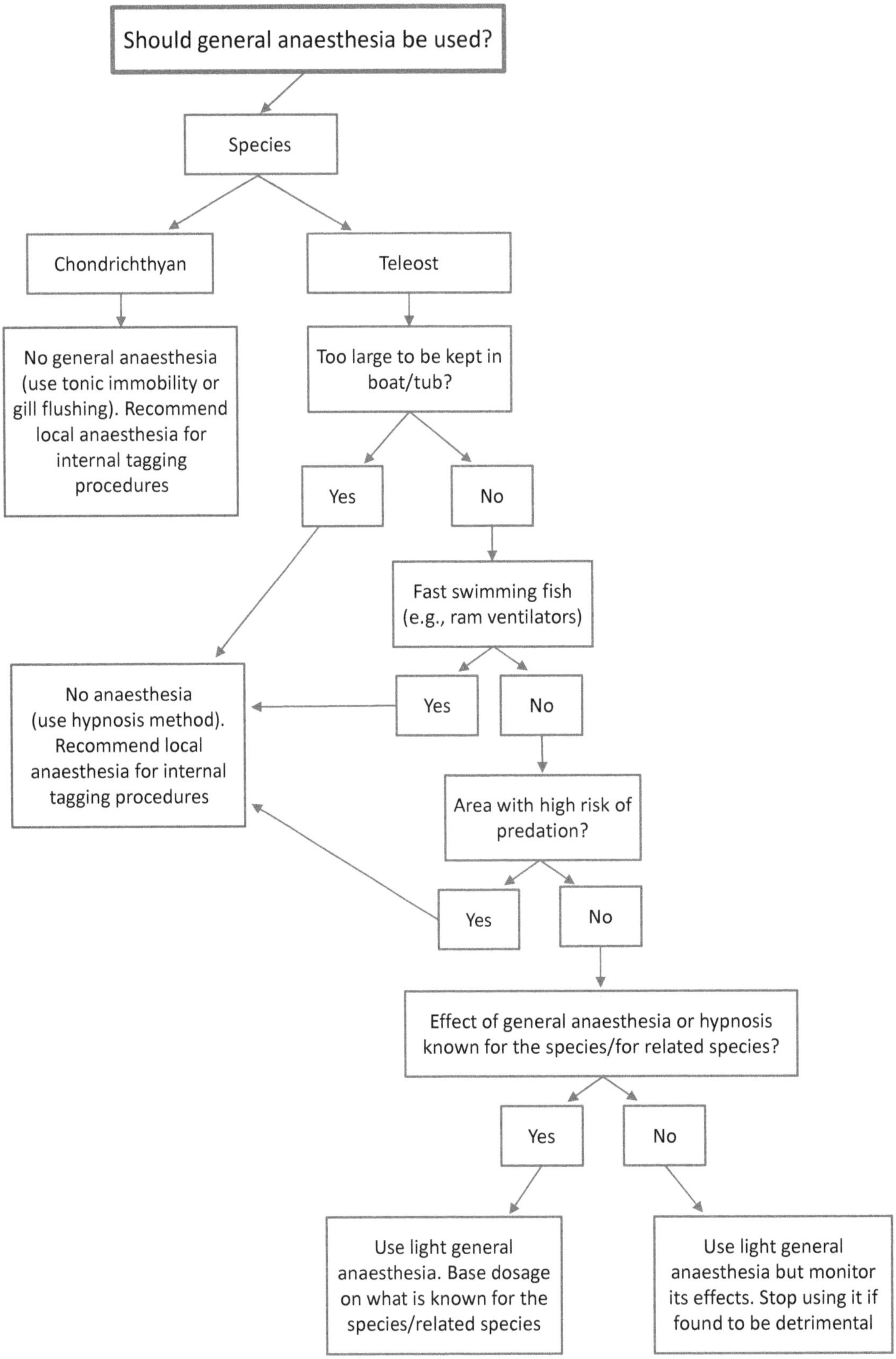

Figure 13.4: Decision flowchart on general and local anaesthesia use for internal tagging procedures. Illustration by Adam Barnett.

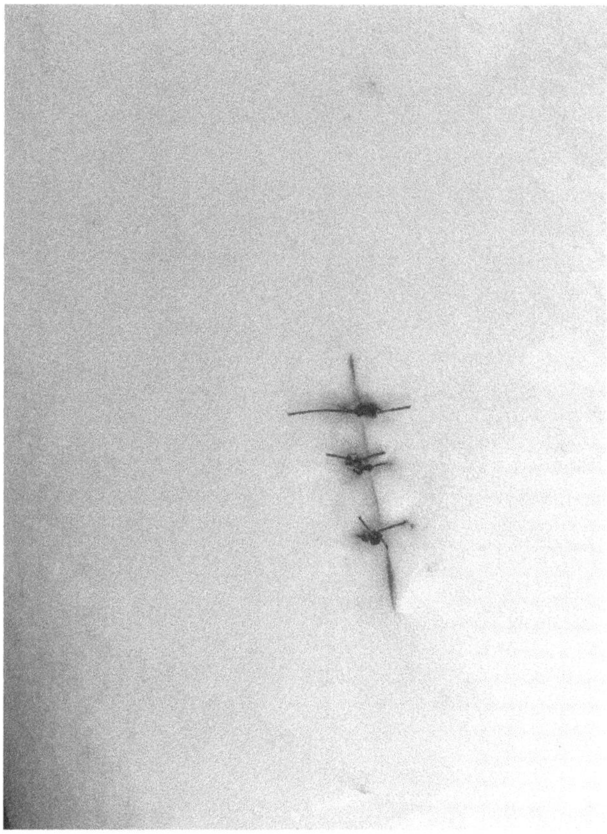

Figure 13.5: Suture site following acoustic tag insertion into a shark peritoneal cavity. Photo by Paul Butcher (NSW DPI).

Monitoring during procedures

A member of the research team responsible for monitoring should always ensure water is continually flowing over or covering gills and the fish is always wet. Changes in colour or mottled skin can be an indication that the teleost or chondrichthyan is not doing well (e.g. may need increased water flow/oxygen). Significant deterioration during procedures should result in the procedures being ceased until the animal can be stabilised. It is also not desirable to place costly tags on animals that will not survive the procedure.

Recovery and release

Teleosts that were placed under light general anaesthesia should be placed in recovery containers on the boat or in cages attached to the boat, and monitored until showing signs of recovery (e.g. regaining equilibrium, responding to touch (e.g. tail grab) and, for fish being released from the recovery container, showing a body flex response when being transferred from container to the water). If recovery cages have doors, open the door to see if the fish swims out on its own. Recovery times can vary considerably between species. For large teleosts or chondrichthyans where a local anaesthetic was applied, free them from restraints, return them from tonic immobility (if applied) and hold them lightly to see if they will swim under their own strength. If the animal appears lethargic/weak or does not show signs of wanting to swim away, gently move it back and forth to ensure water flows over the gills. For large teleosts and sharks tagged in water, the boat can be put into gear and this will flush water across the gills as the boat moves very slowly forward. These animals should only be released when capable of swimming under their own strength. Batoids (rays, skates, sawfish) can be released immediately after surgery as they will sit on the bottom and breathe through buccal pumping.

Passive integrated transponder (PIT) tags

For species consumed by humans, only food-safe polymer PIT tags should be used. Larger PIT tags can be implanted surgically as described above. Smaller PIT tags are applied just under the skin in the dorsal body musculature or into the body cavity (intracoelomic), using a needle and/or applicator gun. The specific location will depend on the fish size and species. Disinfect the applicator needle and PIT tag (e.g. using Betadine®) before deployment. PIT tags are applied at a shallow angle with needle pressure just enough to penetrate the body wall so that the needle enters the muscle or body cavity parallel to the body wall, not perpendicular. Multiple injectors are often needed as the needles have to be disinfected between fish (e.g. soaked in ethanol or rinsed in a 50:50 Betadine® and distilled water solution). PIT tags can be deployed in small juvenile fish, so the 2% rule may need to be considered.

Animal treatment, withdrawal and euthanasia

If a poor/negative response to anaesthesia is evident, stop the procedure and move the animal to a recovery cage/tub to monitor recovery. Flushing gills with water may help recovery. If an internal organ is accidently cut, implanting the transmitter should be abandoned and fish may need to be euthanased if bleeding profusely.

Equipment and maintenance

Equipment for holding fish for tagging may include:

- cradle/tub
- tail ropes (for large fish)
- bilge pump and hose with valve to adjust water pressure
- battery for bilge pump

- anaesthetic (and instrument to measure volumes)
- tub to anaesthetise fish
- recovery cage/tub
- aerator or oxygen for recovery tub
- soft net for handling
- towels (multi-purpose, e.g. cover eyes, keep fish damp or protected from sun).

Medical items may include:

- needle drivers/holders
- sutures
- scalpel-blades or knife
- tweezers
- antiseptic (liquid, e.g. Betadine®)
- filtered/distilled water
- containers for antiseptic baths (decreasing concentration)
- latex gloves
- transmitters.

Specific qualifications, experience and training

Training is required for researchers to be able to conduct invasive procedures on live fish competently. Training should only be provided by experienced practitioners. Using an accepted commercial preparation, such as AQUI-S®, is appropriate where light general anaesthesia for internal procedures on small animals that can be brought onto the boat is required. Advanced knowledge of appropriate dosages based on target species (if known) should be ascertained before fieldwork commences. For local anaesthesia, researchers should liaise and undergo training with a veterinarian (preferably one proficient with fish) before undertaking fieldwork. A dosage plan based on the target species should also be developed in consultation with a veterinarian.

Initial practice in incisions and suturing should be conducted on materials/objects (e.g. bananas, oranges) and dead fish. Trainees should observe an experienced practitioner when they implant transmitters into live fish. When the trainee is competent in all facets of internal tagging, they conduct a series of procedures on live fish under the supervision of the trainer. Once regarded as proficient in implanting transmitters in live fish, the researchers can conduct procedures unsupervised (see CSIRO 2015 for further details on training).

Alternative procedures

Internally implanting transmitters is considered the lower-impact option in most cases, and is the most widely used method in longer-term studies. Benefits include eliminating the potential for biofouling on the tag, which irritates/impacts tagged fish and avoids any capacity for the tag to cause drag on the fish, and increasing tag retention time.

EXTERNAL TAGGING AND PHOTO IDENTIFICATION

Luciana C. Ferreira and Sean Tracey

Context and scope

This GOP describes methods for external tagging and individual identification of teleosts and chondrichthyans. Many of these species are captured and tagged to understand their movement patterns in time and space. These data can be critical for improving understanding of habitat use, seasonal or prey drivers, and elucidating associated oceanographic or ocean chemistry factors that influence movements. Information on movements, growth rates, relative abundance and mortality obtained from tags can also assist in scientific assessments of populations, which are important for fisheries management. Tag types and attachment methods vary depending on the species targeted and the research questions posed (Table 13.9). Jepsen *et al.* (2015) also provide a detailed list of tagging methods for a range of species.

Animal welfare considerations

Anaesthesia

The application of external tags, except for fixed fin mounts, is generally a rapid process. Depending on the capture rate of the target species it is possible to tag large numbers of animals rapidly; this technique is particularly useful for tag and recapture studies that rely on a large sample size of individuals, generally tagged with passive tags, to estimate population size. External tagging usually involves subdermal insertion of stainless steel or plastic dart heads. These activities are also often undertaken by recreational anglers who participate in citizen science programs (Chapter 10) on teleosts and chondrichthyans. For these rapid, minimally invasive procedures, anaesthesia is rarely applied. See Figure 13.4 for guidance on deciding to use local or general anaesthesia for tagging procedures.

Behavioural changes

Animals might flee in the presence of divers during photo identification. Standard operating procedures for animal

Table 13.9: Considerations for methods commonly used for tagging teleosts and chondrichthyans.

Method	Attachment type	Considerations
Photo identification	None	Suitable for animals with distinctive natural colouring or patterning (which shows limited change over time), or scars and deformities. Requires repeat observation *in situ*.
Camera tags (crittercams)	Fin mount (clamp)	Animals require a large dorsal attachment point. Suitable for larger fish and chondrichthyans.
Satellite-linked tags	Fin mount (fixed); intramuscular (towed)	Animals require a large dorsal attachment point that breaks the surface of the water. Suitable for some larger fish and chondrichthyans.
Identification tags (spaghetti, T-bar, rototag)	Intramuscular/intraskeletal	Requires fish to be recaptured. Different tag types should be considered based on size of the animal (e.g. T-bar for small fish, spaghetti tag for larger fish/chondrichthyans, rototags for chondrichthyans).
Acoustic tag	Intramuscular/intraskeletal (may also be deployed internally)	Transmitters send data to a receiver. Tag sizes allow use on a vast range of species and sizes.
Pop-up satellite tag (PSAT)	Intramuscular/intraskeletal	Does not require recapture, but larger tag size and potential drag restricts use to larger fish and chondrichthyans.
Accelerometer and archival tag	Intramuscular/intraskeletal; fin mount (clamp)	Requires fish to be recaptured or tag to shed and be recovered. Often mounted to other tags such as identification or PSAT.

encounter have been developed for some species (e.g. whale sharks; Department of Parks and Wildlife 2013); these procedures should be reviewed by investigators before commencing a study. Short-term behavioural effects may be expected from tag attachment, the risk of which can be minimised by ensuring that tags do not exceed a mass appropriate for the study species. Typically, a tag should not weigh more than 2% of the animal's body mass (Smircich and Kelly 2014). However, larger tag-to-body ratios might be possible for some species, and size and shape of fins, body size and condition (intramuscular attachment) should be also be considered.

Stress and external injury

Some level of stress to the animal is unavoidable during capture, handling and tagging. To reduce stress related to handling and tagging of animal, all tagging procedures must be conducted by experienced investigators. The animal should be monitored constantly, and the procedure ended if excessive stress is observed. Hydrodynamic drag of towed tags may cause changes in swimming efficiency and lead to increased energetic demands. This risk is minimised by using tags that are designed to improve hydrodynamics and minimise effects on swimming. Also, fin-mounted tags using clamps are designed to detach after 24 h or a maximum of weeks. Moderate discomfort is likely to be experienced from intramuscular and fixed fin-mount tag attachments. Discomfort is minimised by affixing external tags to dorsal musculature where connective tissue is thicker or to cartilage (i.e. the dorsal fin of elasmobranchs, which does not contain blood supply or nerve endings).

Air exposure

Tagging procedures should be completed as quickly as possible to reduce stress caused by air exposure. If a procedure is expected to take longer than 3–5 min, gills (for animals tagged on board vessels) should receive constant irrigation.

Increased risk of predation

Animals might experience greater predation risk post-release. This risk can be lowered if stress levels are minimal during the tagging process, and the animal is allowed recovery time in water. These strategies will allow them to move away quickly once released. Avoiding using anaesthetics reduces susceptibility to predation post-release.

Tag retention

Tag loss can affect studies aiming to estimate population size. For electronic tags, which are often expensive, early tag detachment can result in substantial data loss and incur a large financial cost. For conventional tags, a double-tagging component is often added to an experiment to assist in quantifying tag loss rate. However, quantification relies on a sufficiently large sample of recaptured double-tagged fish. For satellite tags, the number of data retrieved from the tag will generally indicate if premature detachment occurred. A combination of conventional and telemetry tagging can also provide insight into tag retention rates (Jepsen *et al.* 2015). Tag retention will vary by attachment method, but also by species with some more likely to shed an external tag than others (Jepsen *et al.* 2015).

General procedures

Procedure for observational tagging

Photographic identification has great potential for mark–recapture analysis in elasmobranchs. The presence of natural markings in some species allows for permanent 'tagging' of individuals. Natural markings include natural colouring patterns on the skin, or scars and deformities. The effectiveness of this method depends on target species and the presence of natural markings, their behaviour, natural environment and population size (Marshall and Pierce 2012). Natural markings of individuals are recorded by photography (still and video), most commonly through diving or free-diving with the animal in-water. Snorkellers or divers approach the free-swimming animal and photograph a standardised area of the body where identifiable markings occur. The area selected for photo identification will depend on the focal species, and include the dorsal and ventral region, or the left and right sides of the body. A standardised area is also needed when using scars and deformities (e.g. deformities of the dorsal fin) for identifying animals.

Procedures for fin-mount attachments

Fin mounts attached with clamps can be used on free-swimming animals or on restrained animals alongside a boat or on board vessels (see Chapters 30 and 31 for capture and restraint details). Stainless-steel clamps are used for short-term deployments of camera tags and accelerometer packages that need to be attached to clamps via a docking pin to the dorsal fin. Clamps conform to the shape of the fin and allow the tag to stay attached without moving or puncturing the animal's skin (Gleiss *et al.* 2009; Chapple *et al.* 2015). The clamp should be attached near the base of the dorsal fin where connective tissue is thickest. Where tags are deployed in-water, divers or snorkellers swim alongside the animal and open the clamp around the dorsal fin to attach it or use a specialised tagging pole. This method allows the animal to swim away immediately after tag deployment. Consideration of shark size is necessary to determine the height of clamp deployment on the fin and ensure the best field of view for a camera tag. The clamp is passively released from the animal after a given amount of time through the use of corrodible links that must be selected in consideration of water temperature, deployment duration and movement rate of the animal tagged. Tags deployed with clamps are encased in packages containing a buoy to allow tag recovery. Consequently, these tag types are often large. Tag size in relation to animal body mass and size (< 0.2%) must be considered.

Procedures for fixed attachments

Animals are restrained alongside the vessel or, for smaller animals, brought on board (see 'Capture and release methods' earlier in this chapter). A fin-mount fixed attachment is the most common attachment for satellite-linked transmitters on sharks as the tag's antenna, and wet and dry sensors must remain out of the water when the shark is on the water's surface (Ferreira *et al.* 2018). Hence, this attachment type is only suitable for species with wide and/or tall dorsal fins. These tag attachment methods may also be used on large teleosts, but have been used less frequently because these species tend to spend less time at the water's surface (required for tags to transmit). Tags are mounted on the dorsal fin using bolts made of corrodible titanium or stainless steel that allow the tag to fall off after battery exhaustion. The tag is secured with neoprene, a steel washer and nuts. The neoprene helps avoid contact between the metal components and the shark's skin, which may cause metal corrosion (Figure 13.6). Fin-mounted tags are unlikely to cause long-term damage on the shark's dorsal fin if attached for ≤ 24 months (Jewell *et al.* 2011). Tag placement must be determined based on the size and shape of the fin of individual to be tagged. Multiple (two to four) holes are drilled into the dorsal fin of the animal guided by configuration of attachment points of tag used (Figure 13.6).

Procedure for intramuscular or intraskeletal attachment

Intramuscular or intraskeletal tags can be attached to animals when they are free swimming (in-water), restrained alongside the vessel, or brought on board the vessel (see Chapters 30 and 31 for capture and restraint details). These tags are primarily attached with a tag applicator (Bradford *et al.* 2009). The primary component of an applicator is a needle (either hollow or solid

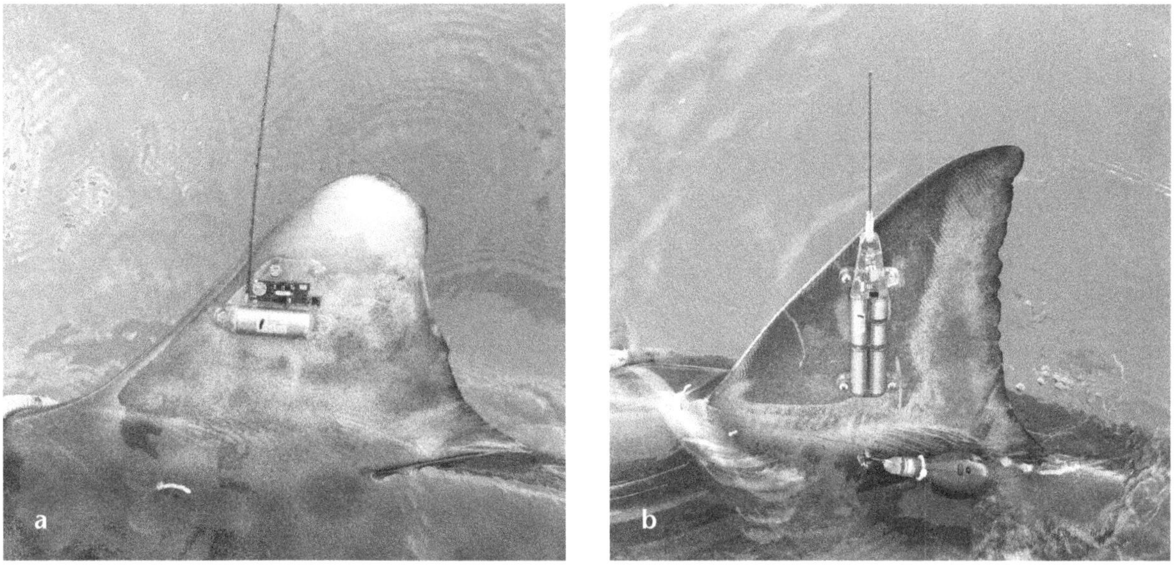

Figure 13.6: External tag attachments for (a) fin-mounted satellite and yellow intramuscular spaghetti identification tags fitted to a tiger shark (*Galeocerdo cuvier*) and (b) fin-mounted satellite and intramuscular pop-up satellite tags (PSAT) (double-tagging) fitted to a great white shark (*Carcharodon carcharias*). Photos by Paul Butcher (NSW DPI).

depending on tag anchor configuration) of sufficient size to hold the tag and length to reach the desired anchor point, but not so long as to cause unnecessary damage to the animal. The decision to attach the tag intramuscularly or intraskeletally will depend on the tag's anchor type. A range of different anchor types have been designed for different species and attachment points. Some attachment methods have additional considerations for the animal, such as the need to remove or lift scales (e.g. when using T-bar anchors).

Intramuscular tags often have a larger flat anchor head than other anchor types; this design will provide some resistance against the muscular tissue and reduce the probability of tag rejection. While the method is based on intramuscular attachment, additional factors, such as applying the tag in areas with denser tissue (often under dorsal fin structure, see Figure 13.6), or in species with thicker skin, can reduce the probability of tag loss. Intraskeletal anchors will generally have some form of hook that will lock around skeletal structure, such as dorsal fin rays (pterygiophores).

Another important consideration when applying an external tag is the length of the applicator. A shorter applicator (or tagging pole) allows for more accurate and controlled placement of the tag, facilitating greater potential for tag retention and reduced potential impact on the animal. However, in many cases, particularly with larger fish, sharks or when operating from larger vessels, a longer tag pole may be required for crew and animal safety (to prevent a large animal thrashing around close to the boat, potentially causing damage to itself, crew or the vessel).

Animal treatment, withdrawal and euthanasia

Signs of distress (unusual movements, and changes in breathing rates, colour of gills and activity, and swimming ability) should be monitored by a team member during the procedure. If the animal appears excessively distressed based on these triggers, work should cease immediately, and the animal be released or monitored until it recovers. If the animal is injured to the point where it would have a poor chance of survival if returned to the water, it should be euthanased (see 'Lethal biological sampling' within this chapter).

Equipment and maintenance

Specific equipment depends on the method selected. For observational tagging, only camera equipment may be required; however, for tagging general equipment may include:

- fin-mount and intramuscular attachment
- battery operated drill
- tether, tag and tag head
- tag applicator
- antiseptic (liquid, e.g. Betadine®)

- 70% ethanol for sterilising
- latex gloves
- cradle/tub
- tail ropes (for large fish)
- bilge pump and hose with valve to adjust water pressure
- recovery cage/tub
- aerator or oxygen for recovery tub
- soft net for handling
- towels (multi-purpose, e.g. to cover eyes, and to keep fish damp or protected from sun).

Specific qualifications, experience and training

Handling and tagging large animals should only be undertaken by experienced practitioners or trainees under the supervision of more-experienced personnel, until they are deemed competent. Snorkelling or diving experience is required for in-water observational studies, as well as knowledge about the behaviour of the targeted species and local environmental conditions.

Workplace health and safety

Health and safety considerations are the same as those detailed in 'Non-lethal biological sampling' earlier in this chapter.

Alternative procedures

Currently, no methods are available for acquiring data on fish movements without handling and tagging animals. Alternative procedures for observational-based studies could include baited remote underwater video stations (BRUVS; Chapter 14), remotely operated vehicles (ROVs) and drones (Chapter 6 and 12). However, images and videos collected by these remote systems are sometimes impeded by body position, distance and angle in relation to camera.

TRANSPORT, HANDLING AND HOUSING

Samantha J. Nowland, Rob L. Jones and Andrea Taylor

Context and scope

This general operating procedure (GOP) describes ethical techniques for transport, handling and housing teleosts and chondrichthyans, predominantly for keeping under aquaria and laboratory conditions. It includes topics such as:

- animal welfare considerations
- transport, handling, acclimation and housing procedures
- disease and biosecurity considerations
- return to the wild and euthanasia
- equipment and maintenance
- qualifications, experience and training
- workplace health and safety
- alternative procedures or lower-impact methods.

Animal welfare considerations

The importance of fish welfare in research has increasingly been recognised in the past 20 years (Jones 2019). There are critical points during transport, handling and acclimation to minimise risk to animals. Teleosts and chondrichthyans can be subject to external injury, internal injury, osmoregulatory and temperature stress, oxygen depletion or oversaturation, and general handling stress.

External injury

Common risks of handling include loss of mucous and/or scales, cuts and scrapes.

Using an Environet^{TM} for small animals or a sling/stretcher for large animals will minimise injury to fins, eyes, scales, tail, gills and mucous layers. Wearing wet cotton gloves or wetting hands when handling teleosts or chondrichthyans will also help prevent loss of mucus. Prophylactic antibiotic injection (Chapter 16) and application of povidone–iodine (10%) can be used to prevent infections and aid healing.

Osmoregulatory stress

Rapid salinity changes cause osmoregulatory stress in teleosts and chondrichthyans, so salinity of transport water should match that of capture water. Teleost blood salinity is 8–9 parts per thousand (ppt) so reducing salinity gradually can relieve osmoregulatory stress for euryhaline fish (those species able to tolerate a wide range of salinity). Non-euryhaline fish should usually be kept above 15 ppt, dependent on species (R. Jones, pers. comm.). However, chondrichthyan blood salinity is 35–37 ppt so decreasing salinity is not advised (Hammerschlag 2006).

Temperature stress

Excessive temperature change must be avoided during transport. It should be monitored and managed with ice and/or heating if necessary. Reducing temperature by up to 7°C (depending on species) can be beneficial for reducing transport stress (Wedemeyer 1997), but raising it is not advisable. For chondrichthyans, a temperature change of more than 1 or 2°C is not advisable.

Oxygen depletion or oversaturation

Dissolved oxygen (DO) must be continuously or regularly monitored to ensure transport water matches that of source water. As a rule, 100% saturation is optimal, and up to 200% is acceptable during transports (Harmon 2009). For chondrichthyans, increasing DO to 130–150% saturation will provide mild sedation during transport and handling (Smith *et al.* 2004; Smith *et al.* 2017). DO can be increased using compressed oxygen and a diffuser stone, combined with water movement and sufficient water surface area.

Handling stress

Handling stress can be caused by capture (e.g. chasing with a net or catching on a line), hypoxia during removal from the water and water quality deterioration from confinement in a small space. The neurological response to stress leads to rapid hormone production (e.g. cortisol) triggering metabolic and osmotic disturbances (Harmon 2009). Chondrichthyans produce 1-α-hydroxycorticosterone in response to stress (Evans *et al.* 2010). For the long-term health of the fish, it is important to reduce as many of the above-mentioned stressors as possible. Some chondrichthyans, such as rays, secrete excessive mucus and organic waste when stressed. Therefore, it is important to implement water exchanges and/or filtration during transport. External stimuli and handling should be kept to a minimum, and the transportation container and equipment should have easy access for frequent monitoring.

Transport

Teleosts and chondrichthyans can be transported in bags or tanks/containers by boat, vehicle and aircraft, depending on size, numbers and transport logistics. It is important to have receiving water ready and conditioned. DO must be maintained at or above 100% saturation. Adequate air movement above the water must be maintained so that accumulation of carbon dioxide (which will decrease the water pH) does not occur. Temperature and salinity should be held within the optimum range appropriate for the species without any rapid changes, and insulated containers should be utilised for transportation.

Transport will almost always induce some level of stress, which can cause animals to excrete waste rapidly. In turn this causes a spike in ammonia, so water exchanges or ammonia binders should to be considered for longer transports or those with high biomass. Where possible, fasting for 24–48 h before transport will reduce this waste excretion. Water changes during any transport must be planned for and undertaken as required.

Regular water testing is essential to ensure good water quality is maintained. Buffers can be added to the water to increase pH if it begins to decrease towards unsafe levels for the species. A lid or cover should be used in tanks/container transports to ensure animals cannot jump out, and provide a darkened environment, which will also reduce stress.

Handling in captivity

Teleosts have a protective mucous layer to prevent the entry of pathogens through the skin. Care must be taken to minimise damage to the mucus or injury to the skin, which may cause death or a delay in recovery because of secondary bacterial infections. Methods to minimise damage include:

- using wet hands and, where practical, slings with a smooth, wet surface for moving teleosts out of the water, instead of nets
- using appropriately sized nets with no rough surfaces, such as Environets™
- minimising time out of water by ensuring sufficient numbers of staff are present for each animal movement and taking the time to brief all staff before undertaking movements
- treating any transport injuries with a topical application of 10% povidone-iodine, and an injectable antibiotic if appropriate (see Chapter 16)
- for smaller teleosts, water conditioner (e.g. API® Stress Coat™ at 0.5 mgL^{-1}) can be used to reduce stress and promote healing.

Handling chondrichthyans is consistent with the above procedure, with the addition of hand protection. When working with large chondrichthyans, chain mail or neoprene gloves should be worn.

Acclimation

Acclimation, where gradual water changes can be implemented throughout transportation and at the final location for housing is vital to prevent physiological stress and fatality (Smith *et al.* 2004). Water parameters such as DO, salinity, temperature and ammonia at destination should be kept within optimal ranges for the species, and be as close as logistically possible to that of transport water.

All animals should be kept in quarantine appropriate to the level of biosecurity risk of the animal source to prevent entry of potential pathogens to other animals at the facility. Prophylactic treatments can be considered to reduce parasite load and prevent infections from minor handling injuries on a case-by-case basis.

Low light and cooler temperatures can be helpful to alleviate stress. Gradual adjustment of salinity to reduce osmoregulatory stress can be used and started within the first 48 h, depending on the species (see Table 13.10). Holding tanks should be kept clean via regular removal of debris on the bottom and sides of the tank. Common marine parasites can rapidly increase in numbers in debris outside the host, before reinfecting it. Cleaning tanks regularly will help to break this life cycle, lower parasite load and prevent large infestations from developing.

Housing teleosts and chondrichthyans

Housing requirements will vary enormously, ranging from an open (flow through) system to a closed (recirculating) system. It is essential that water quality is maintained within optimum physicochemical parameters for the species housed. Stocking densities must be appropriate for the species and should take into account natural schooling preferences, aggression/cannibalism factors, ontogeny and behaviour to provide sufficient space for natural swimming behaviour (Spotte 1991). Cannibalistic teleosts should be kept with conspecifics of a similar size to minimise stress on smaller teleosts. Tanks can be fitted with structures, such as hides, to mitigate aggression and alleviate stress. Hides can promote competition if insufficient numbers are available for all the animals in a group and can make it more difficult to clean the tank, so they are more likely to be useful in tanks with smaller numbers of animals. Care should be taken to ensure no sharp edges or objects in the tank can cause injury.

If freshwater is used to manufacture artificial seawater or contain freshwater species it should be analysed for contaminants and filtered or treated before use (Smith *et al.* 2017; Smith *et al.* 2004). Natural or artificial lighting should be used to provide 12 h day/night photoperiods. A daily logbook should be kept, recording measurements of water quality factors such as DO, salinity, temperature, pH, nutrient concentrations (e.g. ammonia) and observations such as animal behaviour, health and feeding. It is essential to understand normal behaviour of your species in order to notice any changes that may indicate stress or disease.

Teleosts and chondrichthyans should be fed a diet as similar as possible to their natural diet (if known), or a diet appropriate for the species after a weaning transition period. They should not be fed live vertebrates. Common marine food, such as fish, crustaceans, cephalopods and worms, should be sourced from a local, reputable supplier with good seafood handling practices and should be frozen. Frozen food should be fed shortly after defrosting to minimise nutrient loss, and vitamin supplements are recommended to replace those lost in the freeze–thaw process. Where possible, wild teleosts can be weaned onto commercially available artificial diets. These diets offer a standardised food supply with optimised nutrient profiles developed for a range of different teleosts, and eliminate the biosecurity risk of frozen foods. For chondrichthyans, vitamin and mineral supplements, especially iodine, are required to prevent the development of deficiencies, especially goitre, in closed systems (Jones 2018).

Disease and biosecurity

Teleosts' or chondrichthyans' entry into a facility must follow appropriate translocation regulations and operate within the facilities biosecurity policy. Newly introduced animals must be quarantined to prevent risk to other animals within the facility, and strict monitoring must be undertaken and recorded. This period should be for a minimum of 14 days, but 30 days is ideal.

If signs of adverse health are observed in a single animal, biosecurity measures must be implemented. At a

Table 13.10: Suggested salinity adjustments to reduce osmoregulatory stress in teleosts and chondrichthyans.

Class	Recommendation
Euryhaline teleosts	Most teleost blood salinity is 8–9 ppt. Moving the salinity 3 ppt per day towards fish blood salinity from the capture water salinity will reduce their need to excrete salts.
Non-euryhaline teleosts	Non-euryhaline marine fish have a lower tolerance for salinity change and salinity should only be reduced to 15 ppt or higher, depending on species.
Chondrichthyans	Salinity must be maintained at full strength seawater; however, some species are an exception.

minimum, the animals should be removed from the population (aquaria) and quarantined in separate aquaria with increased water flow (100% per hour), daily vacuums and separate quarantine equipment. Daily observations must be recorded and, in the case of morbidity or death, samples should be submitted for diagnosis if a notifiable disease is suspected. Parasites, infections and disease are common in housed teleosts and chondrichthyans, which are often treated with medication and freshwater dips (Dean *et al.* 2005; Smith *et al.* 2004; Smith *et al.* 2017).

Considerations for return to the wild and euthanasia

Returning animals to the wild needs to be considered in the experimental design phase, as the teleosts or chondrichthyans will need to be kept in a biosecure environment for the duration of the research. Translocation regulations may not permit release depending on the location of source and release. If necessary, teleosts and chondrichthyans should be euthanased by an overdose of an anaesthetic agent such as AQUI-S®. The *ikejime* (brain spike) method (Diggles 2006) may be used but only by suitably trained and qualified personnel. An ice slurry is only appropriate for small bodied (< 5 cm) tropical teleosts and not at all for chondrichthyans (Jones and Daly 2014).

Equipment and maintenance

Typical items may include:

- transport vessels (bags or tanks/tubs) and housing aquaria appropriate for species
- water supply matching the physicochemical parameters required for individual species
- water monitoring equipment such as DO meter, refractometer, thermometer and ammonia test kit
- nets or slings/stretchers for transfer
- gloves/personal protection
- data recording equipment
- chemicals potentially required such as AQUI-S®, ammonia locker, povidone–iodine and antibiotics
- compressed oxygen bottles, regulators, line and stone or ceramic diffusers
- battery operated air stones.

Specific qualifications, experience and training

Competency requirements for animal researchers when transporting, handling and housing teleosts and chondrichthyans may include the appropriate vehicle or vessel licences (e.g. coxswains), the appropriate licence or permit to collect animals, skills/experience handling the study species, knowledge of species-specific disease control zones, and ethics approval for the research project.

Workplace health and safety

Personnel should undertake all appropriate risk assessments, which may include basic hazard identification, job safety analysis, risk register and incident reporting. Some examples of specific hazards when dealing with animals in the laboratory or aquaria may include cuts, bites, and stings (from handling animals), electric shock (from pumps and heaters in water), and zoonotic disease (introduced pathogens).

Alternative procedures

Researchers should consider if study questions could be answered with remote monitoring equipment or catch and release methods (e.g. tagging or sampling teleosts and chondrichthyans).

REFERENCES

Ángeles Esteban M (2012) An overview of the immunological defenses in fish skin. *ISRN Immunology* **2012**, 853470. doi:10.5402/2012/853470

Anderson B, Belcher C, Slack J, Gelsleichter J (2018) Evaluation of the use of portable ultrasonography to determine pregnancy status and fecundity in bonnethead shark *Sphyrna tiburo*. *Journal of Fish Biology* **93**, 1163–1170. doi:10.1111/jfb.13831

Ayvazian SG, Wise BS, Young GC (2002) Short-term hooking mortality of tailor (*Pomatomus saltatrix*) in Western Australia and the impact on yield per recruit. *Fisheries Research* **58**, 241–248. doi:10.1016/S0165-7836(01)00387-3

Balázs G, Vörös J, Lewarne B, Herczeg G (2020) A new non-invasive in situ underwater DNA sampling method for estimating genetic diversity. *Evolutionary Ecology* **34**, 633–644. doi:10.1007/s10682-020-10053-1

Barker D, Allan GL, Rowland SJ, Pickles JM (2002) *A Guide to Acceptable Procedures and Practices for Aquaculture and Fisheries Research.* 2nd edn. NSW Fisheries Animal Care and Ethics Committee, Nelson Bay.

Barnett A, Redd KS, Frusher SD, Stevens JD, Semmens JM (2010) Non-lethal method to obtain stomach samples from a large marine predator and the use of DNA analysis to improve dietary information. *Journal of Experimental Marine Biology and Ecology* **393**, 188–192. doi:10.1016/j.jembe.2010.07.022

Bradford RW, Hill P, Davies C, Grewe P (2016) A new tool in the toolbox for large-scale, high-throughput fisheries mark-recapture studies using genetic identification. *Marine and Freshwater Research* **67**, 1081–1089. doi:10.1071/MF14423

Bradford RW, Hobday AL, Evans K, Lansdell M (2009) CMAR code of practice for tagging marine animals. CSIRO Marine and Atmospheric Research Paper 028. CSIRO, Hobart.

Barton BA (2002) Stress in fishes: A diversity of responses with particular reference to changes in circulating corticosteroids. *Integrative and Comparative Biology* **42**, 517–525. doi:10.1093/icb/42.3.517

Butcher PA, Broadhurst MK, Hall KC, Cullis BR, Raidal SR (2012) Assessing barotrauma among angled snapper (Pagrus auratus) and the utility of release methods. *Fisheries Research* **127–128**, 49–55. doi:10.1016/j.fishres.2012.04.013

Campbell MJ, McLennan MF, Sumpton WD (2014) Short-term survival of discarded pearl perch (*Glaucosoma scapulare* Ramsay, 1881) caught by hook-and-line in Queensland, Australia. *Fisheries Research* **151**, 206–212. doi:10.1016/j.fishres.2013.12.005

Campbell TW (2015) Blood sample collection and preparation in fish. In *Exotic Animal Hematology and Cytology*. (Ed. TW Campbell) pp. 183–186. John Wiley & Sons, Milton.

Chapple TK, Gleiss AC, Jewell OJ, Wikelski M, Block BA (2015) Tracking sharks without teeth: a non-invasive rigid tag attachment for large predatory sharks. *Animal Biotelemetry* **3**, 14. doi:10.1186/s40317-015-0044-9

Chin A, Mourier J, Rummer JL (2015) Blacktip reef sharks (*Carcharhinus melanopterus*) show high capacity for wound healing and recovery following injury. *Conservation Physiology* **3**, 1–9. doi:10.1093/conphys/cov062

Close B, Banister K, Baumans V, Bernoth EM, Bromage N, Bunyan J, Erhardt W, Flecknell P, Gregory N, Hackbarth H, Morton D, Warwick C (1997) Recommendations for euthanasia of experimental animals: Part 2. DGXT of the European Commission. *Laboratory Animals* **31**, 1–32. doi:10.1258/002367797780600297

Cooke SJ, Wilson AD, Elvidge CK, Lennox RJ, Jepsen N, Colotelo AH, Brown RS (2016) Ten practical realities for institutional animal care and use committees when evaluating protocols dealing with fish in the field. *Reviews in Fish Biology and Fisheries* **26**, 123–133. doi:10.1007/s11160-015-9413-y

Cooke SJ, Woodley CM, Eppard MB, Brown RS, Nielsen JL (2011) Advancing the surgical implantation of electronic tags in fish: a gap analysis and research agenda based on a review of trends in intracoelomic tagging effects studies. *Reviews in Fish Biology and Fisheries* **21**, 127–151. doi:10.1007/s11160-010-9193-3

Cooke SJ, Suski CD (2004) Are circle hooks an effective tool for conserving marine and freshwater recreational catch-and-release fisheries? *Aquatic Conservation* **14**, 299–326. doi:10.1002/aqc.614

Cortés E (2007) Chondrichthyan demographic modelling: an essay on its use, abuse and future. *Marine and Freshwater Research* **58**, 4–6. doi:10.1071/MF06191

CSIRO (2015) *CSIRO Code of Practice for Tagging Marine Animals*. 2nd edn. CSIRO, Melbourne.

Dapp DR, Huveneers C, Walker TI, Drew M, Reina RD (2016*a*) Moving from measuring to predicting bycatch mortality: predicting the capture condition of a longline-caught pelagic shark. *Frontiers in Marine Science* **2**, 126. doi:10.3389/fmars.2015.00126

Dapp DR, Walker TI, Huveneers C, Reina RD (2016*b*) Respiratory mode and gear type are important determinants of elasmobranch immediate and post-release mortality. *Fish and Fisheries* **17**, 507–524. doi:10.1111/faf.12124

Dean MN, Nietfeld TE, Conklin DS (2005) Husbandry notes on the lesser electric ray. *North American Journal of Aquaculture* **67**, 58–65. doi:10.1577/FA03-064.1

Department of Parks and Wildlife (2013) *Whale Shark Management with Particular Reference to Ningaloo Marine Park*. Department of Parks and Wildlife, Perth.

Diggles BK (2016) Development of resources to promote best practice in the humane dispatch of finfish caught by recreational fishers. *Fisheries Management and Ecology* **23**, 200–207.

Ellis JR, McCully Phillips SR, Poisson F (2017) A review of capture and post-release mortality of elasmobranchs. *Journal of Fish Biology* **90**, 653–722. doi:10.1111/jfb.13197

Evans AN, Rimoldi JM, Gadepalli RSV, Nunez BS (2010) Adaptation of a corticosterone ELISA to demonstrate sequence-specific effects of angiotensin II peptides and C-type natriuretic peptide on 1-α-hydroxycorticosterone synthesis and steroidogenic mRNAs in the elasmobranch interrenal gland. *The Journal of Steroid Biochemistry and Molecular Biology* **120**, 149–154. doi:10.1016/j.jsbmb.2010.03.025

Ferreira LC, Mansfield KL, Thums M, Meekan MG (2018) Satellite tracking technologies and their application to shark movement ecology. In *Shark Research: Emerging Technologies and Applications for the Field and Laboratory*. (Eds JC Carrier, MR Heithaus and CA Simpfendorfer) pp. 357–377. CRC Press, Boca Raton, FL.

Gallagher AJ, Serafy JE, Cooke SJ, Hammerschlag N (2014) Physiological stress response, reflex impairment, and survival of five sympatric shark species following experimental capture and release. *Marine Ecology Progress Series* **496**, 207–218. doi:10.3354/meps10490

Gleiss AC, Norman B, Liebsch N, Francis C, Wilson RP (2009) A new prospect for tagging large free-swimming sharks with motion-sensitive data-loggers. *Fisheries Research* **97**, 11–16. doi:10.1016/j.fishres.2008.12.012

Gould A, Grace BS (2009) Injuries to barramundi *Lates calcarifer* resulting from lip-gripping devices in the laboratory. *North American Journal of Fisheries Management* **29**, 1418–1424. doi:10.1577/M08-232.1

Graves JE, Marcek BJ, Goldsmith WM (2016) Effects of air exposure on post release mortality rates of White Marlin caught in the US offshore recreational fishery. *North American Journal of Fisheries Management* **36**, 1221–1228. doi:10.1080/02755947.2016.1204390

Guitreau AM, Eilts BE, Novelo ND, Tiersch TR (2012) Fish handling and ultrasound procedures for viewing the ovary of submersed, non-anesthetized, unrestrained channel catfishes. *North American Journal of Aquaculture* **74**, 182–187. doi:10.1080/15222055.2012.655852

Hammerschlag N (2006) Osmoregulation in elasmobranchs: a review for fish biologists, behaviourists and ecologists. *Marine and Freshwater Behaviour and Physiology* **39**, 209–228. doi:10.1080/10236240600815820

Hammerschlag N, Sulikowski J (2011) Killing for conservation: The need for alternatives to lethal sampling of apex predatory sharks. *Endangered Species Research* **14**, 135–140. doi:10.3354/esr00354

Harmon TS (2009) Methods for reducing stressors and maintaining water quality associated with live fish transport in tanks: a review of the basics. *Reviews in Aquaculture* **1**, 58–66. doi:10.1111/j.1753-5131.2008.01003.x

Heupel MR, Simpfendorfer CA (2010) Science of slaughter: Nned for lethal sampling of sharks. *Conservation Biology* **24**, 1212–1218. doi:10.1111/j.1523-1739.2010.01491.x

Hughes JM, Stewart J, Collins D (2019) Experimental hyperbaric chamber trials reveal high resilience to barotrauma in Australian snapper (*Chrysophrys auratus*). *Fisheries Research* **212**, 172–182. doi:10.1016/j.fishres.2018.12.024

Jepsen N, Thorstad EB, Havn T, Lucas MC (2015) The use of external electronic tags on fish: an evaluation of tag retention and tagging effects. *Animal Biotelemetry* **3**, 49. doi:10.1186/s40317-015-0086-z

Jewell OJD, Wcisel MA, Gennari E, Towner AV, Bester MN, Johnson RL, Singh S (2011) Effects of Smart Position Only (SPOT) tag deployment on white sharks *Carcharodon carcharias* in South Africa. *PLoS One* **6**, e27242. doi:10.1371/journal.pone.0027242

Jones R, Daly J (2014) *Humane Euthanasia Techniques for Ornamental Fish*. Pet Industry Association of Australia, Norwest.

Jones RL (2018) Vitamin mineral supplements for sharks and rays. The Aquarium Vet. <http://www.theaquariumvet.com/wp-content/uploads/2018/09/Discussion-Paper-Vitamin-Supplements-for-Sharks-and-Rays.pdf>.

Jones RL (2019) Aquatic animal welfare module. The Aquarium Vet. <http://www.theaquariumvet.com/education/>.

Kashiwagi T, Maxwell E, Marshall A, Christensen A (2015) Evaluating manta ray mucus as an alternative DNA source for population genetics study: Underwater-sampling, dry-storage and PCR success. *PeerJ* **3**, e1188. doi:10.7717/peerj.1188

Kessel ST, Fraser J, Van Bonn WG, Brooks JL, Guttridge TL, Hussey NE, Gruber SH (2017) Transcoelomic expulsion of an ingested foreign object by a carcharhinid shark. *Marine and Freshwater Research* **68**, 2173. doi:10.1071/MF17022

Kessel ST, Hussey NE, MacLatchey D (2015) Tonic immobility as an anaesthetic for elasmobranchs during surgical implantation procedures. *Canadian Journal of Fisheries and Aquatic Sciences* **72**, 1287–1291. doi:10.1139/cjfas-2015-0136

Key B (2016) Why fish do not feel pain. *Animal Sentience* **3**, 2016.003.

Leary S, Underwood W, Anthony R, Cartner S, Corey D (2013) *AVMA Guidelines for the Euthanasia of Animals: 2013 Edition.* American Veterinary Medical Association, Schaumberg, IL.

Lieber L, Berrow S, Johnston E, Hall G, Hall J, Gubili C, Sims DW, Jones CS, Noble LR (2013) Mucus: aiding elasmobranch conservation through non-invasive genetic sampling. *Endangered Species Research* **21**, 215–222. doi:10.3354/esr00524

Marshall AD, Pierce SJ (2012) The use and abuse of photographic identification in sharks and rays. *Journal of Fish Biology* **80**, 1361–1379. doi:10.1111/j.1095-8649.2012.03244.x

Murray MJ (2010) Endoscopy in Sharks. *The Veterinary Clinics of North America. Exotic Animal Practice* **13**, 301–313. doi:10.1016/j.cvex.2010.01.008

Neiffer DL, Stamper AM (2009) Fish sedation, anesthesia, analgesia, and euthanasia: considerations, methods, and types of drugs. *ILAR Journal* **50**, 343–360. doi:10.1093/ilar.50.4.343

Novelo ND, Tiersch TR (2012) A review of the use of ultrasonography in fish reproduction. *North American Journal of Aquaculture* **74**, 169–181. doi:10.1080/15222055.2012.672370

Phelan M, Campbell D, Humphrey J (2008) Implications of barotrauma and hook type on catching and releasing black jewfish. In *Assessment of the Implications of Target Fishing on Black Jewfish (*Protonibea Diacanthus*) Aggregations in the Northern Territory.* (Ed. M Phelan) pp. 63–92. Northern Territory Government, Department of Industry, Fisheries and Mines, Darwin.

Raby GD, Packer JR, Danylchuk AJ, Cooke SJ (2014) The understudied and underappreciated role of predation in the mortality of fish released from fishing gears. *Fish and Fisheries* **15**, 489–505. doi:10.1111/faf.12033

Readman GD, Owen SF, Knowles TG, Murrell JC (2017) Species specific anaesthetics for fish anaesthesia and euthanasia. *Scientific Reports* **7**, 7102. doi:10.1038/s41598-017-06917-2

Reilly JS (Ed.) (2001). *Euthanasia of Animals Used for Scientific Purposes.* Australian and New Zealand Council for the Care of Animals in Research and Teaching (ANZCCART), Adelaide.

Rose JD, Arlinghaus R, Cooke SJ, Diggles BK, Sawynok W, Stevens ED, Wynne CD (2014) Can fish really feel pain? *Fish and Fisheries* **15**, 97–133. doi:10.1111/faf.12010

Skomal G, Bernal D (2010) Physiological responses to stress in sharks. In *Sharks and Their Relatives: Biodiversity, Adaptive Physiology, and Conservation* (Eds JC Carrier, JA Musick and MR Heithaus) pp. 459–490. CRC Press, Boca Raton, FL.

Sloman KA, Bouyoucos IA, Brooks EJ, Sneddon LU (2019) Ethical considerations in fish research. *Journal of Fish Biology* **94**, 556–577. doi:10.1111/jfb.13946

Smircich MG, Kelly JT (2014) Extending the 2% rule: The effects of heavy internal tags on stress physiology, swimming performance, and growth in brook trout. *Animal Biotelemetry* **2**, 16. doi:10.1186/2050-3385-2-16

Smith MD, Warmolts D, Thoney D, Hueter R (2004) *The Elasmobranch Husbandry Manual: Captive Care of Sharks, Rays and Their Relatives.* Ohio Biological Survey, Columbus, OH.

Smith MD, Warmolts D, Thoney D, Hueter R, Murray M, Excurra J (2017) *The Elasmobranch Husbandry Manual II: Recent Advances in the Care of Sharks, Rays and their Relatives.* Ohio Biological Survey, Columbus, OH.

Sneddon LU (2018) Comparative physiology of nociception and pain. *Physiology (Bethesda, MD)* **33**, 63–73. doi:10.1152/physiol.00022.2017

Spotte SH (1991) *Captive Seawater Fishes: Science and Technology.* Wiley, New York, NY.

St John J, Syers CJ (2005) Mortality of the demersal West Australian dhufish, *Glaucosoma hebraicum* (Richardson 1845) following catch and release: The influence of capture depth, venting and hook type. *Fisheries Research* **76**, 106–116. doi:10.1016/j.fishres.2005.05.014

Sumpton WD, Brown IW, Mayer DG, McLennan MF, Mapleston A, Butcher AR, Welch DJ, Kirkwood JM, Sawynok B, Begg GA (2010) Assessing the effects of line capture and barotrauma relief procedures on post-release survival of key tropical reef fish species in Australia using recreational tagging clubs. *Fisheries Management and Ecology* **17**, 77–88. doi:10.1111/j.1365-2400.2009.00722.x

Swenson EA, Rosenberger AE, Howell PJ (2007) Validation of endoscopy for determination of maturity in small salmonids and sex of mature individuals. *Transactions of the American Fisheries Society* **136**, 994–998. doi:10.1577/T06-193.1

Towner A, Smale M, Jewell O (2012) Boat-strike wound healing in *Carcharodon carcharias.* In *Global Perspectives on the Biology and Life History of the White Shark* (Ed. M Domeier) pp. 77–84. CRC Press, Boca Raton, FL.

Veldhuizen LJL, Berentsen PBM, de Boer IJM, van de Vis JW, Bokkers EAM (2018) Fish welfare in capture fisheries: A review of injuries and mortality. *Fisheries Research* **204**, 41–48. doi:10.1016/j.fishres.2018.02.001

Wagner GN, Cooke SJ, Brown RS, Deters KA (2011) Surgical implantation techniques for electronic tags in fish. *Reviews in Fish Biology and Fisheries* **21**, 71–81. doi:10.1007/s11160-010-9191-5

Wargo Rub AM, Jepsen N, Liedtke TL, Moser ML, Weber ES, III (2014) Surgical insertion of transmitters and telemetry methods in fisheries research. *American Journal of Veterinary Research* **75**, 402–416. doi:10.2460/ajvr.75.4.402

Wedemeyer GA (1997) Effects of rearing conditions on the health and physiological quality of fish in intensive culture. In *Fish Stress and Health in Aquaculture* (Eds GK Iwama, AD Pickering, JP Sumpter and CB Schreck). pp. 35–71. Cambridge University Press, New York, NY.

Wells RMG, McNeil H, MacDonald JA (2005) Fish hypnosis: induction of an atonic immobility reflex. *Marine and Freshwater Behaviour and Physiology* **38**, 71–78. doi:10.1080/10236240400029341

Wendelaar Bonga SE (1997) The stress response in fish. *Physiological Reviews* **77**, 591–625. doi:10.1152/physrev.1997.77.3.591

Westmoreland LSH, Archibald KE, Christiansen EF, Broadhurst H, Stoskopf MK (2019) The mesopterygial vein: a reliable venipuncture site for intravascular access in batoids. *Journal of Zoo and Wildlife Medicine* **50**, 369–374. doi:10.1638/2018-0137

Whittamore JM, Bloomer C, Hanna GM, McCarthy ID (2010) Evaluating ultrasonography as a non-lethal method for the assessment of maturity in oviparous elasmobranchs. *Marine Biology* **157**, 2613–2624. doi:10.1007/s00227-010-1523-4

Williams LJ, Herbig JL, Szedlmayer ST (2015) A cage release method to improve fish tagging studies. *Fisheries Research* **172**, 125–129. doi:10.1016/j.fishres.2015.06.030

Williams SM, Holmes BJ, Pepperell JG (2015) The novel application of non-lethal citizen science tissue sampling in recreational fisheries. *PLoS One* **10**, e0135743. doi:10.1371/journal.pone.0135743

Williamson MJ, Dudgeon C, Sladge R (2018) Tonic immobility in zebra shark, *Stegostoma fasciatum*, and its use for capture methodology. *Environmental Biology of Fishes* **101**, 741–748. doi:10.1007/s10641-018-0734-2

14 Research methods for freshwater animals

Nicole Flint, Alison J. King, Ian Wooden, Melody Serena, Sascha Healy, Deborah S. Bower, David L. Morgan, Scott A. Hardie, Tarmo A. Raadik, David T. Roberts and Joanne Ocock

INTRODUCTION

This chapter reviews general considerations and procedures for the capture and handling of freshwater animals, including fish, reptiles, amphibians and mammals. The study of freshwater animals can range from observational studies to sophisticated capture-based research where animals are released after observations, held for other procedures or euthanased. Investigators can use the general operating procedures (GOPs) described in this chapter as a guide while also drawing on their own and other experienced researchers' knowledge and skills to develop detailed project-specific protocols. Protocols for field monitoring and sampling procedures for freshwater animals are also described in other documents, which can be considered in tandem with the GOPs presented here. For example, DES (2018) describes procedures for sampling fish with a range of equipment types in Queensland, DPI (2015) provides a guide for acceptable procedures and practices in fish research in New South Wales, and DSEWPC (2011) outlines national survey guidelines for Australian threatened fish. Methods for biological sampling, tagging, transport and handling of freshwater fishes are similar to the corresponding methods for marine and estuarine fishes (see Chapter 13), so are not reiterated in this chapter. Researchers need to ensure that the biological requirements of their particular study species are met. Additional considerations specific to freshwater fishes are provided in Chapter 32. Other chapters that are also relevant to freshwater research, include Chapter 4 (eDNA monitoring), Chapter 12 (tagging and identification of marine mammals), and Chapter 16 (veterinary procedures). Methods for capturing and monitoring aquatic birds are detailed in Chapters 15 and 35, and crustaceans in Chapter 28.

NETTING FISH AND TADPOLES

Nicole Flint, Alison J. King, Sascha Healy, Joanne Ocock, Deborah S. Bower, Ian Wooden, David Morgan, Scott A. Hardie, Tarmo A. Raadik, David T. Roberts and Melody Serena

Target taxa

Methods described in this GOP are applicable to tadpoles (Chapter 27) and freshwater fishes (Chapter 32).

Context and scope

This GOP describes procedures and considerations for the capture of tadpoles and freshwater fishes with fyke, seine, gill, dip and larval fish nets. All methods are commonly used for freshwater research in Australia. Netting is one of many methods used to catch vertebrates in freshwater environments and is an efficient way to sample large numbers of animals and a diversity of species. Cryptic or rare fish species are more likely to be detected when using a combination of these methods across the diel (24 h) cycle. These methods are often supplemented with spotlighting, underwater video, electrofishing or bait traps (see other GOPs in this chapter). Nets can be selective, with factors such as mesh size, deployment location and deployment time modified to target particular species or size classes (particularly for fish).

Animal welfare considerations

Netting involves the capture and restraint of fish and tadpoles until they are removed from the net and released. Generally, fish and tadpoles are retained in the net with little stress or damage and can be released unharmed. In worst-case scenarios, entrapment of fish and tadpoles in nets and post-capture handling can cause physical damage (e.g. scale loss, bruising, tissue damage or lacerations), increase the risk of predation, stress and air exposure, and result in unintentional mortality of target species. Non-target animals, such as turtles, snakes, adult frogs, water birds, and mammals such as rakali (water rats, *Hydromys chrysogaster*) and platypus (*Ornithorhynchus anatinus*) can also be caught and potentially injured or killed. These risks can be reduced substantially through targeted net deployment times, specific net types and mesh sizes for target animals, observing or checking the gear (equipment) at appropriate intervals during deployment, and careful net hauling and animal handling practices.

Handling

Handling and removing fish from nets can be difficult and should be done carefully and quickly by experienced researchers (or under the supervision of experienced investigators). For some fish species or situations, it may be less stressful for both the researchers and animals if the fish are anaesthetised before handling (see Chapters 13 and 16), although anaesthesia introduces additional risks (Chapter 16) and is often unnecessary if invasive procedures are avoided. Once fish are removed from nets, they should be placed immediately into well-aerated (ideally) water before additional handling. Large fish or turtles are often removed first by members of the survey team (to protect smaller animals from injury and predation) while other team members continue to process smaller fish and tadpoles. When handling fish, investigators will often wear wet cotton gloves to reduce injury to fish skin and the mucosal layer. Fish should be handled quickly and efficiently so the time that they are held out of water is minimised (DPI 2015). Containers of aerated stream water are often required to hold catches for processing. Multiple containers can be useful for large numbers of small fishes or when a range of size classes is captured. Subsampling large catches if processing time is extended can assist with reducing handling time for abundant species (often tadpoles or small fish).

A single-use glove is recommended when handling tadpoles (or frogs) to reduce transmission of pathogens, such as chytrid fungus (Murray *et al.* 2011). All glove types (latex, nitrile and vinyl) are likely to be lethal to some tadpole species, but vinyl appears to carry less risks (Cashins *et al.* 2008); gloves should be rinsed with water from the study site before handling specimens. An alternative option if gloves are not suitable is washing hands with ≥ 70% alcohol, allowing them to dry, then rinsing thoroughly with water between each animal to remove the alcohol (Murray *et al.* 2011). Single-use plastic sealable bags or a sorting tray can also be used to hold and identify multiple individual tadpoles (DECC 2008; Murray *et al.* 2011). Since handling can stress tadpoles and make them more susceptible to infection, they should only be handled when essential (Murray *et al.* 2011).

External injury

Fish skin, fins, mouth, operculum, gills and eyes can be injured by nets. Contact nets, such as gill nets, are most likely to cause external injuries (Veldhuizen *et al.* 2018). Gill nets are often cut by investigators to facilitate the rapid release of captured animals either into a holding tank or back into the waterway (avoiding placing nets and their catch onto dry or hot ground); a net repair kit should be carried in case this situation arises.

Predation and crushing

If predatory animals (e.g. large fish, sharks, crocodiles, turtles, rakali, some birds and crayfish) are present, the predation risk to trapped animals is increased. Even medium-sized fish can prey on smaller fish that are trapped in nets. This risk can be reduced by checking nets regularly, using gear appropriate for the target species and sizes, and excluding predatory animals where possible (e.g. using exclusion screens in the entrance of fyke nets) (see Morgan *et al.* 2021a). Nets (particularly fyke nets) used to capture tadpoles or small fish should be checked more frequently at sites with a higher risk of predation. When clearing fyke nets, large fish and predators, such as turtles and crayfish, are often removed first to decrease stress and predation risk to smaller fish and tadpoles (Ocock *et al.* 2018). Larger individuals (e.g. large eels) can crush smaller fish in fyke nets if kept in the net. Allowing larger individuals to escape (e.g. via a cod end opening) above water can reduce the risk of injury to smaller animals.

Capture stress

Stress levels of some fish are reportedly higher after capture in gill nets than other fishing methods, such as electrofishing (Harrell and Moline 1992) and jigging (Toledo-Guedes *et al.* 2016). Capture duration is an important factor that influences post-release survival of fish caught in nets (Bell and Lyle 2016). Shorter net soak times or seine hauls (which limit the time animals spend in nets) can be implemented to reduce capture duration. When gill netting, survival rates of captured fish can be increased by monitoring nets and removing fish as they are captured.

Air exposure

Completing post-capture processing (the time the animal spends out of water) as quickly as possible reduces the stress on fish and tadpoles caused by air exposure. Longer exposure increases the chance of asphyxiation, although the time after which asphyxiation occurs differs between species (Lambooij *et al.* 2012) and with air temperature. For example, higher temperatures increase stress caused by air exposure in cold water fish species (e.g. as demonstrated for European grayling, *Thymallus thymallus*; Pinder *et al.* 2019).

Risks to non-target species

Most by-catch in nets set for fish and tadpoles comprises non-target fish species and crustaceans. Fish by-catch can be reduced by using appropriate gear types for the target species and their size or by installing by-catch reduction devices. To prevent air-breathing animals (e.g. adult frogs, platypus, turtles, crocodiles, rakali, snakes and water birds) drowning in fyke nets, the cod end of the net needs to be raised at least 20 cm above the water surface, and potentially supplemented by a large float placed inside the cod end to maintain an airspace. Extra care may be needed when deploying floats in windy conditions, changing water levels or varying flows to ensure they do not twist and progressively reduce the amount of air space in the cod end (or isolate the cod end from the rest of the net). An 'escape ring' of a specified diameter can also be inserted into the cod end to allow air-breathing vertebrates and large eels to escape. If some turtles in the study area are likely to be too large to fit through all of a fyke net's hoops, an air space should be maintained in each net compartment with the use of a float. When fyke nets are used to sample small fish, by-catch can also be excluded by fitting an exclusion screen to the net entrance (e.g. < 50 mm square mesh to exclude platypus (Grant *et al.* 2004); or fine mesh to sample only small fish such as galaxiids (Hardie *et al.* 2006)). Air-breathing vertebrates can drown rapidly when captured in gill nets, and are at higher risk of mortality in fyke nets set in fast-flowing, turbulent or cold water. Refer to 'Capturing freshwater turtles, snakes and platypus' later in this chapter for additional advice about mitigating animal welfare risks for turtles or platypus, particularly at sites where these species are abundant.

General procedures

Preparation

Investigators should identify the most suitable nets for their target species, including type, dimensions and mesh size, as differently sized cohorts may be captured more effectively using different gear. For example, larval fish might be best collected using light traps or plankton nets, small juveniles may be best targeted using seine or fyke nets, while large fish that occupy different habitats or niches may require gill nets (Chapman *et al.* 2006; Ebner and Morgan 2013). Depending on the environment, other equipment may also be vital to sampling success. For example, a boat may be required to deploy or retrieve nets, or to allow safe access to tropical rivers where estuarine crocodiles (*Crocodylus porosus*) may occur. Before commencing sampling, investigators should check local water gauging stations for suitable hydrological conditions over the trapping period (i.e. water levels, flows). The study site's physical features may also affect study design, including the type of nets selected and the location of suitable places to deploy a boat (if required), and to deploy and retrieve nets. If required, fish holding containers with aerators can be prepared in a shady area for processing the catch.

Procedure for fyke nets

Fyke netting is a passive sampling technique where fish and tadpoles swim into the mouth of the net and are captured via a series of smaller compartments or hoops (Figure 14.1a). This approach means that some species or individuals may not be sampled, depending on their activity patterns and how they use different habitats. Fyke netting is often used for smaller-bodied fish species, tadpoles and cryptic species that are active at night (Hardie *et al.* 2006; Beatty *et al.* 2014; Lintermans 2016; Wassens *et al.* 2016), so nets may be set overnight to optimise catch rates. Fyke netting is generally best suited to still or slow-flowing habitats or sheltered areas in wind-swept environments (e.g. large lakes), as high flow or current and large amounts of floating debris result in nets becoming ineffective because of clogging, rolling or dislodgement. Nets can be double- or single-winged, and in flowing waters they can be deployed facing downstream or upstream. In standing and flowing waters, fyke nets are often deployed so that the wings intersect the shoreline to capture fish moving in littoral areas, and to determine the direction of their movement (e.g. if fish are moving upstream for spawning). Fyke nets can also be set fully submerged in deep locations (e.g. > 5 m) to target benthic fishes (Hardie *et al.* 2011), although doing so is not standard practice, and should only be conducted where air breathing animals are not at risk and correct deployment using a boat is difficult. It may be necessary to use a boat in deep water habitats or where operating without a boat is dangerous (e.g. in northern Australian rivers where crocodiles are often present; Figure 14.1b).

Fyke nets are often deployed by being tied to wooden or metal stakes that are driven into the substrate, so that the nets are lying on the substrate and set relatively tightly across their length. Where hard substrata (e.g. rocky habitats) prevent the use of stakes, fyke nets can be set using lead weights and floats or tied to natural habitat features (e.g. snags). The use of weights and floats (and rope) also allows nets to be set in deep water. Funnels within hoops must be at least partially submerged to allow fish to swim through and in all cases requirements for preventing risks to by-catch (see 'Animal welfare considerations') need to be carefully considered. When targeting tadpoles, adult frogs may be encountered as by-catch so a small air space needs to be left between each hoop and the water surface (Wassens *et al.* 2016).

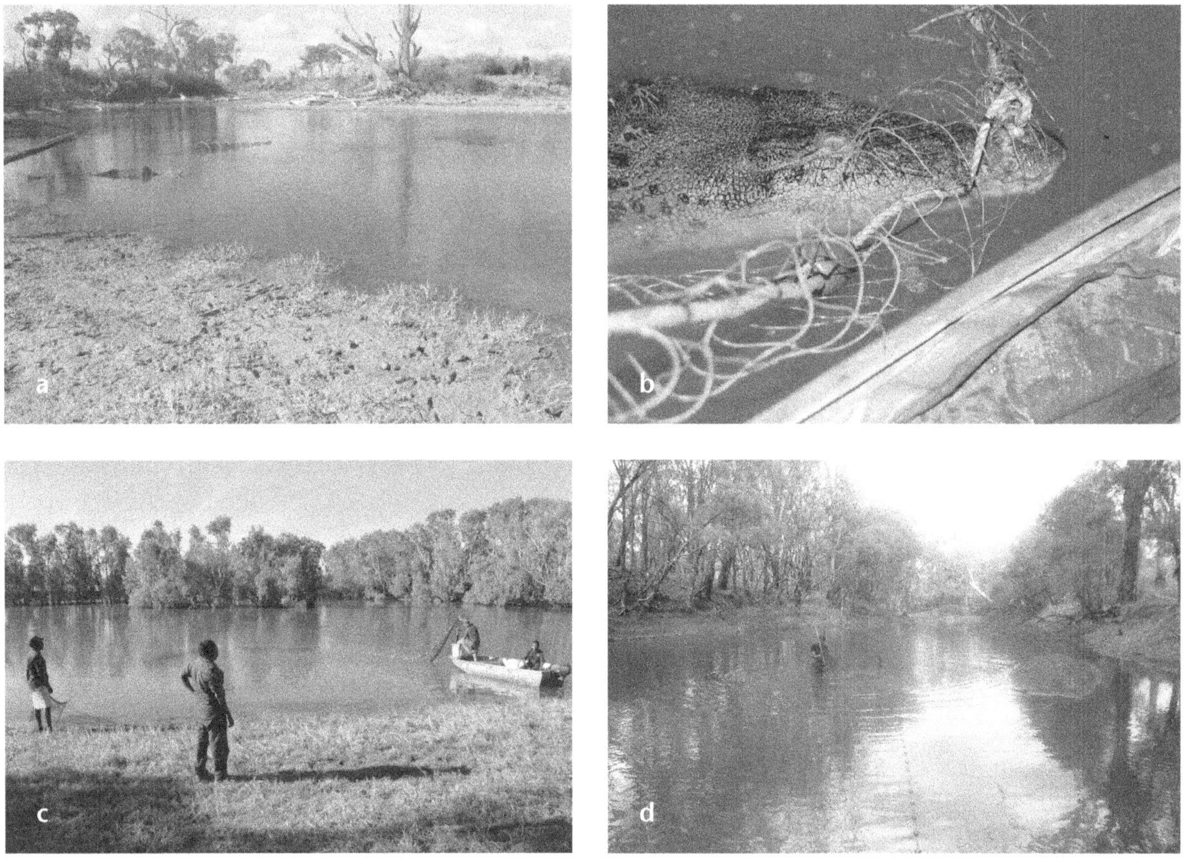

Figure 14.1: (a) Multiple fyke nets set in a waterway. Photo by Iain Ellis/ NSW DPI Fisheries. (b) The estuarine crocodile (*Crocodylus porosus*) is an unwanted by-catch species when netting in northern Australia. Photo by David Morgan. (c) Nyikina Mangala Rangers deploying a seine net from a boat in the Kimberley. Photo by David Morgan. (d) Seine netting from the bank of a shallow waterway. Photo by Nicole Flint.

Mesh size, hoop size, net length and the number of wings must be suitable for the site, conditions and target species (DES 2018). Time of year for sampling should take into account the timing of recruitment of target species into sampled habitats if young-of-the-year are captured. Additionally, the potential for variation in the catchability of fish during spawning aggregations and attraction to or avoidance of passive methods, such as fyke nets (Hardie *et al.* 2005; Hardie *et al.* 2006), needs to be considered carefully. Fishing effort associated with fyke netting is often measured (and standardised) by recording the set and haul times to calculate the soak time of nets (e.g. overnight, 12 h) (Beatty *et al.* 2014). When retrieving nets, the wings should be brought to the first hoop, then the first hoop lifted clear of the water and shaken gently to move captured animals into the next hoop. Hoops are lifted sequentially and shaken until the catch is at the cod end of the net, which is then untied to release the catch into holding containers of aerated stream water for recovery and processing.

Procedure for seine nets

Seine nets are mesh walls that have a lead line on the bottom of the net and a float line at the top, and may have a pocket in the middle to retain animals. They are often used to sample the entire water column for small freshwater fish in shallow creeks, wetlands, pools and edge habitats (Figure 14.1c, d). Seine nets are probably less effective than fyke nets for detecting tadpoles in wetland complexes (Wassens *et al.* 2016). Seines can be hauled against the flow (or in still, minimal, or no-flow conditions) by two people (Figure 14.1d), with the foot rope on the lead line held against the substrate. Sampling efficiency is reduced if the area is not free of large woody debris or rocks (the inability to sample habitat structure is a limitation of this method). Investigators draw the lead (bottom) line ahead of and inside the float (top) line of the seine to guide fish into the back of the net (e.g. pocket) and minimise escape during hauling. Nets can vary in mesh size, length and depth (drop) depending on the target species, site conditions and monitoring objectives. Smaller meshes (≤ 3 mm) are useful for capturing small and juvenile fish, but hauling a small mesh net is slower (because of resistance against hauling the net), so fast-moving species often avoid the net.

Fishing effort associated with seine netting is often measured (and standardised) by recording the area sampled (e.g. area of 20 m^2). Once the seine haul is completed, investigators haul the net to the shore to process the catch. If few fish are caught, they can be processed directly from the wet net; larger catches can either be processed from the net while it remains in the water or first placed into aerated holding containers. Boats can be used for modified seine or trawl net sampling, where one operator stays on the shore and the boat is used to move the seine out into deeper water before it is dragged back to the shore. In this case, the lead line is not held down manually so it can either be further weighted or be assumed to be travelling along the substrate.

Procedure for gill nets

Gill nets are mesh walls with a float line at the top and sometimes a lead line to weight the bottom, and can be made to be buoyant (float at the top) or negatively buoyant (rest on the substrate). Mesh is most often monofilament or nylon, although cotton mesh is sometimes used. Nets vary in their length, drop and mesh size. Gill nets are often used to sample medium- to large-bodied fish and will not capture fish that are much narrower than the mesh size or tadpoles. Mesh size is selected to target the species required or a range of mesh sizes (in panels) is used to sample the fish community (DES 2018). Mesh shape can also be varied to target species with differing cross-sectional shapes. For example, a shorter, wider mesh is more efficient for wider-bodied fish such as Murray cod. Nets with up to a 3 m drop can be set in deep water (e.g. reservoirs and large rivers) and shallow water can be sampled using a smaller drop size. Net length may also vary in accordance with a waterway's physical attributes.

The float line of gill nets should be tied off at each end. Using a boat makes it much easier to deploy and retrieve a gill net, even if one end is anchored on shore. Gill nets are not suitable for high-flow environments and often become snagged in waterways with abundant instream structure or debris. Research teams should carry equipment to retrieve snagged sections of mesh to prevent ghost netting (i.e. unretrieved nets, or net sections, that continue to capture fish while unsupervised).

Depending on survey requirements and permit conditions, gill nets must be checked visually or manually at appropriate intervals while they are set. In some jurisdictions, fishing permit conditions may require gill nets to be checked at regular intervals; for example, in Queensland, DES (2018) recommends checking nets every 30 min. If several nets are deployed, they should be retrieved in the same order. Fishing effort associated with gill netting is often measured (and standardised) by recording the soak time, net length and mesh size (see Lear *et al.* 2019; Morgan *et al.* 2021b). Personnel remove fish from the net as it is retrieved and place them into a holding container of aerated water, keeping the rest of the net in the water. To avoid removing scales and damaging the body and fins, trapped fish can be pushed gently headfirst through the mesh. Fish removal should be done by experienced investigators (or under their supervision) and investigators often cut the gill net to remove an animal that is badly entangled.

Nets need to be checked regularly, and if large numbers of fish of one species are collected (e.g. schooling species such as bony herring, *Nematalosa erebi*) the nets should be removed to avoid local depletion or impacts on susceptible species. Large predators, such as crocodiles, sharks and sawfish, often roll in gill nets and can become entangled, and are also hazardous to investigators trying to remove them. In these circumstances, if gill nets need to be used, care should be taken to reduce netting time and investigators should be stationed at the net to observe any captures and immediately remove them. Investigators should avoid using weighted gill nets at sites where platypus occur or restrict use to daylight hours when platypus activity is reduced and the animals are more likely to detect and avoid nets (see 'Capturing freshwater turtles, snakes and platypus' for more details).

Procedure for dip nets

Dip, sweep or pond nets consist of an open-faced net on a hoop attached to a pole. Nets differ in mesh size, hoop diameter and pole length. Dip nets are sometimes useful for targeting tadpoles, small-bodied fish or fish larvae in shallow water. The use of spotlights at night is an effective means of attracting fish when dip netting. Dip nets can be used at multiple depths and locations using an exaggerated sweeping movement to capture tadpoles (DECC 2009; Wassens *et al.* 2013). Sweep time (e.g. 1 min) or sampled area (e.g. 5 m^2) can be used to semi-quantify sampling effort across replicate samples at sites. If schools of fish, larvae or tadpoles are scooped with a dip net, personnel transfer them to a container of stream water for processing. Water in the holding container may need to be aerated more gently than for larger fish, as small fish and tadpoles can be damaged by strong water currents. Larval fish may require euthanasia and preservation for accurate taxonomic identification.

Procedure for larval fish nets

Larval fish nets (similar to plankton nets but with slightly larger mesh, often 300–500 μm) can be used as an active capture method when towed from a boat or anchored as passive driftnets in flowing waterways. A smaller version can be thrown into the water and retrieved by pulling back towards the shore with the tow rope. Large stronger-swimming fish and air-breathing animals are unlikely to be encountered as by-catch in larval fish nets as they can avoid the net or swim back through the opening. Exclusion screens (e.g. a 50 mm bar trellis or a reversed mesh cone installed at the mouth of the net) can also be used to prevent large fish entering passively deployed larval nets. To measure fishing effort, nets are either towed or deployed for a set period (e.g. towing for 10 min) and, in some cases, flow meters are positioned in the mouth of the net to calculate the volume of water sampled for catch estimates (Neal *et al.* 2012). The contents of the net can be rinsed into the narrow end of the net, then tipped into a holding container of stream water via a removable collection cup. Water in the holding container may need to be aerated more gently than for larger fish, as small fish and tadpoles can be damaged by strong water currents.

Animal treatment, withdrawal and euthanasia

Fish can be captured efficiently in nets and many species can have good survival outcomes. Non-target fish with minor scale loss, lacerations or fin damage can still be released. If necessary, fish can be gently 'swum' manually through the water to wash oxygenated water over their gills until they regain equilibrium and swim off independently. Fish and tadpoles with life-threatening injuries (e.g. cuts to the abdomen, badly torn gills, signs of advanced disease, stress or lack of recovery) may need to be euthanised by (or under the supervision of) an experienced researcher (see Chapter 32). Exotic species may have to be euthanised under permit conditions and not returned to the waterway (see Chapter 32); researchers need to understand legal permit requirements for the jurisdiction they are working in. Veterinary assistance is seldom warranted for fish or tadpoles.

Investigators need to consider whether flow or weather conditions are predicted to change substantially during fieldwork. Nets may have to be removed if water levels rise or fall unexpectedly, a fish migratory event is in progress (demonstrated by abnormally large numbers of fish being captured), or non-target species (e.g. freshwater turtles, platypus, threatened non-target fish species) are captured. In particular, weighted gill nets present a high mortality risk to air-breathing vertebrates, including platypus (Grant 2012), so appropriate risk management may include removing nets proactively if vulnerable species are detected in the vicinity.

Equipment and maintenance

Equipment will vary depending on the species or taxon, local environment and study objectives (Table 14.1). Personnel rinse, clean and dry nets between sites and remove any debris. Care should be taken when drying large nets to ensure that birds or other terrestrial animals do not become entangled. Pest or weed species, or pathogens should not be transferred between sites. Nets and other equipment may need to be sterilised between sites. Personnel mend damage to nets as necessary before storing, and thoroughly clean and disinfect all equipment, shoes and vehicles between tadpole sampling sites to minimise the risk of transferring disease (e.g. amphibian chytrid fungus; see Chapter 27).

Specific qualifications, experience and training

Capturing wild fish for research requires knowledge of where and when to fish, and experience in using the equipment (Cooke *et al.* 2016). No formal training is required for using nets to capture fish and tadpoles, but investigators should be confident and competent with sufficient experience in operating the net to do so safely and efficiently. Competent personnel are able to recover, process and release animals efficiently, reducing the risk of stress-related injury or death. New investigators should be accompanied and trained by an experienced supervisor to ensure competency as determined by the organisation. Teams need to be able to identify catch and by-catch and to demonstrate competence with the specific methodology proposed. Familiarity with the triggers to change the method is required.

Workplace health and safety

Injury from animal spines or bites

Fish spines, turtle claws and animal bites can cause injuries requiring medical attention. Wearing heavy duty wet cotton gloves, covered footwear and a long-sleeved shirt reduces the risks of injury to both the animal and the handler. Some freshwater fish species, including bullrouts (family Tetrarogidae) and most catfishes (family Ariidae and Plotosidae), have venomous spines, and the freshwater whipray (*Urogymnus dalyensis*) possesses a

Table 14.1: Suggested equipment and materials for netting methods.

Deploying and retrieving nets	Removing and processing animals	Maintenance, repairs and other	Field hygiene kit for frogs and tadpoles
• Copies of permits and approvals • Information signs with permit details • Appropriate type and size (length, drop and mesh size) nets selected for the species and site • Ropes, floats, stakes and anchors/weights to secure nets • Watch or stopwatch to time deployments • Equipment to retrieve snagged nets • Boat, motor/oars and safety gear (often required for gill nets and towed larval fish nets)	• Sturdy cotton gloves (wet) for handling fish • Non-latex gloves for handling tadpoles (must be proven or rendered safe for the species) • Needle-nose pliers to lift net away from fish • Fine-point scissors and knife to cut net to release animals if needed • Several large holding containers, portable aerator with spare batteries • Clean non-chlorinated water in sealed containers, in case site water is unsuitable to use for holding • Anaesthetic for handling or euthanasia • Separate gloves and containers for handling and mixing anaesthetics or other chemicals • Preservation equipment (e.g. alcohol) • Bags, jars or vials required for samples, including labels • Field identification guide(s) and camera • Data sheets, pencils, pens, waterproof marker • Data collection equipment (e.g. scales, rulers, fish measuring boards) • Equipment to mark animals (e.g. tags)	• Net repair kit, including extra mesh • Spare nets • First aid kit • For night sampling: torches, headlamps, net lights • Personal protective equipment (e.g. life jacket, waders, dive boots, long-sleeved shirts, hat, sunscreen, insect repellent). Insect repellent and sunscreen may be detrimental to amphibians so ensure hands and equipment that may contact frogs or tadpoles are kept free of these chemicals	Source Murray *et al.* (2011): • Plastic box to separate equipment • Small Styrofoam™ esky • Disposable gloves (non-latex), noting they must be proven or rendered safe for the species before use • 70% alcohol for handwashing • Spray or wash bottle of disinfectant • Scrubbing brush for cleaning mud off footwear and vehicles • Bucket for mixing and soaking items in disinfectant • Plastic bags for hygienic temporary animal handling • Sharps container

stinging barb. First aid kits should include a thermos of hot (not scalding) water to alleviate pain from stings; medical attention should be sought when required. Adult male platypus produce venom delivered by spurs located on the hind legs and may be caught unintentionally when targeting fish and tadpoles. Refer to Chapter 17 for information about its effects and how to lift and carry platypuses safely.

In tropical and subtropical areas, estuarine crocodiles, freshwater crocodiles (*C. johnstoni*) and sharks (e.g. *Carcharhinus leucas* and *Glyphis* spp.) pose a serious risk to personnel undertaking water-based activities. Organisations with researchers working in these areas often require specific training in safe behaviour and sampling practices. Safety requirements should be addressed through risk assessments. There may be sites where the risk posed by estuarine crocodiles or sharks precludes safe research. Snake bite when working in or near water is also a risk, which occurs infrequently, but has serious consequences.

Injury from nets

Nets and ropes should be coiled when not in use to avoid trip and entanglement hazards. Long gill nets can be heavy when full and care must be taken to avoid injury when hauling. Seining from shore requires investigators to walk through the water and care must be taken, especially in turbid or fast-flowing water. Entanglement is also a risk during setting and hauling if long nets are not handled carefully or if investigators are inexperienced. Snagging on clothing or fingers is a common netting problem that should be carefully managed. Swimming and diving to retrieve snagged nets can carry serious operator risks and are not recommended.

Alternative procedures

Passive survey techniques (including observation, snorkelling, cameras, sonar and eDNA) that involve minimal or no interference with natural behaviour are becoming more popular and increasing in variety (see 'Low-impact techniques for monitoring and detecting freshwater animals' within this chapter). However, these methods are not suitable for studies that require handling (e.g. to obtain measurements, biopsies or body condition assessments); this issue limits their range of research applications (see Ebner and Morgan 2013).

TRAPPING FISH AND TADPOLES

Nicole Flint, Alison J. King, Sascha Healy, Joanne Ocock, Deborah S. Bower, David L. Morgan, Ian Wooden, Scott A. Hardie, Tarmo A. Raadik, David T. Roberts and Melody Serena

Target taxa

Methods described in this GOP are applicable to tadpoles (Chapter 27), and large- and small-bodied freshwater fish (Chapter 32).

Context and scope

This GOP details trapping procedures for tadpoles and fish in freshwater environments using common passive trap types, including box, fishway and light traps, and drum nets. Box and light traps use bait or chemical lures to attract target taxa; drum nets and fishway traps do not. The selection of one method over another depends on the study objectives, including the need to sample particular species or life-history stages.

Animal welfare considerations

Passive trapping poses a lower risk of contact injury to animals than some other capture methods (e.g. netting). Nevertheless, several risks to animals are associated with these trapping methods, which can be minimised through short deployment times, monitoring traps during deployment, and appropriate hauling and handling practices. Many of the animal welfare considerations associated with netting of fish and tadpoles, related to handling, predation and crushing by larger animals caught in the same trap, and air exposure, are shared by the techniques detailed in this GOP.

Handling

Refer to 'Netting fish and tadpoles' earlier in this chapter.

External injury

Similar to netting, fish skin, fins, gills and eyes can occasionally be injured during trapping, although injury is less likely using methods detailed in this GOP than for some netting methods (Veldhuizen *et al.* 2018). Traps can be cut open if captured animals appear stressed and need to be released quickly. Investigators should keep sturdy scissors, and a repair kit or spare traps on hand. Some large trap types (e.g. fishway traps) are made from robust material, such as stainless steel, which potentially increases the risk of external injuries such as abrasions, scale loss and lacerations. Design elements can be included to reduce this risk, such as compartments to keep fish in water during trap removal and emptying phases, and rubber matting on the trap's floor to reduce abrasions while traps are cleared. Suspending the traps partially in water while removing trapped animals progressively can also reduce the risk of injury by allowing the animals to remain submerged.

Predation and crushing

Refer to 'Netting fish and tadpoles' earlier in this chapter.

Capture stress

Little is known about how trapping affects stress levels in fish or tadpoles. A review of commercial fishing techniques (in marine environments) identified 85 articles on fish capture injuries and mortality, only nine of which referred to traps (Veldhuizen *et al.* 2018). Of those studies, the variables associated with fish injury included changes in water temperature, capture depth and fishing duration. Oxygen depletion is a possible cause of mortality if traps are set in deep water or overnight. Traps that provide some level of refuge from exposure (e.g. direct sunlight) will reduce the risk of stress, as does ensuring that the trap does not alter water conditions. For example, traps constructed of black steel can heat up, and traps that exclude water flow can reduce dissolved oxygen concentrations.

Air exposure

Refer to details under 'Netting fish and tadpoles' earlier in this chapter.

Risks to non-target species

Fish by-catch can be reduced by using appropriate trap types for the target species or by installing by-catch reduction devices. Non-target air-breathing animals (including adult frogs, platypus, turtles, crocodiles, rakali, snakes and water birds) are at risk of drowning in traps that have an entrance large enough for an animal to enter, but not easily escape. Traps fitted with internal entrance funnels pose an especially high risk to species, such as platypus, that consistently try to locate an exit in the trap's outer perimeter (Serena *et al.* 2016). Various forms of by-catch exclusion devices can be incorporated into traps, including coarse mesh over openings to exclude larger-bodied animals or air-breathing vertebrates. An air space should be maintained in traps set at sites where air-breathing fauna are at risk of being captured. Traps should also be checked sufficiently often to preclude by-catch being unduly stressed by factors such as hunger, crowding or hypothermia.

General procedures

Before sampling, investigators should determine the most appropriate traps to meet the objectives of the study and consider the need for additional equipment. For example, a boat may be required for deploying or retrieving traps in deeper waters, or for use in tropical rivers where estuarine crocodiles pose a threat to investigators. Consulting gauging stations and completing reconnaissance site visits before setting traps will ensure investigators understand the study site's water level variations and physical features before commencing sampling. If required, holding containers with aerators can be set up in a shady location to process animals removed from traps.

Procedure for box traps

Collapsible box traps (also called bait traps or sometimes bait nets) are small rectangular traps made of fine mesh, with funnelled entrance holes at each end and a zippered bait compartment. They provide a passive capture technique useful for catching smaller fish and tadpoles (Figure 14.2a, b). Box traps can be set during the day or overnight. If set overnight, they can be used to capture nocturnal species and those that are more active at dawn and dusk (crepuscular species). Night deployment carries a risk of trapped animals being exposed to potentially lethal low dissolved oxygen concentrations in some wetland systems, so operators need to be familiar with the physicochemical properties of the waterbody. Deployment duration is generally greater than 1 h; total deployment time is recorded to allow effort to be calculated and standardised among samples (where required). Commonly used baits include dried or wet pet food (e.g. cat food, chicken pellets, meat) placed in the zippered compartment, chemical lights (e.g. glowsticks) placed inside the trap (Bower *et al.* 2014; DES 2018), or both. Box traps are effective in capturing common small-bodied fish without the use baits (Balcombe and Gloss 2000).

Box traps can be used in various water depths depending on the location, study site and target species. The entrances on either end of the trap must be submerged. Investigators typically record variables such as location details of each trap, water depth and habitat type. Tadpole and fish trapping detectability is influenced by surrounding habitat complexity, so setting traps at

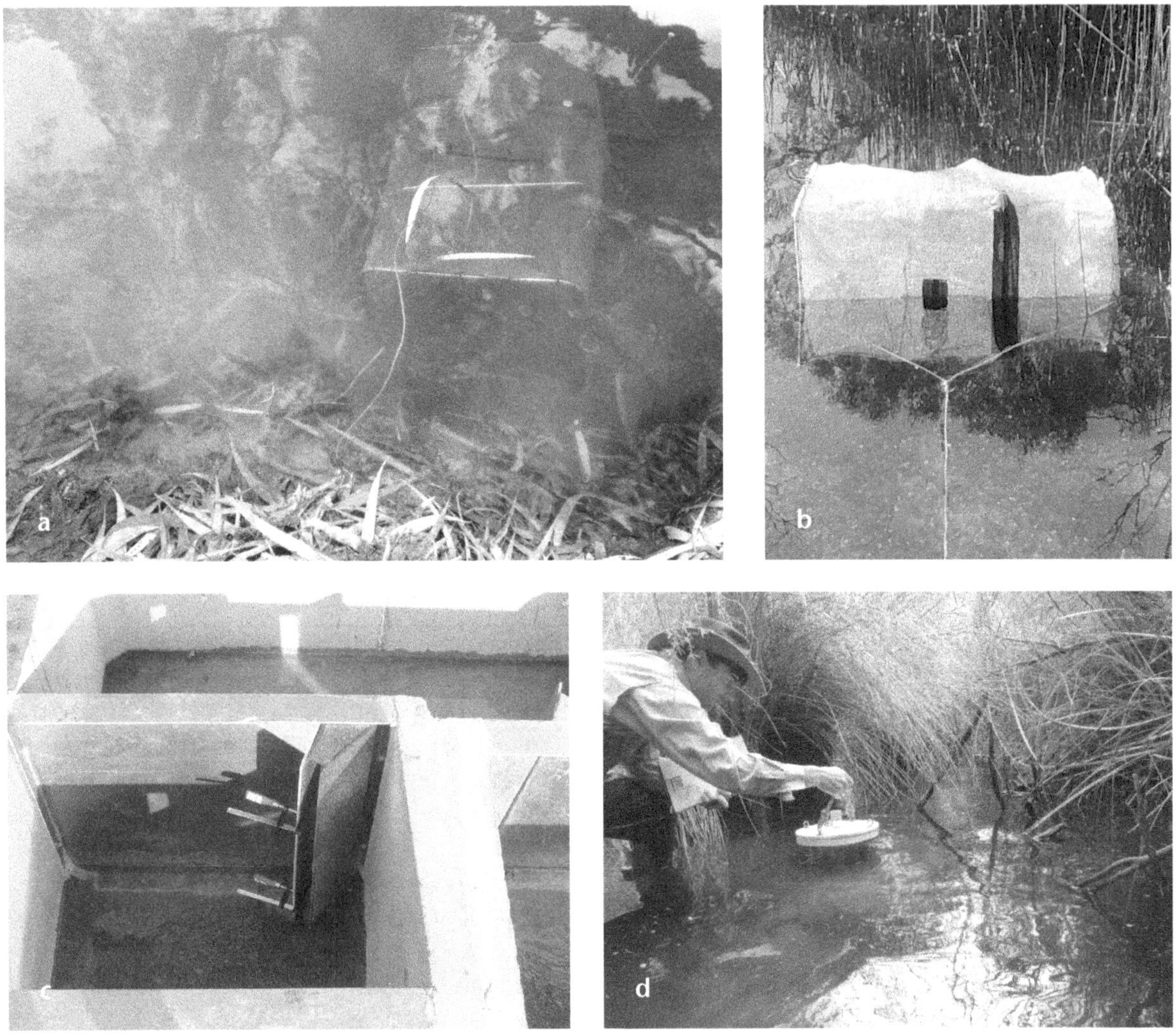

Figure 14.2: (a) Box trap baited with dry cat food and deployed in the shallows to capture small fish. Photo by Nicole Flint. (b) Box trap partly submerged in vegetation for tadpole monitoring; note air space above the surface (which can also be achieved with a float) and placement on side to ensure bait is submerged. Photo by Sascha Healy. (c) Funnel fishway trap (Goodga River, WA). Photo by David Morgan. (d) Larval fish light trap deployed and retrieval. Photo by Stephen Beatty.

sites varying in water depths and habitat structure can reduce capture bias (Sanders *et al.* 2015). Traps can be set from the bank or from a boat. Traps need to be placed far enough apart to be independent of each other and can be anchored by tying them with rope to bankside vegetation, a float or a stake (DES 2018). When setting traps for tadpoles (which need to air-breathe from time to time), or if hatchling turtles are present at the study site, ensure that an air space is maintained above the surface of the water. As traps are collected, fish and tadpoles are gently tipped or scooped into a holding container filled with aerated stream water (or clean unchlorinated water if stream water is unsuitable). Tadpoles can be difficult to see in traps, so investigators check traps meticulously to avoid missing small individuals, and remove them carefully to avoid damage.

Procedure for drum nets

Drum nets are collapsible string mesh cylinders (~1.5 m diameter) with a funnel entrance supported by steel hoops at either end. Some variants are fitted with wings or a larger framed entrance mouth (frog mouth drum net). Drum nets are deployed with ropes attached to poles driven into the substrate upstream and downstream of the trap and are typically used in flowing waters with the entrance orientated downstream to capture fish moving upstream. Optimal performance with this equipment is achieved when targeting migrating fish during periods of increased flow. In these conditions, location and setting the net properly is critical for maximising catch rates. While infrequently used for research, drum nets may sometimes be beneficial for targeting large-bodied migrating fish. Typically, stretch mesh sizes of 50–150 mm are used. Unless the mesh size is sufficiently large to allow any trapped air-breathing animals to escape, drum nets pose a high risk of their drowning. In general, drum nets should be used only when other alternatives are unavailable to answer the study objectives, and regularly checked.

Procedure for fishway traps

Customised traps can be used to determine the effectiveness of fishways installed on weirs and barrages. An example image is provided from the Goodga River Fishway, a vertical-slot fishway composed of a series of cells separated by baffles to reduce flows (Figure 14.2c). The fish move upstream through runs and into resting pools through funnels designed to minimise downstream movement (Morgan and Beatty 2006). To retain their shape and position, and to allow for multiple deployments, fishway traps may be constructed of stainless-steel mesh, and can be designed to fit within fishway pools to block the exit or entrance (e.g. O'Connor *et al.* 2019). Specialised equipment, such as cranes or winches, are often needed for deployment and retrieval of fishway traps because of their large size. Investigators check and clear traps regularly, determined by the study design or fish community likely to be encountered. Traps often also need to be placed proximal to the flow in the fishway to ensure fish will enter the traps and not bypass the entrances.

Procedure for light traps

Light traps (Figure 14.2d) are effective for capturing larval and juvenile fish and can be effective for tadpoles, including in areas with dense vegetation or where gear avoidance may be an issue (Gyekis *et al.* 2006). Light traps set overnight commonly capture a wider range of species than larval driftnets (e.g. Humphries *et al.* 2002, but see King *et al.* 2020 for tropical systems). They consist of one or more transparent plastic external compartments with an internal plastic tube housing a light source, and a narrow gap around all sides to allow larval fish to enter. Commercial units may be of a rectangular, cylindrical or quatrefoil design. The waterproof light source can consist of a chemical light (glowstick), or an energy efficient white light, such as a light-emitting diode (LED). Applying mesh around the trap entrances will reduce unwanted by-catch (mostly small-bodied adult fish and crustaceans) and the potential for predation on trapped larvae, but can also reduce the ease in which larvae enter the traps. Traps are typically left unattended overnight (set at dusk) and collected in the morning. Deployment and retrieval by boat may be required, especially in deep water sites. Following collection of traps, larvae can be gently rinsed and tipped into a holding container of stream water. Water in the holding container may need to be aerated more gently than for larger fish, as small fish and tadpoles can be damaged by strong water currents. Larval fish typically require euthanasia and preservation for accurate taxonomic identification.

Animal treatment, withdrawal and euthanasia

Survival rates for trapped fish are often high (e.g. 90% survival of endangered pygmy perch *Nannoperca oxleyana*; Knight *et al.* 2007) if the fish are removed from traps and released quickly. Fish with minor lacerations or fin damage can still be released. Alternatively, if required, fish can be gently 'swum' manually through the water to wash oxygenated water over their gills until they regain equilibrium and swim off independently. Fish and tadpoles with life-threatening injuries (e.g. deep cuts to the abdomen, badly torn gills, signs of advanced disease or stress), may need to be euthanased by (or under the supervision of) an experienced researcher (see Chapter 32). Non-native (introduced) fishes may be required to be killed under permit conditions and not returned to the waterway (see Chapter 32). Veterinarian assistance is seldom warranted for fish or tadpoles. Submerged traps should be removed promptly, and trapping protocols reviewed if non-target species (e.g. freshwater turtles, platypus, non-target fish) die or are injured in traps.

Equipment and maintenance

Equipment and maintenance considerations (including cleaning and disinfection protocols) are similar to those covered within 'Netting fish and tadpoles', but see Table 14.2 for other suggested equipment and materials.

Specific qualifications, experience and training

Refer to 'Netting fish and tadpoles' earlier in this chapter.

Workplace health and safety

Refer to 'Netting fish and tadpoles' in this chapter.

Table 14.2: Suggested equipment and materials required for trapping fish and tadpoles.

Deploying and retrieving traps	Removing and processing animals	Maintenance, repairs and other	Field hygiene kit for frogs and tadpoles
• Copies of permits and approvals • Information signs with permit details • Appropriate traps selected for the species and site (tagged with identification details) • Ropes, floats, stakes and anchors/weights to secure traps • Watch or stopwatch to time deployments • Equipment to retrieve snagged traps • Boat, motor/oars and safety gear (if required)	• Sturdy cotton gloves (wet) for handling fish • Non-latex gloves for handling tadpoles (must be proven or rendered safe for the species) • Scissors, pliers and knife to cut trap to release animals if needed • Large holding containers, portable aerators with spare batteries • Clean non-chlorinated water in sealed containers, in case site water is unsuitable to use for holding • Anaesthetic for handling or euthanasia • Separate gloves and containers for handling and mixing anaesthetics or other chemicals • Preservation equipment (e.g. alcohol) • Bags, jars or vials required for samples, including labels • Field identification guide(s) and camera • Data sheets, pencils, pens, waterproof marker • Data collection equipment (e.g. scales, rulers, fish measuring boards) • Equipment to mark animals (e.g. tags)	• Trap repair kit • Spare traps • First aid kit • For night sampling: torches, headlamps, trap/rope lights • Personal protective equipment (e.g. life jacket, waders, dive boots, long-sleeved shirts, hat, sunscreen, insect repellent). Insect repellent and sunscreen may be detrimental to amphibians so ensure hands and equipment that may contact frogs or tadpoles are kept free of these chemicals	Source Murray *et al.* (2011): • Plastic box to separate equipment • Small Styrofoam™ esky • Disposable gloves (non-latex), noting they must be proven or rendered safe for the species before use • 70% alcohol for handwashing • Spray or wash bottle of disinfectant • Scrubbing brush for cleaning mud off footwear and vehicles • Bucket for mixing and soaking items in disinfectant • Plastic bags for hygienic temporary animal handling • Sharps container

Alternative procedures

Refer to 'Netting fish and tadpoles' in this chapter.

ELECTROFISHING

Ian Wooden

Target taxa

This GOP addresses key principles for electrofishing for all fish occurring in freshwater environments (Chapter 32); some electrofishing units can also be used to capture fish in estuarine waterbodies.

Context and scope

Electrofishing is an active sampling tool commonly used in fish research for its ability to sample a diversity of species and size classes efficiently across a variety of freshwater habitats (Yoder and Smith 1999). Electrofishing uses an electrical current that is passed through the water to inhibit the swimming ability of fish and allow them to be caught in a dip net. Application of the correct electrical waveform can attract fish through forced swimming (galvanotaxis) followed by muscle relaxation (galvanonarcosis), allowing the fish to be captured easily. Boat-, bank- or backpack-mounted electrofishing apparatus are used in many freshwater habitats. Highly specialised electrofishing equipment can also be used in estuarine conditions (Lieschke *et al.* 2019). Researchers should consider sampling objectives, physical constraints, biological characteristics of target species, equipment and operational requirements to optimise sample efficiency and minimise potential adverse impacts from electrofishing on investigators and aquatic animals. Electrical equipment designed for seining, fish anaesthesia, general handling and guiding are not covered in this GOP.

Animal welfare considerations

Risks to fish

When used correctly, electrofishing can be a very low impact technique. The risks of electrofishing to fish are well documented (Snyder 2003). Risks can be managed by ensuring that only investigators with suitable experience and training, who can identify ideal water quality conditions and appropriate electrofishing settings, undertake the procedure. Researchers or institutes often have their own guidelines for the safe use of electrofishing (Nielsen 1998). In general, impacts on fish welfare when electrofishing can be immediate or delayed and include:

- mortality (Dolan and Miranda 2004)
- haemorrhage (Miranda and Kidwell 2010)

- vertebral fractures (Clément and Cunjak 2010; Culver and Chick 2015)
- tissue injury (branding) (Snyder 2003)
- asphyxiation
- cardiac disturbance (Schreer *et al.* 2004)
- reduced spawning success (Muth and Ruppert 1996)
- physiological stress as a result of capture and handling (Mesa and Schreck 1989)
- reduced growth.

Investigators must develop controls to minimise the risk of injury to fish, which include a detailed context-specific standard operating procedure (SOP). The SOP will detail correct selection of electrical waveform and intensity (power), which can be a balance between the physiological and biological characteristics of target animals and water electrical conductivity (sampling efficiency), post-capture handling techniques and consideration of species-specific tolerance to electrofishing in the sample design.

Risks to non-target species

Animals, both aquatic and terrestrial, occurring in a sample area may potentially be affected by electrofishing and could result in physical injury and behaviour disruptions (Reynolds 1996). Aside from fish, welfare risks to non-target animals are not well documented, but include frogs (Allen and Riley 2012), platypus (Grant and Temple-Smith 2003; Pettigrew and Wilkens 2003), salamanders (Kyrsko and Nickerson 2003) and cetaceans (Thomas *et al.* 2019). Electrofishing operations should only be employed by appropriately trained staff. Operations need to consider the minimum required electrofishing power to elicit a response from fish that also reduces the risk of injury to animals. Appropriate selection of sampling periods reduces risks by considering times of day and seasons that could predispose non-target animals to electrofishing. For example, investigators often avoid crepuscular periods and sample outside of the non-target species breeding season. Avoiding energising an area where non-target species are observed can further reduce risk. Wading and boating operations associated with electrofishing can also damage or disturb habitat and animals (e.g. freshwater mussels), so investigators must take care to minimise these impacts while sampling.

General procedures

Electrofishers used by Australian fish researchers are backpack, bank- and boat-mounted (NSW Fisheries 1997). In a backpack electrofishing unit, the pulsator is generally worn on a trained electrofishing operator's back, above water level, so sampling areas must be shallow and wadable (Figure 14.3a). The anode is usually a ring-shaped section at the end of a long, insulated pole, which is moved through the water ahead of the operator. The cathode trails behind the operator and is typically a long, braided steel cable. Bank-mounted units have higher power capacity than backpack units, use a similar anode as the backpack units with a cathode plate deployed in the water, and can also be used in wadable waterways. Boat-mounted electrofishers (Figure 14.3b) are also high-powered units, with boom-mounted anodes usually protruding from the bow, and usually use the boat as the cathode. Boat-mounted electrofishing allows fish to be sampled from larger and deeper habitats (*cf.* backpack and bank-mounting electrofishing)

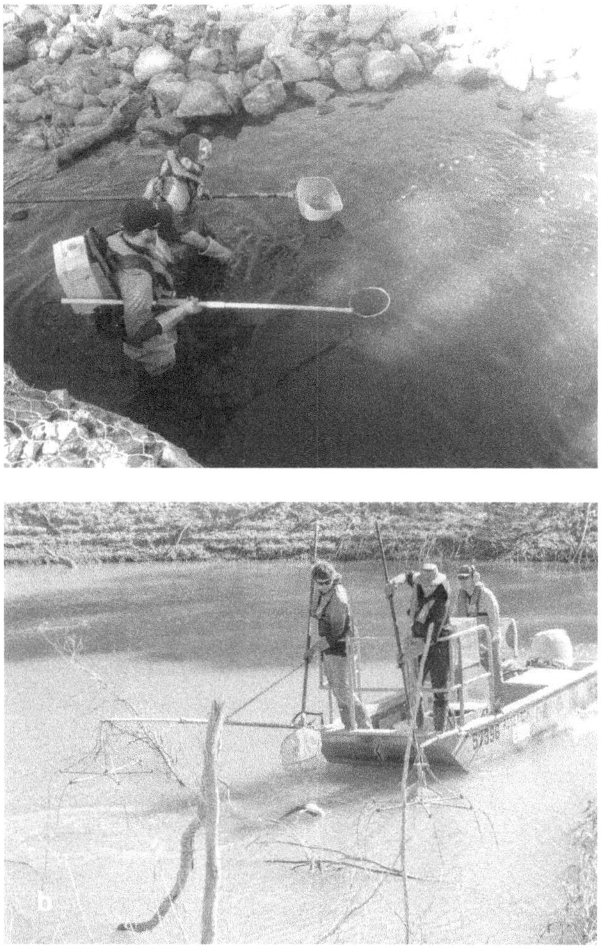

Figure 14.3: (a) Backpack electrofishing in a shallow pool. (b) Boat-based electrofisher and crew working on the Darling River. Photos by Ian Wooden/NSW DPI Fisheries.

Affected fish usually swim towards the anode and are caught using dip nets by additional trained operators and placed into containers of aerated water for recovery; more cryptic species may need to be actively retrieved from among habitat. The effectiveness and safety of electrofishing is influenced by a range of factors. Institutions often develop a SOP for electrofishing, to ensure appropriate sampling design, standardised effort, effective capture, staff safety and minimisation of harmful impacts while using the technique. Researchers train with experienced investigators before accreditation to be competent in the technique and post-capture processing requirements. It is essential that researchers account for the contributing effects of equipment, operator training, sample environment, experimental design, electrofishing set-up and target species when undertaking electrofishing operations. Investigators should comply with the *Australian Code of Electrofishing Practice* (NSW Fisheries 1997) and any updates to this code.

Equipment

The choice of electrofishing equipment is dependent on sampling site characteristics, including site access, depth, flow velocity, target species size, and the electrofishing unit's power capability. Environmental conditions, particularly water conductivity, will directly influence the equipment's ability to generate the required power for effective electrofishing (Miranda 2009). Operators learn how to manage these considerations through specialised workplace and workshop training modules. Where multiple electrofishing units are available, researchers ensure that they are calibrated, effective and safe, by undertaking field mapping and servicing the equipment regularly. To reduce the risk of injury to staff and animals, professionally constructed and tested electrofishing equipment is used.

Operator training

Inexperienced electrofishing operators need to be trained by experienced personnel to control equipment and guide electrofishing operations. Doing so ensures correct practices, including establishing effective electrical waveforms, good communication between operators, and efficiently and safely capturing and handling fish. The netters that accompany backpack, bank and boat-mounted electrofishing operators help to reduce injuries to target and by-catch species, by minimising exposure time of animals in the electric field. Netters working with electrofishing operators avoid reintroducing netted fish into the electrified field or into future sampling areas, to reduce the risk of overexposure. Efficiency of netters and fishers can be variable, being dependent on training and experience, so implementation of training and standardised sampling teams is of utmost importance to this sampling technique.

Environment

A range of environmental parameters influence electrofishing efficiency substantially. Water conductivity, temperature, dissolved oxygen, turbidity, depth, water velocity and habitat complexity influence catchability and risk of injury to study animals. When developing an electrofishing SOP and survey design, researchers should consider the likely effects of each of these factors on the sampling data and animals.

Sample design

Sample designs using electrofishing require procedures to ensure standardised effort, effective capture and minimisation of harmful impacts to animals. Factors to consider include duration of electrofisher application (effort), season, time of day, reach or sample length, sample path and habitats that are fished. An understanding of the habitats (e.g. snags, backwaters, aquatic plant beds) within a sample area that are likely to provide refuge for target species is critical for sampling efficiency and standardising catch data across sites. Effort associated with electrofishing is often measured (and standardised) by recording reach length, fishing time (unit 'on' time) and/or total sampling period. Increasingly, investigators are including electrofishing power standardisation in their protocols to improve the robustness of sample data. Avoiding temperature extremes and spawning periods will contribute to minimising impacts on sensitive fish and non-target species, and help standardise results.

Electrical waveform

Electrofishing success and rate of animal injury are influenced strongly by the intensity and shape of the electrical waveform applied during sampling (Reynolds 1996). Researchers often conduct pilot sampling programs to determine a standardised approach to equipment parameters and sampling design, balance effective sampling with reduced fish injury, and facilitate repeatable capture efficiency. Increased values of electrical intensity, pulse duration and frequency can result in increased electrofishing-induced injuries to aquatic animals, with frequency cited as the most critical factor (Reynolds 1996; Snyder 2003). An effective SOP will guide the electrofishing operator through a process that identifies the minimal power required to elicit a capture response in target fish species/communities.

Target species and developmental stage

The susceptibility of fish to electrofishing capture (Price and Peterson 2010; Lyon *et al.* 2014) or injury differs between species because of anatomical differences (e.g. vertebral count, tissue, scaling, environmental tolerance), body size, physiology, behaviour patterns (e.g. habitat selection, activity patterns), habitat complexity and water quality parameters. For example, seasonal water temperature may dictate more suitable sampling windows for some fish species. Similarly, capture efficiency and exposure to injury also varies between developmental stage (larva, juvenile, adult). Sweep net electrofishing, which uses a smaller anode ring within a fitted square frame is an effective larval fish sampling technique (King and Crook 2002).

Post capture handling

Well-designed housing, appropriate handling techniques, prophylactic treatments and suitable recovery periods between procedures are commonly used to reduce the impact and stress on collected fishes. Fish may be placed into well-aerated holding containers for recovery and to await processing. If fish are returned to the water after handling, sampling points should be suitably distant from each other to ensure no cumulative sampling or exposure to electrofishing by fishes.

Animal treatment, withdrawal and euthanasia

The effects of electrofishing on fish health has been the subject of considerable research. Much of this research has focused on the relationship between electrical characteristics (waveform) and mortality and injury rates. Mortality rates are generally lower for direct current (DC) electrofishing and reduced electrical intensity. However, mortality rates and susceptibility to electrofishing injury vary between species and their tolerance to sampling conditions. To reduce the likelihood of injury or mortality to fish or non-target animals, only minimum power settings necessary to attract and immobilise target fish effectively should be used and contact of fish with live anodes avoided. Trained operators select appropriate electrofishing settings to minimise risks to fish described in 'Animal welfare considerations'. Qualified operators are trained on appropriate electrical settings to minimise injury.

Visible signs of stress or injury in fish may include branding or darkened marks, bleeding from gills, spinal disfiguration, increased mucus production, discolouration, reddening of fin outer edges, flared gills and operculum, increased opercular rate, surface breathing and loss of equilibrium and lethargy (see 'Animal welfare considerations' within this GOP for more information). Post-capture handling and care are critical for reducing capture stress and mortality. As for other fish capture methods, investigators ensure the provision of well-aerated containers of suitable water to hold captured fish during recovery, aim to minimise numbers of fish and holding times, and release fish once they have fully recovered from the effects of electrofishing. Flow-through recovery tank systems are preferred when possible because water conditions tend to deteriorate with holding time and crowding. Backpack electrofishing crews use large holding buckets with aerators, change water frequently, and minimise captive fish size and numbers while sampling. Fish with minor external damage can still be released following recovery.

Post-release survival of any fish species or life-history stage cannot be assumed based on characteristics of other fish species, so researchers often seek species-specific information and, if none is available, may need to undertake controlled experiments before commencing electrofishing studies on wild populations. Fish with life-threatening injuries (e.g. deep cuts to the abdomen, body deformation, badly torn gills, or signs of advanced disease or stress as described above), may need to be euthanased (see Chapter 32). Factors that may affect the decision to withdraw electrofishing from the study include extremes of water temperature (upper or lower limits of species threshold), visible injury or mortality rates resulting from sampling, or if a fish migratory event is in progress. The presence of threatened species, spawning aggregations or nesting fish in the study may also justify withdrawal from sampling. Furthermore, unsafe environmental conditions, such as heavy rain and electrical storms, may also warrant that sampling cease.

Equipment and maintenance

Maintenance of electrofishing equipment is essential for safe and effective operation. Generators, electrofishing control units, batteries, boats, trailers and ancillary equipment (nets, personal protective equipment or PPE, defibrillators and first aid kits) require regular cleaning, repair and servicing. Operational and safety inspections on electrofishing equipment must be completed annually by qualified commercial providers, while electrofishing operators conduct safety system checks before every use. Aquatic hygiene protocols, including cleaning of boats, electrofishing anodes, nets, tubs waders and trailers, will aid in preventing transfer of biological material and pathogens between sample sites. Typical equipment is detailed in Table 14.3.

Specific qualifications, experience and training

Electrofishing is a high-risk activity that uses electrical voltages, which can be lethal to humans (Reynolds 1996; Lazauski and Malvestuto 1990; Balachandran *et al.* 2013) and should only be conducted by trained and experienced (accredited) personnel. Incorrect operation can also adversely impact aquatic wildlife or yield inaccurate sample data. Research authorities must take appropriate steps to ensure all personnel involved in electrofishing are suitably qualified, including receiving training in electrofishing theory (e.g. US Fish and Wildlife Service 2018), operation, safety procedures and experience with relevant electrofishing gear type(s). As part of the SOP, training documentation and record keeping systems to ensure work, health and safety compliance are developed. Training can also be accessed from equipment manufacturers or external training providers. Operators are often required to hold current certification in first aid, including cardiopulmonary resuscitation (CPR) and defibrillator operation, and undertake regular medical checks. Boat electrofishing operations require crewing and for vessels to be compliant with jurisdictional regulations. Investigators should have appropriate training and experience on the electrofishing vessels available for use. Teams need to be able to identify catch and by-catch and to demonstrate competence with the specific methodology proposed. Familiarity with the triggers to adjust the method or settings is required.

Workplace health and safety

Also refer to 'Netting fish and tadpoles' earlier in this chapter.

Electrical shock

Electrofishing is hazardous with backpack, bank and boat electrofishing units capable of electrifying personnel and by-standers. Electrification can result in heart failure, respiratory arrest and electrical burns. Other potential risks related to electrical shock include bodily contact with electrodes or water within the electric field and shocks from inadequately constructed equipment (NSW Fisheries 1997). Electrofishing operations and equipment should comply with the Australian Code of Electrofishing Practice (NSW Fisheries 1997) and any updates to the code, and with relevant Australian

Table 14.3: General equipment items that may be required for electrofishing operations.

Apparatus	Protective equipment	Additional items
• Electrofishing apparatus (type dependent on sampling requirements and habitat type) • Knotless mesh landing nets with insulated handles suitably sized for target species (knotless to reduce damage to fish skin) • Water quality instrumentation, including conductivity, temperature and dissolved oxygen probes • Either live-well equipment or large holding container (e.g. covered tubs, plastic-handled buckets, water pumps, oxygen cylinders, aerators, transfer hoses) • Fish handling nets and slings • Repair kit for apparatus and spares of any equipment that may become damaged during use • Watch or stopwatch to time fishing effort	• Rubber boots, or non-breathable waders, plus 1000 V rated linesmen gloves must be worn by all electrofishing team members during operations. Waders should generally not be worn in boating operations. • Sturdy cotton gloves (wet) for handling fish • Separate gloves and containers for handling and mixing anaesthetics or other chemicals • Personal protective equipment (e.g. electrical gloves, life jacket, non-breathable waders and belt, gumboots, polaroid sunglasses, fish handling gloves, long-sleeved shirt, hat, sunscreen, insect repellent) • First aid kit and defibrillator • Communication plan and equipment (mobile or satellite phones, EPIRB, etc.)	• Copies of permits and approvals and information signs with permit details • Data collection and recording equipment (e.g. scales, rules, fish measuring boards, notebooks, data sheets, pencils, pens, waterproof markers) • Equipment to mark animals (e.g. tags) • Anaesthetic for fish handling or euthanasia • Sample collection and storage equipment (e.g. vials, alcohol, labels, scissors, forceps, cold storage, otolith removal tools)

electrical standards. The risk of electric shock can be minimised greatly by ensuring only suitably qualified staff operate equipment, that less experienced staff are appropriately supervised, suitable PPE (e.g. electrical gloves and insulated footwear) is always worn, and that all equipment is compliant and regularly maintained. Institutions should require staff to be trained in first aid, including CPR and use of a defibrillator. Even minor electrical shocks are to be treated as serious and patients immediately conveyed to hospital.

Electrofishing operations must be suspended immediately if rain occurs or staff are wet, or if there are electrical storms nearby. Institutions undertaking electrofishing operations have appropriate risk assessments and take measures to ensure staff safety, including the development of training and safety programs (similar to US Fish and Wildlife Service 2016). General public and by-standers are at risk near electrofishing operations. Avoidance, crowd control, adequate communication and signage should be employed by investigators to prevent accidental injury to by-standers. Investigators need to monitor their surrounds and suspend operations in the proximity of others.

Alternative procedures

Electrofishing is an efficient tool for sampling fish assemblages and when conducted correctly may impact wildlife less than some other techniques. Constraints of research objectives, environment (e.g. depth, water conductivity), target fish species, end use and injury minimisation may justify use of alternate methods, including underwater cameras, snorkelling, netting and trapping (see other GOPs within this chapter), eDNA techniques (Chapter 4) or angling (Chapter 13).

CAPTURING FRESHWATER TURTLES, SNAKES AND PLATYPUS

Melody Serena, Deborah S. Bower, Nicole Flint and Alison J. King

Target taxa

This GOP applies to freshwater turtles and aquatic snakes (see Chapter 26) and platypus (see Chapter 17).

Context and scope

This GOP describes netting and trapping techniques and practices for freshwater turtles and aquatic snakes, and platypus. It covers a range of net and trap types that are commonly used for research purposes in Australia and elsewhere, including:

- fyke nets (platypus, turtles, aquatic snakes)
- gill nets (platypus, turtles) and trammel nets (turtles)
- collapsible crayfish traps, crab pots, cathedral traps, hoop nets and drum nets (turtles)
- seine netting (turtles)
- dip netting (turtles)
- hand capture by snorkelling or muddling (turtles, file snakes).

Animal welfare considerations

Risks to platypus

A range of animal welfare risks are associated with capture methods for platypus, which can be mitigated by checking nets frequently, ensuring that nets are set in appropriate locations (i.e. avoiding sites with strong currents or turbulence) and (if possible) not trapping during the breeding season. General risks to consider are detailed in Table 14.4. Specific risks and mitigation options associated with each method are detailed under 'General procedures' within this GOP.

Table 14.4: Capture-related risks to platypus.

Risk	Mechanism
Exhaustion and drowning	Exhaustion may occur if captured animals are forced to cope with strong currents or turbulent water in the end chamber of a fyke net. An active platypus drowns in < 3 min when confined underwater (Grant *et al.* 2004).
Hypothermia	The lower limit of the platypus's thermoneutral zone is ~15°C (Bethge *et al.* 2001).
Hunger	Food travels from a platypus's stomach to its colon in ~5 h (Booth and Connolly 2008).
Stress	Plasma glucocorticoid concentration rises markedly within 30 min of a platypus being captured in a fyke or unweighted gill net (McDonald *et al.* 1992).
Predation	For example, predation is a risk from European red foxes (*Vulpes vulpes*) (if nets are stretched onto land or into very shallow water) or large long-finned eels (*Anguilla reinhardtii*).
Injuries from fighting	Injuries inflicted by adult males may occur if two or more males are confined together during the platypus breeding season in winter and spring.

Risks to turtles

A range of animal welfare risks associated with capturing turtles (as listed in Table 14.5) can largely be mitigated by checking nets or traps frequently. Specific risks and mitigation options associated with each method are detailed under 'General procedures' within this GOP.

Risks to non-target species

Non-target animals captured in fyke nets include fish, birds, rakali, crocodiles, freshwater crayfish (*Cherax* spp., *Euastacus* spp.) and other sizeable crustaceans, water dragons (*Physignathus lesueurii*) and crocodiles. Rakali typically escape from fyke nets quite rapidly by chewing a hole through netting, and so are mainly targeted by setting baited wire mesh cage traps on the banks (e.g. Speldewinde *et al.* 2013). Welfare risks in fyke nets are mainly to ducklings or fish that are injured or killed by larger predatory species. All by-catch should be released when first encountered. Small ducklings must be released as a group with their parent. Fish are the main non-target animals captured in other types of gear set for platypus or turtles and can be difficult to remove unharmed, particularly from gill nets. Personnel should consider not setting gill nets where fish are abundant and likely to be captured as by-catch. Alternatively, if gill nets specifically need to be set, personnel should check them regularly and release fish promptly. If turtle gill nets are weighted, they present a risk of drowning to platypus unable to swim to the surface.

General procedures

Procedure for fyke nets

For platypus, fyke nets are typically set in the afternoon at four or more sites distributed at a minimum spacing of 0.5 km, and remain in the water overnight. Animals do not become entangled in netting, but are directed into a series of non-return chambers by two lateral wings that span the entire width of the channel and extend up the banks for at least 1 m where possible (Figure 14.4). Two nets are normally set as a pair, with one facing upstream and one facing downstream (Serena and Williams 2012). For turtles, fyke nets can be set at any time, but should be monitored closely for rises in water level and to prevent overfilling with target or non-target animals. Bait can be added to the end chamber to increase the probability of turtle (but not platypus) captures.

A substantial air space must be maintained in the final (and ideally every) net chamber by anchoring the end of the net well above the water. Floats can be a useful addition to each chamber to ensure that air is available (Larocque *et al.* 2012). To reduce predation risk, nets are not stretched across land or very shallow water. The end chamber should only be placed in slow-flowing water and ideally at an angle to the current. Nets should not be set if water depth is likely to increase substantially (e.g. because of rainfall) and nets must be checked periodically (including just before dark, if set for platypus) to ensure they

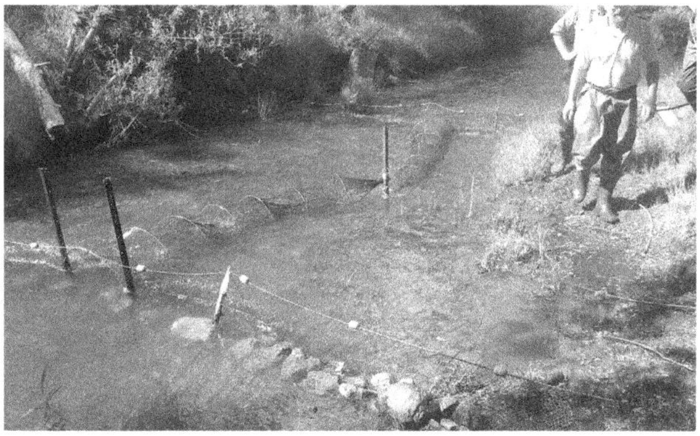

Figure 14.4: A pair of platypus (*Ornithorhynchus anatinus*) fyke nets – the end of each net is staked securely above the water to ensure access to air along its length. Photo by the Australian Platypus Conservancy.

Table 14.5: Risks to freshwater turtles associated with capture.

Risk	Mechanism and mitigation options
Drowning	Some freshwater turtle species develop elevated blood lactate and pronounced acidosis in response to a lack of air (Larocque *et al.* 2012). While the optimal surfacing time of a turtle will vary with temperature, species and size, captured animals must be regularly removed from traps that do not provide an air space.
Stress	Corticosterone levels of freshwater turtles (e.g. *Trachemys scripta*) increase following capture and handling and decline over the next 30 min of restraint (Cash *et al.* 1997).
Predation	Predation on juvenile turtles, for example by large fish (Phillott and Parmenter 2000), can occur if traps are not checked regularly.
Injuries	Physical damage results from crowding in traps.

have not been tampered with and are still correctly set. In places where platypus occur, nets are checked at intervals of < 4 h during the night if water temperature is > 15°C, or < 2 h if water temperature is < 15°C.

Procedure for gill nets

For platypus, gill nets (typically 15–30 m long × 1.2–2.5 m drop) are fitted with floats, but not lead weights, so animals can swim to the surface after becoming entangled. Turtle nets are generally fitted with floats and weights. For both taxa, two or more nets are normally set at the same site in the afternoon and attended constantly until they are removed from the water. Float lines should be carefully monitored for movement indicating a capture has occurred. Protocols to address welfare risks to air-breathing species in gill nets include the following (as detailed by Grant and Carrick (1974) and Grant (2012) for the platypus):

- Do not deploy gill nets in areas where they are likely to become snagged on bottom debris; this situation can result in animals drowning (particularly platypus) and can also create hazards for persons removing nets.
- Check nets visually every 10–15 min (using a spotlight after dark) where platypus may be present; check once per hour for turtles.
- Lift the full length of the net out of the water every hour (ideally from a boat) to check that it hangs freely.
- Avoid using weighted gill nets (e.g. as used for fish sampling) at sites where platypus occur, or restrict netting to daylight hours when platypus activity is reduced and the animals are more likely to detect and avoid nets.

Collapsible crayfish traps, crab pots, cathedral traps, hoop nets and drum nets (turtles)

All turtle traps use funnels to direct individuals into a chamber, or set of chambers. Funnels are designed to reduce the probability that turtles escape, with different designs varying in efficiency. Turtles are attracted to traps by bait, usually meat. Trap success can be improved further with use of a lead net (driftnet) that extends out from the trap for 10 m and directs swimming turtles towards the entrance. Mesh size and funnel design will determine the size and hence age of target taxa that are sampled. Turtles need to breathe, so traps are set with the top few centimetres exposed to air or are checked frequently (not less than once per hour) to remove submerged individuals. Floats inside the trap provide additional security to ensure that air is available to captured animals. Personnel should not set nets if water depth is likely to increase substantially (e.g. from rainfall or water being released from weirs). In high winds or currents, traps can become twisted. They should be regularly checked, stabilised with stakes or removed in such conditions. Traps should be closely monitored when set in areas with unknown turtle densities as they can become overcrowded in high-density situations, resulting in damage to smaller individuals. An air space must be maintained in traps set at sites where other air-breathing animals (platypus, rakali, reptiles or birds) are at risk of entering.

Procedures for seine netting (turtles)

Seine netting is useful in small areas of shallow water (< 1.5 m in depth) without excessive benthic sediment. Two people are positioned at either end of the net to drag it through the water. Additional people can assist by positioning themselves behind the net and helping to keep the line taut. Nets are ineffective in areas with benthic debris because they become entangled and allow turtles to escape. Nets may become overcrowded in high-density situations; to avoid damaging smaller individuals, check nets regularly and remove larger individuals. Nets must also be checked carefully for fish and care should be taken not to place a hauled net onto hot ground in case it still contains undetected fish by-catch.

Procedures for dip netting (turtles, aquatic snakes)

Dip netting is useful in clear water for turtle species that avoid traps (e.g. pig-nosed turtles, *Carettochelys insculpta*). Target animals (turtles and aquatic snakes) are located visually either from the shore or a boat and the dip net is used to scoop the animal from the water. Care must be taken not to injure the target animal with the net or by boat-strike.

Procedures for hand capture, snorkelling, muddling (turtles, aquatic snakes)

Hand captures are useful when water is too shallow for traps, such as in drying water holes (muddling) or when water clarity permits target individuals to be observed (snorkelling or diving). Target individuals are located visually, and captured and restrained by hand (see Chapter 26 for taxa-specific restraint methods). Individuals are processed immediately and released or held in a plastic container in the shade (usually for no more than 30 min).

Animal treatment, withdrawal and euthanasia

Investigators should remove traps and fyke nets if water levels rise unexpectedly or a fish migration event is in progress. All types of nets or traps should be removed if unacceptably large numbers of target animals or by-catch are being captured (i.e. more than can be processed in a reasonable time frame). Platypus may need treatment for injuries caused by previous entanglement in items of litter (e.g. elastic hair-ties, nylon fishing line) looped tightly around the neck or torso (Serena and Williams 2021). Rubbish should normally be removed using small scissors and forceps before releasing the animal promptly back to the water at its capture site to avoid further unnecessary stress. If injury is severe or euthanasia seems warranted, convey the animal without delay to a veterinarian for assessment (see Chapter 17). Turtles will often recover from serious injury. However, in the event that a fishing hook has been swallowed or the individual is likely to be in pain, the animal should be euthanased following appropriate protocols or veterinary assistance sought (see Chapter 26).

Equipment and maintenance

Equipment needs for each method are detailed in Table 14.6. Generally, all that is required for gill netting of turtles and platypus are gill nets (two to four per site, plus rope to anchor nets), a seine net or dip net (turtles only), and small boat and oars. Equipment requirements for turtle hand capture by snorkelling or muddling are relatively straightforward and include a snorkelling mask or diving equipment, and wetsuit or long pants and sleeves, and appropriate footwear for personal protection. All equipment should be cleaned of debris and mud, and disinfected before being taken to another site or catchment. Protocols for managing potential disease risks for turtles are detailed in Chapter 26.

Specific qualifications, experience and training

Specialised skills and experience are needed to capture and handle platypus (Chapter 17), freshwater turtles and aquatic snakes (Chapter 26) safely and effectively. At least one experienced person with extensive knowledge about the biology and behaviour of the target species and prior experience with relevant capture and handling methods must attend capture activities. Teams need to be able to identify by-catch, to demonstrate competence with the specific methodology proposed, and to be aware of the range of situations requiring methods to be terminated or changed.

Workplace health and safety

Injury from animal spines or bites

Adult male platypus can inject venom delivered by spurs located on the lower hind legs (Grant 1995). See

Table 14.6: General equipment requirements for capture of platypus and turtles.

Platypus netting	Turtle capture	Fyke netting	Collapsible turtle traps
• Netting equipment, including any floats, weights or ties required • Headlamps (and possibly extra handheld lamps) • Clean dry cloth bags and plastic hobby boxes to hold animals • Pre-cut pieces of twine to secure tops of holding bags • Equipment to mark and measure animals, obtain tissue samples, etc. • Field guide(s) to identify by-catch species • Personal protective equipment (waders, etc.) • First aid kit, including small sharp scissors and forceps to remove litter	• Capture equipment, including any floats, weights or ties required • Capture bags and plastic tubs • Equipment to mark and measure animals or obtain tissue samples • Field guide(s) to identify by-catch species • Personal protective equipment (e.g. waders and gloves) • First aid kit, including small sharp scissors and forceps	• Fyke nets (two per site) • Metal star pickets to pin wings and cod end • Sledge hammer for driving in star pickets • Information signboards with relevant permit numbers • Waist or chest waders	• Traps (cray, cathedral or hoop drum traps) • Bait (usually meat) • Metal star pickets to pin wings and hoops • Sledge hammer for driving in star pickets • Floats

Chapter 17 for information about its effects and how to lift and carry animals safely. Turtles and fish may pose risks of injury from scratches, bites, or fin spines. Heavy duty wet cotton gloves and a long-sleeved shirt should be worn when handling fish and turtles to reduce risks of injury to both the animal and the handler (see 'Netting fish and tadpoles' within this chapter).

Infection by animal-borne disease

Though a platypus-borne disease has never been known to be transmitted to a human, the species carries several possible zoonoses (Chapter 17). People coming into contact with a platypus, or a used capture bag, should wash their hands or apply hand sanitiser immediately afterwards (or wear single use rubber/latex gloves during handling). Used capture bags should be stored in a disposable plastic bag before being laundered. Several bacteria that occur in freshwater turtles are zoonotic to humans (Chapter 26); therefore, personnel should practise good hygiene protocols, including regular handwashing and use of hand sanitiser, after handling them.

Alternative procedures

Live trapping is an effective means to capture individuals for occupancy and population estimates, and to obtain demographic data or samples needed for studies of morphology, genetics or physiology. Less-invasive alternatives for some types of research may include recording the occurrence or behaviour of animals through direct observation or by using elevated or underwater cameras, obtaining presence/absence data by sampling eDNA (extracting and analysing DNA contained in water samples, see Chapter 4). By recording the frequency of sightings at nominated sites over time, variation in activity (and hence presumed abundance) can be monitored.

LOW-IMPACT TECHNIQUES FOR MONITORING AND DETECTING FRESHWATER ANIMALS

Nicole Flint, Alison J. King, Ian Wooden, Scott A. Hardie and Tarmo A. Raadik

Target taxa

This GOP applies to freshwater fish (Chapter 32) and turtles (Chapter 26), and may also be applicable to marine animals (Chapters 28–31). Some of the visual methods described may be most suitable for larger, or less-cryptic aquatic animals. Direct diurnal observation from the banks can be used to detect and monitor rakali (Williams and Serena 2018) or platypus (Easton *et al.* 2008) without adversely affecting their behaviour.

Context and scope

Capturing and handling of animals are not required for all research applications. In these cases, lower-impact techniques can be useful for activities such as behavioural observations; identifying and monitoring fish spawning or nesting sites; detecting threatened, rare or introduced species; or for situations where capture is unadvisable or impossible. This GOP details procedures and principles for underwater videoing of aquatic animals from baited and unbaited monitoring stations, snorkelling and diving procedures for observing animals, and underwater sonar and acoustic monitoring. Non-invasive methods, such as eDNA (Chapter 4) are also often used in studies of freshwater animals, but currently do not allow estimates of abundance – only the presence of the target species.

Animal welfare considerations

Few impacts of observational research on aquatic animals have been reported. Techniques detailed in this GOP may have an increased likelihood of affecting species at certain times (e.g. during breeding, spawning or when animals are protecting eggs or young). However, in general these techniques are likely to have little to no impact on target and non-target taxa. The behavioural changes in study animals caused by observer effects where the observer may be interacting with the animal (e.g. snorkelling) are a well-documented source of potential sampling error (Thompson and Mapstone 1997; Dearden *et al.* 2010; Ebner and Morgan 2013), and need to be considered and accounted for by investigators. Other more-distant observation techniques such as sonar, cameras and acoustic monitoring are less likely to produce observer effects in animals.

Disruption to activities

Disruption to animal activities for these techniques are minimal. However, some fish species appear wary of underwater equipment, such as cameras (e.g. silver biddy, *Gerres filamentosus*, and mangrove jack, *Lutjanus argentimaculatus*; Ebner and Morgan 2013). In marine environments, coral reef fish changed their behaviour in the presence of snorkellers (Dearden *et al.* 2010). Disturbance to animals during critical behaviours, such as feeding, breeding or nesting, could result in stress, but are unlikely to have any long-term impacts if the disruption time is limited. Study animals may be exposed to an increased risk of predation by some observation methods either by behaving abnormally as a result of the disruption (e.g. if disturbed by snorkellers or divers), or through predators being alerted to their presence (e.g. attraction of predators to baited video monitoring sites).

Habituation

If study animals become habituated to baits, or the presence and activities of observers, their natural behaviour could be affected with potential longer-term impacts. For example, fish that are habituated to people or baited monitoring equipment may become easier targets for anglers. Habituation may also affect study results. For example, underwater video recording of coral reef fish assemblages recorded significantly lower diversity and abundance during snorkelling disturbances (Dearden *et al.* 2010).

General procedures

Video monitoring

Image capture techniques, including remote underwater video stations, either baited (BRUVS) or unbaited (RUVS), are becoming more common in studies of species assemblages in Australian freshwater environments (Ebner and Morgan 2013; King *et al.* 2018). Video monitoring is effective in freshwater environments where visibility is high, but its effectiveness decreases in turbid waters and probably also in habitats with dense vegetation (Ebner and Morgan 2013). Video stations are deployed during daylight hours, either by wading in shallow waters (where it is not dangerous to do so), or by boat in deeper water or tropical rivers where crocodiles are present. Underwater cameras are housed in a plastic- or metal-framed construction that can be weighted or anchored to the substrate (fixed), or in a moving configuration from a boat (King *et al.* 2018). If baited, a mesh bag is typically used to hold fresh bait, such as fish or prawns, and is stationed within view of the camera. Operating times vary by study and according to the battery capabilities of the camera, and can be used to standardise deployments. A benefit of video monitoring over direct observation is that cameras can be deployed at sites that would be difficult or dangerous for snorkellers to access (King *et al.* 2018).

Footage captured by underwater cameras is downloaded for visual analysis. Analysis is generally undertaken manually, but improvements in image recognition (Donaldson *et al.* 2020) and counting software are occurring rapidly, allowing for automated animals counts and identification. Video camera techniques have the inherent advantage of providing a permanent record of fish observations, enabling identifications to be verified later if required or archived for future reference. However, high image quality, including suitable image resolution, is critical for ensuring useful data.

Snorkelling and diving

Snorkelling or diving along transects, often referred to as underwater visual census (UVC), can be effective for detecting and monitoring fish species and can be employed in clear freshwaters if safe to do so (Ebner *et al.* 2015). Visual census is often used in clear marine waters, such as around coral reefs. When conducted by an experienced researcher the method can provide more-rigorous data on the presence and absence of small-bodied species in streams than video monitoring (Ebner *et al.* 2015). Snorkelling in freshwater is often conducted along transects or in defined sample areas (e.g. river reaches) by single or multiple investigators, with support staff remaining on shorelines or boats. Researchers must be adept at identifying species quickly, as sighting times can be short and distinguishing between some species difficult (Pidgeon 2004).

Various life stages can be targeted by this observational method. For example, snorkel-based monitoring of adults and eggs at benthic spawning sites has been used to study reproductive ecology and inform management of threatened galaxiid fish species in clear-water highland lakes in Tasmania (Hardie *et al.* 2011). Depending on diel patterns of activity and habitat use of target species, snorkelling at night can provide more efficient estimates of abundance and size structure than during the day (Hardie *et al.* 2006). Potential sources of bias include the observational skills of investigators, inconsistency in size estimates and failure to detect species that are present, particularly if they are small or cryptic (DSEWPC 2011). An alternative visual census technique for areas where investigators cannot enter the water, such as where crocodiles pose a risk, is to use a small, modified boat with a Perspex® viewing area (see King *et al.* 2018).

Sonar

High-frequency multi-beam sonar imaging, commonly referred to as imaging sonar, is an emerging tool for monitoring freshwater animals. Currently, the method is used for overall counts or biomass estimates of fish, and to detect movements for connectivity assessments or spawning migrations (e.g. Doehring *et al.* 2011; Egg *et al.* 2018). In some freshwater systems, sonar performs well for detecting numbers of individuals (Egg *et al.* 2018). Length estimates of fish can also be recorded once sonar images are calibrated against a sample of fish (Cook *et al.* 2019). Sonar can be conducted in low-light environments and in turbid waters. Species identification can be challenging in comparison to camera- and net-based methods and requires interpretation by competent and experienced investigators. Sonar equipment can be operated from a boat or a fixed structure, such as a weir or bank. Data are recorded, collected and analysed using specialised software or manually.

Acoustic monitoring

Acoustic monitoring in freshwater environments relies on recording and analysing sounds collected with a hydrophone to extract information about particular species (Desjonquères *et al.* 2020). Researchers are increasingly able to use underwater acoustic monitoring for studies that do not require capture, with the method still undergoing active development and validation (Lindseth and Lobel 2018). Applications of the method include identification of species presence or absence, spawning and environmental conditions. The best-studied species in this emerging monitoring field are coral reef fishes (Lindseth and Lobel 2018); however, recent research has shown acoustic monitoring may also be an effective tool for assessing Australian freshwater assemblages, but this application requires further testing and validation (Desjonquères *et al.* 2020; Linke *et al.* 2020). Fish and macroinvertebrates (Desjonquères *et al.* 2020) can be monitored with this technique, but the method is limited to animals that create sound and by the need for a comprehensive sound library (Linke *et al.* 2020). To gather accurate assemblage data, researchers employing acoustic monitoring should consider sampling at different times of day (Linke *et al.* 2020). However, when evaluating the presence or absence of particular species, researchers could choose to target certain times of day when the species are known to be most active. Similar to image analysis, the limiting factor for acoustic monitoring is the need to analyse recordings manually and annotate acoustic events, and the need for a library of validated aquatic noises (Linke *et al.* 2020).

Animal treatment, withdrawal and euthanasia

The risk of observational research causing injury to animals is very low. While unlikely, animals could be injured by unintentional physical contact with monitoring equipment or through an observer-driven panic response (e.g. to snorkelling). Generally, fish with minor injuries can be released, but fish with life-threatening injuries (e.g. deep cuts to the abdomen, badly torn gills, signs of advanced disease or stress) may need to be euthanased. Veterinarian assistance is seldom required for fish, but may be warranted for other aquatic vertebrates.

Equipment and maintenance

Equipment requirements are specific to the selected technique. Some equipment (e.g. diving equipment, sonar) requires regular maintenance either by the operator or by the supplier. Researchers must be careful not to transfer pests, weeds or pathogens between sites. All equipment, including boats, should be checked carefully for debris, mud and vegetation, which must be removed before the equipment is deployed elsewhere. Equipment should be disinfected between sites. It is good practice to mend and replace parts as necessary before storing equipment.

Specific qualifications, experience and training

Much of the equipment described in this GOP is technically specialised. Researchers should be familiar with the equipment and associated data analyses to maintain data integrity. Researchers need to obtain specialised training for diving and operating boats.

Workplace health and safety

Refer to 'Netting fish and tadpoles' for details of risks associated with animal spines and bites. Some monitoring equipment can be heavy, so standard best practice procedures should be followed when lifting. Procedures such as snorkelling and diving pose drowning and injury risks to operators if not conducted safely and by qualified personnel who are strong swimmers. Institutions and investigators must ensure that protocols are in place to avoid dangerous practices or situations. All personnel should be trained properly in the use of the selected equipment and method.

Alternative procedures

The methods described in this section are inherently low impact compared to techniques that require capturing and handling of animals. Researchers select the low-impact method that is most appropriate for their study objectives and context. For example, video or acoustic monitoring may be lower impact than snorkelling for some study species and situations.

REFERENCES

Allen M, Riley S (2012) *Effects of Electrofishing on Adult Frogs*. Prepared for Casitas Municipal Water District, Arcata, CA.

Balachandran A, Krishnan B, John L (2013) Accidental deaths due to electrocution during amateur electro-fishing. *Journal of Evolution of Medical and Dental Sciences* **2**, 9376–9379.

Balcombe SR, Gloss GP (2000) Variation in carp gudgeon (*Hypseleotris* spp.) catch rate in dense macrophytes. *Journal of Freshwater Ecology* **15**, 389–395. doi:10.1080/02705060.2000.9663757

Beatty SJ, Morgan DL, Lymbery AJ (2014) Implications of climate change for potamodromous fishes. *Global Change Biology* **20**, 1794–1807. doi:10.1111/gcb.12444

Bell JD, Lyle JM (2016) Post-capture survival and implications for by-catch in a multi-species coastal gillnet fishery. *PLoS One* **11**, e0166632. doi:10.1371/journal.pone.0166632

Bethge P, Munks S, Nicol S (2001) Energetics of foraging and locomotion in the platypus *Ornithorhynchus anatinus*. *Journal of Comparative Physiology. B, Biochemical, Systemic, and Environmental Physiology* **171**, 497–506. doi:10.1007/s003600100200

Booth R, Connolly J (2008) Platypuses. In *Medicine of Australian Mammals*. (Eds L Vogelnest and R Woods) pp. 103–132. CSIRO Publishing, Melbourne. doi:10.1071/9780643097971

Bower DS, Pickett EJ, Stockwell MP, Pollard CJ, Garnham JI, Sanders MR, Clulow J, Mahony MJ (2014) Evaluating monitoring methods to guide adaptive management of a threatened amphibian (*Litoria aurea*). *Ecology and Evolution* **4**, 1361–1368. doi:10.1002/ece3.980

Cash WB, Holberton RL, Knight SS (1997) Corticosterone secretion in response to capture and handling in free-living red-eared slider turtles. *General and Comparative Endocrinology* **108**, 427–433. doi:10.1006/gcen.1997.6999

Cashins S, Alford R, Skerratt LF (2008) Lethal effect of latex, nitrile, and vinyl gloves on tadpoles. *Herpetological Review* **39**, 298–301.

Chapman A, Morgan DL, Beatty SJ, Gill HS (2006) Variation in life history of land-locked lacustrine and riverine populations of *Galaxias maculatus* (Jenyns 1842) in Western Australia. *Environmental Biology of Fishes* **77**, 21–37. doi:10.1007/s10641-006-9051-2

Clément M, Cunjak RA (2010) Physical injuries in juvenile Atlantic salmon, slimy sculpin, and blacknose dace attributable to electrofishing. *North American Journal of Fisheries Management* **30**, 840–850. doi:10.1577/M09-165.1

Cook D, Middlemiss K, Jaksons P, Davison W, Jerrett A (2019) Validation of fish length estimations from a high frequency multi-beam sonar (ARIS) and its utilisation as a field-based measurement technique. *Fisheries Research* **218**, 59–68. doi:10.1016/j.fishres.2019.05.004

Cooke SJ, Wilson ADM, Elvidge CK, Lennox RJ, Jepsen N, Colotelo AH, Brown RS (2016) Ten practical realities for institutional animal care and use committees when evaluating protocols dealing with fish in the field. *Reviews in Fish Biology and Fisheries* **26**, 123–133. doi:10.1007/s11160-015-9413-y

Culver EF, Chick JH (2015) Shocking results: assessing the rates of fish injury from pulsed-DC electrofishing. *North American Journal of Fisheries Management* **35**, 1055–1063. doi:10.1080/02755947.2015.1074964

Dearden P, Theberge M, Yasue M (2010) Using underwater cameras to assess the effects of snorkeler and SCUBA diver presence on coral reef fish abundance, family richness, and species composition. *Environmental Monitoring and Assessment* **163**, 531–538. doi:10.1007/s10661-009-0855-3

DECC (2008) 'Hygiene protocol for the control of disease in frogs'. NSW Department of Environment and Climate Change, Information Circular Number 6, Sydney.

DECC (2009) *Threatened Species Survey and Assessment Guidelines: Field Survey Methods for Fauna, Amphibians*. NSW Department of Environment and Climate Change, Sydney.

DES (2018) *Monitoring and Sampling Manual: Environmental Protection (Water) Policy*. Queensland Department of Environment and Science, Brisbane.

DPI (2015) *A Guide to Acceptable Procedures and Practices for Aquaculture and Fisheries Research*. 4th edn. New South Wales Department of Primary Industries, Port Stephens.

Desjonquères C, Gifford T, Linke S (2020) Passive acoustic monitoring as a potential tool to survey animal and ecosystem processes in freshwater environments. *Freshwater Biology* **65**, 7–19. doi:10.1111/fwb.13356

Doehring K, Young RG, Hay J, Quarterman AJ (2011) Suitability of Dual-frequency Identification Sonar (DIDSON) to monitor juvenile fish movement at floodgates. *New Zealand Journal of Marine and Freshwater Research* **45**, 413–422. doi:10.1080/00288330.2011.571701

Dolan CR, Miranda LE (2004) Injury and mortality of warmwater fishes immobilized by electrofishing. *North American Journal of Fisheries Management* **24**, 118–127. doi:10.1577/M02-115

Donaldson JA, Drews Jr P, Bradley MJ, Morgan DL, Baker R, Ebner BC (2020) Countering low visibility in video survey of an estuarine fish assemblage. *Pacific Conservation Biology* **26**, 190–200. doi:10.1071/PC19019

DSEWPC (2011) *Survey Guidelines for Australia's Threatened Fish: Guidelines for Detecting Fish Listed as Threatened under the* Environment Protection and Biodiversity Conservation Act 1999. Australian Government Department of Sustainability, Environment, Water, Population and Communities, Canberra.

Easton L, Williams G, Serena M (2008) Monthly variation in observed activity of the platypus *Ornithorhynchus anatinus*. *Victorian Naturalist* **125**, 104–109.

Ebner BC, Fulton CJ, Cousins S, Donaldson JA, Kennard MJ, Meynecke J-O, Schaffer J (2015) Filming and snorkeling as visual techniques to survey fauna in difficult to access tropical rainforest streams. *Marine and Freshwater Research* **66**, 120–126. doi:10.1071/MF13339

Ebner BC, Morgan DL (2013) Using remote underwater video to estimate freshwater fish species richness. *Journal of Fish Biology* **82**, 1592–1612. doi:10.1111/jfb.12096

Egg L, Pander J, Mueller M, Geist J (2018) Comparison of sonar-, camera- and net-based methods in detecting riverine fish-movement patterns. *Marine and Freshwater Research* **69**, 1905–1912. doi:10.1071/MF18068

Grant T (1995) *The Platypus*. UNSW Press, Sydney.

Grant T (2012) Environmental impact assessment: monitoring from a platypus perspective. In *Science Under Siege: Zoology Under Threat*. (Eds P Banks, D Lunney and C Dickman) pp. 107–113. Royal Zoological Society of New South Wales, Mosman. doi:10.7882/FS.2012.045

Grant TR, Carrick FN (1974) Capture and marking of the platypus, *Ornithorhynchus anatinus*, in the wild. *Australian Zoologist* **18**, 133–135.

Grant TR, Lowry MB, Pease B, Walford TR, Graham K (2004) Reducing the by-catch of platypuses (*Ornithorhynchus anatinus*) in commercial and recreational fishing gear in New South Wales. *Proceedings of the Linnean Society of New South Wales* **125**, 259–272.

Grant TR, Temple-Smith PR (2003) Conservation of the platypus, *Ornithorhynchus anatinus*: threats and challenges. *Aquatic Ecosystem Health & Management* **6**, 5–18. doi:10.1080/14634980301481

Gyekis KF, Cooper MJ, Uzarski DG (2006) A high intensity LED light source for larval fish and aquatic invertebrate floating quatrefoil light traps. *Journal of Freshwater Ecology* **21**, 621–626. doi:10.1080/02705060.2006.9664123

Hardie SA, Barmuta LA, White RWG (2005) Spawning related seasonal variation in fyke net catches of golden galaxias (*Galaxias auratus*): implications for monitoring lacustrine galaxiid populations. *Fisheries Management and Ecology* **12**, 407–409. doi:10.1111/j.1365-2400.2005.00454.x

Hardie SA, Barmuta LA, White RWG (2006) Comparison of day and night fyke netting, electro-fishing and snorkelling for monitoring a population of the threatened golden galaxias (*Galaxias auratus*). *Hydrobiologia* **560**, 145–158. doi:10.1007/s10750-005-9509-9

Hardie SA, Macfarlane KR, Barmuta LA (2011) *Life Histories of Galaxiid Fishes in Arthurs Lake and Great Lake, Tasmania, and Effects of Water Level Fluctuations on their Habitats And Populations.*' Report for Hydro Tasmania. Hydro Tasmania, Hobart.

Harrell RM, Moline MA (1992) Comparative stress dynamics of brood stock striped bass *Morone saxatilis* associated with two capture techniques. *Journal of the World Aquaculture Society* **23**, 58–63. doi:10.1111/j.1749-7345.1992.tb00751.x

Humphries P, Serafini L, King AJ (2002) River regulation and fish larvae: variations through space and time. *Freshwater Biology* **47**, 1307–1331. doi:10.1046/j.1365-2427.2002.00871.x

King AJ, Crook DA (2002) Evaluation of a sweep net electrofishing method for the collection of small fish and shrimp in lotic freshwater environments. *Hydrobiologia* **472**, 223–233. doi:10.1023/A:1016307602735

King A, George A, Buckle DJ, Novak PA, Fulton CJ (2018) Efficacy of remote underwater video cameras for monitoring tropical wetland fishes. *Hydrobiologia* **807**, 145–164. doi:10.1007/s10750-017-3390-1

King AJ, Doidge C, Buckle D, Tyler KJ (2020) Preliminary evidence of spawning phenologies of freshwater fish in a wet-dry tropical river: the importance of both wet and dry seasons. *Marine and Freshwater Research* **71**, 202–212. doi:10.1071/MF18458

Knight J, Glasby T, Brooks L (2007) A sampling protocol for the endangered freshwater fish, Oxleyan Pygmy Perch *Nannoperca oxleyana* Whitley. *Australian Zoologist* **34**, 148–157. doi:10.7882/AZ.2007.012

Krysko K, Nickerson M (2003) Surveying for hellbender salamanders, *Cryptobranchus alleganiensis* (Daudin): a review and critique. *Applied Herpetology* **1**, 37–44. doi:10.1163/157075403766451216

Lambooij E, Digre H, Reimert HGM, Aursand IG, Grimsmo L, van de Vis JW (2012) Effects of on-board storage and electrical stunning of wild cod (*Gadus morhua*) and haddock (*Melanogrammus aeglefinus*) on brain and heart activity. *Fisheries Research* **127–128**, 1–8. doi:10.1016/j.fishres.2012.04.004

Larocque SM, Cooke SJ, Blouin-Demers G (2012) A breath of fresh air: avoiding anoxia and mortality of freshwater turtles in fyke nets by the use of floats. *Aquatic Conservation* **22**, 198–205. doi:10.1002/aqc.1247

Lazauski HG, Malvestuto SP (1990) Electric fishing: results of a survey on use, boat construction, configuration and safety in the USA. In *Developments in Electric Fishing* (Ed. IG Cowx) pp. 327–339. Fishing News Books, Blackwell Scientific Publications, Oxford, UK.

Lear KO, Gleiss AC, Whitty JM, Fazeldean T, Albert J, Green N, Ebner BC, Thorburn DC, Beatty SJ, Morgan DL (2019) Recruitment of a critically endangered sawfish into a riverine nursery is dependent on natural flow regimes. *Scientific Reports* **9**, 17071. doi:10.1038/s41598-019-53511-9

Lieschke JA, Dean JC, Pickworth A (2019) Extending the effectiveness of electrofishing to estuarine habitats: laboratory and field assessments. *Transactions of the American Fisheries Society* **148**(3), 584–591. doi:10.1002/tafs.10158

Lindseth AV, Lobel PS (2018) Underwater soundscape monitoring and fish bioacoustics: a review. *Fishes* **3**, 36. doi:10.3390/fishes3030036

Linke S, Dicker E, Gifford T, Desjonqueres C (2020) Diurnal variation in freshwater ecoacoustics: implications for site-level sampling design. *Freshwater Biology* **65**, 86–95. doi:10.1111/fwb.13227

Lintermans M (2016) Finding the needle in the haystack: comparing sampling methods for detecting an endangered freshwater fish. *Marine and Freshwater Research* **67**, 1740–1749. doi:10.1071/MF14346

Lyon JP, Bird T, Nicol S, Kearns J, O'Mahony J, Todd CR, Cowx IG, Bradshaw CJA (2014) Efficiency of electrofishing in turbid lowland rivers: implications for measuring temporal change in fish populations. *Canadian Journal of Fisheries and Aquatic Sciences* **71**, 878–886. doi:10.1139/cjfas-2013-0287

McDonald IR, Handasyde KA, Evans BK (1992) Adrenal function in the platypus. In *Platypus and Echidnas* (Ed. ML Augee) pp. 127–133. Royal Zoological Society of New South Wales, Mosman.

Mesa MG, Schreck CB (1989) Electrofishing mark recapture and depletion methodologies evoke behavioral and physiological changes in cutthroat trout. *Transactions of the American Fisheries Society* **118**, 644–658. doi:10.1577/1548-8659(1989)118<0644:EMADME>2.3.CO;2

Miranda LE (2009) Standardizing electrofishing power for boat electrofishing. In *Standard Methods for Sampling North American Freshwater Fishes.* (Eds SA Bonar, WA Hubert, DW Willis) pp. 223–230. American Fisheries Society, Bethesda, MD.

Miranda LE, Kidwell RH (2010) Unintended effects of electrofishing on nongame fishes. *Transactions of the American Fisheries Society* **139**, 1315–1321. doi:10.1577/T09-225.1

Morgan DL, Beatty SJ (2006) Use of a vertical-slot fishway by galaxiids in Western Australia. *Ecology Freshwater Fish* **15**, 500–509. doi:10.1111/j.1600-0633.2006.00190.x

Morgan DL, Lear KO, Ebner BC, Beatty SJ (2021a) Net design for selective control of the 'plague minnow' *Gambusia holbrooki* that minimises impact on native fishes. *Journal of Fish Biology.* doi:10.1111/jfb.14895

Morgan DL, Lear KO, Dobinson E, Gleiss AC, Fazeldean T, Pillans RD, Beatty SJ, Whitty JM (2021b) Seasonal use of a macrotidal estuary by the endangered dwarf sawfish (*Pristis clavata*). *Aquatic Conservation* **31**, 2164–2177. doi:10.1002/aqc.3578

Murray K, Skerratt L, Marantelli G, Berger L, Hunter D, Mahony M, Hines H (2011) *Hygiene Protocols for the Control of Diseases in Australian Frogs.* Australian Government Department of Sustainability, Environment, Water, Population and Communities, Canberra.

Muth RT, Ruppert JB (1996) Effects of two electrofishing currents on captive ripe razorback suckers and subsequent egg-hatching success. *North American Journal of Fisheries Management* **16**, 473–476. doi:10.1577/1548-8675(1996)016<0473:EOTECO>2.3.CO;2

Neal JW, Adelsberger CJ, Lochmann SE (2012) A comparison of larval fish sampling methods for tropical streams. *Marine and Coastal Fisheries* **4**, 23–29. doi:10.1080/19425120.2011.651521

Nielsen JL (1998) Scientific sampling effects: electrofishing California's endangered fish populations. *Fisheries* **23**, 6–12. doi:10.1577/1548-8446(1998)023<0006:SSEECE>2.0.CO;2

NSW Fisheries (1997) 'Australian code of electrofishing practice'. NSW Fisheries Management Publication No 1, Standing Committee for Fisheries and Aquaculture, Canberra.

Ocock J, Spencer J, Amos C, Walcott A (2018) *Monitoring Manual OEH Environmental Water Program Standard Methods – Frogs.* NSW Office of Environment and Heritage, Sydney.

O'Connor J, Pickworth A, Fanson B, Lovric D (2019) Assessment of a vertical slot fishway in south-eastern Australia designed to pass numerous species and size classes of fish. *Ecological Management & Restoration* **20**, 151–155. doi:10.1111/emr.12367

Pettigrew JD, Wilkens L (2003) Paddlefish and platypus: parallel evolution of passive electroreception in a rostral bill organ. In *Sensory Processing in Aquatic Environments.* (Eds SP Collin and NJ Marshall) pp. 42–433. Springer, New York, NY. doi:10.1007/978-0-387-22628-6_22

Phillott AD, Parmenter JC (2000) Predation on *Emydura krefftii* and *Chelodina expansa* hatchlings in central Queensland. *Herpetofauna* **30**, 22–25.

Pidgeon R (2004) *A Review of Options for Monitoring Freshwater Fish Biodiversity in the Darwin Harbour Catchment.* Report prepared for Water Monitoring Branch, Natural Resource Management Division, Department of Infrastructure, Planning and Environment, Palmerston.

Pinder AC, Harrison AJ, Britton JR (2019) Temperature effects on the physiological status and reflex impairment in European grayling *Thymallus thymallus* from catch-and release angling. *Fisheries Research* **211**, 169–175. doi:10.1016/j.fishres.2018.11.014

Price AL, Peterson JT (2010) Estimation and modeling of electrofishing capture efficiency for fishes in wadeable warmwater streams. *North American Journal of Fisheries Management* **30**, 481–498. doi:10.1577/M09-122.1

Reynolds JB (1996) Electrofishing. In *Fisheries Techniques.* 2nd edn. (Eds BR Murphy and DW Willis) pp. 221–253. American Fisheries Society, Bethesda, MD.

Sanders MR, Clulow S, Bower DS, Clulow J, Mahony MJ (2015) Predator presence and vegetation density affect capture rates and detectability of *Litoria aurea* tadpoles: wide-ranging implications for a common survey technique. *PLoS One* **10**(11), e0143733. doi:10.1371/journal.pone.0143733

Schreer J, Cooke S, Connors K (2004) Electrofishing-induced cardiac disturbance and injury in rainbow trout. *Journal of Fish Biology* **64**, 996–1014. doi:10.1111/j.1095-8649.2004.00364.x

Serena M, Grant TR, Williams GA (2016) Reducing bycatch mortality in crustacean traps: effect of trap design on platypus and yabby retention rates. *Fisheries Research* **175**, 43–50. doi:10.1016/j.fishres.2015.11.010

Serena M, Williams GA (2021) Factors affecting the frequency and outcome of platypus entanglement by human rubbish. *Australian Mammalogy.* doi:10.1071/AM21004

Serena M, Williams GA (2012) Effect of sex and age on temporal variation in the frequency and direction of platypus (*Ornithorhynchus anatinus*) captures in fyke nets. *Australian Mammalogy* **34**, 75–82. doi:10.1071/AM10056

Snyder DE (2003) Invited overview: conclusions from a review of electrofishing and its harmful effects on fish. *Reviews in Fish Biology and Fisheries* **13**, 445–453. doi:10.1007/s11160-004-1095-9

Speldewinde PC, Close P, Weybury M, Comer S (2013) Habitat preference of the Australian water rat (*Hydromys chrysogaster*) in a coastal wetland and stream, Two Peoples Bay, south-western Australia. *Australian Mammalogy* **35**, 188–194. doi:10.1071/AM12001

Thomas PO, Gulland FMD, Reeves RR, Kreb D, Wang D, Smith B, Malik M, Ryan GE, Phay S (2019) Electrofishing as a potential threat to freshwater cetaceans. *Endangered Species Research* **39**, 207–220. doi:10.3354/esr00962

Thompson AA, Mapstone BD (1997) Observer effects and training in underwater visual surveys of reef fish. *Marine Ecology Progress Series* **154**, 53–63. doi:10.3354/meps154053

Toledo-Guedes K, Ulvan EM, Uglem I (2016) Commercial gillnetting is more stressful for saithe (*Pollachius virens* L.) than jigging: but is fillet quality affected? *Aquatic Living Resources* **29**, 203. doi:10.1051/alr/2016013

US Fish and Wildlife Service (2016) 'Principals and techniques of electrofishing (online) – CSP2C01'. US Fish and Wildlife Service National Conservation Training Centre, America.

US Fish and Wildlife Service (2018) *Service Manual Chapters, Chapter 6 Electrofishing Safety – 241 FW 6.* US Fish and Wildlife Service National Conservation Training Center, Washington, DC.

Veldhuizen LJL, Berentsen PBM, de Boer IJM, van de Vis JW, Bokkers EAM (2018) Fish welfare in capture fisheries: a review of injuries and mortality. *Fisheries Research* **204**, 41–48. doi:10.1016/j.fishres.2018.02.001

Wassens S, Hall A, Spencer J (2016) The effect of survey method on the detection probabilities of frogs and tadpoles in large wetland complexes. *Marine and Freshwater Research* **68**, 686–696. doi:10.1071/MF15183

Wassens S, Jenkins K, Spencer J, Bindokas J, Kobayashi T, Bino G, Watts RJ, Lenon E, Thomas R, Baumgartner L, Hall A (2013) *Monitoring of Ecosystem Responses to the Delivery of Environmental Water in the Murrumbidgee River and Connected Wetlands, 2012–13, Final Report 2.* Commonwealth Environmental Water Office, Institute for Land, Water and Society, Charles Sturt University.

Williams G, Serena M (2018) Distribution of the Australian water-rat *Hydromys chrysogaster* in Victoria: findings from community-based sightings and live-trapping surveys. *Victorian Naturalist* **135**, 71–83.

Yoder CO, Smith MA (1999) Using fish assemblages in a state biological and criteria program: essential concepts and considerations. In *Assessing the Sustainability and Biological Integrity of Water Resources Using Fish Communities.* (Ed. TP Smith) pp. 17–63. CRC Press, Boca Raton, FL.

15 Research methods for birds

Tegan K. Douglas, Michael A. Weston, Claire N. Greenwell, Amanda Lilleyman, Neil A. Hamilton, Simon Cherriman, Nicholas Dunlop, Grainne S. Maguire, Rosalind Jessop, Grace Maglio, Lisa E. O'Neill, John Porter, Deborah Sullivan, Jennifer A. Spencer and David Parker

INTRODUCTION

Over time, birds have been caught for food, husbandry, domestication, ornamentation, to carry messages, control pests and hunt food, as pets and status symbols, and for religious practices (Bub 1991). The diversity of their morphology, biology, and habitats means that a plethora of techniques has been developed for capturing, keeping, and collecting information about them. This chapter details general operating procedures (GOPs) for key contemporary avian-specific research methods. Methods with similar techniques and animal welfare considerations have been combined in the same GOP.

CENSUSES, TRANSECTS, POINT COUNTS, AREA SEARCHES AND GENERAL OBSERVATION

Tegan K. Douglas, Michael A. Weston, Amanda Lilleyman, John Porter and Jennifer A. Spencer

Target taxa

This GOP applies to all bird taxa (Chapters 33–36).

Context and scope

This GOP outlines a range of survey techniques for free-ranging birds where the study aims to identify individual birds in a defined area by sight, call or both. It also addresses flock following (when a flock, rather than an individual, is observed) and observations of (usually marked) individuals' behaviour or use of a particular resource (i.e. a roost site, food or water source). These methods are typically used to determine species presence, abundance or density, and to gather behavioural data about individuals, cohorts, species or communities.

Terrestrial habitats are usually surveyed on foot. However, boats or canoes, quad bikes, all-terrain vehicles, cars, planes, helicopters or drones may be used to survey study areas. Binoculars or spotting scopes aid identification and count accuracy. Habitat is usually traversed in a consistent manner and individual survey events are generally repeated on consecutive days, or at monthly or seasonal intervals. As with most work involving free-ranging birds, early mornings (when many species are particularly active) are most productive, followed by late afternoons. However, surveys may be completed at any time of day (or night) depending on the research question.

The selection of one method over another depends on the size and type of area needing to be covered during each survey event, survey duration, required precision and the purpose of the derived data. Personnel often collect supplementary data during observational studies, including distance from the observer or a marker, timed use of a resource, and interspecific interactions. Observational methods are typically very low impact and are among the most widely used scientific sampling methods for birds.

Animal welfare considerations

Disruption to natural activities

Birds may be disturbed by observers. The distance at which species respond to disturbance through increased vigilance, and/or the initiation of escape, is often considered to indicate their sensitivity to disturbance; species that respond and flush when a disturbance is relatively distant are more sensitive than those that do not react visibly until the disturbance is close to them (Weston *et al.* 2012; Guay *et al.* 2016). Flock following or making repeated behavioural observations of the same individual may cause short-term disruptions to natural activities. Personnel should move quietly and maintain the maximum distance possible to the study subjects while still being able to collect viable data (Figure 15.1). When watching a fixed point (like a waterhole), a hide or hidden position can be used to increase proximity to the study animals and decrease disturbance (Guay *et al.* 2016). When conducting surveys, observers should maintain a distance greater than the birds' alert distance where possible (Weston *et al.* 2012).

For behavioural studies, an upper limit on maximum duration for each observation event is encouraged (Altmann 1974) and should be reduced if observers note repeated visible signs of agitation or disturbance. However, physiological stress can be measured (via increased heart rate, or cortisone levels) well before birds show obvious external signs of stress (Charuvi *et al.* 2020). When conducting point counts, observers should arrive at the monitoring point and stand quietly for a fixed interval before starting the survey to allow birds time to resume normal behaviour. Similarly, those doing vehicle-based surveys should consider the most efficient method to cover the survey area that minimises total disturbance time.

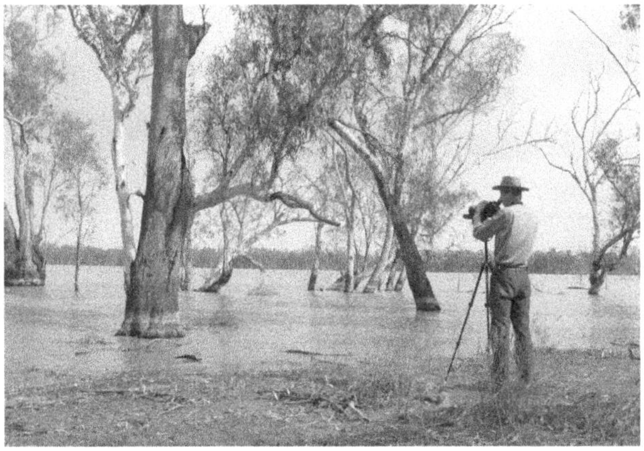

Figure 15.1: An observer counts waterbirds and waders on a lake with a spotting scope. The observer has selected a vantage point that allows clear views of the site at a distance that does not cause disturbance to the birds that may be roosting, nesting or feeding on the water. Photo by David Parker.

Exposure to predators

Repeated visits by personnel to a site are well known to increase predation risks, especially during the breeding season by creating tracks through vegetation, inadvertent widening of trails, trampling of vegetation, interruption to incubation, exposure of nest sites and spreading human scent (Ibanez-Alamo *et al.* 2012; Champagnon *et al.* 2019). Using existing paths (including animal trails) where possible will minimise this risk. Marking survey area boundaries with flagging tape may attract predators such as corvids so it is preferable to identify recognisable habitat features that will reduce trampling and disturbance to the site. Consistently using an appropriate approach to particular features will prevent observers creating multiple tracks.

General procedures

Preliminary planning and observer training

Observational and behavioural surveys can be structured in numerous ways depending on the research question. Stationary point counts, area searches bounded by size or habitat characteristics, and transects are used to answer questions about presence and density, while behavioural, movement and resource-use studies are usually undertaken by locating and following a particular group or individual, or by focusing on particular features in the habitat and recording observations when birds arrive (Bibby *et al.* 2000). The selected method will influence the sampling effort required for statistical rigour, including survey duration and frequency.

Species and site knowledge are important in determining if the proposed method will detect the species in suitable numbers or frequencies to collect the required data, without affecting foraging, roosting or breeding behaviour (Gaunt and Oring 2010; McLeod *et al.* 2013; Weston *et al.* 2020). Where multiple observers are recording data at the same site, consistency in behaviour and recording procedures is key. A pilot or training survey visit with observers will establish consistency in survey protocols, estimating flock sizes, distance assessment, behavioural classification and other measures. This step can also help demonstrate that the survey method can be conducted with minimal disturbance to the target bird community.

General survey procedures – on-ground surveys

Handheld GPS units can assist observers in navigating to selected habitat features and recording the distances covered. Observers should approach each survey area with steady casual movements and minimise noise and movement during the survey. Ideally, surveys should be conducted by a single observer, but multiple observers may be required to collect adequate data or cover large areas, particularly if a simultaneous count is required. Multiple observers should minimise talking and other disturbance for the survey's duration, and depart survey areas quietly. Temporary markers or hides should be removed at the conclusion of the project.

Point and transect counts

Personnel can stand at a predetermined location for a fixed period (e.g. 5 min), recording the birds they see or hear from that point (Davies 2010). For each bird detected, personnel often record exact or incremental distances to the bird by estimation or by measuring the distance with a laser rangefinder. Surveyors can walk a transect or a loop consisting of multiple point counts in a survey session; surveyors will often pause at each point for 1 min before recommencing recording as a 'settling time' for birds. For transect counts, observers can follow a fixed-length or predetermined path slowly, on foot or by vehicle. All bird species and individuals or just bird classes are identified, counted and recorded. Distance from the observer or transect line is usually recorded.

Area searches

During area searches, observers traverse habitat, counting and recording all individuals detected by sight and sound. The area searched usually constitutes the same habitat type throughout. The search can be delimited by both area and survey duration, such as the 20 min, 2 ha area search (Barrett *et al.* 2003), or just by one factor. Modifications to this method include using bird community diversity to determine a results-based stopping rule to end the survey (Watson 2003; 2017). Under this protocol, the stopping rule (e.g. a time bracket where only a limited number of 'new' species are detected) is a proxy for relative survey effort, to ensure that surveys are sufficiently thorough to detect a balance of common and unusual species in the target habitat. Regardless of method all birds encountered are identified, either counted or recorded as present, and the total survey duration is noted.

Territory mapping

For territory mapping, observers move through a grid, noting the specific locations of individuals and groups of birds on the grid, recording movements, territorial displays, disputes and nest locations. Mapping is repeated multiple times to determine home-range size and territory boundaries, allowing estimates of the density of territorial bird species (Bibby *et al.* 2000; Davies 2010).

Behavioural observations: following flocks or individuals

Free-roaming individuals or flocks can be identified at the study site by sight and sound. To avoid disturbance, birds are usually not approached directly, but watched from a distance or with personnel placing themselves in the path of a moving flock to make observations as the birds pass by. This method may include (for example) noting interactions between marked individuals, foraging manoeuvres of focal individuals, heights used in the habitat or calling behaviour. Birds may be physically marked (e.g. with a leg band) or 'marked' simply with the observers' eye. Once the individual is lost from view, the behavioural observations on that individual cease. To avoid introducing bias by only noting the most conspicuous behaviours, the first behaviour observed is typically ignored (Altmann 1974). Often a time limit is applied, such as only recording three foraging manoeuvres, or recording behaviour at 15 s intervals for a maximum of 20 min, or recording all behaviours in one predetermined activity period. Alternatively, the activity of the marked individuals are recorded until they are lost from sight. For bird groups, flock scans are used to record the behaviour category of every individual at fixed time intervals (e.g. every 20 min; Altmann 1974). Sometimes observations of behaviour or habitat use are simply noted as part of area searches or other survey types. When evaluating habitat use or resource selection, personnel may stand or sit within view of a habitat feature, such as a bird bath or roost site, and may follow the individual to continue to record the activity if it moves a short distance away. Depending on the research question, observers may record bird numbers and species composition, interspecific interactions, and timing and duration of visits. Observers may use a hide, or sit at a distance with a spotting scope, to minimise disturbance.

Marked bird resighting

While observers can traverse the habitat to search for marked individuals, most resighting work is done by watching birds approach specific habitat features, such as water points for bush birds or high-tide roosts for shorebirds. Observers sit still in a hide or at a vantage point where they are able to observe birds without disturbing them. Flocks are visually scanned by observers for marked individuals from a distance.

Aerial counts

Aerial surveys provide a rapid method of collecting data over large spatial and long temporal scales (Chapter 6); the method is often used for waterbirds (Kingsford 1999). Aerial surveys may be completed with either fixed-wing or helicopter aircraft, but larger-scale surveys typically use fixed-wing planes because they are more cost-efficient. In Australia, fixed-wing aerial surveys are generally flown at a height of 30–46 m and a speed of 167–204 km h^{-1}, within 150 m of the shoreline, where waterbirds usually congregate (Kingsford *et al.* 2020). Helicopters have added manoeuvrability as well as the capacity to stop for additional ground-based counts, making them suitable for smaller or more irregular-shaped waterbodies, such as inland lake and river systems. Generally, aircraft flight time is minimised to reduce the duration of disturbance. Disturbed birds mostly swim, dive or fly away from the aircraft, but generally resettle with a few minutes (Kingsford 1999). Several different approaches can be used to count birds from an aircraft, including total, proportional and transect counts (Kingsford and Porter 2009). Selection of take-off and landing locations should be planned to minimise disturbance to birds (Weston *et al.* 2020; see also Chapter 6).

Watercraft counts

Watercraft enable access to islands, tidal areas, vegetated wetlands and the birds that inhabit them. Standardisation of methods is critical for these counts, so ideally the same vessel and the same personnel are used for each survey. Observers count birds on both sides of the vessel, including all birds on the water or in flight in a sampling window roughly 100 m either side, ahead and above the boat (Agler *et al.* 1999; Bibby *et al.* 2000). The vessel should move a standard distance from the shoreline, where navigation allows, to ensure that birds roosting or foraging on the waters' edge are recorded. Researchers should consider speed and distance when using boats to count waterbirds, particularly for breeding species, as some are sensitive to large motorised watercraft (Gaunt and Oring 2010).

Colony counts

Personnel planning to undertake counts of birds in breeding colonies should refer to 'Monitoring of colonial birds at breeding colonies' later in this chapter for strategies to minimise potential animal welfare impacts and increase accuracy of counts.

Animal treatment, withdrawal and euthanasia

The techniques outlined in this GOP do not involve capture or handling, so treatment or euthanasia is unlikely to be required. Personnel may witness natural injury or mortality events as part of their data collection. However, these events are not typically considered triggers for intervention. Recording if and when study species appear to become sensitive to the observers' presence, or if an averse or unusual response is detected, may allow the observer to withdraw those particular individuals from the study and consider how surveys at that site can be modified to minimise future disturbance.

Equipment and maintenance

Specific equipment will vary depending on the selected survey method, but are typically simple. Key items may include binoculars, a spotting scope and tripod, notebook, datasheet, smartphone or other data recording device, GPS, camera to record site photographs and/or marked individuals or to confirm species identification where needed, laser rangefinder (for estimating distances), and flagging tape or post markers.

Specific qualifications, experience and training

Qualifications and experience required vary depending on the research question and specific survey technique, and mostly relate to data integrity rather than animal welfare concerns. Previous experience in bird identification in the field is desirable. Ideally, personnel should be able to identify the target species or, for community surveys, most of the species likely to be encountered at the site. Personnel should be versed in strategies for identifying unfamiliar species by sight, sound and behaviour. Personnel must be competent in conducting the selected survey methods, including field navigation where relevant, strategies for estimating distance and being able to identify and code animal behaviour and quantify disturbance, and also be familiar with any tools and equipment used (e.g. adjustment of optical and electronic equipment).

Workplace health and safety

No direct handling of wildlife is required for this method. General health and safety protocols for outdoor work or working in remote areas are required depending on the study location. Observers unfamiliar with the survey area, particularly in remote locations, should be well versed in navigation and location techniques.

Alternative procedures

These techniques are used to gather information on species' presence and absence, density, abundance, population demographics and behaviour. Although some presence/absence data may be collected for vocal species with automated recording units or camera traps (Chapter 5), these methods are generally not appropriate for full species community assessments. No alternative lower-impact methods are available to replace observational surveys. Historical data can be used to supplement the dataset, which is often accessible via open-access, citizen science–based data repositories, such as the Atlas of Living Australia, Birdata, or eBird (Chapter 10).

CALL PLAYBACK AND BROADCAST SURVEYS

Tegan K. Douglas, Claire N. Greenwell, Neil A. Hamilton and Michael A. Weston

Target taxa

This GOP applies to all bird taxa (Chapters 33–36).

Context and scope

This GOP considers all aspects of playing bird calls (call playback or tape lures) for bird capture, monitoring and management activities. Call playback is used to elicit a response, usually from highly gregarious or territorial birds, and is advantageous for detection of nocturnal or cryptic species. As well as assisting species detection (i.e. broadcast surveys), playback is frequently used alongside capture techniques to increase capture rates or target particular species or individuals. Call playback can be used alongside decoys to influence breeding site selection for colonial nesting seabirds.

Depending on research questions, the broadcast calls can be those of the target species or their prey, and may be used alongside visual decoys. Activities using call playback must consider possible disturbance of these vocalisations. Consequently, the choices of playback timing, duration, volume and call type are all important decisions that affect research outcomes and animal welfare. Call playback by itself does not always require approval from an animal ethics committee (AEC) approval depending on the context, but researchers should confirm requirements with an appropriate AEC and other relevant bodies, such as the Australian Bird and Bat Banding Scheme (ABBBS; Drynan 2015).

Animal welfare considerations

Call playback can increase the efficiency of capture or monitoring work. Many agencies have protocols that recommend limiting the use of call playback (Watson *et al.* 2019), but the potential physiological and long-term impacts of the method on animal welfare are not well studied. Personnel should consider the potential impacts on the welfare of their particular target and non-target species based on available evidence (Drynan 2015).

Disruption to normal and breeding activities

Broadcasting bird calls may disrupt normal activities of target and non-target species, depending on the type of vocalisations used. Territorial species could cease other normal activities to concentrate on territorial defence, potentially increasing energy expenditure and stress if the disturbance is prolonged. During the breeding season, excessive playback may reduce breeding success as breeding pairs or incubating females dedicate more time to defence than food provisioning or nest attendance (Debus 1995; DEWHA 2010). When calls of predatory species are broadcast, prey species may increase their vigilance or hide from the anticipated threat. Use of playback should be judicious, and for the minimum amount of time required. Speakers must be turned off between sessions.

Increased predation risk or excessive catch rates

Broadcasting calls of gregarious bird species may attract predators. Personnel should remain vigilant to any sign of predators when using playback for capture work. Playback should be broadcast at a natural volume. Small periods of silence between calls will ensure that any alarm calls emitted by the target animals are not drowned out by the recorded vocalisations. When call playback is used to increase catch rates at mist nets (Chapter 7), care must be taken to monitor catch numbers. If swamped by an influx of birds, personnel must cease call playback and close nets temporarily while processing.

Encouraging poor site selection

When using playback to influence site selection by colonial seabirds, personnel should assess the suitability of the proposed site carefully. In addition to increased predation risk because of broadcast calls, other site-based threats, such as proximity of disturbance and availability of food throughout the breeding period should be evaluated. Calls should only be broadcast during times or conditions when birds would be prospecting sites naturally.

General procedures

Planning

The selected call type must reflect the study question. The decision to use male or female calls, or advertising, foraging or alarm calls, and the geographical location of the source audio will influence species' responses. Seasonal and diel timing of the activity is also critical, as species' responses to calls often vary with these factors (Herzog *et al.* 2002). Using playback during the breeding season can have substantial negative effects on birds and should be used with caution at these times (DEWHA 2010). Additionally, Australia has a paucity of bird call libraries (although see www.acousticobservatory.org), so personnel may also need to collect and catalogue calls from nearby populations before commencing the study.

General considerations

Where playback is being used at night, personnel should minimise background light from equipment. Recordings should be used that have minimal or neutral background noise, and do not include alarm or predator calls. Calls should ideally be broadcast at a sound level that mimics natural call volume without distortion from equipment. Personnel best hear and determine direction of response calls when they are not holding the speaker, so placing speakers several metres away, or working in teams of dedicated operators and listeners, will improve detection capacity.

Effect of playback on other monitoring activities

Where using playback in proximity to automated recording units (Chapter 5), care must be taken to note and time playback, such that playback calls detected on recording devices can be eliminated from later analyses. Variability in the use of call playback in constant effort community banding projects also interferes with accuracy of project metrics such as catch rate calculations.

Playback for capture

In concert with a species-appropriate capture method, a selection of calls can be played on a music player and speaker (or similar) and placed by the trap or net (Bloom *et al.* 2007). Constant calls can be effective for flocking or migratory species. However, intervals of silence between calls may be more effective for territorial birds because they mimic the calling pattern of free-ranging birds and can be used in conjunction with decoys. Where no captures are made in several net rounds, playback should be suspended temporarily or changed. The ABBBS identifies general guidelines on use of tape lures during bird-banding (Drynan 2015).

For mist netting (see Chapter 7) of territorial birds, particularly strongly terrestrial species, multiple speakers can be installed several metres away from either side of the mist net, with personnel located in a hide nearby. Personnel in the hide control which speaker plays the call, switching between them depending on which side of the net the birds are on.

Broadcast surveys for detection and behaviour response studies

Detection surveys combine passive (no playback) and active (playback) components. If target birds are already calling at the start of the survey period, then playback may be unnecessary. A typical procedure (DEWHA 2010 after Debus 1995) is as follows:

- Personnel walk to a survey point (broadcast station) and wait a nominated passive listening time, while scanning the area and acclimating to all audible calls. If unsolicited target calls are heard, playback is not required.
- If no calls are heard during the passive listening period, personnel broadcast target calls in short bursts (the exact time depends on normal call length, but normally 10–20 s), interspersed with larger breaks to listen for responses (30–60 s) for up to five repetitions. Personnel cease playback if the target species is heard or antagonistic behaviour is detected.
- The listening and calling sequence can be repeated at multiple survey points, spaced outside of hearing range of each other.

Acoustic behaviour studies work in a similar fashion, using playback to simulate the presence of other animals, such as potential predators or competing males (e.g. see Kostoglou *et al.* 2017, 2020). Behavioural responses are recorded under a schedule of natural volume of playback, compared against a control of no playback.

Playback for influencing site selection

Call playback is used, sometimes in combination with decoys, to influence 'safe' site selection or to restore former seabird breeding areas by simulating an active colony (Greenwell *et al.* 2021a). Seabirds rely on strong sensory signalling and conspecific audio-visual cues (e.g. call playback and decoys), providing an opportunity to influence behaviour (Friesen *et al.* 2017). Personnel deploy decoys in lifelike spacing and at appropriate locations. Personnel must keep clear of sites while calls are broadcast, so a wireless speaker or long cables work best. Playback timing is matched to times when birds are prospecting and playbacks should mimic active colony sounds. Equipment is not left unattended. Broadcasts are made for a fixed period before being stopped. The response of seabirds to social facilitation (e.g. call playback and decoys) varies among species and populations (Friesen *et al.* 2017) and consequently the duration of stimuli required to encourage site selection will be species-specific.

Animal treatment, withdrawal and euthanasia

Call playback does not involve animal handling, so treatment and euthanasia may only be relevant if other procedures (e.g. capture) are done in conjunction with playback. Researchers should use behavioural and environmental cues to determine whether withdrawal from a site or study is necessary. This scenario may occur where researchers discover an active nest nearby or where playback elicits interest from resident predatory species that may put the study animals at risk. Alternative sites or timing should be considered in these situations.

Equipment and maintenance

In addition to any equipment required for capture (for capture-based studies), typical items required for call playback studies may include an audio player, Bluetooth® or wired speaker or megaphone, spare batteries, weatherproof coverings for speakers and player, decoys, parabolic microphone and sound recorder.

Specific qualifications, experience and training

Personnel should understand the types of calls being broadcast and typical vocalisations of the target species, and have sufficient knowledge of bird behaviour to interpret behavioural responses.

Workplace health and safety

Injury from target or non-target species

While unlikely, animals may respond antagonistically towards call playback, creating a risk of injury to personnel (e.g. if working with large raptors; see Chapter 34). Personnel should halt activities and withdraw if this situation occurs.

Alternative procedures

Using call playback in capture and monitoring work expedites captures and detections. Conducting these activities passively (without playback) may have less immediate effects on the behaviour of target animals, but doing so is likely to increase total capture time and result in raised potential for captures of non-target species.

MONITORING OF COLONIAL BIRDS AT BREEDING COLONIES

Nicholas Dunlop, Claire N. Greenwell, Tegan K. Douglas, Michael A. Weston, John Porter, Rosalind Jessop, Lisa O'Neill and Jennifer A. Spencer

Target taxa

This GOP applies to colonial seabirds and colonially nesting waterbirds (Chapter 35).

Context and scope

This GOP describes the monitoring and capture of colonial nesting birds at their breeding grounds by hand, hand nets, nest traps or mist nets (procedures for mist nets are also detailed in Chapter 7). Targeting birds at breeding colonies provides opportunities to capture otherwise highly mobile species with relative ease. Typically, work at colonies informs investigations of population size, species longevity, movement, natal site fidelity, breeding and general ecology, marine pollution and food web dynamics. Best-practice, low-impact approaches vary among and within species at different stages of the nesting cycle. The extent of impacts also depends on nest location and level of nest-site fidelity. Timing of survey may be crucial as some species have highly specific seasonal timing of breeding; others may have more extended or even year-round breeding (Parker and Rexer-Huber 2016). General survey guidelines are detailed in Magrath *et al.* (2010) for Australian threatened species and Parker and Rexer-Huber (2016) for burrow-nesting species.

Animal welfare considerations

Disruptions to natural activities

The high density of birds at breeding colonies means that incursions by researchers into or near colonies may disturb large numbers of birds, sometimes leaving eggs and chicks temporarily unattended (see Chapter 35). To minimise unnecessary energy expenditure by birds, research activities should be concentrated to avoid flow-on physiological and breeding cycle implications (Bamford *et al.* 2013). When working in bird breeding colonies, where possible researchers should minimise the total time spent in the colony, total number of visits, and number of personnel to minimise potential disturbance of nesting birds. Nest trapping and other colony work is generally best conducted at dawn, dusk or during the peak changeover times (for species with synchronous incubation scheduling). Knowledge of the species behaviour should dictate timing. Processing birds should be done in a timely manner and researchers should suspend capture temporarily where capture rates exceed processing capabilities. For protracted procedures, removing the birds from the colony is likely to have fewer impacts on the overall colony than working *in situ*.

Colony abandonment

Colonial birds are less sensitive to disturbance late in the nesting period, as site tenacity increases closer to the time of hatching (Safina and Burger 1983; Nisbet 2000). Attempts to trap or handle birds at the nest site should be avoided during courtship, pre-laying and early incubation, unless doing so is integral to the research question being addressed. Generally, surface-nesting species with high nest-site fidelity are more tolerant of capture and handling than low site-fidelity species. However, site tenacity can also be reduced by frequent predator incursions or poor foraging conditions, and researchers should be prepared to reassess conditions if 'flighty' behaviour is observed.

Exposure to predators

Working in colonies may increase exposure of birds to predation if predators learn to associate research activities with food (Sutherland 2004). Regular monitoring of traps during trapping sessions and remaining alert to potential risks will help to reduce the potential for exposure to predators. Eggs and chicks may be exposed to predators if adults are flushed into the air and away from nest sites. Researchers should evaluate the potential risk from aerial predators in these situations. In some cases, impacts can be mitigated by working at night. Ultimately, understanding the breeding behaviour of the target species will determine the most suitable time response.

Egg and chick exposure to environment

To minimise egg and chick exposure, attempts to capture, handle or observe nesting birds should not be made during unfavourable weather conditions (e.g. rain, high winds, heat or cold). Exposure time can be reduced by targeting different areas in the colony sequentially. Nest traps should be monitored and removed if incubation does not resume within ~30 min. Taking breaks between trapping sessions and making the most of changeover periods (see published literature on incubation periods for the target species, where available) will help to reduce chick and egg exposure.

Collapsing burrows

Burrow nesting seabird species generally return to their colonies at night and do not interact with researchers during the day. Researchers may inadvertently collapse burrows or disturb habitat if moving about the colony. Burrow collapse may interrupt breeding attempts early in the breeding season or entomb adults, eggs, or chicks later in the season. The research plan should involve consistent access paths to study burrows with some hardening of tracks if necessary. Soil strength may decline seasonally with moisture levels and burrows may collapse more readily late in the season. See Chapter 35 for additional details on mitigating risks of burrow collapse and habitat disturbance at seabird colonies.

Drowning

For colonies nesting in vegetation over or near water, nestlings could fall from nests into the water, or run into water while researchers work in the colony. Under these circumstances, researchers should work as a team, concentrating on a small part of the colony at a time, and always remain vigilant to bird responses to the presence of surveyors. To minimise the risk of processed nestlings leaping into the water upon return to the nest, the bird can be placed on the nest and temporarily covered with a handling bag. Personnel should keep their hand on the bag over the nestling until it settles, before removing the bag and departing. A long-handled net may be used to retrieve flightless nestlings from the water and, where appropriate, return birds to their nests. Contingency plans should be prepared before the commencement of fieldwork to deal with nestlings that cannot be successfully returned to the nest.

Abandonment of eggs and young

Nestlings may be abandoned if they stray from nests (Greenwell *et al.* 2021b). Understanding the colonial behaviour of the target species will help to reduce potential for abandonment. For example, some species exhibit strong nest-site fidelity up until fledging, so young must be returned to nests post-handling to prevent abandonment. The most appropriate time of capture for these species may be early in the nestling stage, when the potential for dispersal is reduced during colony disturbance (Bamford *et al.* 2013). For other species, nest site attachment is reduced with chick age, when strong vocal recognition enables adults and their young to locate each other in the colony (Shugart 1978; Saino and Fasola 1996). In species where chicks become relatively mobile in a short period and develop strong vocal recognition, banding later in the breeding period may reduce the potential for abandonment and reduce disturbance levels in the colony (e.g. Greenwell *et al.* 2021b). Removing adult birds from burrows before chicks hatch should be undertaken with caution, and preferably at the end of the incubation period or while chicks are being actively brooded (Blackmer *et al.* 2004; Sanz-Aguilar *et al.* 2010).

Repeated recaptures and capture of non-target species

Seabirds that are captured and handled at night can be dazzled by head torches and should be placed nearby in a safe location to allow their eyes to adjust on release (Bub 1991; Redfern and Clark 2001). This procedure occasionally results in the same individuals being recaptured on multiple occasions. To reduce handling time and stress, leg bands of marked birds should be checked immediately and recaptures from the same sampling period released immediately. Trapping periods should be limited in their duration. Non-target species occupying the same environment may be captured, particularly if using mist nets. Non-target animals should be cleared from mist nets immediately and released appropriately.

General procedures

Planning

The proposed design and capture methods employed are evaluated by the researchers based on the project aims and breeding ecology of the target bird species. Each activity considers appropriate timing, the likely response of the colony, the most appropriate site access to minimise disturbance, predation potential, non-target disturbance and interactions with local human activities, if relevant.

Burrow counts

One of the most commonly used techniques for estimating seabird abundance is to count nests or burrows, which usually involves measuring the perimeter and area of the colony, sampling plots and extrapolating these numbers to the colony. The possibility of differing densities of birds occurring in differing habitats should be considered when sampling. Burrow occupancy should also be assessed (Parker and Rexer-Huber 2016) as colonies may have a large portion of unoccupied burrows in any season, some burrows may be occupied by non-breeding individuals, or breeding may have already failed in a burrow. Accuracy of occupancy estimates have improved with the use of site-appropriate burrow scopes (Priddel *et al.* 2006).

Colony counts

Some wetland bird species (particularly order Pelecaniformes and families Phalacrocoracidae, Ardeidae and Threskiornithidae) (see Chapter 35) can nest in large numbers in small areas of a wetland. Colony surveys are generally undertaken on foot, or from a kayak or small boat, and waterbirds are observed using binoculars and telescopes. Data collection can include recording the number of nests of each species (and stage of nesting) per nesting tree/nesting vegetation clump within a recorded area of each colony. This information can be used for long-term monitoring to document number of active colony sites and number of nests of each species for a given season. Accuracy is improved by using the same observers where possible across colony counts and using two observers to cross-check nests counts for each nesting tree. More recently, drones have been used to collect high resolution data on colony extent and number of nests for very large ibis colonies in wetlands in inland Australia. These studies considered the height and speed of the drone and limited the total time spent over individual nests (Lyon *et al.* 2018; Francis *et al.* 2020; see Chapter 6). This new technique is improving data reliability for large waterbird colonies, which are often impossible to access on foot to conduct complete colony counts, with counts often based on a combination of assessment from aerial survey and/or ground count for a subsection of a colony site.

Nest trapping

Trapping at nests is often used to capture individual birds or pairs in a colony (Mills and Ryder 1979; Sutherland 2004). Trap design and dimensions vary, but most commonly consist of a baseless walk-in cage with a door or treadle (Figure 15.2; Mills and Ryder 1979). The cage mesh allows clear vision of the clutch and the frame should not have sharp edges. Walk-in traps are placed over the nest so that the nest is located towards the back of the trap, with the door facing the direction investigators intend to approach from. Investigators should note surrounding nests and identify a preferred path to use when returning to check the trap. When first deployed, birds in the immediate vicinity may disperse. However, as investigators exit the colony site, neighbouring birds should return to their nests and resume incubation. At the nest trap, the occupant will typically return to the nest location in a short period. It may walk around or land on top of the trap for a short time before finding the entrance, at which point it will resume incubation. Birds are free to come and go through the entrance and generally do not show any visible signs of distress until investigators return (Sutherland 2004).

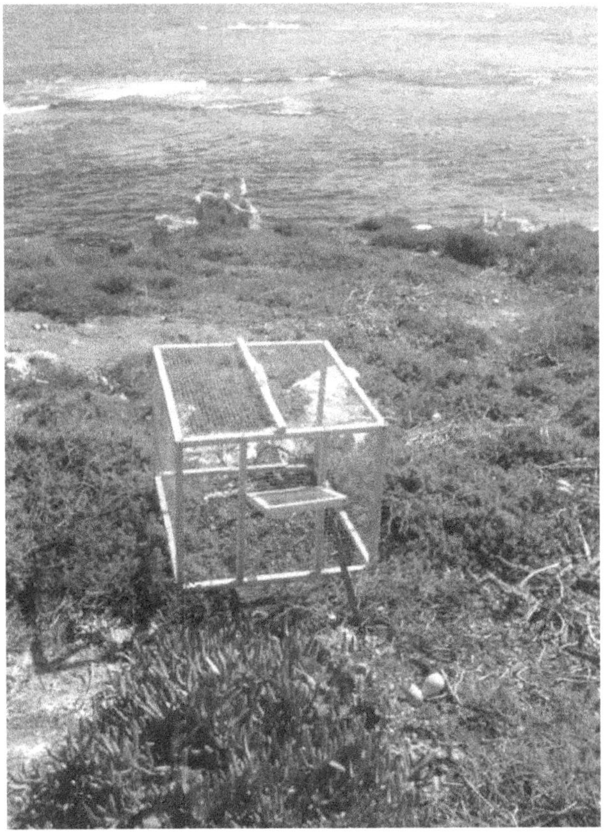

Figure 15.2: Nest trap set on an active silver gull (*Chroicocephalus novaehollandiae*) nest. Note proximity of other active nests, and adult birds in the background. Photo by Sandy J. McNeill.

Traps should be monitored continually to ensure that eggs are not left unincubated for long periods of time (i.e. not ≥ 30 min in temperate weather conditions). Trapped birds may develop trap shyness post-capture, resulting in individuals being unwilling to re-enter a trap. In such cases, the trap should be removed and trapping resumed following change-over of the incubator. Published literature on incubation shift duration for the target species, where available, can guide the timing interval of trap placement. For logistical reasons and to prevent interference (i.e. disturbance of birds at one trap when checking another), the number of traps operated at any one time should not exceed the number that the investigators can check in a timely manner.

Hand capture

Adults and chicks may be removed directly from nests by hand, but care should be taken to ensure that they are returned to their own nest (e.g. Greenwell *et al.* 2021b). When working in dense colonies, nests can be marked with pot plant tags, flagging tape or golf tees (depending on habitat type) to aid this process. In dense colonies, chicks should be placed into individual holding bags (DBCA 2017) and processed away from the colony. The chicks of tree- or shrub-nesting species (i.e. noddies and cormorants) should be banded soon after hatching as older chicks will leap from nests prematurely.

For crèche-forming species, or surface-nesting species where nest site–fidelity diminishes and strong vocal recognition develops between adults and their young, runners (young birds that can leave the nest, but cannot yet fly) may be rounded up during the day or night to cohort mark large numbers of birds (Dunlop 2018). The most appropriate techniques vary between species. This technique is labour intensive and requires a sufficiently large number of people to cover the width of the breeding area at a spacing of approximately ≤ 2 m. Corrals with temporary drift fences may be used to drive and hold the crèches until the birds are processed (Bub 1991; FAO 2007; Johnston *et al.* 2015). Chicks that can run and have developed pin feathers (as a minimum) are suitable for collection. Birds can be placed into calico holding bags or suitable sized crates. Recently hatched downy chicks within nest scrapes must not be collected for bulk processing.

Most burrow-nesting seabirds have strong nest fidelity and may be sampled at any time after laying, with caution. Prospecting birds and non-breeders should not be extracted from burrows. Older chicks and adults can be removed safely from burrows (if the burrow is stable) for processing.

Handheld net capture

Long-handled nets or a shepherd's crook can be used to capture incubating adults in some colonies at the right stage (Bacon and Evrard 1990). If necessary, this method can be combined with night lighting to dazzle the target temporarily (Bub 1991). A sharp point of white-light of medium brightness is best for dazzling adults. More-powerful lights risk damage to the birds' eyesight and alert the colony to the investigator's presence. Red lights are useful for observation but will not assist capture.

Mist-net capture

Mist nets can be used to capture adults in the vicinity of the breeding colony. Protocols for mist netting should follow those outlined in Chapter 7, with consideration for minimising effects on breeding colonies. Where adults are returning to brood young, processing should occur as quickly as possible to minimise impacts mentioned earlier.

Animal treatment, withdrawal and euthanasia

Investigators are responsible for overseeing capture and handling operations and must monitor activities undertaken by less-experienced personnel. When an injured bird is identified and the investigator deems that the injury is treatable and possible, the animal should be taken to a veterinarian promptly. When transport to a veterinarian is not possible or the bird deemed untreatable, injured animals should be euthanased by experienced personnel (see Chapter 35 for protocols for aquatic birds).

Equipment and maintenance

Equipment will vary depending on the species being targeted, their breeding ecology and study objectives. Typical items may include:

- long-handled net
- shepherd's crook
- nest traps; custom-made for the target species
- mist-netting equipment
- thick gloves when handling large Procellariformes
- safety glasses
- calico holding bags or boxes/crates
- head torch
- equipment for recording data
- specific equipment related to study design (e.g. water depth rulers, callipers, scales and animal marking equipment)
- net and/or trap repair equipment
- hand sanitiser and hand washing facilities
- first aid kit
- licences and permits.

Specific qualifications, experience and training

The skills required to undertake bird handling and capture are relatively consistent between species, although sensitivity to human disturbance may vary between species. Personnel should be competent with the technique proposed and familiar with the species or similar taxa, having undertaken similar work. Alternatively, personnel should be trained or supervised by someone who is. To be considered competent, personnel should have undertaken or been involved in at least one study or project using the proposed techniques. Personnel banding birds will need to have appropriate ABBBS qualifications.

Workplace health and safety

Animal bites, scratches and zoonoses

Capture and handling of birds may result in injuries to handlers through bites and scratches. Appropriate handling techniques reduce this risk. Personal protective equipment such as thick gloves and safety glasses may be appropriate for some species. High concentrations of birds within breeding colonies may increase the potential for disease transmission (see Chapter 35). All injuries and scratches should be treated as soon as possible to prevent the risk of infection. Birds have the potential to transmit diseases to human, particularly through faecal contamination. All personnel must practise good hygiene after handling seabirds.

Alternative procedures

Working at breeding colonies provides one of the few opportunities to research healthy seabird and waterbird species. Collection of scats or feathers may be considered for non-individualised biological sampling (Chapter 4). While remote monitoring equipment, such as camera traps (Chapter 5) or drones (Chapter 6), could be used to answer some questions including collecting high resolution colony counts (e.g. Lyon *et al.* 2018) and detailed information on reproductive success (e.g. Brandis *et al.* 2014), these methods are generally not useful for behavioural and population studies of birds where individual identification is necessary (Mills and Ryder 1979).

NEST AND HOLLOW INSPECTIONS, INCLUDING HANDLING OF EGGS AND CHICKS

Simon Cherriman, Tegan K. Douglas and Michael A. Weston

Target taxa

This GOP applies to all bird taxa (Chapters 33–36), but particularly parrots and passerines (Chapter 33) and raptors (Chapter 34).

Context and scope

This GOP outlines research methods for investigating the breeding ecology of terrestrial bird species, where the researcher interacts directly with breeding adults, offspring, nests or nest sites. Nest can comprise burrows, bare scrapes on the ground, mounds, cup- or dome-shaped nests, natural or artificial tree hollows and cavities, or be located on natural or anthropogenic ledges. Nests vary in size, construction material and robustness, and are found in diverse habitat types at varying heights. Nests can contain single eggs or large clutches. Chicks can be precocial or altricial and receive varying amounts of parental care pre- and post-hatching. Inspection of nests is typically undertaken by direct assessment from the ground, tree climbing (e.g. Pay *et al.* 2021) or with an elevated working platform, or indirectly with pole-mounted cameras or similar, depending on requirements and habitat. Eggs and birds are often subjected to other procedures, such as egg candling or floating, morphometric measurements, and applying tags or transmitters. Nests also may be measured or fitted with sensor loggers.

Animal welfare considerations

Abandonment of the nesting attempt or nest destruction

Nest searches or visits to known sites should be avoided during early breeding stages. The probability of abandonment often reduces as breeding progresses (Götmark 1992; Sun *et al.* 2020), so well-incubated eggs or nestlings are less likely to be deserted than incomplete nests or freshly laid clutches. Birds do not abandon eggs or young after 'smelling' the presence of humans, but avian vision is acute and observation of prolonged intrusion at the nest can alter adult behaviour and sometimes prompt desertion, particularly in raptors (Rosenfield *et al.* 2007) (Chapter 34). Secondary breeding attempts are often undertaken in a completely new nest, despite the existing one being intact. Time taken to construct or prepare a new site can delay fledging time of the replacement clutch and affect survivorship as season and resource availability (e.g. food) changes. Nests of some species are permanent fixtures in a well-established, continuously occupied home range. Inadvertent disturbance leading to the deterioration or destruction of these nest sites may affect site occupation by these sedentary species.

Disturbance to nesting adult birds

Nesting birds become stressed if flushed repeatedly from active nests, in severe instances losing body condition, becoming malnourished and unable to rear young successfully, particularly in species where only one sex incubates (Götmark 1992). Disturbance is minimised by understanding the target species' biology and nesting routines before fieldwork commences. Research visits should overlap with times or stages of the breeding cycle that are likely to have the least impact on the birds, including at daily incubation changeover, or later in the breeding cycle, when adults typically spend less time at or near the nest. The sensitivity of nesting adult birds to investigators can vary between sites, with those more remote or isolated from humans exhibiting higher responsiveness (Thibault *et al.* 2020). Conversely, naive species may exhibit lowered responses.

Monitoring visible stress levels is not always possible as parent birds often respond to intrusion by leaving the site to observe intruders from a distance, and sometimes long before the researcher reaches the nest. Even birds that appear to be behaviourally tolerant may actually be experiencing physiological responses to humans (Charuvi *et al.* 2020). Short nest visits minimise this impact. Where species deter intruders with aggressive attacks, the intensity of attacks can increase during cooler weather (Fisher *et al.* 2004), so visits should be undertaken during favourable weather conditions, minimising time spent near the nest. Aggressive nest defence can even cause experienced investigators to unconsciously rush procedures (Kostoglou *et al.* 2020), so particular care is required.

Nestling and egg exposure

Prolonged inspection of nests will result in chilled eggs and potential abandonment. Similarly, young chicks not capable of thermoregulation subjected to prolonged exposure may experience hypo- or hyperthermia. All handling, transport, and processing techniques should eliminate the potential for over-heating and over-cooling of eggs and chicks. Egg flotation can be conducted with tepid or lukewarm water, and eggs dried before being replaced in the nest. Inspections in cold or wet weather should be avoided, activities always undertaken quickly, and the nest site vacated promptly after inspections are complete.

Predation

Research activities may alert predators to cryptic nests, resulting in egg or nestling predation. Corvids are particularly vigilant and may observe human activity to locate potential prey opportunities (Ekanayake *et al.* 2015a, b). Nesting birds repeatedly flushed from nests may catch the attention of aerial predators. Terrestrial predators may follow human scent trails to nests, and benefit from widening of paths, and inadvertent vegetation trampling and clearing. Efficient planning ensures that a minimal number of site visits are made with personnel acting efficiently and discretely near the nest.

Damage to eggs during inspection or handling

Eggs are fragile and should be handled as little as possible. Where handling is necessary to determine laying date or similar (Liebezeit *et al.* 2007), personnel should handle only one egg at a time, carefully placing rather than dropping eggs onto any instruments or containers, and using cushioning or padding to minimise impact with hard surfaces (Figure 15.3). Small cracks and chips can be repaired successfully with glue or nail varnish (Gage and Duerr 2020), but care should be taken to minimise the amount of sealant spread over the surface of the eggs to avoid impeding airflow.

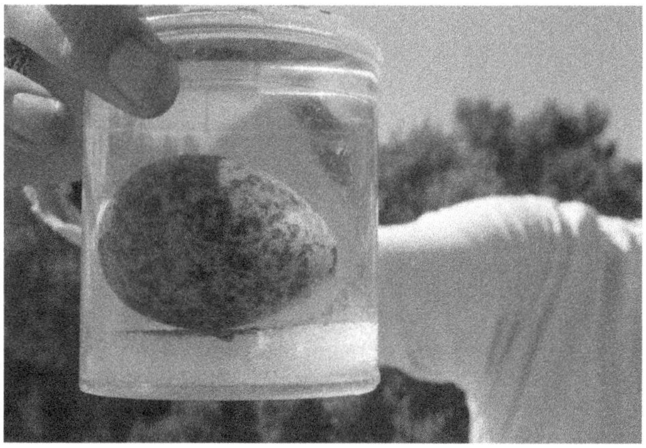

Figure 15.3: Floating a masked lapwing (*Vanellus miles*) egg in tepid water. Note the disc of Styrofoam™ at the bottom on the canister to cushion the egg. Photo by Michael A. Weston.

Reduced provisioning or injury to nestlings

If prolonged procedures interrupt natural feeding rates, supplementary food appropriate to the species can be placed at the nest to offset loss of resources (E. Weston, pers. comm.). Improper handling of nestlings can lead to injury or death. Some nestlings respond to nest intrusion by flapping their wings or lunging forwards in a threat display, causing feather damage if they catch tree limbs or cavity walls. Nestlings should be secured quickly, manually restrained or placed inside a carry bag. Handling bags containing chicks should not contact sharp or hard objects as they are transferred to the ground or processing station. A carry bag can be lowered to the ground clipped to a climbing line. Carry bags should never be attached to the safety harness of a descending climber, as climbing line failures can result in injury.

General procedures

Planning

A detailed fieldwork plan is key to maximising efficiency and minimising time spent at nest sites. Season, weather and timing of the event in relation to the birds' breeding cycle should be considered. Routes to and from nest sites should be determined in advance to reduce disturbance to nesting habitat. All equipment needs to be checked and tested thoroughly before fieldwork, and roles among personnel decided, with group size as small as practical. Personnel should identify activities that should be avoided (such as shouting and other loud noises) to minimise stress to birds and review indicators of bird stress that all personnel are to be alert for.

Nest searching

Bird nests are usually located by systematic surveys undertaken on foot in suitable habitat (see 'Censuses, transects, point counts, area searches and general observation' earlier in this chapter). Nest locations of small or cryptic species are often pinpointed by direct observation of the individuals suspected to be breeding. Occupancy of tree hollows is determined by 'tap and flush' surveys, which are conducted by raking a stick against the tree trunk underneath a potential hollow (DBCA 2015). Aerial surveys for larger nests are possible using light aircraft, helicopters, or unmanned aerial vehicles (UAVs) and drones. The efficiency of UAVs is unclear in these scenarios, as excessive disturbance from their use in lengthy surveys may outweigh potential benefits (Rebolo-Ifrán *et al.* 2019; see Chapter 6 for an evaluation of methods and potential impacts). Once the subject is located, personnel can use binoculars or a spotting scope to observe 'normal' nesting behaviour from a distance, determining breeding stage and nest contents with minimal disturbance. Doing so informs the optimal timing for return visits and detailed inspection.

Physical inspection using indirect means

Low nests within 5 m of the ground (e.g. pigeons, honeyeaters) can be inspected with a simple pole fitted with an angled mirror or camera, extended to the height of the nest, allowing the researcher to view the contents. A similar set-up with telescopic poles can reach nests up to ~20 m. Contents of burrows or cavity nests can be observed with probe cameras (e.g. Seasnake®). Drones have been employed to inspect nests (Junda *et al.* 2015), but this technique is still evolving and is limited to higher nests that are not obscured by canopy foliage. All indirect methods obviate the need for climbing and are rapid (e.g. < 5 min).

Physical inspection and transport of eggs or nestlings

Research requiring handling of eggs or nestlings should be undertaken by qualified personnel with appropriate training and experience, at a time that minimises disturbance to the target species. A cherry picker or elevated working platform can be used to access sites adjacent to roads or tracks. In more-remote landscapes, tree-climbing or rope-access techniques are necessary to access nests in trees and tree hollows, or on cliffs.

Once at the nest, the climber should secure themselves with at least two anchor points in a position that allows easy access to the nest without moving it. A backpack or carry bag is then unclipped from the climber's safety gear and typically placed at the edge of the nest, in supporting foliage or hung adjacent to it. Most nestling birds respond to nest intrusion by sitting or squatting low in the nest and remaining motionless, and so can be easily removed by the investigator lifting them gently with both hands from the nest and placing them into the carry bag in one smooth motion. For example, this method has been used for Tasmanian wedge-tailed eagles (*Aquila audax fleayi*) (Pay *et al.* 2021). However, for hollow-nesting species a telescopic pole with a hoop bag or noose fitted to one end is required to scoop up or 'lasso' nestlings that must be extracted from within (often deep) tree-hollows. A towel-lined carry bag creates a soft lining on which chicks can be placed. Eggs require a smaller container lined with cotton wool or fine cloth to prevent damage during transport. The bag should be lowered (or on cliffs, raised) to assistants at ground level for processing, which can be completed in the open, or in a blind or processing tent.

Processing and handling

Nestlings can be removed from the carry bag for processing, using a size-appropriate hold (Rosenfield *et al.* 2007). In broods of two or more chicks, chicks are usually processed individually, the rest remaining in the dark carry bag or holding bag. Small passerine chicks can be handled and processed by a single researcher, but larger species like cockatoos or raptors may need to be held by an assistant (Figure 15.4). Falconry hoods can help prevent unnecessary stress in young raptors, and in some cases their legs should be tied together to avoid injuries to themselves and personnel. Care must be taken during all transport and handling to maintain even environmental conditions, including avoiding prolonged handling times, to avoid nestling hypo- or hyperthermia.

Once processed, birds should be replaced in the carry bag and hoisted back to the nest by the tree climber who returns them to the nest. Species from open nests should be replaced gently one at a time, and hollow-nesting species lowered carefully into the nest chamber and encouraged out of handling bags. Behaviour of the birds must be monitored throughout. Personnel should leave

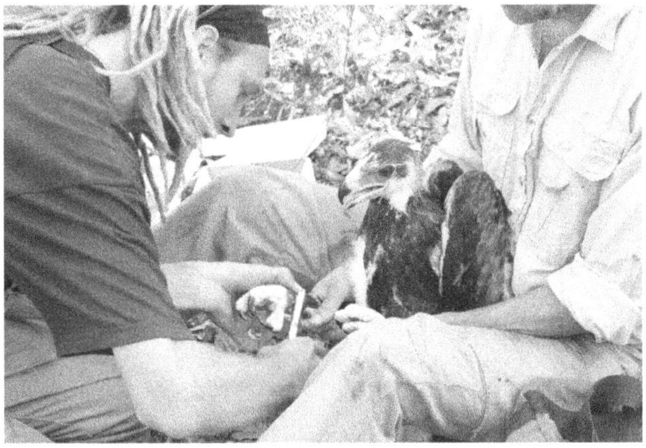

Figure 15.4: Having an experienced assistant hold a raptor, like this wedge-tailed eagle (*Aquila audax*), firmly during banding prevents unnecessary movement and potential injury. Photo by Stuart Rae.

the nest site promptly and normally return to an observation point to watch and ensure that parents return and tend to nestlings.

Animal treatment, withdrawal and euthanasia

Researchers monitor the status of both nestling and adult birds continually. Where experienced personnel deem that treatment is necessary and possible, the animal is either treated *in situ* or, if injuries are severe, taken to a veterinarian. For example, external signs of nestling hyperthermia include gaping (opening the mouth), and treatment (water with or without electrolyte additives) can be given orally with an eye-dropper if necessary. Not all personnel (i.e. working in remote areas) will be able to transport animals to a veterinarian and doing so may result in additional stress and trauma to the animal, so the welfare costs of such intervention must be evaluated against the benefits of treatment. If life-threatening injuries are present when nests are visited or obtained during research procedures, then euthanasia using cervical dislocation (for smaller species) or blunt force trauma (larger birds) may be necessary (see Chapters 33–36). Highly stressed parent birds will conduct repeated attacks with or without alarm vocalisations and principal researchers may decide that withdrawal from the nest and site is needed. When nestlings or eggs are returned to a nest, the behaviour of chicks and parents should be scrutinised from a distance; intervention should only occur only if senior researchers deem that nests have been abandoned.

Equipment and maintenance

General equipment may include binoculars or a spotting scope, carry bag, processing equipment, electrolyte mixture, safety glasses or goggles and gloves. For ground-based monitoring, personnel may require a pole-mounted mirror or camera, and telescopic pole (e.g. Spiderbeam®). Physical nest inspections may require climbing ropes, harness, webbing and appropriate hardware, a helmet, a telescopic pole with a noose or hoop bag, carry bag and handling ropes.

Specific qualifications, experience and training

Researchers should be competent with the specific technique proposed, and familiar with the species or similar taxa having undertaken similar work. Alternatively, personnel should be trained or supervised by someone who is. To be considered competent, personnel should have undertaken or been involved in at least one study or project using the proposed technique, including handling of the target or similar taxa. Climbing personnel should be trained and have advanced experience in the techniques required.

Workplace health and safety

Bites, scratches, stings, disease and allergy risks

Person protective equipment such as hats, face shields and gloves should be considered, depending upon the nest defence tactics of adult birds, including raptors (Chapter 34), and the sharp talons and bills of nestlings. Non-target animals occupying the same habitats as the research species can cause severe injury to field personnel. Beehives are often present in tree hollows and in some building cavities, so thorough assessment of hazards should be made before nest climbing. Personnel should consider the potential for transmission of diseases or parasites from animals to humans (and vice versa) as per the relevant species accounts (Chapters 34–36).

Meticulous hygiene practices, including regular washing of hands, field equipment and carry bags, and immediate treatment of bites or scratches should be followed at all times. Bags for holding birds should only be used once each session or changed between individual birds. Personnel who are known to develop allergies should inform group leaders before the activity commences. People with severe allergies associated with birds, with immune deficiency diseases or on immunosuppressant therapy should not handle birds.

Alternative procedures

Studies that use the methods detailed in this GOP usually seek to answer specific breeding biology questions, so alternative methods are generally insufficient. Fitting nestlings or juveniles with marks and tags can be less stressful than the handling of adults, which (1) require more technical methods of capture that cause greater interruptions to natural behaviour, and (2) are less likely to accept marking devices fitted after advanced development. However, all researchers on projects involving nests should consider alternative approaches, including if data can be collected during the non-breeding season when disturbance will be negligible. Egg handling can be minimised by considering indirect and alternative means of data collection, including use of museum specimens, eggs from abandoned clutches, or inferred from alternative field observations.

SIMPLE CAPTURE METHODS, INCLUDING HAND CAPTURE AND SPOTLIGHTING

Deborah Sullivan, Tegan K. Douglas, Claire N. Greenwell and David Parker

Target taxa

This GOP applies to all bird taxa (Chapters 33–36), but particularly large waterbirds such as pelicans and swans, and burrow-nesting seabirds (Chapter 35).

Context and scope

This GOP details methods for capture of birds by hand, and with simple, handheld tools, such as individual foot snares, hand nets, throw nets, net guns and crooks, with or without spotlights. All methods require researchers to be able to get close to their study animals, and usually only capture one or a small number of birds at a time. These simple capture methods work well for birds that readily habituate or are already habituated to humans (such as those in urban areas), or that readily approach vehicles or boats (e.g. around fisheries and ports). They are also suitable for temporarily flightless or reluctant fliers, including nestlings generally, almost flightless species such as plains-wanderers (*Pedionomus torquatus*), species that undergo simultaneous wing moult (e.g. ducks), nocturnal or crepuscular birds that roost in open areas and are tolerant of human presence during the day such as bush stone-curlews (*Burhinus grallarius*), burrow-nesting birds such as many seabirds, or birds that are encountered at night and dazzled with a spotlight for capture (e.g. the stubble quail, *Coturnix pectoralis*). Researchers can target specific individuals or cohorts at known locations, and encourage them to approach with food or burley, or simply by approaching the target species on foot. Birds may also be encountered semi-opportunistically through 'spotlighting' (see also Chapter 4) by driving/walking after dark through likely habitat, and using car headlights, a handheld torch or head torch to detect bird eyeshine. When spotlighting on foot, researchers can work as a team, to twinkle flocks towards catching personnel, with multiple headtorches to dazzle or distract birds from the catching process. These methods can be used to target particular individuals in a flock, including to capture birds for animal welfare intervention purposes (e.g. entangled, injured, or oiled birds – see Weston *et al.* 2008, 2009). Researchers working in breeding colonies should also see 'Monitoring of colonial birds at breeding colonies' earlier in this chapter.

Animal welfare considerations

Disruption to normal activities

Natural loafing and aggregation locations make effective trapping sites, but personnel must minimise interruption to the normal activities of target species and other birds using the site. Roles should be identified clearly during catch attempts, and excess personnel kept clear of the catch area. In the case of flocking birds, captured birds should be removed from the vicinity of the catch area for processing to avoid disturbing remaining birds. Processing of solitary species (e.g. the plains-wanderer) can be completed at the point of capture to minimise disturbance or stress to the individual. In general, processing should be undertaken by experienced personnel and birds released as quickly as possible.

Stress and injury during capture and handling

Equipment should be maintained and only operated by, or under the direct supervision of, experienced personnel. Gauges of nets and lines must be appropriate for the species being targeted. Hand nets and crooks have smooth, rounded edges, and all nets and netting should be kept in good repair. Birds can be extracted swiftly, but carefully, from nets. Species-appropriate holding methods should be used to quickly transfer captured birds to suitable holding or transport facilities. Researchers should remain vigilant for indicators of stress in target and non-target species at all times. Capture work should be conducted during fair weather, avoiding temperature extremes that may exacerbate bird stress levels.

Drowning risk

Drowning presents a risk where birds are caught on or close to water (Ferris and Gilbert 2014). When a catch attempt is made from a boat, at the water's edge or over water, birds should be lifted immediately out of the water to be secured, and all netting lifted out of the water and checked for by-catch. Catches should be made away from underwater obstacles (like engine rotors) that could inhibit swift extraction. Where handheld net guns are used, nets must be tethered to the launching device and an assistant with a long-handled net should remain on standby to retrieve the bird should it enter the water (with the net attached) after the net is fired.

Disorientation and increased predation risk from spotlight dazzling

Use of spotlights for capture or night-time processing work by torchlight can temporarily dazzle and disorientate birds. Birds subject to bright light during capture and/or processing must be placed in a suitable release location that allows their eyesight to recover (Bub 1991; Redfern and Clarke 2001). Placing birds on the ground, near cover, but away from researcher activities is preferred, although some seabirds can be faced into the wind and allowed to take off from open hands. Personnel should remain alert for evidence of predators during capture and processing, and personnel must have the capacity to hold birds temporarily, or move them to an alternative release site if predators are detected.

Disruption to breeding activities

See 'Monitoring of colonial birds at breeding colonies' and 'Nest and hollow inspections, including handling of eggs and chicks' earlier in this chapter.

Capture and interference by non-target species

Non-target captures are unlikely as personnel activate the capture tool. Throw nets and net guns can capture multiple individuals, so personnel should check them thoroughly after each deployment. For noose poles, the noose is lightly covered/buried with substrate material to eliminate non-target species from exposing or dislodging the line until it is activated by personnel. When capturing birds in a location with high pedestrian traffic, particularly dog walkers (on and off lead), participants should be on standby to direct public away from the trapping area.

General procedures

Planning

Target species and site knowledge will inform appropriate capture methods. The required number of experienced researchers is likely to vary depending on the capture environment, method, and nature of any additional procedures. A minimum of two personnel is preferred. These techniques should be undertaken by or under the direct supervision of competent, experienced investigators who are proficient in the capture and handling of wild birds. Where capture is required for animal welfare purposes, an understanding of the type of injury or entanglement, and target species, will inform capture methods and avoid any further injury or delays to capture (Ferris and Gilbert 2014). For example, beak-entangled Australasian darters (*Anhinga novaehollandiae*) are rarely caught with hand nets, but are routinely captured using handheld net launching devices (Western Australian Seabird Rescue, pers. comm.). Injured birds requiring treatment and/or rehabilitation should be placed into appropriately sized, soft animal crates for transportation immediately following capture.

Individual foot/leg noose

Foot or leg nooses are ideal for capturing large waterbirds that can be lured or 'twinkled', such as pelicans, swans and ducks. Individual foot/leg nooses are constructed from appropriate weight fishing line (35–45 kg for pelicans) and attached to a rod or pole with a 2 mm diameter stainless steel ring creating the running noose. The noose has a 50 cm diameter and should be shallowly buried beneath substrate (e.g. sand). Food can be used to lure the bird and when the target has entered the noose, the rod/pole is pulled quickly for the noose to encircle the leg. Tension should be maintained until the bird is secured safely by additional personnel trained in capture and handling techniques. The noose can then be removed from captured bird.

Beak grab

The beak grab technique is suited to birds that are located at sites frequently used by the public or habituated species (e.g. Australian pelican, *Pelecanus conspiculatus*), where other capture techniques may not be feasible (Ferris and Gilbert 2014). Birds at these sites are often habituated to people and will generally approach closely to obtain food. A fish is required as a lure for this method. The target can be lured close enough for capture by waving a fish towards it. As the bird attempts to take the fish, the researcher catches the lower mandible in their fingers. As they pull the bird towards them, they use their other hand to control the upper mandible. One hand gently holds the bill, leaving a finger placed between upper and lower mandible. The other hand is free to reach around the body of the bird, therefore controlling the wings. The bird should be sitting comfortably with one arm around the body, wings closed and hand controlling the beak. Experienced personnel can perform the whole action swiftly and with minimal movement.

Hand capture

One- or two-handed hand capture can be used for flightless or otherwise approachable animals. When within a close enough range, personnel can swiftly snatch a bird, using a motion that ensnares or surrounds the animal, avoiding pinning or crushing it. Personnel should aim for the body of the bird, and not grasp just the flight or tail

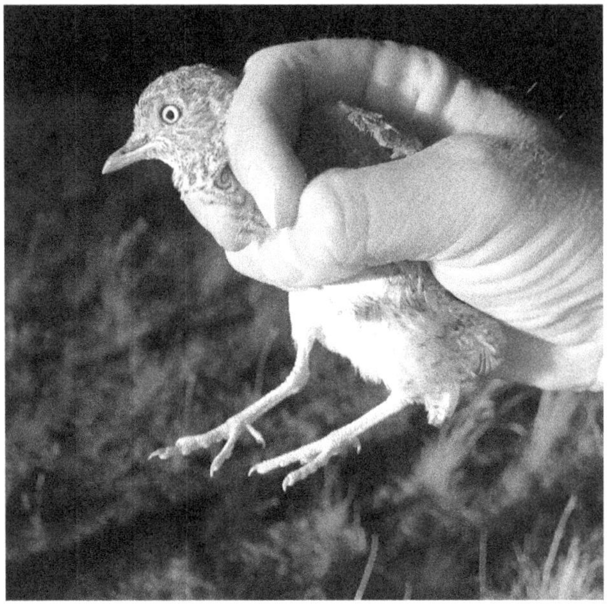

Figure 15.5: Plains-wanderer (*Pedionomus torquatus*) captured by hand with a spotlight and held in an appropriate grip, with its legs free. Photo by David Parker.

feathers, nor, in a rush to secure the bird in hand, restrict movement of the bird's legs. The bird can then be secured in a size-appropriate hold (Figure 15.5), so that it cannot flap or injure itself, and placed into a holding bag for processing.

Hand net

A long-handled net of appropriate gauge can be used to assist capture, with or without a spotlight (Bub 1991). Targets are generally located on the ground, low in the vegetation or on water. The observer should approach obliquely. Surreptitious motions work best, so researchers should take small quiet steps (or approach via a slow crawl) and hold the net parallel to the ground. The net should not be swung in an arc, but slowly moved towards the bird until the pole can be darted forwards and the hoop dropped over the bird. In well-timed captures the bird will not take flight, or will have only just lifted, with researchers angling the net to intercept the bird's flight direction. Swiping nets at birds already in flight should not be done. When using a spotlight, personnel should aim to keep themselves and the nets from casting shadows until the last minute, with one person responsible for directing and moving the spotlight if necessary and the other person responsible for catching the bird. Birds should be extracted immediately from the net and transferred to a holding bag.

Throw net

A circular net with weighted edges that can be cast by hand over birds, in a method similar to that used for capturing fish. When used over water, care should be taken to quickly remove and extract any catches.

Net gun/net launcher

Net guns, as discussed in Chapter 7, are handheld devices that use compressed air (or gunpowder) to propel a small net towards a target, with an effective range of around 6 m (Western Australian Seabird Rescue 2018). Net guns can be used in open areas on land or water and can be fired from boats or vehicles, with different gauge nets used for differently size birds (Buidin *et al.* 2015). They are most effective when fired over birds on the ground, or the water's surface, rather than towards birds in flight, but drowning risk must be assessed (see 'Animal welfare considerations').

Shepherd's crook

The shepherd's crook is best used in situations when other capture techniques are not feasible. A shepherd's crook can be used to guide a bird to a position where handling can be achieved.

Spotlighting

Spotlights (handheld, head torches or fixed to a car) can be used to aid most of the methods mentioned in this GOP when they are conducted at night. White lights of medium brightness with a sharp point work best. The observer should keep the beam of light fixed on the bird while the catcher approaches, making minimal noise and avoiding breaking the beam (Bub 1991). Once personnel are within range of the bird with their chosen capture implement (e.g. hand, net) they lean in to catch the bird with a swift movement. When working in a team, one researcher can hold the light steady, while the other approaches and catches. While red filtered lights are used for general nocturnal/cave observation with minimal interference (see Chapter 4), they are unsuitable for dazzling animals during capture. However, they can be used during the capture of ground-dwelling birds (e.g. plains-wanderer), which are reluctant to fly.

Processing, handling and release

Handling should be minimal and ideally undertaken by one person. Some species may benefit from having their eyes covered, or being held in a cloth bag, while processing (Bub 1991). Personnel should be familiar with the target species to aid correct handling. For example, pelicans are mouth breathers and will become distressed if their beak is closed or body held too tightly, restricting movement of the keel bone, which facilitates breathing. Health and stress levels should be monitored throughout the handling process. Visibly stressed individuals must be released as quickly as possible. Care should be taken with spotlighted birds as their night vision has been compromised temporarily. Birds can be placed on the ground, away from researchers (and lights), so that their eyes can adjust and they can move away in their own time (Redfern and Clark 2001). Birds that prefer to fly can be placed on the raised palm of a team member, facing into the wind for release.

Animal treatment, withdrawal and euthanasia

Investigators are responsible for overseeing capture and handling operations and must monitor activities and personnel. When an injured bird is identified and the lead investigator deems that treatment is appropriate and possible, the animal should be taken to a veterinarian promptly. When transport to a veterinarian is not possible or the bird deemed untreatable, injured animals should be euthanased by experienced personnel (see Section 3 for appropriate methods). Birds captured for welfare reasons should be assessed by veterinarian or treated *in situ* by personnel experienced in common only injuries.

Equipment and maintenance

In addition to the particular capture device being used (i.e. noose and rod, hand net, throw net, net gun or shepherd's crook), the following items materials are commonly required:

- processing equipment tailored for the target species and study design (e.g. callipers, wing ruler, tape measure, eye hood, cloth bag, and sampling equipment depending on study design)
- equipment for recording data
- spare fishing line and stainless-steel ring
- net repair materials
- spare cartridges and nets for net gun
- small scissors
- transport bags/soft animal crate
- binoculars
- first aid kit (human and animal)
- hand sanitiser and hand washing facilities
- personal protective equipment (including eyewear)
- licences and permits.

Fishing line will degrade over time, so nooses should be tested before each use by running fingers along the line to feel for wear or weak points. The running noose should be able to move freely. Appropriately weighted fishing line should be used to avoid leg damage.

Specific qualifications, experience and training

The skills required to undertake these capture methods vary depending on sensitivity of the species to the presence of humans and disturbance, and the nature of the study. Personnel should be competent with the technique proposed, familiar with the species or similar taxa, having undertaken similar work. Alternatively, personnel should be trained or supervised by someone who is. Personnel undertaking capture and banding will require an A-class ABBBS licence (basic capture methods endorsement, minimum). Depending on design, use of the net gun may also require a firearms licence.

Workplace health and safety

Refer to details in 'Nest and hollow inspections, including handling of eggs and chicks' earlier in this chapter. Capture and handling of birds may result in injuries to handlers through bites and scratches. Appropriate handling techniques reduce this risk. Personal protective equipment, including thick gloves and safety glasses, is essential when handling some species that are known to target eyes (e.g. egrets, *Ardea* and *Egretta* spp.). All injuries and scratches should be treated as soon as possible to prevent the risk of infection. Birds have the potential to transmit diseases to human, particularly through faecal contamination and regurgitation. All personnel must practice good hygiene after handling birds. Net guns, if used, must be treated with care and only operated as directed by the manufacturer. They pose risk of injury to both operators and bystanders, so must only be used by or under the direct supervision of experienced personnel, should never be pointed in the direction of people and should always be stored appropriately between uses.

Alternative procedures

Although alternative methods exist for the general capture of these taxa, the simple methods outlined here allow for highly targeted capture efforts, making them suitable for capture of particular individuals, or specific or low numbers of birds. By-catch is minimal and the simple equipment used minimises the potential for equipment malfunction impacting bird or operator welfare. They can also often be utilised in a broader variety of settings than other methods.

FOOT SNARES, NOOSE CARPETS AND BAL-CHATRIS

Grainne S. Maguire, Michael A. Weston, Tegan K. Douglas and Rosalind Jessop

Target taxa

This GOP applies to shorebirds and small ground-dwelling birds (involving the use of foot snares, noose carpets; see Chapters 33 and 35) and raptors, including owls (bal-chatris; see Chapter 34).

Context and scope

This GOP outlines the use of foot snares, noose carpets and bal-chatris to capture free-ranging, ground-frequenting birds. Noose carpets consist of a series of running nooses made from fishing line, attached to a flexible base, which is pegged firmly to the substrate. Noose carpets are typically used to capture shorebirds and other species more likely to walk or run than fly. Bal-chatris are box-, cone- or saucer-shaped traps with an external array of nooses enclosing a lure or decoy, targeting species that catch terrestrial prey (Figure 15.6; Bloom *et al.* 2007). These methods are ideal for targeted capture of individual birds; construction of traps is tailored to specific species. Captured birds are often subject to additional procedures before release. These methods are also used to capture birds for animal welfare purposes (e.g. oiled, injured or entangled birds; see Weston *et al.* 2008, 2009).

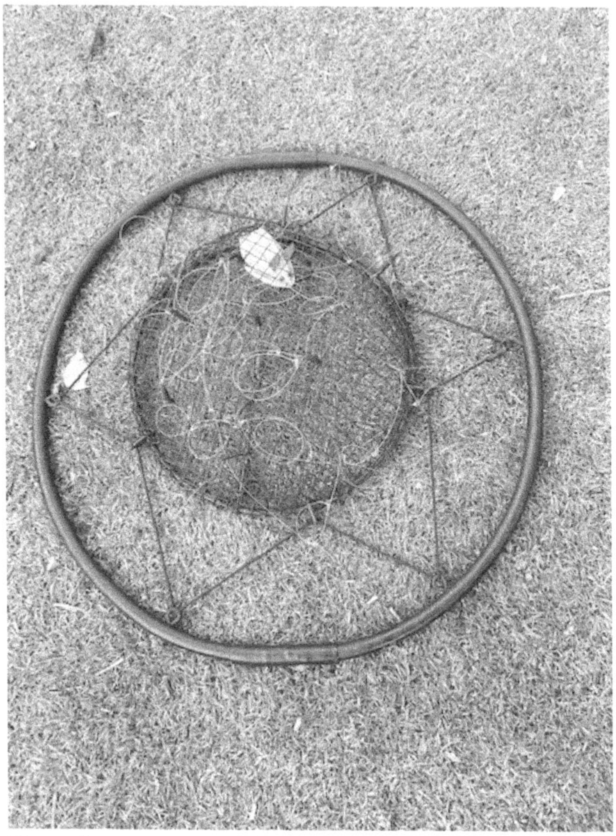

Figure 15.6: A saucer-shaped bal-chatri trap, with a toy mouse in the lure compartment for demonstration. Photo by Neil A. Hamilton.

Animal welfare considerations

Fatalities or injuries from entrapment

Traps are tailored to the target species. The height of a standing noose or foot snare and weight of the fishing line can be planned to minimise risk of strangulation or leg damage. Researchers should monitor traps continually during deployment. Personnel should be familiar with bird behaviour on capture, allowing them to 'read' the situation and approach a captured bird as quickly as possible. Fitness and mobility of the research team are paramount, and personnel should be positioned strategically to reach caught individuals quickly (i.e. no more than 15 s for noose carpets; M. Weston, pers. comm.). On reaching the trap, personnel should secure the bird in a bander's grip or another size-appropriate method before disentangling it. Clothing and equipment pose entanglement and crushing risks, so personnel should avoid having dangling and entangling items on them at the trap. Final checks should ensure nothing is entangled in the trap before lifting bird away from it. Traps and pegs should be removed immediately after use.

Capture of non-target species

A minimum of two people per trap is recommended, as personnel 'twinkling' (moving slowly towards the target animals, to encourage them to walk into the capture area) will potentially be too distant to monitor for non-target species. Noose carpets are pegged down sufficiently so that they do not lift away from the substrate when a bird is captured, based on average body mass of common species occurring at the trap location. Additionally, the carpet has a degree of flexibility to limit jarring legs of any captured birds. Trap placement should discourage non-target species from approaching traps, with non-target captures able to be released immediately. When capturing birds in a location with free-roaming dogs, additional observers should intercept dog owners before they approach the trapping area. With permission, signage erected at access points can be used to warn of research in progress.

Simultaneous multiple captures

Capture teams should consist of at least two people. Typically, one bird per handler is manageable for experienced personnel, but one person will be required to hold birds while the other extracts it from the trap. Where multiple birds become entangled, nooses can strain legs and feet. Traps should be unpegged to reduce any pressure on the birds' legs and feet from the noose/s. To reduce the risk of catching three or more birds simultaneously, flocks are encouraged away from the trap line.

Drowning

Trap placement mitigates the risk of inundation in tidal environments. Traps are set at least 2 m from the active swash zone. Researchers should also set markers well above the area in line with the trap, so if water washes across the trap, the trap can be relocated easily. Traps should be monitored continuously during deployment.

Extreme temperatures

Although captured birds are removed within minutes of capture, trapping when temperatures are < 10°C or > 33°C, and during periods of heavy rain, should be avoided. Forecasts and weather conditions should be monitored continuously on site. Personnel should seek shade or shelter when handling and processing birds to minimise the risk of hypothermia or hyperthermia.

Exposure to predators

Investigators should remain alert for avian and terrestrial predators that may be drawn to lures or captured birds. Personnel should scan for threats during all stages of the capture, including potential incursion by the public, dogs and vehicles. If a threat is detected twinkling should cease or release delayed until the threat has gone.

Use of live lures – fatality, injuries and stress

Where alternative sound and movement decoys (such as wind-up or battery-operated decoys, or articulated specimens (real or artificial) that move in the wind; or audio decoys – small portable speakers that play conspecific or prey species calls) do not work, live prey can be considered, with several animal welfare considerations (Bloom *et al.* 2007). When using live lures, juveniles and domesticated species (such as chickens, doves, mice and rats) are recommended as they are generally less stress prone than wild or adult animals. The compartment in the trap that houses the lure should be sufficiently large that target animals cannot reach in and injure the live lure. Lure animals should be removed as soon as traps are closed and housed in appropriate conditions between sessions (i.e. at a suitable temperature with adequate shade, food and water). Multiple trapping sessions should use different lure animals. Personnel must monitor the condition of lure animals and remove them if they exhibit signs of stress.

Disruptions to natural activities

Trapping only occurs during an active breeding event when the breeding individuals are the target of specific research; otherwise, actively breeding birds should be avoided. Trapping during the laying phase should be avoided at all costs because of the risk associated with handling egg-carrying females (i.e. rupturing the egg internally). Extra precautions should be taken to minimise disturbance to active nests or chicks. Only one of the incubating pair should be captured at a time, leaving the remaining bird to tend to the nest. Strict time limits minimise disruption to the breeding pair, so that nests are not abandoned for more than 40 min at a time. Under less favourable weather conditions this time limit should be reduced to 20 min or alternatively the trap repositioned well away from the nest. When chicks are present, only one of the breeding pair is caught, leaving the remaining partner with the brood.

General procedures

Planning

These techniques should be undertaken by or under the direct supervision of experienced investigators who are proficient in the capture and handling of wild birds. The required number of experienced researchers will vary depending on the capture environment, the anticipated number of captures and the intensity of any additional procedures. A minimum of two personnel is required per noose carpet array. Forecasts and tidal conditions should be checked to ensure conditions are appropriate. If targeting breeding birds breeding stage must be confirmed to minimise interference with breeding success.

Trap setting and duration

A thorough search of the trapping area will ascertain the presence of any active nests (of target and non-target species) or other hazards, particularly for beach-nesting birds. Traps should be positioned well away from these nests and activities not undertaken in proximity to incubating birds. Noose carpets can be pegged securely to the substrate and lightly dusted with sand to camouflage the 'carpet' (Figure 15.7). Noose carpets on beaches can be flanked by 'wings' of seaweed to encourage birds towards the trap. Bal-chatris with live lures should be placed on even ground and pegged securely (Bloom *et al.* 2007). Bal-chatris with artificial decoys can be operated similarly, but may also be dropped onto a track from a slow-moving vehicle under a likely perch to attract scavenging raptors. In this instance, the vehicle drives onwards, but not out of sight, with personnel watching closely to see if a target approaches the trap. With sufficient personnel, multiple traps can be deployed for general capture, but a single trap is best for targeting individuals. Trapping duration varies with objectives, target species and breeding cycle. All efforts should minimise disruption to normal activities, and care should be taken to target only one of the breeding pair on a given day to ensure the pair or family unit are not disturbed for > 40 min.

Twinkling and capture

Birds can be encouraged towards noose carpets by 'twinkling', where one or multiple personnel move slowly towards the target animals, at a pace that encourages them to walk in a particular direction, but not take flight (Standen *et al.* 2018). Continuous assessment of any active nests, condition of the noose carpet, tide/wave height, presence of predators/people/dogs, position of target bird and non-target birds is necessary. The twinkler should walk with appropriate direction and speed to bring birds level with the trap. Relaxed twinkling can occur until birds are within 15 m of the trap, but then pressure needs to be applied to ensure that they cross the trap line. Twinklers should maintain a close enough distance to ensure that they can reach the trap and settle the bird within 10 s of capture. When a non-target conspecific is captured, it is unlikely that the remaining birds will cross the existing trap line, so the trap line will usually need to be moved. Bal-chatris target visual predators, so twinkling is not required, but personnel should generally remain at a distance or in a nearby vehicle while surreptitiously monitoring the trap.

Extraction and processing

Personnel should approach birds from the direction that the bird entered the trap. Personnel can then place their hand over the bird, holding the bird in the bander's grip or a similar appropriate hold. Birds should not be lifted immediately, but rather personnel should feel carefully for entanglements, freeing the legs gently. A bird may be caught by multiple nooses/snares, so personnel should run a hand between the trap and bird to ensure that unseen entanglements have not occurred before lifting the bird. A sheet can be used to cover and calm live lure animals, and all traps and pegs should be removed from

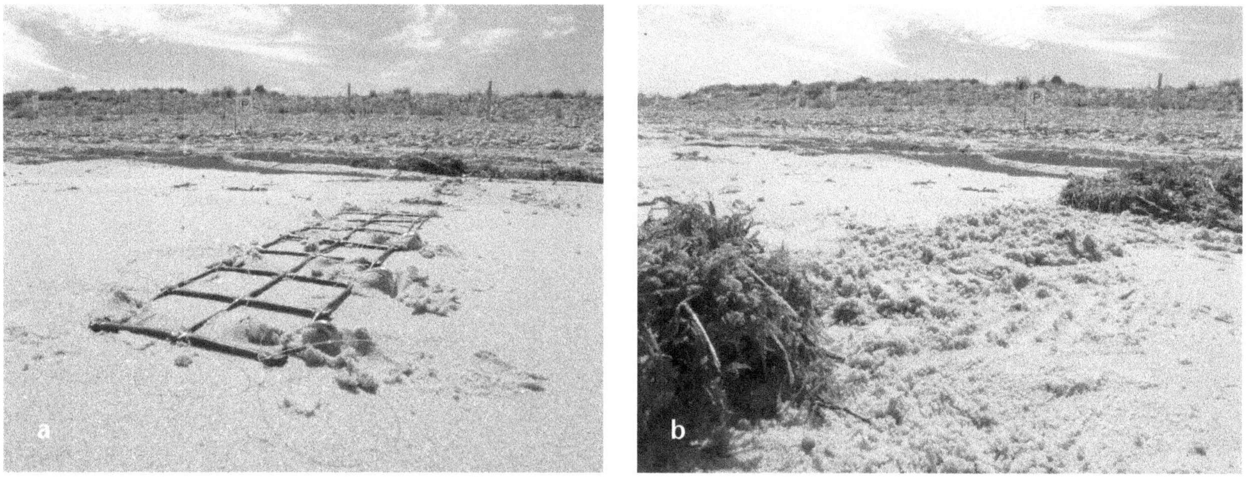

Figure 15.7: Close-up of a segment of a noose carpet for hooded plovers (*Thinornis rubricollis*) (a) pegged into the ground and camouflaged and (b) ready for capture. Photos by Grainne S. Maguire.

the trapping site. When multiple traps are deployed an audit should be conducted before departure. Traps must not be left unattended while processing occurs. Birds can be placed in holding bags for transport to a processing site (see Chapters 33–36 for transport details for different taxa). Lures should be removed from the trap and placed into sheltered holding facilities. Care must be taken to remove all traps at the end of the session as abandoned traps will continue to capture birds.

Animal treatment, withdrawal and euthanasia

If a bird is injured, but the injury does not impair walking or flight, it should be released immediately and monitored. If flight or walking is likely to be impaired and possibly inhibit a bird's survival, the individual should be placed in a clean cloth bag or dark box with non-slip flooring and transported to the nearest veterinarian or animal hospital, or euthanased (depending on the approved protocols). If a captured bird appears stressed at any time (e.g. with signs of lethargy, laboured or slowed breathing, or loss of motor control), processing must cease. The bird can be settled in a bird bag and released as soon as possible.

Equipment and maintenance

Equipment will vary depending on the species or taxa, local environment and study objectives. Fishing line will degrade over time so before each use nooses should be tested by pulling on each loop to check that they are still viable. Frames of traps should be checked for sharp edges. Typical equipment items may include:

- trap(s)
- decoys/lures
- tent pegs (to secure traps)
- spare fishing line (e.g. 0.22 mm, 2.7 kg, Maxima Ultragreen™ (0.009 inch, 6 lbs)) for noose repairs)
- mallet
- small scissors or quick-unpick tool
- bird bags/transport boxes (for captures and lures)
- binoculars
- two-way radios.

Specific qualifications, experience and training

The skills required to undertake trapping using foot snares, noose carpets or bal-chatris vary depending on sensitivity of the study species to the presence of humans and disturbance, and the nature of the study. Personnel should be competent with the technique proposed, familiar with the species or similar taxa, having undertaken similar work. Alternatively, personnel should be trained or supervised by someone who is. Personnel undertaking capture and banding will require an A-class ABBBS licence (basic capture methods endorsement, minimum).

Workplace health and safety

Refer to details in 'Nest and hollow inspections, including handling of eggs and chicks' earlier in this chapter.

Alternative procedures

Few alternative procedures exist for targeted trapping of ground-frequenting birds. If birds have an active nest, walk-in traps or spring traps offer an alternative, albeit with higher welfare risks to the nest itself. Cannon netting (see 'Cannon nets and other large propelled nets' later in this chapter) is another common shorebird capture technique. However, it is generally not feasible for capture in many locations (i.e. sites frequently used by the public) and when targeting low numbers or specific individual birds.

TECHNIQUES FOR INDIVIDUAL BIRD CAPTURE: SWEDISH GOSHAWK, BOW AND TOP-ENTRANCE CAGE TRAPS

Neil A. Hamilton and Tegan K. Douglas and Michael A. Weston

Target taxa

This GOP applies to all bird taxa (Chapters 33–36).

Context and scope

This GOP describes the use of highly targeted traps to catch individuals of a range of avian taxa, including Swedish goshawk, Larsen and other drop-in traps, bow, clap and hoop traps, and tip-top or top-entrance (Figure 15.8) treadle cage traps (Meng 1971; Bub 1991). Although sometimes differing in name and design, these traps all operate with similar principles. They all entice birds to approach the trap from above or beside with lures, bait or decoys. The operator or the bird triggers the trap, with spring-loaded components surrounding the bird in netting, or gravity-aided components, such as fall-away perches, which drop it into a compartment. Traps catch only one individual at a time, although treadle cage traps can be reset to catch multiple individuals. Trap size

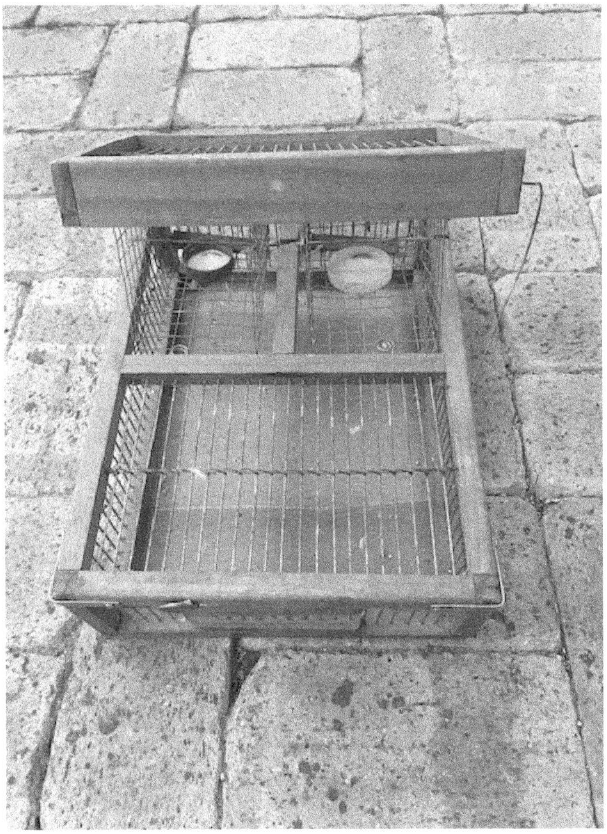

Figure 15.8: A handmade tip-top cage trap for catching small groups of gregarious passerines, such as fairy-wrens (*Malurus* spp.) or finches (*Taeniopygia* spp.). Small feed trays are positioned in each of the catch cages. Photo by Neil. A Hamilton.

and lure combination are matched to the target taxa. These methods are commonly used for visual hunters, such as owls, raptors and large passerines. Live lures (chickens, mice, pigeons, mealworms and other invertebrates) were traditionally used (Bub 1991), although are now often replaced with visual and audio decoys. Traps can also use seed, fresh seeding grasses and flowering plants to attract smaller granivores and nectarivores.

Animal welfare considerations

Fatalities or injuries in the trap

Trap size and construction materials should take into account the target species and be sized appropriately, so that moving mechanisms do not touch the bird as the trap closes. Mesh should be small enough that target animals cannot push their heads through the mesh, and traps should not have sharp edges. Sharp edges (e.g. on new traps) can be filed until smooth. Rounded designs are preferred and padding on the leading edge of the mechanism can minimise injury in the event of misfire. The trap should be heavy enough so that trapped birds cannot open the mechanism partially from the inside and are pegged into the ground or weighted down to minimise movement once caught. Personnel should watch traps from a hide or check them regularly.

Use of live lures: fatality, injuries and stress

See considerations for 'Foot snares, noose carpets and bal-chatris' earlier in this chapter.

Heat stress, exposure or injury

Trap placement should take into account ground temperature and sun exposure for the entirety of the trapping session, for the welfare of the target birds and any live lures. Traps should be checked at regular intervals and birds removed immediately once caught. Gloves can be worn to assist personnel in restraining the captured bird quickly and remove it from the trap.

Attracting predators or by-catch

Live lures, decoys and bait can all attract non-target species. Traps should be placed in areas with as little potential for by-catch as possible, and checked regularly or watched from a hide, to ensure that non-target animals do not approach them. Traps can be set on raised platforms (such as tables or roofs) to discourage terrestrial predators.

Disruptions to normal behaviour

Trapping may affect the welfare of trapped animals by interfering with their natural activities (breeding, feeding, social and territorial interactions), particularly if using audio decoys or callers (see 'Call playback and broadcast surveys' earlier in this chapter). Researchers should avoid trapping for extended periods in the immediate vicinity of active nests. Birds should be released as soon as possible after trapping and processing.

General procedures

Preliminary work

Knowledge of target species is critical for using these traps successfully and without adverse effects. To aid decisions about trap type (such as size, mechanism and lure/decoy/bait type), particularly where little work has been done on the study species previously, novel trap configurations can be trialled under controlled conditions. Pilot studies are best undertaken with captive birds initially, and in cooperation with local zoos or wildlife parks to test suitability with the target or an analogous species.

Site selection

Site knowledge and species habits will determine trap placement. Generally, traps should be placed in a shaded, but relatively open location, where birds can see the lure or decoy and approach from above or beside. Trapping should be undertaken in fine weather, with minimal wind and no extreme temperatures. Generally, early morning or late afternoon provide the best conditions, but timing is species-dependent. Trapping at night is suitable for nocturnal species. Trapping in public areas needs to be undertaken carefully and with consideration of the need for community involvement or awareness (see Chapter 3 for considerations around working in urban areas). Multiple traps can be deployed at once, but the overall number should be dictated by the time taken to complete a round of trap checks.

Trap set-up

Traps can be pegged in place and camouflaged. Ground mesh should be buried with sand or leaf litter, and any pebbles or sticks that may become potential projectiles and cause injury to birds should be removed. Lures or decoys should be installed. For baited traps using seed blocks or trays, tying bait or trays in place with cable tie or soft wire will ensure that seed/mealworms/bait will not tip out of the tray. Before vacating the trapping site, personnel should double-check the sensitivity of trigger mechanisms and confirm that moving parts will not snag on anything when triggered.

Checking traps

Where a hide is not used, traps should be checked at regular intervals – usually every 20–30 min depending on weather conditions (Lowe 1989). Where a hide is used, it should be installed in a position where personnel can view the trap, the lure and the approach of any targets or potential by-catch. When checking the trap, personnel should approach it quickly and quietly, and check the status of the lures each time. When a capture is made, large traps can be covered with a drop sheet to calm birds if necessary. Most traps have a hatch for quick removal of birds. Gloves can help personnel isolate birds in the trap and minimise damage from talons before placing them in a soft holding bag (DBCA 2017).

Trap closure or resetting

If a trap is not being reset, personnel should close it and remove lures or transfer them to holding accommodation before processing any captures. If resetting traps, personnel should check trap condition and make any repairs/adjustments. Any loose bait outside the food tray should be removed to minimise attraction of non-target species. The trap (including lure, decoy or bait) should be removed between trapping sessions and at the end of each trapping, and personnel should ensure that no components are left behind. Bags and covers can be used to store and transport traps to minimise the need for repairs.

Animal treatment, withdrawal and euthanasia

Researchers should monitor the situation continually. Where experienced personnel deem that treatment of the lure or target animal is necessary and possible, the animal should be taken to a veterinarian. Not all personnel will be able to transport animals to a veterinarian and doing so may result in additional stress and trauma to the animal. The principal researcher should plan for this scenario before trapping. Mortally injured animals should be euthanased by experienced personnel (or those under the supervision of experienced personnel) in line with established guidelines; also see details in Chapters 33–36. Necropsy of the animal in the field may be undertaken by experienced personnel if the cause of death is not obvious. Photographs or samples can be taken for follow-up or future research.

Equipment and maintenance

General equipment requirements are detailed in Table 15.1. Traps can comprise a variety of materials and should be suitably coloured to aid camouflage. Rounded edges and soft mesh or nylon netting is preferred. Net gauge should be small enough that birds cannot push their head or body parts through the mesh. Traps should have a latch that holds the trap closed once triggered.

Specific qualifications, experience and training

The skills required to undertake trapping-based studies vary depending on sensitivity of the study species to the presence of humans and disturbance, and the nature of the study. Personnel should be competent with the technique proposed, having undertaken similar work. Alternatively, personnel should be trained or supervised by someone who is. To be considered competent, personnel should have undertaken or been involved in at least one

Table 15.1: Suggested equipment and materials required for the installation and operation of traps.

Setting traps and hides	Checking traps	Processing and releasing animals	Maintenance
• Trap • Pegs • Mallet • Gloves • Lures • Decoys • Bait • Housing for live lures (e.g. food and water) • GPS • Stakes • Camouflage material • Ropes/tie downs • Chair • Binoculars/scope • First aid kit • Licence and permits • Processing tent	• Safety glasses • Gloves • Drop sheet • Handling bags • Transport boxes	• Callipers • Wing ruler • Tail ruler • Scales • Calico bags • Clipboards and data sheets • Bird identification guides • Bird marking implements • Solid container for animal transportation • Electrolyte and dropper • Hand sanitiser	• Cable ties • Gaffer tape • Spare string/mesh • Lubricant oil for trap mechanism • Screwdriver • Hammer • Pliers • Spare nails/screws • Small tool kit

study or project using the proposed techniques. Personnel may require appropriate licence qualification from the ABBBS.

Workplace health and safety

Manual handling and crushing injuries

Personnel follow standard procedures for manual handling. Bulky traps should be carried by multiple personnel. Care should be taken when placing traps, hammering in pegs, and setting triggers to avoid crushing injuries. For additional details refer to 'Nest and hollow inspections, including handling of eggs and chicks' earlier in this chapter.

Alternative procedures

These trapping methods are highly targeted towards focal species. Decisions about trap type (such as size, mechanism and lure/decoy/bait type) should be made to optimise time to capture and minimise by-catch. More-passive methods, such as mist nets (Chapter 7), are often unsuitable for these species, with low target capture rates and high numbers of by-catch common. Decoys can be used as an alternative to live lures. However, decoys may not be a reasonable substitute in all circumstances (i.e. some species are not attracted to decoys). Different types of decoys (or live lures) can be trialled on captive birds before commencing fieldwork.

CORRAL OR DRIVE TRAPS, AND BAITED FUNNEL AND CROW TRAPS

Tegan K. Douglas, Michael A. Weston, Amanda Lilleyman and Rosalind Jessop

Target taxa

The procedures described in this GOP are appropriate for gregarious ground-frequenting birds, such as corvids (Chapter 33), ducks, geese and pelicans (Chapter 35).

Context and scope

This GOP details the use of corral, drive, funnel and crow traps for the capture of flocks of medium to large ground-frequenting birds. Traps consist of static structures of net or mesh over or around a rigid frame. Funnel traps are usually discrete structures, but corral and drive traps are often erected *in situ*, to suit topography and target flock size. A funnel-shaped entrance encourages birds to walk, fly or swim into a smaller, often enclosed, holding area, where they have difficulty detecting the exit. A crow traps is a large cage with a funnel structure on the roof that permits birds to enter, but is difficult for them to exit (Shannon *et al.* 2014). Traps can be baited with grain, carrion or artificial decoys to passively attract captures, or trapping can occur when birds are undergoing their post-breeding moult and are not capable of flight, so personnel can drive or twinkle flocks towards the catching compartment on foot or by kayak. A door or hatch allows ready access to extract birds from the catching compartment, but can also be fixed open to acclimate birds. Traps are usually located on grasslands or near water, on lake edges or dam walls, or modified to sit on floating pontoons. Traps are often purpose built to suit bird and flock size (Bub 1991; Shannon *et al.* 2014). These methods are not suitable for capturing birds at breeding sites, because of the impact of extended total holding time on incubation and chick feeding routines.

Animal welfare considerations

Predation risk

Aggregations of birds in the traps can attract predators, including cats, foxes, raptors and crocodiles. Carefully considered trap placement, erecting traps in open areas away from dense shrubbery, perches, water edges can minimise the risk posed by predators (Bub 1991). As traps often stay in place for extended periods to allow target species to acclimate to their presence, evidence of predators (tracks, scats, prey remains and photographs) before and during trapping should be monitored. Physical exclusion, timing trapping when predators are inactive, and active deterrence of predators between trapping sessions helps deter persistent targeting by predators. Traps are not left unsupervised, even if observers watch from a distance.

Interruption to normal activities

Effective trap placement often coincides with identifying birds' natural loafing and aggregation locations. However, personnel should still aim to minimise interruption to birds' normal activities, such as feeding or bathing. Traps should be checked at regular intervals, with predetermined criteria determined for how frequently birds should be removed, processed and released.

Injury in trap

Traps should not have sharp internal edges, and have rounded edges rather than sharp corners where possible. Personnel should check traps regularly for sharp wires, and loose or torn mesh. Mesh size should be small enough so that birds cannot partially climb through, or get extremities stuck in holes. Trap roofs should be sufficiently tall so that birds can stand upright and in a normal posture, but low enough that they cannot take flight inside the trap. Traps should be installed on level ground and snagging hazards are removed.

Injury during extraction and holding

To minimise risk of injury during extraction, both from other captures and from the trap, removal of birds from the trap should happen quickly, with personnel moving quietly and efficiently. A shade cloth cover placed over the trap can be used to help quiet birds (Bub 1991). Appropriate handling techniques must be employed at all times (Chapters 33 and 35). For smaller catch sizes or calm species, processing can occur *in situ*. However, other species will need to be transferred to suitable temporary holding facilities, where they can be kept out of the weather at species-appropriate densities.

Environmental exposure

Traps leave birds exposed to the elements for extended periods. Even when traps are catching birds in their regular loafing locations, trap mesh will still increase humidity and reduces airflow. Trapping should only be undertaken during fine weather, avoiding high and low temperature extremes, high winds, rain and thunderstorms. Where possible, placing traps on light-coloured substrate or in the shade will reduce convective radiation.

Non-target or interspecific interactions

Baited traps can attract non-target species, including rodents, crabs or cattle. Removal of food between trapping sessions decreases attraction of other species, and thorough checking of trap area before the trapping session identifies the presence of potential non-target species in the vicinity. If antagonistic behaviours are observed between conspecifics caught in a trap, shifting timing of capture work to a different time of year, or adjusting trap size to accommodate natural distancing behaviours of target species may alleviate the issue.

Inundation and drowning risk

Where the funnel component of a drive trap is set in water, entanglement and drowning may occur in submerged trap components. Mesh should be taut, and mesh gauge should be such that birds will not become entangled under the water. Careful, deliberate movements must be used when driving or twinkling birds into the capture area, to avoid spooking them such that they dive or fly towards the net at speed (Bub 1991). Targeting aquatic species on the water's edge requires ongoing monitoring and assessment of changing water levels with tides and river flows. Traps should be placed well above the high tide mark and personnel monitoring traps remotely should also be able to assess water levels. If traps do become inundated, sufficient numbers of personnel must be on hand to 'walk' the trap onto dry land or the trap must have a hatch to allow quick release of trapped birds.

General procedures

Planning

Trap size and placement are tailored to the target species, so species and location knowledge are key to success. Reconnaissance is needed to observe natural behaviours of free-ranging birds, to determine loafing locations, flock sizes and natural spacing. Trapping should be planned for clement weather and outside of the breeding season.

Trap placement and set-up

Skittish species may take time to acclimate to the presence of the trap, so traps can be installed in advance of the capture session and potentially pre-baited, providing that access doors can be latched open to allow free movement. Traps should be placed on level ground and pegged firmly in place into the substrate (Figure 15.9). Personnel should check for sharp edges, loose mesh or dangling wires, or damage to mesh or netting. For baited traps, food should be placed into a tray for easy clean-up, and decoys installed. Multiple traps can be opened, but they must be able to be monitored easily and be readily accessible. A nearby monitoring location should be identified that provides a vantage point to observe the entire trap, possibly with the aid of binoculars or a scope.

Trap checking, driving and capture

Ideally, the trap is placed where it can be monitored from a distance without disturbing the flock. A predetermined capture interval or maximum flock size should be adhered to for passive traps, to avoid extending total holding time. Capture interval and maximum size are based upon project data requirements and tempered by personnel numbers, holding capacity, procedure processing time and total holding time. For drive traps, when a suitable flock has gathered, personnel can twinkle birds into the catch area. When birds are in the compartment, the capture time should be called and personnel should move quickly and quietly to the trap. The capture compartment can be covered with a shade cloth or sheet to calm birds during extraction and processing. Docile species can be removed individually and processed *in situ*, but for more-fractious species or extended procedures captures are removed and transported to keeping cages or boxes before processing. Holding facilities should provide shelter to personnel and captures from prevailing weather. Antagonistic species should be held individually, but otherwise small single-species groups can be held in uncrowded compartments. Compartments should be designed to facilitate natural standing postures of species and can take varied forms, from pet crates and other types of ventilated plastic crates, to collapsible shade cloth compartments dug into the substrate at the processing station (Chapter 35).

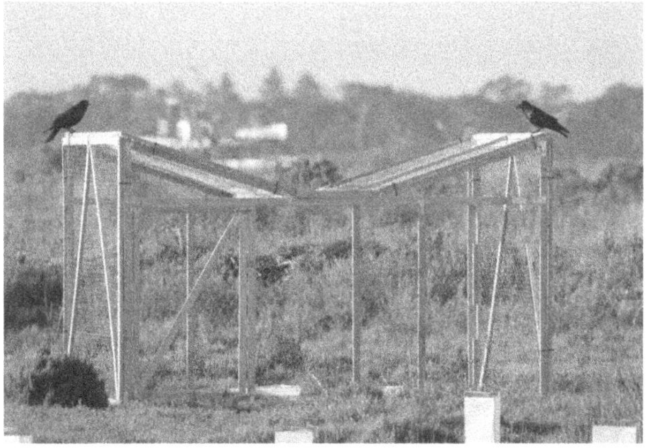

Figure 15.9: Little ravens (*Corvus mellori*) investigate an Australian crow trap. Photo by Michael A. Weston.

Multiple trapping events

If ongoing captures are planned, processing should occur at a nearby location to minimise ongoing capture site disturbance. Designated personnel should be responsible for monitoring the trap while processing occurs. For ongoing capture, after each cohort of targets is removed the trap should be thoroughly checked, maintenance conducted and bait refreshed.

Animal treatment, withdrawal and euthanasia

Investigators are responsible for overseeing capture and handling operations and must monitor activities undertaken by less-experienced personnel. When an injured bird is identified and where the investigator deems that the injury is treatable and possible, the animal should be taken to a veterinarian promptly. When transport to a veterinarian is not possible or if the bird is deemed untreatable, injured animals should be euthanased by experienced personnel on humanitarian grounds. A protocol for euthanasia should be developed before the commencement of the project; see also details in Chapter 35.

Equipment and maintenance

Equipment requirements will vary depending on the study objectives, species and specific method, but typically includes traps (fixed units) or trap construction materials, pickets/stakes, ropes, mallet, mesh/netting, hand nets, holding compartments, processing equipment, a bird hide and two-way radio. Holes in mesh can be repaired *in situ*, and all trap components should be checked for deterioration before and after trapping sessions, with unsound parts repaired or replaced.

Specific qualifications, experience and training

Key recommended competency requirements are listed in Table 15.2.

Workplace health and safety

Refer to details for 'Nest and hollow inspections, including handling of eggs and chicks' earlier in this chapter.

Alternative procedures

Where captures of large numbers of waterbirds are required few lower-impact methods exist. The methods detailed in this GOP facilitate individual identification of birds by capture, and subsequent banding allows the study of dispersal and migration, behaviour and social structure, life span and survival rates, reproductive success individual and subspecies variation, disease status and population dynamics. These data cannot be collected without capturing free-ranging animals.

CANNON NETS AND OTHER LARGE PROPELLED NETS

Rosalind Jessop, Tegan K. Douglas and Amanda Lilleyman

Target taxa

This GOP applies to ground-frequenting flocking birds, such as parrots and starlings (Chapter 33), and shorebirds (waders), ducks and geese, terns and gulls, cormorants and pelicans (Chapter 35).

Context and scope

This GOP describes the capture of birds with cannon and whoosh nets at resting or loafing sites, or pre-baited feeding sites, but does not cover use of projectile nets solely over water (see Chapter 35). Large rectangular nets are set by furling into a line (usually) directly onto the ground behind the catch area. With the back edge tethered and the front edge attached to weighted projectiles (cannon net) or with metal rings threading the sides of the nest onto to guide poles (whoosh net), the net is propelled over the birds gathered in the catching area. Cannon nets fire the projectiles simultaneously from two to four cannons powered by black powder, while whoosh nets use release of springs or bungee cord to launch the net. Catch sizes vary according to study objectives, and catches of up to 1000, but usually 100 to 350 birds can be made safely in many circumstances. This method is sometimes used for control of pest birds because it can catch many birds at once.

Table 15.2: Competency requirements for animal researchers undertaking corral, drive or funnel trapping.

Competency category	Competency requirement	Competency assessment
Catch team leader (catch site selection, catch oversight)	A-class licence (with basic capture methods endorsement as a minimum).	Experience in the environmental conditions of the catch, e.g. tropics, temperate climate, familiar with the mix of species likely to be caught. To be considered competent, personnel must have appropriate ABBBS endorsement and previously participated in or been involved in at least one project for the mix of species.
Trap set-up	A-class licence (basic capture methods endorsement, minimum). Others to be supervised.	To be considered competent, personnel must have appropriate ABBBS endorsement and previously participated in or been involved in at least one project for the mix of species, and with this capture method.
Bird extraction	A-class licence (basic capture methods endorsement, minimum). Others to be supervised.	To be considered competent, personnel must have appropriate ABBBS endorsement and have a wide experience in processing and appropriate handling techniques for the species likely to be caught.
Twinklers/herders	No experience necessary, but must be able to follow instructions from experienced personnel.	Nil.

Animal welfare considerations

Drowning

In wet catches (when catching birds next to water or on the incoming tide) the fired net could drown birds by holding them underwater. Careful planning, site assessment and reconnaissance mitigate drowning risk by informing understanding of catch site characteristics and bird behaviour, tide, swell, wave height and wind at net firing. Team leaders should select appropriate net lengths and mesh sizes for the species and location, check for adverse substrates (e.g. sticky mud) and clear snagging hazards during net setting (Bub 1991). Where wet catches are likely, agile runners are assigned to enter the water to retrieve nets for wet catches and remove projectiles quickly. A suitably sized team (i.e. minimum of one person per 3.5 m of net), with experienced personnel evenly spread, enables efficient 'tenting' of small-mesh nets to quickly walk birds onto sand, or rapid lifting of large-mesh nets to move birds to dry areas in one movement. Nets should not be fired if > 20% of the catch area is inundated unexpectedly.

Collision

Birds may be struck and killed by the flying net, ropes or projectiles. Partial misfire can cause ropes and projectiles to be dragged across the catching area (Bub 1991). Risks can be mitigated by setting nets to suit weather and location conditions, using easily visible distance markers, and testing circuits and wiring before firing. Personnel should know the location of safety markers and monitor nets continuously, and never fire if birds are airborne over catch area, on the net or in the safety zone. A jiggler line (a piece of string with fabric flags, loosely arranged in the danger area immediately in front of a set cannon or whoosh net and trailed back to a hide where it can be slowly reeled in by personnel) can be used to discourage birds from the safety area. Nets should be constructed to incorporate sufficient slack when roped to prevent birds being flattened to the ground.

Injury (crushing, broken bones, lacerations)

Birds can be injured when the net is fired or when they are caught under the net and flapping, and are particularly susceptible to feather abrasion when in peak moult (Coxen *et al.* 2018). Tangled birds can be seriously injured if not extracted properly. Personnel roles during extraction should be preassigned, with birds extracted by qualified personnel, monitoring continuously for bird safety and handling. When lifting or moving nets, care should be taken not to drag birds across substrate, looking for entanglements that might result in injury before movement. In temperate areas, covering material, if used, should be lifted, not dragged, across the birds/net, stretched tight and placed over the birds in the net. In the tropics, shade material must be held above the net at all times, and radiant heat from substrate must be considered. No-one should walk/stand on the net or covering material. Transport boxes and bags should be moved carefully, carried level or with bags carried around the neck or wrist, adhering to species protocols (e.g. individual containment for species like gull-billed terns). The fabric sides of keeping cages need to be kept taut so that birds do not become entangled in the fabric folds, and so that personnel cannot accidentally crush birds when kneeling nearby. Internal mesh flaps of keeping cages are always kept covered with sand to prevent toenail loss.

Thermal stress

Birds can suffer thermal stress during capture, holding or processing. Thermal stress is mitigated by determining upper and lower operating temperature limits for capture sessions appropriate for the geographical location. Shading birds in the net during extraction, or using a covering material can mitigate thermal extremes in the net, but temperatures and birds are still monitored continuously. Shaded keeping cages may be erected in the cool of the day to maintain low internal temperatures, but their placement must enable cages to receive suitable airflow. To mitigate against hypothermia, wet birds should be warmed and allowed to dry before release; wet birds must not be left sitting alone in keeping cages.

Stress and capture myopathy

Birds can suffer stress if overcrowded and excessive or inappropriate handling occurs, with birds most susceptible immediately before migration. To reduce the risk of myopathy, particularly in long-legged species, species should be separated in keeping cages of appropriate height for normal standing posture and at an appropriate density. Researchers should use the least harmful handling techniques, such as keeping legs and feet dangling when processing birds. Birds are always processed in priority order. For example, sensitive species first, longer-legged species or individuals that have been held the longest, with personnel looking for stress indicators, such as closed eyes. Shorebirds are not held for longer than 4 h, although limits for other species vary (de Beer *et al.* 2001). Birds are released by placing them on the ground, allowing them to walk first and then fly, from a blind if necessary. Personnel should check for predators such as raptors before releasing birds.

Disruptions to normal activities and predation

Catching birds at loafing sites allows capture and processing to occur while birds are normally less active. Using keeping cages allows birds to still engage in some loafing activities, such as preening. Processing should take place in a timely manner, and birds released appropriately. Individual or injured birds can be susceptible to attack by raptors immediately on release. Personnel should not release birds immediately after processing if raptors are nearby, instead holding them temporarily until the predator has moved away and then releasing them in groups. Persistent or habituated raptors can be avoided by taking captured birds to an alternative nearby location for release.

By-catch

Nets should not be fired if non-target species are in the catch area that may be damaged by the net firing (i.e. tall birds in a catch targeting shorter birds) or damage other birds in the net. Otherwise, once extracted, by-catch can be released immediately from the capture site without holding or processing, provided it is safe to do so.

General procedures

Planning and preparation

Using propelled nets is a complex procedure that should only be undertaken by experienced researchers with relevant ABBBS accreditation. Firearms licences may be required for storage, transport, and use of black powder when cannon netting. Standen *et al.* (2018) outlines detailed procedures for cannon netting. Several procedural considerations are more relevant for this method than for other capture techniques because of the potential for a large number of birds to be captured in a single event. Team size and skill composition, thorough preparatory work and communication lines, and a clear catch protocol that has been articulated to all personnel are essential elements to effective cannon netting. Assignment of team roles before catches ensures sufficient spread of expertise across roles and clear knowledge of required duties at all stages.

Target species and site knowledge will inform appropriate method, net set-up and placement decisions. However, set-up is done without knowing the eventual catch size and species composition, so sufficient allowance is necessary to house and process large or diverse catches. Tidal heights and weather conditions may vary from forecasts, so the catch protocol should clarify operating limits under different scenarios. Excess birds may be released at the catch site if they cannot be processed within an acceptable timeframe. A general site safety assessment for birds and personnel should be completed before final site selection. Cannons require advance preparation of charges, and all electrical equipment should be tested before each catch, and circuits tested once the net is set. Nets, keeping cages, bungee cords and other equipment should always be checked for wear and repaired if necessary.

Catch set-up

Set-up involves multiple tasks, with one, sometimes two, nets set simultaneously (Standen *et al.* 2018). Specific net placement should consider weather and tide conditions at the likely firing time. Once in place, all net and firing equipment should be double-checked by a single person, for consistency and accountability. Teams should also erect hides and firing positions within easy net access, and set up a processing station nearby with keeping cages and identify release site/s.

Firing the net and extraction

Once set, personnel should vacate the area to position themselves at firing positions, in bird hides, or simply out of sight to allow birds to return. This process may take up to 5 h. Personnel may twinkle birds towards nets (Figure 15.10a, b), but nets should never be fired unless sufficient personnel are able to reach nets and extract birds quickly. Clear communication from the firing position ensures that safety protocols are maintained. Personnel should mobilise quickly after the net has been fired to cover or shade birds, move the net from the water if needed, extract birds (Figure 15.10c) and transfer birds to keeping cages at the processing site. Location of required equipment (keeping cages, covering material and transport boxes) and responsibilities for getting these to the nets should be determined in advance and communicated to the whole team.

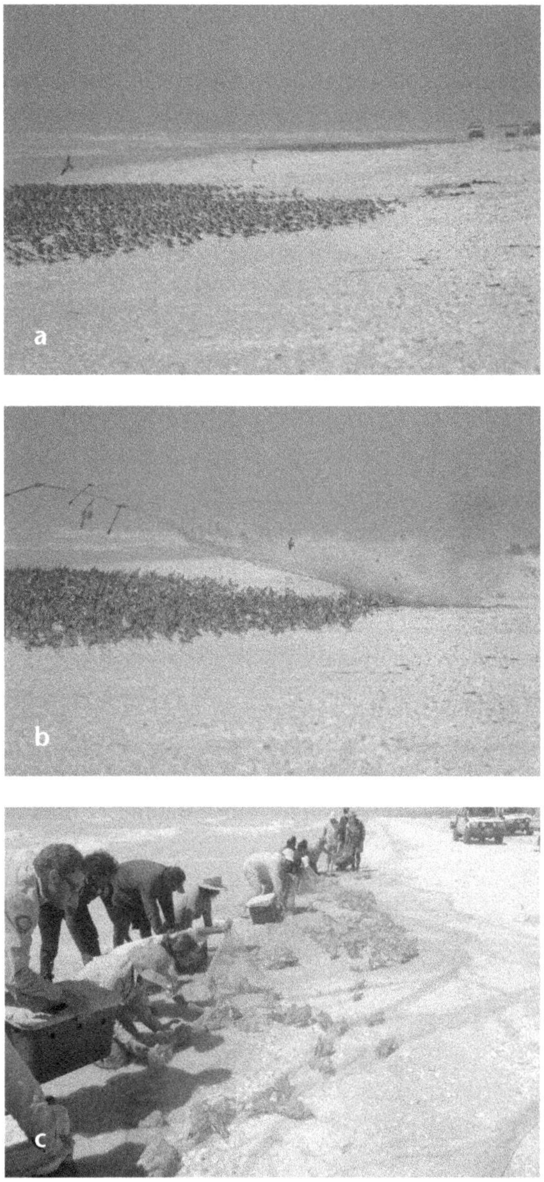

Figure 15.10: (a) Vehicles twinkle from both ends of the beach to concentrate flocks of birds (in this instance, mostly wader species, order Charadriiformes) in front of the set and camouflaged cannon nets. Nets will not be fired if birds are in flight above the catch area or are in the 'danger zone' immediately in front of the furled net. Photo by Prue Wright. (b) When the tide and the twinklers have pushed the birds into the catching area, but no birds are in the firing line, the cannons are fired. The trajectory of the projectiles launches the net over the roosting flocks. All personnel mobilise to the catch area to extract birds. Photo by Prue Wright. (c) The team works together to quickly extract the birds (a mixed flock capture, including bar-tailed godwit, *Limosa lapponica*; common greenshank, *Tringa nebularia*; great knot, *Calidris tenurostris*; red knot, *Calidris canutus*; and curlew sandpiper, *Calidris ferruginea*), experienced personnel securing and disentangling the birds, and placing them in species-specific holding boxes, for transfer to a sheltered processing area. Photo by Olivia Gourley.

Holding and processing

Birds should be transferred to species-specific holding cages at species-specific densities. Small teams can be allocated a species to process, and animal welfare monitored at all stages. Designating an animal welfare officer who checks bird status before release can streamline the process. Keeping cages should be checked thoroughly before removal. No equipment should be left in the catching or processing area once the activity is complete.

Animal treatment, withdrawal and euthanasia

Euthanasia or treatment protocols must be incorporated into the pre-planning of any project. Personnel with appropriate training and experience in euthanasia techniques must be present in the field and the closest suitable veterinary practice identified (if the primary investigators choose to seek treatment for injured birds). Triggers for euthanasia or treatment typically include injuries such as a broken wing or pelvis, capture myopathy (long term), crush injuries, or unresolved head trauma. Refer to Chapters 33–36 for further details on euthanasia techniques.

Equipment and maintenance

Equipment will vary depending on the species or taxon, local environment, and study objectives. Detailed equipment needs are outlined in Standen *et al.* (2018) and Blythman (2017). Since catch efforts are often undertaken in remote locations, sufficient spares, repair materials and tools should be kept on hand. The capacity to communicate with personnel (via handheld or vehicle VHF radio) is also essential.

Specific qualifications, experience and training

The skills required to undertake cannon netting vary depending on the role to be undertaken by the team member. Suggested competency levels for principal researchers are listed in Table 15.3.

Workplace health and safety

Transport of nets, preparing of catching area

Care should be taken when transporting nets as injury can result from manual handling (back injury, strains, sprains). To help limit manual handling, the vehicle should be positioned as closely as possible to work area. Use of several persons to move net and use stretcher will also help reduce the likelihood of injury.

Table 15.3: Competency requirements for animal researchers undertaking cannon net procedure.

Competency category	Competency requirement	Competency assessment
Selection of catch site	A-class licence (with endorsement for cannon netting).	Experience in the environmental conditions of the catch, e.g. tropics, temperate climate, familiar with the mix of species likely to be caught. Personnel should state clearly the nature of their previous experience (including taxa worked with and approximate months/years). To be considered competent, personnel must have appropriate ABBBS endorsement and previously participated in or been involved in at least one project for the mix of species.
Basic set-up tasks: furling, pegging, camouflage	A-class licence (basic capture methods endorsement, minimum). Others to be supervised.	Sufficient A-class licence holders present to supervise others.
Advanced net-setting tasks: wiring cannon, setting angles, checking set-up	A-class licence with cannon net endorsement, firearms licence (some states).	A-class licence with cannon net endorsement.
Hide team support, reporting on species and number of birds present in catching area	A-class licence (basic capture methods endorsement, minimum). Others to be supervised.	Experience in species identification and counting birds in flocks for the geographical location.
Final decision on net fire	A-class licence with cannon net endorsement.	Personnel should have experience in the environmental conditions of the catch, e.g. tropics, temperate climate, familiar with the mix of species likely to be caught. Personnel should state clearly the nature of their previous experience (including taxa worked with and approximate months/years). Experience in at least one project for the mix of species.
Supervise procedures at net, move out of water, extraction, transport	A-class licence with cannon net endorsement.	As above.
Help move net out of water	A-class licence (basic capture methods endorsement, minimum). Others to be supervised.	Personnel should be able to follow instructions.
Help take birds from under net and put in transport boxes, basic tasks	ABBBS licence holder (A or C).	Personnel should have experience in the species identification for the geographical location.
Take birds from net if entangled	ABBBS A-class licence.	Only A-class licence holders.
Transport keeping boxes to keeping cages, transfer birds from transport boxes to keeping cages	A-class licence (basic capture methods endorsement, minimum). Others to be supervised.	No experience, close supervision by A-class licence holders.
Supervision of keeping cages and bird welfare - Keeping Cage Controller	ABBBS A-class licence.	Personnel should have experience in the species identification for the geographical location and be able to identify birds in distress.
Assisting to monitor bird welfare	A-class licence (basic capture methods endorsement, minimum). Others to be supervised.	Personnel should have experience in the species identification for the geographical location and be able to identify birds in distress.
Supervision of processing team (with guidance of Catch Commander)	A-class licence (basic capture methods endorsement, minimum). Others to be supervised.	Personnel should have a wide experience in processing the species likely to be caught.

Using cannon net device

Burns and injuries may occur from accidental firing of cannon or cannon net. Only qualified personnel should undertake tasks as the catch protocol. Visitors must be kept off site by the 'spotter' or supervised closely.

Bites, scratches and disease exposure

Refer to details for 'Nest and hollow inspections, including handling of eggs and chicks' earlier in this chapter. When needed, personnel can wear rubber or latex gloves that can be disinfected or disposed of. Wearing protective eyewear when working with larger gulls and terns is advised. Personnel should not eat, drink, or smoke while handling birds, and should wash hands thoroughly after handling birds.

Alternative procedures

Individual identification of birds by capture and banding allows the study of dispersal and migration, behaviour and social structure, life span and survival rates, reproductive success individual and subspecies variation, disease status and population dynamics. Cannon netting allows the capture of large numbers of birds at once and is relatively quick and efficient if undertaken by experienced personnel. However, researchers should consider if other trapping methods (see other GOPs in this chapter) may be more appropriate for answering research questions and will reduce impacts on target species.

INDIVIDUAL AND COHORT MARKING

Tegan K. Douglas, John Porter, Michael A. Weston and Neil A. Hamilton

Target taxa

This GOP applies to all bird taxa (Chapters 33–36).

Context and scope

This GOP outlines the application of individual or cohort marking techniques for birds (Figure 15.11). It includes markers such as ABBBS-issue, individually numbered leg bands, readable leg and neck bands, cohort and individual coloured leg bands (metal and plastic), engraved and plain leg flags, wing (patagial) tags, and marks such as plumage dyes and leg stains. Flipper bands and tags are no longer considered acceptable for marking wild penguins, although they are still useful for individual identification of captive animals. Passive integrated transponder (PIT) tags are used instead. Chapter 8 details general principles for using PIT tags. Methods for applying flipper tags are not covered in this GOP. Apart from observational surveys, banding is one of the most commonly performed scientific activities that involves capturing birds and releasing them unharmed. The ABBBS database shows that wetland birds and seabirds together comprise more than three-quarters (78%) of the 10 most commonly banded bird species in Australia (Table 15.4). Different marks and markers are appropriate for different taxa dependent on size, morphology, colouration and ecology. Birds retain these for the medium or long term, and sometimes permanently. Repeated captures or resightings of marked birds provide information on longevity, movement and dispersal, acquisition of ageing and sexing characteristics, and facilitate field behavioural studies and citizen science projects on wild bird populations. They are also used to identify individuals held in captivity for research and husbandry.

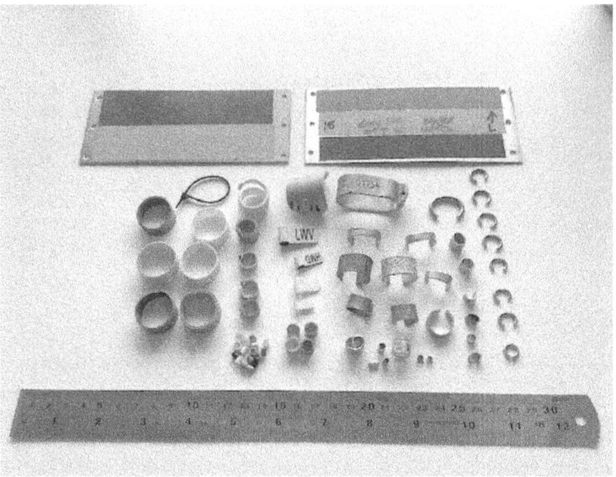

Figure 15.11: A selection of individual and cohort markers (left to right), including colour bands of various sizes, a nasal saddle, engraved and plain leg flags, ABBBS-issue bands and donna bands, with colour bands for emus at the top. Photo by Neil A. Hamilton.

Animal welfare considerations

Marking birds is associated with a range of potential animal welfare impacts (Table 15.5) that can largely be mitigated by ensuring that personnel are experienced, handling time is minimised, and the selected method is appropriate to the species.

Table 15.4: Ten most commonly banded bird species in Australia from highest to lowest numbers banded.

ABBBS data; collated June 2020.

Common name	Number of banding records		
	Wetland bird	Seabirds	Bushbirds
Crested tern		242 985	
Silvereye			174 232
Red-necked stint	168 518		
Silver gull	137 410		
Short-tailed shearwater		123 271	
New Holland honeyeater			106 353
Little penguin		99 889	
Wedge-tailed shearwater		92 692	
Pied cormorant	69 673		
Straw-necked ibis	56 948		
Total	432 549	558 837	280 585
%	34%	44%	22%

Disruption to normal behaviour during capture, processing and release

Researchers should process and release animals quickly and efficiently to minimise interference to natural activities. Where multiple species are caught in the same capture effort, stress-prone species should be processed first. In mixed cohort captures, incubating adults or dependent young should be prioritised over others, with territorial species and dependent young released at the capture site. Birds need to be released during their active period. However, diurnal birds can be held overnight or nocturnal birds held during the day in suitable holding facilities if they cannot be released immediately (de Beer *et al.* 2001).

Injury and stress during handling

Researchers should monitor birds' health and stress levels throughout the marking process. Stress ratings are available for some species (de Rebeira 2006), but handlers must remain alert for visible signs of distress (e.g. excessive flapping of wings, closed eyes, drooping heads). Handling is minimised by having appropriate holding arrangements for multiple birds, with researchers only removing birds from containment for processing. Visibly stressed individuals should be released as quickly as possible, and can be offered an electrolyte solution (on a clean spoon or with an eye-dropper) before release.

Injury caused by applying the marker

Marks and markers must only be applied by, or under the supervision of qualified personnel. Only the appropriately sized marker should be applied to a species (ABBBS 2000). Almost all band-related injuries can be avoided with an efficient processing station (including appropriate storage of marking equipment between sessions), and by researchers paying close attention when applying bands and tags. Individual birds with pre-existing injuries should be assessed carefully before any mark or marker is applied; marking may be abandoned if the primary investigator decides that doing so would worsen the injury. Dyes or paints must be non-toxic and allowed to dry completely before release of the marked individual.

Snagging, damage or increased predation risk

Bands and tags should be fully closed and any joins or seals checked before release. Little evidence is available to suggest that appropriately fitted bands cause snagging risk or impede movement; however, the band/flag/tag may wear in a manner that poses some risk to certain species (Griesser *et al.* 2012). Markers must be constructed of a suitably robust material for the conditions they will be subjected to. Where recaptures or resightings suggest that the mark or marker is affecting survivorship, researchers should reassess the marking method before additional individuals are marked. Deteriorating markers should be removed or replaced on recaptured birds. Dyes or paints should be applied to ventral surfaces or other parts of the body that do not increase visibility to predators.

General procedures

Planning

Researchers should consult with and adhere to advice issued by the ABBBS, which oversees all aspects of bird banding, including the issue of metal bands, reports on moratoria of marking materials for particular species, and tracks the use of colour-banding schema on wild bird populations. Colour combinations of leg flags used on shorebirds and seabirds form part of an international cooperative project that must be adhered to (East Asian Australasian Flyway Partnership 2020). Personnel should review the extensive literature on marking

Table 15.5: Potential animal welfare impacts issues to consider for marking and attaching devices to wetland birds.

Calvo and Furness (1992); Sharp *et al.* (2007).

Animal welfare issue	Potential cause and impacts	Mitigation
Pain	Discomfort (short or long-term) and injury from incorrect application of tags, bands or harnesses.	Training and experience in handling.
Stress and shock (capture myopathy)	From handling and marking. Impacts of capture myopathy may vary from temporary incapacitation to rapid physiological decline and mortality.	Marker design appropriate to species. Training and experience in handling to reduce time. Species-specific handling requirements.
Infection	Arising from skin damage from tags and collars. From transferal of infectious disease by researchers between individuals.	Correct training and fitting of appropriate markers. Proper hygiene controls.
Impaired mobility, chafing, constriction or limb or digit loss or deformity	From poorly designed, incorrectly sized and fitted or damaged bands, collars and harnesses. May cause loss of condition or reduced breeding success. From removal of feathers for sampling or device attachment.	Appropriate markers correctly designed and fitted.
Toxicity	From paints, dyes and other markers.	Evidence of non-toxicity to target species.
Increased aggression or predation	Aggression from conspecifics or predation risk from increased visibility.	Evidence of successful deployment without adverse effects.
Decreased ability to feed or capture prey	From impaired movement or because prey animals may be more aware of the marked animal's presence.	Correct training and fitting of appropriate markers.
Inhibition or alteration of normal behaviours	From altered visual appearance or poorly fitted marker.	Correct training and fitting of appropriate markers.
Entanglement	Of tags, bands collars and harnesses on vegetation, branches or debris resulting in injury or immobilisation.	Correctly fitted species appropriate markers.

studies, including potential for adverse effects on study species, during study design. When using a novel application of marks and markers (e.g. on a previously unstudied species or a temporary marker made from a novel substance), researchers should review the literature thoroughly, and consider testing the method on an analogous captive species or testing the long-term visibility of the marker colour or material under similar environmental conditions in advance of the study. Coloured and engraved markers must be distinguishable under field conditions and distances, and remain so for the duration of the study.

Pre-capture

The 'processing station' or similar should be set up before the first bird is captured. Clean equipment should be laid out for ease of use, and roles within the team determined. For smaller catch efforts, particularly of single species, equipment may be held on hand in a toolbox or similar, for immediate processing *in situ*.

Holding pre-marking

Passerines can be held in soft holding bags (DBCA 2017), suspended on a rope or rack, in shade and out of the wind. Larger birds may be contained more effectively in a box (Bub 1991), or in shade cloth compartments on the ground. Multiple individuals must not be held in the same compartment or container unless they have plenty of space and are unlikely to be antagonistic towards each other. Where birds are delivered to the banding station continuously, researchers should ensure that birds are processed in the order that they arrive.

Marking

Birds that cannot be identified to species should not be marked. Only appropriately sized bands should be applied to each species – nestlings may have larger tarsus widths than adult birds, but must not be given a larger-sized band or flag (ABBBS 2000), even where evidence of nestlings losing bands exists (Lees *et al.* 2017). Likewise, young of dimorphic species that cannot be sexed should not be banded if the female and male require differently sized bands. Generally the marker should be applied before any other processing or procedures are undertaken (Sutherland *et al.* 2004). Smaller birds will be held and processed by the same researcher, while larger species may require one person to hold the bird, and the second to apply the mark. Stress-prone species can be partially covered (in a bag or with a hood), to keep them calm during marking and processing.

Different marker types have different application methods. For leg bands and flags the broad process is as follows:

- Metal ABBBS butt-ended bands are applied by five-hole or two-hole pliers, or flanged/lock-on bands with flat-nosed pliers, following Lowe (1989). They are generally applied in a two-step method, although band material stainless steel bands require a different process, following established guidelines (i.e. Lowe 1989; de Rebeira 2006; FAO 2007).
- Small coated-metal colour bands are applied as above. Larger-flanged aluminium colour bands are riveted on. Split stainless steel wire 'donna' bands (for large parrots) are applied with specialised pliers.
- Small split-ring plastic colour bands are applied using a small metal shoehorn to open the band, resting the concave edge of the shoehorn along the bird's tarsus, before sliding the band off the shoehorn onto the bird's leg.
- Readable bands have a vertical split with a small overlap and are opened with circlip pliers to place on the leg.
- Larger rolled colour bands are applied by unravelling and re-rolling the band, with the outside end rolled in a new loop around the birds' leg, then the remainder of the band rolled around it, like a cassette tape.
- The flanges of leg flags are held open just enough to slide over the leg of the bird.

All plastic bands and flags generally need to have their edges sealed. Depending on the band material, sealing can be done with a dab of Super Glue^{TM}, solvent or a soldering iron. Care should be taken to hold the mark closed while the sealant dries, avoiding contact with feathers, limbs or the handler. All birds fitted with a colour band of any description must also be given a standard ABBBS-issue metal band.

Patagial (wing) tags have been trialled in various sizes and materials, but generally consist of a numbered or lettered metal tag held in place by a rivet through the patagium (Sutherland *et al.* 2004; Martin and Major 2010). Their use on migratory birds, such as ducks and gulls in the Northern Hemisphere, and Carnaby's black-cockatoo in Australia, has resulted in some negative effects (Saunders 1988; Brua 1998; Varland *et al.* 2007; Trefry *et al.* 2013). However, Martin and Major (2010) found that patagial tags were suitable for use on Australian white ibis (*Threskiornis moluccus*) despite recording some negative effects in smaller bird species. Their continued use is the subject of much debate (Trefry *et al.* 2013), and their use versus other marking methods should be assessed carefully.

Neck bands and collars are often used on long-necked birds, such as swans and geese, enabling long-distance identification when birds are swimming (Figure 15.12; MacInnes and Dunn 1988; Johnson and Sibly 1989). Collars consist of durable plastic with a vertical slit that is held open while placed around the birds' necks. When closed the band has a small overlap where sealant is applied to finish. These markers have been used widely in the Northern Hemisphere for decades, primarily on geese and swans (Menu *et al.* 2000; Reed *et al.* 2005). In Australia they have been used on black swans (*Cygnus atratus*) successfully (Guay and Mulder 2009).

Generally, dyes and pains are applied to white or pale parts of the plumage or to legs, with colour and/or numbers providing individual mark combinations. Materials vary but must be non-toxic, and substances should be dry before birds are released to avoid accidental ingestion (Sutherland *et al.* 2004). Other markers, such as nape tags, nasal saddles and disks, streamers and web markers, have been used in the Northern Hemisphere, but their use in Australia remains limited. General principles of PIT tag application are described in Chapter 8, with additional details for aquatic birds in Chapter 35.

Pre-release checks

All markers should be checked before release. Any glue, solvent or dye must be dry. Bands and flags should move smoothly on the limb, without affecting joints. No feathers should be caught in the joins or seals of the markers. For colour combinations and engraved flags, a final check will help to ensure that correct combinations have been used and all necessary data recorded. Colouring metal bands with a black marking pen can reduce their visibility and may help minimise the risk of nest eviction of banded nestlings by adults.

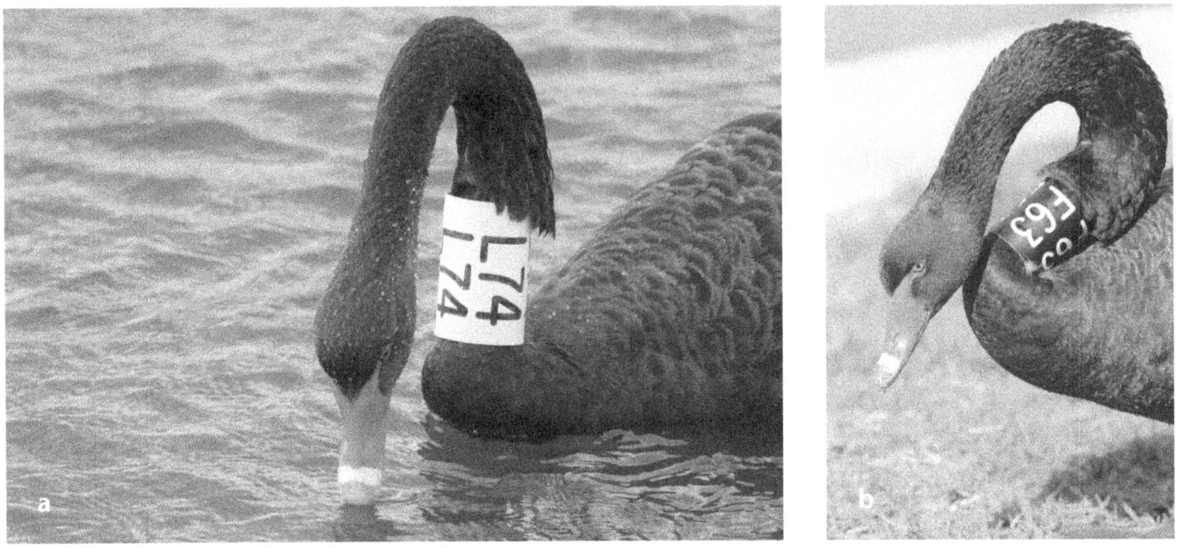

Figure 15.12: Black swans fitted with neck collars. Photos by Michael A. Weston.

Animal treatment, withdrawal and euthanasia

Researchers should monitor the situation continually. Where experienced personnel deem that treatment is necessary and possible, the animal should be taken to a suitably qualified veterinarian. Not all personnel will be able to transport animals to a veterinarian and doing so may result in additional stress and trauma to the animal. Mortally injured animals are euthanased by experienced personnel (or those under the supervision of experienced personnel) in line with established protocols. Necropsy of the animal in the field may be undertaken by experienced personnel if the cause of death is not obvious. Personnel must assess whether birds with pre-existing (healed) injuries, such as missing toes, joint damage or leg scarring, can be marked safely with no effect on survivorship. Where the marker touches an injured join or/limb or would exacerbate the healed scar, and the animal cannot be marked on an alternate limb, the bird should be released without being marked, or in the case of a re-trapped bird, the marker removed and not replaced.

Equipment and maintenance

General equipment requirements are detailed in Table 15.6. Equipment should be kept clean and checked for function and condition before each marking session. Keeping equipment in a toolbox or other container assists with keeping equipment clean and organised.

Suitability of colours, materials and/or flag engraving methods needs to be assessed over time as they become worn and will deteriorate. Re-trapping previously marked

Table 15.6: General equipment requirements for marking birds.

Animal holding and processing	Applying bands	Processing and releasing animals	Trap maintenance
• Callipers • Wing ruler • Tail ruler • Scales • Calico bags • Clipboards and data sheets • Bird identification guides • Bird marking implements • Containers for animal holding • Electrolytes and dropper • Hand sanitiser • Licenses and permits	• Banding pliers • Band sealant • Unbanding pliers • Safety glasses • Gloves • Drop sheet • Handling bags • Transport boxes	• Callipers • Wing ruler • Tail ruler • Scales • Calico bags • Clipboards and data sheets • Bird identification guides • Bird marking implements • Solid container for animal transportation • Electrolytes and dropper • Hand sanitiser	• Cable ties • Gaffer tape • Spare string/mesh • Lubricant oil for trap mechanism • Screwdriver • Hammer • Pliers • Spare nails/screws • Small tool kit

birds provides the opportunity to check for band/flag/tag wear, confirm no injuries have arisen. Recapturing marked individuals provides an opportunity to replace illegible or worn markers, and assess longevity of marker materials in the study environment.

Specific qualifications, experience and training

Personnel should be competent with the technique proposed and familiar with the species or similar taxa having undertaken similar work. Alternatively, personnel should be trained or supervised by someone who is. To be considered competent, personnel should have undertaken or been involved in at least one study or project using the proposed techniques. Personnel undertaking banding will need to have at least an A-class ABBBS licence or be supervised by someone who does. Training in the insertion of PIT tags is required if this technology is used for species unsuited to ABBBS bands.

Workplace health and safety

Refer to details for 'Nest and hollow inspections, including handling of eggs and chicks' earlier in this chapter.

Alternative procedures

If study objectives rely on the identification of individuals or cohorts, then few alternatives exist. Mark and marker type, material and colour can influence animal welfare outcomes substantially, although responses vary markedly between species and studies (Trefry *et al.* 2013). Ultimately, researchers should be aware of the literature available on marking outcomes for their species (if available) and evaluate the likely outcomes from using one mark or marker type over another.

TELEMETRY TAGS AND GEOGRAPHICAL POSITION DATA COLLECTORS

Amanda Lilleyman, Grace Maglio, Tegan K. Douglas, Michael A. Weston, Simon Cherriman, John Porter and Neil A. Hamilton

Target taxa

This GOP applies to passerines and parrots (Chapter 33), raptors (Chapter 34), and shorebirds and seabirds, including penguins (Chapter 35), and quail species.

Context and scope

This GOP describes the attachment of radio-, satellite- and GPS-tracking devices and geolocators to birds. Tracking tags are used to understand fine-scale, local and migratory movements of birds, but can also log physiological and behavioural data. Birds can carry tracking devices on their bodies for many months, depending on the attachment method. Attachment methods vary, but include gluing transmitters directly to the birds' skin, attaching to a leg band, tying them to tail feathers, taping devices to dorsal feathers, and attaching them with leg loop or backpack harnesses (Maglio and Lilleyman 2019). Selection of an attachment method is determined by the bird's body mass, structure and posture, the species' general and movement ecology, and transmitter construction and data collection trigger.

Animal welfare considerations

Time spent in captivity

Researchers should minimise the total time that birds are held, including during pre- and post-processing, and all animal welfare and transmitter fit checks. Birds may require appropriate housing between handling events, so researchers should be aware of husbandry requirements for the species (see the relevant chapters in Section 3) and recognise their behavioural stress cues. Handling and checks should be completed by experienced bird handlers. Enclosures can be built to house study animals temporarily. Personnel should consider appropriate viewing points or camera installation to monitor bird welfare with minimal disturbance. Enclosures need to contain species-appropriate structures (i.e. vegetation, sand, soil and water) and be tall enough to allow birds to retain their natural posture. For example, shorebirds can be housed in keeping cages comprising a frame covered with shade cloth. The base sits directly on sand, providing a natural substrate, and the shade cloth allows airflow. Birds cannot see through the shade cloth, which helps to minimise stress. Shorebirds captured at high tide roosts can be held in captivity for $\leq$ 4 h before they should be released. If birds are to be held in captivity for a longer duration or overnight, they should be fed and watered, and kept in a cool dark space.

Thermal stress

Climatic conditions may affect study animals during handling. Some birds, such as Charadrii (shorebirds), are prone to heat stress, which can develop into leg cramp. This risk can be avoided by providing appropriate housing that allows birds to move around without hurting themselves. Increased handling time results in increased stress, so personnel should only handle birds for the minimum time necessary to complete all processing and apply the tracking device. Having clear procedures and fixed roles within the team helps to avoid excessive or repeated handling of individual birds. When birds are handled their legs should remain free and able to dangle to avoid leg cramp.

Capture myopathy

If capture myopathy occurs, the bird should be housed in a box for rehabilitation. Some individuals can be held in a sling if necessary, fed and watered and provided with physiotherapy for cramped muscles (i.e. as per Rogers *et al.* 2004). Once rehabilitated, birds can be released at the capture site.

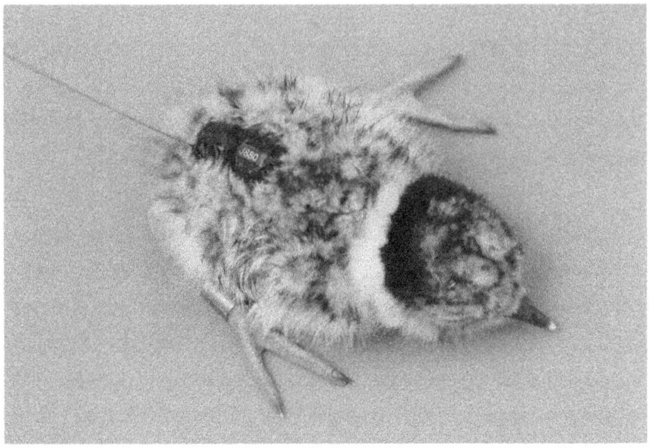

Figure 15.13: Radio transmitter attached to 1 day old hooded plover (*Thinornis rubricollis*) chicks. Photo by Michael A. Weston

Inappropriate tag selection and attachment method

A widely cited general rule for device mass suggests that devices for birds should weigh ≤ 5% of the individual's body mass, although more recently 3% has been suggested as more appropriate (Barron *et al.* 2010; Portugal and White 2018), particularly for migratory species. Main methods of attachment include harness or backpack fittings, glue (Hill and Talent 1990) and/or sutures, collars (Boiko and Wikelski 2019), adhesive tape (Vandenabeele *et al.* 2011), leg mounts and internal implantation (Roshier and Asmus 2009; Douglas *et al.* 2017). Several reviews have reported a wide range of effects of harnesses and devices (as a generalised group) on different bird species (Barron *et al.* 2010; Vandenabeele *et al.* 2011; Lameris *et al.* 2018), which are linked to the type of harness used, but their use for some species remains contentious. Birds with long bills or flexible necks may catch their bills in harness material. Researchers may trial tag attachments on analogous captive species before deploying tags on wild birds. Tag and harness materials should be robust enough to suit the environment that the bird lives in, and tag and harness colour should not impede survivorship. With caution, appropriately sized and correctly fitted transmitters are also suitable for attachment to nestlings (Figure 15.13; Lees *et al.* 2017).

Tag harness incorrectly attached and snagging risk

Transmitters should only be attached by trained personnel. Once the tag is attached the bird should be housed in a quiet place to allow observation. Transmitter type and placement minimise drag and snagging risk, and should not impede movement. For example, dorsal transmitters need to be positioned on the back between the wings to avoid drag while the bird is in flight. Tagged birds should be able to stand normally. A bird that sits or falls backwards might have an inappropriately positioned tag, which should be adjusted.

General procedures

Project planning

Project planning takes into consideration the appropriate transmitter weight for the study species (Casper 2009), but also transmitter type, attachment and capture method. When working on a novel species, a captive trial with an analogous species can assist in identifying potential issues. Transmitters can broadcast signals (radio), collect and store (geolocators and some GPS), or collect, store and transmit (GPS and satellite) information. Decisions on transmitter type are informed by research aims, the likelihood of personnel being in proximity to the bird to download data, or recapturing individuals to remove and retrieve telemetry data. Attachment method decisions are based on minimising impacts on the animals' natural behaviours. Researchers should consider the ability of the study species to chew and damage the transmitter or the means of attachment, or reports of adverse events from previous or similar studies (Mallory and Gilbert 2008; Ingwersen 2013).

Preparing and checking tags

Researchers can prefabricate the tag and attachment to minimise handling time of the birds. This process may include measuring harness straps, gluing elastic band loops, crimping loops, or gluing tags to gauze. Some tags need modifications to accommodate harness loops or to make them more streamlined. Tags should be switched on and tested before deployment to ensure that GPS components are obtaining fixes accurately, or that radio transmitters are broadcasting at their designated frequency. Some devices require a period of *in situ* pre-deployment for geographical ground-truthing. All necessary tag information should be recorded and double-checked.

All measuring and attachment equipment should be checked and on hand prior to the start of tagging process. A designated scribe should record notes on tag checks, measurements, the condition and welfare of the bird throughout processing, and should also monitor total holding time.

Attaching a tag to a bird

Once the bird is ready to be tagged, the researcher applies the tag while an assistant holds the bird. For shorebirds, tags are positioned on the back of the bird above the uropygial gland (oil preening gland), but also see Chan *et al.* (2016) for descriptions of a full-body harness attachment. For parrots, pigeons, and some raptor species, a backpack (chest) harness is attached between the wings where the bend of the wing is located.

For tags with Teflon® or tape harnesses, loops can be slipped over the wings or the legs depending on the harness type, and adjusted so that the harness is located under the feathers and sits flat on the skin. Leg-loop harnesses should be a snug fit within the leg sockets to hold the loops in place (Mallory and Gilbert 2008). Personnel tighten each loop and keep the lengths the same. Once the tension feels right, the ribbon loops should be of equal length and the tag should be centred on the bird's back. Personnel can test loop tension by placing their little finger under the tag. If the finger fits, then the loop is sufficiently tight. The ribbon lengths are held in place and the crimping tool fastens the crimp in position. For elastic band harnesses, one wing or leg should be fitted first; the remaining loop is eased over the other limb. A crochet hook or similar can be used to adjust feathers so that tag and harness sit flat against the skin.

Smaller tags can be glued to birds and will often last several months without affecting feather moult. The bird will shed the skin layer and moult the back feathers, causing the tag to fall off in the process (Lees *et al.* 2017). Personnel should consider the stage of feather moult before gluing radio tags onto birds. When gluing tags to birds, feathers should be trimmed to reveal feather stubs of around 0.5 cm long. Personnel should apply cyanoacrylate glue to one side of the tag and place the tag on the bird's skin and feather stubs. The tag needs to be held in place for 30 s and then given a gentle tug on the transmitter wire to ensure that it is secure.

Transmitters can be attached to tail feathers with thread or electrical tape (Whisson *et al.* 2015). Thread weaves central tail feathers and harness together, with additional dabs of glue holding arrangement fast, whereas tape holds several layers of feathers together to create a stable base for the transmitter to be attached to.

When attaching geolocators, tags can be attached by either gluing the tag to a leg flag or attaching a geolocator to a Velcro® leg mount or band.

All birds fitted with a geo-reference device should also be fitted with an approved individual identification ABBBS band (see 'Individual and cohort marking'). Doing so allows tagged birds to be identified later if recovered, with or without the tracking device. This is particularly important for injured or dead birds, to monitor for any adverse impacts of the tag and/or attachment method.

Pre-release checks

Once the tag has been attached, a final check will help confirm appropriate tension and fit of the device. The bird should be placed in an empty keeping cage. After 5–10 min settling time, the bird should be checked for normal standing and walking behaviour. Sitting down behaviour may indicate that the tag is sitting too far back on the bird and upsetting its centre of gravity. If this situation occurs, personnel should adjust the tag accordingly. If the tag is not sitting correctly on bird, then the team leader will decide if it should be cut off. When glue is used it must not be applied to body or flight feathers. When the bird is ready to be released, personnel ensure that opportunistic predators are not present, and release the bird safely away from team. A burrow-nesting bird should be returned to its burrow and observed for a time to ensure it does not abandon the burrow.

Transmitter detachment or removal

Transmitter attachments incorporate a method for self-detachment by moulting out with old feathers or being designed such that breaks in the harness allow the transmitter to fall free readily. However, any recapture is an opportunity to check for any wear or damage to the bird or transmitter and consider adjustments that need to be made.

Animal treatment, withdrawal and euthanasia

Tags attached to flying birds should typically be ≤ 3% of the bird's body mass, based on their mass at processing (Casper 2009). Researchers assess each bird to be tagged based on its mass and alertness. No tag should be fitted to birds that appear dazed or stressed. If the researcher is attaching radio tags to shorebirds, then they should select birds that have already started their primary flight feather moult as this process indicates that the bird is likely to stay in the local region, which is crucial for local radio tracking. Lead researchers are responsible for the welfare of all birds during fieldwork and decide on the outcome of any injured birds. If any birds are severely injured during catching procedures and cannot be rehabilitated, then those individuals can be euthanised by an appropriate method. Euthanasia should take place at the site of capture if the injury is too severe for rehabilitation, or the bird taken to a veterinarian.

Equipment and maintenance

General equipment requirements are few; but typical items may include a tag of appropriate design and mass, Teflon® ribbon, crimps, pliers, tweezers, datasheets, scissors, a ruler, cyanoacrylate glue, appropriate ABBBS bands and banding equipment.

Specific qualifications, experience and training

Only experienced people should attach tags to birds, particularly when the species is known to be sensitive. Personnel should be competent with the technique proposed, and familiar with the species or similar taxa, having undertaken similar work. Alternatively, personnel should be trained or supervised by someone who is. To be considered competent, personnel should have undertaken or been involved in at least one study or project using the proposed techniques. Personnel should have a wide experience in processing and handling, and be able to identify birds in distress. Personnel may require an A-class ABBBS licence for some activities.

Workplace health and safety

Refer to details for 'Inspection of nests and hollows, including handling of eggs and chicks' earlier in this chapter.

Alternative procedures

Coloured leg bands or engraved leg flags may be attached to birds for observational studies. However, these methods require intensive resighting efforts and the results can be biased depending on where and when the researcher visits. This method is unsuitable for understanding movement or habitat use of birds at night and is not necessarily lower impact than the use of telemetry devices. Where snagging risk is a concern, radio transmitters can be surgically implanted (see Chapter 9). However, this method decreases detection range substantially and is likely to be suitable only for studies of sedentary birds.

COLLECTION OF REGURGITATE, CROP CONTENTS, SCATS AND PELLETS

Tegan K. Douglas and Michael A. Weston

Target taxa

This GOP applies to all bird taxa (Chapters 33–36).

Context and scope

This GOP details methods to collect dietary and pathogen information from birds from regurgitate, prey remains, pellet and scat collection (see also Chapter 4). Researchers gather samples from around nests, roost sites or feeding platforms. Researchers may collect samples opportunistically (i.e. collecting regurgitate, pellets, or scat when encountered during other procedures). Active collection of samples typically involves researchers holding animals until they produce a sample, by inducing regurgitation or lavaging crop samples. Typically, researchers identify food items or pathogens in samples visually or with genetic analyses, or evaluate isotopic or energetic content or the presence of specific compounds (Weston 2007). These methods inform research on avian energetics and physiology, bioaccumulation, disease transmission, general ecology and breeding biology. This GOP should be considered alongside appropriate capture methods, and for working at nests or colonial seabird colonies (see 'Monitoring of colonial birds at breeding colonies', earlier in this chapter).

Animal welfare considerations

Loss of nutrition

Care must be taken not to reduce the ability of individuals to meet their nutritional requirements, when inducing samples. Marking individuals will ensure that the procedure is not performed on the same individual in consecutive sampling events. Alternative means of collecting data from adults that are provisioning chicks should be considered, to avoid reducing effective feeding rates of dependent young.

Interference with normal activities

Researchers should process and release animals quickly to minimise interference with their natural activities. Where holding birds to collect scat samples, a maximum holding time (often around 1 h) should be adhered to so that birds are not deprived of foraging opportunities for extended periods. In mixed cohort captures, incubating adults or dependent young should not be held for faecal sample collection. Birds need to be released during their active period, although it is appropriate to hold diurnal birds overnight or nocturnal birds during the day in suitable holding facilities, if they cannot be released immediately. Burrow-nesting birds should be released back into their own burrow after processing.

Injury and stress during handling

Handling is minimised by having appropriate holding arrangements for multiple birds, with researchers designing and adhering to a protocol that allows for efficient data collection with minimal double-handling. Researchers should monitor birds' health and stress levels throughout the process. Size- and species-appropriate handling methods (e.g. bander's or parrot grip) should always be used. Active collection of crop samples should always be undertaken by two personnel to ensure that the individual bird is held firmly and is not injured during the procedure. Syringes and tubing should not have sharp edges, should be of a size suited to the species, and the procedure should only be performed by experienced personnel.

General procedures

Planning

Species and site knowledge will inform the appropriate time for sampling to occur with minimal disturbance. Less invasive methods (passive or opportunistic collection) should be favoured, particularly if samples do not need to be traced to a particular individual. Circumstances may support a more-invasive method where alternatives do not exist. For example, crop lavage is highly invasive, but may provide a more-accurate dietary assessment for species with diets composed of soft items that do not persist in faecal samples. All collection equipment should be prepared and kept on hand alongside other equipment.

Sample collection

To avoid cross-contamination, samples can be deposited directly into individual vials or other containers. Equipment that comes into contact with samples (e.g. gloves or forceps) should be sterilised between samples with ≥ 70% alcohol or similar. An effective labelling system helps to ensure data integrity – pre-printed stickers can be used to minimise transcription errors on labels.

Passive and opportunistic collection considerations

Passive collection of scats, pellets and prey remains should be undertaken at times that minimise disturbance to the birds that deposited them. Depending on research questions and the types of sample required, samples from breeding sites (individual nests and colonies) may be collected outside the breeding season, or at stages of the breeding cycle where negative effects are likely to be low, such as at pair changeover, when fledglings are not being incubated or immediately post-fledging (see 'Monitoring of colonial birds at breeding colonies' earlier in this chapter, and Dunlop and McNeill 2017). Pellet collection under roosts of nocturnal species is less likely to cause disturbance when done in the morning; collection around water points can be completed at any time. Recently deceased individuals encountered in breeding colonies may also be suitable for regurgitation samples. If samples are likely to be encountered during other activities, researchers should ensure that sufficient equipment is kept on hand to collect and label it in an accurate and sterile manner.

Active collection considerations – scat collection

On capture, birds should be placed in individual holding compartments modified for sample collection (Wooller and Calver 1981). Wooden, plastic or cardboard boxes may be used to create a dark holding space, provided they are of sufficient height to enable birds to standard with normal posture. Boxes should have a removable floor covering (e.g. paper, paper towel or sandpaper). Birds should be left undisturbed in compartments for a predetermined time (usually 1 h is sufficient, but times may vary with the species' gut passage time) before processing and release. Birds should be released even if no sample is produced in the allotted time. Compartments need to be sanitised between individuals and flooring replaced. Flooring retaining the sample can be clipped and placed in a labelled container for appropriate storage.

Active collection considerations – stomach or crop lavage

Only alert individuals that show minimal signs of stress after capture and processing should be considered for crop lavage. To induce samples, birds are held upright in a size-appropriate hold, with their wings folded naturally against the body and head and/or neck held in a straight position (Holt *et al.* 2002). A second researcher uses a lavage or irrigation syringe partially filled with distilled water, fitted with a rounded, pliable length of tubing, inserting it into the bird's oesophagus and down to the crop, avoiding the glottis and the trachea. Injecting a small amount of water into the crop and palpating the syringe plunger will extract a mixture of water containing a food sample from the crop. Care must be taken not to aspirate water or the sample into the bird's lungs. Appropriately sized syringe tubing should be selected with an external diameter appropriate for the bird, an internal diameter greater than the food particle size in the crop, and of sufficient length to reach the bird's crop. Once the sample mixture is captured in the syringe, it should be removed and transferred to a labelled vial. Care must be taken to avoid cross-contamination of syringe contents. Ideally, a new syringe is used for each bird.

Animal treatment, withdrawal and euthanasia

Passive collection does not require animal handling, so treatment and euthanasia are not relevant for those techniques. However, researchers should use behavioural and environmental cues to determine whether withdrawal is necessary because of excessive disturbance to nearby birds. Alternative sites or timing should be considered in these cases. For induced samples, researchers may cease trying to collect a sample from an individual that appears to be excessively stressed (based on the researcher's experience of that species' cues, e.g. excessive panting) or where sample collection cannot occur in a reasonable period of time. Researchers should monitor the situation continually during opportunistic, active and induced collection and watch for cues specific to their species.

Equipment and maintenance

Equipment requirements are minimal for most procedures and may include sample vials or bags, holding containers, lavage syringes and ≥ 70% alcohol or similar for sterilisation purposes.

Specific qualifications, experience and training

Suggested competency levels for principal researchers are listed in Table 15.7.

Workplace health and safety

Refer to details for 'Nest and hollow inspections, including handling of eggs and chicks' earlier in this chapter.

Alternative procedures

Historically, many of these types of samples would have been collected through gut analysis of deceased specimens, which were either donated by third parties or shot as part of the study. The least invasive methods (i.e. passive or opportunistic sampling) should be selected where appropriate. Alternatives like next-generation sequencing could be considered instead of crop lavage (King *et al.* 2015; Cristol-Martínez *et al.* 2016). General isotopic information can be obtained from feather samples, if species-specific prey information is not required (Dunlop and McNeill 2017).

Table 15.7: Competency requirements for animal researchers undertaking collection of scat and crop samples.

Competency category	Competency requirement	Competency assessment
Species identification and stress assessment	Previous experience in bird identification and welfare assessment.	Personnel must be able to identify the species targeted for the project and be familiar with indicators of stress.
Sample collection	Previous experience in sample collection.	Personnel must be competent in collecting and analysing samples, including identifying food items, maintaining data integrity and following hygiene protocols to avoid cross-contamination.
Animal handling	Previous experience in bird handling of the targeted species.	Personnel should be competent with the technique proposed and familiar with the species or similar taxa, having undertaken similar work.
Crop sampling	Previous experience in taking samples from similar species.	Personnel should be competent with the technique proposed and familiar with the species or similar taxa, having undertaken similar work. To be considered competent, personnel should have undertaken or been involved in at least one study or project using the proposed technique.

REFERENCES

ABBBS (2000) *Recommended Band Size List: Birds of Australia and its Territories.* Australian Bird and Bat Banding Scheme, Biodiversity Groups, Environment Australia, Canberra.

Agler BA, Kendall SJ, Irons DB, Klosiewski SP (1999) Declines in marine bird populations in Prince William Sound, Alaska coincident with a climatic regime shift. *Waterbirds* **22**, 98–103. doi:10.2307/1521998

Altmann J (1974) Observational study of behaviour: sampling methods. *Behaviour* **49**, 227–266. doi:10.1163/156853974X00534

Bacon BR, Evrard JO (1990) Horizontal mist net for capture of upland nesting ducks. *North American Bird Bander* **15**, 18–19.

Bamford M, Dunlop N, Gamblin T, Bamford A (2013) *Fauna Sampling Manual. Guide to Sampling Techniques for Wildlife Research in Western Australia.* Conservation Council of Western Australia, Perth.

Barrett G, Silcocks A, Barry S, Cunningham R, Poulter R (2003) *The New Atlas of Australian Birds.* Royal Australasian Ornithologists Union, Melbourne.

Barron DG, Brawn JD, Weatherhead PJ (2010) Meta-analysis of transmitter effects on avian behaviour and ecology. *Methods in Ecology and Evolution* **1**, 180–187. doi:10.1111/j.2041-210X.2010.00013.x

Bibby CJ, Burgess ND, Hill DA, Mustoe SH (2000) *Bird Census Techniques.* 2nd edn. Academic Press, Sydney.

Blackmer AL, Ackerman JT, Nevitt GA (2004) Effects of investigator disturbance on hatching success and nest-site fidelity in a long-lived seabird, Leach's storm-petrel. *Biological Conservation* **116**, 141–148. doi:10.1016/S0006-3207(03)00185-X

Bloom PH, Clark WS, Kidd JW (2007) Capture techniques. In *Raptor Research and Management Techniques.* 2nd edn. (Eds DM Bird and KL Bildstein). pp. 193–220. Hancock House, Surrey, Canada.

Blythman M (2017) *Guidelines for the Approved Control Technique for Introduced Corellas.* Department of Biodiversity, Conservation and Attractions, Perth.

Boiko D, Wikelski M (2019) Moulting sites of Latvian whooper swan *Cygnus cygnus* cygnets fitted with GPS-GSM transmitters. *Wildfowl Journal* **5**, 229–241.

Brandis K, Koeltzow N, Ryall S, Ramp D (2014) Assessing the use of remote camera traps to measure reproductive success in ibis breeding colonies. *Australian Field Ornithology* **31**, 99106.

Brua RB (1998) Negative effects of patagial tags on ruddy ducks. *Journal of Field Ornithology* **69**, 530–535.

Bub H (1991) *Bird Trapping and Bird Banding: A Handbook for Trapping Methods all over the World.* (Trans. F Hamerstrom and K Wuertz-Schaefer). Cornell University Press, New York, NY.

Buidin C, Rochepault Y, Aubry Y (2015) Trapping non-breeding red knot *Calidris canutus* with a gunpowder-propelled net-gun. *Wader Study* **122**, 12–17. doi:10.18194/ws.00007

Calvo B, Furness RW (1992) A review of the use and the effects of marks and devices on birds. *Ringing & Migration* **13**, 129–151. doi:10.1080/03078698.1992.9674036

Casper RM (2009) Guidelines for the instrumentation of wild birds and mammals. *Animal Behaviour* **78**, 1477–1483. doi:10.1016/j.anbehav.2009.09.023

Champagnon J, Carré H, Gili L (2019) Effects of research disturbance on nest survival in a mixed colony of waterbirds. *PeerJ* **7**, e7844. doi:10.7717/peerj.7844

Chan YC, Brugge M, Tibbitts TL, Dekinga A, Porter R, Klaassen RH, Piersma T (2016) Testing an attachment method for solar-powered tracking devices on a long-distance migrating shorebird. *Journal of Ornithology* **157**, 277–287. doi:10.1007/s10336-015-1276-4

Charuvi A, Lees D, Glover HK, Rendall AR, Dann P, Weston MA (2020) A physiological cost to behavioural tolerance. *Behavioural Processes* **181**, 104250. doi:10.1016/j.beproc.2020.104250

Coxen CL, Collins DP, Carleton SA (2018) Capture and injury rates of band-tailed pigeons using whoosh nets. *The Wilson Journal of Ornithology* **130**, 321–326. doi:10.1676/16-069.1

Cristol-Martínez E, Moreno-Moyano LT, Wormington KR, Brown PH, Stanley D (2016) Using Next Generation Sequencing to contrast the diet and explore pest-reduction services of sympatric bird species in Macadamia orchards in Australia. *PLoS One* **11**, e0150159. doi:10.1371/journal.pone.0150159

Davies SJJF (2010) Long-term indices of density of ten woodland passerines at Eyre Bird Observatory. *Corella* **34**, 1–6.

de Beer SJ, Lockwood GM, Raijmakers JHFA, Raijmakers JMH, Scott WA, Oschadleus HD, Underhill LG (Eds) (2001) *SAFRING Bird Ringing Manual.* ADU Guide 5, Avian Demography Unit, The University of Cape Town, Cape Town, South Africa.

de Rebeira P (2006) *Bander's Guide to the Birds of Western Australia.* CPS & AM de Rebeira, Glen Forrest.

Debus SJS (1995) Surveys of large forest owls in northern New South Wales: methodology, calling behaviour and owl responses. *Corella* **19**, 38–50.

DBCA (2015) *How to Monitor and Maintain Artificial Hollows for Carnaby's Cockatoo. Fauna Notes.* Western Australian Department of Biodiversity, Conservation and Attractions, Perth.

DBCA (2017) *Standard Operating Procedure: Animal Handling and Restraint Using Soft Containment.* Department of Biodiversity Conservation and Attractions, Perth.

DEWHA (2010) *Survey Guidelines for Australia's Threatened Birds.* Australian Government Department of Water, Heritage and the Arts, Canberra.

Douglas TK, Cooper CE, Withers PC (2017) Avian torpor or alternative thermoregulatory strategies for overwintering? *The Journal of Experimental Biology* **220**, 1341–1349. doi:10.1242/jeb.154633

Drynan D (Ed.) (2015) New draft policy on the use of tape lures. *Flightlines: Newsletter of the Australian Bird and Bat Banding Scheme,* No. 30, 4. Department of the Environment and Energy, Government of Australia, Canberra. <https://www.environment.gov.au/system/files/resources/6c8488ec-e120-41cc-ad12-4402075680b2/files/flightlines-july-2015.pdf>.

Dunlop JN (2018) *Fairy Tern Conservation in Western Australia.* Conservation Council of Western Australia, Perth.

Dunlop JN, McNeill S (2017) Local movements, foraging patterns, and heavy metals exposure in caspian terns *Hydroprogne caspa* breeding on Penguin Island, Western Australia. *Marine Ornithology* **45**, 115–120.

East Asian Australasian Flyway Partnership (2020) *Coordination of Colour Marking.* East Asian Australasian Flyway Partnership, Incheon, Korea.

Ekanayake KB, Whisson DA, Tan LX, Weston MA (2015a) Intense predation of non-colonial, ground-nesting bird eggs by corvid and mammalian predators. *Wildlife Research* **42**, 518–528. doi:10.1071/WR15080

Ekanayake KB, Sutherland DR, Dann P, Weston MA (2015b) Out of sight but not out of mind: corvids prey extensively on eggs of burrow-nesting penguins. *Wildlife Research* **42**, 509–517. doi:10.1071/WR15108

FAO (2007) Wild birds and avian influenza: an introduction to applied field research and disease sampling techniques. In *Animal Production and Health Manual* (Eds D Whitworth, SH Newman, T Mundkur and P Harris). FAO, Rome.

Ferris R, Gilbert J (Eds) (2014) *First Responders Resource Guide for Seabird Emergencies.* Australian Seabird Rescue, Ballina.

Fisher RJ, Poulin RG, Todd LD, Brigham RM (2004) Nest stage, wind speed, and air temperature affect the nest defence behaviours of burrowing owls. *Canadian Journal of Zoology* **82**, 707–713. doi:10.1139/z04-035

Francis R, Lyons M, Kingsford RT, Brandis K (2020) Counting mixed breeding aggregations of animal species using drones: lessons from waterbirds on semi-automation. *Remote Sensing* **12**, 1185. doi:10.3390/rs12071185

Friesen MR, Beggs JR, Gaskett AC (2017) Sensory-based conservation of seabirds: a review of management strategies and animal behaviours that facilitate success. *Biological Reviews of the Cambridge Philosophical Society* **92**, 1769–1784. doi:10.1111/brv.12308

Gage LJ, Duerr RS (Eds) (2020) *Hand-rearing Birds*. 2nd edn. Wiley, Hoboken, NJ.

Gaunt AS, Oring LW (Eds) (2010) *Guidelines to the Use of Wild Birds in Research*. 3rd edn. The Ornithological Council. <https://birdnet.org/wp-content/uploads/2017/07/guidelines_august2010.pdf>.

Götmark F (1992) The effects of investigator disturbance on nesting birds. In *Current Ornithology Volume 9*. (Ed. DM Power) pp. 63–104. Springer, Boston, MA.

Greenwell CN, Born K, Admiraal R, Hodgson A, Dunlop JN, Loneragan NR (2021a) Social facilitation for conservation planning: understanding fairy tern behaviour and site selection in response to conspecific audio-visual cues. *Endangered Species Research* **45**, 147–157. doi:10.3354/esr01127

Greenwell CN, Dunlop JN, Admiraal R, Loneragan NR (2021b) The secret life of fairy terns: breeding chronology and life history observations of *Sternula nereis nereis* in south-western Australia. *Pacific Conservation Biology*. doi:10.1071/PC20056

Griesser M, Schneider NA, Collis M-A, Overs A, Guppy M, Guppy S, Takeuchi N, Collins P, Peters A, Hall ML (2012) Causes of ring-related injuries in birds – evidence and recommendations from four field studies. *PLoS One* **7**, e51891. doi:10.1371/journal.pone.0051891

Guay PJ, Mulder RA (2009) Do neck-collars affect the behaviour and condition of black swans (*Cygnus atratus*)? *Emu* **109**, 248–251. doi:10.1071/MU09020

Guay PJ, van Dongen WF, Robinson RW, Blumstein DT, Weston MA (2016) AvianBuffer: An interactive tool for characterising and managing wildlife fear responses. *Ambio* **45**, 841–851. doi:10.1007/s13280-016-0779-4

Herzog SK, Kessler M, Cahill TM (2002) Estimating species richness of tropical bird communities from rapid assessment data. *The Auk* **119**, 749–769. doi:10.1093/auk/119.3.749

Hill LA, Talent LG (1990) Effects of capture, handling, banding, and radio-marking on breeding least terns and snowy plovers. *Journal of Field Ornithology* **61**, 310–319.

Holt PS, Vaughn LE, Gast RK, Stone HD (2002) Development of a lavage procedure to collect crop secretions from live chickens for studying crop immunity. *Avian Pathology* **31**, 589–592. doi:10.1080/0307945021000024599

Ibanez-Álamo JD, Sanllorente O, Soler M (2012) The impact of researcher disturbance on nest predation rates: a meta-analysis. *The Ibis* **154**, 5–14. doi:10.1111/j.1474-919X.2011.01186.x

Ingwersen D (2013) Achievements and lessons from three captive releases of regent honeyeaters *Anthochaera phrygia* in north-east Victoria. *Australasian Ornithology Conference*. 4–7. December, Auckland.

Johnson IP, Sibly RM (1989) Effects of plastic neck collars on the behaviour and breeding performance of geese and their value for distant recognition of individuals. *Ringing & Migration* **10**, 58–62. doi:10.1080/03078698.1989.9676009

Johnston GR, Waterman MH, Manning CE (2015) Movement and mortality of Australian pelicans (*Pelecanus conspicillatus*) banded at inland and coastal breeding sites in South Australia. *Pacific Conservation Biology* **21**, 271–276. doi:10.1071/PC14925

Junda J, Greene E, Bird DM (2015) Proper flight technique for using a small rotary-winged drone aircraft to safely, quickly, and accurately survey raptor nests. *Journal of Unmanned Vehicle Systems* **3**, 222–236. doi:10.1139/juvs-2015-0003

King RA, Symondon WOC, Thomas RJ (2015) Molecular analysis of faecal samples from birds to identify potential crop pests and useful biological agents in natural areas. *Bulletin of Entomological Research* **105**, 261–272. doi:10.1017/S0007485314000935

Kingsford RT (1999) Aerial survey of waterbirds on wetlands as a measure of river and floodplain health. *Freshwater Biology* **41**, 425–438. doi:10.1046/j.1365-2427.1999.00440.x

Kingsford RT, Porter JL (2009) Monitoring waterbird populations with aerial surveys–what have we learnt? *Wildlife Research* **36**, 29–40. doi:10.1071/WR08034

Kingsford RT, Porter JL, Brandis KJ, Ryall S (2020) Aerial surveys of waterbirds in Australia. *Scientific Data* **7**, 1–6. doi:10.1038/s41597-020-0512-9

Kostoglou K, van Dongen WF, Lees D, Maguire GS, Weston MA (2017) Acoustic cues from within the egg do not heighten depredation risk to shorebird clutches. *Behavioral Ecology* **28**, 811–817. doi:10.1093/beheco/arx040

Kostoglou K, van Dongen WF, Weston MA (2020) Parental defence in shorebirds is mediated by embryonic calling, ambient temperature and predator latency. *Journal of Ornithology* **161**, 1153–1165. doi:10.1007/s10336-020-01787-4

Lameris TK, Müskens GJ, Kölzsch A, Dokter AM, Van der Jeugd HP, Nolet BA (2018) Effects of harness-attached tracking devices on survival, migration, and reproduction in three species of migratory waterfowl. *Animal Biotelemetry* **6**, 7. doi:10.1186/s40317-018-0153-3

Lees D, Sherman CD, Maguire GS, Dann P, Weston MA (2017) Implications of radio-tracking for the survival of masked lapwing chicks. *Corella* **41**, 37–41.

Liebezeit JR, Smith PA, Lanctot RB, Schekkerman H, Tulp I, Kendall SJ, Tracy DM, Rodrigues RJ, Meltofte H, Robinson JA, Gratto-Trevor C, Mccaffery BJ, Morse J, Zack SW (2007) Assessing the development of shorebird eggs using the floatation method: species-specific and generalised regression models. *The Condor* **109**, 32–47. doi:10.1093/condor/109.1.32

Lowe KW 1989. *The Australian Bird Bander's Manual*. Australian Bird and Bat Banding Schemes, Australian National Parks and Wildlife Service, Canberra.

Lyons M, Brandis K, Callaghan C, McCann J, Mills C, Ryall S, Kingsford R (2018) Bird interactions with drones, from individuals to large colonies. *Australian Field Ornithology* **35**, 51–56. doi:10.20938/afo35051056

MacInnes CD, Dunn EH (1988) Components of clutch size variation in Arctic-nesting Canada geese. *The Condor* **90**, 83–89. doi:10.2307/1368436

Maglio G, Lilleyman A (2019) Best practice methods and advances in tagging birds for research. Workshop held at the *Australasian Ornithological Conference*, Darwin 1 July 2019.

Magrath M, Weston M, Olsen P, Antos M (2010) *Survey Guidelines for Australia's Threatened Birds*. Department of the Environment, Water, Heritage and the Arts, Canberra.

Mallory ML, Gilbert CD (2008) Leg-loop harness design for attaching external transmitters to seabirds. *Marine Ornithology* **36**, 183–188.

Martin JM, Major RE (2010) The use of cattle ear-tags as patagial markers for large birds – a field assessment on adult and nestling Australian white ibis. *Waterbirds* **33**, 264–268. doi:10.1675/063.033.0218

McLeod EM, Guay PJ, Taysom AJ, Robinson RW, Weston MA (2013) Buses, cars, bicycles and walkers: the influence of the type of human transport on the flight responses of waterbirds. *PLoS One* **8**, e82008. doi:10.1371/journal.pone.0082008

Meng H (1971) The Swedish goshawk trap. *The Journal of Wildlife Management* **35**, 832–835. doi:10.2307/3799794

Menu S, Hestbeck JB, Gauthier G, Reed A (2000) Effects of neck bands on survival of greater snow geese. *The Journal of Wildlife Management* **64**, 544–552. doi:10.2307/3803252

Mills JA, Ryder JPP (1979) Trap for capturing shore and seabirds. *Bird-Banding* **50**, 121–123. doi:10.2307/4512436

Nisbet ICT (2000) Disturbance, habituation and management of waterbird colonies. *Waterbirds* **23**, 312–332.

Parker GC, Rexer-Huber K (2016) 'Guidelines for designing burrowing petrel surveys to improve population estimate precision'. Agreement on the Conservation of Albatrosses and Petrels. <https://www.acap.aq/resources/acap-conservation-guidelines/2830-guidelines-for-designing-burrowing-petrel-surveys/file>.

Pay JM, Katzner TE, Hawkins CE, Koch AJ, Wiersma JM, Brown WE, Mooney NJ, Cameron EZ (2021) High frequency of lead exposure in the population of an endangered Australian top predator, the Tasmanian wedge-tailed eagle (*Aquila audax fleayi*). *Environmental Toxicology and Chemistry* **40**, 219–230. doi:10.1002/etc.4914

Portugal SJ, White CR (2018) Miniaturization of biologgers is not alleviating the 5% rule. *Methods in Ecology and Evolution* **9**, 1662–1666. doi:10.1111/2041-210X.13013

Priddel D, Carlile N, Fullagar P, Hutton I, O'Neill L (2006) Decline in the distribution and abundance of flesh-footed shearwaters (*Puffinus carneipes*) on Lord Howe Island, Australia. *Biological Conservation* **128**, 412–424. doi:10.1016/j.biocon.2005.10.007

Redfern CPF, Clark JA (2001) *Ringers' Manual.* British Trust for Ornithology, Thetford, UK.

Reed ET, Gauthier G, Pradel R (2005) Effects of neck bands on reproduction and survival of female greater snow geese. *The Journal of Wildlife Management* **69**, 91–100. doi:10.2193/0022-541X(2005)069<0091:EONBOR>2.0.CO;2

Rogers DI, Battley PF, Sparrow J, Koolhaas A, Hassell CJ (2004) Treatment of capture myopathy in shorebirds: a successful trial in northwestern Australia. *Journal of Field Ornithology* **75**, 157–164. doi:10.1648/0273-8570-75.2.157

Rosenfield RN, Grier JW, Fyfe RW (2007) Reducing Management and Research Disturbance. In *Raptor Research and Management Techniques* (Eds DM Bird and KL Bildstein). 2nd edn. pp. 193–220. Hancock House, Surrey, Canada.

Roshier DA, Asmus MW (2009) Use of satellite telemetry on small-bodied waterfowl in Australia. *Marine and Freshwater Research* **60**, 299–305. doi:10.1071/MF08152

Safina C, Burger J (1983) Effects of human disturbance success in the black skimmer. *The Condor* **85**, 164–171. doi:10.2307/1367250

Saino N, Fasola M (1996) The function of embryonic vocalization in the little tern (*Sterna albifrons*). *Ethology* **102**, 265–271. doi:10.1111/j.1439-0310.1996.tb01124.x

Sanz-Aguilar A, Tavecchia G, Minguez E, Massa B, Valvo FL, Ballesteros GA, Barberá GG, Amengual JF, Rodriguez A, McMinn M, Oro D (2010) Recapture processes and biological inference in monitoring burrow-nesting seabirds. *Journal of Ornithology* **151**, 133–146. doi:10.1007/s10336-009-0435-x

Saunders DA (1988) Patagial tags: do benefits outweigh risks to the animals? *Australian Wildlife Research* **15**, 565–569. doi:10.1071/WR9880565

Shannon K, Weston MA, Whisson DA (2014) Sex bias in captured little raven *Corvus mellori* varies with entry aperture size in a modified Australian crow trap. *Corella* **38**, 22–23.

Sharp T, Saunders G, Mitchell B (2007) *Marking of Pest Animals Used in Research. Standard Operating Procedures for the Humane Research of Pest Animals in Australia.* NSW Department of Primary Industries, Orange.

Shugart GW (1978) The development of chick recognition by adult caspian terns. *Proceedings of the Colonial Waterbird Group* **1**, 110–117. doi:10.2307/1520907

Standen R, Jessop R, Minton C (2018) *Cannon-netting Induction Manual.* Australasian Wader Studies Group, Mt Eliza, Victoria.Sun A, Whelan S, Hatch SA, Elliott KH (2020) Tags below three percent of body mass increase nest abandonment by rhinoceros auklets, but handling impacts decline as breeding progresses. *Marine Ecology Progress Series* **643**, 173–181. doi:10.3354/meps13341

Sutherland WJ (2004) Bird ecology and conservation: a handbook of techniques. *Journal of Chemical Information and Modeling* **53**, 1689–1699.

Sutherland WJ, Newton I, Green RE (2004) *Bird Ecology and Conservation: A Handbook of Techniques.* Oxford University Press, Melbourne.

Thibault M, Weston MA, Ravache A, Vidal E (2020) Flight-initiation response reflects short-and long-term human visits to remote islets. *The Ibis* **162**, 1082–1087. doi:10.1111/ibi.12810

Trefry SA, Diamond AW, Jesson LK (2013) Wing marker woes: a case study and meta-analysis of the impacts of wing and patagial tags. *Journal of Ornithology* **154**, 1–11. doi:10.1007/s10336-012-0862-y

Vandenabeele SP, Wilson RP, Grogan A (2011) Tags on seabirds: how seriously are instrument-induced behaviours considered? *Animal Welfare (South Mimms, England)* **20**, 559–571.

Varland DE, Smallwood JA, Young LS, Kochert MN (2007) Marking techniques. In *Raptor Research and Management Techniques.* 2nd edn. (Eds DM Bird, DM and KL Bildstein) pp. 221–236. Hancock House, Surrey, Canada.

Watson DM (2003) The 'standardized search': an improved way to conduct bird surveys. *Austral Ecology* **28**, 515–525. doi:10.1046/j.1442-9993.2003.01308.x

Watson DM (2017) Sampling effort determination in bird surveys: do current norms meet best-practice recommendations? *Wildlife Research* **44**, 183–193. doi:10.1071/WR16226

Watson DM, Znidersic E, Craig MD (2019) Ethical birding call playback and conservation. *Conservation Biology* **33**, 469–471. doi:10.1111/cobi.13199

Western Australian Seabird Rescue (2018) *New tool to help wildlife.* <https://wasr.org.au/in-the-media/new-tool-to-help-wildlife/>.

Weston M (2007) The foraging and diet of non-breeding hooded plovers *Thinornis rubricollis* in relation to habitat type. *Journal of the Royal Society of Western Australia* **90**, 89–95.

Weston MA, Dann P, Jessop R, Fallaw J, Dakin R, Ball D (2008) Can oiled shorebirds and their nests and eggs be successfully rehabilitated? A case study involving the threatened hooded plover *Thinornis rubricollis* in south-eastern Australia. *Waterbirds* **31**, 127–132. doi:10.1675/1524-4695(2008)31[127:COSATN]2.0.CO;2

Weston MA, Liu X, Tsuzuki T, Fallaw J, Dann P (2009) Forensic fibre analysis to determine the origins of leg-entangling threads on shorebirds: a case study. *Bulletin - Wader Study Group* **116**, 46–48.

Weston MA, McLeod EM, Blumstein DT, Guay PJ (2012) A review of flight-initiation distances and their application to managing disturbance to Australian birds. *Emu-Austral Ornithology* **112**, 269–286. doi:10.1071/MU12026

Weston MA, O'Brien C, Kostoglou KN, Symonds MR (2020) Escape responses of terrestrial and aquatic birds to drones: Towards a code of practice to minimize disturbance. *Journal of Applied Ecology* **57**, 777–785. doi:10.1111/1365-2664.13575

Whisson DA, Weston MA, Shannon K (2015) Home range, habitat use and movements by the little raven (*Corvus mellori*) in a coastal peri-urban landscape. *Wildlife Research* **42**, 500–508. doi:10.1071/WR15039

Wooller RD, Calver MC (1981) Feeding segregation with an assemblage of small birds in the karri forest understorey. *Australian Wildlife Research* **8**, 401–410. doi:10.1071/WR9810401

16 Veterinary procedures for Australian wildlife

Jordan O. Hampton, Sarah J. Gill, Derek Spielman, Andrew Peters, Simone Vitali, Wayne Boardman, Tim Portas and Graeme Coulson

INTRODUCTION

Advanced veterinary techniques are increasingly being incorporated into Australian wildlife research, including where manual restraint is inadequate for safe handling of animals, to address animal welfare needs when painful or invasive procedures are performed, and when invasive biological samples (especially blood) are required to answer a research question. These techniques have played an increasing role in wildlife research, driven by intensifying animal welfare scrutiny, an expansion of the role of wildlife veterinarians, and a growing appreciation for the importance of wildlife diseases for conservation and public health. Underpinning guidelines are provided here for several important veterinary techniques that are applied to wildlife.

SEDATION AND GENERAL ANAESTHESIA

Jordan O. Hampton, Tim Portas and Wayne Boardman

Target taxa

Sedation and general anaesthesia are commonly used for a variety of wildlife species, including mammals (Chapters 17–25), reptiles (Chapter 26), amphibians (Chapter 27), fish (Chapters 30–32), and birds (Chapters 33–36) (West *et al.* 2014). Here, the focus has been placed on general themes that apply to terrestrial vertebrates. Fish anaesthesia is not discussed in detail in this section, with taxa-specific information provided in Chapters 30–32. Anaesthesia has not been discussed for invertebrates (Chapters 28–29).

Context and scope

This GOP describes general principles of wildlife anaesthesia and methods of providing sedation and anaesthesia to different groups of Australian vertebrates. It provides general guidance and further reading, but limited species-specific information. Sedation and anaesthesia may be used to provide chemical restraint to permit the safe handling of dangerous animals, reduce stress associated with capture, handling and manipulation, or provide analgesia during painful or invasive procedures (West *et al.* 2014). Wild animals may be sedated or anaesthetised once they are in-hand or chemical restraint may be used to capture them (see 'Chemical immobilisation' in this chapter). In terms of animal welfare and human safety, chemical restraint may provide better outcomes in certain species and situations, such as handling of crocodiles (*Crocodylus* spp.) (Olsson and Phalen 2013), or a useful adjunct to manual restraint in others, such as translocation of macropods (Batson *et al.* 2016). However, chemical restraint of wildlife can cause mortalities and is associated with several types of negative animal welfare impact (Hampton *et al.* 2021).

Animal welfare considerations

Several categories of potential animal welfare impacts may be associated with chemical restraint: (1) anaesthetic complications caused by the suppressive effects of the drug on body systems (especially in stressed or sick animals), or by errors in anaesthetic administration (e.g. overdose, underdose, mis-injection); (2) thermoregulation challenges (i.e. hyperthermia and hypothermia); (3) capture myopathy (see 'Chemical immobilisation' in this chapter); and (4) short-term post-anaesthesia behavioural changes.

Anaesthetic complications

It is often possible to titrate induction doses for domestic animals to minimise adverse effects. However, when anaesthesia is administered via remote injection (see 'Chemical immobilisation' in this chapter), drugs are often delivered at the higher end of their dose range to achieve rapid induction (Hawkins *et al.* 2019) and to avoid the need to 'top up', which prolongs recovery. However, high drug doses create risks of animals entering planes of anaesthesia deeper than desired and that may manifest (depending on veterinary drugs used) as bradycardia, hypotension, hypertension, hypoventilation, hypoxaemia, hypothermia and prolonged recovery (Mayberry *et al.* 2014). Furthermore, it is usually not possible to assess fully a wild animal's fitness for chemical restraint before the event; this issue makes them more susceptible to undesirable anaesthetic outcomes.

Hyperthermia and hypothermia

Monitoring body temperature and/or anticipating thermoregulatory requirements are fundamental for appropriate management of wildlife under chemical restraint. Anaesthesia interferes with an animal's capacity to thermoregulate, meaning that body temperature disturbances (hyperthermia and hypothermia) commonly occur unless animals are monitored closely. While hyperthermia is particularly common with remote immobilisation (Hampton *et al.* 2021) (see 'Chemical immobilisation'), hypothermia more commonly occurs in cold conditions and during long procedures involving deep planes of anaesthesia. When field immobilisation procedures are performed under cold conditions (e.g. at night in winter), hypothermia risk should be addressed by wrapping animals in wool blankets and positioning them on insulated surfaces (see 'General procedures' in this GOP). Where possible, field research timing should be planned to coincide with the most appropriate environmental conditions, including ambient temperature.

Violent recoveries

The risk of stress and self-inflicted injury should be mitigated by careful planning of recovery conditions (e.g. recovery of animals in soft bags, in a quiet darkened environment), and a thorough understanding of the physiological effects of the anaesthetic drug used. A degree of struggling can be anticipated as animals recover from anaesthesia (Woolnough *et al.* 2012). However, violent, 'stormy' or unsteady recoveries are most commonly associated with inappropriate selection of drugs and doses, and inadequate post-anaesthetic care (Mayberry *et al.* 2014).

Short-term behavioural changes

Non-lethal negative effects of chemical restraint may extend to altered levels of activity and mobility for several days post-procedure (Brogi *et al.* 2019). Pre-anaesthetic planning should take into account any implications of recovery time for the welfare of animals after the procedure (Mayberry *et al.* 2014).

General procedures

Most of the principles of veterinary anaesthesia for domestic animals are applicable to Australian native animals, but some specialised considerations apply (Vogelnest and Portas 2019). One approach to chemical restraint will not suit all contexts. Initial considerations include the species involved, the procedures required, the skillset of the research staff, the budget available and the options permitted under legislation. Other site-specific factors also need to be considered. For example, different considerations are required for remote field work compared to procedures performed in indoor facilities.

Route of administration

Wild animals may be sedated or anaesthetised via three main routes: (1) induction via inhalational anaesthesia (intubation, use of an inhalation anaesthetic induction chamber, or facemask ('masking down') (Figure 16.1a); (2) hand or pole injection on restrained animals (intravenous or intramuscular); and (3) via remote injection (see 'Chemical immobilisation').

Drug selection

Many combinations of veterinary anaesthetics and sedatives may be applicable in particular situations (West *et al.* 2014); this breadth of combinations cannot be covered in detail here. In brief, most contemporary approaches use

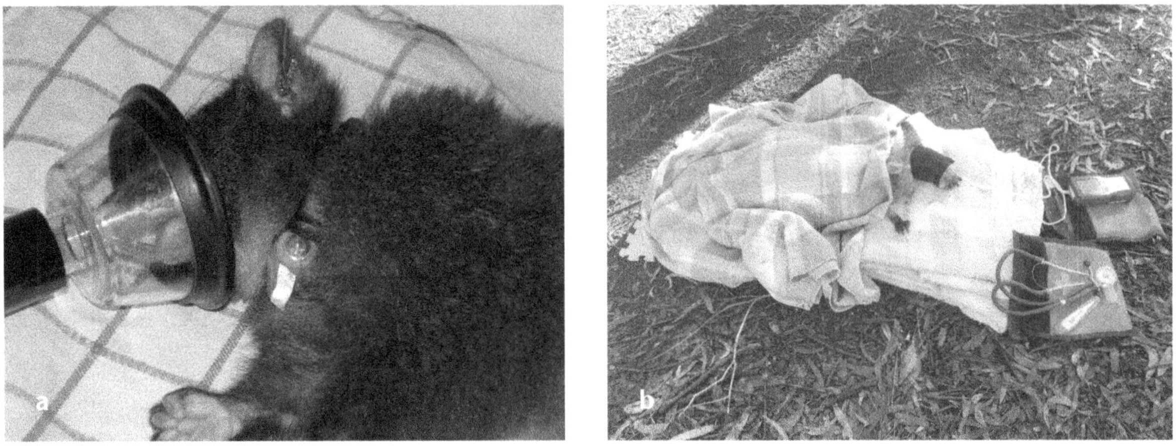

Figure 16.1: Managing anaesthesia in two different marsupial species. (a) A western ringtail possum (*Pseudocheirus occidentalis*) maintained under inhalational general anaesthesia using a facemask and isoflurane. Photo by Judy Clarke. (b) An eastern grey kangaroo (*Macropus giganteus*), heavily sedated via remote injection of tiletamine–zolazepam, being monitored and kept warm while recumbent. Photo by Jordan O. Hampton.

isoflurane for gaseous anaesthesia (Bryant *et al.* 2010), or injectable sedatives and anaesthetics that typically include tiletamine–zolazepam (Zoletil®) (Figure 16.1b), medetomidine and ketamine. Less commonly used injectables include diazepam, midazolam, xylazine, alfaxalone, azaperone and butorphanol. Many of these drugs are classed as Schedule 4 (S4) agents (e.g. tiletamine–zolazepam) and can be accessed by non-veterinarians under specific conditions that vary by jurisdictions. However, several of these drugs are classed as Schedule 8 (S8) agents (e.g. ketamine) and can only be accessed by veterinarians, and so are inaccessible to most researchers. Finally, some Schedule 6 (S6) drugs are available for fish anaesthesia (e.g. iso-eugenol or AQUI-S®), see Chapter 13.

Inhalational anaesthesia

Gaseous anaesthesia is widely used for Australian wildlife, but requires specialised equipment (Lewis 2004). The most commonly used inhalational anaesthetic for wildlife is isoflurane in oxygen, which may either be used as the sole anaesthetic agent (Bino *et al.* 2018) or can be used to maintain anaesthesia after initial induction with injectable sedation (Clarke *et al.* 2013). In birds and small mammals, facemask induction (Figure 16.1a) using isoflurane gives rapid induction and recovery with high margins of safety. However, facemask induction is not practical for larger mammals such as kangaroos as they will struggle and fail to be anaesthetised safely. It is also of limited use for reptiles, which can breath-hold for long periods. Induction chambers are of more use for species such as platypuses (*Ornithorhynchus anatinus*) (Bino *et al.* 2018).

Dosage calculation

Once a chemical restraint regime has been decided on for any scenario, the next step is to determine how much drug should be administered. An appropriate quantity (dose) of a drug must be administered to produce a desirable pharmacological response without overdosing and causing physiological injury. These known chemical quantities will repeatably induce a therapeutic effect in any given animal species, but large differences in effective dosage exist between species. Doses for gaseous anaesthesia are typically given as the percentage of an inhalational agent in inspired air (e.g. 2.5% isoflurane), while injectable dosages are typically measured in milligrams of drug per kilogram of bodyweight (mg/kg). For this reason, small animals should be weighed before anaesthesia where possible. Hand injection typically requires lower dosages than remote injection (see 'Chemical immobilisation') (Ryeng *et al.* 2002).

Animal treatment, withdrawal and euthanasia

Chemical restraint should be considered where the benefits of such restraint outweigh the potentially negative impacts on animal welfare, or where potentially painful or invasive procedures are intended to be undertaken. Euthanasia should be considered where an animal is deemed to be suffering or deteriorating and ready access to a qualified veterinarian or veterinary facility is not possible. Before commencing fieldwork, researchers should ensure that they are familiar with the appropriate methods of field euthanasia pertaining to the species they are working with.

Equipment and maintenance

Equipment required for sedation or anaesthesia include:

- injectable veterinary drugs (personnel should ensure that they have more than required)
- anaesthetic or sedative delivery equipment (e.g. gaseous anaesthesia circuit, remote delivery equipment, syringes and needles)
- anaesthetic monitoring equipment (i.e. thermometer, stethoscope, pulse oximeter) (Figure 16.1b)
- data sheets and veterinary chemical use logbooks
- equipment to aid thermoregulation – water for dousing in hot weather, foam mats and woollen blankets or external heat sources in cold weather
- equipment for anaesthetic support – supplementary oxygen, oxygen concentrator, IV fluids
- euthanasia equipment
- post-mortem equipment (e.g. formalin pots for histopathology) for animal mortalities.

Specific qualifications, experience and training

The sedation and anaesthesia of wildlife is a specialised field in veterinary medicine (West *et al.* 2014). Legislation pertaining to who may legally anaesthetise wildlife and under what conditions vary by jurisdiction in Australia (Table 16.1). In general, sedation or general anaesthesia of wildlife should only be undertaken by or under the direct supervision of a registered veterinarian. Consultation with veterinarians experienced with the taxon under consideration is strongly advised before formulating protocols for any project.

Workplace health and safety

Wildlife anaesthesia poses some important hazards to field biologists. Safety risks include (1) needle-stick injuries from sharps; (2) being bitten, scratched or kicked by recovering animals: and (3) zoonotic hazards, such as blood- or saliva-borne pathogens (e.g. Q fever, Australian bat lyssavirus). Anyone handling veterinary drugs should wear gloves and eye protection. All staff should be trained in appropriate responses to accidental human exposure to the drugs being used. Animal handlers should be vaccinated against diseases considered high risk for their level of exposure and should wash hands after operations. Personnel should have a current Senior First Aid Certificate, and at least one team member should have advanced training. The National Wildlife Biosecurity Guidelines contain more-detailed information about wildlife biosecurity risks and mitigation (Wildlife Health Australia 2018) and should be referred to in the planning and implementation of a wildlife anaesthetic procedure.

Alternative procedures

If chemical restraint is not essential for animal welfare reasons in any given context, alternative capture methods that use manual restraint can be considered (Olsson and Phalen 2013). The length of the procedure will play an

Table 16.1: Competency requirements for animal researchers undertaking sedation or anaesthesia of wild animals.

Competency	Competency requirement	Competency assessment
Handling captured animals	Experience in handling target or similar species.	Demonstrated practical experience under the supervision of a person experienced in handling captured animals of the target or similar species. Personnel should be deemed suitably competent by an experienced handler before handling animals on their own.
Performing sedation or anaesthesia	Considered an 'act of veterinary medicine' in many Australian jurisdictions. Acts of veterinary medicine requires registration as a veterinarian or accreditation.	Demonstrated practical experience under the supervision of a veterinarian.
Using Schedule 4 veterinary chemicals	Working under the direct supervision of a veterinarian OR possession of accreditation to perform acts of veterinary medicine (jurisdiction-specific) OR a research permit allowing access to prescription medicines.	Demonstrated practical experience under the supervision of a veterinarian.
Using Schedule 8 or 9 veterinary chemicals	Registration as a veterinarian.	N/A

important role in determining whether physical or chemical restraint is more appropriate. For example, manual restraint of a small macropod for 5–10 min may yield desirable animal welfare outcomes under the appropriate environmental and procedural circumstances, whereas prolonged manual restraint is likely to be associated with complications such as exertional myopathy (McMahon *et al.* 2013). However, no realistic alternatives to general anaesthesia are available for undertaking most invasive procedures (see 'Analgesia and antibiotics' in this chapter). The advice of a veterinarian experienced in the veterinary care of the species in question is essential to making sound, welfare-based decisions about the need for chemical restraint.

CHEMICAL IMMOBILISATION: DARTS AND POLE SYRINGES

Jordan O. Hampton and Graeme Coulson

Target taxa

Chemical immobilisation is commonly used for the safe handling of a wide variety of larger mammals, including koalas (*Phascolarctos cinereus*) (Chapter 20), macropods (Chapter 21), eutherian carnivores (Chapter 22), and ungulates (Chapter 24), pinnipeds (Chapter 25) and, occasionally, large birds such as emus (*Dromaius novaehollandiae*) (Chapter 36; Cushing and McClean 2010). Remote chemical immobilisation (darting) is usually restricted to large-bodied mammals (> 20 kg) such as ungulates, macropods and pinnipeds. However, specialised darting methods have been adapted for species < 5 kg, such as feral cats (*Felis catus*) (McGregor *et al.* 2016).

Context and scope

This GOP describes methods of chemically immobilising large-bodied mammals for capture, including macropods and koalas, terrestrial ungulates, pinnipeds and smaller mammals such as possums and eutherian carnivores. Drugs and their recommended dosages are covered in 'Sedation and general anaesthesia'.

Animal welfare considerations

Several categories of potential animal welfare impacts are associated with chemical immobilisation: (1) stress from being pursued before darting; (2) ballistic (dart trauma) injuries; (3) darting, but failing to capture an animal; (4) thermoregulation challenges, i.e. hyperthermia and hypothermia; e) anaesthetic complications (see 'Sedation and general anaesthesia'); f) capture myopathy; g) infection at injection sites; h) injection into non-target areas; and i) short-term post-capture behavioural changes.

Pursuit before darting

Considerable exertion can be caused by pursuit; chase time is well described in animal welfare literature and many programs attempt to restrict this duration to < 5 min to minimise the risks of hyperthermia and capture myopathy (Breed *et al.* 2019). Mode of pursuit (i.e. via vehicle; helicopter or fixed-wing aircraft; boat) may influence stress and exertion of pursued animals (see Chapter 6 for considerations relating to aerial pursuits). Refer to 'Capturing ungulates with corral and pen traps' in Chapter 7 for further discussion on the risks of capture myopathy.

Ballistic injuries

Risk of traumatic dart impact injuries is inherent to all remote injection methods. The high kinetic energy transferred by darts can lead to broken bones, and injuries are common when non-target anatomical sites are accidentally darted (e.g. the cranium or thorax). Having appropriately trained and licenced personnel undertaking the procedure, at a suitable distance, will help minimise the likelihood of these injuries occurring.

Failure to capture

Remote chemical immobilisation attempts often fail. Animals that are darted with barbed or cuffed darts, but are not captured (i.e. left with an embedded dart), will experience a protracted period of pain, and an elevated risk of subcutaneous and intramuscular infection. The risk of excessive stress (and capture myopathy) as a result of extended pursuit should be evaluated against the impacts of pain and infection risk. Animals that are immobilised, but not located before recovery may experience other welfare issues (listed below).

Anaesthetic complications

Refer to 'Sedation and general anaesthesia' earlier in this chapter.

Hyperthermia and hypothermia

Hyperthermia is particularly common with immobilisation methods that involve pursuit, particularly helicopter darting (Woolnough *et al.* 2012). High environmental temperatures, direct sunlight and drugs that interfere with thermoregulation are also risk factors. Planned (non-emergency) immobilisation operations should be timed to avoid hot seasons and the heat of the day (e.g. undertaken either in the early morning or late afternoon). However, late afternoon operations often involve releasing animals in darkness. Hyperthermic animals should be removed from direct sunlight (if possible) and active cooling should be used, usually water dousing.

Capture myopathy

Capture myopathy is a common metabolic disease of animals subjected to protracted stress and/or exertion. The prognosis for recovery is poor once clinical signs are present and often requires euthanasia. Capture myopathy is associated with extended pursuit, prolonged restraint without anaesthesia, unsuccessful induction efforts requiring multiple rounds of darting, and extended anaesthetic procedures (Breed *et al.* 2019). Personnel need to have a good understanding of the physiology of their study species and abandon pursuit efforts if the risk of myopathy increases.

Secondary infection

Darting can lead to deep wounds that predispose animals to subcutaneous and intramuscular infections, especially when barbed darts are used (Hampton *et al.* 2021). Wounds should be treated appropriately once the animal is immobilised.

Short-term behavioural changes

Non-lethal negative effects of immobilisation may result in altered levels of activity and mobility for several days post-capture. Where possible, animals should be monitored following release. Personnel should avoid immobilisation attempts when predators are known to be in the area.

General procedures

Equipment selection

Immobilisation drugs can be directly injected by hand, through a pole syringe, or can be remotely delivered using a dart that must be fired from a projector. Projectors include dart rifles, dart pistols, crossbows and blowpipes. For situations where an animal can be safely approached within 5 m, but hand injection is not safe or feasible, a pole syringe can be used. Pole syringes consist of a hypodermic syringe fitted to a light-weight extension pole (Figure 16.2a). They are used to safely inject animals caught in snares, traps, or pens, animals not fully immobilised after darting, or animals habituated to human presence (e.g. eastern grey kangaroos, *Macropus giganteus*; King *et al.* 2011). Pole syringes have also been used from vehicles after chasing animals with heightened flight responses (e.g. banteng, *Bos javanicus*; Bradshaw *et al.* 2005). Pole syringes present advantages to other methods, including negligible noise, low risk to cohort animals, and minimal cost. Pole syringes are not classified as firearms under state or territory legislation.

For all other animals that require chemical immobilisation, darting is necessary. Darts used for remote injection are effectively 'flying syringes', but have very different ballistic characteristics to bullets. Darts can be fired via crossbows (now rarely used), blowpipes, or dart rifles, with darts being fired on foot, from a hide, from a stationary vehicle, or from a moving vehicle, boat or helicopter (Figure 16.2b). Dart volumes range from 0.5–10 mL

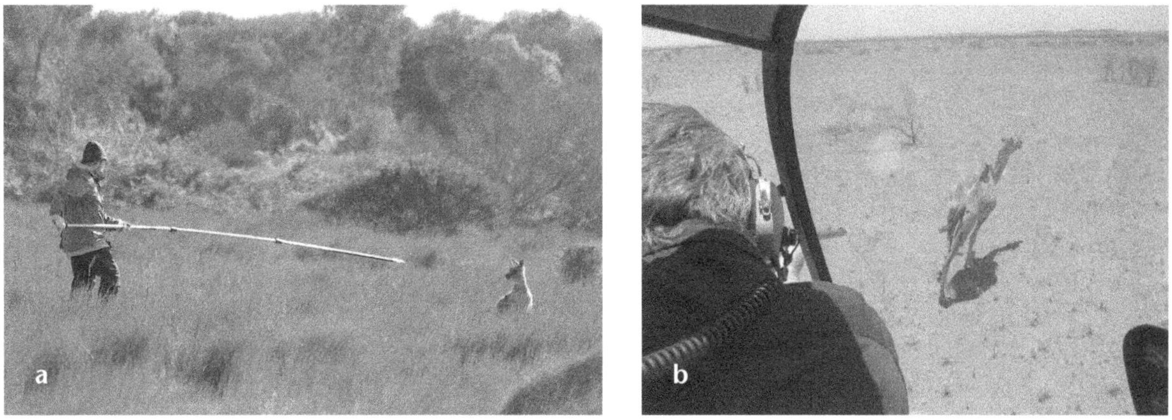

Figure 16.2: Different methods of chemical immobilisation. (a) An eastern grey kangaroo (*Macropus giganteus*) approached with an extendable pole syringe. Photo by Graeme Coulson. (b) A feral camel (*Camelus dromedarius*) darted from a helicopter. Photo by Jordan O. Hampton.

and two different dart types are available: charge-powered and pressurised. The maximum effective range of darting is rarely > 40 m.

Drug selection and dosage calculation

The recommended dosages of drugs chosen for wildlife anaesthesia are not covered in detail here (see 'Sedation and general anaesthesia'). Historically, paralytic agents (neuro-muscular blockers) were used to immobilise wildlife (Woolnough *et al.* 2012), but contemporary methods use sedatives and anaesthetics such as tiletamine-zolazepam, medetomidine and ketamine. Several agents used for darting are Schedule 8 (S8) chemicals (e.g. ketamine) and can only be accessed by veterinarians (see 'Specific qualifications and experience'). Some contemporary darting methods use highly potent opioids that are Schedule 9 (S9) chemicals, e.g. thiafentanil (Cushing and McClean 2010), which are prohibited for most researchers. Ground-based darting typically requires dosage increases of around 50% above hand or pole syringe injection. Higher dosages still are required for helicopter darting because of the increased stress and agitation of animals from these types of pursuits (see Chapter 6), which affects anaesthetic efficacy. A common approach to minimise the risk of adverse events is to use a dose at the upper limit of the recommended dose range to avoid the necessity of repeat darting or 'topping-up', which greatly complicate the procedure, extend duration and heighten risks involved with recovery.

Approach strategies

The flight distance of most wild animals is greater than the effective range of dart rifles, so strategies have to be adopted to either allow the researcher to get closer to the animal or to entice the animal to come closer to the researcher. Strategies commonly used include working at night using spotlight, thermal or night vision, the use of hides and tree stands, or first trapping the animals (see Chapters 7, 12, 13, 14 and 15 for a range of capture methods). In ground-based darting, the distance to the animal must be accurately measured (usually with a laser range finder), a stable darting position adopted (Zabek *et al.* 2015) and the target animal must be stationary.

Induction period

The period from first drug administration to a satisfactory level of immobilisation is known as the induction period (typically 3–10 min). It is important to keep the animal in sight and remain quiet during this interval. Transmitter darts have been used for animals with heightened flight responses, e.g. feral horses (*Equus caballus*) (Zabek *et al.* 2015).

Approaching and handling a recumbent animal

Once an injected animal has become recumbent, a capture team can approach it. If an animal is recumbent, but appears alert, personnel should always approach quietly from behind the animal. The first priority when approaching is to restrain the animal safely so that it cannot rise unexpectedly. A blindfold should be fitted to the animal as soon as possible. Sometimes physical restraint equipment may be required for dangerous species or individuals that are not deeply anaesthetised. Once the animal is securely restrained, the immobilisation team should proceed with the required procedures as quickly as possible.

Anaesthetic monitoring and support

Refer to 'Sedation and general anaesthesia' earlier in this chapter.

Recovery and release

All research procedures (e.g. collar fitting; sample collection) must be completed before preparing an animal for release. Some chemical regimes (e.g. tiletamine–zolazepam) lack reversal agents and may require researchers to wait for prolonged periods with recovering animals, sometimes for several hours (McGregor *et al.* 2016). Other immobilisation drugs do have reversal agents (e.g. atipamezole for medetomidine; Woolnough *et al.* 2012; Zabek *et al.* 2015), which enable faster recoveries. Blindfolds must be removed before animals are released from physical restraint, along with any equipment used to make handling safe, e.g. hobbles for deer (Hampton *et al.* 2019). Animals can have unsteady recoveries in which they fall over, thrash or stumble, so personnel should monitor the animal for a period once it is released to ensure that injuries requiring treatment do not occur.

Animal treatment, withdrawal and euthanasia

Chemical immobilisation may be associated with adverse animal welfare events that require major treatment or euthanasia. The following presentations generally require euthanasia: (1) fractured limbs from dart impact; (2) penetrated thorax from dart impact; (3) capture myopathy; (4) failure to recover from anaesthesia after > 4 h; and (5) fractured bones or major lacerations suffered during unsteady recoveries. Hyperthermic animals require treatment by cold water dousing; hypothermic animals require treatment by warming via woollen blankets or external heat sources such as warm water bottles; and hypoxaemic animals require treatment via administration of supplemental oxygen (see 'Sedation and general anaesthesia') (Hampton *et al.* 2021), although oxygen bottles are not always carried in the field. If animals are darted with barbed or cuffed darts and are not captured (i.e. left with an embedded dart), attempts should be made to capture the animals via a different means.

Equipment and maintenance

In addition to the equipment listed in the previous section, 'Sedation and general anaesthesia', the following is required specifically for remote chemical immobilisation:

- dart rifle, blow pipe or syringe pole
- power source for dart rifle (e.g. CO_2 bulbs – ensure that an oversupply is on hand)
- darts of appropriate volumes (ensure you have more than you need)
- veterinary drugs (ensure you have more than you need)
- laser range finder and binoculars
- data sheets and veterinary chemical use logbooks
- spare batteries for electronic equipment (ensure you have more than you need).

Specific qualifications, experience and training

As with sedatives, anaesthetics, analgesics and antibiotics (see 'Sedation and general anaesthesia' and 'Analgesia and antibiotics'), all veterinary drugs used for chemical immobilisation are classified under schedules that specify the level of regulation over the drug's availability (Table 16.2). Immobilisation has an additional layer of legislative restrictions because all dart guns are legally classified as firearms and require appropriate licensing and specialised training (Table 16.2; see also 'Capturing wombats and macropods by stunning and netting' in Chapter 7).

Workplace health and safety

See details under 'Sedation and general anaesthesia'. Anyone loading darts (especially pressurised darts) should wear gloves and eye protection. Where available, antidotes/reversal agents should always be carried in the field.

Alternative procedures

Many alternative capture methods can be used in place of chemical immobilisation, notably specialised manual restraint techniques, including use of net guns for deer (Hampton *et al.* 2019). A range of potential techniques are detailed in Chapters 7, 12, 13, 14 and 15.

Table 16.2: Competency requirements for animal researchers undertaking chemical immobilisation of wild animals.

Competency category	Competency requirement	Competency assessment
Handling captured animals	Experience in handling target or similar species.	Demonstrated practical experience under the supervision of a person experienced in handling captured animals of the target or similar species. Personnel should be deemed suitably competent by an experienced handler before handling animals on their own.
Operating a dart gun	A relevant firearms licence. Completion of a chemical immobilisation training course. Experience in darting. Regular practice at a rifle range to maintain competence.	Demonstrated practical experience under the supervision of a person experienced in darting. Personnel should be deemed suitably competent by an experienced darter before darting animals on their own.
Using Schedule 4 veterinary chemicals	Working under the direct supervision of a veterinarian OR possession of accreditation to perform acts of veterinary medicine (jurisdiction-specific) OR a research permit allowing access to prescription medicines. Completion of a chemical immobilisation training course.	Demonstrated practical experience under the supervision of a veterinarian.
Using Schedule 8 or 9 veterinary chemicals	Registration as a veterinarian.	N/A

ANALGESIA AND ANTIBIOTICS

Jordan O. Hampton, Andrew Peters and Sarah J. Gill

Target taxa

The use of analgesia and antibiotics applies to all Australian wildlife, but focus has been placed here on native and introduced mammals (Chapters 17–25), reptiles (Chapter 26), amphibians (Chapter 27) and birds (Chapters 33–36).

Context and scope

In this GOP, the use of analgesic and antibiotic medications for wildlife are described in the context of field research. Analgesia refers to the use of medication to relieve pain. Antibiotics refer to the use of antimicrobial substances (most commonly those active against bacteria) as medication. The techniques required for some situations will not be accessible to all wildlife researchers and the involvement of an experienced wildlife veterinarian will be required in all cases. Relatively few scenarios commonly encountered by wildlife researchers would warrant the use of analgesic and antibiotic medications. These chemicals are mostly used in veterinary hospitals, rehabilitation centres and zoos (Le Souëf *et al.* 2015). However, for some specialised applications (e.g. surgery), they may be warranted.

Animal welfare considerations

At least two categories of potential animal welfare impacts are associated with the use of analgesic and antibiotic medications for wildlife: (1) harm caused by not using medication (pain and risk of infection) and (2) harm caused by using medication (pain caused by injections, side-effects and inappropriate dosing).

General procedures

Veterinary chemicals used and their recommended dosages in different species are beyond the scope of this chapter, but are detailed in reference texts (Divers and Mader 2005; National Health and Medical Research Council 2014; Whiteside 2014; Vogelnest and Portas 2019).

Analgesia

For occasions where an animal is experiencing pain or discomfort as a result of an invasive procedure, a best-practice approach is to include the administration of adequate analgesia (Whiteside 2014). This process comes with the proviso that the pharmacological effect and effective dosing of available analgesics are known for that species (National Health and Medical Research Council 2014) and that those analgesics can be practicably and safely administered. Pharmacokinetic studies have not been undertaken for most analgesic drugs in the majority of Australian wildlife species (National Health and Medical Research Council 2014), so most analgesic doses are extrapolated from related species. Inherent risks are associated with the use of analgesia in species for which little evidence of their effectiveness or safety exists. These risks must be balanced against the potential benefit of providing analgesia. Use of analgesia is influenced by an assessment of the likely pain associated with a procedure. For instance, it is uncommon to provide analgesia to a wild animal during venipuncture (for blood collection) (see 'Blood collection and processing'), but commonly used during surgical implantation of a telemetry device (Bryant *et al.* 2010). Knowledge of pain and the perception of pain in many taxa is scant, but evolving (Hawkins *et al.* 2019). A precautionary approach (i.e. assume pain is associated with invasive procedures) is advisable in the absence of empirical evidence to the contrary.

In brief, non-steroidal anti-inflammatory drugs (NSAIDs) such as meloxicam are the class of veterinary chemicals most commonly used; the routes of administration most commonly employed in wildlife are intramuscular (Bryant *et al.* 2010) or subcutaneous (Le Souëf *et al.* 2015) injection. NSAIDs have also been used to improve animal welfare outcomes during lethal control (poisoning) of introduced species, such as red foxes (*Vulpes vulpes*) (Marks *et al.* 2009). Local anaesthetics (e.g. lignocaine) are rarely used for wildlife, but may be employed when performing locally painful procedures, such as skin biopsy (Chinnadurai *et al.* 2016) or some marking techniques (see Chapter 8). Many other analgesic approaches exist; it is advisable to consult a wildlife veterinarian when planning analgesia for wildlife.

Antibiotics

The use of antibiotics in wildlife has ethical considerations beyond animal welfare, which must be carefully considered. Antibiotic use in free-ranging wildlife is associated with potentially important but poorly understood risks, the most prominent of which is the development and spread of antimicrobial resistance (AMR) in the environment (Vittecoq *et al.* 2016). In all situations where antibiotics are used, the principles of good antimicrobial stewardship must be understood and adhered to (Fishman 2006), although the risks of AMR development associated with occasional antibiotic use in wild animals are much lower than those associated with routine use in livestock etc. Scant knowledge is available of the safety and pharmacological activity, including effective dosing regimens, of most antibiotics in most wildlife species. Also, several antibiotics are known to cause potentially lethal disruption of normal gastrointestinal flora (dysbiosis). This consideration is particularly important for mammalian herbivores because of the substantial potential to cause dysbiosis if oral antibiotics are given (Vogelnest 2015).

Administering antibiotics to wildlife for a sufficient duration to achieve effective therapy and to avoid AMR development are also associated with practical constraints. As a general rule, antibiotics should not be used unless compelling justification indicates a need to do so. The following situations may meet this criterion subject to veterinary assessment: management of injuries or disease associated with bacterial infection in wildlife held in captivity for at least the duration of therapy (Le Souëf *et al.* 2015; Booth and Nyari 2020), prophylactic use during field procedures (Coulson *et al.* 2008), and treatment of darting injuries (see 'Chemical immobilisation').

Animal treatment, withdrawal and euthanasia

Analgesics and antibiotics should only be used on wildlife when a compelling reason indicates the need to do so, where the potential risks are considered and outweighed by the likely benefits, and in consultation with a veterinarian. There may be situations associated with the use of analgesics and antibiotics that warrant euthanasia in extreme cases. The inability to provide adequate management of painful conditions caused by anthropogenic interventions would be one such situation. However, any such deliberation would depend on the severity of the condition and the ease with which euthanasia could be performed.

Equipment and maintenance

Depending on what medications are to be administered and to which species, a variety of delivery methods is available. The most common route of delivery for wildlife is via intramuscular or subcutaneous injection. Medication can also be administered via the oral route, but this method is less frequently used in wildlife than in domestic animals. Oral medication can be administered to birds via crop needles or crop tubes (Baldrey 2020). For each case, variables such as species, frequency of administration, treatment length, ability to monitor effects, restraint and other factors will influence what medication is used and the delivery route (Vogelnest and Portas 2019). Administration of medication typically requires:

- appropriate veterinary chemicals at an appropriate concentration and within the expiry date
- refrigeration – some antibiotics and analgesics require storage at ~4°C
- sterile hypodermic needles of appropriate gauge and length
- sterile syringes
- skin disinfectant and gauze or cotton swabs
- oral medication delivery materials (e.g. crop needle/tube, oesophageal tube).

Administering equipment must never be reused on two or more separate individual animals without medical sterilisation of the equipment in between those uses.

Specific qualifications, experience and training

Analgesic and antibiotic use should be considered judiciously and following the guidance of a veterinarian. Veterinarians play an important role in informed antimicrobial decision-making and stewardship (Vittecoq *et al.* 2016). Ideally, a qualified veterinarian with expertise in analgesia and antibiotic use in the species or taxonomic group under consideration should be involved in all research projects. All details of doses, administration routes and side effects should be provided by the registered consulting veterinarian.

As with sedatives and anaesthetics (see 'Sedation and general anaesthesia' and 'Chemical immobilisation'), all veterinary chemicals used for analgesia or antibiosis are classified under schedules that specify the level of regulation over their availability. Nearly all antibiotics are classed as Schedule 4 chemicals, meaning that they are prescription-only medications (Table 16.3). Storing, prescribing, dispensing and using medications carry legal responsibilities and researchers and veterinarians must be familiar with all relevant legislation, which varies between jurisdictions (Cook and Grimes 2005).

Workplace health and safety

See details under 'Sedation and general anaesthesia'.

Table 16.3: Competency requirements for animal researchers administering antibiotics or analgesics to wild animals.

Competency category	Competency requirement	Competency assessment
Handling captured animals	Experience in handling target or similar species.	Demonstrated practical experience under the supervision of a person experienced in handling captured animals of the target or similar species. Personnel should be deemed suitably competent by an experienced handler before handling animals on their own.
Using Schedule 4 veterinary chemicals	Working under the direct supervision of a veterinarian OR possession of accreditation to perform acts of veterinary medicine (jurisdiction-specific) OR a research permit allowing access to prescription medicines.	Demonstrated practical experience under the supervision of a veterinarian.

Alternative procedures

If administering medication to animals is deemed to be highly dangerous for the animal or staff, the most obvious alternatives are to forgo dosing (if the need is not urgent) or euthanasia of the injured animal if the condition is severe.

BLOOD COLLECTION AND PROCESSING

Derek Spielman, Sarah J. Gill and Jordan O. Hampton

Target taxa

The general principles of blood collection and the techniques for doing so apply to most vertebrate taxa (see Section 3).

Context and scope

Blood sampling is a basic technique that may be used for several wildlife research applications. Analysis of blood samples is a specialised field of veterinary medicine, but some general background is provided here. Blood contains three components: red blood cells, white blood cells, and either plasma from anticoagulated blood or serum from coagulated blood. Centrifuging moves red cells to the bottom of a sample, plasma to the top and the white blood cells (buffy coat) form a thin (~0.5–1 mm thick) greyish line between these layers. Blood sampling may be employed to look for immunological evidence of exposure to infectious diseases (Huaman *et al.* 2020), to assess exposure to a toxin (Hivert *et al.* 2018) or biomarker (Cowled *et al.* 2006) or, more commonly, to infer an animal's health status (McMichael *et al.* 2015). For animals with nucleated red blood cells (birds, reptiles, amphibians and fish), blood may be also used to collect DNA for genetic studies (Szczys *et al.* 2005; Weston *et al.* 2020).

Animal welfare considerations

Pain and distress during the procedure

Blood is generally collected from live animals, but may also be collected from freshly killed animals; this is common for introduced species subjected to culling, e.g. deer (Huaman *et al.* 2020). When applied to live animals, blood collection is invasive. Personnel require training in restraint and venipuncture, and some taxa require sedation or general anaesthesia (see 'Sedation and general anaesthesia') to obtain a good sample and reduce risks to the animal and handler (Tsai *et al.* 2015). During handling and blood collection, animals will experience stress and some pain, which can be minimised by ensuring that personnel are properly trained in all methods or supervised by experienced colleagues.

Physiological considerations

Withdrawing blood from an animal can affect its physiology and even lead to death if too much blood is collected, or bleeding is profuse (uncommon). Often, only tiny blood volumes can be collected from small wild animals. The maximum permissible blood volume collected per day is 10% of the circulating blood volume, which in most animals is 5–10% of their body mass. Thus, 0.5% of the total body mass is generally the maximum permissible volume of blood to be collected. For large introduced mammals (e.g. deer), this volume may be > 10 mL (Huaman *et al.* 2020), but for many birds and reptiles it may be < 1 mL (Weston *et al.* 2020). Most DNA studies require very little blood, so maximum volumes allowed for animals < 7 g is 1/3 of a standard capillary tube, for animals 7–15 g it is 1/2 of a standard capillary tube, and for animals > 15 g it is 1 standard capillary tube.

General procedures

The most appropriate methods of blood collection vary with species, individual animal characteristics (e.g. age and sex), the volume of blood required and research requirements.

Preparation of the puncture site and data recording

Personnel should assemble required equipment before restraining the animal. Prior to venipuncture, the intended puncture site should be prepared. Preparation may include shaving or clipping the site (mammals) or disinfecting the intended puncture site. Diluted chlorhexidine solution (1:40) can be used for this purpose. Alcohol (≥ 70%) is also suitable and is better at wetting the hair of mammals, which helps to visualise the vein. Personnel should allow the alcohol to air-dry to avoid contaminating the sample. Alcohol should not be used on frogs as it is an irritant. Geckos and other small animals can absorb the alcohol through their skin so it must be used with care.

Needle dimensions

Needle size can be critical to the success of blood collection, as well as to the trauma caused to the animal. Using a needle that is too large for the targeted vein makes the process extremely challenging. Conversely, smaller gauge needles are more likely to damage blood cells as the blood is collected – a gentle steady technique is required to minimise this risk whatever the needle size. For many small species (especially birds and reptiles), very small needles must be used (Figure 16.3a, b). For example, a 27 G needle was used for the tarsal vein of the hooded plover (*Charadrius cucullatus*) (Weston *et al.* 2020). Small-gauge butterfly catheters also facilitate

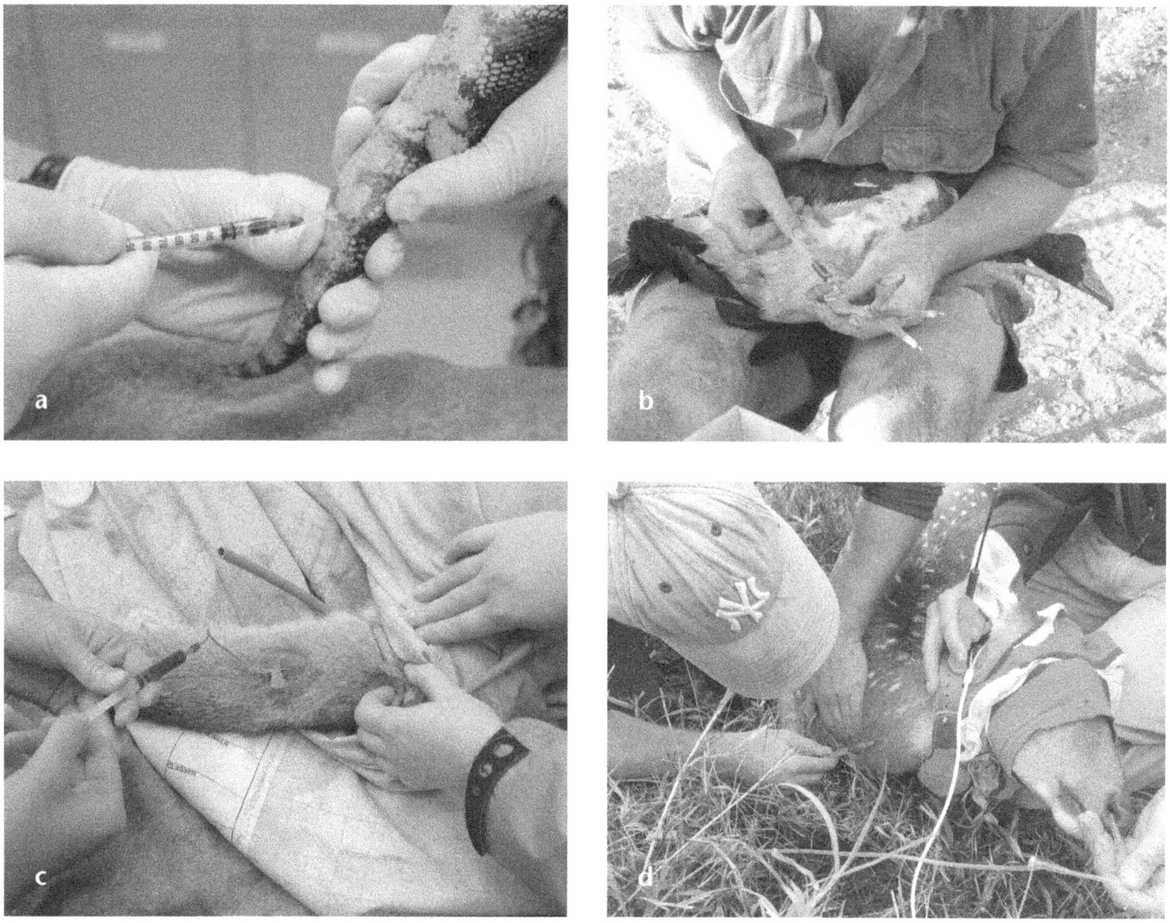

Figure 16.3: Venipuncture sites for blood collection from Australian wildlife species. (a) The ventral coccygeal vein of an eastern blue-tongued lizard (*Tiliqua scincoides scincoides*). Photo by Andrea Reiss, Wildlife Health Australia. (b) The median metatarsal vein of a magpie goose (*Anseranas semipalmata*). Photo by Jordan O. Hampton. (c) The lateral tail vein of a tammar wallaby (*Notamacropus eugenii*). Photo by Derek Spielman. (d) The jugular vein of a chital deer (*Axis axis*). Photo by Jordan O. Hampton.

gentle collection of blood in small animals (Figure 16.3c). Conversely, for ungulates, large needles ≤ 20 G are regularly used (Figure 16.3d).

Appropriate veins

Body size and blood vessel anatomy vary enormously for the range of species covered in this GOP. As a result, considerable variation exists for which veins are used most commonly for blood collection in each taxon (see Table 16.4 for general recommendations for a range of taxa). Each vein has a specific anatomical name that will mean little to readers unfamiliar with that species. Researchers contemplating blood collection in a new species for the first time should consult species-specific references. Some general comments are possible, but should be treated only as broad guidelines. For example, the ventral coccygeal vein is commonly used for snakes. For birds, wing veins and leg veins, such as the median metatarsal vein (Figure 16.3a), are often used. For smaller mammals, several different veins may be used; for example, peripheral ear veins are used for Tasmanian devils (*Sarcophilus harrisii*) (Hivert *et al.* 2018). For large mammals, especially ungulates, the jugular vein is often the preferred site.

Haemostasis

Personnel should apply moderate pressure immediately following withdrawal of the needle or when sufficient

Table 16.4: Appropriate locations and equipment for the collection of blood samples from a range of Australian taxa.

Species	Sites	Restraint	Needle	Comments
Platypus	Venous sinus of the dorsal bill, jugular vein	Anaesthesia advised to avoid bill laceration.	23–25 G needle or butterfly catheter, bevel directed abaxially (away from the axis or central line)	The jugular vein can be difficult to locate because of loose skin. Using butterfly catheters reduces the risk of laceration.
Echidna	Venous sinus, jugular, cephalic or femoral veins	Anaesthesia is advised.	23–25 G needle or butterfly catheter	The echidna's venous sinus is smaller than in the platypus.
Kangaroos and wallabies	Lateral caudal vein, recurrent tarsal vein, cephalic vein, jugular vein	Manual restraint is generally sufficient in small macropods.	20–25 G butterfly catheters recommended, appropriate to the animal size	The head should be covered at all times.
Large possums and large gliders	Jugular, cephalic, lateral caudal, ventral caudal, ear and femoral veins, and tibial artery	Anaesthesia recommended.	22–26 G	
Pygmy possums and small gliders	Tibial artery, jugular and lateral caudal veins	Anaesthesia advised.	29 G needle and tuberculin syringe for the tibial artery	Extra care should be taken to minimise haematoma. If collecting from the tibial artery, apply digital pressure following needle withdrawal.
Wombats	Femoral, radial, cephalic or median metatarsal vein	Anaesthesia required.	20–22 G	The thick skin can hamper visualisation and palpation of blood vessels.
Koala	Cephalic vein	Manual restraint.	22–25 G	Larger volumes of blood can be collected from the femoral or jugular veins but this requires anaesthesia.
Large dasyurids	Cephalic, femoral, jugular and ventral caudal veins	Manual restraint.	22–25 G	
Small dasyurids and murids	Lateral caudal vein, jugular, saphenous and sublingual veins and orbital sinus	Manual restraint or general anaesthesia.	23–27 G	
Bandicoots and bilbies	Jugular, saphenous and lateral caudal veins	Manual restraint or general anaesthesia.	22–26 G	

blood has been obtained from a needle prick. Excessive pressure limits blood flow within the damaged vein, impairing formation of the clot and delaying haemostasis. Aids to control excessive bleeding should be kept readily available (e.g. antiseptic powders or tissue glue). Silver nitrate sticks (styptic pencils) are caustic and should not be used on skin.

Blood collection tubes

A variety of blood collection tubes commercially available. The appropriate type for any research project invariably depends on the question being answered and the conditions of the field work. The most important distinction is between tubes containing anticoagulant that prevents blood from clotting and those that do not. Generally speaking, anticoagulant tubes are required for haematological analysis of blood, whereas clotted samples yield serum and can be used for biochemistry and serology (Huaman *et al.* 2020). The anticoagulants typically used include EDTA (lavender-top tubes) and heparin (green-top tubes). EDTA is suitable for haematology, some toxicant studies (Hivert *et al.* 2018) and sample storage in most species. Exceptions include some birds, most reptiles and many amphibians (Fudge 2000) in which the erythrocytes often lyse in EDTA.

Collecting, storing and shipping blood tubes

For plain tubes, once a clot has formed and contracted, personnel should aspirate serum (centrifugation will increase yield, but is not essential), and place it in a labelled screw-top vial. Some serum tubes now contain a chemical separator that separates the serum from the blood clot. For anticoagulant tubes, personnel should repeatedly gently invert the tubes for 5 min to ensure that the cells are fully suspended. If required, a thin smear is made (see below). Blood samples should be kept cool, but not in direct contact with a freezer brick. Collection tubes should be labelled with the animal's identification code, date and sample type (plasma, buffy coat or whole blood). For haematological and biochemical analysis of blood (whole blood, serum or plasma), samples must arrive at the laboratory within 72 h. Samples should be kept chilled (2–4°C) but must not be frozen. For genetic studies using polymerase chain reaction (PCR), samples can be frozen at –20°C or –80°C. Freeze–thaw cycles must be minimised; if the sample cannot be kept frozen in transit, then it can be kept chilled for up to 5 days (Clark 2004).

Interpretation of blood results

In general, measurement of haematological, biochemical and serological parameters from blood samples are left to specialised staff in dedicated laboratories and will not be covered here. Suffice to say that haematology is a complex discipline with important differences between wildlife taxa, for example between mammals (Clark 2004) and birds (Clark et al. 2009).

Preparation of thin blood smears

One example of a useful blood analysis technique that can be performed with minimal equipment is a blood smear. Thin blood smears can be used for Giemsa staining (glass slides) and light microscopy (haematology). To do so, place two or three small drops (~2 mm in diameter) of blood ~0.5 cm from the labelled end of the glass slide. Personnel should use a commercial spreader slide with bevelled edges or a second clean microscope slide. The edge of the spreader should be placed on top of the slide at a 45° angle, just beyond the blood drops. The spreader slide is drawn back towards the blood drops and the drops allowed to spread along the spreader's edge. Once the blood is spread along the entire edge, the spreader should be moved forward immediately at a 45° angle in a steady motion, and the thin smear air-dried quickly. This technique requires clean slides, training and practice (Clark 2004).

Animal treatment, withdrawal and euthanasia

When compared to other veterinary procedures applied to wildlife, blood collection is associated with relatively infrequent adverse animal welfare events. Severe haematomas and secondary infections because of venipuncture may require treatment. Neither presentation is likely to be sufficiently severe to warrant euthanasia.

Equipment and maintenance

Equipment required for blood collection includes:

- gloves
- hair clippers for mammals
- 70% alcohol or diluted chlorhexidine solution
- appropriately sized needles and syringes
- blood tubes of chosen volume contained appropriate anticoagulant.
- refrigeration or freezing facilities
- glass slides and coverslips for blood smears
- spreader slide with bevelled edges for blood smears
- capillary (microhaematocrit) tubes and pipettes for blood smears

- gauze swabs
- antiseptic powder or tissue glue
- marker pen and pencil for labelling tubes and slides
- a portable centrifuge can be useful when collecting clotted blood in plain tubes as it allows serum to be drawn off and frozen if blood can not be transferred to a laboratory within 24 h.

Specific qualifications, experience and training

Blood collection methods are invasive and highly technical and should only be undertaken by veterinarians or other trained personnel.

Workplace health and safety

See details under 'Sedation and general anaesthesia'. These methods are associated with a risk of transmission of zoonoses or anthropozoonoses. Personnel should follow suitable hygiene practices, use only sterile and unused needles and syringes, and clean all other equipment meticulously between animals. Personnel working with certain species may require vaccinations (e.g. Q fever; Australian bat lyssavirus) before conducting work. Used needles or shattered glass slides should be disposed of in sharps containers and not left unsecured.

Alternative procedures

Collection of blood samples is necessary for health evaluations and for answering a range of questions about animal physiology and health, which typically cannot be answered with any other technique.

REFERENCES

Baldrey V (2020) Guide to using antibiotics in pet birds. *In Practice* **42**, 394–404. doi:10.1136/inp.m3092

Batson WG, Gordon IJ, Fletcher DB, Manning AD (2016) The effect of pre-release captivity on post-release performance in reintroduced eastern bettongs *Bettongia gaimardi*. *Oryx* **50**, 664–673. doi:10.1017/S0030605315000496

Bino G, Kingsford RT, Grant T, Taylor MD, Vogelnest L (2018) Use of implanted acoustic tags to assess platypus movement behaviour across spatial and temporal scales. *Scientific Reports* **8**, 5117. doi:10.1038/s41598-018-23461-9

Booth R, Nyari S (2020) Clinical comparison of five anti-chlamydial antibiotics in koalas (*Phascolarctos cinereus*). *PLoS One* **15**, e0236758. doi:10.1371/journal.pone.0236758

Bradshaw C, Traill L, Wertz K, White W, Gurry I (2005) Chemical immobilisation of wild banteng (*Bos javanicus*) in northern Australia using detomidine, tiletamine and zolazepam. *Australian Veterinary Journal* **83**, 616–617. doi:10.1111/j.1751-0813.2005.tb13273.x

Breed D, Meyer LC, Steyl JC, Goddard A, Burrough R, Kohn TA (2019) Conserving wildlife in a changing world: understanding capture myopathy – a malignant outcome of stress during capture and translocation. *Conservation Physiology* **7**, coz027. doi:10.1093/conphys/coz027

Brogi R, Brivio F, Bertolucci C, Benazzi M, Luccarini S, Cappai N, Bottero E, Pedrazzoli C, Columbano N, Apollonio M (2019) Capture effects in wild boar: a multifaceted behavioural investigation. *Wildlife Biology* **2019**, 1–10. doi:10.2981/wlb.00497

Bryant G, Eden P, De Tores P, Warren K (2010) Improved procedure for implanting radiotransmitters in the coelomic cavity of snakes. *Australian Veterinary Journal* **88**, 443–448. doi:10.1111/j.1751-0813.2010.00633.x

Chinnadurai SK, Strahl-Heldreth D, Fiorello CV, Harms CA (2016) Best-practice guidelines for field-based surgery and anesthesia of free-ranging wildlife. I. Anesthesia and analgesia. *Journal of Wildlife Diseases* **52**, S14–S27. doi:10.7589/52.2S.S14

Clark P (2004) *Haematology of Australian Mammals*. CSIRO Publishing, Melbourne.

Clark P, Boardman W, Raidal S (2009) *Atlas of Clinical Avian Hematology*. John Wiley & Sons, Oxford, UK.

Clarke J, Warren K, Calver M, de Tores P, Mills J, Robertson I (2013) Hematologic and serum biochemical reference ranges and an assessment of exposure to infectious diseases prior to translocation of the threatened western ringtail possum (*Pseudocheirus occidentalis*). *Journal of Wildlife Diseases* **49**, 831–840. doi:10.7589/2011-12-345

Cook DL, Grimes DT (2005) Harmonisation of control of use legislation for veterinary medicines. *Australian Veterinary Journal* **83**, 124–125. doi:10.1111/j.1751-0813.2005.tb11606.x

Coulson G, Nave CD, Shaw G, Renfree MB (2008) Long-term efficacy of levonorgestrel implants for fertility control of eastern grey kangaroos (*Macropus giganteus*). *Wildlife Research* **35**, 520–524. doi:10.1071/WR07133

Cowled BD, Lapidge SJ, Smith M, Staples L (2006) Attractiveness of a novel omnivore bait, PIGOUT®, to feral pigs (*Sus scrofa*) and assessment of risks of bait uptake by non-target species. *Wildlife Research* **33**, 651–660. doi:10.1071/WR06054

Cushing A, McClean M (2010) Use of thiafentanil-medetomidine for the induction of anesthesia in emus (*Dromaius novaehollandiae*) within a wild animal park. *Journal of Zoo and Wildlife Medicine* **41**, 234–241. doi:10.1638/2009-0143R1.1

Divers SJ, Mader DR (2005) *Reptile Medicine and Surgery*. Elsevier Saunders, St Louis, MO.

Fudge A (2000) Avian blood sampling and artifact considerations. In *Laboratory Medicine: Avian and Exotic Pets*. (Ed. A Fudge) pp. 1–8. Saunders, Philadelphia, PA.

Hampton JO, Amos M, Pople T, Brennan M, Forsyth DM (2021) Minimising mortalities in capturing wildlife: refinement of helicopter darting of chital deer (*Axis axis*) in Australia. *Wildlife Research* **48**, 304–313. doi:10.1071/WR20106

Hampton JO, Finch N, Watter K, Amos M, Pople T, Moriarty A, Jacotine A, Panther D, McGhie C, Davies C, Mitchell J, Forsyth DM (2019) A review of methods used for the capture of wild deer in Australia. *Australian Mammalogy* **41**, 1–11. doi:10.1071/AM17047

Hawkins MG, Guzman DSM, Paul-Murphy J (2019) General principles of analgesia and anesthesia in wildlife. In *Medical Management of Wildlife Species: A Guide for Practitioners*. (Eds SM Hernandez, HW Barron, EA Miller, RF Aguilar and MJ Yabsley) pp. 45–73. John Wiley and Sons, Hoboken, NJ.

Hivert L, Clarke J, Peck S, Lawrence C, Brown W, Huxtable SJ, Schaap D, Pemberton D, Grueber CE (2018) High blood lead concentrations in captive Tasmanian devils (*Sarcophilus harrisii*): a threat to the conservation of the species? *Australian Veterinary Journal* **96**, 442–449. doi:10.1111/avj.12753

Huaman JL, Pacioni C, Forsyth DM, Pople A, Hampton JO, Carvalho TG, Helbig KJ (2020) Serosurveillance and molecular investigation of wild deer in Australia reveals seroprevalence of *Pestivirus* infection. *Viruses* **12**, 752.

Fishman N (2006) Antimicrobial stewardship. *American Journal of Infection Control* **34**, S55–S63.

King W, Wilson M, Allen T, Festa-Bianchet M, Coulson G (2011) A capture technique for free-ranging eastern grey kangaroos (*Macropus giganteus*) habituated to humans. *Australian Mammalogy* **33**, 47–51. doi:10.1071/AM10029

Le Souëf A, Holyoake C, Vitali S, Warren K (2015) Presentation and prognostic indicators for free-living black cockatoos (*Calyptorhynchus* spp.) admitted to an Australian zoo veterinary hospital over 10 years. *Journal of Wildlife Diseases* **51**, 380–388. doi:10.7589/2014-08-203

Lewis JC (2004) Field use of isoflurane and air anesthetic equipment in wildlife. *Journal of Zoo and Wildlife Medicine* **35**, 303–311. doi:10.1638/03-072

Marks CA, Gigliotti F, Busana F (2009) Assuring that 1080 toxicosis in the red fox (*Vulpes vulpes*) is humane. II. Analgesic drugs produce better welfare outcomes. *Wildlife Research* **36**, 98–105. doi:10.1071/WR05018

Mayberry C, Bencini R, Mawson P, Maloney S (2014) Sedation of western grey kangaroos (*Macropus fuliginosus ocydromus*) with tiletamine-zolazepam. *Animal Welfare (South Mimms, England)* **23**, 141–144. doi:10.7120/09627286.23.2.141

McGregor H, Hampton JO, Lisle D, Legge S (2016) Live-capture of feral cats using tracking dogs and darting. *Wildlife Research* **43**, 313–322. doi:10.1071/WR15134

McMahon C, Wiggins N, French V, McCallum H, Bowman D (2013) A report of capture myopathy in the Tasmanian pademelon (*Thylogale billardierii*). *Animal Welfare (South Mimms, England)* **22**, 1–4. doi:10.7120/09627286.22.1.001

McMichael L, Edson D, McLaughlin A, Mayer D, Kopp S, Meers J, Field H (2015) Haematology and plasma biochemistry of wild black flying-foxes (*Pteropus alecto*) in Queensland, Australia. *PLoS One* **10**, e0125741. doi:10.1371/journal.pone.0125741

National Health and Medical Research Council (2014) *A Guide to the Care and Use of Australian Native Mammals in Research and Teaching.* National Health and Medical Research Council, Canberra.

Olsson A, Phalen D (2013) Comparison of biochemical stress indicators in juvenile captive estuarine crocodiles (*Crocodylus porosus*) following physical restraint or chemical restraint by midazolam injection. *Journal of Wildlife Diseases* **49**, 560–567. doi:10.7589/2012-06-160

Ryeng KA, Larsen S, Arnemo JM (2002) Medetomidine-ketamine in reindeer (*Rangifer tarandus tarandus*): effective immobilization by hand-and dart-administered injection. *Journal of Zoo and Wildlife Medicine* **33**, 397–400. doi:10.1638/1042-7260(2002)033[0397:MKIRRT]2.0.CO;2

Szczys P, Hughes C, Kesseli R (2005) Novel microsatellite markers used to determine the population genetic structure of the endangered roseate tern, *Sterna dougallii*, in Northwest Atlantic and Western Australia. *Conservation Genetics* **6**, 461–466. doi:10.1007/s10592-004-4975-6

Tsai P-P, Schlichtig A, Ziegler E, Ernst H, Haberstroh J, Stelze HD, Hackbarth H (2015) Effects of different blood collection methods on indicators of welfare in mice. *Lab Animal* **44**, 301–310. doi:10.1038/laban.738

Vittecoq M, Godreuil S, Prugnolle F, Durand P, Brazier L, Renaud N, Arnal A, Aberkane S, Jean-Pierre H, Gauthier-Clerc M (2016) Antimicrobial resistance in wildlife. *Journal of Applied Ecology* **53**, 519–529. doi:10.1111/1365-2664.12596

Vogelnest L (2015) Marsupialia (Marsupials). In *Fowler's Zoo and Wild Animal Medicine, Volume* 8. (Eds RE Miller and ME Fowler.) pp. 255–274. Elsevier, St Louis, MO.

Vogelnest L, Portas T (2019) *Current Therapy in Medicine of Australian Mammals.* CSIRO Publishing, Melbourne.

West G, Heard D, Caulkett N (Eds) (2014) *Zoo Animal and Wildlife Immobilization and Anesthesia.* John Wiley & Sons, Hoboken, NJ.

Weston MA, Clarke K, Maguire GS, Sumner J (2020) Morphological and molecular evidence of population divergence in a widespread shorebird across its southern mainland Australian distribution. *Conservation Genetics* **21**, 757–770. doi:10.1007/s10592-020-01286-2

Whiteside DP (2014) Analgesia. In *Zoo Animal and Wildlife Immobilization and Anesthesia.* (Eds G West, D Heard and N Caulkett.) pp. 83–108. Wiley Blackwell, Ames, IA.

Wildlife Health Australia (2018) *National Wildlife Biosecurity Guidelines.* Wildlife Health Australia, Sydney.

Woolnough AP, Hampton JO, Campbell S, Lethbridge MR, Boardman WS, Sharp T, Rose K (2012) Field immobilization of feral 'Judas' donkeys (*Equus asinus*) by remote injection of medetomidine and ketamine and antagonism with atipamezole. *Journal of Wildlife Diseases* **48**, 435–443. doi:10.7589/0090-3558-48.2.435

Zabek MA, Wright J, Berman DM, Hampton JO, Collins CW (2015) Assessing the efficacy of medetomidine and tiletamine–zolazepam for remote immobilisation of feral horses (*Equus caballus*). *Wildlife Research* **41**, 615–622. doi:10.1071/WR14108

Section 3

SPECIES PROFILES

Introduction

Bradley P. Smith, Helen P. Waudby, Corinne Alberthsen and Jordan O. Hampton

This section details specific considerations for using Australian wildlife for scientific, management and teaching purposes. It covers all native and introduced Australian fauna, either as single species or within a larger taxonomic group. Fishes and crustaceans have been included in view of the growing body of knowledge around the cognitive and social complexities of these taxa and their ability to feel pain (e.g. Franks *et al.* 2021 and references therein). Many species hold cultural and spiritual significance for Indigenous Australians (Aslin and Bennett 2000; Weir 2012). It was not possible to represent the diversity of Indigenous names and perspectives for species across geographies and language groups adequately. However, the adoption of Indigenous names, and appreciation of all cultural perspectives and knowledge in wildlife research and management are paramount to conducting research holistically and effectively in many landscapes (Wilson *et al.* 2010; Walsh *et al.* 2014).

While many of the research methods outlined in Section 2 can be used across species, the design of research projects often requires adaptation and customisation depending on the species of interest. As such, this section provides a guide to species-specific considerations for researchers and animal ethics committee (AEC) members who may be planning or evaluating wildlife research or education activities, rather than a hard set of rules. Details such as conservation or taxonomic status, and species' distributions, are not included unless they affect practical considerations. Each profile includes a brief overview of the species' characteristics, including their biology and behaviour. These profiles also discuss animal welfare considerations around capture and handling, which often include veterinary considerations (chemical restraint, other medications, infectious diseases and euthanasia). An attempt is made to describe all of the ways (direct and indirect) in which wildlife research may harm animals and provide recommendations for mitigating these impacts, for example stressing that for any wild animal euthanased *in situ*, researchers need to ensure that any chemical agents used do not pose a secondary toxicity risk to wild scavengers (i.e. carcasses should be appropriately disposed of).

While the risk of pathogen transmission in wildlife research is not a new one, the COVID-19 pandemic has highlighted the threat of zoonoses to researchers and anthropozoonoses to wildlife. We recommend that all wildlife researchers review their capture and handling protocols carefully in view of the risks of pathogen transmission, including potential zooanthroponoses (refer to WHA 2021 for an example relating to bats).

Each species profile follows the same template (modelled on those developed by NHMRC 2014), but individual profile content reflects the nature of the individual species or taxa being described. Readers are also directed to relevant general operating procedures detailed in Section 2. These profiles are intended to be brief and readers are encouraged to consult the literature and experts for more-detailed information, where necessary.

Some veterinary procedures detailed in these profiles will need to be performed by a veterinarian (particularly when administration of restricted drugs is required); others can be performed by experienced personnel or under the supervision of a veterinarian. Readers should confirm the experience and legal/licensing requirements for their procedures during the planning stage of their research. For many species, details on the recommended drug doses and administration routes are provided, but this information is not intended to replace more detailed veterinary texts or the advice of a practising veterinarian. Rather, these considerations are included (and covered more generally in Chapter 16) to provide researchers with a starting point for planning studies, and for AEC members reviewing applications.

ACKNOWLEDGEMENTS

We are grateful to Dr Derek Spielman, Dr Peter Holz, Dr Sarah Gill and Dr Vere Nicolson for reviewing the veterinary considerations for all chapters in this section.

REFERENCES

Aslin HJ, Bennett DH (2000) Wildlife and world views: Australian attitudes toward wildlife. *Human Dimensions of Wildlife* **5**, 15–35. doi:10.1080/10871200009359177

Franks B, Ewell C, Jacquet J (2021) Animal welfare risks of global aquaculture. *Science Advances* **7**, eabg0677. doi:10.1126/sciadv.abg0677

NHMRC (2014) *A Guide to the Care and Use of Australian Native Mammals in Research and Teaching.* National Health and Medical Research Council, Canberra.

Walsh F, Christophersen P, McGregor S (2014) Indigenous perspectives on biodiversity. In *Biodiversity: Science and Solutions for Australia.* (Eds S Morton, A Sheppard and M Lonsdale) pp. 81–100. CSIRO Publishing, Melbourne.

Weir JK (2012) *Country, Native Title and Ecology.* ANU ePress, Canberra.

WHA (2021) *Bat Health Focus Group.* Wildlife Health Australia. <https://wildlifehealthAustralia.com.au/ProgramsProjects/BatHealthFocusGroup.aspx>.

Wilson GR, Edwards MJ, Smits JK (2010) Support for Indigenous wildlife management in Australia to enable sustainable use. *Wildlife Research* **37**, 255–263. doi:10.1071/WR09130

17 Monotremes

Melody Serena, Peggy D. Rismiller and Joanne H. Connolly

INTRODUCTION

Two monotreme species are found in Australia: the platypus (*Ornithorhynchus anatinus*) and the short-beaked echidna (*Tachyglossus aculeatus*). Monotremes are distinguished from marsupials and eutherians by a suite of distinctive features, including hatching their young from small leathery-shelled eggs and the occurrence of electroreceptors in the bill (platypus) or beak (echidna). Some attributes can present challenges to field researchers, including a low body temperature (making animals susceptible to heat stress) and a diet that precludes providing a bait reward in nets or traps. Though both species lack teeth as adults, the male platypus is equipped with venomous spurs and echidnas are covered in sharp (though non-venomous) spines.

PLATYPUS

Melody Serena and Joanne Connolly

Characteristics

The platypus is readily identified by its superficially duck-like bill, dense brown fur, strongly webbed front feet and broad tail (a major fat repository). The genitals are contained within the abdomen so males and females are most readily distinguished by a pointed spur, around 10–20 mm long, located on a male's inner ankle. The spur is connected by a duct to a venom-secreting gland. Venom production peaks just before and during the breeding season in late winter and spring, implying that it is mainly used to compete for mates (Grant 2007). Platypus venom is not life-threatening to humans but can cause localised tissue damage, severe swelling and pain that are best relieved by a regional nerve block (Fenner *et al.* 1992). Adult males are typically larger than females (total male length = 400–630 mm, mass = 0.8–3.0 kg; total female length = 370–550 mm, mass = 0.6–1.7 kg) (Van Dyck *et al.* 2013).

Biology and behaviour

Platypus occupy rivers, creeks, lakes and ponds at all elevations along the south-eastern and eastern coast of mainland Australia (from western Victoria to about Cooktown, Queensland), and occur on King Island and across most of Tasmania. Apart from vagrants occasionally sighted in the lower Murray River, the species is effectively extinct in mainland South Australia, where only a few animals were reported at the time of European settlement. A small, introduced population is found offshore on Kangaroo Island (Grant 1992). No subspecies are recognised.

Platypus forage exclusively in the water, mainly on small benthic invertebrates (Marchant and Grant 2015). Animals are most active at night, but also feed diurnally. Population densities are typically low, although more than 10 animals can sometimes occur per kilometre of river channel (Serena and Grant 2017). Home ranges of neighbouring adults usually overlap and can be up to 15 km long (males) or 4–5 km long (females) (Serena and Williams 2013). Platypus mainly rest in burrows located near the water's edge that are difficult to detect visually (Serena *et al.* 1998; Thomas *et al.* 2019).

Mating occurs in late winter or spring, commencing around 2–3 months earlier in Queensland than in Tasmania. Females lactate for up to 4 months, rearing one to three juveniles without male assistance. The percentage of females raising young can vary considerably (e.g. ranging from 17 to 71% of females in the upper Shoalhaven River; Serena and Grant 2017).

Capture and handling

Platypus surveys are conducted by direct visual observation, detecting platypus DNA in water samples, using time-lapse cameras and/or by setting nets (fyke nets if water is ≤ ~0.5 m deep; rectangular mesh gill nets if water is ≥ 1 m deep). Netting is often required for research, but can compromise animal welfare (e.g. animals can drown in nets). To minimise this risk, mesh nets must be unweighted and continually attended, and should not be deployed if they are likely to be snagged by woody debris or weighed down by large numbers of captured fish. Similarly, an air space must be maintained in a fyke net's final chamber and ideally along the net's entire length. Unlike mesh nets, fyke nets are normally set at multiple sites and attended only periodically, so captured platypus may experience both stress and hunger given that food exits the gut in ~5 h (Booth and Connolly 2008). Depending on water temperature, animals held in fyke nets can also become severely hypothermic. Accordingly, platypus fyke nets should be checked at intervals of ≤ 4 h (and no more than 2 h if water temperature at dusk is less than 15°C, the presumed lower limit of the platypus's thermoneutral zone; Bethge *et al.* 2001). Capture methods for platypus are covered in more detail in Chapter 14.

A captured platypus should be transferred immediately to its own clean, dry cloth bag, about the size of a pillowcase or slightly longer, fastened securely at the top. If a platypus is to be held captive for more than a few minutes, it should be transferred to a second dry bag after the first bag has absorbed surface moisture from its fur. The bag should be placed in an open-topped box to restrict movement further. To prevent overheating, animals should not be exposed to air temperatures above 27°C (Booth and Connolly 2008). A lethargic platypus may be stressed and should be released immediately after checking for possible lesions caused by prior litter entanglement. See Booth and Connolly (2008) for advice on housing a platypus during extended transport or longer-term captive husbandry.

To reduce stress, a conscious platypus's eyes should be covered during handling, all procedures on a conscious animal should be completed within 10 min, and the animal should be released back to the wild at the site of capture as soon as possible (ideally immediately after processing). To avoid handlers being spurred, an adult male (or animal of unknown sex) should only be lifted or held by gripping the end half of its tail (Figure 17.1) and should never be supported from below, even if contained within a bag.

Marking is undertaken by implanting a microchip tag subcutaneously between the shoulder blades, directing the point of the needle towards the animal's head and pinching a fold of skin so the needle is perpendicular to the skin surface. Physical condition is most often assessed by using a standard five-point scale based on tail thickness and pliability (Grant and Carrick 1978; illustrated in Booth and Connolly 2008), although the ratio of body

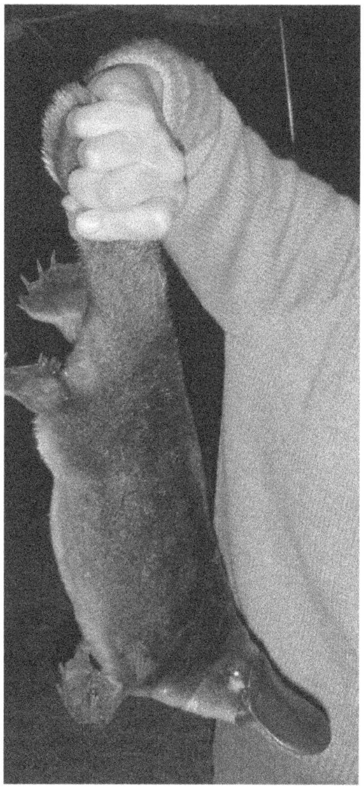

Figure 17.1: An adult male platypus (*Ornithorhynchus anatinus*) can be safely lifted by gripping the end half of its tail. Photo by Tom Claridge.

mass to bill width or ultrasonographic measurements of tail fat depth can also be used (MacGregor *et al.* 2016). Age classes (three in males, two in females) are assigned based on the size and shape of the venom-delivering spur in males or the occurrence of related vestigial structures in females (Williams *et al.* 2013).

Veterinary considerations

Personnel should have a good working knowledge of platypus biology and behaviour and be demonstrably competent with the proposed methodology. Minor field procedures (including measuring and marking animals, administering oxytocin to determine lactational status and collecting samples of faeces, urine, hair, venom or toe webbing) can be performed on appropriately restrained, conscious animals. Miniature radio transmitters can be glued to a shaved patch of rump skin of conscious animals without difficulty (Thomas *et al.* 2019). In the case of toe webbing (used for DNA studies), a 2 × 2 mm section of skin webbing is cut from the edge of a front foot using sharp, sterile scissors after disinfecting the site with 70% alcohol. Alternative sources of DNA include whole blood, blood spots on filter paper or tail hair follicles. For other procedures, the use of analgesia, sedation or anaesthesia is recommended (Holz 2014).

Analgesia, sedation and anaesthesia

Local anaesthesia (lignocaine or bupivacaine) may be used for analgesia during invasive but localised procedures such as punch biopsies (Bino *et al.* 2018; Vogelnest and Portas 2019). Sedation (diazepam at 0.5–1 mg/kg via intramuscular injection) may be used to minimise stress during procedures such as blood sampling, radiography and attaching external tracking devices.

Anaesthesia is usually gaseous (inhalational) rather than injectable. A surgical plane of anaesthesia (see Chapter 16) is required for abdominal insertion of tracking devices (Bino *et al.* 2018) or when the platypus is placed on its back for ultrasonography (Macgregor 2015). Inhalational anaesthesia with 5% isoflurane or sevoflurane in oxygen can be induced using a T-piece and a face mask that can enclose either the bill or the entire head and usually takes effect in 1–2 min. Anaesthesia is maintained with 1.5–2% isoflurane in oxygen (Booth and Connolly 2008). Vital signs during anaesthesia should be monitored carefully (see Table 17.1); sudden onset of apnoea/bradycardia is common during induction or recovery, but is generally not life-threatening (Booth and Connolly 2008; Macgregor 2015). Recovery from gaseous anaesthesia is normally rapid (righting reflex returns within 3–5 min) and platypus can generally be released after 1 h (Booth and Connolly 2008).

Platypus have an unusual diving-adapted physiology that may inconsistently be evident during anaesthesia. Sedatives and analgesics should only be administered by people with appropriate training in these procedures. Inhalation anaesthetics and drugs used for euthanasia should only be administered by, or under the supervision of, a suitably qualified veterinarian with appropriate species-specific experience.

Blood collection

Blood can be collected from a conscious platypus (without chemical restraint) if the animal is firmly physically restrained (Figure 17.2). Blood is collected using a 25 G needle or 25 G butterfly catheter and a 1–3 mL syringe from a venous sinus located just beneath the skin of the bill margin. The needle is inserted to a depth just past the bevel and rotated so the bevel faces laterally (Figure 17.2) (Holz 2014).

Euthanasia

Two-stage euthanasia is recommended whereby intramuscular sedation is followed by intracardiac pentobarbitone injection (150 mg/kg) after sedation has taken effect

Table 17.1: Physiological reference values for adult platypus.

Attribute	Value
Body Temperature	32.08 ± 0.75°C[a]
Respiratory rate	20–50 breaths/min[a]
Conscious heart rate	140–230 beats/min[b]
Diving heart rate	10–120 beats/min during dives[b]
Isoflurane anaesthesia heart rate (stable)	180–220 beats/min[a], 114–162 beats/min[c]
Sudden onset apnoea/bradycardia under isoflurane anaesthesia	10–12 beats/min[a], 30–72 beats/min (occasionally a 10 s gap)[c]

[a] Booth and Connolly (2008); [b] Grant (2007); [c] Macgregor 2015

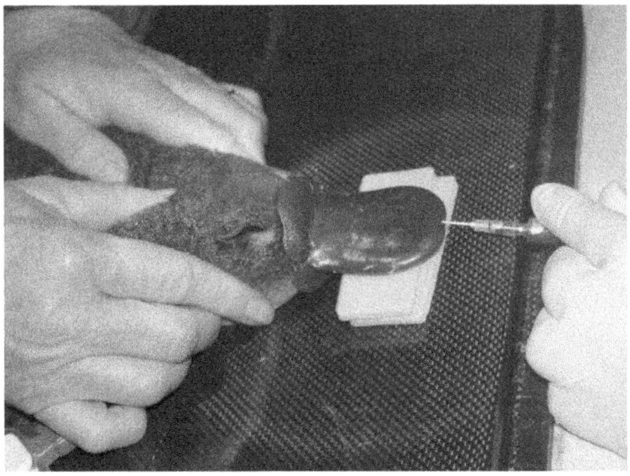

Figure 17.2: Drawing blood from the bill of an anaesthetised platypus (*Ornithorhynchus anatinus*). Photo by Joanne Connolly.

(NHMRC 2014). Death should be confirmed using standard procedures: confirming the absence of a corneal reflex, confirming the absence of breathing, using a stethoscope to confirm the absence of heartbeat, and confirming the presence of fixed and fully dilated pupils, relaxed jaw tone, and flaccid tongue for at least 5 min. Any animal euthanased with pentobarbitone represents a secondary toxicity risk to wild scavengers and should be disposed of via deep burial.

Infectious pathogens

Only a small number of infectious agents and parasites (many of which are non-pathogenic) have been reported for the platypus (Table 17.2). However, to avoid cross-infecting captured animals, holding bags should not be used more than once in each fieldwork session and should be machine-washed and dried in sunlight before reuse; platypus anaesthetic face masks should be disinfected after each use. Following direct contact with an animal or used holding bag, researchers should wash their hands thoroughly or use hand-sanitiser (or wear disposable rubber/latex gloves that are discarded after each use).

General operating procedures

General operating procedures relevant to platypus research may include direct visual observation (including spotlighting) and evaluation of eDNA (Chapter 4), camera trapping (Chapter 5), citizen science approaches (Chapter 10), direct capture by netting (Chapter 14), marking with microchips (Chapter 8), radiotelemetry (Chapter 9) and several medical procedures (Chapter 16).

SHORT-BEAKED ECHIDNA

Peggy Rismiller and Joanne Connolly

Characteristics

The short-beaked echidna is a small- to medium-sized, stocky, terrestrial, egg-laying mammal. It is easily distinguished from all other Australian mammals by its domed, spine-covered body, skin-covered beak and backward-rotated hind limbs that produce a unique rolling gait. Hairs cover the legs and belly and surround the spines. Echidnas have no teeth, but a long (up to 18 cm) worm-like tongue can be extruded through the small mouth opening under the tip of the beak. The eyes are small and external ear flaps generally are not present, but the ear slits are large. Front and back limbs have five toes, with one to three grooming claws on each hind foot. Arrangement of the muscles attached to the short, stout limbs gives the echidna enormous strength for digging and climbing.

It is not possible to sex an echidna by external features, as genitals are located internally. In some subspecies, both males and females may retain a spur on the inner hind foot and both can contract abdominal muscles to form a pseudo-pouch. Echidnas are not sexually dimorphic in size. Body mass of adult males and females varies from 2.5–7 kg with body length ranging from 30 to 50 cm (Griffiths 1978).

Biology and behaviour

Short-beaked echidnas occupy most terrestrial habitats in every Australian state and territory, and parts of south-eastern New Guinea. Five subspecies are recognised (one each in New Guinea, Tasmania and on Kangaroo Island; two on the Australian mainland), distinguished by pelage density, spine length and number of grooming claws.

Echidnas feed on a wide range of invertebrates, including beetles, worms, ants, termites and various larvae (Griffiths 1978; Rismiller 1999; Sprent and Nicol 2016). They are extremely mobile, occupying overlapping home ranges that each comprise up to 200 ha (Rismiller and McKelvey 2009; Nicol *et al.* 2011). Echidnas can be both diurnally and nocturnally active, depending on the locality and season. They have a low active body temperature (31–33°C) and avoid activity during the heat of the day in summer because they do not sweat or pant. Echidnas can enter torpor (an inactive state) throughout the year (Rismiller and Grutzner 2019; Nicol and Andersen 2000).

Table 17.2: Known infectious agents in the platypus.

From Hall (2019). 'Z' indicates a zoonosis.

Category of infection	Infectious agent of disease	Disease in platypus
Fungi	*Mucor amphibiorum*	Chronic skin and sometimes lung ulcers; death
	Trichophyton mentagrophytes var. *mentagrophytes* (Z)	Hair loss on the tail
	Unknown fungal organisms	Skin granulomas
Bacteria	*Leptospira* sp. (Z)	Subclinical kidney infection
	Salmonella spp. (Z)	Diarrhoea; systemic disease
	Corynebacterium ulcerans	Skin ulcers
	Dermatophilus congolensis	Scabs on skin
	Aeromonas hydrophila, *E. coli*	Aspiration pneumonia; death
	Ehrlichia ornithorhynchi	Subclinical infection of white blood cells (neutrophils)
Viruses	Adenovirus-like agent	Cytomegalic inclusion disease; subclinical kidney infection
	Putative *Papilloma* virus	Papules on webbing of feet
Protozoa	*Theileria ornithorhynchi*	Intracellular infection of red blood cells (often subclinical); anaemia
	Trypanosoma binneyi	Present in blood plasma; subclinical infection
	Toxoplasma gondii	Subclinical infection of heart
	Coccidia	Subclinical infection of small intestine
Trematodes (flukes)	*Mehlisia ornithorhynchi*	Subclinical infection of small intestine
	Maritrema ornithorhynchi	Subclinical infection of small intestine
	Moreauia mirabilis	Subclinical infection of small intestine
Nematodes (roundworms)	Rhabditoid and filarioid spp.	Subclinical infection of skin
Cestodes (tapeworms)	*Spirametra erinacei*	Lung plerocercoids
Ticks	*Ixodes ornithorhynchi*	Skin irritation; transmit blood parasites
Mites	Trombiculid mites	Irritation of skin, external ear canal
Fleas	*Pygiopsylla hopli*, *Pygiopsylla zethi*	Skin irritation
Annelids	Leeches	Skin irritation; transmit blood parasites

Echidnas are solitary except during the winter breeding season when a single female may be followed by one or more males. After 1–4 weeks of courtship, a female generally mates with only one male (Morrow *et al.* 2009; Rismiller and Grutzner 2019). A single egg is laid 23 days later (Rismiller and McKelvey 2000) and hatches after a further 10.5 days (Griffiths 1978). In most subspecies, the young are carried in a pseudo-pouch for up to 50 days before being deposited in a nursery burrow. The female returns to suckle her young for 2 h every 5 days until it is weaned and completely independent at 200–210 days (Rismiller and McKelvey 2009). Sexual maturity occurs at the age of 5–7 years (Rismiller and McKelvey 2003). Mature females reproduce once every 3–5 years (Rismiller and McKelvey 2000).

Capture and handling

Traps are not used to capture echidnas as they are not attracted to baits. Field studies consequently rely on searching for and capturing echidnas by hand. The safest and easiest way to pick up an echidna is to kneel behind the animal and insert one or both hands around the shoulders and front legs as it digs down to evade capture. When the echidna relaxes, the handler can push further under the animal's shoulders until the soft underbelly is felt, and then lift the echidna steadily from the ground. The echidna's natural reaction is to move forward and curl around the hands, which should provide a firm grip for the echidna and handler while protecting the animal from spiking itself. Alternatively, depending on the substrate, an echidna can be rolled on its back by inserting a hand under one side of the animal and lifting. If gloves are worn, handlers should avoid using heavy leather gloves that reduce dexterity and interfere with feeling an animal's movements. Handlers should never use a shovel or grab and pull an echidna by the hind legs as these actions can cause injuries.

A captured echidna should be placed in a tightly woven hessian/jute bag (around 1 × 0.6 m in size) as spines can get stuck and break in a loosely woven bag. The bag should be secured tightly during transport in a vehicle. A large, heavy duty plastic stacker box (e.g. 65 × 42 × 38 cm with a lid that clips on one side and is bolted on the other) is ideal for safely transporting an echidna in a vehicle or housing an echidna for a short period (< 48 h). For short-term transport, the bagged echidna can simply be placed in the box. If an echidna is being held overnight, a series of 3–5 mm smooth air holes should be drilled in two sides and a 10 cm layer of leaf litter and soil placed in the box so that the animal can burrow down. Echidnas are skilled at escaping, so if the echidna is not secured in a bag it should not be placed in a cardboard box, wooden crate or Styrofoam™ cooler, even for a short period.

Care should be taken to keep the captured echidna cool (ideally at an ambient temperature of 20–28°C). The animal's low active body temperature means that exposure to high temperatures will result in stress and possible death. Echidnas are also very sensitive to sound, so all procedures should be conducted quietly. See Jackson (2003) for advice about housing an echidna during extended transport and longer-term captive husbandry.

Echidnas can be marked for visual identification by slipping coloured tubing over spines on designated parts of the body – for example, white tail left (WTL) and red rump right (RRR) (Rismiller and McKelvey 2000). For permanent identification a microchip tag can be inserted subcutaneously, mid-body on the ventral side where hair and spines intersect (Rismiller and McKelvey 2000, 2003). Direction of insertion of microchips is towards the head.

Veterinary considerations

Sedation and anaesthesia

Minor procedures such as body condition assessment, faecal collection, injections, weighing or marking can be performed by trained researchers using physical restraint alone. All other procedures, including thorough physical examination, most types of sample collection (e.g. blood and oral swabs) and radiography are best performed when animals are sedated or anaesthetised.

Ketamine (5 mg/kg) plus medetomidine (0.05 mg/kg) or a 6 mg/kg dose of tiletamine–zolazepam can be given via intramuscular injection for sedation or anaesthetic induction before isoflurane maintenance (Johnston *et al.* 2006; Vogelnest and Portas 2019). However, in most circumstances, gaseous anaesthesia using isoflurane or sevoflurane (induction 5% in oxygen; maintenance 1–2% in oxygen) is the preferred method for anaesthesia, using an induction chamber or face mask (see Chapter 16) as echidnas cannot be intubated. A hollow cylinder of appropriate length for the beak of an echidna (such as the 10 mL syringe case used by Johnston *et al.* 2006) can serve as a face mask, placed with care to avoid occluding the nostrils. The echidna's pulse rate is difficult to detect by feel, so anaesthetic depth is assessed by using a stethoscope to monitor heart rate (normally 96 ± 13 beats per minute at rest) and by observing respiratory rate (normally 11 ± 3 breaths per minute at rest (Jackson 2003). Transient atypical periods of apnoea, sometimes with bradycardia, can occur in anaesthetised individuals (Rissman 2000).

Blood collection

The best site to sample blood is a venous sinus marked by a soft swelling on the dorsal beak, just behind the nostrils (Johnston *et al.* 2006; Holz 2014). After swabbing the beak with 70% alcohol (taking care to keep alcohol from entering the nasal cavity), blood (0.5–2 mL) is collected using a 25 G needle or 25 G butterfly catheter and 1–3 mL syringe. To avoid collapsing the sinus, do not exert too much pressure on the syringe (Figure 17.3; Chapter 16).

Euthanasia

Pentobarbitone at a standard euthanasia dose (150 mg/kg intracardiac) in a heavily sedated or anaesthetised echidna is recommended (NHMRC 2014). Death should be confirmed using standard protocol: absence of heartbeat and rhythmic breathing, absence of a corneal reflex along with a fixed and fully dilated pupil, relaxed jaw tone, and flaccid tongue, observed for at least 5 min. Any animal euthanased with pentobarbitone represents a secondary toxicity risk to wild scavengers and should be disposed of via deep burial.

Infectious pathogens

A low number of infectious agents and parasites have been identified in echidnas (Table 17.3). Many are

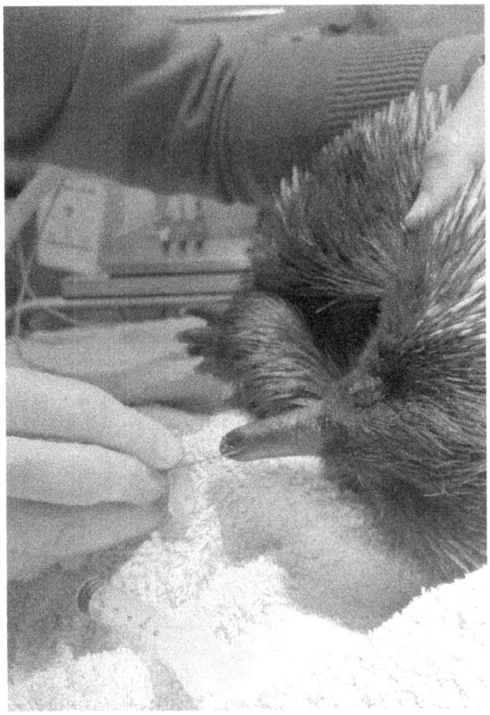

Figure 17.3: Collecting blood from the venous sinus in the echidna's beak (*Tachyglossus aculeatus*). Photo by Matthew De Cicco.

non-pathogenic and their clinical significance remains unknown. To avoid cross-infecting captured animals, only use holding bags or boxes once per field session and wash these thoroughly and dry in sunlight before reuse; echidna anaesthetic face masks should be disinfected after each use. Following contact with an animal or used holding bag, researchers should wash their hands thoroughly or use hand-sanitiser (or wear disposable rubber/latex gloves that are discarded after each use).

General operating procedures

General operating procedures relevant to echidna research may include visual observation and spotlighting (Chapter 4), camera trapping (Chapter 5), citizen science approaches (Chapter 10), marking with microchips (Chapter 8), tracking (Chapter 9) and a range of medical procedures (Chapter 16).

ACKNOWLEDGEMENTS

Thanks to Tom Grant and Rosemary Booth for providing valuable feedback on early drafts of this chapter.

Table 17.3: Infectious disease agents in the short-beaked echidna.

From Hall (2019) and Vogelnest and Portas (2019). Possible zoonoses are identified by a 'Z'.

Category of infection	Infectious agent	Disease in echidnas
Viruses	Herpesvirus	Multisystemic infections, hepatitis, death
	Poxvirus	Dermatitis
	Adenovirus	Cytomegalic lesions (subclinical) in kidneys
Bacteria	*Salmonella* spp. (Z)	Fatal septicaemia, can be subclinical carrier
	Edwardsiella spp.	Bronchopneumonia
	Proteus spp.	Possible septicaemia, enteritis, peritonitis
	Aeromonas spp.	Possible septicaemia, enteritis, peritonitis
	Fusobacterium spp.	Oesophagitis, gastritis
	Staphylococcus spp.	Generalised chronic or focal dermatitis
	Streptococcus spp.	Septicaemia, focal hepatitis, pulmonary oedema
	Mycobacterium spp.	Generalised, chronic, fatal infections
	Corynebacterium spp.	Oesophagitis, gastritis
Fungi	*Nannizzia gypsea* (*Microsporum gypseum*)	Dermatopathy (ringworm) with quill fracture
	Trichoderma spp.	Dermatopathy with quill fracture
	Malassezia spp.	Circular hair loss (with secondary pyoderma in young animals)
	Candida albicans	Oesophagitis, gastritis
	Cryptococcus neoformans	Lung granulomas

Category of infection	Infectious agent	Disease in echidnas
Protozoa	*Theileria tachyglossi*	Incidental finding, significance unknown
	Babesia tachyglossi	Incidental finding, significance unknown
	Toxoplasma gondii	Neurological abnormalities, pneumonia, non-suppurative encephalitis, hepatitis, splenitis, nephritis
	Emeria tachyglossi	Coccidia causing enteritis (small intestine), possibly multisystemic, fatal
	Emeria echidnae	Coccidia causing enteritis (small intestine), possibly multisystemic, fatal
	Octosporella hystrix	Enteritis
	Anaplasma marginali-like	Incidental finding, significance unknown
	Hepatozoan tachyglossi	Incidental finding in debilitated individual
	Atoxoplasma-like	Common incidental finding, possibly with multisystemic coccidiosis
Cestodes (tapeworms)	*Spirametra erinacei* (*S. erinaceieuropaei*)	Chronic masses (subcutaneous and lung)
	Echidnotaenia tachyglossi	Incidental finding, significance unknown
	Linstowia echidnae	Incidental finding, significance unknown
Nematodes (roundworms)	*Parastrongyloides* spp.	Enteritis, possibly fatal if > 500 worms
	Nicollina spp.	Enteritis, possibly fatal if > 500 worms
	Tachynema spp.	Enteritis, possibly fatal if > 500 worms
	Tasmanema mundayi	Enteritis, possibly fatal if > 500 worms
	Ophidascaris robertsi	Larvae recorded from lung
	Dipetalonema spp.	Recorded from subcutaneous tissue
Ticks	*Ixodes* spp.	Anaemia if > 20 ticks, disease vector, dermatitis, possible paralysis
	Haemaphysalis humerosa	Anaemia if > 20 ticks, Q fever vector
	Amblyomma spp.	Anaemia if > 20 ticks, disease vector, dermatitis
	Aponomma tachyglossi	Anaemia if > 20 ticks, disease vector, dermatitis
	Aponomma concolor	Anaemia if > 20 ticks, disease vector, dermatitis
Fleas	*Echidnophaga* spp.	Possible skin effects
	Pulex irritans	Possible skin effects
	Bradiopsylla echidnae	Possible skin effects
	Stephanocircus dasyure	Possible skin effects
Mites	*Odontocarus echidnus*	Possible skin effects

REFERENCES

Bethge P, Munks S, Nicol S (2001) Energetics of foraging and locomotion in the platypus *Ornithorhynchus anatinus*. *Journal of Comparative Physiology. B, Biochemical, Systemic, and Environmental Physiology* **171**, 497–506. doi:10.1007/s003600100200

Bino G, Kingsford RT, Grant T, Taylor MD, Vogelnest L (2018) Use of implanted acoustic tags to assess platypus movement behaviour across spatial and temporal scales. *Scientific Reports* **8**, 5117–5128. doi:10.1038/s41598-018-23461-9

Booth R, Connolly J (2008) Platypuses. In *Medicine of Australian Mammals*. (Eds L Vogelnest and R Woods) pp. 103–132. CSIRO Publishing, Melbourne. doi:10.1071/9780643097971

Fenner PJ, Williamson JA, Myers D (1992) Platypus envenomation – a painful learning experience. *The Medical Journal of Australia* **157**, 829–832. doi:10.5694/j.1326-5377.1992.tb141302.x

Grant TR (1992) Historical and current distribution of the platypus, *Ornithorhynchus anatinus*, in Australia. In *Platypus and Echidnas* (Ed. ML Augee) pp. 232–254. Royal Zoological Society of New South Wales, Mosman.

Grant TR (2007) *Platypus*. 4th edn. CSIRO Publishing, Melbourne.

Grant TR, Carrick FN (1978) Some aspects of the ecology of the platypus, *Ornithorhynchus anatinus*, in the upper Shoalhaven River, New South Wales. *Australian Zoologist* **20**, 181–199.

Griffiths M (1978) *The Biology of the Monotremes*. Academic Press, New York, NY.

Hall J (Ed.) (2019). *Proceedings: Wildlife Health and Pathology Short Course, Taronga Zoo*, February 2019. Taronga Conservation Society Australia, Mosman.

Holz P (2014) Monotremata (Echidna, Platypus). In *Zoo Animal and Wildlife Immobilization and Anaesthesia*. 2nd edn. (Eds G West, D Heard and N Caulkett) pp. 517–519. John Wiley and Sons, Hoboken, NJ.

Jackson S (2003) Echidna. In *Australian Mammals: Biology and Captive Management*. (Ed. S Jackson) pp. 33–51. CSIRO Publishing, Melbourne.

Johnston SD, Madden C, Nicolson V, Cowin G, Pyne M, Booth R (2006) Venipuncture in the short-beaked echidna. *Australian Veterinary Journal* **84**, 66–67. doi:10.1111/j.1751-0813.2006.tb13132.x

Macgregor JW (2015) Conservation of the platypus (*Ornithorhynchus anatinus*): development of a framework to assess the health of wild platypus populations. PhD thesis. Murdoch University, Australia.

Macgregor JW, Holyoake C, Munks S, Connolly JH, Robertson ID, Fleming PA, Lonsdale RA, Warren K (2016) Assessing body condition in the platypus (*Ornithorhynchus anatinus*): a comparison of new and old methods. *Australian Journal of Zoology* **64**, 421–429. doi:10.1071/ZO16071

Marchant R, Grant TR (2015) The productivity of the macroinvertebrate prey of the platypus in the upper Shoalhaven River, New South Wales. *Australian Journal of Zoology* **66**, 1128–1137. doi:10.1071/MF14301

Morrow G, Andersen NA, Nicol SC (2009) Reproduction strategies of the short-beaked echidna – a review with new data from a long-term study on the Tasmanian subspecies (*Tachyglossus aculeatus setosus*). *Australian Journal of Zoology* **57**, 275–282. doi:10.1071/ZO09037

National Health and Medical Research Council (2014) *A Guide to Care and Use of Native Mammals in Research and Teaching*. Commonwealth of Australia, Canberra. <www.nhmrc.gov.au/guidelines/publications/ea29>.

Nicol SC, Andersen NA (2000) Patterns of hibernation of echidnas in Tasmania. In *Life in the Cold: Proceedings of the Eleventh International Hibernation Symposium*. (Eds G Heldmaier and M Klingenspor) pp. 21–29. Springer, Berlin.

Nicol SC, Vanpe C, Sprent J, Morrow G, Andersen NA (2011) Spatial ecology of a ubiquitous Australian anteater, the short-beaked echidna (*Tachyglossus aculeatus*). *Journal of Mammalogy* **92**, 101–110. doi:10.1644/09-MAMM-A-398.1

Rismiller PD (1999) *The Echidna, Australia's Enigma*. Hugh Lauter Levin Associates, Southport, CT.

Rismiller PD, Grutzner F (2019) *Tachyglossus aculeatus* Monotremata: Tachyglossidae). *Mammalian Species* **51**, 75–91. doi:10.1093/mspecies/sez012

Rismiller PD, McKelvey MW (2000) Frequency of breeding and recruitment in the short-beaked echidna, *Tachyglossus aculeatus*. *Journal of Mammalogy* **81**, 1–17. doi:10.1644/1545-1542(2000)081<0001:FOBARI>2.0.CO;2

Rismiller PD, McKelvey MW (2003) Body mass, age and sexual maturity in short-beaked echidnas, *Tachyglossus aculeatus*. *Comparative Biochemistry and Physiology A* **136**, 851–865. doi:10.1016/S1095-6433(03)00225-3

Rismiller PD, McKelvey MW (2009) Activity and behaviour of lactating echidnas (*Tachyglossus aculeatus multiaculeatus*) from hatching of egg to weaning of young. *Australian Journal of Zoology* **57**, 265–273. doi:10.1071/ZO09031

Rissman RA (2000) Chemical immobilisation of the short-beaked echidna (*Tachyglossus aculeatus*): comparative physiological effects of seven different anaesthetic agents in echidna (alphaxalone, isoflurane, ketamine, medetomidine, medetomidine-ketamine, tiletamine/zolazepam and xylazine). MVetSci thesis. The University of Sydney, Australia.

Serena M, Grant TR (2017) Effect of flow on platypus (*Ornithorhynchus anatinus*) reproduction and related population processes in the upper Shoalhaven River. *Australian Journal of Zoology* **65**, 130–139. doi:10.1071/ZO17025

Serena M, Thomas JL, Williams GA, Officer RCE (1998) Use of stream and river habitats by the platypus, *Ornithorhynchus anatinus*, in an urban fringe environment. *Australian Journal of Zoology* **46**, 267–282. doi:10.1071/ZO98034

Serena M, Williams GA (2013) Movements and cumulative range size of the platypus (*Ornithorhynchus anatinus*) inferred from mark-recapture studies. *Australian Journal of Zoology* **60**, 352–359. doi:10.1071/ZO12121

Sprent JA, Nicol SC (2016) Diet of the short-beaked echidna (*Tachyglossus aculeatus*) in the Tasmanian Southern Midlands. *Australian Mammalogy* **38**, 188–194. doi:10.1071/AM15023

Thomas JL, Parrott ML, Handasyde KA, Temple-Smith P (2019) Burrow use by juvenile platypuses (*Ornithorhynchus anatinus*) in their natal home range. *Journal of Mammalogy* **100**, 1182–1190. doi:10.1093/jmammal/gyz078

Van Dyck S, Gynther I, Baker A (2013) *Field Companion to the Mammals of Australia*. New Holland Publishers, Sydney.

Vogelnest L, Portas T (Eds) (2019) *Current Therapy in Medicine of Australian Mammals*. CSIRO Publishing, Melbourne.

Williams GA, Serena M, Grant TR (2013) Age-related change in spurs and spur sheaths of the platypus *Ornithorhynchus anatinus*. *Australian Mammalogy* **35**, 107–114. doi:10.1071/AM12011

18 Marsupial carnivores

Chris R. Pavey, Jenny Molyneux, Gerhard Körtner, J. Anthony Friend, Rebecca Vaughan-Higgins, Bronwyn A. Fancourt, Jaime Heiniger and Helen P. Waudby

INTRODUCTION

Dasyurids (marsupial carnivores) occur in Australia and New Guinea, constituting the order Dasyuromorphia. The order consists of three families: the Dasyuridae (containing the most species); the Myrmecobiidae, containing one species, the numbat (*Myrmecobius fasciatus*); and the Thylacinidae, containing the now extinct thylacine (*Thylacinus cynocephalus*). Dasyurids, also sometimes known as dasyurid marsupials or carnivorous marsupials, are united by their predatory lifestyle and mode of reproduction. The size range of the group is considerable, from the world's smallest marsupial, the long-tailed planigale (*Planigale ingrami*) at 2.6 g, to the thylacine at 35 kg. Dasyurids are superficially similar in morphology to placental carnivores. This similarity resulted in many groups having common names derived from their eutherian counterparts. Examples include 'marsupial rat' for the kowari (*Dasyuroides byrnei*), 'native cat' for quolls (*Dasyurus*), 'marsupial mouse' for antechinuses (*Antechinus* spp.) and dunnarts (*Sminthopsis* spp.), and 'banded anteater' for the numbat.

SMALL DASYURIDS

Jenny Molyneux, Chris R. Pavey, Gerhard Körtner and Helen P. Waudby

Characteristics

All dasyurids share a similar body plan with only minor variations in morphology. They typically possess prominent ears and eyes, a pointed snout, unspecialised limbs and teeth designed for biting and cutting. The kultarr (*Antechinomys laniger*), a small dasyurid found in Australia's arid zone, is the sole species with long hind limbs. Within the smaller dasyurids, body masses range from around 2.6 g for the long-tailed planigale to around 231 g for the brush-tailed phascogale (*Phascogale tapoatafa*).

Biology and behaviour

Small dasyurids occur across mainland Australia and Tasmania, occupying all environments except freshwater systems. Most species are terrestrial, although phascogales and some antechinus species are mostly arboreal.

Home-range size varies widely, typically being greater in larger species and in males (within species). For example, male brush-tailed phascogales (230 g) have an average home range of 106 ha, whereas female (155 g) ranges average 41 ha (Soderquist 1995; Körtner *et al.* 2019). Smaller species, such as Giles' planigale (*Planigale gilesi*), have home ranges of < 1 ha (Warnecke *et al.* 2012).

Most species are strictly nocturnal. In winter, some arid zone species are active during the day; the fat-tailed false antechinus (*Pseudantechinus macdonnellensis*) is partially diurnal (Pavey and Geiser 2008), while the kaluta (*Dasykaluta rosamondae*) is almost exclusively diurnal (Körtner *et al.* 2010). Activity patterns can vary with breeding condition, as displayed in male antechinuses, which increase diurnal activity during the peak of breeding seasons when seeking females (Körtner and Geiser 1995). Diurnal shelter locations vary with environment. Arid species that occupy sand deserts (mulgaras, dunnarts, ningauis) typically shelter underground in burrows that provide thermal buffering. Planigales typically occupy soil cracks as do some dunnart species (Warnecke *et al.* 2012; Waudby and Petit 2017). Phascogales mostly shelter in tree hollows and crevices.

Small dasyurids feed primarily on invertebrates. Species occupying rainforest have the most diverse diets. For example, the black-tailed dusky antechinus (*Antechinus arktos*) and brown antechinus (*A. stuartii*), in south-east Queensland, feed on insects (adults and larvae), springtails, arachnids, crustaceans, millipedes, centipedes and terrestrial snails (Gray *et al.* 2016). Most species occasionally consume vertebrate prey with the importance of vertebrates in the diet increasing with body size. The mulgaras and kowari prey on birds, reptiles and mammals, including rodents and other dasyurids (Pavey *et al.* 2018).

Most (probably all) small dasyurids, particularly the desert-dwelling species, can enter daily torpor. Daily torpor is similar to hibernation, but is short term (i.e. < 24 hours) and characterised by reduced body temperature (to about 10–20°C), metabolic rate and water loss. The ability to enter torpor reduces the energy requirements of small mammals, including their need for food and water; this ability is a considerable advantage during cold conditions and times of food scarcity (Geiser 2004). Animals may enter torpor when captured in traps overnight, particularly during cool conditions.

The life histories of small dasyurids are diverse, varying in terms of the life span of the male, onset and duration of the breeding season and age at maturity (Baker and Dickman 2018). The family is renowned for the reproductive strategy of antechinus and phascogales, the kaluta and northern quoll, which display a post-mating die-off of all males at 11 months of age. The life strategy of these species, known as semelparity (a single reproductive episode before death), is simple, with mating occurring during a short period in spring. All males die soon after their first breeding season as a result of stress (high levels of corticosteroids) and associated disease. In contrast, females survive for 2 or 3 years. *Pseudantechinus* species vary this strategy, with a portion of males surviving and breeding successfully in a second breeding season. Mulgaras can enter oestrus for a second time during the same season if necessary (usually in response to unsuccessful mating or death of young), while many arid-zone species (including planigales, ningauis, kowari, kultarr, and some dunnarts) typically breed twice in a season.

Capture and handling

As a result of their small sizes, short life spans and varied diets, small dasyurid marsupials require specialised care. Specific requirements vary among groups. If capture is necessary, choice of trap type and deployment strategy should be based on knowledge of the life-history traits of the target species. The most common trap types are aluminium folding box traps (typically Elliott traps) and pitfall traps. Ground-dwelling species have also occasionally been captured with funnel traps. Captured animals can be housed for short periods in appropriately sized calico bags. Bags should be inverted or sewn to reduce exposure to seams and the chance of animals catching and becoming tangled in loose threads or loops. Care should be taken to ensure that animals are maintained at an appropriate body temperature. Animals that are in torpor when removed from traps should be allowed to rouse from that state before release –by either warming them if quick release is required (heat from hands may be sufficient, although longer applications of a heat source may be required) or allowing them to rouse naturally using their own internal body heat and as ambient temperatures increase (generally, an option if animals are being housed during the day). Animals should not be released while in torpor because they are particularly susceptible to predation while in that state.

Cages for transport should be of a size appropriate to the species, allowing the animal sufficient space to turn easily, but not be thrown around while in transport. All cages should be non-abrasive and have sufficient ventilation outlets. For long periods of travel, bedding (e.g. cut up grass or coconut fibre matting) can be provided to keep the animal comfortable and calm. Animals should be transported individually, except for females with pouch young, who should remain together.

Physical restraint for short periods can be achieved by 'scruffing' the animal between the shoulder blades or, if longer examination is required, grasping the base of the tail between the thumb and index finger and using the remaining fingers to restrain the body. If greater restraint is needed to examine dentition, a three-finger pincer grasp around the head with the body supported in the palm is suitable. To reduce stress, it is preferable for the animal to remain in the bag as much as possible during examination. Specific care should be taken when handling kultarrs as their long hind legs are easily damaged during handling. If handled correctly and calmly, small dasyurids are usually quiet and can be examined easily (in some cases scruffing may not be required at all).

Long-term housing should provide suitable nesting sites and meet the habitat requirements of individual species. For example, phascogales should be provided with climbing structures and high nesting boxes to support their arboreal behaviour. Social organisation specific to a species' requirements should also be maintained. Overcrowding may lead to greater levels of aggression in a captive population and the killing of young. The introduction of new individuals should be monitored with care and sufficient nesting sites provided to reduce aggression. In breeding populations of some species, such as red-tailed phascogales (*Phascolgale calura*), males should only be housed with females during the breeding season to reduce aggression towards young. Many species are temperature sensitive, undergoing periods of torpor when cold. Heating or cooling should be provided as appropriate to ensure adequate access to a broad temperature gradient relative to requirements.

Fresh water and food should be provided if a dasyurid is held captive. Diet should be varied and include live invertebrates, dog kibble, egg and mincemeat, supplemented with calcium and vitamins. Dasyurids that sometimes eat vertebrates, such as mulgaras, should be provided with cut up day-old mice or chicks at least once per week. Feathers should be removed to avoid compaction in the gut. Weaner mice should be cut up to minimise the visual association between pouch young and food. Any meat products should be frozen for a minimum of 1 week before being fed to animals to reduce the possibility of toxoplasmosis infection from the parasite *Toxoplasma gondii* (Attwood *et al.* 1975).

Individual identification of dasyurids is difficult with pelage and size being uniform within sexes and species, so individuals usually need to be marked to facilitate identification of recaptured individuals. For marking within a trapping session, clipping hair or paint marking will allow the identification of recaptured individuals. As most species groom regularly, paint marking should be placed on locations on the body that the animal cannot easily access, such as between the shoulder blades. For more-permanent identification, pinna (ear) notching or microchipping are preferred methods. Tattooing tails may also be an option. Historically, toe clipping and pinna tattooing (larger species only) have also been used for marking, although methods such as toe clipping are falling out of favour for use in mammals (Jung *et al.* 2020).

Whether inserting a microchip or notching the ear, the sites involved should be cleaned with ≥ 70% alcohol before and after the procedure to reduce the chance of infection. A small amount of veterinary bonding agent can be used to seal the site after tag insertion, if desired. Microchips should be fitted subcutaneously between the shoulder blades and inserted only by individuals who have been trained to undertake the procedure on small animals. The small size and thin skin of dasyurid marsupials, particularly smaller species, necessitate a high level of competence to ensure that the tag is inserted correctly. Pinna notching and microchipping can be done without sedation or anaesthesia, although a numbing agent may be used first if desired.

Tracking using telemetric devices is often valuable to determine movement patterns; however, this methodology is difficult to apply to small dasyurid marsupials because of the group's size. If used, telemetry devices should generally weigh ≤ 10% of the individual animal's body mass to ensure the device does not have a negative impact on the animal's ability to move and behave freely (see discussion in Chapter 9). Current models of satellite trackers are usually too heavy for use in these taxa. If used, telemetry devices can be attached with a collar or backpack system or glued to the back for short term deployments. Collars should be removed once no longer needed, and equipped with a weak link to ensure that they fall off in case the animal cannot be recaptured. Backpacks and glue-on transmitters should align with the animal's profile to minimise interference with movement, particularly for species that access burrows and other confined spaces. The short life span of small dasyurids and quick growth of young, mean that only adults should be fitted with telemetry devices to ensure they do not become restrictive as the animal grows. Telemetry devices should not be attached to females with pouch young because of the animal's higher energetic demands at this life stage. Alternative tracking methods, such as spooling (Molyneux *et al.* 2018), fluorescent pigment tracking and trailing animals after release (McLean 2015), have been used on various species in this group.

Veterinary considerations

Sedation and anaesthesia

Animals should only be sedated or anaesthetised if undertaking a major invasive examination (i.e. performing surgery). Should anaesthesia be required, the preferred method of gaseous administration is by inhalation rather than injection. Isoflurane in oxygen offers a wide safety margin for mammals. Induction is usually at 4% and maintenance at 1–2%. For longer procedures, all marsupial carnivores should be intubated (requiring placement of an endotracheal tube) (Chapter 16).

Blood collection

Small blood samples can be collected with capillary tubes after pricking an ear vein or one of the two lateral veins near the base of the tail with a 27 G needle (Johnstone *et al.* 2012).

Euthanasia

Depending on the species, euthanasia via pentobarbitone injection (intravenous or intracardiac) to an anaesthetised animal can be used (Reilly 2001) where personnel have the appropriate licences and training. Any animal euthanased with pentobarbitone represents a secondary toxicity risk to wild scavengers and should be disposed of via deep burial (or collected as a voucher specimen). Physical euthanasia (stunning followed by cervical dislocation) can be used for some species where circumstances necessitate (e.g. in remote areas).

Infectious pathogens

Endoparasites include a variety of trematodes, tapeworms and roundworms that may occur across the entire body, although intestinal worms are most common (Beveridge and Spratt 2003). Unsurprisingly, understanding of endoparasite prevalence is inconsistent within the group, with knowledge based disproportionally on some more-common or readily studied species (e.g. *Antechinus agilis*). Records of ectoparasites are common across species, particularly those in high rainfall areas, including a variety of ticks, lice, mites and fleas. As in many Australian native mammal species, *Toxoplasma gondii*, transmitted from cats, poses risks to dasyurids and can cause severe clinical signs and death (Attwood and Woolley 1970). Minor irritations to humans can be caused by parasites carried by dasyurids and bacterial infections from scratches or bites can be painful if left untreated.

General operating procedures

Suitable trapping methods for small dasyurids include pitfall, aluminium box, cage and sometimes funnel traps (Chapter 7). Appropriate marking methods include microchipping, ear tagging, ear notching and possibly tattooing (Chapter 8). A range of tracking methods (Chapter 9), and low-impact and indirect methods of detection or study, such as measurement of dens and burrows, scat collection, assessment of tracks and other traces (Chapter 4), camera trapping and hair trapping (Chapter 5), are also appropriate, depending on the species and study objectives. Medical procedures are detailed in Chapter 16.

LARGE DASYURIDS

Gerhard Körtner, Chris R. Pavey, Bronwyn Fancourt and Jaime Heiniger

Characteristics

The large dasyurids include four quoll species and the Tasmanian devil (*Sarcophilus harrisii*). Their basic body plan is shared with smaller dasyurids (prominent eyes and ears, pointed snouts, teeth designed for biting and cutting). Body masses range from around 500 g for adult male northern quolls (*Dasyurus hallucatus*) to up to 14 kg in Tasmanian devils.

Biology and behaviour

Large dasyurids once occurred across mainland Australia and Tasmania. However, all species have declined in geographical range as a result of habitat destruction, introduced predators, cane toads and disease. All species are listed as threatened. The Tasmanian devil and eastern quoll (*D. viverrinus*) are now confined to Tasmania, the western quoll (*D. geoffroii*) to south-west Western Australia, the northern quoll to sections of its former range in northern Australia and the spotted-tailed quoll (*D. maculatus*) to eastern Australia, including Tasmania.

These species occupy diverse environments across Australia, from rainforests to sand deserts. Quolls are swift movers on the ground and efficient climbers, whereas the Tasmanian devil is mostly terrestrial once adult. Most quolls and the Tasmanian devil are crepuscular (active at twilight) and nocturnal; however, spotted-tailed quolls can exhibit cathemerality (irregular intervals of activity during the day or night). Daytime shelters include hollow logs, burrows, caves and rock piles.

Within this group, the proportion of vertebrates in the diet increases with body size. The smaller species, the northern and eastern quolls, exhibit a high degree of insectivory (Fancourt *et al.* 2018), whereas the larger spotted-tailed quoll is a predator of mainly small- and medium-sized mammals, and the Tasmanian devil is a specialised scavenger (Jones and Barmuta 1998). As in other animal groups, home range increases with increasing body mass, but is also resource driven to an extent (Körtner *et al.* 2019). Males have a much larger home range than females. Although generally solitary, the home range of several males can overlap extensively. In contrast, females in some species tend to express some form of territoriality (Firestone *et al.* 1999).

The larger dasyurids are relatively short lived. Some populations of northern quoll exhibit semelparity, where all males die shortly after the first and only mating season (Oakwood *et al.* 2001). Even the spotted-tailed quoll, roughly the size of a domestic cat, rarely lives longer than 3 years in the wild and only a few years longer in captivity (Körtner *et al.* 2004). Although polyoestrus, quolls and devils raise only one litter per year (Figure 18.1) and breeding is broadly synchronised, occurring at around the same time each year (Tyndale-Biscoe 2005). Maximum litter size is determined by the number of teats in the pouch, which typically ranges from four in the Tasmanian devil up to eight in the northern quoll. All species appear to be polygamous and a female might mate with several males, resulting in multiple paternity within a litter (Glen *et al.* 2009).

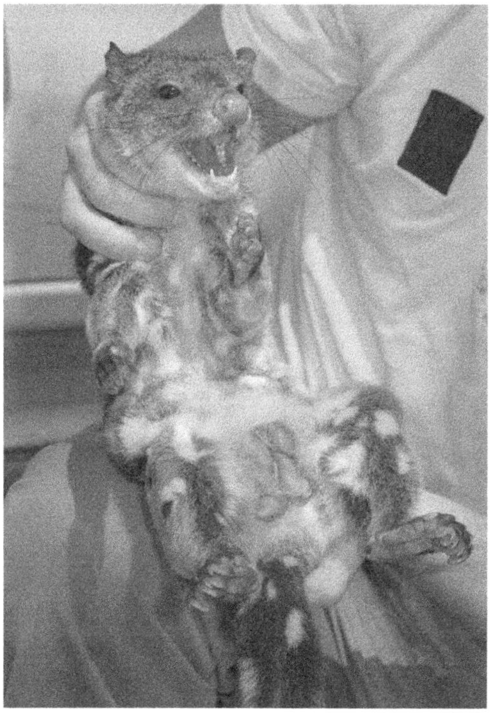

Figure 18.1: A female spotted-tailed quoll (*Dasyurus maculatus*) with pouch young. Photo by Gerhard Körtner.

Capture and handling

All large dasyurid species are relatively easy to detect with hair tubes (Ruibal *et al.* 2010) and baited (Hohnen *et al.* 2013) or lured camera traps (Fancourt *et al.* 2015). However, live trapping is still required when morphometric data are required, tissue or blood samples are to be collected or telemetry collars are to be fitted. The broadly synchronised breeding of large dasyurids means that it is relatively easy to avoid stages of the breeding season when offspring are presumed most vulnerable; the breeding season should be avoided unless breeding itself is the subject of the study. Dasyurids are not known to evict pouch young when stressed in a trap, but pouch young can be accidentally dislodged (although they can usually be reattached carefully). Although not supported by empirical evidence, it is assumed that trapping females can be most detrimental after the still helpless and blind juveniles are first deposited in a den. Trapping success is usually highest shortly before and during the mating season because of the increased mobility of males at this time; this increased mobility can also lead to male-biased trapping success (Körtner *et al.* 2004).

Cage traps covered to provide protection from sun, rain and wind are suitable for capturing most large dasyurids. A meat-based lure should be used. Quolls and devils can exert considerable force with their jaws and break through weakly constructed weld mesh and/or fracture teeth. Furthermore, attempts to escape can result in injuries to the animal with superficial abrasions to the muzzle being common. Traps made using a smaller mesh size can ameliorate such injuries. To reduce potential damage to teeth, assist in sterilising against disease transmission (see below) and provide increased insulation from cold temperatures in Tasmania, large diameter polyvinyl chloride (PVC) pipe traps are used for devils and quolls.

A trail-based trapping program can be adopted to capture most of the species covered in this sub-chapter. However, for some species, such as the northern quoll, traps may need to be carried into rocky outcrops or suitable habitat away from trails. Optimal spacing between traps will vary according to the target species' activity range. For example, the home range of large dasyurids, such as the spotted-tailed quoll, can encompass many square kilometres (Körtner *et al.* 2019), and so it might take several weeks for a quoll to visit a specific area within its home range and be captured (Körtner *et al.* 2016). By comparison, the eastern quoll has a small home range (0.35–0.44 km^2; Godsell 1983) that overlaps with several other individuals, and so multiple individuals can be captured easily using a few traps located in proximity to each other. Accordingly, trapping surveys for highly trappable (and retrappable) species, such as the eastern and northern quoll, should be limited to around 3–5 nights.

Traps must be checked at least daily. For larger species (i.e. spotted-tailed quolls and devils), the risks from overheating or hypothermia because of delays in checking traps are less relevant than in the smaller dasyurids, for several reasons. First, relative surface area decreases with body size. Therefore, less heat is absorbed into a larger body volume. Fur insulation is also more efficient in larger species (Schmidt-Nielsen 1972), reducing the risk of rapid overheating. Second, the mass-specific metabolic rate is lower in larger animals (Riek 2008), meaning that body energy stores, such as fat, last considerably longer. While small dasyurids, such as planigales, need to eat an amount of food close to their body mass per day, quolls and devils have proportionally much lower energy requirements and can survive several days without feeding, although energy requirements increase substantially in lactating females (Green and Eberhard 1979). In wetter and cooler areas, hypothermia is unlikely to affect larger species, such as the devil. Again, the favourable surface-area-to-volume (SAV) ratio in large-bodied animals (Schmidt-Nielsen 1972) improves insulation and body energy stores generally last longer. However, the absence of substantial fat stores and the higher SAV ratio in the smaller eastern quoll means more care is required when trapping in cold environments, such as Tasmania.

Quolls and devils have an undeserved reputation for being aggressive and difficult to handle, but the opposite is usually the case. An opaque, sturdy fabric capture bag can be used to extract animals from the trap, restrain animals and keep them calm during handling. For devils, single-use close-weave hessian sacks are appropriate. However, to prevent disease transmission between individuals, sacks should not be reused on more than one animal. A funnel-shaped bag with a Velcro® or zipper closure along the side is ideal for restraining spotted-tailed quolls, while smaller fabric bags such as calico are suitable for smaller quoll species. If the animal has to be extracted from the bag or the head region is to be inspected, it should be held securely around the neck while the body is pinned to the ground (Figure 18.2). Handling an animal by its tail should be avoided. Where possible, fabric capture bags should not be reused for multiple individuals without cleaning to minimise transmission of parasites and pathogens between individuals.

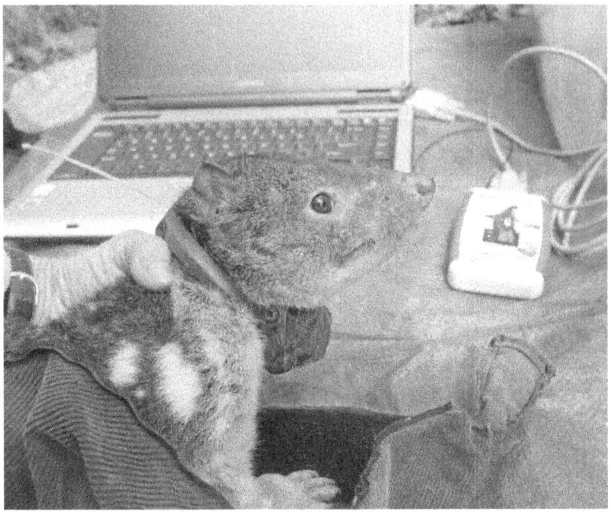

Figure 18.2: A male spotted-tailed quoll with radio transmitter attached. Photo by Gerhard Körtner.

Large dasyurids can be marked with microchips without anaesthesia while restrained in a capture bag. The same applies to fitting transmitter collars (Körtner *et al.* 2016) (Figure 18.2). Tattooing of pouch young has been tested as a means of permanent marking (Soderquist and Dickman 1988). For quolls, their individual spot patterns provide a viable alternative to marking individuals. Photographs taken from either side provide a reference; this approach is also an option for identifying individuals from camera trap images (Hohnen *et al.* 2013; Rowland *et al.* 2020).

If animals have to be moved off site, a bag, covered trap or cat carrier is ideal for transportation of quolls, while devils can be transported in PVC pipe traps. For smaller species, some traps may also suffice as housing for a day or so in captivity; however, holding relatively large animals for longer periods will require designated enclosures. Quolls and devils are adept climbers and can also dig under fences, so a sturdy wire enclosure with roof and floor is required. The enclosure should include a nest box and, for prolonged periods in captivity, some environmental enrichment and the opportunity to bask in the sun during cold days. Generally, these solitary animals should be housed as individuals except for breeding purposes. Food is mostly meat based. Quolls rarely drink, but clean water should always be provided.

Veterinary considerations

Sedation and anaesthesia

Quolls and devils should only be sedated or anaesthetised if undertaking a major invasive examination or procedure (i.e. surgery). The approaches for sedating and anaesthetising quolls and devils are the same as those for small dasyurids; however, no anaesthesia is required for minimally invasive procedures, such as collecting ear tissue biopsies or blood samples.

Blood collection

Small blood samples can be collected with capillary tubes after pricking an ear vein. Larger blood samples can be taken from the jugular vein, either under physical restraint (for calm animals) or anaesthesia (Hivert *et al.* 2018; Chapter 16).

Euthanasia

Two-stage euthanasia by anaesthetising with an inhalant anaesthetic (e.g. isoflurane) followed by an intravenous or intracardiac injection of pentobarbitone is recommended (Reilly 2001). Any animal euthanased with pentobarbitone represents a secondary toxicity risk to wild scavengers and should be disposed of via deep burial. Though not preferred, physical euthanasia methods (such as shooting) may be required in remote field situations.

Infectious pathogens

Quolls and devils carry a diversity of internal and external parasites that are generally poorly described (Obendorf 1993). Besides generalised external parasites, such as ticks and fleas that move between several species, large dasyurids carry a host-specific flea (*Uropsylla tasmanica*) that is the only known flea species to complete its whole life cycle on the host's body (Pearse 1981). The larvae of *Uropsylla* bury under the skin of the host, often in large numbers, causing considerable skin irritations, inflammation and occasional bald patches (Vilcins *et al.* 2008), with large burdens leading to anaemia. Among internal parasites, nematodes and tapeworms regularly inhabit the intestinal tracts. Two species of nematodes are known to form ulcers in the stomach wall that can lead to internal bleeding (Mawson 1968). *Toxoplasma gondii* infection can be prevalent in quoll populations where feral cats roam. However, infection does not lead to disease (toxoplasmosis), nor does it appear to have any direct or indirect impact on either devils or quolls (Fancourt *et al.* 2014).

The most high-profile disease in this group is devil facial tumour disease (DFTD), a fatal transmissible cancer affecting the Tasmanian devil (McCallum *et al.* 2009). While this cancer is mainly spread during aggressive contacts between devils, transmission via capture and handling devices cannot be excluded. Traps must be sterilised between captures, single-use handling bags must not be reused on multiple animals, and all processing equipment must be disinfected with a veterinary-grade disinfectant between animals. The disease highlights the value of preventative disinfection of all equipment used in the capture and handling of the larger dasyurids.

General operating procedures

Cage traps are a common trapping method for large dasyurids, although PVC pipe traps are the preferred trap type for devils (and sometimes quolls) in Tasmania (Chapter 7). Aluminium box traps are sometimes used to capture northern quolls (e.g. Ibbett *et al.* 2018), but trapped quolls may become saturated and stressed during wet weather and overheat in hot weather in these types of traps (J. Heiniger, pers. comm.). Appropriate marking methods include microchipping and tattooing, although ear notching and ear tagging are also sometimes used (Chapter 8). A range of low-impact and indirect methods of detection or study, such as measurement of dens and burrows, scat collection, assessment of tracks and other traces (Chapter 4), and camera trapping (Chapter 5), are also appropriate, depending on the species and study objectives. Various tracking methods may also be used for these species (Chapter 9). Veterinary procedures are detailed in Chapter 16.

NUMBAT

J. Anthony Friend and Rebecca Vaughan-Higgins

Characteristics

The numbat (*Myrmecobius fasciatus*) is a medium-sized marsupial with a head-body length of 20–25 cm and tail length of 15–18 cm. Adult males weigh 400–750 g, and females 300–650 g. Numbats possess morphological specialisations related to their diet of termites: a pointed snout, eyes near the top of their narrow, flat head, 50–52 reduced teeth and a long vermiform (worm-like) tongue that can extend at least 5 cm beyond the tip of the snout. The numbat's characteristic 'bottle-brush' tail is held aloft while foraging or moving about; their dark-reddish brown rump is banded by four to 11 white stripes that assist with camouflage.

Biology and behaviour

Numbats are currently found in Western Australia, South Australia and New South Wales. The previously wide range across southern Australia has contracted severely since the early 1800s. By the mid-1980s the species was confined to just two isolated populations in south-western Australia, but since then control of foxes and cats, and successful translocations have bolstered numbers, and eight populations are present across these three states.

Numbats are active only by day and use relatively large home ranges of 25 to > 100 ha (Christensen *et al.* 1984; Friend 2008; Hayward *et al.* 2015). Individuals of the same sex occupy exclusive home ranges, but males and females overlap to some degree (Friend 2008). Individuals are generally solitary except during the short mating season, and from August to November when females have dependent unattached young. The diet is composed almost entirely of termites, extracted by the numbat with its long tongue from their shallow soil galleries or from under fallen sticks and bark. Wild numbats feed on at least 25 termite species at Dryandra, Western Australia, eaten in proportion to their abundance (Calaby 1960).

Numbats use hollow logs and trees as boltholes to escape from predators, for resting during the day and for nesting at night. Consequently, telemetry collars should have a low physical profile (Figure 18.3) to minimise risk to the animals as they push through narrow cracks in logs. Both males and females also sleep in burrows that they construct or renovate, with a terminal chamber packed with soft nest material, such as shredded bark, leaves or flowers. Burrows are favoured in cooler weather and from early August by females to deposit and care for their young (Christensen *et al.* 1984; Friend 2008).

In Western Australia, mating occurs from late December to late January and males expend considerable energy moving large distances in search of receptive females. As females in oestrus are only receptive for ~48 h, capture and removal of individuals from the field even for short periods can reduce the likelihood of successful mating. Numbat capture should be avoided at this time.

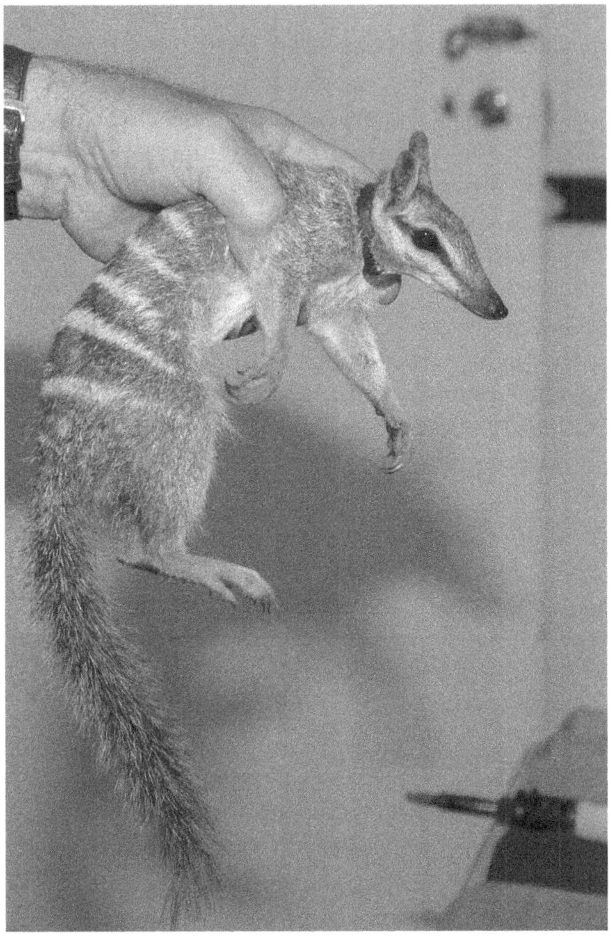

Figure 18.3: Numbat (*Myrmecobius fasciatus*) with radio transmitter attached. Photo by John Lawson.

Females carry young attached to their teats from late January to early August. While the young are firmly attached for most of this time, they are most at risk of becoming detached during handling soon after birth (January to mid-February) and when they are large (July and early August), at which time they can leave the nipple when nesting at night. Capture of females during these periods is not recommended or should be undertaken only by experienced numbat handlers.

While numbats may use several nests over a short period most of the year, extreme care should be taken in approaching a denning site where a female is caring for her young after deposition. The female will move her young when danger is perceived, even in response to a minor disturbance. While several burrows and suitable hollow logs and trees will be used by each female, the act of moving the young poses substantial risk to the female and young, especially from birds of prey. The deployment of camera traps near burrows should also be undertaken with extreme care as some females will move their young in response to camera placement, particularly if the camera is too close. Principles of ethical camera trap use (see Chapter 5) should be followed if they are used.

Capture and handling

Conventional live-trapping techniques are ineffective for capturing wild numbats. Currently, the only practical method is to search for individuals from a slowly moving vehicle during the day, move on foot towards a sighted animal, and keep it in sight until it enters a hollow log. Removal from the log can often be undertaken using a hose and net as described by Hayward *et al.* (2015). Alternatively, a cage trap with the back replaced by mesh to admit light and air can be attached to the log entrance, after blocking other potential escape holes. Excavation of numbats from nest burrows is very disruptive and should be a last resort.

Numbats can be marked by inserting microchips subcutaneously in the interscapular area (see Chapter 8). Numbats have tough skin, which resists microchip insertion, so isoflurane gaseous general anaesthesia is recommended if microchipping. The insertion site should be disinfected before insertion and closed using an absorbable suture to prevent transponder loss. Pelage markings are individually recognisable, so maintaining a photo library of individuals will also allow ready identification. Tips on handling numbats are given in Power and Monaghan (2003). As with other small- to medium-sized marsupials, numbats may be easily handled in a bag, exposing parts of interest as needed. However, they may also be held out of the bag for examination using one hand with a firm grip across the shoulders and around the upper thorax (Figure 18.3) and appear less stressed by this process than many mammals. Wild numbats are usually quite docile if held firmly and are generally less prone to struggle than are captive animals. It is unusual for a numbat to attempt to bite the handler.

Numbats should not be held for longer than a few hours during field studies. Their specialised diet means that transition to an artificial diet requires time, which is impractical in the field. Consequently, investigations that require holding of numbats for greater than a few hours should use captive animals. When returning an animal to the wild after handling or during translocation to a new site, release should be directly into a hollow log that has been checked for predators, rather than into the open. Release of numbats after dark is not recommended; it is preferable to hold an animal overnight for release the next day, making sure that it is insulated against heat loss. Numbats can be held in cotton bags for transport over short distances. Power and Monaghan (2003) provide details of approved boxes for transport by air.

Veterinary considerations

Sedation and anaesthesia

Gaseous anaesthesia is most commonly used for induction and maintenance. Induction is achieved with 5% isoflurane in oxygen administered via a well-fitting facemask, with a blindfold used to cover the eyes to minimise arousal. Numbats often hold their breath during induction, which can slow the process. However, numbats can be easily maintained on a mask for short procedures (< 10 min in duration). For longer procedures, numbats should be intubated. Recovery is often rapid following cessation of isoflurane administration. Like all small mammals (see Chapter 16), maintaining body temperature throughout procedures completed under anaesthesia is critical because of the likelihood of heat loss from the numbat's high surface-area-to-volume ratio. Sedation of numbats is uncommon, although the principles are similar to those for small dasyurids (Vitali and Monaghan 2009).

Blood collection

Blood collection is difficult because of the thick skin, lack of visible vessels and poor blood flow, especially in the field when numbats may be hypothermic, so general anaesthesia is recommended. Active warming of extremities with heat packs may be required to minimise peripheral vasoconstriction. The best blood collection sites are the femoral, jugular and brachiocephalic veins (see Vitali and Monaghan 2009 for detailed instructions).

Euthanasia

A two-step procedure is recommended for euthanasia of numbats, involving induction with gaseous anaesthesia or an injectable agent, followed by intravenous or intracardiac pentobarbitone. Animals euthanased with pentobarbitone represent a secondary toxicity risk to wild scavengers and should be disposed of via deep burial. Other generally acceptable methods for chemical euthanasia are as for rats and mice as described in Reilly (2001). If no field anaesthesia option is available and no veterinary practice is close, then blunt force trauma should be used. Cervical dislocation is acceptable only on very young individuals weighing < 150 g.

Table 18.1: Diseases and parasites of the numbat based on captive numbat records from wild-caught individuals and captive-bred individuals from the Native Species Breeding Program at Perth Zoo.

Type of pathogen	Details
Parasitic	***Ectoparasites*** Mites: *Mesolaelaps australiensis* Ticks: *Ixodes vestites, I. myrmecobii, Amblyomma triguttatum* Fleas: *Echidnophaga myrmecobiid, E. perilis* (Calaby 1960)
	Endoparasites Nematodes (phylum Acanthocephala): *Multisentis myrmecobius* (thorny-headed worm; Smales 1997) associated with gastrointestinal pathology, including inguinal hernias and gastrointestinal torsion (Haigh and Friend 1999) in wild and captive individuals.
	Protozoa *Toxoplasma gondii* is yet to be diagnosed in captivity over a 20 year period (Perth Zoo, unpublished data), but susceptibility is presumed.
Bacterial	*Campylobacter coli* detected on faecal culture from several clinically normal numbats (Vitali and Monaghan 2009).
	Clostridial necrotic enteritis associated with two deaths in captivity.
	Erysipelothrix rhusiopathiae isolated from a wild numbat on necropsy (Vaughan-Higgins *et al.* 2013).*
	Listeria monocytogenes caused neurological signs in captivity.*
	Mycobacterium intracellulare associated with foot lesions and *M. chelonae abscessus* associated with pustular skin lesions on the ventrum in captive numbats (Gaynor *et al.* 1990).
	Salmonella of varying serotypes including *muenchen, S. cholerae-suis* (var. Australia and var. *decatur*), *S. wandsbek* and *S. Indiana* diagnosed on routine faecal culture in wild and captive individuals. Cultured in animals with mucoid or malodorous faeces and shedding may be associated with periods of stress (Power and Monaghan 2003).*
Fungal	Cryptococcal pneumonia diagnosed at necropsy in a captive individual (*Gaynor et al.* 1990).
Viral	No reports of viral disease were found.
Mixed aetiology	***Skin disease*** In captivity, obesity and excessive moisture in enclosure substrate are risk factors for development. Many cases resolve spontaneously, but unresponsive cases require investigation (Vitali and Monaghan 2009). Bacterial dermatitis may include exudative lesions, hair loss, scurf and scale production.
	Cardiopulmonary diseases Pleurisy with pyothorax (possibly secondary to oesophageal perforation), cryptococcal pneumonia (Gaynor *et al.* 1990), focal granulomatous mycobacterial pneumonia, epicarditis and possible carcinoma leading to chylothorax, and atherosclerosis of the aorta and carotid vessels have been reported in captivity (Vitali and Monaghan 2009).

* Zoonotic infection.

Infectious pathogens

Vitali and Monaghan (2009) review numbat diseases in detail (Table 18.1). Other diseases of relevance to numbat research in captivity include degenerative joint disease (osteoarthritis of the hips and hock in captive aged individuals), gastrointestinal disease, genitourinary disease, trauma and tumours.

General operating procedures

Appropriate marking methods include microchipping (Chapter 8) under anaesthesia (Chapter 16). Relevant telemetry methods are detailed in Chapter 9. A range of low-impact and indirect methods of detection or study, such as measurement of dens and burrows, scat collection, assessment of tracks and other traces (Chapter 4), and camera monitoring (Chapter 5) may also be appropriate, depending on the study objectives.

REFERENCES

Attwood HD, Woolley PA (1970) Toxoplasmosis in dasyurid marsupials. *Pathology* **2**, 77–78. doi:10.1016/S0031-3025(16)39577-0

Attwood HD, Woolley PA, Rickard MD (1975) Toxoplasmosis in dasyurid marsupials. *Journal of Wildlife Diseases* **11**, 543–551. doi:10.7589/0090-3558-11.4.543

Baker A, Dickman CR (2018) *Secret Lives of Carnivorous Marsupials.* CSIRO Publishing, Melbourne.

Beveridge I, Spratt DM (2003) Parasites of carnivorous marsupials. In *Predators with Pouches.* (Eds M Jones, C Dickman and M Archer) pp. 383–396. CSIRO Publishing, Melbourne.

Calaby JH (1960) Observations on the banded ant-eater *Myrmecobius f. fasciatus* Waterhouse (Marsupialia), with particular reference to its food habits. *Proceedings of the Zoological Society of London* **135**, 183–207. doi:10.1111/j.1469-7998.1960.tb05841.x

Christensen P, Maisey K, Perry DH (1984) Radiotracking the numbat, *Myrmecobius fasciatus*, in the Perup Forest of Western Australia. *Wildlife Research* **11**, 275–288. doi:10.1071/WR9840275

Fancourt BA, Hawkins CE, Cameron EZ, Jones ME, Nicol SC (2015) Devil declines and catastrophic cascades: is mesopredator release of feral cats inhibiting recovery of the eastern quoll? *PLoS One* **10**, e0119303. doi:10.1371/journal.pone.0119303

Fancourt BA, Hawkins CE, Nicol SC (2018) Mechanisms of climate change-induced species decline: spatial, temporal and long-term variation in the diet of an endangered marsupial carnivore, the eastern quoll. *Wildlife Research* **45**, 737–750. doi:10.1071/WR18063

Fancourt BA, Nicol SC, Hawkins CE, Jones ME, Johnson CN (2014) Beyond the disease: is *Toxoplasma gondii* infection causing population declines in the eastern quoll (*Dasyurus viverrinus*)? *International Journal for Parasitology. Parasites and Wildlife* **3**, 102–112. doi:10.1016/j.ijppaw.2014.05.001

Firestone KB, Elphinstone MS, Sherwin WB, Houlden BA (1999) Phylogeographical population structure of tiger quolls *Dasyurus maculatus* (Dasyuridae: Marsupialia), an endangered carnivorous marsupial. *Molecular Ecology* **8**, 1613–1625. doi:10.1046/j.1365-294x.1999.00745.x

Friend JA (2008) Numbat *Myrmecobius fasciatus*. In *The Mammals of Australia.* 3rd edn. (Eds S van Dyck and R Strahan), pp. 163–165. Reed New Holland, Sydney.

Gaynor WT, Cousins DV, Friend JA (1990) Mycobacterial infection in numbats (*Myrmecobius fasciatus*). *Journal of Zoo and Wildlife Medicine* **21**, 476–479.

Geiser F (2004) The role of torpor in the life of Australian arid zone mammals. *Australian Mammalogy* **26**, 125–134. doi:10.1071/AM04125

Glen AS, Cardoso MJ, Dickman CR, Firestone KB (2009) Who's your daddy? Paternity testing reveals promiscuity and multiple paternity in the carnivorous marsupial *Dasyurus maculatus* (Marsupialia: Dasyuridae). *Biological Journal of the Linnean Society* **96**, 1–7. doi:10.1111/j.1095-8312.2008.01094.x

Godsell J (1983) Ecology of the eastern quoll, *Dasyurus viverrinus* (Dasyuridae: Marsupialia). PhD thesis. Australian National University, Australia.

Gray EL, Burwell CJ, Baker AM (2016) Benefits of being a generalist carnivore when threatened by climate change: the comparative dietary ecology of two sympatric semelparous marsupials, including a new endangered species (*Antechinus arktos*). *Australian Journal of Zoology* **64**, 249–261. doi:10.1071/ZO16044

Green B, Eberhard I (1979) Energy requirements and sodium and water turnovers in two captive marsupial carnivores, the Tasmanian devil (*Sarcophilus Harrisii*) and the native cat (*Dasyurus viverrinus*). *Australian Journal of Zoology* **27**, 1–8. doi:10.1071/ZO9790001

Haigh SA, Friend JA (1999) Veterinary aspects of several threatened Western Australian mammal species. *Australian Association of Veterinary Conservation Biologists Newsletter* **16**, 5–6.

Hayward MW, Poh ASL, Cathcart J, Churcher C, Bentley J, Herman K, Kemp L, Riessen N, Scully P, Diong CH, Legge S, Carter A, Gibb H, Friend JA (2015) Numbat nirvana: conservation ecology of the endangered numbat (*Myrmecobius fasciatus*) (Marsupialia: Myrmecobiidae) reintroduced to Scotia and Yookamurra Sanctuaries, Australia. *Australian Journal of Zoology* **63**, 258–269. doi:10.1071/ZO15028

Hivert LG, Clarke JR, Peck SJ, Lawrence C, Brown WE, Huxtable SJ, Schaap D, Pemberton D, Grueber CE (2018) High blood lead concentrations in captive Tasmanian devils (*Sarcophilus harrisii*): a threat to the conservation of the species? *Australian Veterinary Journal* **96**, 442–449. doi:10.1111/avj.12753

Hohnen R, Ashby J, Tuft K, McGregor H (2013) Individual identification of northern quolls (*Dasyurus hallucatus*) using remote cameras. *Australian Mammalogy* **35**, 131–135. doi:10.1071/AM12015

Ibbett M, Woinarski JCZ, Oakwood M (2018) Declines in the mammal assemblage of a rugged sandstone environment in Kakadu National Park, Northern Territory, Australia. *Australian Mammalogy* **40**, 181–187. doi:10.1071/AM17011

Johnstone CP, Lill A, Reina RD (2012) Does habitat fragmentation cause stress in the agile antechinus? A haematological approach. *Journal of Comparative Physiology. B, Biochemical, Systemic, and Environmental Physiology* **182**, 139–155. doi:10.1007/s00360-011-0598-7

Jones ME, Barmuta LA (1998) Diet overlap and relative abundance of sympatric dasyurid carnivores: a hypothesis of competition. *Journal of Animal Ecology* **67**, 410–421. doi:10.1046/j.1365-2656.1998.00203.x

Jung TS, Boonstra R, Krebs CJ (2020) Mark my words: expert's choice of marking methods used in capture-mark-recapture studies of small mammals. *Journal of Mammalogy* **101**, 307–317. doi:10.1093/jmammal/gyz188

Körtner G, Geiser F (1995) Body temperature rhythms and activity in reproductive Antechinus (Marsupialia). *Physiology & Behavior* **58**, 31–36. doi:10.1016/0031-9384(94)00384-H

Körtner G, Gresser S, Mott B, Tamayo B, Pisanu P, Bayne P, Harden B (2004) Population structure, turnover and movement of spotted-tailed quolls on the New England Tablelands. *Wildlife Research* **31**, 475–484. doi:10.1071/WR03041

Körtner G, Holznagel N, Fleming PJS, Ballard G (2016) Home range and activity patterns measured with GPS collars in spotted-tailed quolls. *Australian Journal of Zoology* **63**, 424–431. doi:10.1071/ZO16002

Körtner G, Rojas AD, Geiser F (2010) Thermal biology, torpor use and activity patterns of a small diurnal marsupial from a tropical desert: sexual differences. *Journal of Comparative Physiology. B, Biochemical, Systemic, and Environmental Physiology* **180**, 869–876. doi:10.1007/s00360-010-0459-9

Körtner G, Trachtenberg A, Geiser F (2019) Does aridity affect spatial ecology? Scaling of home range size in small carnivorous marsupials. *Naturwissenschaften* **106**, 42. doi:10.1007/s00114-019-1636-7

Molyneux J, Pavey CR, James AI, Carthew SM (2018) Habitat use by the brush-tailed mulgara (*Dasycercus blythi*). *Australian Journal of Zoology* **65**, 335–345. doi:10.1071/ZO17032

Mawson PM (1968) Two species of nematoda (Spirurida: Spiruridae) from Australian dasyurids. *Parasitology* **58**, 75–78. doi:10.1017/s0031182000073431

McCallum H, Jones M, Hawkins C, Hamede R, Lachish S, Sinn DL, Beeton N, Lazenby B (2009) Transmission dynamics of Tasmanian devil facial tumor disease may lead to disease-induced extinction. *Ecology* **90**, 3379–3392. doi:10.1890/08-1763.1

McLean AL (2015) Conservation biology of an endangered semi-arid marsupial, the sandhill dunnart (*Sminthopsis psammophila*). PhD thesis. The University of Adelaide, Australia.

Oakwood M, Bradley AJ, Cockburn A (2001) Semelparity in a large marsupial. *Proceedings. Biological Sciences* **268**, 407–411. doi:10.1098/rspb.2000.1369

Obendorf DL (1993) Diseases of dasyurid marsupials. In *The Biology and Management of Australasian Carnivorous Marsupials.* (Eds M Roberts, J Canio, G Crawshaw and M Hutchins) pp. 39–46. Metropolitan Toronto Zoo and the Monotreme and Marsupial Group of the American Association of Zoological Parks and Aquariums, Toronto, Canada.

Pavey CR, Burwell CJ, Körtner G, Geiser F (2018) Trophic ecology of marsupial predators following reshaping of predator assemblages in arid Australia. *Journal of Mammalogy* **99**, 1128–1136. doi:10.1093/jmammal/gyy100

Pavey CR, Geiser F (2008) Basking and diurnal foraging in the dasyurid marsupial *Pseudantechinus macdonnellensis. Australian Journal of Zoology* **56**, 129–135. doi:10.1071/ZO08032

Pearse AM (1981) Aspects of the biology of *Uropsylla tasmanica* Rothschild (Siphonaptera). MSc thesis. The University of Tasmania, Australia.

Power VL, Monaghan C (2003) Numbats. In *Australian Mammals: Biology and Captive Management.* (Ed. SM Jackson) pp. 99–125. CSIRO Publishing, Melbourne.

Riek A (2008) Relationship between field metabolic rate and body weight in mammals: effect of the study. *Journal of Zoology* **276**, 187–194. doi:10.1111/j.1469-7998.2008.00482.x

Reilly JS (Ed) (2001) *Euthanasia of Animals Used for Scientific Purposes.* 2nd edn. Australian & New Zealand Council for the Care of Animals in Research and Teaching (ANZCCART), Adelaide.

Rowland J, Hoskin CJ, Burnett S (2020) Camera traps are an effective method for identifying individuals and determining the sex of spotted-tailed quolls (*Dasyurus maculatus gracilis*). *Australian Mammalogy* **42**, 349–356. doi:10.1071/AM19017

Ruibal M, Peakall R, Claridge A, Murray A, Firestone K (2010) Advancement to hair-sampling surveys of a medium-sized mammal: DNA-based individual identification and population estimation of a rare Australian marsupial, the spotted-tailed quoll (*Dasyurus maculatus*). *Wildlife Research* **37**, 27–38. doi:10.1071/WR09087

Schmidt-Nielsen K (1972) *How Animals Work.* Cambridge University Press, London, UK.

Smales LR (1997) *Multisentis myrmecobius*, gen. et sp. nov. (Acanthocephala: Oligacanthorhynchidae), from the numbat, *Myrmecobius fasciatus*, and a key to genera of the Oligacanthorhynchidae. *Invertebrate Systematics* **11**, 301–307. doi:10.1071/IT95023

Soderquist TR (1995) Spatial organization of the arboreal carnivorous marsupial *Phascogale tapoatafa. Journal of Zoology* **237**, 385–398. doi:10.1111/j.1469-7998.1995.tb02769.x

Soderquist TR, Dickman CR (1988) A technique for marking marsupial pouch young with fluorescent pigment tattoos. *Australian Wildlife Research* **15**, 561–563. doi:10.1071/WR9880561

Tyndale-Biscoe H (2005) *Life of Marsupials.* CSIRO Publishing, Melbourne.

Vaughan-Higgins RJ, Bradfield K, Friend JA, Riley TV, Vitali SD (2013) Erysipelas in a numbat (*Myrmecobius fasciatus*). *Journal of Zoo and Wildlife Medicine* **44**, 208–211. doi:10.1638/1042-7260-44.1.208

Vilcins IM, Old JM, Körtner G, Deane EM (2008) Ectoparasites and skin lesions in wild-caught spotted-tailed quoll (*Dasyurus maculatus*) (Marsupialia: Dasyuridae). *Comparative Parasitology* **75**, 271–277. doi:10.1654/4339.1

Vitali S, Monaghan C (2009) Numbats. In *Medicine of Australian Mammals* (Eds L Vogelnest and R Woods) pp. 383–395. CSIRO Publishing, Melbourne.

Warnecke L, Körtner G, Burwell CJ, Turner JM, Geiser F (2012) Short-term movement patterns and diet of small dasyurid marsupials in semiarid Australia. *Australian Mammalogy* **34**, 49–54. doi:10.1071/AM10052

Waudby HP, Petit S (2017) Thermoregulatory value of cracking-clay soil shelters for small vertebrates during extreme desert conditions. *Integrative Zoology* **12**, 237–249. doi:10.1111/1749-4877.12225

19 Wombats, bandicoots, bilbies, possums and gliders

Karleah K. Berris, Laura Ruykys, Ross L. Goldingay, Damian S. Morrant, Jasmin G. Packer, Kris Descovich, Alison Matthews, Amy Coetsee, Vere Nicolson, Alan Horsup, Katherine Moseby, Hayley Louise Jose, Sarah J. Gill and David A. Taggart

INTRODUCTION

Wombats, bandicoots, bilbies, possums and gliders comprise a suite of marsupial species that are herbivorous, omnivorous, insectivorous or nectarivorous. Many species covered in this chapter provide important ecological services through their foraging habits, including bioturbation and pollination. Some species, such as wombats and bilbies, construct burrows that are beneficial refuges to other wildlife. These species also show morphological adaptations to their burrowing, digging or arboreal lifestyles.

WOMBATS

Laura Ruykys, Karleah K. Berris, Kris Descovich, Alison Matthews, Vere Nicolson, Alan Horsup and David A. Taggart

Characteristics

Three species of wombat occupy two genera: the bare-nosed (or common) wombat (*Vombatus ursinus*), southern hairy-nosed wombat (*Lasiorhinus latifrons*) and northern hairy-nosed wombat (*L. krefftii*). Hairy-nosed wombats are distinguishable from bare-nosed wombats by their softer, silkier fur above and paler fur below, square muzzle, fine hairs on their nose, and pointed, erect ears (Van Dyck and Strahan 2008). Wombat body mass is not sexually dimorphic. The northern hairy-nosed wombat is the largest of the three species, with adults averaging 31.5 kg. Adult bare-nosed wombats average 26 kg and southern hairy-nosed wombats 25 kg (range 23–38 kg). Bare-nosed wombats have a rear-opening pouch and hairy-nosed wombats a pouch that opens ventrally. All species have two teats, a tail so short it is almost indistinguishable, a unique gastric gland in the stomach, and hook-shaped sperm that are very different to those of most other marsupials except for their close relative, the koala (Van Dyck and Strahan 2008).

Biology and behaviour

The bare-nosed wombat occurs in temperate areas of south-eastern Australia, extending from southern Queensland to Tasmania. The southern hairy-nosed wombat previously occurred from southern New South Wales to south-eastern Western Australia. The species' distribution is now fragmented and mainly concentrated in five populations in semi-arid South Australia, as well as south-eastern Western Australia, and just across the South Australian border. In South Australia, important subpopulations occur on the Nullarbor Plain, Gawler Ranges, Murraylands, and Yorke and Eyre peninsulas. The northern hairy-nosed wombat previously occurred in an inland arc from the Riverina area of southern New South Wales to inland central Queensland; however, it is presumed to have been only patchily distributed throughout its range before the arrival of Europeans in Australia (Swinbourne *et al.* 2017). It is now one of the world's rarest mammals. The main threats to wild wombats are drought (including effects associated with climate change), infectious disease, competition from European rabbits (*Oryctolagus cuniculus*), control actions (shooting, poisoning, fumigation, burrow ripping) by landholders, land-use changes and habitat loss, and road accidents (vehicle collisions) (Swinbourne *et al.* 2017; Taggart *et al.* 2020).

Wombats are nocturnal, fossorial and cryptic in nature, which has somewhat hampered research on wild populations. Warrens are central to their survival, providing protection from environmental extremes, predators and dehydration. All species are major soil engineers within the Australian landscape, with their burrows also providing protection to other non-burrowing, vertebrate species. Their diet is dominated by low-quality grasses with high-fibre and high-silica content (up to 95% of the diet) and forbs (Evans *et al.* 2003). Wombats have particularly low energy, protein and water requirements, and an exceptionally low field metabolic rate. This helps them to maintain condition even during times of low food availability, and to spend minimal time above ground feeding. Their mostly nocturnal activity is likely related to ambient temperature and humidity and possibly light intensity. In some locations, wombats may emerge during the day to bask or graze close to their warrens if the temperature is low, or in overcast conditions (Finlayson *et al.* 2005).

All three species are more tolerant of cold than of hot weather and can become heat stressed if they do not have the capacity to cool down. During the day, wombats will move to different areas of the burrow to micromanage their exposure to ambient temperature and humidity (Tyndale-Biscoe 2005). Wombats are mostly solitary and use extensive scent marking to identify their presence to other individuals (Finlayson *et al.* 2005); however, hairy-nosed wombats have been recorded to share burrow systems at times. Wombats' home range varies depending on the species and location (2–25 ha for 95% minimum convex polygon (MCP) in hairy-nosed wombats; average ~5–190 ha MCP recorded in bare-nosed wombats). Home ranges are centred around their warrens and some wombats use multiple warrens, allowing them to range over larger areas (Matthews 2011).

Breeding in bare-nosed wombats may occur at any time of the year; however, hairy-nosed wombats show seasonality in births (mid-July to December for southern hairy-nosed wombats; November to March for northern hairy-nosed wombats). Single young are born to all three species; this has a pouch life of up to 9 months, followed by 3–9 months at foot. Breeding and juvenile survival are highly dependent on rainfall and vegetation growth. Animals reach sexual maturity at ~3 years of age (Van Dyck and Strahan 2008; Taggart *et al.* 2020). Wombats are typically long-lived species (15–25 years in the wild) that produce an average of two young every 3 years. Juveniles and subadult animals are highly susceptible to drought (Taggart *et al.* 2020).

Capture and handling

Wombats are large and strong. Therefore, they require suitably experienced personnel for trapping and handling. Wombats can be caught in large and sturdy weld-mesh cage traps (800 × 450 × 450 mm) with inward-swinging doors that are set near the burrow entrance, or via opportunistic hand capture using a long-handled net (1620 mm handle with an 840 mm diameter hoop). Capture by stunning has also been used successfully in open habitats (Taggart *et al.* 2003) and is covered in detail in Chapter 7.

Ejection of pouch young and capture myopathy have never been observed during capture and trapping. Trap-related health risks for wombats are primarily associated with (1) hyperthermia, which can occur relatively easily in wombats as they do not sweat; and (2) stress associated with trap placement in, or close to, burrows/warrens. Traps placed directly into burrow entrances may cause high levels of stress. Wombats may avoid them and can remain underground for long periods (≤ 14 days), which denies them access to food or other resources and is particularly risky for lactating females with or without pouch young. Construction of fencing around warrens, 1–2 m beyond the burrow spoil mounds, is generally thought to be a better technique (Figure 19.1). Traps

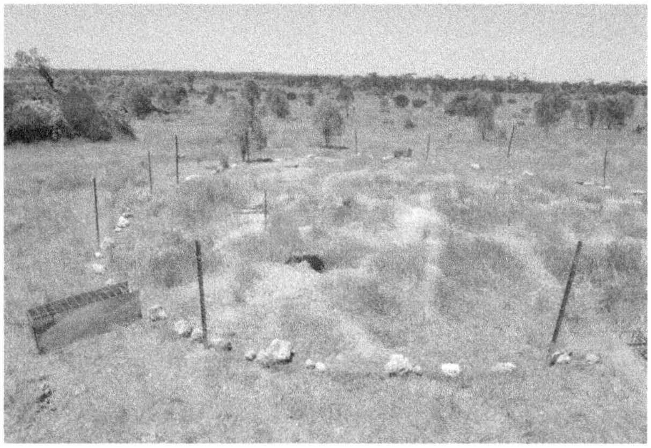

Figure 19.1: Fenced wombat warren with cage traps positioned at openings in the fence to capture wombats as they attempt to exit the fenced area. Photo by David Taggart.

should be wired securely into the fence, with the entrance to the trap flush with the fence and directly over a wombat trail leading away from the burrow entrance. The fence should have a 30–40 cm skirt on the inside that is held to the ground securely by pegs or rocks, to prevent wombats digging out.

Cage trapping is most effective from dusk until dawn, as these are the times when wombats are most active. Traps should be checked early and regularly across periods of animal activity and closed during periods of inactivity. Trapping during hot weather is inappropriate. Trapping wombats from warrens can take 2–7 days. Cage traps should be removed from the warren after a maximum of 8 days.

Because of their size and strength, wild wombats should be anaesthetised for handling, physical examination, measurement, marking and attachment of tracking collars. Physical examination should follow the procedures of Jackson (2003). To hold an un-anaesthetised wombat (not recommended for wild wombats), the animal should be picked up from behind with one arm under the armpit and across the chest, with the other arm supporting the rump (Jackson 2003).

For handling and short-distance transport in cooler weather, wombats can be transported in large hessian sacks or pet packs; however, care must be taken to ensure that animals do not overheat. For longer distances in cooler weather, transportation crates can be constructed using marine plywood (approximate dimensions: 90 × 90 × 60 cm), or large pet crates can be used, with suitable bedding such as straw (Treby 2005). Sufficient ventilation is important during transportation to help animals maintain a thermoneutral body temperature. Because of their low energetic requirements, wombats do not need to be fed if the transport period is ≤ 24 h. Southern and bare-nosed wombats are kept in numerous zoological collections, so captive management is relatively well documented, although breeding success is poor and unreliable (Jackson 2003; Treby 2005; Bryant and Reiss 2008).

Wombats can be individually marked with a microchip (passive integrated transponder (PIT) tag) implanted between the scapulae, parallel to the long axis of the body (see Chapter 8). Insertion should be performed under anaesthesia because of the thickness of a wombat's skin. A small, coloured, reflective cattle ear tag may be fitted to assist in identifying individuals from a distance; however, if netting such animals, care must be taken that the tag does not become caught on netting and ripped out (NHMRC 2014).

Wombats can carry telemetry (e.g. VHF, GPS and/or satellite) neck collars relatively well (Finlayson *et al.* 2005; Matthews 2011). Collars must be fitted quite tightly because of their stocky neck and head being relatively similar in size (Finlayson *et al.* 2005). Collars should comprise double thickness seatbelt webbing (25 mm wide) or a material of a similar soft, flexible and strong nature; otherwise, neck lesions will result. Collars made of material that is too flimsy will be rapidly destroyed by a wombat. Wider collars are more easily thrown by the wearer. Collar attachment should account for wombats' strong claws and for their underground and digging habits, ensuring that prominent gaps are not present around the neck that could result in the animal becoming ensnared when digging and manoeuvring. It is best to fit wombat collars when animals are under anaesthesia and when they are in very good condition (winter and spring) to avoid any risk of strangulation. Expert advice should be sought from suitably experienced personnel before commencing tracking studies.

Although wombats are resilient, signs of mild stress during handling can include loud vocalisations and teeth gnashing. Substantial stress can also be experienced during short-term captivity, particularly during warm weather, without overt behavioural change. Therefore, handling times, particularly for animals that are not anaesthetised, should be kept to a minimum. Wombats have been observed in a torpor-like behavioural state, although true torpor, as indicated by sufficiently low body temperatures, has not been recorded (Descovich *et al.* 2017). During this torpor-like behaviour, wombats are unresponsive to external stimuli and may be mistaken as deceased. Care should be taken if approaching a wombat in this state as, once roused, they may become agitated and aggressive if not habituated to human presence.

Veterinary considerations

Sedation and anaesthesia

To anaesthetise wombats, an intramuscular injection of tiletamine–zolazepam may be administered at a dose of 3–5 mg/kg (NHMRC 2014). Delivery of the same drug regimen by dart at close range has been used as a capture technique with mixed success (Matthews 2011). To achieve a surgical plane of anaesthesia or to abolish chewing movements, supplementary anaesthesia with an inhalation agent such as isoflurane in oxygen may be required (see Chapter 16). Alternatively, for juvenile animals and captive wombats that can be reliably handled, gaseous anaesthesia can be used for induction and maintenance, using isoflurane in oxygen (5% induction, 1% maintenance) via a facemask while animals are manually restrained (Bryant and Reiss 2008; NHMRC 2014). Endotracheal intubation in wombats has resulted in complications with trauma to the mucosa of the trachea; therefore, oxygen and isoflurane delivered via facemask may be more appropriate for invasive surgery. The advantages of gaseous anaesthesia include much quicker recoveries. The use of long-acting neuroleptic agents in wombats has resulted in profound and prolonged tranquilisation for periods of weeks and is therefore not recommended.

Blood collection

Blood is most commonly collected from the cephalic vein of anaesthetised wombats (Reiss *et al.* 2008; Death *et al.* 2011).

Euthanasia

Two-stage euthanasia is recommended, whereby anaesthesia (for example, an intramuscular injection of tiletamine–zolazepam) is followed by pentobarbitone (150 mg/kg) delivered via the intravenous or intracardiac route (NHMRC 2014). Any animal euthanased with pentobarbitone represents a secondary toxicity risk to wild scavengers and should be disposed of via deep burial. If pentobarbitone is unavailable and an animal requires emergency euthanasia in the field, a shot to the brain using an appropriate firearm is acceptable. Captive bolts have also been used (Hing *et al.* 2019).

Infectious pathogens

Causes of death in wild wombat populations may not be well understood because their fossorial lifestyle means bodies may not be discovered; furthermore, the animals are nocturnal and cautious, making observation difficult. There are, however, several diseases known to affect wombats in the wild. Sarcoptic mange is an infectious disease caused by the microscopic, burrowing mite *Sarcoptes scabiei*. Clinical signs include erythema (skin reddening), alopecia (hair loss) and parakeratosis (skin crusting). Bare-nosed and southern hairy-nosed wombats are affected; it is also likely that the disease could also affect northern hairy-nosed wombats. In bare-nosed wombat populations, mange is both enzootic and epizootic, with significant mortality and substantial decreases in local abundance. In southern hairy-nosed wombats, mange appears to be epizootic (i.e. temporarily prevalent and widespread in a population) rather than enzootic (regularly affecting animals), but there can be sudden increases in incidence with severe effects on individuals in some populations or colonies (Ruykys *et al.* 2009). Sarcoptic mange can be transferred to other animals, including humans.

Toxoplasmosis, caused by the protozoan parasite *Toxoplasmosis gondii*, is common in bare-nosed wombats and can be characterised by neuropathic signs such as a head tilt, abnormal diurnal behaviour, blindness and circling. Serological surveys have found many wild bare-nosed wombats to be seropositive and usually asymptomatic.

Adiaspiromycosis and pneumonia are caused by soil-dwelling fungi of the genus *Emmonsia*. Although not common in wombats, fatal cases have been recorded in all species. Bacterial pneumonia has also been reported. Several other potential bacterial, viral, fungal, protozoal and ectoparasitic pathogens have been recorded in wombats; however, none appears to cause disease at the population level, and some do not appear to be pathogenic (Bryant and Reiss 2008).

General operating procedures

A range of low-impact and indirect methods of detection or study, such as measurement of dens and burrows, scat collection, assessment of tracks and other traces (Chapter 4), camera and hair trapping, and conservation detector dogs (Chapter 5) may be used to study wombats depending on study objectives. Wombats are typically trapped with cage traps (Chapter 7), and marked with microchips or ear tags (Chapter 8). Radiotelemetry with collar attachments may also be used for wombats (Chapter 9). Medical procedures, including anaesthesia, are detailed in Chapter 16. Additional considerations for wombat husbandry and captive management are detailed in Treby (2005) and Jackson (2003).

BANDICOOTS AND BILBY

Karleah K. Berris, Jasmin G. Packer, Amy Coetsee, Hayley Louise Jose and Katherine Moseby

Characteristics

Bandicoots and bilbies are members of the order Peramelemorphia, which is endemic to Australia, New Guinea and nearby islands (Van Dyck and Strahan 2008). *Isoodon*, *Perameles*, *Echymipera* and *Macrotis* species are extant within Australia, but the sole species in the genus

Chaeropus is extinct. Phylogeny and taxonomy of *Peramelemorphia* has not been completely resolved; however, molecular findings indicate that bilbies (*Macrotis lagotis*) and the pig-footed bandicoot (*Chearopus*) families are likely to be distinct from other Australian bandicoots (Warburton and Travouillon 2016).

Bandicoots and bilbies are small to medium-sized marsupials, ranging in size from 230 g (average body mass of the western barred bandicoot, *P. bougainville*) to 2.5 kg (a large male bilby) (Seebeck *et al.* 1990; Van Dyck and Strahan 2008). Sexual dimorphism occurs in most species, with males generally larger than females in *Isoodon*, *Echymipera* and *Macrotis* species. Most bandicoots and bilbies have long, pointed snouts that enhance their strong sense of smell, relatively short fore limbs and hind limbs that are adapted for strong propulsion (Warburton and Travouillon 2016). Both bandicoots and bilbies show adaptations of their fore limbs for scratch digging, and some also for excavation of burrows, which reduces their manual dexterity (Warburton and Travouillon 2016).

Biology and behaviour

Bandicoots and bilbies were widely distributed across Australia before European settlement, occurring in arid, semi-arid, temperate and tropical habitats. Australian members of the order Peramelemorphia have undergone dramatic declines in abundance and range since European settlement; this is reflected in several recorded extinctions (e.g. the desert bandicoot, *P. eremiana*; lesser bilby, *M. leucura*; and southern pig-footed bandicoot, *C. ecaudatus*) and the threatened conservation status of most remaining species. Bandicoots and bilbies have arguably suffered more severe population declines than any other group of Australian marsupials since European settlement. This decline is mainly a result of habitat loss and predation by the introduced red fox (*Vulpes vulpes*) and feral cat (*Felis catus*; Seebeck *et al.* 1990).

Extant bandicoot and bilby species appear to be opportunistic omnivores, with seasonal and spatial variation in diet recorded for some species, such as bilbies. Dietary items include invertebrates, plant material (bulbs, fruits, roots and seeds) and fungi (Warburton and Travouillon 2016). Several species of bandicoots and bilbies could be described as ecologically flexible, with varied diets and previous distributions that encompassed many different habitat types. Species belonging to this group play important ecological roles through their propensity for scratch digging during foraging. Their digging behaviour aids in dispersal of mycorrhizal fungal spores, the turnover of soil and creation of microhabitats in freshly disturbed (spoil heap) and protected (pit) conditions that can enhance plant germination (Fleming *et al.* 2014). Bilby burrows are also used by other species as a refuge. Hence, many species of Peramelemorphia have been termed 'ecosystem engineers'.

Bandicoots and bilbies range from crepuscular to primarily nocturnal and mostly solitary. Home-range areas vary greatly depending on species and climatic zone, with mean home-range sizes of ~1–16 ha recorded in *Isoodon* species, and ~2 to 51 ha recorded in bilbies (MCP; Moseby and O'Donnell 2003; McRae 2004). For both bandicoots and bilbies, females tend to have smaller home ranges than males (McRae 2004). During the day, bandicoots shelter in diurnal dens or nests in leaf litter or dense vegetation, while bilbies retreat to underground burrows that they have excavated.

Reproduction in bandicoots and bilbies is characterised by a short gestation period (12.5 days in eastern barred bandicoots, *Perameles gunnii*, to 14 days in bilbies) and potentially high reproductive output under favourable environmental conditions (Seebeck *et al.* 1990). Breeding can occur year-round or seasonally depending on the climatic zone and habitat type, and both bandicoots and bilbies have been observed to have multiple litters of young in a year (Seebeck *et al.* 1990; Warburton and Travouillon 2016). Mean litter sizes of bandicoots of 1.8 to five young per litter have been recorded (J. Packer, unpublished data; Warburton and Travouillon 2016). Bilbies generally have one or two young per litter, although litters of three are occasionally reported (Southgate *et al.* 2000). Pouch life in bandicoots is generally shorter than in bilbies (55–60 days in *Isoodon* spp., up to 90 days in bilbies; Warburton and Travouillon 2016). Most bandicoot species and bilbies have been observed to have as many as four litters in a year under good environmental conditions. Young can become reproductively active from 3–6 months of age. Rapid onset of sexual maturity and the ability to breed prolifically means many species are able to take advantage of favourable environmental conditions, and reintroductions are generally successful if threats from exotic predators can be managed effectively.

Capture and handling

Medium wire cage traps (60 × 29 × 25 cm) are suitable for the capture of bandicoots and bilbies of a range of sizes, either baited or set in the entrance to active burrows (bilbies). Elliott (Type A) traps are also suitable for juvenile, subadult and small adult bandicoots; however, Elliott traps would exclude larger individuals or species. Wire cage traps should be positioned under vegetation to reduce exposure to weather, sunlight and predation, and covered with plastic, hessian or a shade cloth to reduce exposure to sun and/or rain while still maintaining adequate ventilation. Stressed animals in cages will increase their activity, sometimes injuring their noses and claws. Checking traps at night or just before sunrise (or afternoon for bandicoots active during the day) can minimise stress. Cages are usually baited with a mixture of peanut butter and oats, although additional additives can be integrated such as apple, carrot, honey, golden syrup, linseed oil or sardines. Additionally, biodegradable and biosecure material (e.g. hessian squares) can be placed in traps as bedding and for enrichment. Time spent in traps should be limited as much as possible and traps closed in inclement weather. Bilbies can be trap shy and difficult to trap, especially in the wild. In these cases, placing traps in the entrance to burrows (McGregor and Moseby 2014) or using pen traps can increase trap success. Pen traps are constructed from 90 cm high wire mesh that is placed in a ring around the resident burrow with holes cut out at ground level so cage traps can be placed flush with the inside of the mesh pen (see Figure 19.1 for a similar example used for wombats). Bilbies and some species of bandicoots (such as the western barred bandicoot) can also be successfully captured at night using spotlights and handheld fishing nets. Spotlighting can occur on foot or in a vehicle. When a bilby or bandicoot is spotted it can be chased by up to three people with nets, who place the net in front of the animal so it runs into the net. Care must be taken not to injure the animal so experienced netters are needed.

Bandicoots and bilbies tend to be calm if handled gently and often do not struggle or bite. They can sometimes bolt from the trap into the catch bag and can kick out with their back legs while being handled. Bandicoots and bilbies are calmer if their heads are covered. Therefore, it is recommended they are handled in a dark calico or cotton trap bag. The individual should be held so that contact is maximised with a firm surface, such as the handler's body or lap. Alternatively, the handler can use a two-hand hold, where one hand is placed around the shoulders and back of the neck, with the other around the hips to support the weight and to prevent injury to the handler and animal. Animals should never be held solely by the tail or legs because they are fragile. Generally, bandicoots and bilbies are not anaesthetised for handling unless more-invasive procedures are being undertaken (e.g. blood sampling). Some species of bandicoots, such as the western barred bandicoot, are susceptible to stress during handling, which can be fatal if capture myopathy occurs. The western barred bandicoot should be handled gently with minimal restraint and processed as quickly as possible.

Passive integrated transponders (PIT) tags can be used to identify individuals. PIT tags should be inserted by syringe under the skin between the scapulae, or slightly above the hind limb on southern brown bandicoots because of their tough skin between the shoulder blades. Bilbies have thin skin and care must be taken not to use too much force to implant the microchip. In comparison, some bandicoot species (the western barred bandicoot, southern brown bandicoot) have tough skin and lose fur easily when personnel are trying to pinch the skin for microchip placement. Ear notching can also be a useful method for identifying individuals; although tears on ears can make these marks difficult to differentiate over time.

Bandicoots and bilbies have had issues with their front legs becoming caught in telemetry collars, because of their propensity to dig with their front feet. Telemetry collars can also be difficult to attach to bandicoots because of their tapering head. Therefore, transmitters affixed to the base of tail using either tape or an adhesive have been used as an alternative short-term option (< 5 days – 3 months) as has gluing transmitters to the fur on the back or rump. Glue attachments on the fur generally last < 2 weeks before falling off. Some transmitters have been surgically implanted into the peritoneal cavity, but doing so requires intensive and ongoing veterinary support and can lead to health issues. Transmitters can be successfully attached to bilby tails for up to 3 months before they fall off, but they can be reattached regularly and left on for up to 1 year. Bilby tail transmitters must be applied by skilled handlers as the tail must be shaved before attachment and any pressure on the tail from the transmitters can lead to ulcers and tail damage. Special tape and a specific wrapping method are required; this is best learned from an expert who has conducted previous telemetry studies with bilbies. It is recommended that expert advice be sought before carrying out telemetry studies.

For transport, individual transport boxes should be used: usually plastic pet crates, which can be cushioned with shredded paper and transported by air-conditioned car in hot weather. Cardboard can be placed over most of the holes in the side of the pet crate to make a dark environment and reduce stress. In some cases, animals have been transported in catch bags inside pet crates. Bilbies and bandicoots can also be transported in individual wooden boxes with straw with dimensions of ~50 × 20 × 20 cm. For longer transport distances, bandicoots and bilbies can be held overnight in their pet packs with some food (e.g. mealworms and chopped vegetables). For short-term housing, a minimum enclosure space of 16–20 m^2 has been used for eastern barred bandicoots. Enclosures should have a solid concrete base to prevent animals digging out; however, sufficient softer substrate should be provided to mitigate damage to claws and noses. Captive management of bandicoots and bilbies is well documented (e.g. Jackson 2003).

Veterinary considerations

Sedation and anaesthesia

Anaesthesia is usually not required for animal handling, processing or fitting of telemetry transmitters. Anaesthetics may be used to minimise pain and distress during procedures such as blood collection (NHMRC 2014). Inhalation of isoflurane in oxygen (4–5% induction, 2–3% maintenance) via a facemask has been used to anaesthetise bandicoots (Packer 2014). Further information on anaesthesia can be found in Lynch (2008) and Chapter 16.

Blood collection

Blood can be collected from bandicoots and bilbies in two general ways. First, blood can be collected from the jugular or femoral vein of anaesthetised animals using 25 G needles and syringes. Second, small volumes (≤ 0.5 mL) of blood can be collected from non-anaesthetised animals under manual restraint by nicking a marginal (lateral) ear vein and allowing blood to travel down a heparinised microhaematocrit tube into a blood collection tube (Lynch 2008).

Euthanasia

Bandicoots and bilbies are commonly euthanased via a two-stage injection approach, involving sedation via intramuscular tiletamine–zolazepam (5 mg/kg), followed by pentobarbitone (150 mg/kg) delivered by intravenous or intracardiac injection (NHMRC 2014). Any animal euthanased with pentobarbitone represents a secondary toxicity risk to wild scavengers and should be disposed of via deep burial. Euthanasia via physical methods (gunshot or blunt force trauma to the back of the skull) is only generally used in emergency situations in remote locations where chemical agents are not accessible.

Infectious pathogens

Bandicoots and bilbies carry various ectoparasites such as fleas, ticks and mites. There is little evidence that they carry zoonotic diseases that pose a direct risk to humans when good hygiene practices are followed. Toxoplasmosis is the main significant disease reported for this taxon. Toxoplasmosis has been reported in both *Isoodon* and *Perameles* genera, and in bilbies. Eastern barred bandicoots with toxoplasmosis have been recorded to display unnatural daytime movements, incoordination, staggered movements and possibly blindness (Seebeck *et al.* 1990). Toxoplasmosis deaths have been reported in this species.

General operating procedures

A range of low-impact and indirect methods of detection or study, such as measurement of dens and burrows, scat collection, and assessment of tracks and other traces (Chapter 4), camera and hair trapping, and conservation detector dogs (Chapter 5) may be used to study these taxa depending on study objectives. These species are typically trapped with cage or aluminium box traps (Chapter 7), and marked with microchips or by ear notching (Chapter 8), but see also Jose and Packer (2020). Various tracking methods may be used for these taxa (Chapter 9). Medical procedures, including anaesthesia, are detailed in Chapter 16.

POSSUMS AND GLIDERS

Ross L. Goldingay, Damian S. Morrant and Sarah J. Gill

Characteristics

In Australia, the possums and gliders comprise six marsupial families and ~31 possum and glider species (Acrobatidae, Petauridae, Phalangeridae, Pseudocheiridae and Tarsipedidae; see Van Dyck and Strahan 2008; Van Dyck *et al.* 2013; Cremona *et al.* 2021). Possums and gliders range in size from the little pygmy possum (8 g) up to the spotted cuscus (5 kg). They have characteristically sharp claws and an opposable, nail-less toe, with large pads on the hind foot to aid climbing. All gliders and nearly all possums are arboreal and occupy forest or heathland; however, some are semi-terrestrial, including the mountain pygmy possum (*Burramys parvus*), rock ringtail possum (*Petropseudes dahli*) and scaly-tailed possum (*Wyulda squamicaudata*). Possums and gliders are highly adapted to their arboreal/climbing lifestyle. Possums have fully or partially prehensile tails, and gliders have a furred membrane of skin between the front and hind feet, called a patagium, which acts like a wing when outstretched. Australia has three distinct types of gliding possums, each more closely related to a non-gliding species than each other, indicating that this form of locomotion has evolved independently at least three times. Two species of the matchbox-sized feathertail gliders (*Acrobatidae*), five species of the small- to medium-sized gliders (*Petauridae*) and currently one species of the larger folivorous greater glider (*Pseudocheiridae*) are recognised.

Biology and behaviour

Gliders occur across northern Australia, down a wide zone in eastern and southern Australia, and into South Australia. None occurs through the interior of the continent or the south-west, and until the introduction of the sugar glider > 100 years ago, none occurred in Tasmania. The possums include the diminutive honey possum (*Tarsipes rostratus*) in south-western Australia, pygmy possums (*Burramys* and *Cercartetus* spp.), ringtail possums (*Pseudocheirus* spp.), brushtail possums (*Trichosurus* spp.), lemuroid possum (*Hemibelideus lemuroides*), cuscuses (four genera in Australia), the threatened Leadbeater's possum (*Gymnobelideus leadbeateri*), and the distinctive, and often-noisy, striped possum (*Dactylopsila trivirgata*). Some species have broad geographical ranges beyond Australia, whereas others are endemic and confined within a single region. Leadbeater's possum, for example, is patchily distributed within a 70 × 80 km^2 area in the Victorian Central Highlands, and a small, isolated population ~50 km east of Melbourne.

Possums and gliders vary in size, diet, and spatial requirements. Smaller species tend to occupy smaller ranges compared to larger species; however, diet also has a profound influence. Species that feed on foliage tend to occupy smaller areas than those that do not. This contrast is most evident between the 1500 g, folivorous greater glider (*Petauroides volans*), which has a home range ~1–5 ha, and the 600 g exudivorous yellow-bellied glider (*Petaurus australis*) with a home range of ~50 ha. Surprisingly, the tiny pygmy possums are highly mobile. One mountain pygmy possum was recorded to have covered 500 m in 3 min (Broome 2001). In comparison, the much larger yellow-bellied glider has been recorded travelling 600 m in 20 min. The eastern pygmy possum (*C. nanus*) frequently traverses 300–500 m in a night, and the western pygmy possum (*C. concinnus*) has been tracked 4.7 km in a single night, sometimes travelling at rates that human observers struggled to match (Morrant and Petit 2012).

Possums and gliders may be herbivorous, insectivorous, nectarivorous, or omnivorous. Some species are dietary specialists that rely almost entirely on, for example, nectar and pollen (honey possum) or leaves (greater glider). The greater glider, mountain brushtail possum (*T. cunninghami*) and ringtail possums are folivores. Common brushtail possums (*T. vulpecula*) consume foliage from a range of plants but will also feed on fruit and insects (Johnson and Hemsley 2008). Striped possums may be considered insectivores because their diet mostly comprises ants, termites, crickets and the wood-boring larvae of beetles and moths (Rawlins and Handasyde 2002). The yellow-bellied glider is extreme in that at the northern and south-western ends of its range eucalypt sap comprises > 80% of its diet (Carthew *et al.* 1999), whereas in other parts of their range, eucalypt nectar, insect honeydew and manna may be relatively more important.

Possums and gliders have a range of social systems. Species like the eastern pygmy possum are solitary, and adult females raise their young alone. When the young attain a certain size the mother stops occupying the maternal nest and the young subsequently disperse. In contrast, the petaurid gliders live in family groups that may consist of an adult pair and young, in multi-female groups, and occasionally multi-male groups. One squirrel glider group that occupied a nest box in Brisbane comprised 13 separate individuals, including three breeding females (one with two pouch young and two lactating), two adult males, one subadult female, three subadult males, and four nestlings (two females and two males). Ten social groups of yellow-bellied glider on the Atherton Tableland, studied over 1 year, comprised five adult pairs, three multi-female (with one male) and two multi-male (with one female) groups (Goldingay *et al.* 2001).

One other notable aspect of social organisation in the possums and gliders is the use of vocalisations. A primary function of calling is as a territorial advertisement. Group territories are often exclusive, and trespassing animals are often repelled and in extreme cases killed. The most vocal of the possums and gliders is the yellow-bellied glider, which vocalises at a rate of 5–15 calls per hour for the first few hours after dark and at a lower rate while foraging for the rest of the night, more than any other marsupial (Goldingay 1994).

Capture and handling

Some possums are semi-terrestrial, which enables ground-based trapping techniques, including pitfall trapping for pygmy possums (e.g. Pestell and Petit 2007; Morrant and Petit 2012) and cage traps for common brushtail possums (Johnson and Hemsley 2008; Packer 2014). Cat squeeze cages can be used to restrain less-compliant species, such as brushtail possums, for example to administer an injection. However, many species remain in trees and require more-specialised capture techniques. An alternative to traps, which can reliably provide access to some species, is the deployment of artificial nest boxes (Rueegger *et al.* 2013; Goldingay *et al.* 2020). Permanent ladders (> 6 m high) can be attached to trees, to access horizontal brackets fixed to their trunks where nest boxes are fastened. This method, pioneered by Smith (1984) for capturing Leadbeater's possums, has also been employed to target trees used for sap feeding by yellow-bellied gliders (Goldingay *et al.* 2001). Smaller possum and glider species (e.g. pygmy possums and small gliders) may also be caught in cage, pipe (Winning and King 2007) or aluminium box traps mounted in trees and baited with an appropriate attractant. Mountain pygmy possums are trapped with aluminium box (Elliott) traps (Broome 2001).

Darting can be used to capture animals in trees, with nets deployed beneath the animals to break their fall when they succumb to the medication (Rawlins and Handasyde 2002). Greater gliders may be captured by firing a rifle at the branch where they sit, which forces a 'parachute' descent after which they can be captured by hand (Kehl and Borsboom 1984). Ringtail possums are often difficult to trap because they are not attracted to most bait types and do not readily enter traps. For these species, 'hook and net' techniques where the animal is shaken from the tree and caught in a net may be useful (see Chapter 7 for a discussion of the technique). Depending on study objectives, possums and gliders can be studied with spotlighting and observation, including stagwatching (Smith *et al.* 1989; see also Chapter 4).

Most species can be handled by trained personnel with minimal difficulty. For example, pygmy possums are docile and easily handled, and in some instances may be in torpor when removed from traps. However, the claws and teeth of larger possum and glider species can be sharp, and immobilisation in a cloth bag is recommended. Brushtail and ringtail possums can be held with one hand around the neck and shoulders and the other around the tail or rump.

Animals can be identified using a range of standard methods, including ear tags, microchips, ear notches or tattooing. Topical anaesthesia can be used to reduce pain during these procedures. Microchips should be implanted subcutaneously between the scapulae and in smaller species should be inserted under anaesthesia (Johnson and Hemsley 2008). Telemetry collars can be attached without anaesthesia, although some researchers choose to use anaesthetics for practical reasons or to minimise negative animal welfare impacts. Small species, such as pygmy possums, can be radio tracked by attaching VHF transmitters to their pelage using a small volume of surgical glue (Morrant and Petit 2012).

Possums and gliders should be provided with food if held in captivity for extended durations. An appropriate food should be chosen based on published literature and knowledge of the species' diet.

Veterinary considerations

Sedation and anaesthesia

As with most marsupials, intramuscular tiletamine–zolazepam is the most common approach for chemical restraint of possums (Viggers and Lindenmayer 1995). Alternatively, benzodiazepines (e.g. diazepam 0.5–1 mg/kg) or opioids (e.g. butorphanol 0.4–1 mg/kg) may be administered intramuscularly for sedation to allow minor invasive procedures or transport (Vogelnest and Portas 2019). General anaesthesia may be induced, via a facemask (see Figure 16.1a in Chapter 16), with gaseous isoflurane (5%) in oxygen and maintained at 1–2%. Larger species may be intubated with an endotracheal tube. Anaesthetic induction of smaller species may also be performed using an induction chamber (Vogelnest and Portas 2019).

Blood collection

Blood is generally collected from the lateral tail vein of anaesthetised possums (Clarke *et al.* 2013).

Euthanasia

When required, two-stage euthanasia is generally used, whereby a sedative (usually tiletamine–zolazepam) is administered intramuscularly (Vogelnest and Portas 2019), followed by an intravenous or intracardiac injection of pentobarbitone (Reilly 2001; NHMRC 2014). Larger, more-aggressive animals such as brushtail and ringtail possums, and gliders, may need to be placed in a sack or bag to permit sedation, or alternatively placed in an anaesthetic chamber (Vogelnest and Portas 2019). Any animal euthanased with pentobarbitone represents a secondary toxicity risk to wild scavengers and should be disposed of via deep burial. Intraperitoneal injection of concentrated barbiturates is generally only acceptable in an anaesthetised animal (Reilly 2001). Pygmy possums and honey possums should be euthanased using similar gaseous or chemical methods as are used for rodents. Physical euthanasia methods, which may be necessary in remote areas, are difficult to apply reliably, unless the animal can be adequately restrained (Reilly 2001).

Infectious pathogens

Possums and gliders carry a range of pathogens that pose a threat to conspecifics and other animals, including humans. Bites and scratches can be inflicted during handling of possums and gliders, although reports of associated infections are rare. Many of the diseases of possums and gliders are potential zoonoses, including leptospirosis, yersiniosis, salmonellosis and dermatophytosis (Johnson and Hemsley 2008). Two particularly significant pathogens are *Francisella tularensis* (tularaemia), which is rare in Australia, and *Mycobacterium bovis* (bovine tuberculosis), which is absent from Australia but widespread in brushtail possums in New Zealand (Johnson and Hemsley 2008). An important emerging zoonosis transmitted by brushtail and ringtail possums is Buruli ulcer, caused by *M. ulcerans*, which manifests as progressive skin ulcers in humans (Carson *et al.* 2014). The disease is mostly known as a tropical disease but has been at the centre of recent outbreaks in south-east Australia.

General operating procedures

Research methods and procedures relevant to studying possums and gliders are covered in more detail in Section 2. Suitable techniques may include direct observation (usually with spotlighting and sometimes stag-watching) (Smith *et al.* 1989), assessment of tracks and traces, scat analysis, and installation and monitoring of nest boxes (Chapter 4). Other detection methods may include acoustic monitoring, call playback, camera trapping and conservation detector dogs (Chapter 5). Trapping techniques typically include pitfall, aluminium box, cage or pipe trapping, and the 'hook and net' technique may be useful for capturing some species (Chapter 7). Marking methods may include microchipping, ear tagging, ear notching and tattooing (Chapter 8). A range of tracking methods may apply to these species (Chapter 9). Citizen science approaches may also be used (Chapter 10), and also a range of veterinary procedures (Chapter 16).

REFERENCES

Broome LS (2001) Density, home range, seasonal movements and habitat use of the mountain pygmy possum *Burramys parvus* (Marsupialia: Burramyidae) at Mount Blue Cow, Kosciuszko National Park. *Austral Ecology* **26**, 275–292. doi:10.1046/j.1442-9993.2001.01114.x

Bryant B, Reiss A (2008) Wombats. In *Current Therapy in Medicine of Australian Mammals*. (Eds L Vogelnest and R Woods) pp. 329–358. CSIRO Publishing, Melbourne

Carthew S, Goldingay R, Funnell D (1999) Feeding behaviour of the yellow-bellied glider (*Petaurus australis*) at the western edge of its range. *Wildlife Research* **26**, 199–208. doi:10.1071/WR98021

Carson C, Lavender CJ, Handasyde KA, O'Brien CR, Hewitt N, Johnson PD, Fyfe JA (2014) Potential wildlife sentinels for monitoring the endemic spread of human buruli ulcer in South-East Australia. *PLoS Neglected Tropical Diseases* **8**, e2668. doi:10.1371/journal.pntd.0002668

Clarke J, Warren K, Calver M, de Tores P, Mills J, Robertson I (2013) Hematologic and serum biochemical reference ranges and an assessment of exposure to infectious diseases prior to translocation of the threatened western ringtail possum (*Pseudocheirus occidentalis*). *Journal of Wildlife Diseases* **49**, 831–840. doi:10.7589/2011-12-345

Cremona T, Baker AM, Cooper SJB, Montague-Drake R, Stobo-Wilson AM, Carthew SM (2021) Integrative taxonomic investigation of *Petaurus breviceps* (Marsupialia: Petauridae) reveals three distinct species. *Zoological Journal of the Linnean Society* **191**, 503–527. doi:10.1093/zoolinnean/zlaa060

Death CE, Taggart DA, Williams DB, Milne R, Schultz DJ, Holyoake C, Warren KS (2011) Pharmacokinetics of moxidectin in the southern hairy-nosed wombat (*Lasiorhinus latifrons*). *Journal of Wildlife Diseases* **47**, 643–649. doi:10.7589/0090-3558-47.3.643

Descovich KA, Johnston S, Lisle A, Nicolson V, Janssen T, Brooks P, Phillips CJC (2017) Long-term measurement of body temperature in the southern hairy-nosed wombat (*Lasiorhinus latifrons*). *Australian Mammalogy* **39**, 48–55. doi:10.1071/AM15041

Evans MC, Green B, Newgrain K (2003) The field energetics and water fluxes of free-living wombats (Marsupialia: Vombatidae). *Oecologia* **137**, 171–180. doi:10.1007/s00442-003-1322-4

Finlayson G, Shimmin G, Temple-Smith PD, Handasyde K, Taggart DA (2005) Burrow use and ranging behaviour in the southern hairy-nosed wombat (*Lasiorhinus latifrons*) in the Murray Lands, South Australia. *Journal of Zoology* **265**, 189–200. doi:10.1017/S095283690400620X

Fleming PA, Anderson H, Prendergast AS, Bretz MR, Valentine LE, Hardy GES (2014) Is the loss of Australian digging mammals contributing to a deterioration in ecosystem function? *Mammal Review* **44**, 94–108. doi:10.1111/mam.12014

Goldingay RL (1994) Loud calls of the yellow-bellied glider (*Petaurus australis*)- territorial behaviour by an arboreal marsupial? *Australian Journal of Zoology* **42**, 279–293. doi:10.1071/ZO9940279

Goldingay RL, Quin D, Churchill S (2001) Spatial variability in the social organisation of the yellow-bellied glider (*Petaurus australis*) near Ravenshoe, north Queensland. *Australian Journal of Zoology* **49**, 397–409. doi:10.1071/ZO00084

Goldingay RL, Rohweder D, Taylor BD (2020) Nest box contentions: are nest boxes used by the species they target? *Ecological Management & Restoration* **21**, 115–122. doi:10.1111/emr.12408

Hing S, Hampton JO, Gibson TJ (2019) Animal welfare and the killing of wildlife by captive bolt in Australia. *Australian Zoologist* **40**, 170–180. doi:10.7882/AZ.2018.035.

Jackson S (2003) *Australian Mammals: Biology and Captive Management.* CSIRO Publishing, Melbourne.

Johnson R, Hemsley S (2008) Gliders and possums. In *Medicine of Australian Mammals.* (Eds L Vogelnest and R Woods) pp. 395–437. CSIRO Publishing, Melbourne.

Jose H, Packer JG (2020) *Technical Report: Small Mammal Mark–Recapture Trapping Protocol.* University of Adelaide, Adelaide. doi:10.13140/RG.2.2.18607.56481

Kehl J, Borsboom A (1984) Home-range, den tree use and activity patterns in the greater glider (*Petauroides volans*). In *Possums and Gliders.* (Eds AP Smith and ID Hume) pp. 229–236. Surrey Beatty and Australian Mammal Society, Sydney.

Lynch M (2008) Bandicoots and bilbies. In *Current Therapy in Medicine of Australian Mammals.* (Eds L Vogelnest and R Woods) pp. 439–464. CSIRO Publishing, Melbourne.

Matthews A (2011) Climate change influences on the distribution and resource use of common wombats *Vombatus ursinus* in the Snowy Mountains, Australia. PhD thesis. Charles Sturt University, Australia.

Moseby KE, O'Donnell E (2003) Reintroduction of the greater bilby, *Macrotis lagotis* (Reid) (Marsupialia: Thylacomyidae), to northern South Australia: survival, ecology and notes on reintroduction protocols. *Wildlife Research* **30**, 15–27. doi:10.1071/WR02012

McGregor HM, Moseby KE (2014) Improved technique for capturing the greater bilby (*Macrotis lagotis*) using burrow cage traps. *Australian Mammalogy* **36**, 259–260. doi:10.1071/AM14011

McRae P (2004) Aspects of the ecology of the greater bilby, *Macrotis lagotis*. MSc thesis. The University of Sydney, Australia.

Morrant DS, Petit S (2012) Strategies of a small nectarivorous marsupial, the western pygmy-possum, in response to seasonal variation in food availability. *Journal of Mammalogy* **93**, 1525–1535. doi:10.1644/12-MAMM-A-031.1

National Health and Medical Research Council (2014) *A Guide to the Care and use of Australian Native Mammals in Research and Teaching.* National Health and Medical Research Council, Commonwealth of Australia, Canberra.

Packer JG (2014) Invasive non-native plants retain native mammal communities in novel ecosystems. PhD thesis. The University of Adelaide, Australia.

Pestell AJL, Petit S (2007) Methods and ethical considerations of pitfall trapping for the western pygmy possum (*Cercartetus concinnus* Gould) (Marsupialia: Burramyidae), with observations on capture patterns and nest sites. *Wildlife Research* **34**, 296–305. doi:10.1071/WR06090

Rawlins DR, Handasyde KA (2002) The feeding ecology of the striped possum *Dactylopsila trivirgata* (Marsupialia: *Petauridae*) in far north Queensland, Australia. *Journal of Zoology* **257**, 195–206. doi:10.1017/S0952836902000808

Reilly JS (Ed) (2001) *Euthanasia of Animals Used for Scientific Purposes.* 2nd edn. Australian & New Zealand Council for the Care of Animals in Research and Teaching (ANZCCART), Adelaide.

Reiss A, Portas T, Horsup A (2008) Hematologic and serum biochemical reference values for free-ranging northern hairy-nosed wombats. *Journal of Wildlife Diseases* **44**, 65–70. doi:10.7589/0090-3558-44.1.65

Rueegger NN, Goldingay RL, Brookes LO (2013) Does nest box design influence use by the eastern pygmy-possum? *Australian Journal of Zoology* **60**, 372–380. doi:10.1071/ZO12117

Ruykys L, Taggart DA, Breed WG, Schultz D (2009) Sarcoptic mange in southern hairy-nosed wombats (*Lasiorhinus latifrons*): distribution and prevalence in the Murraylands of South Australia. *Australian Journal of Zoology* **57**, 129–138. doi:10.1071/ZO09010

Seebeck JH, Brown PR, Wallis RL, Kemper CM (Eds) (1990) *Bandicoots and Bilbies.* Surrey Beatty and the Australian Mammal Society, Sydney.

Smith AP (1984) Demographic consequences of reproduction, dispersal and social interaction in a population of Leadbeater's possum (*Gymnobelideus leadbeateri*). In *Possums and Gliders.* (Eds AP Smith and ID Hume) pp. 359–373. Surrey Beatty and Australian Mammal Society, Sydney.

Smith AP, Lindenmayer D, Begg RJ, Macfarlane MA, Seebeck JH, Suckling GC (1989) Evaluation of the stag-watching technique for census of possums and gliders in tall open forest. *Australian Wildlife Research* **16**, 575–580. doi:10.1071/WR9890575

Southgate RI, Christie P, Bellchambers K (2000) Breeding biology of captive, reintroduced and wild greater bilbies, *Macrotis lagotis* (Marsupialia: Peramelidae). *Wildlife Research* **27**, 621–628. doi:10.1071/WR99104

Swinbourne MJ, Taggart DA, Peacock D, Ostendorf B (2017) Historical changes in the distribution of hairy-nosed wombats (*Lasiorhinus* spp.): a review. *Australian Mammalogy* **39**, 1–16. doi:10.1071/AM15046

Taggart DA, Finlayson GR, Richings N, Shimmin G, Dibben R, Adcock J, Temple-Smith PD (2003) Environmental factors affecting the capture of southern hairy-nosed wombats (*Lasiorhinus latifrons*) by stunning. *Wildlife Research* **30**, 539–546. doi:10.1071/WR01105

Taggart DA, Finlayson GR, Sparrow E, Dibben R, Dibben J, Campbell L, Peacock D, Ostendorf B, White C, Temple-Smith PD (2020) Environmental factors influencing hairy-nosed wombat abundance in semi-arid rangelands. *The Journal of Wildlife Management* **84**, 921–929. doi:10.1002/jwmg.21858

Treby D (2005). Husbandry manual for the common wombat, *Vombatus ursinus*, northern hairy-nosed wombat, *Lasiorhinus krefftii*, and southern hairy-nosed wombat, *Lasiorhinus latifrons*. Master of Philosophy thesis. The University of Queensland, Australia.

Tyndale-Biscoe H (2005). Wombats: vegetarians of the underworld. In *Life of Marsupials.* (Ed. H Tyndale-Biscoe) pp. 269–285. CSIRO Publishing, Melbourne.

Van Dyck S, Gynther I, Baker A (2013) *Field Companion to the Mammals of Australia.* New Holland Publishers, Sydney.

Van Dyck S, Strahan R (Eds) (2008) *The Mammals of Australia.* 3rd edn. Reed New Holland, Sydney.

Vogelnest L, Portas T (2019) *Current Therapy in Medicine of Australian Mammals.* CSIRO Publishing, Melbourne.

Viggers KL, Lindenmayer DB (1995) The use of tiletamine hydrochloride and zolazepam hydrochloride for sedation of the mountain brushtail possum, *Trichosurus caninus* Ogilby (*Phalangeridae*, Marsupialia). *Australian Veterinary Journal* **72**, 215–216. doi:10.1111/j.1751-0813.1995.tb03523.x

Warburton NM, Travouillon KJ (2016) The biology and palaeontology of the Peramelemorphia: a review of current knowledge and future research directions. *Australian Journal of Zoology* **64**, 151–181. doi:10.1071/ZO16003

Winning G, King J (2007) A new trap design for capturing squirrel gliders and sugar gliders. *Australian Mammalogy* **29**, 245–249. doi:10.1071/AM07029

20 Koalas

Aditi Sriram, Derek Spielman, Kita Ashman, Desley Whisson, Lachlan Wilmott and George Madani

INTRODUCTION

The koala (*Phascolarctos cinereus*) is the sole member of the family Phascolarctidae in the order Diprotodontia. The koala is one evolutionary significant unit with no subspecies (Kjeldsen *et al.* 2016). This chapter details key characteristics of koalas and practical considerations for studying them, including a section that details clinical methods specific to koalas.

KOALA

Aditi Sriram, Kita Ashman, Desley Whisson, Lachlan Wilmott and George Madani

Characteristics

Koalas are medium-sized arboreal marsupials displaying clinal variation in size across their geographical range. Southern koalas are ~30% larger than those in the north with mean adult masses of females and males ranging from 5.1 to 6.5 kg in northern populations and 8–12 kg in the cooler south (Martin and Handasyde 1999), respectively. Sexual dimorphism is pronounced with males being up to 50% larger and heavier than females. In profile, males can be distinguished from females by their squarer head shape compared to the more-aquiline features of females. Breeding males have an obvious stained sternal gland and a pair of external testes. The flattened bare nose in males extends higher on the face than in females. Koalas have strong and muscular bodies with disproportionately long limbs, well-insulated fur and a vestigial indiscernible tail. The fore feet are forcipate (shaped like forceps) with two opposable thumbs; the hind feet are syndactylous (second and third hind digits are united) with the hallux (big toe) being opposable and clawless. All other digits have strongly recurved claws that aid gripping and climbing. Vertically slit irises and forward-facing eyes combined with fluffy ears make koalas highly appealing to the public and a popular Australian icon.

Biology and behaviour

Koalas are endemic to Australia and have a vast, but disjunct, distribution across eastern Australia, occurring in eucalypt forests and woodlands across south-eastern Australia from Cooktown in northern Queensland to in and around Adelaide in South Australia (Martin and Handasyde 1999). Koalas are more abundant at lower elevations, particularly in the foothills of the Great Dividing Range and coastal plains, but also extend into drier woodlands and associated riparian environments further west within their range (Martin and Handasyde 1999). Land clearing, infectious diseases, fire and historic hunting have reduced koala numbers severely. Australia's koala population is now fragmented with remaining subpopulations isolated or poorly connected. Reintroductions and translocations have returned them to former parts of their range, but have also resulted in poor genetic diversity and populations requiring management in parts of South Australia and western Victoria (Menkhorst 2008; Whisson and Ashman 2020).

Koalas are specialised folivores with a primary diet of eucalypt leaves. Dietary preferences vary regionally depending on available *Eucalyptus* spp. and the biochemistry, fibre, nitrogen and water content of leaves (Moore and Foley 2000). Within their home range, koalas eat several primary feed species where available, as well as secondary species. Eucalypt leaves have a high fibre content and little nutritional value and require considerable energy to digest. Consequently, koalas have a low metabolic rate that is approximately half that of other mammals and are generally inactive to conserve energy, sleeping up to 18 h per day (Ryan *et al.* 2013).

Koalas are mostly nocturnal and solitary. Mean home-range sizes vary from < 1 ha where there are highly preferred food trees to ~300 ha in poorer areas (Martin and Handasyde 1999). Koalas tend to change trees daily, often descending to the ground in the evening. Animals average nightly movements of around 200 m, but can cover up to 2.5 km in one night (Matthews *et al.* 2016). They do not build nests or use tree hollows; however, they preferentially select taller and older trees, which provide greater shade in warm weather (Crowther *et al.* 2014). Koalas derive most of their nutritional and hydration needs from leaves, but have also been observed licking water from stem flow in trees during and following rain (Mella *et al.* 2020).

Female koalas are induced ovulators, sexually reproductive from 24 months, and produce one young (very occasionally twins) per season (Martin and Handasyde 1999). Breeding occurs in spring and summer heralded by the commencement of bellowing from males combined with scent marking from their sternal glands. During this time males will increase daily movements, spending more time travelling along the ground; fights between competing dominant males can lead to fatal injuries. Gestation lasts between 34 and 36 days with lactating young remaining in the pouch for the first 6 months of its life (Martin and Handasyde 1999). From 6 months onwards the pouch young begins to climb out of the pouch intermittently and clamber around the mother's body; by 9 months of age, it leaves the pouch permanently and will ride on the mother's back. Young are generally weaned at around 12 months of age. Wild koalas have been recorded living up to 18 years, although 12 years is more typical. Females tend to live longer than males who succumb to misadventure more often because of increased movement and fighting associated with breeding (Martin and Handasyde 1999).

Capture and handling

Specialised capture techniques developed for koala capture include flagging (Radford *et al.* 2006) (Figure 20.1),

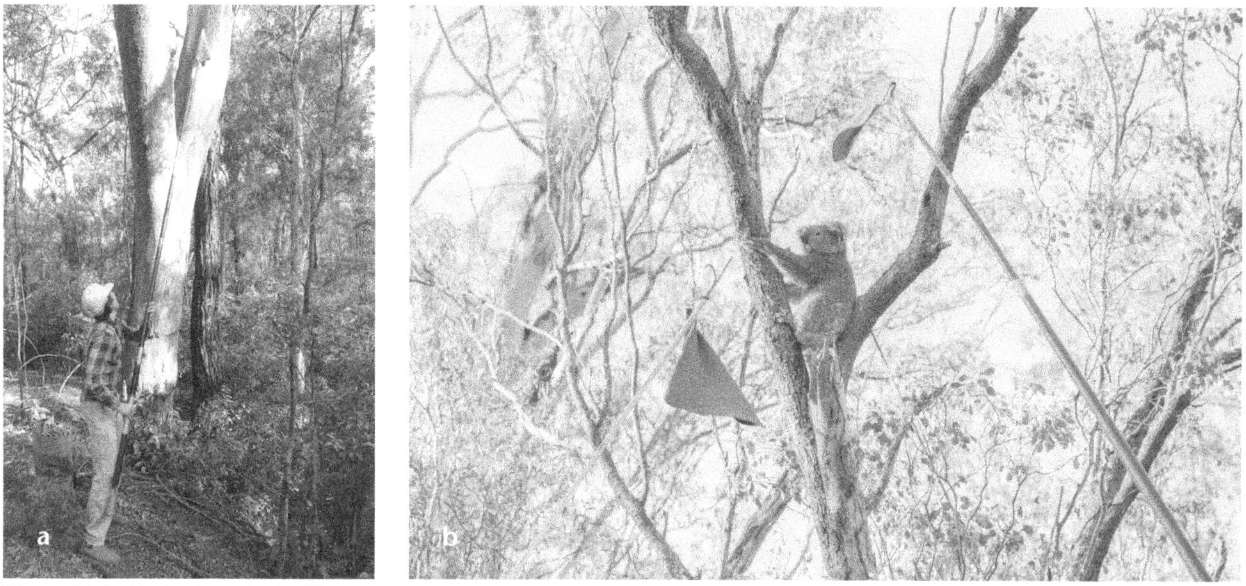

Figure 20.1: Methods for koala (*Phascolarctos cinereus*) capture: (a) An extendable pole with a cloth flag attached operated by personnel on the ground. Photo by Aditi Sriram. (b) Flagging method where flags attached to extendable poles are used to direct the koala's descent. Photo by George Madani.

safety line (noose) and flag (Madani *et al.* 2020), darting (Lynch and Martin 2003) and koala traps (Phillips 2011; Ashman and Whisson 2020). An assessment of the capture site (topography, vegetation and canopy structure) will determine the feasibility, safety and animal welfare risks of any capture method. Active capture methods (flagging, safety line and flag, darting) and passive capture methods (koala trap) vary in their advantages and limitations. Availability of equipment, personnel experience and research purpose (frequency of capture, likelihood of euthanasia) should be considered when developing a plan for koala captures. Darting is used uncommonly and won't be described further.

Flagging is an active method of koala capture where a 'flag' (piece of fabric or plastic) connected to an extendable pole is waved above the koala's head. The poles are operated by personnel on the ground if the koala is within reach or by a tree climber. The koala perceives the flags as a threat and descends the tree. When the koala is within range of a catcher, it can be manipulated gently into a catch bag. The height and complexity of the tree and terrain are limitations to flagging. Flagging koalas in tall, dense vegetation may increase the likelihood of a fall if the koala attempts to escape by jumping between branches (Radford *et al.* 2006). In this environment, experienced personnel should be able to read the animal's behaviour/intent and avoid prolonged capture attempts of animals that appear highly stressed, injured or unwell. In areas where koalas are habituated to human presence or capture, flagging may be unsuccessful as the koalas can become familiar with and less responsive to the flag.

A minimum of two people is required for capture when using the noose and flag technique: a tree climber, if the koala cannot be reached with an extendable pole from the ground, and the ground-based catcher who assists with flagging, holding the safety line and bagging the koala. The safety line (noose) and flag technique require the use of one or two long (≥ 5 m), extendable, aluminium or fibreglass poles. A rope noose with a stopper knot is attached to the end of the pole and placed over the koala's head and around its neck. The noose is fitted with a stopper knot so it only tightens to the approximate circumference of the koala's neck. The safety line is manipulated by the catcher and prevents the koala from ascending the tree or moving away from the catcher. It is not used to pull the koala down the tree. The koala is then coaxed down the tree by waving a flag above its head. The catchers must ensure the safety line does not become entangled during the process; it may be necessary to disentangle the line several times during capture. Once in reach, the koala can be placed in a catch bag in the tree and lowered to the ground or flagged down to the ground and captured in a catch bag. See Madani *et al.* (2020) for a detailed description of the methodology. Reports of capture-related injuries in koalas are few. In a review of the use of the safety line (noose) and flag method, minor adverse events were reported in < 1% of captures (Madani *et al.* 2020).

Trapping is a passive method of koala capture where a temporary fence, with a single point of exit into a cage trap, is constructed around the base of the tree. The fence is constructed using a series of Corflute® panels of at least 900 mm in height, joined side by side with duct tape or cable ties. The fence should be placed at least 2 m from the base of the tree and include a single panel with an opening through which the cage trap entrance can be attached. A large collapsible, treadle-based cage trap (128 × 42 × 42 cm) is recommended as it allows the trap to be opened at either end to remove the koala from the trap. The top and sides of the trap should be covered with cloth or Corflute® panels to provide protection from inclement weather.

Once the trap is set, a motion-sensing camera may be deployed on the tree facing the trap entrance. Trap trigger devices such as X-trail cameras (model X-Trail 4GR 12MP HD Cellular Trail Camera) have an inbuilt cell booster that enables multimedia messaging of images from the motion-sensing camera to mobile phone devices for immediate alerts when the camera is triggered by a koala entering the trap. Such devices reduce welfare impacts of trapping as well as improving cost efficiency by reducing the frequency of trap checks. If a trap trigger device is not deployed, traps should be checked at 2 h intervals and should not be deployed in extreme weather (heat or rain). Once a koala has entered the trap, one end of the trap may be opened, and a noose rope can be placed over the koala's head and around its neck. The catcher (with the noose rope in hand) should then stand behind the open trap and allow the koala to walk out of the trap. The koala may then be placed in a catch bag for processing. Dense vegetation and overlapping canopies restrict the use of traps as koalas may move between trees rather than descend the tree into the trap. Passive methods of capture, such as koala traps, are considered safer. Minor injuries, such as abrasions from contact with the trap, are infrequent (Ashman and Whisson 2020).

Table 20.1: General equipment requirements for the capture of koalas.

Flagging	Safety line and flag	Koala traps
• Extendable poles; height dependent on height of tree. • Flags attachable to extendable poles. • Calico or canvas capture bags (diameter 45–60 cm and depth 60–90 cm). • Specialist climbing gear to ascend trees for captures that cannot be achieved from the ground.	• Two extendable poles with a hook and point attachment (extendable to a least 5 m). • Flags attachable to extendable poles. • Rope (safety line) with loop and stopper knot to create a noose. The safety line must be soft and long enough to ensure that the ground-based catcher has enough length to reach twice the height of the koala in the tree in case the animal falls and needs to be lowered quickly to the ground. • Calico or canvas capture bags (diameter 45–60 cm and depth 60–90 cm). • Specialist climbing gear to ascend trees for captures that cannot be achieved from the ground.	• Trap wall (e.g. Corflute® panels), at least 900 mm high. • Duct tape or cable ties to secure trap wall panels. • Koala cage trap. • Cloth or cover to place over the top of the trap.

Equipment required varies with the method of capture. Equipment for tree climbing is specialised and personnel-specific. A first aid kit and personal protective equipment specific to each capture method should be included in the field kit. General equipment requirements are detailed in Table 20.1

Koalas should be handled by experienced personnel (or under their direct supervision) and handling times minimised. Koalas have strong, recurved claws that must be disengaged carefully from the tree during handling. Large canvas or calico bags are ideal for capturing and handling koalas (DPIE 2020). When removing koalas from a tree, the catch bag is worked under the rump and above the head. The claws should be carefully disengaged from the tree and the koala placed in the catch bag (Figure 20.2). Once in the bag, the koala can be weighed, restrained within the bag for examination or transported short distances.

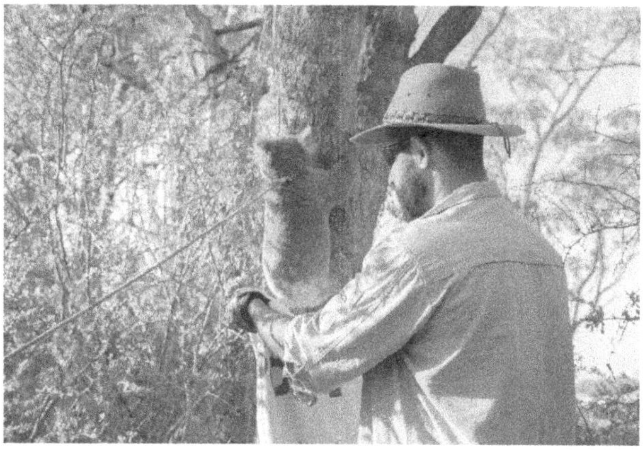

Figure 20.2: Koala (*Phascolarctos cinereus*) descending a tree following its capture by safety line (noose) and flag method. The koala can be gently manipulated into the catch bag by placing the bag under the rump and working it over the head of the koala. Photo by George Madani.

Koalas generally remain calm if restrained properly. Koalas can be restrained in a sitting position, facing away from the handler, with their body supported on the handler's lap or on the ground. The right wrist and ankle are held together in one hand and the left wrist and ankle in the other. Keeping the head covered with the catch bag or a towel will help calm the koala. Alternatively, koalas can be restrained and examined within the catch bag with their head, arms or legs exposed out of the bag as required. Koalas should not be lifted or held around the chest as they tend to panic when their paws are unrestrained and they are unable to grip anything (Blanshard and Bodley 2008); it also leaves the handler vulnerable to bites and scratches.

Koalas can be transported short distances in a catch bag ensuring they are supported during transportation (i.e. on a person's lap) (DPIE 2020). Well-ventilated, purpose-built wooden crates or transport boxes are ideal for longer-distance transport. A rolled-up towel can be provided for the koalas to latch on to during transportation (DPIE 2020). Ambient temperature should be monitored during transportation to prevent hypo- or hyperthermia.

While reports of obvious injury are rare, the risk of injury to the koala can be minimised by ensuring that capture duration is kept short and personnel are experienced in the selected capture method. Koalas have a low metabolic rate and limited energy reserves. Consequently, it is important to ensure that stress and energy expenditure are minimised during captures (Madani *et al.* 2020). During capture, personnel should aim to minimise noise, and limit people and vehicular traffic to avoid disturbance. As with all wildlife species, some stress to captured animals is unavoidable (Narayan *et al.* 2013). However, knowledge of and experience with koala captures will allow personnel to modify or abort captures in response to koala behaviour. Koalas may display various signs of stress during capture including:

- vocalisation
- urination/defaecation
- increased respiratory rate
- ear flicking
- clawing at or thrashing within the trap
- panting or open mouth breathing.

Panting or open-mouth breathing is a sign of severe stress in koalas and a consistent indicator that capture attempts should be aborted (Radford *et al.* 2006). Little is known about capture-related stress and its effects on koala physiology. Radford *et al.* (2006) reported that most captured animals displayed transient signs of stress (as listed above); however, no indications of clinical compromise were observed on examination post-capture. McDonald *et al.* (1990) found no evidence of a marked short-term adrenocortical response to the stress of capture in most wild koalas, but Narayan *et al.* (2013) found that handled koalas had 200% higher faecal cortisol metabolite levels than their non-handled counterparts. While studies that have monitored koalas following capture have not suggested any short-term detrimental effects of capture, no study has evaluated the direct or long-term effects of capture and associated stress in koalas. Any animals showing abnormal behaviour during capture or upon release (panting, lethargy or abnormal gait) should be monitored and if necessary, recaptured for further assessment.

In ambient temperatures > 30°C, prolonged capture attempts should be avoided because of the risk of hyperthermia. Koalas have insulating (thick) fur and a limited ability to shed heat (Hanger and Gillett 2019). Koalas experiencing heat stress may display signs such as panting, salivating on wrists and/or progressive lethargy. Captured koalas displaying these signs should be cooled by applying cold water to the feet, the ears and the inguinal region and released as soon as possible (Hanger and Gillett 2019). Capture during heavy or persistent rainfall should also be avoided as handling koalas in wet conditions can disrupt the insulating properties of their fur increasing the risk of hypothermia (NHMRC 2014).

Females with back young have been captured successfully with active and passive capture techniques (Hanger and Gillett 2019; Ashman and Whisson 2020; Madani *et al.* 2020). The small back young usually remains on the mother during capture. Older young may leave the mother voluntarily and remain in the tree during or before capture (DPIE 2020). Elongated teats noted during pouch checks of a female indicate the koala has dependent young. Trees nearby should be searched for the young, which must be monitored closely. The young and mother should be reunited as soon as possible (Hanger and Gillett 2019).

When capturing multiple animals, biosecurity should be another important consideration to avoid the transmission of parasites and pathogens (Wildlife Health Australia 2018; DPIE 2020). Equipment must be cleaned of organic matter and disinfected with 60–70% alcohol or a glutaraldehyde- or chloramine-based disinfectant, before use between animals. Catch bags should be cleaned, then washed in hot water and detergent and dried thoroughly between capture sites. Personnel should implement good hygiene practices, including using gloves and/or thorough hand washing before and after handling koalas (DPIE 2020).

Microchips and ear tags are permanent methods of identification and are used widely in koala management and monitoring. Microchips should be inserted subcutaneously between the shoulder blades. Ear tags are colour coded and individually numbered. Numbered sheep ears tags are appropriate and can be applied using a compatible applicator (DPIE 2020). Ear tags are applied midway along the circumference of the ear. The fur may be clipped and tag site cleaned then disinfected before application. Prominent blood vessels, visible following clipping, should be avoided (see Chapter 8). Where a tissue biopsy sample is required, a biopsy punch can be used to collect tissue from the ear, while also creating a tag ring for placement of an ear tag.

Telemetry devices attached to collars, anklets and ear tags are used to monitor koalas. Rubbing, strangulation and constriction injuries have been reported with the use of collars and anklets, resulting from poor application or design of the devices. Koalas with devices should be monitored frequently and regularly to enable intervention to remove problematic devices and provide treatment when required (see Chapter 9).

Veterinary considerations

While reported incidents of injuries in koalas from capture are few (Ashman and Whisson 2020; Madani *et al.*

2020), capture poses animal welfare risks. Koalas injured during capture should be assessed by experienced personnel to determine if veterinary intervention is required. Veterinary assessment is recommended for koalas found with substantial injuries (e.g. bone fractures), illness (e.g. severe clinical chlamydial disease) or an atypical body condition score (i.e. if lower relative to other koalas in the area). At release, if the koala appears unsteady, has difficulty climbing or displays unusual behaviours, the animal should be monitored and recaptured for further assessment if necessary. Refer to details under 'Collection of biological samples' later in this chapter for more information.

Euthanasia

The recommended method of euthanasia in koalas is via overdose of barbiturates administered intravenously. Extravasation of barbiturates causes irritation and pain (NHMRC 2014). Therefore, where possible, the animal should be sedated (see the next sub-chapter, 'Collection of biological samples') or anaesthetised before euthanasia to improve venous access and reduce stress associated with restraint. Captive bolts have also been used for koala euthanasia, and avoid all of the difficulties associated with access to scheduled veterinary chemicals, injection routes and secondary toxicity risks (Hing *et al.* 2019). In remote locations or where personnel do not have the appropriate qualifications to administer drugs, a shot to the brain with a firearm can be employed as a method of euthanasia (although it precludes a thorough necropsy and histopathological investigation). Licensing requirements should be consulted before using firearms. Any animal euthanased with pentobarbitone represents a secondary toxicity risk to wild scavengers and should be disposed of via deep burial.

Infectious pathogens

As with many wildlife species, koalas can carry zoonotic agents, but this risk is relatively low and few cases of disease transmission between koalas and humans have been reported (Blanshard and Bodley 2008). *Sarcoptes scabei*, the mite causing sarcoptic mange, can be found in free-ranging koalas, can cause self-limiting disease in humans (Blanshard and Bodley 2008; Speight *et al.* 2017). The risk of transmission can be reduced by the use of appropriate hygiene and personal protective equipment.

Chlamydia and koala retrovirus (KoRV) are two major pathogens affecting koalas. *Chlamydia pecorum* is implicated as the primary cause of chlamydial disease in koalas and is a major challenge to clinical and population management (Quigley and Timms 2020). Regional differences in the strain, prevalence and manifestation of disease caused by chlamydia should be considered when working across various populations and is particularly relevant to translocations (Quigley and Timms 2020). Koala retrovirus refers to a group of viruses specific to koalas. KoRV is associated with cancers and immunosuppressive disorders in koalas, although a definite causative relationship has not been established (Quigley and Timms 2020). Prevalence and disease vary with the different subtypes of KoRV and research into understanding disease mechanisms and its complex epidemiology continue.

General operating procedures

Other research methods and procedures relevant to studying koalas are detailed elsewhere in this book, including observation, assessment of scats and traces (Chapter 4), camera traps and acoustic recorders (Chapter 5), aerial surveys (Chapter 6), microchipping and ear tagging (Chapter 8), tracking methods (Chapter 9), citizen science approaches (Chapter 10), and several other veterinary procedures (Chapter 16).

COLLECTION OF BIOLOGICAL SAMPLES

Derek Spielman and Aditi Sriram

Context and scope

This general operating procedure (GOP) provides guidelines for the collection of diagnostic samples in koalas, including chemical immobilisation techniques to facilitate sample collection. Collection of biological samples and clinical data should be considered during koala captures to maximise the benefit and information gained during captures. As capture, sedation and sampling are invasive and pose risks for koalas, they should only be conducted by trained and experienced personnel. Sedatives/anaesthetics for koalas must be administered by or under the supervision of a registered veterinarian. Anaesthetic agents vary in their duration of action, depth of anaesthesia and mode of delivery (see Chapter 16). Alfaxalone (1–3 mg/kg delivered intravenously) is recommended for use in the field as it provides a reliable and smooth induction and recovery. Gaseous anaesthetic agents, such as isoflurane combined with oxygen, are commonly used as they allow for titration of anaesthetic

Table 20.2: Body condition scoring procedures for koalas.

Koala Health Hub (2019); adapted from Jackson (2003).

Description	Definition	Score
Strong muscle tone. Spine of scapula is palpable on careful palpation. Convex muscle mass on either side of scapula.	Excellent	5
Good muscle tone. Slightly convex muscles on either side of scapula. Spine of scapula easily palpable.	Good	4
Flat to slightly convex muscles on either side of scapula. Spine of scapula prominent on palpation.	Fair	3
Slightly dishing or concave muscle on either side of scapula. Spine of scapula very obvious on palpation. Edges of scapula bone palpable.	Poor	2
Noticeable dishing of muscles on either side of scapula. At times almost no muscles palpable on either side of scapula.	Emaciated	1

depth and duration, and quicker recoveries (Hanger and Gillett 2019). Koalas should be monitored closely during induction and recovery and only released once determined to be fully conscious and ambulatory.

Animal welfare considerations

Risks associated with anaesthesia

Animal welfare considerations relating to the capture of koalas are outlined earlier in this chapter. An important consideration during anaesthesia of koalas is the animal's health status and potential predisposing conditions, which may increase anaesthetic-associated risk (Chapter 16). Koalas with signs of disease, poor body condition (Table 20.2), injury or other clinical signs are not ideal candidates for sedation or anaesthesia. Where possible, animals should be individually assessed, and health status and anaesthetic risk considered beforehand. Induction and recovery from anaesthesia must be monitored closely. A recovery protocol and necessary equipment must be available to respond to complications (DPIE 2020).

General procedures

Use of sedation/anaesthesia in koalas

Chemical restraint is commonly used to facilitate sample collection in koalas (Table 20.3). It reduces the stress associated with handling and restraint (see Chapter 16). Various drug regimens can be used for sedation and anaesthesia in koalas; the choice of drugs varies depending on duration and depth of immobilisation and health status of the animal. Sedation or anaesthesia must be delivered by, or under the supervision of, a veterinarian, depending on state or territory legislation regarding acts of veterinary medicine. Koalas should be monitored closely during induction and recovery and only released once determined to be fully conscious and ambulatory (DPIE 2020).

Table 20.3: Common injectable agents for sedating and anaesthetising koalas.

Koala Health Hub (2019); adapted from Vogelnest and Woods (2008) and Gillett (2015). IM = intramuscular; IV = intravenous.

Drug	Dosage and route
Diazepam	0.5–1.0 mg/kg IM
Midazolam	0.2–0.5 mg/kg IM
Alfaxalone	1.0–3.0 mg/kg IM or 0.5–1.5 mg/kg IV
Tiletamine–zolazepam	5–10 mg/kg IM
Tiletamine–zolazepam and medetomidine	3.5 mg/kg + 0.05 mg/kg IM
Isoflurane or sevoflurane in oxygen	Variable, delivered via mask or through intubation

In healthy, free-ranging koalas, chemical restraint will be required for the following procedures:

- *Body temperature*: to record rectal temperature in koalas; a thermometer is inserted into the rectum via the cloaca. A koala's normal rectal temperature ranges from 35.5 to 36.5°C.
- *Oral examination*: sedation allows for a thorough oral examination in koalas while ensuring personnel safety. Personnel examine the oral cavity for teeth wear, signs of periodontal disease and the buccal cavity for food impaction. Tooth wear can also be used as an indicator of relative age in koalas (Blanshard and Bodley 2008).
- *Pouch check*: the pouch can be checked for the presence of a joey, lactation stage (recently weaned or lost joey) and pouch condition (dirty or clean).

- *Lymph nodes*: palpation of the inguinal, axillary and submandibular lymph nodes. Enlarged lymph nodes are indicative of underlying disease processes and may require further investigation.
- *Sample collection*: samples collected to assess general health (blood samples), samples for disease investigation (chlamydia, KoRVA) and genetic sampling require invasive techniques. Chemical immobilisation is recommended to ensure diagnostically valuable samples are collected, with minimal stress to the koala.

Where sedation is not possible (i.e. precluded by recovery time, animal health status or insufficient expertise), invasive sampling will be precluded, but observational data can be collected.

Biological sampling in koalas

Diagnostic sampling in koalas includes and is not limited to:

- conjunctival, nasal, oropharyngeal, urogenital and penile swabs for chlamydia, herpesvirus and KoRVA diagnosis
- blood or tissue samples for genetic testing
- blood samples for general health assessment (biochemistry, haematology, serology).

Table 20.4 lists key diagnostic tests and methods. Swabs used for diagnostic sampling must be sterile, dry and small. The swabs must be firmly rubbed against the target tissue to ensure adequate cellular material is collected on the swabs. However, care must be taken to minimise trauma to the tissues as it can result in substantial discomfort. Detailed protocols, data collection sheets and descriptions on technique and sample processing can be found at www.koalahealthhub.org.au/sampling-protocols/. It is important to ensure samples collected are labelled clearly and include the sample type, collection date and individual animal identification.

Animal treatment, withdrawal and euthanasia

Refer to 'Veterinary considerations' earlier in this chapter.

Equipment and maintenance

Sedation and anaesthesia require the use of veterinary equipment and will vary with procedures to be performed and method (refer to Chapter 16). Equipment required for diagnostic sampling include disposable gloves, and sterile small (~2 mm diameter tip), aluminium- or plastic-shafted, rayon-tipped swabs. Swabs with liquid or gel transport media should not be used as these contain substances that interfere with the diagnostic test.

Specific qualifications, experience and training

Sedation and anaesthesia should only be performed by or under the direct supervision of a veterinarian. Biological

Table 20.4: Key diagnostic tests and summarised methods for koalas.

Diagnostic test	Considerations
Conjunctival swab	The koala's eyelids are lifted (Figure 20.3a), and the swab rubbed against the conjunctival fornix and the inner surface of the upper and lower eyelid (Figure 20.3b). Ensure that the swab does not rub against the globe.
Rectal swab	The cloaca is everted with gentle pressure, the rectal opening identified and the swab inserted ~2–5 cm into the rectum.
Female urogenital sinus	This procedure requires sedation and should only be performed by experienced personnel. Female koalas have a single opening for both their digestive and reproductive tracts (the common vestibule – sometimes called a cloaca). The vagina must be located and the swab inserted carefully into the vaginal passage. Check the swab as it is pulled out to ensure it has no faecal matter on it. Faecal matter indicates that the rectum was probably swabbed erroneously and the procedure should be repeated with a new swab.
Penile urethra	This procedure requires sedation and should only be performed by experienced personnel. The penis can be extruded by applying pressure on either side of the cloaca. Once extruded the swab can be inserted 1–2 cm into the penile urethra (Figure 20.4).
Genetic sampling	Ocular and urogenital swabs collected for disease testing are not ideal for genetic analysis. For genetic sampling, use EDTA blood, or tissue punched from ear-tag placement. The Australian Museum has been nominated as a repository of koala genetic material. If research includes genetic analysis, one sample should be retained by the project and one sent to the Australian Museum. Instructions on the collection and submission of genetic samples to the Australian Museum can be found in the Code of Practice for Injured, Sick and Orphaned Koalas (OEH 2018).

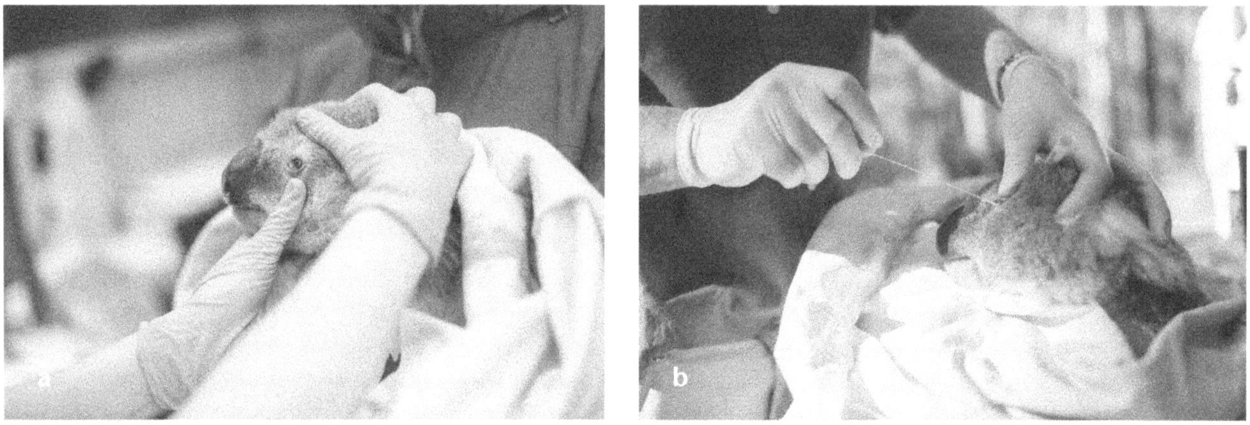

Figure 20.3: (a) Ocular examination in a sedated koala (*Phascolarctos cinereus*). (b) Collecting a conjunctival swab sample from a sedated koala. Photos by Lachlan Wilmott.

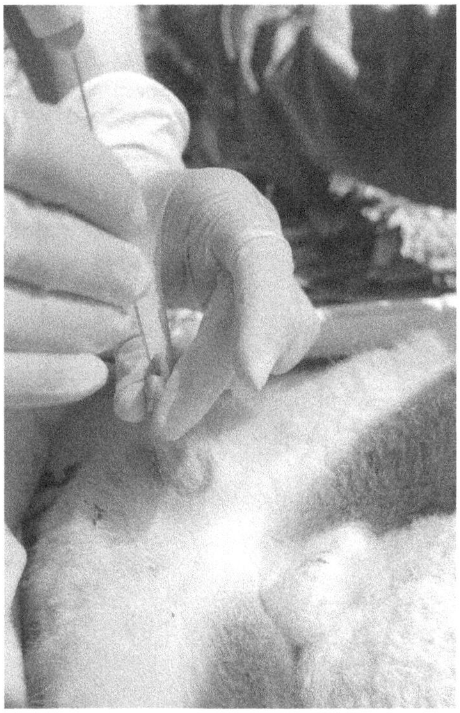

Figure 20.4: Penile urethral swab collection in a sedated male koala (*Phascolarctos cinereus*). Photo by Aditi Sriram.

sampling of koalas requires knowledge of anatomy and techniques, and should be performed by personnel trained for the task.

Workplace health and safety

Hazards when capturing and handling koalas are detailed in earlier sections of this chapter Work health and safety considerations specific to sedation, anaesthesia and sample collection in koalas also include needle-stick injuries and zoonotic diseases. Personnel should use disposable gloves when examining an anaesthetised animal and employ hygiene procedures.

Alternative procedures

No alternative methods are available to collect biological samples from koalas for health screening purpose.

ACKNOWLEDGEMENTS

The authors and editors are grateful to Dr Damien Higgins from the Koala Health Hub for providing access to their resources and for reviewing the chapter.

REFERENCES

Ashman KR, Whisson DA (2020) Developing guidelines for the use of traps to capture koalas. *Australian Mammalogy* **42**, 380–384. doi:10.1071/AM20018

Blanshard W, Bodley K (2008) Koalas. In *Medicine of Australian Mammals*. (Eds L Vogelnest and R Woods) pp. 227–327. CSIRO Publishing, Melbourne.

Crowther MS, Lunney D, Lemon J, Stalenberg E, Wheeler R, Madani G, Ross KA, Ellis M (2014) Climate-mediated habitat selection in an arboreal folivore. *Ecography* **37**, 336–343. doi:10.1111/j.1600-0587.2013.00413.x

DPIE (2020) *Best Practice Guidelines for the Use of Koalas in Scientific Research*. Department of Planning, Industry and Environment, Sydney.

Gillett A (2015) Koala triage, trauma and trauma care. Proceedings of the 4th AVA/NZVA Pan Pacific Conference, Brisbane.

Hanger J, Gillett A (2019) Veterinary involvement in the research and management of free-ranging koala populations. In *Current Therapy in Medicine of Australian Mammals*. (Eds L Vogelnest and T Portas) pp. 507–514. CSIRO Publishing, Melbourne.

Hing S, Hampton JO, Gibson TJ (2019) Animal welfare and the killing of wildlife by captive bolt in Australia. *Australian Zoologist* **40**, 170–180. doi:10.7882/AZ.2018.035

Jackson S (2007) *Australian Mammals: Biology and Captive Management.* CSIRO Publishing, Melbourne.

Kjeldsen SR, Zenger KR, Leigh K, Ellis W, Tobey J, Phalen D, Melzer A, Fitzgibbon S, Raadsma HW (2016) Genome-wide SNP loci reveal novel insights into koala (*Phascolarctos cinereus*) population variability across its range. *Conservation Genetics* **17**, 337–353. doi:10.1007/s10592-015-0784-3

Koala Health Hub (2019) Koala Health Hub. Sydney School of Veterinary Science, Faculty of Science, University of Sydney, Sydney. <http://koalahealthhub.org.au>.

Lynch M, Martin R (2003) Capture of koalas (*Phascolarctos cinereus*) by remote injection of tiletamine-zolazapam (Zoletil®) and medetomidine. *Wildlife Research* **30**, 255–258. doi:10.1071/WR02022

Madani G, Ashman K, Mella V, Whisson D (2020) A review of the 'noose and flag' method to capture free ranging koalas. *Australian Mammalogy* **42**, 341–348. doi:10.1071/AM19064

Martin R, Handasyde K (1999) *The Koala: Natural History, Conservation, Management.* 2nd edn. UNSW Press, Krieger Publishing Corporation, Malabar, FL.

Matthews A, Lunney D, Gresser S, Maitz W (2016) Movement patterns of koalas in remnant forest after fire. *Australian Mammalogy* **38**, 91–104. doi:10.1071/AM14010

McDonald IR, Than KA, Handasyde KA, Michaelides J (1990) Factors affecting plasma adrenocortical hormone concentrations of koalas. In *Biology of the Koala.* (Eds AK Lee, KA Handasyde and GD Sanson) pp. 289–294. Surrey Beatty, Sydney.

Mella V, Orr C, Hall L, Velasco S, Madani G (2020) First insight into natural koala drinking behaviour. *Ethology* **126**, 858–863. doi:10.1111/eth.13032

Menkhorst P (2008) Hunted, marooned, re-introduced, contracepted: a history of koala management in Victoria. *In Too Close for Comfort: Contentious Issues in Human-Wildlife Encounters.* (Eds D Lunney, A Munn and W Meikle) pp. 73–92. Royal Zoological Society of NSW, Mosman.

Moore B, Foley W (2000) A review of feeding and diet selection in koalas (*Phascolarctos cinereus*). *Australian Journal of Zoology* **48**, 317–333. doi:10.1071/ZO99034

Narayan EJ, Webster K, Nicolson V, Mucci A, Hero JM (2013) Non-invasive evaluation of physiological stress in an iconic Australian marsupial: the koala (*Phascolarctos cinereus*). *General and Comparative Endocrinology* **187**, 39–47. doi:10.1016/j.ygcen.2013.03.021

NHMRC (2014) *A Guide to the Care and Use of Australian Native Mammals in Research And Teaching.* National Health and Medical Research Council, Canberra.

Office of Environment and Heritage (OEH) (2018) *Code of Practice for Injured, Sick and Orphaned Koalas.* NSW Office of Environment and Heritage, Sydney.

Phillips S (2011) Development of a lightweight, portable trap for capturing free-ranging koalas *Phascolarctos cinereus. Australian Zoologist* **35**, 747–749. doi:10.7882/AZ.2011.025

Quigley B, Timms P (2020) Helping koalas battle disease – recent advances in Chlamydia and koala retrovirus (KoRV) disease understanding and treatment in koalas. *FEMS Microbiology Reviews* **44**, 583–605. doi:10.1093/femsre/fuaa024

Radford SL, McKee JEFF, Goldingay RL, Kavanagh RP (2006) The protocols for koala research using radio-collars: a review based on its application in a tall coastal forest in New South Wales and the implications for future research. *Australian Mammalogy* **28**, 187–200. doi:10.1071/AM06027

Ryan MA, Whisson DA, Holland GJ, Arnould JPY (2013) Activity patterns of free-ranging koalas (*Phascolarctos cinereus*) revealed by accelerometry. *PLoS One* **8**, e80366. doi:10.1371/journal.pone.0080366

Speight KN, Whiteley PL, Woolford L, Duignan PJ, Bacci B, Lathe S, Boardman W, Scheelings TF, Funnell O, Underwood G, Stevenson MA (2017) Outbreaks of sarcoptic mange in free-ranging koala populations in Victoria and South Australia: a case series. *Australian Veterinary Journal* **95**, 244–249. doi:10.1111/avj.12598

Vogelnest L, Woods R (Eds) (2008) *Medicine of Australian Mammals.* CSIRO Publishing, Melbourne.

Whisson DA, Ashman KR (2020) When an iconic native animal is overabundant: the koala in southern Australia. *Conservation Science and Practice* **2**, e188. doi:10.1111/csp2.188

Wildlife Health Australia (2018) National Wildlife Biosecurity Guidelines (version 1.0). Sydney, NSW. <https://wildlifehealthAustralia.com.au/Portals/0/Documents/ProgramProjects/National_Wildlife_Biosecurity_Guidelines.PDF>.

21 Macropods

Graeme Coulson, Clare Death, Euan Ritchie and Karl Vernes

INTRODUCTION

Macropods comprise the diprotodont marsupial suborder Macropodiformes. Three extant families are represented: the monospecific Hypsiprymnodontidae (musky rat-kangaroo), Potoroidae (eight species of potoroos and bettongs) and Macropodidae (43 species of wallabies and kangaroos). The Macropodidae comprises two subfamilies: the monospecific Lagostrophinae (banded hare wallaby) and the Macropodinae, which encompasses all other species (Eldridge and Coulson 2015; Eldridge and Frankham 2015).

KANGAROOS, WALLABIES AND POTOROIDS

Characteristics

Almost all macropods hop. The sole exception is the musky rat-kangaroo (*Hypsiprymnodon moschatus*), which moves with a quadrupedal bound. Tree-kangaroos also hop, but can walk bipedally when required. The body form of macropods reflects their unusual bipedal hopping gait: hind limbs are longer and stronger than fore limbs, and the pelvic region is much more robust than the thorax, giving macropods a low centre of gravity and a flexible upper body. The tree kangaroos (*Dendrolagus* spp.) are the exception, having well-developed fore limbs of similar length to their hind limbs. In all species, the fourth toe is the most elongated and is armed with a strong claw; the second and third digits are small and syndactylous, used for grooming. Only the musky rat-kangaroo has retained the first toe. Tree kangaroos and rock-wallabies (*Petrogale* spp.) have broad foot pads, with strong, sharp claws in tree kangaroos but greatly reduced claws in rock-wallabies. In all species, the digits of the fore paws are relatively small and similar in size, each with a sharp claw. The tail is narrow and prehensile in the Hypsiprymnodontidae and Potoroidae. Although unable to grip, the tail is elongated in the banded hare wallaby and most macropodines, and is particularly long in tree kangaroos and rock-wallabies. The tail is quite muscular in the largest species.

Relative morphological proportions vary across taxa depending on the degree of sexual dimorphism. The Hypsiprymnodontidae, Potoroidae and Lagostrophinae are sexually monomorphic, so both sexes have dainty fore limbs and large hind limbs. In contrast, most macropodine species have indeterminate growth, continuing to grow through their lives. Macropod males grow faster than females, so most species are sexually dimorphic; the larger species have a greater degree of dimorphism and are the most dimorphic of all terrestrial mammals. Males of the largest species, the red kangaroo (*Osphranter rufus*) can weigh more than 90 kg whereas females are less than 40 kg. Males of the larger species also show pronounced development of the fore limbs and pectoral girdle, reflecting the role of fore limbs as weapons in male–male combat. A few species, such as the red kangaroo, antilopine wallaroo (*Osphranter antilopinus*) and euro (*O. robustus*), have colour dimorphism as well (Eldridge and Coulson 2015).

Macropods have a relatively long head with a tapered muzzle, which is shortened in some taxa such as bettongs (*Aepyprymnus* and *Bettongia* spp.), hare wallabies (*Lagorchestes* spp.) tree kangaroos and the quokka (*Setonix*). All macropods are diprotodonts, having one large pair of procumbent incisors in the lower jaw opposing the incisor arcade in the upper jaw. Only the Hypsiprymnodontidae and Potoroidae have functional canine teeth; tree kangaroos and some hare-wallabies have vestigial upper canines. The Lagostrophinae and Macropodinae have a long diastema between the incisor arcade and the molar row at the rear of the jaw. The larger species have molar progression in the upper and lower jaws, such that molars erupt sequentially at the back of the jaw and progressively drift forward into occlusion, where they become worn and are eventually shed, being replaced by the next molar in the row. Most species have a maximum of four (sometimes five) molars in each quadrant of the jaw, but the nabarlek (*Petrogale concinna*) has an unlimited number in its lifetime.

Biology and behaviour

Macropods occur throughout Australia. Multiple species may be present in the same locality but exhibit differences in terms of body size, habitat, activity and sociality (Kaufmann 1974). The smallest species, including the Potoroidae and many small macropodines, such as the spectacled hare wallaby (*Lagorchestes conspicillatus*), are strictly nocturnal, occupy dense habitat, and are solitary and intolerant of conspecifics. Medium-sized species, such as the tammar wallaby (*Notamacropus eugenii*) and bridled nail-tailed wallaby (*Onychoglaea fraenata*), are mostly nocturnal and stay close to dense habitat, sometimes forming loose aggregations in rich foraging patches. The largest species, such as the grey kangaroos (*Macropus* spp.) and the antilopine wallaroo, are more crepuscular and gregarious, moving into open habitat to forage in coordinated groups and fleeing to cover when disturbed (Eldridge and Coulson 2015). There are exceptions to these general patterns. For example, the diminutive musky rat-kangaroo is solitary, but forages by day on the rainforest floor. The burrowing bettong or boodie (*Bettongia lesueur*) is nocturnal, but shelters by day in large communal burrows. The swamp wallaby (*Wallabia bicolor*) and whip-tailed wallaby are both medium-sized wallabies, but the former is largely nocturnal, solitary and restricted to denser habitat, whereas the latter is crepuscular, gregarious and occupies more-open grassy woodland.

Macropods are essentially sedentary, occupying a stable home range throughout their lives. Home-range size is strongly correlated with sex, body size and habitat productivity (Fisher and Owens 2000): a female long-nosed potoroo (*Potorous tridactylus*) in damp forest would range over 1–2 ha, whereas the range of a female red kangaroo in the arid zone could cover 6000 ha. Home ranges of individuals overlap in all species, although some potoroids have core areas that are defended against neighbouring individuals. Males typically have larger home ranges than females, so male ranges overlap those of multiple females. Males are also the dispersing sex, leaving the maternal home range when they reach sexual maturity and sometimes covering long distances before establishing a new home range.

The musky rat-kangaroo and the potoroids are omnivorous, feeding on a wide range of fruit, seeds, fungi, roots and invertebrates (Eldridge and Frankham 2015). However, the musky rat-kangaroo is primarily insectivorous, whereas the potoroids feed mostly on truffle-like underground fruiting bodies of fungi. All of these small species use their fore limbs to dig for food items, and the bettongs in particular are significant ecosystem engineers because of the large volume of soil they turn over while foraging. The smallest macropodines are browsers, consuming mostly stems and leaves of trees and shrubs, as well as some fungi; the largest are grazers, consuming mainly grasses. Many macropodines that are intermediate in body size are mixed feeders, feeding on browse and grasses in varying proportions. Again, the swamp wallaby is an exception to this pattern, being intermediate in size but having a predominantly browsing diet, which also includes a considerable diversity of fungi. The dentition of macropods corresponds to these dietary preferences: the small omnivores have generalised dentition, the browsers have large premolars to cut stems and high-crowned molars to crush leaves, and the grazers have molar progression to compensate for the abrasive grasses in their diet.

Like all marsupials, macropods give birth to a tiny (< 1 g), undeveloped young after a brief gestation, then nurture it in a pouch, suckling from a teat for some months. The young then begin to leave the pouch for brief excursions, and then leave permanently, but continue to suckle from the same teat outside the pouch until eventually weaned. The musky rat-kangaroo typically gives birth to two young at a time, while all other macropods have a single young. However, cohorts often overlap when one young is attached to teat in the pouch while its older sibling suckles on its chosen teat from outside the pouch.

Many macropod species undergo oestrus around the time of giving birth, and the resultant embryo develops into a 32-cell blastocyst, then enters an extended period of diapause. The length of diapause is controlled by lactation in most species, so the blastocyst resumes development when suckling by the current pouch young lessens as it begins to leave the pouch, or if the pouch young dies. In some species, such as the tammar wallaby, diapause is released by the change in day length after the summer equinox. A few species, such as the western grey kangaroo (*Macropus fuliginosus*), never undergo diapause.

Breeding is strictly seasonal in a few macropod species, such as the tammar wallaby, and Bennett's wallaby (*N. rufogriseus rufogriseus*), the Tasmanian subspecies of the red-necked wallaby. Other species, like the eastern grey kangaroo (*M. giganteus*), have a seasonal birth peak, although births can occur throughout the year. Many species have no seasonal pattern and can breed continuously, as seen in the agile wallaby (*N. agilis*), or breeding may be triggered by rainfall events, as exemplified by the red kangaroo.

Capture and handling

Macropods are strong, but often flighty, requiring specialised capture, handling, housing and transport techniques. The powerful hind limbs of even the smallest macropods are capable of delivering dangerous kicks to handlers. Tree kangaroos and males of large terrestrial species also have strong fore limbs armed with sharp claws. All macropods, including pouch young, can inflict painful bites. The powerful hind limbs generate considerable propulsive force, so macropods can make explosive movements when their feet are in contact with the ground. They can readily clear obstacles and evade handlers, and can receive severe injuries if they collide with fences or other structures. Traps designed for macropods must be as small as possible to limit forceful movement and hard surfaces must be cushioned (see Figure 21.1. for an example).

All macropods can be safely held by the base of their tail, although the tails of potoroos (*Potorous* spp.) are

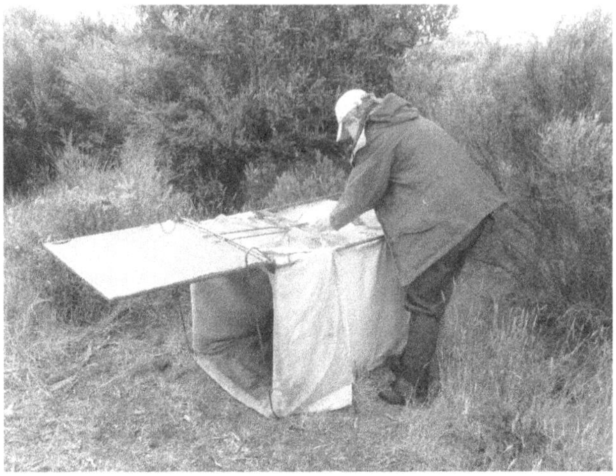

Figure 21.1: Soft-walled, double-layered trap for medium-sized macropods (designed for swamp wallabies, *Wallabia bicolor*) and described in detail by Di Stefano *et al.* (2005). The inner bag can be removed without needing to handle the trapped wallaby directly, improving animal and handler safety. Pictured here baited with carrots. Photo by Clare Death.

quite small. This form of restraint should be minimised by using sedation or anaesthesia, but may be appropriate for short-term control. Macropods do not use their tails defensively, but the muscular tails of the largest species may flail around when an animal is struggling, posing an injury risk to handlers.

Larger species are particularly prone to capture myopathy because of stress and elevated body temperature caused by pursuit, confinement and restraint. The irreversible effects of myopathy are worsened when stress is prolonged, but any stress generates some risk (Shepherd 1981). Accordingly, the larger species should rarely be handled without sedation or anaesthesia.

Female macropods will instinctively eject pouch young when pursued or constrained. Larger pouch young are more likely to be ejected, but even small, unfurred young may be ejected if the mother is severely stressed. Potoroids and rock wallabies are the most likely to eject their young, so must be handled with great care. Stressed animals confined in a trap or box with an ejected pouch young could quickly trample the young and cause severe injury with their sharp claws. In some species it may be helpful to secure large young in the pouch with masking tape or similar, which the mother can remove after release and recovery. Macropods can be transported in specially constructed boxes, pet bags or hessian sacks, preferably suspended in sacks. Animals should not be transported when ambient temperatures are high unless an air-conditioned vehicle is used (Vogelnest and Portas 2008).

A range of methods can be used for long-term marking and tracking of macropods. Individuals of all species can be identified with ear tags made of metal, plastic or composite materials (Figure 21.2). Some species (e.g. potoroos) are prone to tearing tags out of their ears, usually when fighting. Collars bearing alphanumeric characters or geometric symbols can also be used for most species. However, potoroos do not tolerate collars well and care must be taken when fitting collars to minimise hair loss and abrasion. Indeterminate growth of most macropod species must be considered when fitting collars for tracking or identification purposes. Breakaway or drop-off designs may be required to avoid constriction, particularly for males of the larger species. Individuals can be marked temporarily with non-toxic paints and dyes, or by clipping patterns in the fur. Camera traps can be used to record marked individuals, augmenting or completely replacing direct sightings. In a few cases, where populations of large, crepuscular species are habituated to people, it is possible to identify most individuals using sketches and photographs of natural markings.

Telemetric devices are commonly used to track movement and activity of macropods. VHF radio transmitters can be glued onto the fur for short-term tracking or integrated into a collar for longer-term applications. Similarly, GPS receivers can be attached with glue to the animal or carried on a collar (Henderson *et al.* 2018). The weight and bulk of the transmitter assembly that a macropod can carry depend on the size of the species and the sex of the animal; smaller animals can carry only relatively lightweight transmitters, with limitations on signal range and operating life, whereas males of the largest species can carry a more-robust assembly with high performance capabilities.

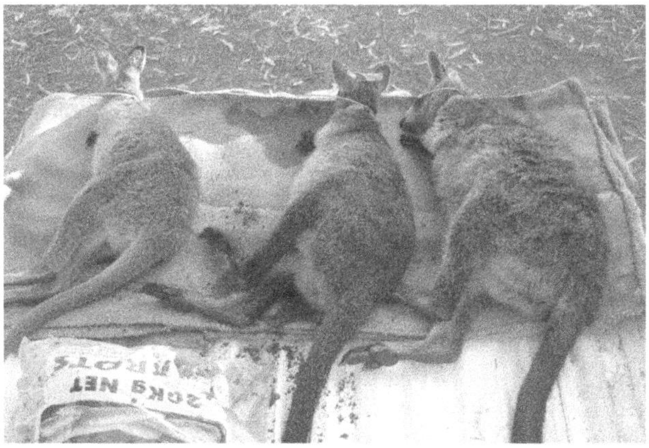

Figure 21.2: A red-necked wallaby (*Notamacropus rufogriseus*) left, and two swamp wallabies (*Wallabia bicolor*), fitted with ear tags and radio collars under anaesthesia with tiletamine–zolazepam. Photo by Graeme Coulson.

Veterinary considerations

Sedation and anaesthesia

Sedation can assist in preventing adverse animal welfare events in macropods subject to capture, handling, transportation and release. Suggested dosing regimens have been recently collated by Vogelnest and Portas (2019). Injectable diazepam (0.1–2.0 mg/kg intramuscularly) is a commonly used tranquiliser across macropod species, with a wide safety margin but variable responses between species and individuals (Vogelnest 2019). It is not sufficiently potent to allow immobilisation or deep sedation. Short-, intermediate- and long-acting neuroleptic tranquilisers can be administered to reduce stress during more-prolonged activities such as transport or introductions (Vogelnest 2019).

The most frequently used injectable field anaesthetic in macropods, as with other marsupials, is tiletamine–zolazepam, generally given at 4–10 mg/kg via intramuscular injection, with the dose depending on the route of administration (hand injection, syringe pole or dart). Tiletamine–zolazepam is considered reliable and safe, but has the disadvantage of a prolonged recovery (Vogelnest and Portas 2019). Placing the recovering animal in or under a hessian or cloth sack or woollen blanket (Figure 16.1b in Chapter 16), and observing the animal until its coordination has returned enough to move away, enables a safe release. Multiple other injectable drug combinations, some with reversal agents, have been successfully used in macropods and are outlined by Vogelnest and Portas (2019).

Gaseous anaesthesia (isoflurane or sevoflurane in oxygen) can also be used for induction or maintenance via a face mask. Tracheal intubation is generally difficult in macropods and not recommended, unless procedures are long or involve the head and neck (Vogelnest 2019). Marsupial studies have demonstrated significant species variation in the metabolism of analgesic drugs, and a combination of local anaesthetic, anti-inflammatories and opioids can be beneficial when managing pain (Bodley 2019). Anaesthetised macropods should have their eyes covered and their nose and mouth angled downwards relative to the neck, to allow saliva or food to drain (Vogelnest 2019). Vital signs should be monitored throughout all procedures. In the field, struggle during capture or restraint must be avoided as this may result in pain and injury to the animal, as well as posing a safety risk to the handler.

Blood collection

Blood is typically collected from the lateral tail vein of sedated or anaesthetised macropods (Figure 16.3c in Chapter 16).

Euthanasia

Methods used for euthanasia may vary according to availability of drugs and equipment, as well as the location, species, size, age and mobility of the macropod requiring euthanasia (AVA 2012). The method of handling and degree of restraint required needs to be taken into consideration when evaluating the appropriate euthanasia method for macropods. The most widely accepted euthanasia method for macropods is an intravenous overdose of the barbiturate anaesthetic, pentobarbitone, following physical or chemical restraint (Vogelnest and Portas 2019). Use of barbiturates may not be appropriate where the carcass will pose a threat to scavenger animals. Any animal euthanased with pentobarbitone represents a secondary toxicity risk to wild scavengers and should be disposed of via deep burial.

The use of firearms may be appropriate for euthanasia in free-ranging macropods if personnel are appropriately trained and licensed; where a shot to the brain of an injured animal is impractical or unsafe, a shot to the heart is permissible (Commonwealth of Australia 2008). The use of a captive bolt may be an alternative, but this method also requires training and the animal must be tightly restrained or immobile (Hing *et al.* 2019). In the event that other options are not available in the field and, as a last resort, a heavy blow to the base of the skull with sufficient force to destroy the brain can result in rapid death if properly applied, but is likewise dependent on the knowledge and experience of the operator (Commonwealth of Australia 2008).

When a female macropod is euthanased, any dependent young (pouch young or young-at-foot) must either be euthanased or taken into care, if deemed appropriate. Euthanasia options for pouch young include captive bolt (Hampton 2019), blunt trauma (Sharp *et al.* 2015) or chemical euthanasia as described for adult kangaroos.

Infectious pathogens

Basic hygiene precautions are recommended when handling macropods because zoonoses pose a risk to humans (Hulst 2019). Of particular concern is Q fever (*Coxiella burnetti*). This is caused by a bacterium vectored by ticks and is endemic in many livestock and macropod populations (Graves and Islam 2016). Most macropods are asymptomatic, but humans risk contracting debilitating Q fever through exposure to aerosols of macropod body fluids or faeces, or by inhalation of contaminated dust. Those working with macropods should be vaccinated.

Wild macropods harbour an unusually wide array of gastrointestinal helminth parasites (Beveridge *et al.* 2010). Although abundance can be very high (i.e. tens of thousands of worms), these burdens are rarely pathogenic except when individual hosts become overwhelmed by poor forage and/or adverse weather conditions (Vogelnest and Portas 2019). Wild macropods can also be infested by a wide range of ectoparasites including lice, mites, biting flies and ticks, which generally do not cause clinical signs in the host, but care should be taken as some ticks transmit zoonotic bacteria (e.g. *Rickettsia australis*), the causative agent of Queensland tick typhus in humans (Hulst 2019).

Captive macropods are generally more prone to disease, although disease outbreaks can occur in wild populations at times. Macropod progressive periodontal disease (lumpy jaw) is a common disease in captive macropods, where it is associated with chronic stress and environmental contamination due to crowded spaces and damp substrates (Rendle *et al.* 2020). This disease is rare in free-ranging macropods, but severe outbreaks occasionally occur (e.g. Borland *et al.* 2012). Macropod herpesviruses are more likely to be present in captive populations, where latent infections can be activated by stress. Prevention of transmission through appropriate biosecurity practices, and an understanding of underlying factors that increase susceptibility (e.g. habitat destruction, in-breeding, concurrent disease), is important (Devlin and Stalder 2019).

Orbiviruses, which are vectored by biting midges that breed after heavy rain, have caused occasional widespread outbreaks of blindness among larger macropods in inland areas (Hooper *et al.* 1999). While this manifestation of disease is generally not fatal, macropods may die from collisions with objects or inability to forage effectively. Orbiviruses have also been associated with epizootics of sudden death in captive macropods (McLelland 2019).

Tree kangaroos housed in tropical regions risk contracting Melioidosis (caused by the bacterium *Burkholderia pseudomallei*) when the soil substrate of the pen is wet for long periods; this can be alleviated by housing animals in pens with hard (e.g. concrete) floors.

General operating procedures

A range of low-impact and indirect methods of detection or study, such as scat collection, and assessment of tracks and other traces (Chapter 4), camera and hair trapping, and conservation detector dogs (Chapter 5) may be used to study macropods. Some species can be caught with cages, draw-string traps (Chapter 7) or by darting with tranquiliser guns (Chapter 16). Citizen science approaches have also been applied to the study of some macropod species (Chapter 10). Depending on the species, macropods can be marked with microchips or ear tags (Chapter 8) or sometimes collars. Radiotelemetry with collars, implanted devices or glued on to the animal may be used to track macropod movements (Chapter 9). Veterinary procedures, including sedation, anaesthesia and blood collection are detailed in Chapter 16.

REFERENCES

AVA (2012) Euthanasia of injured wildlife. <https://www.ava.com.au/policy-advocacy/policies/euthanasia/euthanasia-of-injured-wildlife/>.

Beveridge I, Spratt DM, Johnson PM (2010) Diversity and distribution of helminth parasites in macropodoid marsupials. In *Macropods: The Biology of Kangaroos, Wallabies, and Rat-kangaroos.* (Eds GM Coulson and MDB Eldridge) pp. 231–241. CSIRO Publishing, Melbourne.

Bodley K (2019) Appendix 4. Drug formulary. In *Current Therapy in Medicine of Australian Mammals.* (Eds L Volgelnest and T Portas) pp. 702–727. CSIRO Publishing, Melbourne.

Borland D, Coulson G, Beveridge I (2012) Oral necrobacillosis ('lumpy jaw') in a free-ranging population of eastern grey kangaroos (*Macropus giganteus*) in Victoria. *Australian Mammalogy* **34**, 29–35. doi:10.1071/AM10031

Commonwealth of Australia (2008) *National Code of Practice for the Humane Shooting of Kangaroos and Wallabies for Non-commercial Purposes.* Department of Environment and Heritage, Canberra. <https://www.environment.gov.au/system/files/resources/133025f9-b11c-4083-8960-4bd8e3bed4a8/files/code-conduct-non-commercial.pdf>.

Devlin J, Stalder K (2019) Marsupial herpesviruses. In *Current Therapy in Medicine of Australian Mammals.* (Eds L Volgelnest and T Portas) pp. 353–358. CSIRO Publishing, Melbourne.

Di Stefano J, Moyle R, Coulson G (2005) A soft-walled double-layered trap for capture of swamp wallabies *Wallabia bicolor. Australian Mammalogy* **27**, 235–238. doi:10.1071/AM05235

Eldridge MDB, Coulson GM (2015) Family Macropodidae (Kangaroos and Wallabies). In *Handbook of the Mammals of the World. Vol. 5 Monotremes and Marsupials.* (Eds DE Wilson and RA Mittermeier) pp. 630–735. Lynx Edicions, Barcelona, Spain.

Eldridge MDB, Frankham GJ (2015) Family Potoroidae (Bettongs and Potoroos). In *Handbook of the Mammals of the World. Vol. 5 Monotremes and Marsupials.* (Eds DE Wilson and RA Mittermeier) pp. 600–628. Lynx Edicions, Barcelona, Spain.

Fisher DO, Owens IP (2000) Female home range size and the evolution of social organization in macropod marsupials. *Journal of Animal Ecology* **69**, 1083–1098. doi:10.1046/j.1365-2656.2000.00450.x

Graves SR, Islam A (2016) Endemic Q fever in New South Wales, Australia: a case series (2005–2013). *The American Journal of Tropical Medicine and Hygiene* **95**, 55–59. doi:10.4269/ajtmh.15-0828

Hampton JO (2019) Gunpowder-powered captive bolts for the euthanasia of kangaroo pouch young. *Australian Mammalogy* **41**, 250–254. doi:10.1071/AM18009

Hing S, Hampton JO, Gibson TJ (2019) Animal welfare and the killing of wildlife by captive bolt in Australia. *Australian Zoologist* **40**, 170–180. doi:10.7882/AZ.2018.035

Henderson T, Vernes K, Körtner G, Rajaratnam R (2018) Using GPS technology to understand spatial and temporal activity of kangaroos in a peri-urban environment. *Animals (Basel)* **8**, 97. doi:10.3390/ani8060097

Hooper PT, Lunt RA, Gould AR, Hyatt AD, Russell GM, Kattenbelt JA, Blacksell SD, Reddacliff LA, Kirkland PD, Davis RJ, Durham PJK (1999) Epidemic of blindness in kangaroos – evidence of a viral aetiology. *Australian Veterinary Journal* **77**, 529–536. doi:10.1111/j.1751-0813.1999.tb12127.x

Hulst F (2019) Zoonoses. In *Current Therapy in Medicine of Australian Mammals.* (Eds L Volgelnest and T Portas) pp. 267–284. CSIRO Publishing, Melbourne.

Kaufmann JH (1974) The ecology and evolution of social organization in the kangaroo family (Macropodidae). *American Zoologist* **14**, 51–62. doi:10.1093/icb/14.1.51

McLelland D (2019) Macropods. In *Current Therapy in Medicine of Australian Mammals.* (Eds L Volgelnest and T Portas) pp. 433–450. CSIRO Publishing, Melbourne.

Rendle J, Jackson B, Hoorn SV, Yeap L, Warren K, Donaldson R, Ward SJ, Vogelnest L, McLelland D, Lynch M, Vitali S (2020) A retrospective study of Macropod Progressive Periodontal Disease ("lumpy jaw") in captive macropods across Australia and Europe: Using data from the past to inform future macropod management. *Animals (Basel)* **10**, 1954. doi:10.3390/ani10111954

Sharp TM, McLeod SR, Leggett KEA, Gibson TJ (2015) Evaluation of a spring-powered captive bolt gun for killing kangaroo pouch young. *Wildlife Research* **41**, 623–632. doi:10.1071/WR14094

Shepherd NC (1981) Capture myopathy in the red kangaroo (*Macropus rufus*). In *Wildlife Diseases of the Pacific Basin and Other Countries.* (Ed. ME Fowler) pp. 239–247. Wildlife Disease Association, Sydney.

Vogelnest L (2019) Capture, physical and chemical restraint. In *Current Therapy in Medicine of Australian Mammals.* (Eds L Volgelnest and T Portas) pp. 121–150. CSIRO Publishing, Melbourne.

Vogelnest L, Portas T (2008) Macropods. In *Medicine of Australian Mammals.* (Eds L Vogelnest and R Woods) pp. 133–22. CSIRO Publishing, Melbourne.

Vogelnest L, Portas T (2019) *Current Therapy in Medicine of Australian Mammals.* CSIRO Publishing, Melbourne.

22 Eutherian carnivores

Bronwyn A. Fancourt, Benjamin L. Allen, Stephen M. Jackson, Paul D. Meek, Frances Zewe, Guy Ballard, Linda Behrendorff, Andrew W. Claridge and Peter J.S. Fleming

INTRODUCTION

Three species of introduced free-ranging eutherian carnivores occur in Australia: two canid species and one felid species. The largest wild canid includes dingoes, feral domestic dogs and cross-breeds (*Canis* spp.). Current evidence suggests that dingoes first arrived in Australia > 3500 years ago, with feral modern domestic dogs establishing in the last 230 years. While the classification of dingoes and wild dogs remains intensely debated in Australia, the nomenclatural and taxonomic classification of dingoes, feral domestic dogs and their hybrids has no bearing on their ethical treatment. In the context of this chapter, the term 'dingo' refers to all free-ranging modern dogs and dingoes. A smaller canid, the European red fox (*Vulpes vulpes*), was deliberately introduced to Australia during the mid-1800s (Rolls 1969), and by the early 1900s had established across most of mainland Australia. The feral domestic cat (*Felis catus*) is the only free-ranging felid species occurring in Australia. Domestic cats first came to Australia with European settlers in 1788, but the establishment of feral populations took several decades, with feral cats first recorded in Tasmania during the 1840s and in mainland Australia during the 1850s. While the two canids are common across much of the Australian mainland (though the dingo and fox are absent from Tasmania), feral cats are now ubiquitous across mainland Australia and Tasmania.

DINGOES AND OTHER WILD DOGS

Benjamin L. Allen, Stephen M. Jackson, Guy Ballard, Linda Behrendorff, Andrew W. Claridge, Peter J.S. Fleming and Paul D. Meek

Characteristics

The dingo is a medium-sized canid, with adults usually weighing between 10 and 25 kg, averaging ~16 kg. Adults generally stand ~55 cm to the shoulder and measure ~123 cm from nose to tail tip (Smith 2015). Males are usually larger than females, with variations in size depending on the environment and prey availability. Dingoes typically have three basic coat colours, with most being a ginger or sandy colour, followed by white/cream and black and tan. Hybrid coats, including patchy, sable and brindle are also common where hybridisation with domestic dogs has occurred. Most dingoes often have white points on their toes, feet, tail and chest, although the colour combinations and presence of white patches varies between individuals and is not a reliable indicator of genetic status/hybridisation. The phenotype of feral domestic dogs and dingo–dog hybrids varies greatly according to ancestry (Cairns *et al.* 2021). Dingoes live and breed for up to 14 years in the wild or up to 20 years in captivity (Smith 2015).

Biology and behaviour

Dingoes are distributed across most of Australia, except for some parts of south-eastern and south-western Australia. Feral domestic dogs occur in Tasmania, but

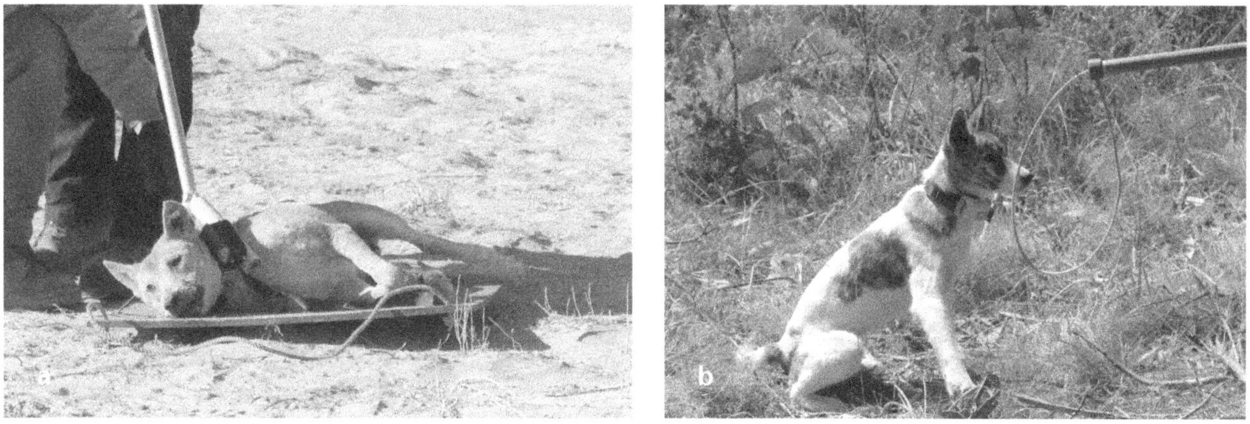

Figure 22.1: (a) Captured wild dog (*Canis* sp.) restrained with a Y-pole. Photo by Paul Meek. (b) Recaptured dog in a foothold trap, about to be restrained with a noose/catch pole. Photo by Andrew Claridge.

dingoes are absent (Fleming *et al.* 2014). Dingo home-range size varies among regions, ranging from < 1 km^2 in some peri-urban areas (McNeill *et al.* 2016) to > 1000 km^2 in arid deserts (Newsome *et al.* 2013). They are generalist, opportunistic carnivores that prefer small- to medium-sized prey weighing < 10 kg (e.g. reptiles, rodents, rabbits, bandicoots, wallabies) when available, although they also eat fruit and other plant material, invertebrates and even large species of kangaroos and ungulates (Doherty *et al.* 2019). Sometimes they are cannibalistic (Meek and Brown 2017; Smith *et al.* 2020).

Dingoes typically form mixed-sex groups of four to eight adults and subadults. Breeding pairs utilise den sites (described in more detail in Chapter 4), producing between one and 10 pups (average five) during each annual breeding season, which peaks in July, but can occur earlier or later (Allen *et al.* 2015; Cursino *et al.* 2017). Dingoes are active throughout the day and night, but large individual variation occurs in activity patterns and space use, depending on the weather, availability of prey and breeding activities. Observations of adult dingo activity peak in autumn (March–May), when abundance is at its lowest. Dingo activity is typically lowest in late winter and spring (August–October) during whelping, when abundance is at its highest (Allen *et al.* 2013).

Capture and handling

Dingoes can be captured with padded-jaw or soft-catch foothold traps (Meek *et al.* 1995), cage traps, Collarum® neck snares or soft-net traps, and by chemical immobilisation via darts (although some devices may not be permitted in all states or territories). Pups can be captured by hand before they develop an innate fear of humans, although the animal welfare implications of disturbing dens and young animals should be considered (see Chapter 4).

Dingoes can be restrained by hand or using a Y-pole or a noose/catch pole (Figure 22.1), and then pinned to the ground on their side. For minimally invasive procedures (e.g. collaring, ear tagging, microchip implantation and cephalic vein blood collection), animals can be temporarily strapped to a restraining board (Figure 22.2) or physically restrained by an operator, without sedation. Some operators prefer to temporarily keep the dingo's mouth closed while processing; this can be achieved using a commercially available domestic dog muzzle or similar restraint. The animal's head can be covered with a towel or hessian bag, to reduce stress and assist in protecting

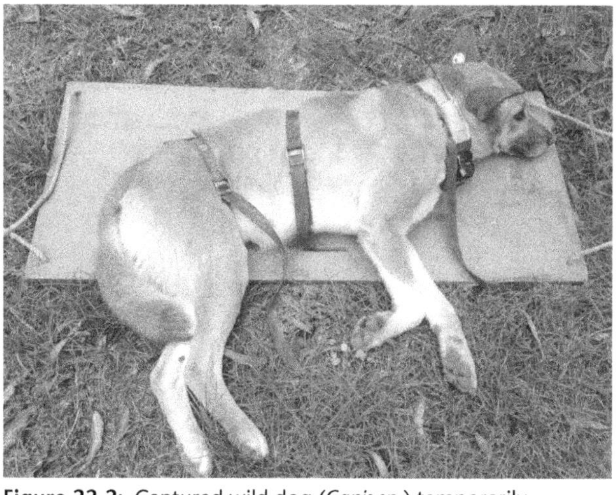

Figure 22.2: Captured wild dog (*Canis* sp.) temporarily strapped to restraining board to facilitate fitting of telemetry collar, marking and sample collection. Numbered tag in the left ear. Photo by Frances Zewe.

the operator from being bitten. The dingo must always be able to breathe freely, and operators should avoid rapid movements and loud or otherwise distressing noises.

Several methods can be used to mark dingoes (see Chapter 8). Passive integrated transponder (PIT) tags, or microchips, implanted subcutaneously between the scapulae (shoulder blades) are often used. While these tags offer a permanent form of identification, animals typically need to be recaptured to scan the tag and confirm identification. Tattoos can be applied to the inside of the ear. Although tattoos are inexpensive, the animal needs to be recaptured to confirm identification. Furthermore, tattoos can fade over time and become difficult to read. Individually numbered, coded or coloured ear tags can be seen from a distance and can allow individual identification without the need to recapture the animal. However, tags may be lost, and numbers and colours can fade or become unclear over time. Individually numbered, coded or coloured collars can also be used. Like ear tags, collars can be seen from a distance, allowing individual identification without needing to recapture the animal. Collars should be removed on completion of the study where possible.

Captive dingoes require a complex environment that provides opportunities to explore and engage in 'natural' behaviours and provides refuge from negative social interactions (Jackson 2003). Enclosures should be furnished with logs, boulders, vegetation and shelters. The legislated *Standards for Exhibiting Australian Mammals in New South Wales* requires an enclosure area of at least 220 m^2, but 300 m^2 is suggested as optimal, to keep one or two dingoes in captivity for public display. An additional 20 m^2 must be added per additional animal (i.e. for each animal greater than two). A 25 m^2 holding yard is also required for up to four animals. Dingoes can be excellent climbers and diggers, so fences should be at least 2 m high with an inward-facing 1 m overhang at the top of the fence to prevent climbing. The fence should also have a 1 m horizontal wire skirt on the inside of the fence at its base to prevent the animals from digging out. Environmental enrichment should be provided to stimulate the animals and help prevent boredom.

Dingoes should be transported in a box that allows them to stand and lie down comfortably (~150 × 80 × 100 cm high). The box must be well ventilated, have a non-slip floor, and provide sufficient space and materials for the animals to lie comfortably. Only one animal should be placed in each box, unless they are young individuals that are part of the same litter. Animals should not be fed during transportation to reduce the likelihood of vomiting. If water is required, a deep sturdy dish should be provided (Jackson 2003).

Veterinary considerations

Sedation and anaesthesia

Sedation and general anaesthesia should be considered for handling wild-caught dingoes if invasive procedures are to be performed. For other contexts, manual restraint alone (e.g. using a restraint board) may suffice (Robley *et al.* 2010). Adequate sedation decreases stress and the risk of injury to the animals and researcher and allows gentle handling. Sedatives appropriate for domestic dogs are also appropriate for dingoes; however, higher doses are invariably required for wild animals when compared to their domestic counterparts (see Chapter 16). Examples of injectable, intramuscular anaesthetic medications used to restrain wild dogs and dingoes for research purposes typically consist of combinations of medetomidine, tiletamine–zolazepam and ketamine. A reversable agent (atipamezole) is available for medetomidine and permits rapid recoveries (Morrant *et al.* 2017).

Blood collection

Blood is typically collected from the jugular or cephalic vein of sedated or anaesthetised carnivores.

Euthanasia

As for many wild mammals, two-stage injectable euthanasia is commonly used. The preferred method of euthanasia for dingoes is intravenous (IV) injection of pentobarbitone. Adequate restraint is required for IV injection, so initial sedation is recommended. If IV injection is not possible, deep sedation or general anaesthesia can be followed by intracardiac injection of pentobarbitone (AVMA 2020). The intraperitoneal route of administration is not appropriate for dingos due to pain associated with injection and slow onset of action (AVMA 2020). Appropriate personnel training and careful attention to relevant legislation is required for the use of pentobarbitone. Any animal euthanased with pentobarbitone represents a secondary toxicity risk to wild scavengers and should be disposed of via deep burial.

Physical methods of euthanasia include shooting for restrained animals at close range (< 5 m). Captive bolts can also be used for dingoes that are adequately restrained, but this method has not been well described in the literature (Reilly 2001).

Infectious pathogens

Dingoes are susceptible to the same ectoparasites, endoparasites, and bacterial, viral, fungal and protozoal infections as other canids (Jackson 2003). They can transmit several zoonotic diseases (Henderson 2009). Of particular concern are tapeworms (particularly hydatids, caused by *Echinococcus granulosus*; Jenkins 2005). Zoonotic endoparasites include roundworms, hookworms and protozoa (*Cryptosporidium* and *Giardia*). Zoonotic ectoparasites include scabies mite (*Sarcoptes scabiei*), fleas and a notable fungal zoonoses, ringworm. Dingoes are susceptible to viral infections including canine distemper, canine parvovirus, canine viral hepatitis and canine herpesvirus.

General operating procedures

General operating procedures may include visual observations, assessments of signs (scats, tracks) and measurement of dens (Chapter 4), hair collection and camera trapping (Chapter 5), cage and foothold traps (Chapter 7), microchipping and ear tags (Chapter 8), telemetry devices (Chapter 9), sedatives and general anaesthetics, tranquiliser darts and poles and collection of blood samples (Chapter 16). Additionally, several nationally recognised standard operating procedures (SOPs) have been developed specifically for dingoes (see www.pestsmart.org.au).

RED FOXES

Paul D. Meek, Stephen M. Jackson, Frances Zewe, Benjamin L. Allen, Andrew W. Claridge, Bronwyn A. Fancourt and Peter J.S. Fleming

Characteristics

The European red fox's pelage is typically orange and white, but varies with genetics, habitat and altitude. For example, high country foxes can be bright orange, silver, and less often, black. Adults stand ~35 cm to the shoulder and measure ~100 cm from nose to tail tip. Adult body mass ranges between 4.7 and 8.3 kg for males and between 4.0 and 6.8 kg for females (Van Dyck and Strahan 2008).

Biology and behaviour

Foxes are widespread across Australia with the exception of far-northern Australia, Tasmania and most small islands (Van Dyck and Strahan 2008). Foxes are dietary generalists and, while largely carnivorous, will also eat vegetation (e.g. berries) (Coman 1973; Short *et al.* 1999; Molsher *et al.* 2000; Roberts *et al.* 2006; White *et al.* 2006). They exploit diverse habitats and ecosystems, including coastal, agricultural, forested and arid habitats. They can thrive in urban and peri-urban environments where they coexist with humans and domestic pets (Coman *et al.* 1991; Meek and Saunders 2000; Marks and Bloomfield 2006; White *et al.* 2006). Home ranges vary from 1 to 270 km^2 across habitat types, with males occupying larger areas than females (Coman *et al.* 1991; Meek and Saunders 2000; Marks and Bloomfield 2006; Carter *et al.* 2012). Home ranges overlap and, where resources are abundant, they are shared among family groups (e.g. urban areas). Similarly, density varies from 0.1 to > 7 foxes km^{-2} (Saunders *et al.* 2010), although densities as high as 13 foxes km^{-2} have been reported in suburban Melbourne (Marks and Bloomfield 1999). Foxes are mostly nocturnal, although this is highly variable. They are mostly solitary, except during the breeding season (spring and summer) when they pair and raise young (Saunders *et al.* 1995). Litters are born in dens (see Chapter 4) and vary in size from one to five, with young weaned in summer and dispersing in late summer (Saunders *et al.* 1995; Marlow *et al.* 2000).

Capture and handling

Foxes are usually captured with padded-jaw or soft-catch foothold traps (Meek *et al.* 1995; Fleming *et al.* 1998), but also using cage traps baited with food lures. Other methods include tranquiliser darting and soft-net traps (Sharpe and Saunders 2008).

Foxes should be restrained using a Y-pole and/or a noose/catch pole (Figure 22.1), and then ideally strapped to a retraining board with the animal's head covered to reduce stress (Figure 22.3). Restraining boards minimise the risk of injury to animals and operators when conducting procedures such as fitting telemetry collars or

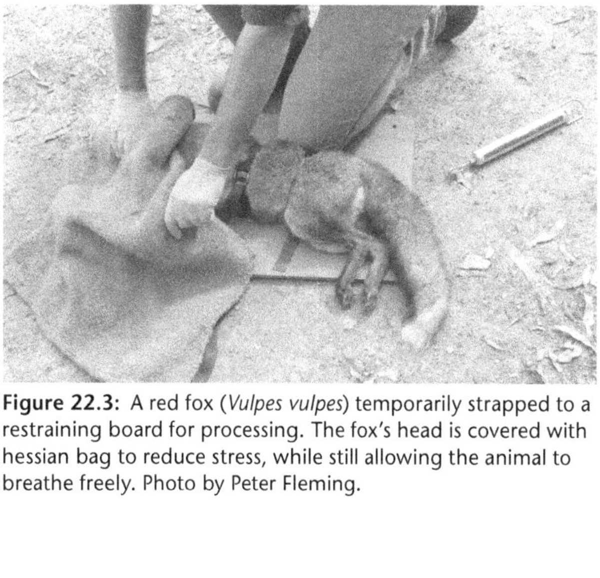

Figure 22.3: A red fox (*Vulpes vulpes*) temporarily strapped to a restraining board for processing. The fox's head is covered with hessian bag to reduce stress, while still allowing the animal to breathe freely. Photo by Peter Fleming.

ear tags. Foxes, more so than dingoes, require constant attention on the restraining board from a dedicated handler. Foxes must be able to breathe freely and should be shaded to avoid overheating, and operators should avoid rapid movements and loud or otherwise distressing noises.

Several methods have been used to mark foxes, including passive integrated transponder (PIT) tags or microchips, implanted subcutaneously between the scapulae, as described for dingoes. Button ear tags (sheep size or smaller) are used for male and female identification and can include transponders for identification of individuals. Reflective colour coding on telemetry collars, including the whip antennae, has been successfully used to identify individuals (Meek and Saunders 2000).

When transporting over short distances (up to 2 km), a fox can be constrained in a hessian bag, or tear-proof breathable bag, with a secure tie to prevent escape. Over longer distances, foxes should be transported in a box that allows the animal to stand and/or lay down. Only one fox per box is recommended and the box must be well ventilated, crush proof, and ideally constructed from timber, with a non-slip floor, and latch or lock to prevent escape. Food and water should not be provided unless necessary. Animals should not be exposed to extreme or unsafe temperatures and should be sheltered from excessive noise, light and visual stimuli.

It is illegal in some jurisdictions to keep foxes without a permit. In New South Wales, the *Exhibited Animals Protection Act 1986* requires an enclosure of at least 100 m^2 for up to two animals, with an extra 10 m^2 for each additional animal. A 25 m^2 holding yard is also required, with 7 m^2 for each additional animal when more than two are contained. Enclosures must be fully enclosed as foxes are agile climbers. Wire mesh should be extended along the ground for at least 1 m around the inside enclosure to prevent foxes from digging under fences. The mesh size on wire fences must be small enough to prevent pups from escaping (wire gauge 3 mm, 50 × 50 mm mesh); alternatively, solid walls can be used over which a roof must be installed. Gates or access points must have a lock, and must not open directly to the outside, to prevent escape. A sight barrier is required, and dens should be contained within the enclosure to allow foxes to hide and escape inclement weather. Environmental enrichment must be provided for stimulus and to prevent boredom.

Veterinary considerations

Sedation and anaesthesia

Trapped foxes can be safely handled through use of chemical immobilisation. For this purpose, anaesthetic and sedative agents are used, namely combinations of medetomidine, tiletamine–zolazepam and ketamine (Bertelsen and Villadsen 2009). A reversable agent (atipamezole) is available for medetomidine and permits rapid recoveries. Where anaesthesia is used, foxes should be kept in a ventilated hessian bag or sturdy travel cage, placed in a cool location, and allowed to fully awaken before release. Refer to 'Capture and handling' for foxes, and 'Euthanasia' as outlined for dingoes for more details.

Blood collection

Blood is typically collected from the jugular or cephalic vein of sedated or anaesthetised foxes.

Euthanasia

Foxes can be euthanased using the same methods outlined for dingoes and other wild dogs, namely shooting or two-stage chemical euthanasia. Any animal euthanased with pentobarbitone represents a secondary toxicity risk to wild scavengers and should be disposed of via deep burial.

Infectious pathogens

Foxes carry a range of ectoparasites, endoparasites and infectious diseases, many of which are zoonotic. The occurrence and prevalence of these agents depend on many factors, including the location and health status of the animal (Dybing *et al.* 2013; Jenkins *et al.* 2014). These pathogens are largely the same as those listed for dingoes and wild dogs.

General operating procedures

General operating procedures relevant to the study of foxes may include visual observations (with or without spotlighting), assessments of signs (scats, tracks) and measurement of dens (Chapter 4), hair collection and camera trapping (Chapter 5), foothold traps (Chapter 7), PIT tags and ear tags (Chapter 8), external telemetry devices (Chapter 9), sedatives and general anaesthetics, tranquiliser darts and poles and collection of blood samples (Chapter 16). Additionally, several nationally recognised SOPs have been developed specifically for foxes (see www.pestsmart.org.au).

FERAL CATS

Frances Zewe, Bronwyn A. Fancourt, Linda Behrendorff, Andrew W. Claridge, Peter J.S. Fleming and Paul D. Meek

Characteristics

Feral cats are unowned free-ranging cats that are not dependent on humans for survival. Adult male cats (toms) can weigh up to 7.3 kg; females (queens) are typically smaller (up to 5 kg) (Van Dyck and Strahan 2008). Coat length is variable and there are many coat patterns (e.g. tabby, tri-colour or tortoiseshell) and colours (e.g. grey, black, ginger, white).

Biology and behaviour

Domestic cats are found across 99.8% of the Australian land mass, including Tasmania and several islands (Abbott 2002; Legge *et al.* 2017). Although queens are sexually mature from four months of age, feral queens typically reproduce from 10 to 12 months. Queens are induced ovulators (i.e. ovulate in response to an external stimulus during, or immediately prior, to mating) and can produce up to three litters annually, although two litters of four or five kittens per year is more typical (Jones and Coman 1982). Litters are born and reared in dens such as European rabbit (*Oryctolagus cuniculus*) burrows, hollow logs or dense vegetation. Feral cats are opportunistic, generalist, and obligate carnivores, with acute senses and refined coordination for hunting their prey. Prey ranges in size from insects, small mammals, birds and reptiles (Catling 1988; Martin *et al.* 1996; Paltridge 2002) up to small wallabies ~4 kg (Fancourt 2015). Feral cats are active day and night. Dietary composition can vary with environmental conditions and prey availability (Catling 1988; Molsher *et al.* 1999; Paltridge 2002). Feral cat home-range size varies with productivity and population density (Bengsen *et al.* 2016), with females and males in semi-arid, low productivity areas ranging up to 42 km^2 and 165 km^2 respectively (Wilson 2020).

Capture and handling

Feral cats can be captured using cage traps or padded-jaw or soft-catch foothold traps (Figure 22.4). Trained cat-tracking dogs can also be used to bail or drive cats up a tree, where the cat can then be hand netted or darted using a tranquiliser gun (McGregor *et al.* 2016).

Feral cats are often fractious, so appropriate handling is essential for cat welfare and handler safety. Sedation or anaesthesia of cats via intramuscular injection of sedative or anaesthetic agents in the field is commonly used to facilitate safe animal handling (e.g. Molsher 2001; Fancourt *et al.* 2021). Captured cats can be restrained using a catch pole or cage crush to facilitate sedation. Cats can also be placed on capture boards and restrained as described for foxes and dingoes, although sedation is preferable to minimise risk to humans and the cats. Care should be taken to avoid placing excessive pressure on the neck of cats to avoid laryngospasm.

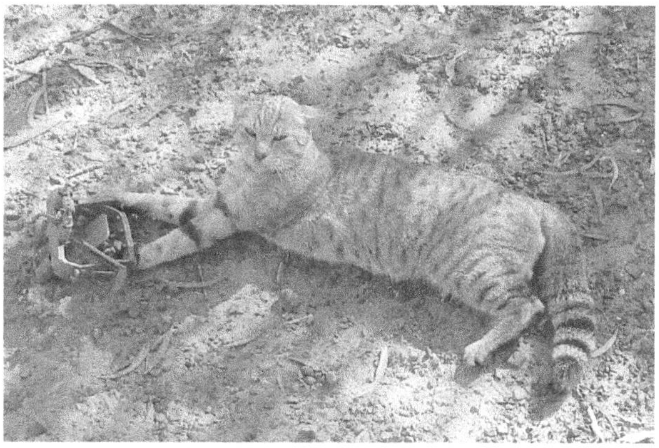

Figure 22.4: Feral cat (*Felis catus*) captured in a padded-jaw foothold trap. Photo by Bronwyn Fancourt.

Passive integrated transponder (PIT) tags, or microchips, implanted subcutaneously between the scapulae, as described for dingoes and foxes can be used to mark cats individually. External identification tags, such as small ear tags or identification collars, can also be applied to cats as described for dingoes and foxes.

Feral cats can be temporarily housed (e.g. during recovery from sedation) in a ventilated animal carrier or cage kept away from noise and visual stimuli and temperature extremes. Hot-water bottles with covers can be used to keep cats warm during field recovery in cool environments. For transporting short distances, a feral cat can be constrained in a hessian or tear-proof breathable bag with secure tie-off to prevent escape. Over longer distances, transport requires a box or sturdy covered travel cage that allows the animal to stand and/or lay down. Only one cat should be transported per box and the box must be well ventilated, crush proof, and have a non-slip floor, and be fitted with a latch or lock to prevent escape. Food and water should not be provided unless necessary. Animals should be sheltered from light and visual stimuli and not exposed to extreme temperature conditions.

Veterinary considerations

Sedation and anaesthesia

Feral cats are difficult and dangerous to handle with physical restraint alone so chemical restraint is invariably used to allow their handling. Sedation is commonly used for short-term field procedures including microchipping, tissue or blood sampling, morphologic measurements, and fitting telemetry devices (Molsher 2001; Fancourt *et al.* 2021). As with dingoes, this species has the advantage that sedatives appropriate for domestic cats are also appropriate for feral cats. However, like dingoes, higher doses are invariably required for wild animals when compared to their domestic counterparts. Injectable, intramuscular veterinary chemicals used to restrain feral cats for research purposes typically include medetomidine, tiletamine–zolazepam and ketamine, or combinations thereof. A reversable agent (atipamezole) is available for medetomidine and permits rapid recoveries.

Blood collection

Blood is typically collected from the jugular vein of anaesthetised feral cats.

Euthanasia

As for many wild mammals, two-stage injectable euthanasia is commonly used: intravenous or intracardiac injection of pentobarbitone following heavy sedation with inhalant anaesthesia (isoflurane) can also be used for fractious cats before euthanasia with an injectable euthanasia agent (AVMA 2020). Any animal euthanased with pentobarbitone represents a secondary toxicity risk to wild scavengers and should be disposed of via deep burial.

The only physical euthanasia method commonly used is shooting, especially for restrained animals at close range (< 5 m), e.g. a feral cat in a cage or foot-hold trap, or those chased up a tree by a detector dog.

Infectious pathogens

Transmission of the zoonotic toxoplasmosis (*Toxoplasma gondii*) is a particular risk when handling feral cats, particularly for immunocompromised or pregnant operators. When handling live or deceased feral cats, oocysts can be transmitted via faecal contamination. Where operators with open wounds handle cats, or where injuries such as scratches or bites are inflicted by cats, bacterial infections can occur, such as those caused by cat scratch fever (*Bartonella henslae*) and several others; see Gerhold and Jessup (2013).

Other zoonotic pathogens of concern for operators that are transmitted by feral cats include endo- and ectoparasites: hookworms (*Ancylostoma* and *Uncinaria* spp.), tapeworms (*Taenia taeniaeformis* and *Spirometra erinacei*), ringworm, scabies mite (*Sarcoptes scabiei*), protozoa (e.g. *Cryptosporidium* spp.) and the fungal dermatophytes that cause ringworm (Gerhold and Jessup 2013). Feral cats are susceptible to viral infections such as feline immunodeficiency virus, feline panleukopenia virus, feline leukemia virus, feline herpes virus, feline calicivirus and feline coronavirus.

General operating procedures

General operating procedures relevant to the study of feral cats may include visual observations, assessments of signs (scats, tracks) and measurement of dens (Chapter 4), hair collection and camera trapping (Chapter 5) and cage and foothold traps (Chapter 7). Microchips and ear tags may be used to mark cats (Chapter 8) and a range of external telemetry devices (Chapter 9) used to track them. Sedatives and general anaesthetics, tranquiliser darts and poles and collection of blood samples (Chapter 16) may all be used in the study of feral cats. Additionally, several nationally recognised SOPs have been developed specifically for cats (see www.pestsmart.org.au).

REFERENCES

Abbott I (2002) Origin and spread of the cat, *Felis catus*, on mainland Australia, with a discussion of the magnitude of its early impact on native fauna. *Wildlife Research* **29**, 51–74. doi:10.1071/WR01011

Allen BL, Allen LR, Engeman RM, Leung LK-P (2013) Intraguild relationships between sympatric predators exposed to lethal control: predator manipulation experiments. *Frontiers in Zoology* **10**, 39. doi:10.1186/1742-9994-10-39

Allen BL, Higginbottom K, Bracks JH, Davies N, Baxter GS (2015) Balancing dingo conservation with human safety on Fraser Island: the numerical and demographic effects of humane destruction of dingoes. *Australasian Journal of Environmental Management* **22**, 197–215. doi:10.1080/14486563.2014.999134

AVMA (2020) *AVMA Guidelines for the Euthanasia of Animals: 2020 Edition*. American Veterinary Medical Association, Schaumburg, IL.

Bengsen AJ, Algar D, Ballard G, Buckmaster T, Comer S, Fleming PJS, *et al.* (2016) Feral cat home-range size varies predictably with landscape productivity and population density. *Journal of Zoology* **298**, 112–120. doi:10.1111/jzo.12290

Bertelsen MF, Villadsen L (2009) A comparison of the efficacy and cardiorespiratory effects of four medetomidine-based anaesthetic protocols in the red fox (*Vulpes vulpes*). *Veterinary Anaesthesia and Analgesia* **36**, 328–333. doi:10.1111/j.1467-2995.2009.00464.x

Cairns KM, Newman KD, Crowther MS, Letnic M (2021) Pelage variation in dingoes across southeastern Australia: implications for conservation and management. *Journal of Zoology* **314**, 104–115. doi:10.1111/jzo.12875

Carter A, Luck GW, McDonald SP (2012) Ecology of the red fox (*Vulpes vulpes*) in an agricultural landscape. 2. Home range and movements. *Australian Mammalogy* **34**, 175–187. doi:10.1071/AM11041

Catling PC (1988) Similarities and contrasts in the diets of foxes, *Vulpes vulpes*, and cats, *Felis catus*, relative to fluctuating prey populations and drought. *Wildlife Research* **15**, 307–317. doi:10.1071/WR9880307

Coman B (1973) The diet of red foxes, *Vulpes vulpes* L., in Victoria. *Australian Journal of Zoology* **21**, 391–401. doi:10.1071/ZO9730391

Coman B, Robinson J, Beaumont C (1991) Home Range, Dispersal and Density of Red Foxes (*Vulpes vulpes* L.) In Central Victoria. *Wildlife Research* **18**, 215–223. doi:10.1071/WR9910215

Cursino MS, Harriott L, Allen BL, Gentle M, Leung LK-P (2017) Do female dingo–dog hybrids breed like dingoes or dogs? *Australian Journal of Zoology* **65**, 112–119. doi:10.1071/ZO17005

Doherty TS, Davis NE, Dickman CR, Forsyth DM, Letnic M, Nimmo DG, *et al.* (2019) Continental patterns in the diet of a top predator: Australia's dingo. *Mammal Review* **49**, 31–44. doi:10.1111/mam.12139

Dybing NA, Fleming PA, Adams PJ (2013) Environmental conditions predict helminth prevalence in red foxes in Western Australia. *International Journal for Parasitology. Parasites and Wildlife* **2**, 165–172. doi:10.1016/j.ijppaw.2013.04.004

Fancourt BA (2015) Making a killing: photographic evidence of predation of a Tasmanian pademelon (*Thylogale billardierii*) by a feral cat (*Felis catus*). *Australian Mammalogy* **37**, 120–124. doi:10.1071/AM14044

Fancourt BA, Augusteyn JD, Cremasco P, Nolan B, Richards S, Speed J, Wilson C, Gentle MN (2021) Measuring, evaluating and improving the effectiveness of invasive predator control programs: feral cat baiting as a case study. *Journal of Environmental Management* **280**, 111691. doi:10.1016/j.jenvman.2020.111691

Fleming PJS, Allen BL, Allen LR, Ballard G-A, Bengsen A, Gentle MN, *et al.* (2014) Management of wild canids in Australia: free-ranging dogs and red foxes. In *Carnivores of Australia: Past, Present and Future.* (Eds AS Glen and CR Dickman.) pp. 105–149. CSIRO Publishing, Melbourne.

Fleming PJS, Allen LR, Berghout MJ, Meek PD, Pavlov PM, Stevens P, Strong K, Thompson JA, Thomson PC (1998) The performance of wild-canid traps in Australia: efficiency, selectivity and trap-related injuries. *Wildlife Research* **25**, 327–338. doi:10.1071/WR95066

Gerhold RW, Jessup DA (2013) Zoonotic diseases associated with free-roaming cats. *Zoonoses and Public Health* **60**, 189–195. doi:10.1111/j.1863-2378.2012.01522.x

Henderson WR (2009) *Pathogens in Vertebrate Pests in Australia.* Invasive Animals Cooperative Research Centre, Canberra.

Jackson SM (2003) Dingoes. In *Australian Mammals: Biology and Captive Management.* (Ed. SM Jackson.) pp. 381–407. CSIRO Publishing, Melbourne.

Jenkins DJ (2005) Hydatid control in Australia: where it began, what we have achieved and where to from here. *International Journal for Parasitology* **35**, 733–740. doi:10.1016/j.ijpara.2005.03.001

Jenkins DJ, Urwin NAR, Williams TM, Mitchell KL, Lievaart JJ, Armua-Fernandez MT (2014) Red foxes (*Vulpes vulpes*) and wild dogs (dingoes (*Canis lupus dingo*) and dingo/domestic dog hybrids), as sylvatic hosts for Australian *Taenia hydatigena* and *Taenia ovis*. *International Journal for Parasitology. Parasites and Wildlife* **3**, 75–80. doi:10.1016/j.ijppaw.2014.03.001

Jones E, Coman B (1982) Ecology of the feral cat, *Felis catus* (L.), in south-eastern Australia II. Reproduction. *Wildlife Research* **9**, 111–119. doi:10.1071/WR9820111

Legge S, Murphy BP, McGregor H, Woinarski JCZ, Augusteyn J, Ballard G, *et al.* (2017) Enumerating a continental-scale threat: How many feral cats are in Australia? *Biological Conservation* **206**, 293–303. doi:10.1016/j.biocon.2016.11.032

Marks CA, Bloomfield TE (1999) Distribution and density estimates for urban foxes (*Vulpes vulpes*) in Melbourne: implications for rabies control. *Wildlife Research* **26**, 763–775. doi:10.1071/WR98059

Marks CA, Bloomfield TE (2006) Home-range size and selection of natal den and diurnal shelter sites by urban red foxes (*Vulpes vulpes*) in Melbourne. *Wildlife Research* **33**, 339–347. doi:10.1071/WR04058

Marlow NJ, Thomson PC, Algar D, Rose K, Kok NE, Sinagra JA (2000) Demographic characteristics and social organisation of a population of red foxes in a rangeland area in Western Australia. *Wildlife Research* **27**, 457–464. doi:10.1071/WR99035

Martin G, Twigg L, Robinson D (1996) Comparison of the diet of feral cats from rural and pastoral Western Australia. *Wildlife Research* **23**, 475–484. doi:10.1071/WR9960475

McGregor HW, Hampton JO, Lisle D, Legge S (2016) Live-capture of feral cats using tracking dogs and darting, with comparisons to leg-hold trapping. *Wildlife Research* **43**, 313–322. doi:10.1071/WR15134

McNeill A, Leung L, Goullet M, Gentle M, Allen B (2016) Dingoes at the doorstep: home range sizes and activity patterns of dingoes and other wild dogs around urban areas of north-eastern Australia. *Animals (Basel)* **6**, 48. doi:10.3390/ani6080048

Meek PD, Brown SC (2017) It's a dog eat dog world: observations of dingo (*Canis familiaris*) cannibalism. *Australian Mammalogy* **39**, 92–94. doi:10.1071/AM16018

Meek PD, Jenkins DJ, Morris B, Ardler AJ, Hawksby RJ (1995) Use of two humane leg-hold traps for catching pest species. *Wildlife Research* **22**, 733–739. doi:10.1071/WR9950733

Meek PD, Saunders G (2000) Home range and movement of foxes (*Vulpes vulpes*) in coastal New South Wales, Australia. *Wildlife Research* **27**, 663–668. doi:10.1071/WR98030

Molsher R, Newsome A, Dickman C (1999) Feeding ecology and population dynamics of the feral cat (*Felis catus*) in relation to the availability of prey in central-eastern New South Wales. *Wildlife Research* **26**, 593–607. doi:10.1071/WR98058

Molsher RL (2001) Trapping and demographics of feral cats (*Felis catus*) in central New South Wales. *Wildlife Research* **28**, 631–636. doi:10.1071/WR00027

Molsher RL, Gifford EJ, McIlroy JC (2000) Temporal, spatial and individual variation in the diet of red foxes (*Vulpes vulpes*) in central New South Wales. *Wildlife Research* **27**, 593–601. doi:10.1071/WR99015

Morrant DS, Johnson CN, Butler JR, Congdon BC (2017) Biodiversity friend or foe: land use by a top predator, the dingo in contested landscapes of the Australian Wet Tropics. *Austral Ecology* **42**, 252–264. doi:10.1111/aec.12427

Newsome TM, Ballard G-A, Dickman CR, Fleming PJS, van de Ven R (2013) Home range, activity and sociality of a top predator, the dingo: a test of the Resource Dispersion Hypothesis. *Ecography* **36**, 914–925. doi:10.1111/j.1600-0587.2013.00056.x

Paltridge R (2002) The diets of cats, foxes and dingoes in relation to prey availability in the Tanami Desert, Northern Territory. *Wildlife Research* **29**, 389–403. doi:10.1071/WR00010

Robley A, Gormley A, Forsyth DM, Wilton AN, Stephens D (2010) Movements and habitat selection by wild dogs in eastern Victoria. *Australian Mammalogy* **32**, 23–32. doi:10.1071/AM09030

Reilly JS (Ed) (2001) *Euthanasia of Animals Used for Scientific Purposes.* 2nd edn. Australian & New Zealand Council for the Care of Animals in Research and Teaching (ANZCCART), Adelaide.

Roberts MW, Dexter N, Meek PD, Hudson M, Buttemer WA (2006) Does baiting influence the relative composition of the diet of foxes? *Wildlife Research* **33**, 481–488. doi:10.1071/WR05009

Rolls EC (1969) *They All Ran Wild. The Story of Pests on the Land in Australia.* Angus and Robertson, Sydney.

Saunders G, Coman B, Kinnear JE, Braysher M (1995) *Managing Vertebrate Pests: Foxes.* Australian Government Publishing Service, Canberra.

Saunders GR, Gentle MN, Dickman CR (2010) The impacts and management of foxes *Vulpes* in Australia. *Mammal Review* **40**, 181–211. doi:10.1111/j.1365-2907.2010.00159.x

Sharpe T, Saunders G 2008. *A Model for Assessing the Relative Humaneness of Pest Animal Control Methods.* NSW Department of Primary Industries, Orange.

Short J, Calver MC, Risbey DA (1999) The impact of cats and foxes on the small vertebrate fauna of Heirisson Prong, Western Australia. I. Exploring potential impact using diet analysis. *Wildlife Research* **26**, 621–630. doi:10.1071/WR98066

Smith BP (Ed.) (2015) *The Dingo Debate: Origins, Behaviour and Conservation.* CSIRO Publishing, Melbourne.

Smith BP, Morrant DS, Vague A-L, Doherty TS (2020) High rates of cannibalism and food waste consumption by dingoes living at a remote mining operation in the Great Sandy Desert, Western Australia. *Australian Mammalogy* **42**, 230–234. doi:10.1071/AM19033

Van Dyck SM, Strahan R (Eds) (2008) *The Mammals of Australia.* Reed New Holland, Sydney.

White JG, Gubiani R, Smallman N, Snell K, Morton A (2006) Home range, habitat selection and diet of foxes (*Vulpes vulpes*) in a semi-urban riparian environment. *Wildlife Research* **33**, 175–180. doi:10.1071/WR05037

Wilson C (2020) Spatial ecology of feral cats (*Felis catus*) and the implications for effective management. BSc (Hons) thesis. The University of New England, Australia.

23 Bats

Lindy F. Lumsden, Damian S. Morrant, Julie Broken-Brow, Peter H. Holz, Adam McKeown, Sarah J. Gill and Eric Vanderduys

INTRODUCTION

Bats are the only mammals capable of true flight. They are nocturnal and, with the exception of flying-foxes, most species are not visible during the day and are difficult to see and hear. These characteristics present challenges for studying them and, in the past, little was known of their ecology and behaviour. However, in recent decades advances in techniques for researching bats have advanced considerably, leading to a dramatic increase in knowledge of these fascinating, but often maligned animals.

Previously, the order Chiroptera was split into two suborders: the Megachiroptera, which included flying-foxes and fruit bats, and the Microchiroptera, which included a range of echolocating, mostly insect-eating bats. These suborders were colloquially known as megabats and microbats respectively. However, recent phylogenetic research has revised this classification with many of the insectivorous bats now considered more closely related to flying-foxes (Teeling *et al.* 2002). These taxa are now classified as Yinpterochiroptera, represented in Australia by the families Pteropodidae (flying-foxes and fruit bats), Megadermatidae (ghost bat), Rhinonycteridae (leaf-nosed bats), Hipposideridae (leaf-nosed bats) and Rhinolophidae (horseshoe bats); and Yangochiroptera (Emballonuridae (sheath-tailed bats), Molossidae (free-tailed bats), Miniopteridae (bent-winged bats) and Vespertilionidae (evening bats)). However, techniques used to study the horseshoe, leaf-nosed and ghost bats are the same as those for the families in Yangochiroptera. Consequently, for the purposes of this chapter, the requirements of the flying-foxes and fruit bats are considered separately to the smaller, echolocating, insect-eating bats. 'Megabats' and 'microbats' are retained as descriptive terms for this distinction.

MICROBATS

Lindy F. Lumsden, Julie Broken-Brow and Peter H. Holz

Characteristics

Australia supports eight insectivorous microbat families. These families contain 68 extant species found in Australia. However, additional subspecies are recognised, which may be elevated to full species in the future (see Armstrong *et al.* 2020 for a list of species). Microbats range in size from the large (150 g) ghost bat (*Macroderma gigas*) to the minute (3 g) northern pipistrelle (*Pipistrellus westralis*). Flight and foraging behaviour vary with wing morphology and echolocation. Bat diversity increases with latitude, with tropical northern Australia supporting the highest diversity of microbats. Many bat species are common and widespread. However, nine species are listed as threatened nationally under the federal *Environment Protection and Biodiversity Conservation Act 1999*, and many others listed as threatened under state/territory legislation. Other species may also be in decline, but limited data are available on long-term population trends for most species, which precludes comprehensive evaluations of status.

Biology and behaviour

The ability to fly means that this diverse group can exploit a range of niches, and they are found in every Australian habitat (excluding sub-Antarctic islands) from the arid interior, temperate forests and woodlands to tropical rainforests. All Australian microbats are nocturnal, with the echolocation of most not able to be heard by human ears, and are typically concealed in roosts during the day, necessitating a range of study techniques. All species echolocate and many studies now use ultrasonic recordings to identify their distinctive high frequency calls.

Little is known about the life history of many microbat species. They are typically long lived. For example, the southern bent-winged bat (*Miniopterus orianae bassanii*) has been recorded as living up to 22 years (Lumsden and Gray 2001). Most species give birth to one young, although some species have twins. In temperate areas usually only one breeding season occurs per year, with the young born early in summer when insects are abundant. In the tropics, birthing has been recorded throughout the year for some species. Females typically leave their young in the roost while they forage, returning several times during the night to suckle them (Lumsden *et al.* 2021). Species that roost in tree hollows or under bark typically shift roosts every few days, cycling through multiple roosts in a localised area. This involves moving their young between roosts, and so occasionally bats carrying young are trapped. Some cave-roosting species congregate in larger numbers, especially at maternity sites that provide the optimal microclimate for raising young, while other species roost in crevices, caves or overhangs alone or in small groups.

Microbats vary their activity levels daily and seasonally. In both temperate and tropical regions bats often enter short periods of torpor during the day. In temperate areas, these periods of torpor lengthen over winter to conserve energy when prey availability is low, with individuals only leaving their roosts every week or so to forage and/or drink. To prepare for this winter torpor period, individuals gain considerable bodyweight in autumn (sometimes increasing in mass by 50%). Bats can eat large quantities of insects each night, consuming up to half to three-quarters of their own body mass. Activity levels can also vary in response to nightly weather conditions, with cold, wet and windy conditions usually avoided.

Capture and handling

This section outlines the main techniques and considerations for undertaking field-based research on microbats. Increasingly, studies now use more indirect techniques, such as acoustic detection. However, not all questions can be answered using indirect approaches, with trapping, handling and marking procedures still required for many studies.

Harp trapping is the most common technique for catching microbats in Australia. Harp traps are available in two-, three- or four-bank designs (e.g. Faunatech Austbat P/L harp traps). Individuals that do not detect the trap's strands of fine, taut fishing line, collide with the fishing line and slide down into the holding bag where they are largely protected from the elements and predators. Harp traps can be highly effective if set in flight paths or at roosts. If set near roosts, such as cave or mine entrances or buildings, they should be kept under constant supervision so that bats can be removed quickly if large numbers are caught; if set in flight paths they can be left unattended, and just checked several times a night. As the bats are unrestrained (compared to mist-net captures), stress levels for most species appear to be low, and trap death rates are very low. Horseshoe bats and leaf-nosed bats are the exception, with these species more susceptible to stress. If trapping for these species (especially at roosts) individuals need to be removed and released quickly. Traps set at roosts should be positioned several metres from the roost exit itself. Trapping should not be conducted on more than one night at a time when set at roosts, whereas traps set away from roosts can remain in place for two consecutive nights, after which time capture rates usually diminish. Trapping success is greatest on nights that are still, calm and not raining. If the weather turns, particularly if the temperature drops markedly or it starts raining heavily, traps should be closed.

Mist nets are also commonly used to trap bats, especially in the tropics and arid regions of Australia. In arid areas, this technique is often used at water bodies, while in the tropics nets are typically set along flight paths either on the ground or elevated in the canopy. Mist nets should not be set at the entrances to caves or mines unless the number of bats using the roost is known to be low, to avoid the risk of catching more bats than can be quickly extracted. As bats can chew their way out of the fine monofilament nets typically used for catching bats within minutes, or become excessively tangled, mist nets need to be under constant supervision. As bats are removed from the nets they can be hung in cloth bags nearby, ensuring they are off the ground or other areas that risk inadvertent squashing.

Trip lines are used less frequently than harp traps and mist nets, but can be an effective addition to mist netting in arid or semi-arid environments. This technique takes advantage of the surprisingly good swimming ability of microbats, with personnel collecting them after they have tripped on the tightly strung fishing line, fallen into the water and swam to shore. Trip lining should only be used on waterbodies with a surface dimension of a maximum of 30 m in any direction, and with banks clear of vegetation. This technique is most effective on warm nights and should not be undertaken if the temperature is below 15°C.

Acoustic lures are an emerging technique in Australia, and significantly increase trap success for some species (Hill *et al.* 2015). The lures attract bats with social or echolocation calls played from an ultrasonic speaker set near a trap or mist net. Little is known about animal welfare impacts associated with the use of these devices, so further investigations are needed. Guidelines are available for their use in the UK (Collins 2016); until guidelines are developed for Australia, these should be followed. For example, distress calls should not be used in the sequence of calls, the lure should be turned off when personnel are extracting bats from traps or nets, the lure should be moved between traps during the night and should not be left playing for extended periods of time in the one location. Lures should also not be used within 50 m of a known roost. A key benefit of lures is that the required number of the target species can often be caught more quickly, and so can reduce the overall number of trapping nights required.

Bats can be extracted during the day from roosts, such as bat boxes. Bat boxes have a slit entrance at the bottom and a hinged lid at the top. When approaching a box, noise should be minimised to reduce the risk of flushing bats, including noise from people at the base of the tree, and especially when personnel position the ladder against the tree and climb the ladder. Once personnel reach the box, a rag can be used to block the entrance and the bats extracted by hand through the opened lid. As bats tend to roost near the top of the box, personnel should exercise caution when opening and closing the lid to avoid injuring the bats or allowing them to escape (Godinho *et al.* 2020). Bats can be placed into cloth holding bags, with roost mates kept together. After bats have been processed, they can be held until dusk and released to fly near the boxes. During the breeding season, groups of bats that include dependent young need to be returned to their boxes soon after processing. In these situations, the entrance to the box should be blocked with a rag to prevent bats taking flight during the day. The rag can then be quietly removed on dusk, from the ground, by gently pulling on a string attached to the bag. Bat boxes should not be checked more than once a month to reduce disturbance (Godinho *et al.* 2020).

A non-invasive, commonly used technique for studying microbats is acoustic detectors, which can be used passively or actively. When deployed passively, as long as lights are not visible on the detector nor sound audible, and the physical positioning of the detector does not impede flight (e.g. where bats are exiting a cave or mine roost), there is no impact on bats. Detectors can be left in place for weeks to years to record nightly activity levels. When used actively, the observer carries the detector and follows bats or walks a transect. The only potential impact is disturbance from the physical presence of the observer, which can be minimised by limiting movement and keeping lights low and shining onto the ground rather than into the air, unless light is needed to help distinguish species in flight to assist identification (e.g. based on flight patterns and size).

Extensive libraries of locally collected reference calls are required to enable call identification. To collect reference calls, bats are trapped, identified to species and their calls recorded on release. As it is critical to ensure that the known-identity bat is the one being recorded, it needs to be distinguished from any other bats flying at the time. This is often achieved by attaching a light tag (refer to Chapter 9). The tag only needs to remain attached for long enough for the bat to settle down into search-phase call mode, so it can be stuck very lightly to the fur. Alternatively, infrared or thermal cameras can be used to follow the bat. Higher-quality reference calls are obtained when the bat is released into an open space near the trapping site; this also gives the bat time to orientate itself in flight before negotiating obstacles such as trees. The person recording the calls can follow the bat to maximise the length of the call sequence.

Over a third of Australia's microbats roost in caves, or cave-like structures, such as disused mines, tunnels, culverts, rock crevices and rock overhangs. Depending on the purpose of the research and the likely level of disturbance, observations of bats in caves and cave-like structures can be undertaken during the day, on dusk as the bats are exiting, or at night. Entering during the day while the bats are roosting can cause substantial disturbance (Bush *et al.* 2016). Therefore, whenever possible, observations should be undertaken while the bats are emerging from the roost on dusk. Doing so is especially important when the purpose is to estimate population numbers, as fly-out counts are an effective and low-disturbance approach, particularly if large numbers of bats are present in the roost. Typically, the exit flight is filmed using a thermal imaging camera, or infrared camera with infrared illuminators, and hence this can be done with no or very little visible light during the exit flight, leaving the bats to fly out normally. The equipment and observers should be positioned to the side of the cave opening to not impede the flight path. Light is minimised by shrouding all camera screens and keeping any computer monitors shut or filtered with red light.

After the roost exit, observers can enter the cave if required (e.g. to estimate the number of remaining adults, or pups in maternity sites or place acoustic detectors inside the cave). Sometimes it may be necessary to enter the cave during the day. Whenever a cave is entered, during the day or at night, noise should be kept to a minimum and observers should remain inside for as little time as possible. The use of red, rather than white, headlights reduces disturbance further. Photographs of roosting bats should be taken with infrared or thermal cameras (Figure 23.1). White light flash should not be used. Observations should, where possible, avoid causing bats to take flight. When observers leave a cave or mine during the day, care should be taken to ensure that any flying bats between the observers and the exit can fly back past the observers rather than being 'pushed' out of the cave or mine. Observers should crouch at the side of the tunnel with lights off and wait for the bats to fly past. Entry into caves or mines in temperate areas should be avoided where possible during winter, or at least minimised, to prevent disturbance to the bats while they are in extended periods of torpor. Disturbance at these times causes bats to use valuable fat reserves to raise their body temperatures.

For techniques that require capture, bats can be held in cloth bags ~30 × 20 cm in size, with a maximum of 10 bats per bag. Bag seams should be on the outside to prevent claw entanglements in cotton thread. Ideally each bag should contain individuals from just one species, especially if carnivorous species, such as the greater broad-nosed bat (*Scoteanax rueppellii*), are trapped. If multiple species are kept together, they should be clustered with similarly sized species. Gloves should always be worn when handling microbats. Heavy duty nitrile gloves (> 0.19 mm thickness) should be used rather than thinner nitrile gloves (~0.1 mm) as the latter are not puncture proof. For larger species, and when removing bats from mist nets, double gloves are recommended, with a thin leather, suede or cotton glove used over the nitrile glove. Handling should be as gentle and light as possible, cupping the bat in an enclosed hand (Figure 23.2), rather than physically restraining it by pinning its wings back. The more loosely the bat is held, while still being contained within the hand, the quieter it usually sits.

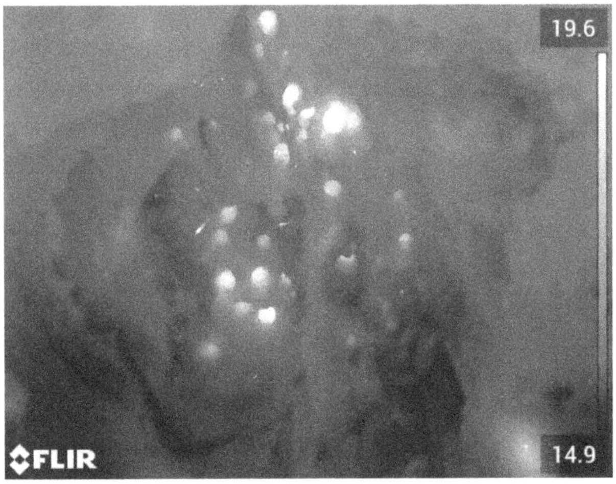

Figure 23.1: A thermal imaging camera reduces disturbance by enabling cave-roosting bats to be observed without any visible light. Photo by Lindy Lumsden.

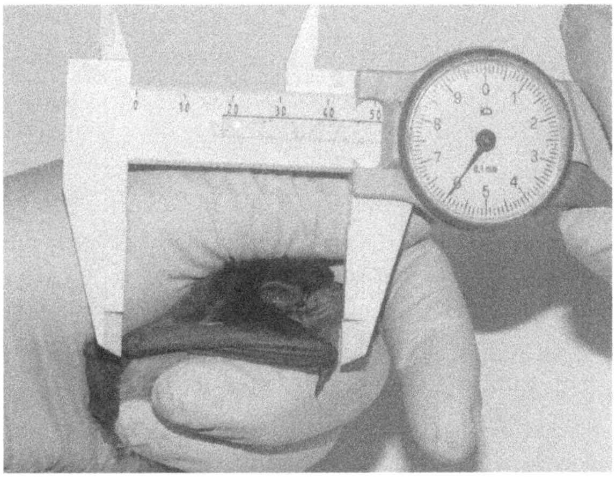

Figure 23.2: Microbats will usually sit calmly, and enable measurements such as the forearm to be taken, if they are loosely enclosed in a cupped hand with the thumb and feet able to grip onto fingers. Photo by Lindy Lumsden.

Individuals are typically identified to species, aged, weighed, measured, and their sex and reproductive condition assessed based on external appearance. This process usually takes only around 2 min per individual. Measurements of ears and wing membranes should only be taken with plastic callipers/rulers to avoid inadvertent punctures. For certain species, any handling may cause death from stress (including, but not limited to, Semon's leaf-nosed bat (*Hipposideros semoni*) and the large-eared horseshoe bat (*Rhinolophus robertsi*)); these species should be identified immediately and released within moments using minimal noise and lights.

A range of methods can be used to mark microbats; the most appropriate technique will depend on the aims of the research. Most techniques may cause some impact on a small proportion of the bats marked. However, if done correctly the risk can be minimised. Ear notching should not be used for marking any microbat species as it may interfere with echolocation.

When it is important to know if a bat has been caught previously over just a short period of time, individuals can be marked temporarily by fur clipping. A small patch of fur can be trimmed (~5 × 5 mm in size), revealing the lower section of the fur sheaths, which are often a different colour to the tips. A small number of individuals can be distinguished by trimming fur in different positions on the back (e.g. left shoulder versus right rump) or alternatively, if identifying individuals is not necessary, all markings can be on the rump. This mark will be obvious for several weeks to several months. The risk of toxicity from other forms of temporary markers such as nail polish or correction fluid is unknown. However, ingestion is likely to occur as bats groom themselves extensively, and because of their small size any toxic effects are likely to be magnified. Therefore, it is recommended that fur clipping is used instead wherever possible.

All bat banding in Australia is coordinated by the Commonwealth Government's Australian Bird and Bat Banding Scheme (ABBBS, www.environment.gov.au/science/bird-and-bat-banding), which provides bands to authorised researchers and requires the submission of the resulting banding data. A permit is only required from the ABBBS if banding is to be undertaken; permits for bat trapping without banding are managed by the state government wildlife agencies. To obtain a bat banding licence, researchers need to have been trained by an A-class bat bander and have a registered project with a sufficiently rigorous design such that the resulting data will be meaningful. Banders need to be experienced not just in the application of a band, but also in how to remove a band that may be causing an injury. Some bat species do not tolerate forearm bands (e.g. members of the Molossidae, Emballonuridae and Rhinolophidae families; Baker *et al.* 2001) and a moratorium is currently in place on the banding of some species.

Passive integrated transponder (PIT) tags are encapsulated microchips, which are injected subcutaneously, enabling individuals to be identified using handheld readers or passively through loop antennas at roosts (e.g. van Harten *et al.* 2019, 2020). The bat should be held gently on a flat surface with its head covered while the tag is injected from the distal edge of the shoulder scruff to rest between the scapulae. Sealing the entrance hole with one drop of surgical adhesive (e.g. 3M Vetbond™) can reduce the risk of tag loss with few negative impacts except for a small patch of fur loss (van Harten *et al.* 2020). PIT tagging can be undertaken safely and quickly by suitably trained individuals, within a few minutes. Bats typically remain calm during the procedure and can fly off in minutes. Anaesthesia is unnecessary to insert a PIT tag and not recommended, to avoid any negative animal welfare impacts associated with anaesthesia and to reduce the length of time the animals need to be held.

Tattooing is a widely accepted method of long-term marking in other mammalian groups. However, for bats, it has been less common because of the prevalence of banding. Recently, with moratoriums on banding some species, researchers have returned to tattooing. Tattoos have been identified on individuals for up to 10 years, and found to be safe, quick and effective at long-term marking of individuals. The bat can be restrained on a flat surface by the handler, with its head covered and its dorsal surface upmost. Its right wing is stretched out and the wrist joint held firmly to prevent any wing movement (Figure 23.3). The tattooist should hold the top of the propatagium flat against a paper towel; this shows any venation to be avoided. This part of the wing membrane is not heavily veined, and no significant bleeding has been recorded from tattooing in this area. The membrane can be prepared with a disinfectant skin preparation (e.g. F10 Skin Prep®) applied with a cotton pad; the skin preparation also acts as a lubricant for the tattoo gun to improve clarity of marks. A unique predetermined number can be tattooed (height of no more than 5 mm) using a human tattoo gun into the central dorsal surface of the propatagium in human-grade 'ultra-black' ink. The

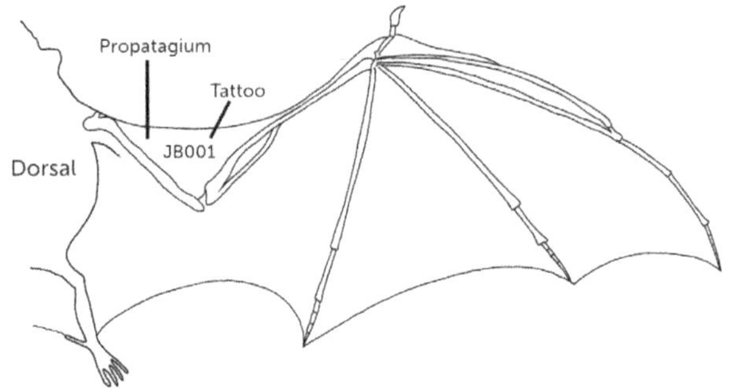

Figure 23.3: Diagram of a bat's right wing showing the position of a tattoo on the dorsal surface of the propatagium (drawing by Julie Broken-Brow and Dirk Mahoney).

pressure applied will affect the 'take up' of the ink and tattoo longevity, so the tattooist must be adequately trained in order to practise the correct pressure. After the number is tattooed, the area should be wiped and disinfected again to remove any excess ink and to prevent infection. The bat can then be immediately released, with the procedure typically taking < 1 min.

Radio tracking can be used for determining roosting and foraging locations. The miniaturisation of transmitters, with some VHF tags now weighing as little as 0.2 g, means that all species can now be tracked. However, larger transmitters are advantageous if mass allows as they can be detected from greater distances and the batteries last longer. Recently, GPS tags have become small enough to use on larger species of microbats, with a combined GPS and VHF package weighing just 1.5 g. GPS transmitters of this size need to be retrieved to download the data, with the VHF transmitter assisting in either finding the shed transmitter or the bat still carrying the transmitter.

Ideally, transmitters should weigh < 5% of the bat's body mass (Aldridge and Brigham 1988). However, bats can carry heavy weights for short periods of time, as illustrated by females carrying large young in flight, and transmitters of up to 10% of the bat's body mass have been used successfully without obvious impacts (Bradbury *et al.* 1979; Lumsden *et al.* 2002). Transmitters should be attached to the dorsal surface of the bat, just below the shoulder blades, after first either trimming a patch of fur the size of the transmitter, or parting the fur to expose some skin. A non-toxic, contact, silicon-based adhesive designed for application to human skin (such as Uro-Bond IV®) should be used. This glue remains rubbery, even when dry, allowing some flex when the bat moves. A thin layer of glue is spread across the base of the transmitter, and on the bat, and after a couple of minutes, once the glue starts to bubble, the two surfaces are brought together. It is important to keep the bat very still during this process so it should be held on a flat surface with its head covered. Once the transmitter is attached, the bat should be held in a cloth bag for a further 15–30 min to ensure the glue has firmly set before it is released. When the transmitter falls off or is groomed off, it typically leaves a bald patch of skin, with the fur subsequently regrowing. Methacrylate glues (e.g. Super Glue™, Vetbond™) are not recommended as they can be more toxic, dry rigidly and so restrict movement, and spread throughout the fur resulting in an even larger bald patch when the transmitter detaches. If the transmitter needs to be removed before it falls off naturally, personnel can use an adhesive remover (e.g. Urocare® or Zoff™ Adhesive Remover). Small VHF transmitters often only stay attached for several days to 2 weeks and so radio-tracked bats should be followed intensively to maximise the amount of data collected (e.g. roosts located every day, individuals followed at night).

Light tags (e.g. Cyalume™ capsules) enable the flight pattern of a bat to be followed without the need for additional lighting. This technique is especially useful when collecting echolocation reference calls to ensure the bat being recorded is the known-identity individual that was released. Tags are usually visible for ~15–20 m. Tags come sealed to prevent any risk of leakage and resulting ingestion of the illumination chemicals. The most commonly used light tags are 2.5 cm long and weigh ~0.2 g, which for most bat species is far less than 5% of their body mass. Tags are attached lengthwise to either the bat's dorsal or ventral surface. Various attachment methods have been used including non-toxic glue, which attaches to the fur and skin, and sticky tape attached to a small tuft of fur. As the bats only need to be seen for a few minutes, a very temporary attachment method is preferable. Tags typically fall off in less than an hour if attached lightly, and often much sooner as individuals can groom them off within minutes after release. Although the attached light could increase the risk of predation by owls, the authors are not aware of any cases of observed predation of a tagged bat.

Genetic samples are usually taken by collecting small amounts of wing tissue, using a small metal biopsy punch (2–4 mm in diameter). The optimal location is close to the body where the wing membrane is thickest and has good healing properties (Weaver *et al.* 2009). The bat is held in one hand with the other used to spread the wing over a pliable plastic mat. A swab of ethanol is used to disinfect the cutting board and both sides of the wing membrane. The biopsy punch and fine forceps are disinfected in ethanol. A second person places the punch over the wing, avoiding veins and tendons, and with a quick push of the punch removes a small amount of tissue. Bat wing membranes heal very quickly from both natural and research-induced wounds, with even large holes seen in wild-caught bats healing quickly. The small holes resulting from genetic sampling heal completely in approximately 2 weeks (Weaver *et al.* 2009). Holes of this size are not considered detrimental to flight. If the procedure is done quickly and carefully, the biopsy can be obtained in around 10 s. No obvious indication of pain has been observed during these procedures if veins and tendons in the wing membrane are avoided. It is not generally thought to be necessary to use local or general anaesthesia when taking bat wing punches. An alternative to wing tissue sampling is the collection of fur. The follicles are required for DNA analysis and so the fur needs to be plucked rather than cut. A tuft of fur is required, and can be collected by pulling out a few shafts at a time from the back of the neck or shoulder region, repeating this action multiple times.

All bats should be released at, or near, the point of capture. Releases should occur at night to avoid the risk of predation by diurnal birds (Speakman *et al.* 1994). In the past, bats have sometimes been placed under bark or in a tree hollow during the day. However, this method should be avoided wherever possible as bats will typically emerge soon after and take flight. Bats should preferably be released on the same night of capture, but if doing so is not possible, they should be held during the day in a cool, humid (particularly for tropical bats) and quiet location and released the following night on dusk. Bats should be warm before attempting release as they may have entered torpor during the day. Personnel should invert the cloth bag in which the bats were held and let them fly off naturally. Some species, especially the free-tailed and sheath-tailed bats, need height to enable them to take flight, so the bag should be held up high on an outstretched arm, and where possible on an elevated platform, such as a vehicle. Long-eared bats will typically fly off quickly while other species, especially free-tailed bats, may take some time. If they are reluctant to fly, despite being warm and active, they can be placed on a tree trunk and allowed to crawl up the trunk to fly off at their own pace. While it might be tempting to throw a bat into the air, this movement should only be undertaken if the bats are very warm and active, but just unwilling to fly, and only if reference calls are required. If the bat is too cold it will fall to the ground. If bats are held for any length of time either during processing or if caught during inclement weather, or if held overnight, they may need to be fed before release, such as with mealworms, to make up for lost foraging opportunities.

Ideally, bats should be processed and released at the site of capture, resulting in no need for transportation. However, if they do need to be transported, they can be housed in securely tied cloth bags and hung from attachment points in the car such as a cargo barrier, or hung in a soft pet carry case with mesh sides. Bats should be kept in well-ventilated areas, and not in enclosed airtight containers (e.g. eskies). Bags of bats should never be placed on a car seat, to avoid the risk of inadvertent crushing. Bats should be kept cool, humid (particularly in the tropics) and out of the sun; during hot weather it may be necessary to use air-conditioning in the car.

If bats need to be temporarily housed before being released back into the wild, they can be kept in enclosures such as soft pet mesh-sided carry cases with materials such as towels or polar fleece to provide hanging spaces for them to roost and hide. If the bats are to be housed for longer than several days, they will need an enclosure large enough to be able to fly, such as a fully enclosed mesh picnic shelter. An enclosure that is ~3.5 × 3.5 × 2 m high will provide sufficient flight space for most species; however, a larger enclosure is needed for the fast-flying free-tailed and sheath-tailed bats. Water should be provided in small dishes that are shallow enough to reduce the risk of drowning. Mealworms are the easiest food to feed microbats. Individuals will initially need to be handfed as most do not recognise non-flying insects as prey. Bats should be fed by gently holding them in one hand and offering them the innards of a mealworm, by breaking off one end and smearing the innards over the bat's lips until it starts to eat. The bat can progressively be encouraged to also consume the exoskeleton of the mealworm. Bats can eat large quantities (e.g. 10–30 mealworms depending on their size and that of the mealworms), so bats should be fed until they are satiated. Feeding once a day should be sufficient as long as the bat is eating well. Mealworms should be supplemented with additives such as Wombaroo Carnivore Mix® to provide a balanced diet. For further details on captive care refer to Jackson (2003).

Veterinary procedures

Analgesia, sedation and anaesthesia

Gaseous rather than injectable anaesthesia is usually used for bats. Microbats can be anaesthetised by administering isoflurane (5% for induction and 2.5% for maintenance) (NHMRC 2014). A small facemask can be constructed from a rubber surgical glove that is punctured to accommodate the bat's face and stretched over the end of a plastic cylinder, such as a syringe case, with the other end connected to the anaesthetic machine hose (see Chapter 16). Sedation is not needed for routine handling or marking of microbats. Analgesics that can be used to relieve pain in injured microbats include butorphanol, buprenorphine and meloxicam (NHMRC 2014).

Blood collection

Blood is typically collected under manual restraint. The skin area should be disinfected first to prevent infection. Blood can be collected via four main methods: (1) by lancing a blood vessel (often the wing veins: propatagial or brachial) and collecting blood in a heparinised haematocrit tube; (2) puncturing the same vessels with a 25 G needle and collecting the resulting blood bead with a micropipette; (3) venipuncture of the median vein (running over the ventral aspect of the humerus) in larger microbats; and (4) venipuncture of the uropatagial vein in the tail membrane of smaller species, using a heparinised or EDTA-coated syringe (Smith *et al.* 2010). Around 5–10% of the blood volume can be safely collected: this equates to approximately 6 µL of blood/gram of bat (see Chapter 16).

Euthanasia

It is very rare that euthanasia is needed when undertaking research on microbats. If required (e.g. in the case of approved specimen collection or terminally injured bat), the preferred method is two-stage chemical euthanasia. Isoflurane-induced anaesthesia is followed by intravenous or intraperitoneal pentobarbitone. Any animal euthanased with pentobarbitone represents a secondary toxicity risk to wild scavengers and should be disposed of via deep burial. Alternatively, an injectable sedative (usually tiletamine-zolazepam) can be administered and, once anaesthetised, the bat can be euthanased by manually applying blunt force trauma, cervical dislocation or decapitation. These techniques must only be undertaken by trained individuals. Hypothermia (e.g. placing the bat in a freezer) should not be used.

Infectious pathogens

Microbats can be subject to several infectious diseases, some of which are zoonotic (Olsson and Woods 2008; Cox-Witton 2019). Australian bat lyssavirus (ABLV) is a fatal (to both humans and bats) zoonosis found in yellow-bellied sheath-tailed bats (*Saccolaimus flaviventris*). Other species of Australian microbats have been recorded with antibodies to the virus, and so all species should be considered potential carriers of the virus. All personnel handling bats must be vaccinated against ABLV (using the rabies vaccination), and maintain the recommended titre level of antibodies.

Ectoparasites, including bat flies, mites, ticks and nematodes, are common but minimal clinical signs are present for bats. Bat fly bites may cause mild skin irritation in people. Histoplasmosis (*Histoplasma capsulatum*) is a fungal disease associated with bat caves and guano. Bats are usually asymptomatic. It is a zoonotic disease with clinical signs in people ranging from no symptoms to a mild flu-like illness, or potentially fatal pneumonia.

The coronavirus that causes COVID-19, while linked to bats overseas, has not been recorded in any Australian wildlife (Wildlife Health Australia 2020a). It is, however, possible that the virus could be transmitted from humans to bats, and appropriate precautions should be taken, including preventing anyone with COVID-19 from handling bats, and regularly cleaning equipment.

White-nose syndrome caused by the fungus *Pseudogymnoascus destructans* is a disease of cave-dwelling microbats that has killed millions of individuals in North America. It is currently believed to be absent from Australia, but could pose a significant risk to temperate cave-dwelling bats if inadvertently introduced (Holz *et al.* 2018).

General operating procedures

Research methods that may be relevant to the study of microbats include direct observation and scat collection/analysis (Chapter 4), acoustic monitoring and camera trapping (Chapter 5), drone observations (Chapter 6), capture with mist nets, harp traps and trip lines (Chapter 7), PIT tagging and tattooing (Chapter 8), radiotelemetry (Chapter 9) and citizen science approaches (Chapter 10). Several veterinary procedures may also be used during the study of microbats (Chapter 16).

MEGABATS

Damian S. Morrant, Adam McKeown, Eric Vanderduys, Lindy F. Lumsden, Peter H. Holz and Sarah J. Gill

Characteristics

Nine species of flying-foxes, fruit bats, tube-nosed bats and blossom bats constitute the Pteropodidae family in Australia. Some of these species also occur extralimitally in New Guinea and offshore islands. The otherwise New Guinean large-eared flying-fox (*Pteropus macrotis*) occurs in the extreme north of Torres Strait, within Australian territory. This is based on unequivocal photographic evidence: there are no specimens from Australia (Van Dyck and Strahan 2008). Megabats are distinguished from insectivorous and carnivorous bats by their external appearance and dietary preference (Olsson and Woods 2008; Van Dyck and Strahan 2008).

Biology and behaviour

Megabats play an important role in the maintenance of biodiversity and ecosystem health. Their mobility makes them effective seed and pollen dispersers, supporting forest maintenance and regeneration, and facilitating healthy gene pools among the plants that they feed on (Fujita and Tuttle 1991; Van Dyck and Strahan 2008). However, their mobility and adaptability to urban environments and the tendency of the four mainland flying-fox species (*Pteropus* spp.) to form large daytime 'camps' can lead to conflict with humans, and active management of the camps is often undertaken (Welbergen *et al.* 2020). Every effort should be taken to minimise disturbance during management activities, and particularly during the breeding season, at times of population stress (e.g. cyclones, heatwaves), and where threatened species may be impacted.

Megabats feed on floral nectar, pollen and fruit. The larger flying-fox species consume both nectar and fruit, depending on seasonal availability, while smaller species, such as little red flying-foxes (*Pteropus scapulatus*) and eastern blossom bats (*Syconycteris australis*), mostly feed on nectar, which they lap up with long, brush-tipped tongues (Van Dyck and Strahan 2008).

Flying-foxes can travel thousands of kilometres a year in search of foraging resources and, in doing so, occupy numerous roosts spread over large areas. For example, a grey-headed flying-fox (*Pteropus poliocephalus*) tracked for 1629 days traversed at least 12 337 km between central Queensland and Melbourne, using 123 roosts during this time (Welbergen *et al.* 2020). Little red flying-foxes are nomadic and move *en masse* from roost to roost covering huge distances as they follow the irregular and patchy flowering of their food trees (Van Dyck and Strahan 2008). Flying-foxes are adaptable and highly mobile, and in many parts of Australia have adopted an urban lifestyle, benefitting from the planting of flowering trees and shrubs, cultivated fruit, and clean and abundant drinking water.

Megabats roost hanging upside-down from their hind feet, with their wings wrapped around their body. The head may be tucked into the chest or hang vertically. Roost selection is driven by availability of suitable roosting trees, fruit and nectar availability within their foraging range, occurrence of parasites, threat from predators, proximity to water, and historical flying-fox occupation (Van Dyck and Strahan 2008). Camps are often located in tall dense vegetation near water bodies. Flying-foxes roost, mate, give birth, and rear their young, in large noisy colonies. These camps may contain thousands of animals and include more than one species. Little red flying-foxes sometimes roost in dense masses in camps of > 1 M animals, occupying trees, dead timber and any other feature that provides a perch.

Animals move among roosts, reusing some over many years. Larger camps can be occupied throughout much of the year, particularly those where bats breed and rear young. Traditionally, these roosts were rarely occupied year-round. However, many urban camps are now used continually, although numbers vary seasonally and regular turnover of individuals occurs (e.g. Meade *et al.* 2019; Department of Agriculture, Water and the Environment 2020). Camps tend to decrease in size as the pup-rearing season progresses and young flying-foxes gain their independence, and can be abandoned from the end of the pup-rearing season until the next breeding season commences. Where this 'window of opportunity' occurs it presents an opportunity to undertake research or management activities such as installation of recording equipment, collection of environmental samples, installation or modification of natural or artificial roosts, or simply undertaking of routine landscape management. As the breeding season progresses, numbers steadily increase, with males noisily contesting courtship territory and courting, and females securing territory where they can bear and raise their young.

The roosting ecology of the smaller megabat species is markedly different from the large ones. Blossom bats typically roost alone among leafy tree canopies in rainforest. They often move roost sites every day within a localised area, and use different areas of the forest seasonally responding to temperature variations (Law 1993). Both blossom bat species can enter torpor when under stress from low temperatures or insufficient food. Eastern tube-nosed bats (*Nyctimene robinsoni*) also typically occupy solitary roosts in canopies; however, they have been observed roosting in groups of up to five in the same tree. They may use some roosts for months and even years (Spencer and Fleming 1989; Van Dyck and Strahan 2008). Bare-backed fruit bats (*Dobsonia magna*) roost in caves, abandoned mines, houses, dense vegetation, and under boulder piles. Roosts are always covered by an overhang or are otherwise in near darkness. In Australia bare-backed fruit bats have not been recorded in colonies greater than ~100, but in Melanesia and Indonesia their camps can number in the thousands (Van Dyck and Strahan 2008).

Megabats invest heavily in reproduction and spend much of their time engaged in courtship and raising offspring. Females care for their young for up to 6 months after birth, depending on the species, and may be pregnant again shortly after young are independent. Females typically give birth to only one young per year. Tube-nosed bats are born from October to December, as are most Australian flying-foxes. Black flying-foxes fit this seasonal breeding pattern in eastern Australia; however, in northern Australia they breed from July to August. Little red flying-foxes are half a year out of phase from the other Australian flying-fox species, with most pups born from April to May. Bare-backed fruit bats are born from September to November. Blossom bats give birth in October or November with sometimes a second birthing peak in February to April (Van Dyck and Strahan 2008).

Capture and handling

The primary means of catching megabats is via mist nets suspended in the canopy or suspended between two telescopic poles (Olsson and Woods 2008). Shorter mist nests are better, as long nets tend to droop. Nets should be situated on the edge or inside the camp in a clear 'lane' that bats in flight would likely follow. Nets should be elevated as high as possible, preferably higher than where the bats are roosting, and should ideally be positioned in dark, shadowy areas so as not to be illuminated by ambient light. For this reason, it is also preferable to avoid catching around the full moon. Catching can be done at dusk or early morning; however, early morning is preferable because the fly-in period is much longer than fly-out, animals have recently fed, and the chance of interactions with bystanders is lower. Personnel should allow room to secure any poles used, and clear an area under the netting lane to minimise tangles. Personnel need to be aware of overhead threats such as powerlines, loose rocks and rotten branches, and implement 'exclusion zones' where warranted, to improve human safety.

Nets must be monitored continuously, as animals will quickly become tangled, requiring excessive time and net cutting to remove the animal. When a bat or any other animal hits the net it should immediately be lowered to ground level. Two people are required to extract bats from nets: one person wearing thick, puncture proof gloves restrains the animal, while the other untangles it from the net. Non-target animals should be checked for injuries and released immediately where appropriate. Target animals should be placed in a pillowcase or similar and hung in a cool, dry place until processing. Ideally animals should be bagged and hung within 5 min of capture. Captured animals should be checked regularly (e.g. every 20 min) for responsiveness or undue stress. Additionally, some species may be captured during the day with a landing net, for example little red flying-foxes, which often roost close to the ground. The animal can be swept into the net, which is then taken to ground level where it is removed and processed in the same way as for captures in mist nets. Mega harp traps, comprising two banks of vertical, nylon-covered wire cables strung between yacht masts, can also be used to catch flying-foxes (Tidemann and Loughland 1993).

Species that are solitary and particularly prone to stress (e.g. tube-nosed bats) should be handled as little as possible and placed in a dark, quiet enclosure to recover after handling, before being released (Olsson and Woods 2008). Megabats must be able to hang upside down from their feet, with clearance beneath their heads, during housing and transport (Figure 23.4a). Where injuries or other circumstances prevent animals from hanging, or cause them to fall from their roost, they should be wrapped in material (e.g. sheet or towel) and supported on a downward angle (Figure 23.4b; Northern Territory Government 2018).

Various combinations of coloured nail varnish can be applied to claws for temporary identification of individuals. Longer-lasting marking methods for megabats include PIT tags, tattooing of the patagium or ears, ear notching, forearm or thumb bands, and necklaces (Jackson 2003). PIT tags should be inserted subcutaneously, on the dorsal

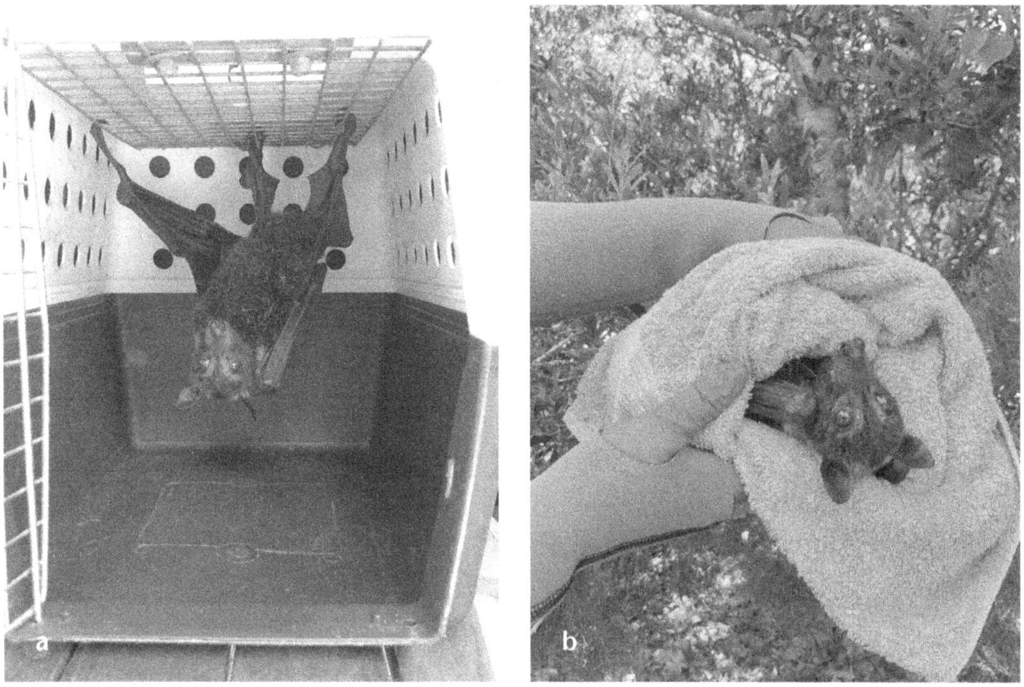

Figure 23.4: (a) A spectacled flying-fox (*Pteropus conspicillatus*) hanging freely in a carry case and (b) handled in a towel with the neck supported, on a downward angle. Photos by tolgabathospital.org.

midline between the scapulae, with the needle directed towards the animal's head. Tissue glue should be applied to the needle hole afterwards, to prevent the PIT tag from falling out (Olsson and Woods 2008). Banding of wildlife in Australia is regulated by the Australian Bird and Bat Banding Scheme (ABBBS), and banders must obtain licences under the ABBBS.

Veterinary considerations

Analgesia, sedation and anaesthesia

Anaesthetic considerations are almost identical to those for microbats. Namely, gaseous anaesthesia is usually administered via facemask. Inhalational induction and maintenance with isoflurane is effective for short procedures (Jonsson *et al.* 2004). Sedation is not usually needed for routine handling or marking of megabats. Analgesics that can be used to relieve pain in injured megabats include butorphanol, buprenorphine and meloxicam (NHMRC 2014). Injections can be administered to bats subcutaneously at the scruff of the neck in a similar manner to domestic animals (see Chapter 16).

Blood collection

Blood is typically collected from the wing veins: propatagial or brachial under anaesthesia (Boardman *et al.* 2020).

Euthanasia

It is rare that euthanasia is needed when undertaking research on megabats. However, if required, the preferred method is the same as for microbats: two-stage chemical euthanasia consisting of isoflurane induction followed by intravenous pentobarbitone. This technique should only be undertaken by trained individuals. Any animal euthanased with pentobarbitone represents a secondary toxicity risk to wild scavengers and should be disposed of via deep burial.

Infectious pathogens

Megabats can carry and transmit several infectious pathogens, some of which are of significance to human health (see Olsson and Woods 2008 for a more comprehensive review of megabat diseases). These pathogens include ABLV, Hendra virus, Menangle virus, *Leptospira* spp. (leptospirosis), and *Salmonella* spp. (salmonellosis). The following discussion is based on the most up-to-date advice available at the time of writing, but could change if additional information becomes available through further research. Readers should obtain current information if it is possible that they will come into contact with bats. The two pathogens, both viruses, that are generally of greatest concern for humans are ABLV and Hendra virus.

Australian bat lyssavirus (ABLV) is closely related to the rabies virus and can be transmitted to humans if infected bat saliva enters the body, usually via a bite or scratch, but also via saliva contact with mucous membranes (eyes, nose or mouth) or pre-existing breaks in the skin. It can cause serious illness, resulting in delirium, paralysis, convulsions and death. ABLV is fatal if not treated before symptoms start, and three people have died as a result of infection since it was first identified in Australia in 1996 (Olsson and Woods 2008). Most records of ABLV are from the four Australian mainland species of flying-foxes. However, any bat in Australia, regardless of species, should be assumed to be a potential carrier of the virus. Although ABLV is more likely to be transmitted by sick or injured bats, healthy animals may also be infectious. Sick, injured or orphaned bats should not be handled, unless absolutely necessary for welfare or research purposes. Personnel who handle bats should wear gloves, have the rabies vaccination, which protects against ABLV, and have their blood tested every 2 years to check their immunity. Anyone potentially exposed to ABLV should wash the wound thoroughly with soap and water for at least 15 min, apply an antiseptic with anti-virus action after washing, and seek medical advice as soon as possible (Olsson and Woods 2008; DoH 2020).

Hendra virus is an emerging zoonosis that causes severe and often fatal disease. To date it has been identified as causing severe and frequently fatal illness in domestic horses and humans. Close contact with nasal and oral secretions during care or necropsy of ill or dead horses is the only known means by which humans can contract Hendra virus. There is no current evidence that Hendra virus can be transmitted directly from flying-foxes to humans, from humans to horses, or that it is airborne. Antibody surveys indicate that all mainland species of Australian flying-foxes may carry the virus. A vaccine has been developed against Hendra virus in horses, and vaccination is considered to be an effective means of mitigating the risk of horses becoming infected and to reduce the likelihood of human exposure (Olsson and Woods 2008; DoH 2020). There is no specific treatment for Hendra virus in humans. Intensive care is provided to infected people, and the administration of monoclonal antibodies is being investigated.

As megabats can inflict scratches and bites that may harbour zoonotic pathogens, they should only be handled by experienced personnel, or under their supervision, and only by people with up-to-date ABLV vaccination and effective immunity (Olsson and Woods 2008). Appropriate personal protection such as gloves, long sleeves, covered footwear, eye protection and safety masks should be worn, and plenty of sanitiser, soap and water should be available. Hats, umbrellas or tarpaulins can be used when working beneath a roost, to shield workers' faces from bat excreta. Heavy-duty, thick nitrile gloves should be worn at all times. Additionally, welders, puncture-proof and/or leather rigger's gloves should be worn to enhance handler safety when handling megabats. Where fine dexterity is required (e.g. when removing a bat from a mist net), fingerless gloves can be worn over a double layer of thick nitrile gloves while a second person with thicker gloves holds the animal (Wildlife Health Australia 2020b). Megabats can also be restrained by being wrapped in a towel, to contain the wings and head. One hand holds the animal's feet and the other its head through the towel.

General operating procedures

Research methods that may be relevant to the study of megabats include direct observation and scat analysis (Chapter 4), acoustic monitoring and camera trapping (Chapter 5), drone observations (Chapter 6), capture with mist nets and harp traps (Chapter 7), PIT tagging and tattooing (Chapter 8), radiotelemetry (Chapter 9), citizen science approaches (Chapter 10) and methods for deterring wildlife (Chapter 11). Several veterinary procedures may also be used during the study of megabats (Chapter 16).

REFERENCES

Aldridge HDJN, Brigham RM (1988) Load carrying and maneuverability in an insectivorous bat: a test of the 5% 'rule' of radio-telemetry. *Journal of Mammalogy* **69**, 379–382. doi:10.2307/1381393

Armstrong KN, Reardon TB, Jackson SM (2020) A current taxonomic list of Australian Chiroptera. Australasian Bat Society website. Version 2020–06–09. <http://ausbats.org.au/species-list/4593775065>.

Baker GB, Lumsden LF, Dettmann EB, Schedvin NK, Schulz M, Watkins D, Jansen L (2001) The effect of forearm bands on insectivorous bats (Microchiroptera) in Australia. *Wildlife Research* **28**, 229–237. doi:10.1071/WR99068

Boardman WS, Baker ML, Boyd V, Crameri G, Peck GR, Reardon T, Smith IG, Caraguel CG, Prowse TA (2020) Seroprevalence of three paramyxoviruses; Hendra virus, Tioman virus, Cedar virus and a rhabdovirus, Australian bat lyssavirus, in a range expanding fruit bat, the Grey-headed flying fox (*Pteropus poliocephalus*). *PLoS One* **15**, e0232339. doi:10.1371/journal.pone.0232339

Bradbury J, Morrison D, Stashko E, Heithaus R (1979) Radio-tracking methods for bats. *Bat Research News* **20**, 9–17.

Bush A, Lumsden L, Ingeme Y (2016) The efficacy and risk of disturbance of monitoring Southern Bent-wing Bats at non-breeding caves. *Australasian Bat Society Newsletter* **46**, 33.

Collins J (Ed) (2016) *Bat Surveys for Professional Ecologists: Good Practice Guidelines*. 3rd edn. The Bat Conservation Trust, London, UK.

Cox-Witton K (2019) Bats. In *Current Therapy in Medicine of Australian Mammals.* (Eds L Vogelnest and T Portas) pp. 555–565. CSIRO Publishing, Melbourne.

Department of Agriculture, Water and the Environment (2020) *National flying-fox monitoring viewer.* Australian Government, Canberra. <https://www.environment.gov.au/webgis-framework/apps/ffc-wide/ffc-wide.jsf>.

Department of Health (DoH) (2020) *Lyssavirus (ABLV).* Australian Government, Canberra. <https://www.healthdirect.gov.au/lyssavirus-ablv>.

Fujita MS, Tuttle MD (1991) Flying foxes (Chiroptera: Pteropodidae): Threatened animals of key ecological and economic importance. *Conservation Biology* **5**, 455–463. doi:10.1111/j.1523-1739.1991.tb00352.x

Godinho LN, Lumsden LF, Coulson G, Griffiths SR (2020) Flexible roost selection by Gould's wattled bats (*Chalinolobus gouldii*) using bat boxes in an urban landscape. *Australian Journal of Zoology* **67**, 269–280. doi:10.1071/ZO20022

Hill DA, Armstrong KN, Barden PA (2015) Preliminary assessment suggests that acoustic lures can increase capture rates of Australian echolocating bats. *Australian Mammalogy* **37**, 104–106. doi:10.1071/AM14019

Holz PH, Lumsden LF, Marenda MS, Browning GF, Hufschmid J (2018) Two subspecies of bent-winged bats (*Miniopterus orianae bassanii* and *oceanensis*) in southern Australia have diverse fungal skin flora but not *Pseudogymnoascus destructans. PLoS One* **13**, e0204282. doi:10.1371/journal.pone.0204282

Jackson S (2003) Bats. In *Australian Mammals: Biology and Captive Management.* (Ed. S Jackson) pp. 297–350. CSIRO Publishing, Melbourne.

Jonsson NN, Johnston SD, Field H, De Jong C, Smith C (2004) Field anaesthesia of three Australian species of flying fox. *The Veterinary Record* **154**, 664. doi:10.1136/vr.154.21.664

Law B (1993) Roosting and foraging ecology of the Queensland blossom bat (*Syconycteris australis*) in north-eastern New South Wales: flexibility in response to seasonal variation. *Wildlife Research* **20**, 419–431. doi:10.1071/WR9930419

Lumsden L, Gray P (2001) Longevity record for a Southern Bent-wing Bat *Miniopterus schreibersii bassanii. Australasian Bat Society Newsletter* **16**, 43–44.

Lumsden LF, Bennett AF, Silins JE (2002) Location of roosts of the lesser long-eared bat *Nyctophilus geoffroyi* and Gould's wattled bat *Chalinolobus gouldii* in a fragmented landscape in south-eastern Australia. *Biological Conservation* **106**, 237–249. doi:10.1016/S0006-3207(01)00250-6

Lumsden LF, Griffiths SR, Silins JE, Bennett AF (2021) Roosting behaviour and the tree-hole requirements of bats: insights from the lesser long-eared bat *Nyctophilus geoffroyi* and Gould's wattled bat *Chalinolobus gouldii* in south-eastern Australia. *Australian Journal of Zoology*, online early. doi:10.1071/ZO20072

Meade J, van der Ree R, Stepanian PM, Westcott DA, Welbergen JA (2019) Using weather radar to monitor the number, timing and directions of flying-foxes emerging from their roosts. *Scientific Reports* **9**, 10222. doi:10.1038/s41598-019-46549-2

National Health and Medical Research Council (NHMRC) (2014) *A Guide to the Care and Use of Australian Native Mammals in Research and Teaching.* National Health and Medical Research Council, Canberra.

Northern Territory Government (2018) *Caring for flying foxes.* Northern Territory Government, Darwin. <https://nt.gov.au/environment/animals/caring-for-wildlife/caring-for-flying-foxes>.

Olsson A, Woods R (2008) Bats. In *Medicine of Australian Mammals.* (Eds L Vogelnest and R Woods) pp. 465–502. CSIRO Publishing, Melbourne.

Smith CS, De Jong CE, Field HE (2010) Sampling small quantities of blood from microbats. *Acta Chiropterologica* **12**, 255–258. doi:10.3161/150811010X504752

Speakman JR, Lumsden LF, Hays GC (1994) Predation rates on bats released to fly during daylight in south-eastern Australia. *Journal of Zoology* **233**, 318–321. doi:10.1111/j.1469-7998.1994.tb08593.x

Spencer HJ, Fleming TH (1989) Roosting and foraging behavior of the Queensland Tube-nosed Bat, *Nyctimene robinsoni* (Pteropodidae): Preliminary radio-tracking observations. *Wildlife Research* **16**, 413–420. doi:10.1071/WR9890413

Teeling EC, Madsen O, Van Den Bussche RA, de Jong WW, Stanhope MJ, Springer MS (2002) Microbat paraphyly and the convergent evolution of a key innovation in Old World rhinolophoid microbats. *Proceedings of the National Academy of Sciences of the United States of America* **99**, 1431–1436. doi:10.1073/pnas.022477199

Tidemann CR, Loughland RA (1993) A harp trap for large megachiropterans. *Wildlife Research* **20**, 607–611. doi:10.1071/WR9930607

Van Dyck S, Strahan R (2008) Suborder Megachiroptera: megabats. In *The Mammals of Australia* (Eds S Van Dyck and R Strahan) pp. 424–447. Reed New Holland, Sydney.

van Harten E, Reardon T, Lumsden LF, Meyers N, Prowse TAA, Weyland J, Lawrence R (2019) High detectability with low impact: optimizing large PIT tracking systems for cave-dwelling bats. *Ecology and Evolution* **9**, 10916–10928. doi:10.1002/ece3.5482

van Harten E, Reardon T, Holz PH, Lawrence R, Prowse TAA, Lumsden LF (2020) Recovery of southern bent-winged bats (*Miniopterus orianae bassanii*) after PIT-tagging and the use of surgical adhesive. *Australian Mammalogy* **42**, 216–219. doi:10.1071/AM19024

Weaver KN, Alfano SE, Kronquist AR, Reeder DM (2009) Healing rates of wing punch wounds in free-ranging little brown myotis (*Myotis lucifugus*). *Acta Chiropterologica* **11**, 220–223. doi:10.3161/150811009X465866

Welbergen JA, Meade J, Field HE, Edson D, McMichael L, Shoo LP, Praszczalek J, Smith C, Martin JM (2020) Extreme mobility of the world's largest flying mammals creates key challenges for management and conservation. *BMC Biology* **18**, 101. doi:10.1186/s12915-020-00829-w

Wildlife Health Australia (2020a) COVID-19 and Australian bats – information for bat carers, researchers and others interacting with bats. <https://www.wildlifehealthAustralia.com.au/Portals/0/Documents/ProgramProjects/COVID-19_Aust_bat_carers_researchers_Oct2020.pdf>.

Wildlife Health Australia (2020b) Personal protective equipment (PPE) information for bat handlers. <https://wildlifehealthAustralia.com.au/Portals/0/Documents/ProgramProjects/PPE_Info_for_Bat_Handlers.pdf>.

24 Ungulates, lagomorphs and rodents

Tasmin L. Rymer, Andrew J. Bengsen, Misha K. Rowell, Jordan O. Hampton, Phoebe A. Burns, Cara Penton, Helen P. Waudby, Tarnya E. Cox, Aaron Greenville and Corinne Alberthsen

INTRODUCTION

Ungulate species found in Australia include horses (*Equus caballus*), donkeys (*E. asinus*), Asian water buffalo (*Bubalis bubalis*), cattle (*Bos tarus/indicus*), goats (*Capra aegagrus hircus*), six deer species (Cervidae), dromedary camels (*Camelus dromedarius*) and pigs (*Sus scrofa*). All of these species, except for the dromedary camel, are hoofed mammals, and none are native to Australia. Lagomorphs are small mammals defined by their unique dentition, namely the two pairs of continuously growing incisors on the upper jaw. The lagomorph species found in Australia are the European hare (*Lepus europaeus*) and the European rabbit (*Oryctolagus cuniculus*), neither of which is native to Australia. Rodents are characterised by a single pair of continuously growing incisors on the upper and lower jaws. Currently, Australia has at least 54 species of native rodents (across seven groups) and four species of introduced rodents.

TERRESTRIAL UNGULATES

Andrew J. Bengsen and Jordan O. Hampton

Characteristics

Ungulates comprise a diverse monophyletic group of seven extant orders, including hoofed mammals, elephants and cetaceans. All terrestrial ungulates in Australia, except the dromedary (referred to as the camel), are hoofed mammals. They range in size from the goat (c. 25–40 kg) to the Asian water buffalo (up to 1200 kg). The body form of the pig is considered most similar to that of ancestral ungulates and has the least specialised morphology. Many ungulate species are behaviourally and morphologically adapted to avoid predators. They typically form herds, and many species display highly vigilant or flighty behaviours. Long, narrow limbs with reduced distal mass and high flexion provide speed through both long stride length and rapid stride rate. Most terrestrial ungulates in Australia are descended from domestic stock.

Biology and behaviour

Home range and movement characteristics vary greatly among, and sometimes within, species. Pigs, for example, tend to have small home ranges and sedentary habits where resources are plentiful and reliable (Saunders and Kay 1996; Mitchell *et al.* 2009). In contrast, camels usually range over large areas, in patterns consistent with searching for and exploiting ephemeral resources, especially water (Wells and Lethbridge 2020). Some species in highly seasonal habitats, such as buffalo in northern Australian floodplains or pigs and deer in alpine areas, concentrate their activity in different habitats at different times of the year (Saunders and Kay 1996; Campbell *et al.* 2020; Davies *et al.* 2020).

All ungulates are herbivorous and are either mostly grazers or browsers. Pigs are more omnivorous than other ungulates, commonly consuming animal material, such as carrion or small ground-dwelling fauna. The bovids, deer and camels are ruminants, whereas horses, donkeys and pigs are monogastric and rely on hindgut fermentation or large volumes of food to achieve adequate nutrition.

Ungulates in Australia are social animals. Most occur in herds that can reach > 100 individuals when conditions and resources are suitable, although groups of < 20 individuals are common in many species. Sambar deer (*Rusa unicolor*) are mostly encountered alone or in small groups. Social organisation and group structure can vary throughout the year, most predictably in species with strong seasonal breeding (e.g. fallow, *Dama dama*, and red deer, *Cervus elaphus*). In these species, adults are sexually segregated throughout much of the non-breeding season, and males and females often use different habitat types (Bentley 1998). Most species use vocalisations or gland secretions for communication.

Capture and handling

The invasive nature of terrestrial ungulate species in Australia influences all aspects of their management, including the reasons why they are captured or killed, and the methods used to do so. Australian ungulates are captured for a variety of reasons, including fitting of telemetry devices, killing (culling) and administration of fertility control. Terrestrial ungulates are transported and housed less frequently than other Australian mammals, but are occasionally transported and slaughtered (e.g. horses), and/or used as 'Judas' animals (i.e. individuals of a gregarious species tracked via telemetry to facilitate culling of their social groups) (Hampton and Hyndman 2019). Consequently, little published information is available on nutrition/feeding for terrestrial ungulates held in captivity in Australia, with the exception of livestock contexts, including for some deer species (e.g. chital deer, *Axis axis*; English 1992).

Compared to native Australian mammal species (e.g. macropods), ungulates are difficult to capture because of their larger size and typically cryptic behaviour (they are difficult to detect until present in high numbers). However, some large ungulate species have been managed as livestock (e.g. cattle; Asian water buffalo), leading to the development of commercially viable capture methods. Of all Australian terrestrial ungulates, deer are the most difficult to capture, with some species (e.g. sambar deer) lacking any recognised capture methods that have been successfully applied in Australia (Hampton *et al.* 2019). For many larger species, the use of chemical restraint is often required because of the potential for human injury during handling. Bovids and deer have horns or antlers that can make handling them particularly dangerous. Aircraft play a prominent role in capture, particularly for large species inhabiting sparsely treed habitats (Boardman *et al.* 2014a; Bengsen *et al.* 2021). Helicopters are used widely for mustering, darting and net gunning. Capture methods commonly used include cage trapping (Figure 24.1a), aerial darting (Figure 24.1b), aerial net gunning (Figure 24.1c) and mustering (Figure 24.1d).

Several procedural documents exist to guide the capture of commonly managed ungulates in Australia (see www.pestsmart.org.au). However, the same limitations that apply to all procedural documents are relevant here (Hampton *et al.* 2016). Of note, some standard operating procedures (SOPs) cite peer-reviewed studies as validation of the capture methods they prescribe (e.g. Boardman *et al.* 2014a, b), but others do not (e.g. Sharp 2012) and recommend capture methods for which substantial animal welfare concerns exist (e.g. use of dogs to capture introduced pigs; Orr *et al.* 2019). In other cases, SOPs prescribe capture methods associated with contested animal welfare outcomes that are illegal for research, but dubiously legal for operational use (i.e. use of neuromuscular blocking agents to capture 'Judas' donkeys; Hampton and Hyndman 2019).

Veterinary considerations

Sedation and anaesthesia

Chemical immobilisation (Table 24.1) is widely used for capture of terrestrial ungulates via darting. Immobilisation regimes are typically a combination of α-2 agonist sedatives (e.g. xylazine), dissociative anaesthetics (tiletamine and ketamine) and benzodiazepine tranquilisers (e.g. zolazepam). The same veterinary chemicals are also often administered via hand injection (or syringe poles) to ungulates under physical restraint. For example, pigs are often immobilised this way to fit telemetry devices once caught in cage traps (Figure 24.1a; Mitchell *et al.* 2009). Other drug classes are used less for capture because of difficulty of access associated with prohibitive scheduling (i.e. Schedule 9) for the potent opioids (e.g. etorphine). Neuromuscular blockers are still used for operational capture of ungulates in at least one context ('Judas'

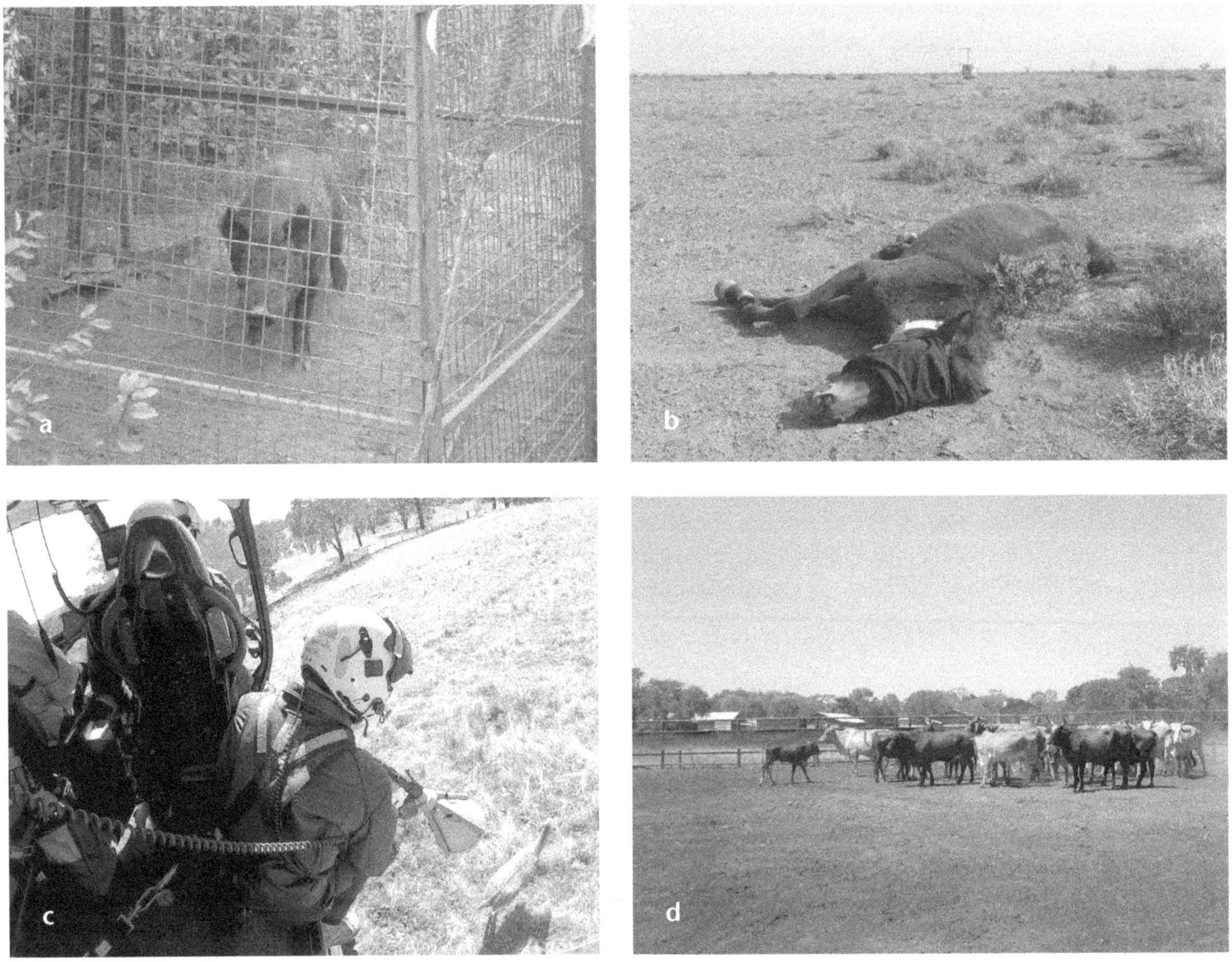

Figure 24.1: Examples of methods used to capture wild terrestrial ungulates in Australia. (a) Cage trapping of a pig (*Sus scrofa*). (b) Aerial darting of a horse (*Equus caballus*). (c) Aerial net gunning of a fallow deer (*Dama dama*). (d) Mustering and yarding of feral cattle (*Bos taurus/indicus*). Photos a, b and d by Jordan O. Hampton; photo c by Andrew J. Bengsen.

donkeys), but this method is associated with substantial animal welfare concerns (Hampton and Hyndman 2019). Few veterinary chemicals are used for wild ungulates outside of immobilisation, with uncommon exceptions such as trials of fertility control.

Blood collection

Blood is typically collected from the tail vein of physically restrained ungulates, the jugular vein of anaesthetised animals (Figure 16.3d) and from the heart of recently killed animals immediately after death (see Chapter 16).

Euthanasia

Physical euthanasia is most commonly applied to wild ungulates. Shooting is most widely used as it can be used safely for recumbent or mobile animals. Most shooting methods used for euthanasia recommend aiming for the brain of the animal from a short distance. Rimfire and centrefire rifles (bullets) and shotguns (shot) have been used for this purpose. Captive bolts are used widely for killing livestock and have been used for wild ungulates (Hing *et al.* 2019), but challenges are associated with restraining dangerous animals unless they are first chemically immobilised. Captive bolts allow physical euthanasia to be applied without the safety risks associated with the firing of projectiles. They rely on tethered ('captive') projectiles that are applied directly to the animal's cranium. Chemical euthanasia is rarely used for wild ungulates because of the difficulties associated with non-veterinarians accessing pentobarbitone and environmental toxicity risks associated with large animals that are difficult to bury.

Table 24.1: Published immobilisation dosages for some Australian terrestrial ungulates.

Hampton (2019).

Species	Drug	Dose (mg/kg)	Route of administration
Asian water buffalo	Thiafentanil Azaperone	0.02 0.2	Helicopter darting
Banteng	Detomidine Tiletamine–zolazepam	0.14 3.0	Syringe pole
Cattle	Xylazine Ketamine	0.6 3.6	Ground-based darting
Chital deer	Medetomidine Tiletamine–zolazepam	0.15 2.6	Helicopter darting
Donkey	Medetomidine Ketamine	0.14 4.1	Helicopter darting
Dromedary camel	Medetomidine Ketamine	0.2 2.5	Helicopter darting
Fallow deer	Xylazine Ketamine	4.0 4.0	Hand injection in trapped animals
Goat	Xylazine	1.7	Helicopter darting
Hog deer	Haloperidol	0.6	Hand injection in trapped animals
Horse	Medetomidine Tiletamine–zolazepam	0.15 3.6	Ground-based darting
Pig	Xylazine Tiletamine–zolazepam	2.2 2.2	Syringe pole
Red deer	Xylazine Tiletamine–zolazepam	4.2 2.8	Ground-based darting
Rusa deer	Xylazine Carfentanil	0.5 0.1	Hand injection in trapped animals

Infectious pathogens

Infectious diseases in wild ungulates are well known because of their capacity to transmit agents to commercial livestock (Cripps *et al.* 2019). Much attention has focused on the capacity of Australia's wild ungulates to act as reservoirs for exotic diseases of economic importance to Australia's livestock industries, such as foot and mouth disease. Surveys of disease prevalence have been completed for some wild ungulate populations. Fortunately, Australia is free of most of the world's most damaging diseases of wild ungulates, including chronic wasting disease (deer) and African swine fever (pigs). However, some pathogens of zoonotic potential are found in wild Australian ungulates, including the bacterium causing Q fever (*Coxiella burnetii*; all ungulates) and brucellosis (*Brucella suis*; pigs; Orr *et al.* 2019). One other context in which wild ungulates may be the source of zoonotic diseases involves faecal contamination of peri-urban human drinking water catchments by introduced pigs and sambar deer (Bennett *et al.* 2015).

General operating procedures

Several research methods and procedures relevant to studying terrestrial ungulates are covered in more detail elsewhere in the book, including direct observation (with or without spotlighting), scat collection and evaluation of tracks and traces (Chapter 4), camera and hair trapping (Chapter 5), and aerial survey methods (Chapter 6). Corrals and pen traps are detailed in Chapter 7. Marking methods typically include ear tagging (Chapter 8) and telemetry devices attached with collars are sometimes deployed to study movements (Chapter 9). Citizen science approaches could also apply to the study of ungulates in some cases (Chapter 10). A range of veterinary procedures apply to the study of ungulates, including capture with tranquiliser guns and poles (Chapter 16).

LAGOMORPHS (RABBITS AND HARES)

Misha K. Rowell, Tasmin L. Rymer and Tarnya E. Cox

Characteristics

Lagomorphs have two pairs of continuously growing incisors on the upper jaw, 16 deciduous teeth and 28 permanent teeth separated from the incisors by a large diastema. They lack canines. Two species have been introduced to Australia: the European hare and the European rabbit. Hares are larger than rabbits, both in body length (up to 750 mm compared to 400 mm) and mass (up to 5 kg compared to 2 kg). Hares are a grizzled yellow-brown colour on the back, and rufous on the shoulders, legs, neck and throat, giving an overall flecked appearance. They have a white belly, and black-tipped tail and ears. Their ears and legs are long, and hares have a high-standing gait. In contrast, rabbits are most commonly grey-brown above; however, black and ginger morphs can occur. Rabbits have a pale belly, lack black tips on their ears, and have shorter ears and legs than hares. The feet of rabbits are covered in hair.

Biology and behaviour

Hares are found in southern and eastern parts of South Australia, Victoria, the Australian Capital Territory, New South Wales and Queensland, and also in northern Tasmania. Rabbits are found in all states and territories, but have a limited distribution in the very northern regions and central Western Australia. Both species prefer habitats with mild, wet winters and hot, dry summers, although both are highly adaptable, and can occupy other climactic zones (Stott and Harris 2006). Favoured areas comprise well-drained, loosely compacted soils. Both species are herbivorous, feeding primarily on foliage, berries, vegetables, seeds, grains, twigs and nuts.

Hares are mostly solitary, with a home range up to 4 km. They do not use warrens/burrows, instead resting in depressions/forms in the ground among long grasses, rocks or logs. Under high densities, rabbits live in territorial social groups comprising a dominant male and multiple females (Gibb 1990). Rabbits are either surface dwelling, using above-ground harbours, such as felled timber and dense thickets (e.g. lantana), or may occupy warrens. Using warrens helps rabbits avoid predators and temperature extremes. Rabbits can also live under buildings and machinery, and rubbish piles. Rabbits can be highly territorial, particularly during the breeding season. Little social interaction occurs between adults of different warrens, and sometimes even within warren systems (Marsh *et al.* 2011). Juvenile rabbits are more social, both within their home warren and across warren systems. Territories of social groups of rabbits are small (< 1 ha). Under low densities, and outside of the breeding season, group living and territoriality decline. Dominant females build nests near the middle of a warren, while subordinates make isolated burrows away from the warren (Gibb 1990).

Mean monthly pregnancy rate and litter size of hares peaks in spring and declines over summer (Stott and Harris 2006). Body mass and condition determine the onset of sexual maturity, but most females reproduce at 6–7 months old (Stott and Harris 2006). Hares have an average of 2.8 leverets. Fertility declines with age, but litter size increases (Stott and Harris 2006). Leverets are precocial at birth, but suckle until they are 38–58 days (Stott and Harris 2006). Rabbits are fertile at 3–4 months, and typically produce one litter (three to nine kits) per month during the breeding season (15–45 young per year; Gibb 1990). Early litter sizes are small (one to three kits), with full litter size (five to nine kits) not achieved until individuals are ~10 months of age. Kits remain in the nest for 20–21 days until weaned (Gibb 1990; see also Chapter 4).

The hare population in Australia is at a low density, but has historically reached plague proportions (Stott and Harris 2006). Hares live up to 12 years (Hackländer and Schai-Braun 2018). Rabbits can live up to 9 years (Macdonald and Barrett 2001). In Australia, rabbits experience a 60–80% mortality rate (adults and juveniles, respectively), with most juvenile rabbits not surviving 12 months. The main factors influencing mortality include climactic extremes, food availability, predation and disease (e.g. myxomatosis, rabbit haemorrhagic disease and coccidiosis).

Capture and handling

Lagomorphs can be trapped using padded-jaw traps, soft net traps and wire cage traps (e.g. Wiretainers Pty Ltd: 31 × 31 × 61 cm) baited with oats, diced carrot or cruciferous vegetables. Traps must be located in safe areas and conditions (e.g. not exposed to severe weather), and checked at least once daily. For transport, an individual can be placed in a cage covered by a bag/fabric to minimise stress or placed into calico/cotton bags if transportation is for a short distance. Trapping and transporting should proceed as quickly as possible to reduce injury/stress. Lagomorphs can be handled by scruffing the neck firmly with one hand, and supporting the hindquarters and back with the other. Alternately, the animal can be handled/carried by placing the head between the arm/elbow and body while maintaining control of, and supporting, the hindquarters.

Rabbits can be housed individually (in hutches) or in groups (in pens; maximum of 15 individuals). Wild adult rabbits should never be housed with individuals from outside of their social group (warren) and rabbits from within the same warren should be monitored closely for signs of aggression. Hares should be housed individually. Rabbits and hares kept in captivity should be provided daily with:

- water *ad libitum*
- 110–150 g food and hay
- enrichment (e.g. shelters)
- bedding materials (e.g. wood shavings, paper or wood pellets or straw)
- a visual health inspection.

Cages and pens should be cleaned weekly. When housed individually, animal identification tags can be used. In group housing, individuals may need to be marked. Marking methods are as described for rodents.

Veterinary considerations

Analgesia, sedation and anaesthesia

Injectable and gaseous anaesthesia are commonly used for lagomorphs. Injectable agents used for lagomorphs include the benzodiazepine tranquiliser diazepam, the neuroleptic acepromazine, the α-2 agonist xylazine and the dissociative anaesthetic ketamine. Intramuscular injections should be given in the quadriceps muscles, but multiple injections can be given in the dorsal thorax/lumbar area. If multiple injections are given, ≥ 2 cm should be left between injection sites (University of South Florida 2018). Intramuscular injections typically require 10–15 min to take effect, and duration of sedation should not exceed 1 h (University of South Florida 2018).

Gaseous anaesthesia using isoflurane and following standard procedures (e.g. Curtin University 2018) can also be safely used (Chapter 16). For anaesthesia, a heating pad is recommended to prevent hypothermia, and ophthalmic ointment can be used to protect the eyes. Where possible, the animal should be weighed before anaesthesia to allow dosages to be accurately determined (Curtin University 2018).

In captivity, animals should be kept on oxygen after anaesthesia until breathing normally. On waking, animals should be moved to a recovery cage. Food, water and treats should be provided. Metoclopramide can be used to prevent gut stasis, which can be life threatening (Curtin University 2018).

Local anaesthetics such as lignocaine and bupivacaine can be injected intradermally. Bupivacaine provides up to 8 h of local analgesia, while lignocaine spray is traditionally used as a local anaesthetic before venipuncture (Curtin University 2018).

Blood collection

Blood can be collected from the ear of sedated or physically restrained animals. The ear should be cleaned using warm water and a chlorhexidine solution, and then tension applied before inserting a 24–20 G angiocatheter bevel-up into the blood vessel directed towards the ear base. The amount of blood drawn depends on the body mass (see Chapter 16). After the catheter is removed, pressure should be applied to the site until bleeding has stopped (University of South Florida 2018).

Euthanasia

Several methods can be used to euthanase rabbits and hares. In the field, shooting is most widely used, with rimfire rifles and shotguns effective. If the animal is in captivity, chemical methods can be more readily used because of their small body size. However, caution needs to be taken to minimise pain and stress before euthanasia. Two-stage chemical euthanasia is widely used, typically consisting of injectable sedation followed by intravenous pentobarbitone. Any animal euthanased with pentobarbitone represents a secondary toxicity risk to wild scavengers and should be disposed of via deep burial. Cervical dislocation can be used on animals < 1 kg.

Infectious pathogens

Lagomorphs are susceptible to several infectious diseases (Table 24.2). *Myxoma* virus, which causes myxomatosis, is fatal, although wild rabbits in some parts of Australia have developed a degree of resistance (Gibb 1990). This virus is no longer released as a biocontrol agent (Williams *et al.* 1995), although it still circulates through the wild rabbit population. *Myxoma* virus is transmitted by biting insects, and no vaccine is available in Australia. Rabbit haemorrhagic disease virus (RHDV), which causes rabbit

Table 24.2: Known infectious agents in lagomorphs, including potential zoonoses.

Causative agent	Disease/illness	Spread	Zoonotic
Viruses			
Lagovirus spp.	Rabbit haemorrhagic disease	Aerosols	N
Myxoma virus	Myxomatosis	Biting insects	N
Bacteria			
Brucella spp.	Brucellosis	Oral route or direct contact	Y
Francisella tularensis	Tularemia	Biting insects or direct contact	Y
Listeria monocytogenes	Listeriosis or febrile gastroenteritis	Oral route	Y
Yersinia pseudotuberculosis	Pseudotuberculosis/Yersinosus	Faecal-oral route	Y

haemorrhagic disease (also known as rabbit calicivirus disease) is used to control wild rabbits. Outbreaks can be caused by deliberate release of the virus through baited carrots or oats during control programs, or by the transmission of wild circulating strains by bush and blow flies (*Calliphoridae*). A vaccine for RHDV is available for domestic rabbits.

Lagomorphs also harbour internal and external parasites (Wibbelt and Frölich 2005). The zoonotic potential is indicated for each, although zoonotic potential is unknown or unreported for many (Table 24.3).

General operating procedures

Research methods and procedures relevant to studying lagomorphs include cage trapping (Chapter 7), microchipping and tattooing (Chapter 8), tracking methods (Chapter 9), citizen science approaches depending on study objectives (Chapter 10) and a range of veterinary procedures (Chapter 16).

RODENTS

Tasmin L. Rymer, Misha K. Rowell, Phoebe A. Burns, Cara Penton, Aaron Greenville, Helen P. Waudby and Corinne Alberthsen

Characteristics

Rodents are characterised by a single pair of continuously growing incisors on the upper and lower mandibles. The front outer surface of these incisors possesses a thick coating of enamel while the back is coated by softer dentine, which causes them to wear to a sharpened point over time. Rodents lack canines and, in some cases, premolars, and usually have three molars. A large diastema separates the incisors and cheek teeth. Australian rodents show great variation in mass (e.g. < 10 g for the delicate mouse, *Pseudomys delicatulus*, and around 1275 g for rakali or water rats, *Hydromys chrysogaster*; Van Dyck and Strahan 2008).

All Australian rodents fall within the subfamily Murinae (Breed and Ford 2007). In Australia, at least 68 native species (in 14 genera) existed before the arrival of Europeans (c. 1600). Since then, around 14 species have become extinct, including the recent extinction of the Bramble Cay mosaic-tailed rat (*Melomys rubicola*) in 2016. The extant species are allocated to seven groups (Roycroft 2020; Roycroft *et al.* 2020).

Biology and behaviour

Australian rodents occupy all habitats, including deserts, rainforests, grasslands and alpine areas (Van Dyck and Strahan 2008). Some species are dietary specialists (e.g. rakali), while others, like the canefield rat (*Rattus sordidus*), are dietary generalists. Some species, like giant white-tailed rats (*Uromys caudimaculatus*), are solitary, while others, like western pebble-mice (*P. chapmani*), are social (Van Dyck and Strahan 2008). Home-range sizes, breeding, reproduction and behaviour are also highly diverse (Van Dyck and Strahan 2008). Many desert-dwelling species are irruptive in the months following above-average rainfall (Greenville *et al.* 2012), and historically some species, such as the long-haired rat (*R. villossisimus*), were reported to reach 'plague' proportions (Greenville *et al.* 2013). Numbers fall as predation rates increase and the food produced by rainfall recedes. Outside of these years (which can be few and far between), many desert species can be difficult to detect, persisting only in small numbers in refuge habitats (Greenville *et al.* 2013; Pavey *et al.* 2017).

Table 24.3: Known internal and external parasites of lagomorphs, indicating zoonotic potential.

Parasite		Zoonotic potential
Internal		
Amoebae	*Entamoeba cuniculi*	Unknown
Cestodes	*Echinococcus granulosus; Taenia serialis*	Y
	Taenia pisiformis	Unknown
Coccidia	*Eimeria exigua; E. flavescens; E. intenstinalis; E. irresidua; E. magna; E. media; E. neoleporis; E. perforans; E. piriformis; E. stiedae; Sarcocystis cuniculi; S. leporum*	Unknown
	Toxoplasma gondii	Y
Flagellates	*Chilomastix cuniculi; Enteromonas* sp.; *Giardia duodenalis; Monocercomonas cuniculi*	Unknown
Microsporidia	*Encephalitozoon cuniculi*	Y
Nematodes	*Nematodirus* spp.; *Obeliscoides cuniculi; Passalurus ambiguous; P. rufescens; Strongyloides papillosus; Retortamonas cuniculi*	Unknown
	Dirofilaria immitis; Gongylonema pulchrum	Y
Trematodes	*Fasciola hepatica*	Y
External		
Fleas	*E. myremecobii; Spilopsyllus cuniculi*	Unknown
	Ctenocephalides spp.; *Echidnophaga gallinacean; Pulex irritans*	Y
Lice	*Haemodipsus ventricosus; Haemodipsus* spp	Unknown
Mites	*Cheyletiella* spp.; *Demodex cuniculi; Psoroptes cuniculi*	Unknown
	Cheyletiella parasitivorax; Leporacarus gibbus; Notoedres cati; Sarcoptes scabiei; trombiculids	Y
Tongue worms (Pentastomida)	*Linguatula serrata*	Y
Ticks	*Amblyomma* sp.; *Dermacentor* sp.; *Ixodes* spp.; *Ornithidoros turicata; Rhipicephalus sanguineus*	Y

Capture and handling

Handlers should be mindful that some species and individuals are more prone to stress than others (e.g. introduced house mice, *Mus musculus*, and native Forrest's mice, *Leggadina forresti*; Petit *et al.* 2012). In general, handling should be minimised where possible.

A diversity of methods can be used for capturing wild rodents. Methods that rely on an attractant or bait (typically a peanut butter–based bait), include aluminium box traps of an appropriate size for the target taxa and wire cage traps for larger species. Where possible, the distance between the treadle or trigger mechanism and the door should be greater than the head–tail length of the target species. This spacing helps to prevent tails being pinned in trap doors, potentially causing skin loss and partial self-amputation of tails in *Pseudomys* species. Box and cage traps can be mounted on tree boles with wooden braces if targeting arboreal/scansorial species (Laurance 1994). Semi-aquatic species, such as the rakali, can be captured in cage traps baited with sardines (e.g. Leigh and Breed 2020). Great care should be taken to ensure that trapped animals are buffered against cold and heat, as some species (e.g. house mice) can succumb to these extremes readily (Waudby *et al.* 2019). If traps are left open during the day, care must be taken to ensure they are not located in direct afternoon sunlight. Eutherian carnivores are capable of opening box traps (by bending back the metal around the door so that it springs open) and may remove individuals from pitfall traps. Rodents are more readily exposed to potential predators in cage traps, although in most cases predators cannot reach trapped species. However, smaller predators, such as northern quolls (*Dasyurus hallucatus*), can reach through cage traps and kill trapped species (Dunlop *et al.* 2017).

Predator interactions can elevate trap stress. Hessian sacks placed around cage traps may obstruct northern quolls. Alternatively, sleeves for cages made of tarpaulin may also be effective and practical to minimise predator-related trap deaths.

Unbaited dry pitfall traps with or without drift net fences can be used to target species not often caught in baited traps; deeper pipe-style pitfalls may be more effective than shallower bucket-style traps for capturing some species, such as hopping mice (*Notomys* spp.) (Waudby *et al.* 2019), as they can escape. Sunflower seeds or another appropriate food source should be added to pitfall traps in areas where small rodents (e.g. silky mice, *P. apodemoides*) occur, as these animals require regular food intake to maintain their body temperature, and can perish overnight in unbaited traps. Towards the end of a rodent irruption in arid regions, adding food to pitfalls can minimise stress and trap death, as natural food resources are in rapid decline. Occasional predation of small rodents in pitfall traps by animals caught in the same trap is sometimes inevitable.

Rodents may experience heart attack if extremely stressed and/or their chest cavity is overly constricted during handling. Animals should be released immediately back into the bag if excessive stress (e.g. loud vocalisations, intense struggling, sudden limpness) is observed. Rodents should not be handled by the tail as doing so can detach the tail sheath (i.e. the skin), particularly in species from the *Zyzomys* and *Pseudomys* genera. Animals can be handled in cloth bags, but personnel should monitor the bags continuously as rodents can chew through the cloth. Eyes should be covered with part of the bag where possible, and only the body part required for processing/sampling left out of the bag. Typically, calico bags turned inside out (so that the seams are not entangled in claws) with tie tops are suitable. Drawstring bags are not recommended as rodents may squeeze through the gap at the top. Triangular linen bags, with Velcro® straps, can be used to immobilise larger rodents. Dark coloured cloth bags are preferable for nocturnal species

The handler's grip should be firm, but not constrictive. The aim of handling is to minimise movement (and therefore potential injury to the animal) and prevent the animal from turning to bite the handler. For small- to medium-bodied rodents, the whole animal can be restrained in a single hand, with the middle, fourth and fifth fingers encircling the lower body, and the thumb and index finger gently restraining the head. Care should be taken to avoid constricting the ribs or applying pressure to the superficial arteries/veins on the sides of the head/neck. Alternatively, the index and middle fingers can secure the head by moving up and over the shoulder blades, with the thumb, fourth and fifth fingers encircling and securing the lower body. For small species, rodents can also be restrained (cautiously) with a pistol-grip hold or 'scruffed' by gathering loose skin between the thumb and forefinger from the top of the animal's head and down the back. If done properly, this method can allow quick assessment of reproductive status (Petit *et al.* 2012). However, scruffing should not be used for species with delicate skin that can be easily torn (e.g. *Zyzomys* spp.). Handlers should avoid simply pinching the skin at the back of the neck to restrain animals because this method is typically ineffective for restraint, allowing the animal to thrash around and turn to bite the handler. Some species, such as Arnhem rock rats (*Z. maini*) and Kimberley rock rat (*Z. woodwardi*) do not cope well with being handled in general, so handling should be avoided where possible for these species.

For large-bodied rodents, two hands can be used, one to secure the neck and head and the other to secure the hind limbs. Caution should be taken when handling rodents as their teeth are sharp, and they have substantial bite force (Samuels 2009). Species that can bite through the bag easily are sometimes better handled on a hard surface (e.g. a lid or table) during processing.

Extra considerations should be taken if more-intensive handling is required (e.g. attaching radio-tracking collars or microchipping) for rodents. Some northern Australian rodents (e.g. *Conilurus* and *Mesembriomys* spp.) get distressed with intensive handling near dawn. Tree-dwelling rodents often return to den sites several hours before dawn, thus requiring earlier processing and handling (e.g. 1–2 h before dawn) to reduce stress and restraint required by handlers. Earlier processing is also recommended for other species susceptible to heart attacks from handling (i.e. *Z. maini* and *Z. woodwardi*). If the animal becomes weak or limp, or shows signs indicating a high level of stress (e.g. excessive struggling or vocalisations), handling should stop and the rodent should be placed back into the cloth bag. Food can be provided in the cloth bag and if improvement is not observed, the animal should be released when safe to do so, providing that it is able to move to shelter.

If transportation is necessary, animals should be kept in a securely tied bag, and placed inside a larger hard container with a secure lid. Rodents can be housed for short periods (i.e. up to 12 h) in relatively small enclosures/containers (e.g. a box, aquaria or cage), providing they can move and turn around comfortably, and the container is well aerated. Containers should be kept at a comfortable temperature, protected from the elements, and placed in a darkened area if possible. Water should be readily available. Appropriate bedding and cover should be provided. If holding for more than 6 h, food appropriate to the species should be offered. In most cases, a combination of seeds and fruit/vegetables is suitable. For omnivorous species, meal worms can be included. Rakali should be given fish or similar. If animals are retained in captivity permanently, consideration should be given to appropriate housing/shelter (e.g. rakali require areas of water at least 100 × 100 × 50 cm; arboreal species require vertical and horizontal branches; Jackson 2003). Burrowing and tree-dwelling nocturnal species are not usually exposed to above-ground daytime temperatures and may be highly susceptible to heat stress.

Choice of marking method depends on required longevity of marks, sensitivity of the study species to marking and handling (Petit *et al.* 2012), and study design. If identification is required for short periods, a non-toxic, indelible marker can be used to write numbers on or mark the tail/ears. Marks require refreshing every 2 or 3 days. Alternatively, non-toxic hair dye can be used to mark the fur. Hair dye lasts ~ 6–8 weeks. Scissors or clippers (for large-bodied rodents) or small nose-hair scissors (for small-bodied rodents) can be used to remove hair/fur for short-term identification. Small patches of fur should be removed from an area that allows for quick and easy identification (e.g. on the rump). This technique allows identification of recaptured individuals for up to 4–6 weeks.

Tattooing or micro-tattooing can be used to mark ears, feet or tails. Micro-tattooing does not necessarily require anaesthesia. A general or local anaesthetic is required for tattooing. Needles must be sharp and sterile. Individual numbering systems can be used, but codes should be simple to limit the number of locations tattooed and allow easy identification. These techniques are more suited for animals that will be kept in captivity for a period following capture, although tattooing has been used successfully to mark and identify wild rodents, and appeared to reduce marking-related deaths in some species, compared to ear notching (Petit *et al.* 2012). Ear notching, punching and tagging can generally be conducted quickly in the field by experienced personnel and the resulting removed tissue can be kept for DNA analysis. Scissors or clippers (for large-bodied rodents), or small nose-hair trimmers or invertebrate dissection scissors (for small-bodied rodents) can be used for notches. Specialised tools, such as an ear punch or tag punch can be used for creating ear punches or inserting tags. Ear punching is not suitable for individuals < 2 weeks of age. Ear tagging may not suitable for smaller rodent species with high levels of communal grooming, as the tags are prone to being pulled out.

Veterinary considerations

Analgesia, sedation and anaesthesia

Appropriate medication for sedation, anaesthesia, and analgesia are listed in Table 24.4. Because of their ubiquity as laboratory animals, much veterinary information on rodents pertains to experimental animal management rather than wildlife management. Some information in

Table 24.4: Suggested drug and route of administration for therapeutic treatment of rodents.

Therapeutic treatment	Drug and route of administration
Sedative	Tiletamine–zolazepam, intramuscular
Anaesthetic	Ketamine and xylazine, intraperitoneal
	Tiletamine–zolazepam, intraperitoneal
	Alfaxalone and xylazine, intraperitoneal
	Isoflurane, gaseous
Analgesic	Buprenorphine, subcutaneous (effective for 8 h)
	Meloxicam, subcutaneous (effective for 24 h)
	Carprofen, intraperitoneal or subcutaneous (effective for 24 h)

Table 24.5: List of diseases transmitted by rodents, with known seropositive prevalence in rodents in Australia, the causative agent, and symptoms of infection in humans.†

Causative agent	Disease	Symptoms
Acanthocephalians		
Moniliformis moniliformis	*Moniliformis moniliformis* infection	Often asymptomatic. Can cause abdominal pain, diarrhoea, dizziness, oedema, vertigo, irritability and anorexia. Infection is very rare.
Bacteria		
Brucella spp.	Brucellosis	Severe flu-like symptoms, sweating, joint and muscle pain, nausea, vomiting, decreased appetite, abdominal pain, constipation or diarrhoea, and hepato- and/or splenomegaly.
Coxiella burnettii	Q fever	Acute flu-like symptoms, high fever, chills, sweats, coughing, chest pain, headache, clay-coloured stools, diarrhoea, nausea, abdominal pain, jaundice, muscle pain, shortness of breath and heart failure.
Clostridium piliforme	Tyzzer's disease	Necrotic lesions on the liver, watery diarrhoea, emaciation, depression, black/tarry faeces, lethargy and hypothermia. Can lead to death.
Leptospira spp., including *L. serovars*	Leptospirosis	Flu-like symptoms, such as fever, chills, headache, nausea or vomiting, diarrhoea, loss of appetite, conjunctivitis, joint and muscle aches and pains, sweats and fatigue. Can lead to death.
Mycoplasma pulmonis	*Mycoplasma pulmonis infection*	Can potentially be transmissible to humans, but information lacking. Probably asymptomatic.
Orientia tsutsugamushi	Scrub typhus	Rash, pneumonia and fatal encephalitis.
Rickettsia typhi or other members of the *Rickettsia*, such as *R. australis*, *R. honei* and *R. felis*	Murine typhus fever, rat typhus, tick typhus or spotted fever	Headache, fever, muscle and joint pain, stiff neck, nausea and vomiting, rash, confusion, stupor, seizures, mental confusion and vertigo/imbalance.
Salmonella typhimurium	Mouse typhoid disease	Nausea, vomiting, stomach pain, fever, chills, headache, diarrhoea and bloody stools.
Spirillum minus or *Streptobacillus moniliformis*	Relapsing fever, rat-bite fever or Haverhill fever	Inflammation, ulcers and a purple/red rash. Symptoms of infection from *S. minus* include swollen or inflamed lymph nodes in the neck, groin and underarms. Those from *S. moniliformis* include chills, fever, vomiting, headaches, swollen joints, back pain, and muscle aches. Infection by *S. moniliformis* can be fatal if untreated because of malignant endocarditis, meningoencephalitis or septic shock. One human fatality in Australia.
Yersinia pestis†	Plague (pneumonic, septicaemic, bubonic)	Fever, headache, shortness of breath, chest pain, coughing, disseminated intravascular coagulation, vomiting, and swollen and painful lymph nodes.
Fungi		
Trichophyton schoenleinii	Tinea favosa	Crusty, yellow, compact, cup-shaped 'scutula' around hairs on the skin, which have an unpleasant odour.

Causative agent	Disease	Symptoms
Nematodes		
Angiostrongylus cantonensis	Angiostrongyliasis (eosinophilic meningitis)	Severe headaches, eosinophilic meningitis and death.
Calodium hepatica	Hepatic capillariasis	Persistent fever, hepatomegaly and leucocytosis with eosinophilia. Extreme cases lead to liver failure and death.
Capillaria spp.	Capillariasis	Acute or subacute hepatitis with peripheral leucocytosis and eosinophilia, hepatomegaly, and persistent fever. Infection is rare.
Eucoleus aerophilus	Pulmonary capillariasis	Bronchitis, coughing, mucoid or blood-tinged sputum, fever, dyspnea, and eosinophilia. Infection is very rare.
Strongyloides spp.	Strongyloidiasis	Often asymptomatic. Abdominal pain, bloating, heartburn, intermittent episodes of diarrhoea and constipation, a dry cough, skin rashes, arthritis, kidney problems, and heart conditions.
Platyhelminthes		
Haplorchis pumilio	*Haplorchis pumilio* infection	Asymptomatic. Diagnosis via shedding of cercariae.
Heterophyes nocens	Heterophyiasis	Epigastric pain, indigestion and abdominal discomfort, diarrhoea, abdominal pain and vomiting.
Hymenolepis diminuta and H. nana	Hymenolepiasis	Often asymptomatic. *H. diminuta* can cause abdominal pain, irritability, itching and eosinophilia. *H. nana* can cause toxaemia, intestinal inflammation, diarrhoea, abdominal pain, anorexia, nausea, weakness, loss of appetite, headaches, itchy buttocks and difficult sleeping.
Opisthorchis spp.	Opisthorchiasis	Often asymptomatic. Indigestion, abdominal pain, nausea, diarrhoea or constipation, and eosinophilia.
Procerovum varium	Ocular granuloma and inflammation	Redness, itching, and swelling/inflammation of the anterior chamber and subconjunctiva of the eye.
Raillietina celebensis	*Raillietina* infection	Often asymptomatic. Can cause gastrointestinal disturbances, irritability, and nausea. Infection is very rare.
Stellantchasmus falcatus	*Stellantchasmus falcatus* infection	Possibly asymptomatic. Confusion with other flukes, so symptoms unclear.
Spirometra spp.	Sparganosis	Often asymptomatic. Can cause pain, oedema, inflammation and slow growing migratory subcutaneous nodules in the tissues, which can lead to death. Infection is very rare.
Protozoans		
Cryptosporidium spp. Including *C. parvum*	Cryptosporidiosis	Acute, watery diarrhoea. Other symptoms include nausea and vomiting, and abdominal pain.

(Continued)

Table 24.5 *Continued*

Causative agent	Disease	Symptoms
Toxoplasmosis gondii	Toxoplasmosis	Swollen lymph glands, especially around the neck, muscle aches and pains, headache, fever, inflammation of the lungs, heart muscle and eye
Trypanosoma lewisi	Trypanosomiasis	Fever, coughing, convulsions, anaemia, lassitude, anorexia and loss of appetite. Infection is rare.
Viruses		
Encephalomyocarditis virus (EMCV)	Encephalomyocarditis (febrile syndrome)	Fever, pale appearance, poor appetite, malaise, nausea, headache, retro-ocular pain, sweats, weight loss, joint and muscle pain, photophobia, chills, vomiting and abdominal pain.
Foot and mouth disease virus (FMDV)	Foot and mouth disease	Sore throat, fever, inflamed throat, and blisters on hands, feet and tongue. Infection is very rare.
Lymphocytic choriomeningitis mammarenavirus	Lymphocytic choriomeningitis	Mild form of meningitis. Headache, nausea or vomiting, fever, decreased appetite, general malaise, neck stiffness, an aversion to bright light, joint aches and pains, muscle aches, stiff neck, drowsiness or confusion, rash, sore throat, stomach pains and diarrhoea.
Reovirus serotype 3 (Reo 3)	Meningitis, primary biliary cirrhosis	Often asymptomatic. Fatigue, itchy skin, fever, chills, sweats, dry mouth and eyes, abdominal pain, muscle wasting, abdominal and leg swelling, jaundice, enlarged liver and spleen, weight loss and confusion.

† Plague occurred in the early 1900s, but only a few cases have been reported since.

the table has been added on medication strategies for captive rodents with the acknowledgment that rodents captured in the field are unlikely to be held in captivity for an appreciable duration.

Blood collection

Caution should be exercised when collecting blood from wild rodents because of their unknown health, nutritional and hydration status. Approximately 10% of an animal's circulating blood volume can be collected in a one-off sampling event without replacement fluids being provided (Parasuraman *et al.* 2010; Chapter 16). Depending on size and species, blood can be collected from the jugular, cephalic or saphenous veins (Heard 2014).

Euthanasia

For rodents < 300 g, carbon dioxide (CO_2) inhalation is sometimes used for euthanasia (although the animal welfare implications of this practice for euthanasing laboratory rats are contentious, e.g. Turner *et al.* 2020) and can be undertaken in the field with appropriate equipment (e.g. Ellis 2017). Two-stage chemical euthanasia can be used, whereby pentobarbitone can be administered via the intravenous, intracardiac or intraperitoneal route following anaesthetic induction (NHMRC 2014). Any animal euthanased with pentobarbitone represents a secondary toxicity risk to wild scavengers and should be disposed of via deep burial. Other euthanasia methods are acceptable with reservations (Reilly 2001): (1) cervical dislocation (rodents < 150 g only); (2) decapitation; and (3) blunt force trauma to the base of the skull for animals > 150 g in the field.

Infectious pathogens

Rodents are vectors for several infectious diseases in Australia, some of which are transmissible to humans (Table 24.5).

General operating procedures

Research methods and procedures relevant to studying rodents are covered in more detail elsewhere in this book, including observation (without spotlighting), assessment of tracks and other traces, collection of scats and evaluation of dens, burrows or hollows (Chapter 4). Other detection methods may include camera and hair trapping, and conservation detector dogs (Chapter 5). A range of capture methods apply to rodents depending on their size and habits, including pitfall, aluminium box, cage and arboreal pipe trapping (Chapter 7). Marking methods may include microchipping, ear tagging, ear notching and tattooing (Chapter 8). Several tracking methods may apply depending on the target species (Chapter 9). For some large and more visible species, such as rakali, citizen science approaches may be useful (Chapter 10). Several veterinary procedures may be used for studying rodents (Chapter 16).

REFERENCES

Bennett A, Haydon S, Stevens M, Coulson G (2015) Culling reduces fecal pellet deposition by introduced sambar (*Rusa unicolor*) in a protected water catchment. *Wildlife Society Bulletin* **39**, 268–275. doi:10.1002/wsb.522

Bengsen AJ, Hampton JO, Comte S, Freney S, Forsyth DM (2021) Evaluation of helicopter net-gunning to capture wild fallow deer (*Dama dama*). *Wildlife Research* Online early. doi:10.1071/WR21007

Bentley A (1998) *An Introduction to the Deer of Australia with Special Reference to Victoria.* Australian Deer Research Foundation, Melbourne.

Boardman WS, Lethbridge MR, Hampton JO, Smith I, Woolnough AP, McEwen MM, Miller GW, Caraguel CG (2014a) Evaluation of medetomidine-ketamine and medetomidine-ketamine-butorphanol for the field anesthesia of free-ranging dromedary camels (*Camelus dromedarius*) in Australia. *Journal of Wildlife Diseases* **50**, 873–882. doi:10.7589/2014-03-059

Boardman WS, Lethbridge MR, Harper M, Woolnough AP (2014b) *CAM004: Field Immobilisation of Camels.* Invasive Animals CRC, Canberra.

Breed B, Ford F (2007) *Native Mice and Rats.* CSIRO Publishing, Melbourne.

Campbell HA, Loewensteiner DA, Murphy BP, Pittard S, McMahon CR (2020) Seasonal movements and site utilisation by Asian water buffalo (*Bubalus bubalis*) in tropical savannas and floodplains of northern Australia. *Wildlife Research* **48**, 230–239. doi:10.1071/WR20070

Cripps JK, Pacioni C, Scroggie MP, Woolnough AP, Ramsey DS (2019) Introduced deer and their potential role in disease transmission to livestock in Australia. *Mammal Review* **49**, 60–77. doi:10.1111/mam.12142

Curtin University (2018) *Standard Operating Procedure: Rabbit Anaesthesia.* Curtin University, Perth.

Davies C, Wright W, Hogan FE, Davies H (2020) Detectability and activity patterns of sambar deer (*Rusa unicolor*) in Baw Baw National Park, Victoria. *Australian Mammalogy* **42**, 312–320. doi:10.1071/AM19029

Dunlop JA, Rayner K, Doherty TS (2017) Dietary flexibility in small carnivores: a case study on the endangered northern quoll, *Dasyurus hallucatus*. *Journal of Mammalogy* **98**, 858–866. doi:10.1093/jmammal/gyx015

Ellis MV (2017) Development of a compact system for field euthanasia of small mammals. *Journal of Mammalogy* **98**, 1211–1214. doi:10.1093/jmammal/gyx072

English AW (1992) Management strategies for farmed chital deer. In *The Biology of Deer.* (Ed. RD Brown) pp. 189–196. Springer, New York, NY.

Gibb JA (1990) The European rabbit *Oryctolagus cuniculus*. In *Rabbits, Hares and Pikas-Staus Survey and Conservation Action Plan.* (Eds JA Chapman and JEC Flux) pp. 116–120. IUCN, Gland, Switzerland.

Greenville AC, Wardle GM, Dickman CR (2012) Extreme climatic events drive mammal irruptions: regression analysis of 100-year trends in desert rainfall and temperature. *Ecology and Evolution* **2**, 2645–2658. doi:10.1002/ece3.377

Greenville AC, Wardle GM, Dickman CR (2013) Extreme rainfall events predict irruptions of rat plagues in central Australia. *Austral Ecology* **38**, 754–764. doi:10.1111/aec.12033

Hackländer K, Schai-Braun S (2018) *Lepus europaeus* Pallas, 1778 European Hare. In *Lagomorphs: Pikas, Rabbits, and Hares of the World.* (Eds AT Smith, CH Johnston, PC Alves and K Hackländer) pp. 187–190. Johns Hopkins University Press, Baltimore, MD.

Hampton JO (2019) *Chemical Immobilisation of Australian Animals.* Ecotone Wildlife, Inverloch.

Hampton JO, Finch NA, Watter K, Amos M, Pople T, Moriarty A, Jacotine A, Panther D, McGhie C, Davies C, Mitchell J (2019) A review of methods used to capture and restrain introduced wild deer in Australia. *Australian Mammalogy* **41**, 1–11. doi:10.1071/AM17047

Hampton JO, Hyndman TH (2019) Underaddressed animal-welfare issues in conservation. *Conservation Biology* **33**, 803–811. doi:10.1111/cobi.13267

Hampton JO, Hyndman TH, Laurence M, Perry AL, Adams P, Collins T (2016) Animal welfare and the use of procedural documents: limitations and refinement. *Wildlife Research* **43**, 599–603. doi:10.1071/WR16153

Heard D (2014) Rodents. In *Zoo Animal and Wildlife Immobilization and Anaesthesia.* 2nd edn. (Eds G West, D Heard and N Caulkett) pp. 893–903. John Wiley and Sons, Hoboken, NJ.

Hing S, Hampton JO, Gibson TJ (2019) Animal welfare and the killing of wildlife by captive bolt in Australia. *Australian Zoologist* **40**, 170–180. doi:10.7882/AZ.2018.035

Jackson S (2003) *Australian Mammals: Biology and Captive Management.* CSIRO Publishing, Melbourne.

Laurance WF (1994) Rainforest fragmentation and the structure of small mammal communities in tropical Queensland. *Biological Conservation* **69**, 23–32. doi:10.1016/0006-3207(94)90325-5

Leigh CM, Breed WG (2020) A demographic study of the water-rat (*Hydromys chrysogaster*) on the River Torrens in Adelaide, South Australia. *Australian Mammalogy* **42**, 277–282. doi:10.1071/AM19049

Macdonald DW, Barrett P (2001) *Mammals of Europe.* Princeton University Press, Princeton, NJ.

Mitchell J, Dorney W, Mayer R, McIlroy J (2009) Migration of feral pigs (*Sus scrofa*) in rainforests of north Queensland: fact or fiction? *Wildlife Research* **36**, 110–116. doi:10.1071/WR06066

Marsh MK, Hutchings MR, McLeod SR, White PC (2011) Spatial and temporal heterogeneities in the contact behaviour of rabbits. *Behavioral Ecology and Sociobiology* **65**, 183–195. doi:10.1007/s00265-010-1024-y

National Health and Medical Research Council (2014) *A Guide to the Care and Use of Australian Native Mammals in Research and Teaching.* National Health and Medical Research Council, Canberra.

Orr B, Malik R, Norris J, Westman M (2019) The welfare of pig-hunting dogs in Australia. *Animals* **9**, 853. doi:10.3390/ani9100853

Pavey CR, Addison J, Brandle R, Dickman CR, McDonald PJ, Moseby KE, Young LI (2017) The role of refuges in the persistence of Australian dryland mammals. *Biological Reviews of the Cambridge Philosophical Society* **92**, 647–664. doi:10.1111/brv.12247

Petit S, Waudby HP, Walker AT, Zanker R, Rau G (2012) A non-mutilating method for marking small wild mammals and reptiles. *Australian Journal of Zoology* **60**, 64–71. doi:10.1071/ZO11088

Parasuraman S, Raveendran R, Kesavan R (2010) Blood sample collection in small laboratory animals. *Journal of Pharmacology & Pharmacotherapeutics* **1**, 87–93. doi:10.4103/0976-500X.72350

Reilly JS (Ed) (2001) *Euthanasia of Animals Used for Scientific Purposes.* 2nd edn. Australian & New Zealand Council for the Care of Animals in Research and Teaching (ANZCCART), Adelaide.

Roycroft EJ (2020) Phylogenomics, molecular evolution and extinction in the adaptive radiation of murine rodents. PhD thesis. The University of Melbourne, Australia.

Roycroft EJ, Moussalli A, Rowe KC (2020) Phylogenomics uncovers confidence and conflict in the rapid radiation of Australo-Papuan rodents. *Systematic Biology* **69**, 431–444. doi:10.1093/sysbio/syz044

Samuels JX (2009) Cranial morphology and dietary habits of rodents. *Zoological Journal of the Linnean Society* **156**, 864–888. doi:10.1111/j.1096-3642.2009.00502.x

Saunders G, Kay B (1996) Movements and home ranges of feral pigs (*Sus scrofa*) in Kosciusko National Park, New South Wales. *Wildlife Research* **23**, 711–719. doi:10.1071/WR9960711

Sharp T (2012) *PIG004: Use of Judas Pigs Standard Operating Procedure.* Invasive Animals Cooperative Research Centre, Canberra.

Stott P, Harris S (2006) Demographics of the European hare (*Lepus europaeus*) in the Mediterranean climate zone of Australia. *Mammalian Biology* **71**, 214–226. doi:10.1016/j.mambio.2006.02.009

Turner PV, Hickman DL, Van Luijk J, Ritskes-Hoitinga M, Sargeant JM, Kurosawa TM, Agui T, Baumans V, Choi WS, Choi Y-K, Flecknell PA, Lee BH, Otaegui PJ, Pritchett-Corning KR, Shimada K (2020) Welfare impact of carbon dioxide euthanasia on laboratory mice and rats: a systematic review. *Frontiers in Veterinary Science* **7**, 411. doi:10.3389/fvets.2020.00411

University of South Florida (2018) *Standard Operating Procedure: Production of Polyclonal Antibodies in Rabbits.* University of South Florida, Tampa, FL.

Van Dyck S, Strahan R (2008) *The Mammals of Australia.* Reed New Holland Publishers, Sydney.

Waudby HP, Petit S, Gill MJ (2019) The scientific, financial and ethical implications of three common wildlife-trapping designs. *Wildlife Research* **46**, 690–700. doi:10.1071/WR19084

Wells CR, Lethbridge M (2020) Intensive and extensive movements of feral camels in central Australia. *The Rangeland Journal* **42**, 195–210. doi:10.1071/RJ19054

Wibbelt G, Frölich K (2005) Infectious diseases in European brown hare (*Lepus europaeus*). *Wildlife Biology in Practice* **1**, 86–93. doi:10.2461/wbp.2005.1.11

Williams CK, Parer I, Coman BJ, Burley J, Braysher ML (1995) *Managing Vertebrate Pests: Rabbits.* Australian Government Publishing Service, Canberra.

25 Marine mammals

Vanessa Pirotta, Rebecca McIntosh, Rachael Gray, Helene Marsh and Michael Lynch

INTRODUCTION

Marine mammals are distributed throughout the world's oceans. Considered sentinel species of marine ecosystem health because of their high trophic position, they fill important ecological roles in the marine environment. The marine waters of Australia are home to a variety of marine mammals, ranging from coastal species such as fur seals and sea lions to migratory giants such as whales. Marine mammals are protected in Australian waters under national legislation, such that any scientific research causing an impact on marine mammals usually requires animal ethics approval. This requirement is to ensure human–wildlife interactions are minimised and animal welfare is prioritised.

CETACEANS (WHALES, DOLPHINS AND PORPOISES)

Vanessa Pirotta and Michael Lynch

Characteristics

'Cetacean' is the collective term for whales, dolphins and porpoises. They are air-breathing marine mammals, with strong muscular tails, found throughout the world's oceans. Cetaceans can be divided into two broad groups: baleen whales and toothed whales. Baleen whales (Mysticeti) include the blue and humpback whales. They have two blowholes, are toothless and have hair-like structures known as baleen to filter feed. Toothless whales also use low-frequency communication to talk to each other over long distances. In contrast, toothed whales (Odontoceti) include sperm whales, beaked whales, beluga whales, narwhals, dolphins and porpoises. Toothed whales have a single blowhole and use high-frequency sounds via echolocation (biological sonar) to communicate and locate food. Forty-five whale, dolphin and porpoise species occur in Australian waters, including the Australian Antarctic Territory (Australian Federal Government 2020). This number includes coastal, migratory and infrequently sighted species. This sub-chapter focuses on two well-studied cetaceans: the humpback whale (*Megaptera novaeangliae*) and the bottlenose dolphin (*Tursiops* spp.), but the principles outlined here are broadly applicable to all species.

Biology and behaviour

Humpback whales

Humpback whales are a migratory species growing up to 17 m long and weighing up to 40 tonnes. They are characterised by large pectoral fins and the hump-like shape they create as they arch their back to dive. Humpback whales frequent Australian waters during winter, where they travel the west and east coasts to northern Australian waters to breed each year. They are commonly sighted along the coast exhibiting acrobatic aerial displays. They are known to breach, tail slap and spy hop. Within the breeding grounds, male humpback whales produce complex songs to attract prospective mates.

Two Southern Hemisphere humpback whale populations migrate annually from high-latitude feeding waters off Antarctica to low-latitude breeding grounds in northern Australia (Chittleborough 1965). The west coast population is known as breeding Stock D (Group IV), and travel along the west coast of Australia to the Kimberley region to breed and calve (Jenner *et al.* 2001). The east coast population breeding is known as Stock E1 (Group V), and travel along the east coast of Australia to breed and typically calve in the Great Barrier Reef (Pirotta *et al.* 2020).

Humpback whales spend most of the austral summer feeding in Antarctic waters on their primary food source, Antarctic krill (*Euphausia superba*). They have also been observed feeding in Australian waters (Pirotta *et al.* 2021). During the late autumn/early winter months, both populations travel to warmer northern Australian waters to breed and give birth. Humpback whales are social animals and are usually seen migrating in pods of two or three, although sometimes larger pods are observed.

Within the breeding grounds, mothers are mostly seen with newborn calves. Mothers may also give birth during their northward migration before reaching these areas (Paterson and Paterson 1984; Pirotta *et al.* 2020). Female humpback whales have a gestation period of 11–12 months and typically give birth to a calf every 2–3 years or, in some cases, in successive years (Chittleborough 1965). A humpback whale calf will stay with its mother generally for a year, after which it is referred to as a 'yearling' humpback whale. Along the migration paths on the west and east coasts of Australia and within the breeding grounds, large pods may form (more than five individuals) in pursuit of one or more female humpback whales. These congregations are generally known as competition pods or heat runs where males will become aggressive towards each other in competition to mate with females. Males are also known to sing a 'whale song' in the breeding grounds to acoustically attract females. Males may mate with multiple females and do not provide parental care to their offspring.

Bottlenose dolphins (Tursiops spp.)

Bottlenose dolphins occur in Australian coastal and offshore waters, growing up to 2–4 m in length and weighing 150–650 kg (Shirihai and Jarrett 2006). Bottlenose dolphins are social, often being found in large groups and sometimes swimming with migrating humpback whales. Three known *Tursiops* species occur in Australian waters: the common bottlenose dolphin (*T. truncatus*), which occurs in deeper offshore environments, the Indo-Pacific bottlenose dolphin (*T. aduncus*), which is the most commonly studied of the three species, and the Burrunan dolphin (*T. australis*) found in southern Australian coastal waters.

Coastal and offshore bottlenose dolphins are highly social and usually found in groups of two or more individuals. Bottlenose dolphins have a range of behaviours, including porpoising (jumping out of the water), bow riding, tail lobbing, chuffing and swimming in pods. Resident populations around Australia (typically of *T. aduncus* and *T. australis*) occur in localised areas, with little movement beyond a small home range. The home ranges of offshore species (typically *T. truncatus*) are larger and occur in deeper waters.

The diet of bottlenose dolphins consists of fish, krill and squid (Shirihai and Jarrett 2006). Bottlenose dolphins have diverse feeding behaviours, particularly in Western Australia (*T. aduncus*). These dolphins are known to intentionally strand or beach when fishing, use marine sponges as mouth shields when digging, 'kerplunking' – a behaviour where dolphins scare fish by tail slapping in shallow waters – and 'conching', where dolphins use conch shells to catch fish (Allen *et al.* 2011).

Bottlenose dolphins calve every 2–6 years in warmer months but this may be year-round in some areas. Males may mate with multiple females, and provide no parental care to their offspring. Females have a gestation period of around 12 months. Calves are dependent on their mothers for 6–12 months (Shirihai and Jarrett 2006). Mothers will provide milk to their calves and protection by swimming closely to their young. They generally remain in large groups.

Capture and handling

Cetaceans are powerful, and can be large, fast and difficult to access. Studying them can be challenging and requires specialised methods. Several standard methods exist to acquire biological, behavioural and acoustic data from wild, free-ranging cetaceans. Common methods include:

- biopsy/sloughed skin (shed skin) collection (e.g. for genetic/molecular sampling or testing for organic pollutants via a biopsy gun, crossbow or pole from the bow of a vessel) – sloughed skin can be collected at the surface depending on activity (e.g. breaching)

- tagging and tracking movements with satellite/high resolution/acoustic tags
- drone research used for photogrammetry data and the collection of respiratory samples (e.g. lung microbiota/viruses sampling from migrating humpback whales; Pirotta *et al.* 2017)
- acoustic monitoring (e.g. hydrophones and acoustics listening stations)
- photography (e.g. photo identification of individuals using natural markings, mark–recapture methods using photographs and assessing impacts of entanglement and/or body condition)
- faecal matter collection
- land-/vessel-based observations and theodolite tracking of whale movements (Pirotta *et al.* 2020) (Figure 25.1)
- abundance surveys (e.g. to determine the abundance of blue and humpback whales via capture–recapture and line-transect methods).

In some areas of the world small, free-swimming cetaceans are captured with seine nets deployed from fast-moving boats, but this technique is rarely used in Australia. Capture and immobilisation of small cetaceans in Australia is largely limited to very young (e.g. abandoned dolphin calves) or very debilitated individuals. In these cases, individuals can often be approached closely to allow restraint. Cetaceans in Australia are typically only transported for rescue and rehabilitation purposes. In most circumstances, doing so is only possible for individuals up to ~5 m in length. The size of larger cetaceans precludes physical restraint. However, interventions to free entangled individuals are not uncommon. Currently, in Australia, a technique of attaching large buoys from a small and highly manoeuvrable vessel to tire the whale is favoured. Once the whale's speed has been impaired, a closer approach can be used to try and cut the entanglement using hooked knives mounted on extension poles.

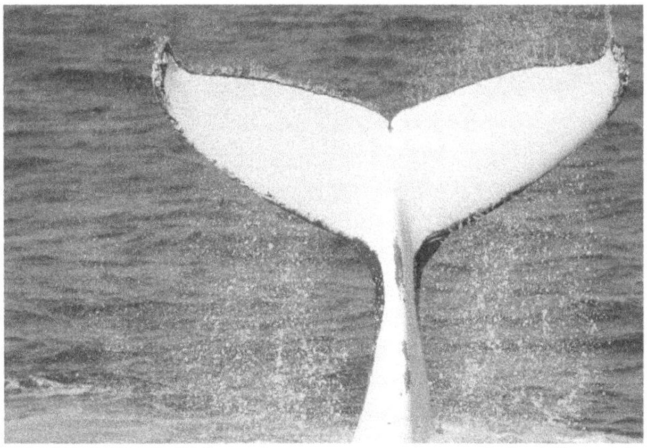

Figure 25.1: Photo identification of whale tail flukes is used to identify individual humpback whales. Each tail fluke pattern and shape is unique to individual whales. Photo by Vanessa Pirotta.

Rescued dolphins may be tagged and fitted with a GPS/satellite tag on the dorsal fin or back to track their movements post-release. Two main types of satellite tags are used for studying/monitoring cetaceans: (1) suction cup tags, and (2) sub-dermal/barb tags designed to anchor (imbed) in the skin/blubber layer for the collection of long-term data. Tags are placed on free-swimming cetaceans using a pole (usually suction cups) or via rifle/crossbow or custom-modified pneumatic line throwers.

Veterinary considerations

As the capture of wild cetaceans for scientific purposes is rare, and these are fully aquatic animals, therapeutics are rarely used except to help injured or harmed individuals (e.g. during entanglements or stranded/beached events).

Sedation and anaesthesia

The administration of sedatives, anaesthetics, analgesics (pain relief medication, most likely in captive/rescue situations) should be administered by a qualified veterinarian (with specific marine mammal experience) or trained personnel under direct supervision of a veterinarian. Sedatives are most frequently used to facilitate euthanasia during stranding events, see below.

Blood collection

Marine mammals can be challenging species for blood collection. Techniques described are specialised and should generally only be attempted by experienced veterinarians. For cetaceans, blood samples are typically taken from the veins of the tail fluke: the dorsal and ventral fluke periarterial vascular rete (Dold and Ridgway 2014).

Euthanasia

Euthanasia is a valuable animal welfare management tool when dealing with stranded cetaceans. Large cetaceans present a challenge in regard to euthanasia. Accepted methods for cetacean euthanasia involve both chemical and physical methods. Chemical methods usually employed for small to medium cetaceans are the administration of an intramuscular sedative (commonly medetomidine or midazolam) followed by a barbiturate (pentobarbitone) administered intravenously, usually into the veins of the tail fluke (Blyde 2019, as cited in Vogelnest and Woods 2019). The sedation is important to avoid vigorous tail flurry at the point of death. Any animal euthansed with pentobarbitone represents a secondary toxicity risk to wild scavengers and should be disposed of via deep burial.

To avoid the relay toxicity risks associated with pentobarbitone use (and the large volumes necessary for cetaceans), intracardiac injection with a saturated potassium chloride (KCl) solution has been used as a chemical euthanasia alternative. Use of KCl rather than a barbiturate means the carcass will not become a source of environmental toxin to scavenging animals. KCl acts by interfering with normal blood ion concentrations and stops the beating of the heart. There are considerable animal welfare concerns associated with this mode of death, so it is imperative that cetaceans are profoundly sedated, or ideally under general anaesthesia, before this method is used (Harms *et al.* 2014). Due to the extensive subcutaneous fat layer (blubber) of cetaceans, custom-made needles of ~1 m in length are required for intracardiac injections in large species (e.g. adult baleen whales; Harms *et al.* 2014). If intracardiac injection is not achieved, the sedation will hasten the death of the animal by depressing respiratory effort.

The most commonly used physical method of euthanasia is the use of firearms (Blyde 2019, as cited in Vogelnest and Woods 2019). This method is only suitable for individuals < 6 m in length and must be performed with a knowledge of appropriate ballistics and anatomical landmarks for this task. In brief, specialised non-deforming (solid) bullets are required in centrefire calibres > 0.30 in order to achieve the penetration required to pass through the skull (Hampton *et al.* 2014). It is essential the delivery of both chemical and physical euthanasia is provided by trained and experienced personnel. Explosives have been used for the euthanasia of large cetaceans but with variable success (Coughran *et al.* 2012) and significant risks to all nearby so should not be attempted.

Infectious pathogens

Cetaceans can carry and transfer pathogens between individuals and throughout populations (Table 25.1). For a comprehensive review, refer to Blyde and Vogelnest (2008). Some diseases carried by cetaceans have the potential to infect humans (e.g. mycobacteriosis, brucellosis) so appropriate personal protective equipment and practices should be employed when attending stranded animals.

Of concern for zoonoses when performing necropsies (or if any is consumed by humans) are *Salmonella* spp.,

Table 25.1: Examples of infectious disease reported from wild and captive cetaceans.

Adapted from Blyde (2019) in Vogelnest and Woods (2019).

Disease	Type	Name	General description
Infectious	Viral	Cetacean morbillivirus	Global distribution. Identified in several species, such as pilot whales.
		Herpesviruses	Lesions on body.
		Poxvirus	Lesions on body. Reported in captive and free-ranging toothed whales globally.
		Papillomaviruses	Small cutaneous wart-like lesions on the skin, tongue, penis and vagina.
	Bacterial	Nocardia	Bacteria present in soil, water and marine sediments causing localised and systemic disease.
		Streptococcus	Bacterial pathogen, e.g. *Streptococcus agalactiae.* Reported causing necrotising fasciitis and abscesses in captive bottlenose dolphins.
		Brucellosis	Causes encephalitis, hydrocephalus and vestibulocochlear nerve pathology.
	Fungal	Lacaziosis	Chronic mycotic disease of the skin
		Other fungi	*Coccidioides* spp., *Cryptococcus* spp., *Blastomyes* spp., *Histoplasma* spp., *Aspergillus* spp. and *Zygomycetes* spp.
	Parasitic diseases	Lung nematodes	Nematodes found in the lungs of free-ranging neonatal cetaceans at necropsy.
		Nasitrematinae	Trematodes that inhabit the cranial sinuses and upper airways of toothed cetaceans.

Staphylococcus spp., *Leptospira* spp., *Erysipelothrix* spp. plus *Brucella* spp. *Mycobacterium* spp., *Toxoplasma gondii, Mycoplasma* spp. and poxviruses.

General operating procedures

Research methods and procedures relevant to studying cetaceans are covered in more detail elsewhere in the book and may include aerial survey methods (Chapter 6), observational studies, capture methods, collection of biological samples and marking methods and attachment of various devices (Chapter 12). Several veterinary procedures may apply to the study of cetaceans (Chapter 16).

DUGONGS

Helene Marsh

Characteristics

The dugong (*Dugong dugon*) is one of the only four extant members of the mammalian order Sirenia (seacows). It is a grey, medium-sized marine mammal that spends its entire life in the sea. Adults can grow to 3.3 m long and weigh up to ~570 kg. Neonates are typically ~1.2 m long and weigh 25–35 kg (Marsh *et al.* 2011).

Biology and behaviour

Dugongs are the most abundant marine mammal in the coastal waters of northern Australia where they occur from Moreton Bay near Brisbane to Shark Bay in Western Australia (Marsh *et al.* 2011). They are also occasionally sighted in New South Wales inshore waters in summer. Dugongs are associated with subtropical and tropical seagrass meadows close to busy ports as well as in remote areas.

Dugong space use is highly individualistic and information is required from at least 10 animals to obtain useful information for a population. GPS-satellite tracking demonstrates that some animals are relatively sedentary for months at a time, while others make directed movements of up to several hundred kilometres in a few days (Marsh *et al.* 2011). Most information on dugong space use has been obtained from GPS-satellite tracking and time–depth recorders (Cleguer *et al.* 2020). The stimulus for most dugong movements is unknown. In the subtropics in winter, local movements can be associated with water temperature (Marsh *et al.* 2011; Zeh *et al.* 2018). Despite their capacity to make large-scale movements, the evidence for fine-scale dugong population structure along the south-east Queensland coast (Seddon *et al.* 2014) suggests that most movements are ranging movements without associated breeding.

The dugong is a seagrass community specialist (Marsh *et al.* 2011). Animals have been recorded eating the leaves and rhizomes of most of the species of seagrasses that occur in their Australian range with the exception of some high biomass temperate species at high latitude range limits. Dugongs variously exhibit one of two feeding modes: (1) cropping leaves, and (2) excavating entire plants and leaving distinctive feeding trails in the seagrass meadow. In some areas and times, dugongs crop algae and eat invertebrates. Dugong feeding has been recorded in water depths to 35 m but mostly occur in waters less than ~15 m deep. Dugongs commence eating seagrass a few days after birth but also suckle from their mothers for at least 18 months.

Dugongs are long lived (maximum life span > 70 years) and slow breeding (Marsh *et al.* 2011). Females typically give birth to one calf at a time at minimum intervals of ~3 years potentially from about age 8 years; however, breeding is deferred during food shortages resulting from seagrass loss following extreme weather events (Marsh *et al.* 2011); at such times mortality can also be high (Meager and Limpus 2014). The only long-term social unit recorded is the cow and her calf. Although large herds are regularly recorded in some areas, especially in Moreton Bay near Brisbane, herd structure appears fluid and the aggregations are considered feeding assemblages rather than social units (Marsh *et al.* 2011). Mating occurs at the end of winter in the subtropics (Lanyon *et al.* 2019). Breeding seasonality is less obvious in the tropics (Marsh *et al.* 2011).

Capture and handling

As a result of their 'threatened' status under state and Commonwealth legislation and frequent occurrence in marine parks or Indigenous Protected Areas, dugong research typically requires multiple government permits, as well as animal ethics permits and agreements with Traditional Owners. A permit is also required to import or export dugong specimens into or from Australia. Animal ethics permits are also required for observational studies, such as aerial surveys (typically conducted from an altitude of ~150 m) or research using drones (from minimum altitudes of 20–30 m).

Dugongs lack a dorsal fin, breach the water surface for only a few seconds to breathe, mostly occur in turbid water, and typically lack unique features that are recognisable over time from photographs. Several researchers have used skin scraping to obtain samples of dugong dermis for genetic analysis without needing to catch the animals (Lanyon *et al.* 2019).

Hundreds of dugongs have been caught and released in Moreton Bay, generally without incident (Lanyon *et al.* 2019). However, some dugongs have degenerative diseases, including cardiomyopathy (Owen *et al.* 2012) and several animals have died during capture attempts. Several deaths during capture for research have been attributed to predisposing conditions. Given that it is impossible to ensure that animals do not have such conditions before capture, it is important for researchers to:

1. engage effectively with local stakeholders
2. have the social licence to use the methods proposed by ensuring that locals, stakeholders and Traditional Owners fully understand them
3. minimise the risk to the local population by ensuring that it is > 100 animals (dugongs are such slow breeders that any research with a risk of causing human-induced mortality should be avoided in small populations; Marsh *et al.* 2011), and
4. minimise the risk of mortality by ensuring that:
   - animals are in good condition (i.e. capture should not be attempted after extensive seagrass loss as a result of an extreme weather event (Marsh *et al.* 2011)), and
   - only unaccompanied adults are targeted.

Dugongs are usually captured using the technique detailed by Lanyon *et al.* (2006), which requires close pursuit of an individual dugong in shallow water via an outboard-powered dinghy or personal watercraft (Cleguer *et al.* 2020). Fuentes *et al.* (2013) developed a dermal hold-fast technique that enables dugong capture without chasing and is suitable for deeper and/or turbid water captures. This technique, which has been permitted and implemented for community-based tracking in Torres Strait, New Caledonia and the Northern Territory, is only appropriate for research partnerships with Indigenous dugong-capture experts because of the cultural protocol required.

Each animal should be monitored closely using a veterinary protocol (Flint and Bonde 2017) to ensure that it remains in good condition before, during and after capture and release. Recommended maximum pursuit times should be strictly observed. Once captured, the dugong is typically supported in the water at the side of the processing boat for tagging (typically using both turtle and passive integrated transponder (PIT) tags), genetic sampling, sexing and measuring. Many individuals have also been successfully translocated to a vessel for detailed health assessments and physiological studies (Lanyon *et al.* 2019). GPS-satellite transmitters are attached to the dugong by a tailstock belt and tether. The tether has a weak link to enable rapid detachment if caught in benthic biota or floating objects and a corrodible link to ensure detachment over time. In areas with an acoustic array, dugongs can be tracked within the vicinity of the array using small acoustic transmitters mounted in a tailstock belt (Zeh *et al.* 2015).

Dugongs have been successfully transported in a moistened sling stretcher to a captive facility via a truck or aircraft. Dugongs are difficult animals to maintain in captivity for prolonged periods, and typically fewer than five animals are held in captivity in the world at any time. Neonatal dugongs are particularly challenging because they require regular feeding with both milk and seagrass (see Blanshard 2000), and it is current practice in Australia to euthanase any neonate that strands without its mother. Some oceanaria have successfully maintained dugongs on a diet of lettuce; others rely on seagrass collected from the wild. Dugongs have never bred in captivity and males and females sometimes have to be separated because of the male's violent behaviour.

Veterinary considerations

Sedation and anaesthesia

There is a paucity of information on dugong therapeutics and few veterinarians in Australia will have significant experience with this group. However, the therapeutics of manatees (*Trichechus* spp.) has been somewhat developed and provides a valuable reference source when considering interventions in dugongs. It is essential that veterinarians and dugong ecologists consult closely when considering veterinary interventions as this approach will enable clinical approaches to be tailored to what will produce the best outcome for the animal.

Many field research procedures commonly applied to dugongs (e.g. telemetry device attachment) are done under physical, rather than chemical, restraint (Sheppard *et al.* 2006). If chemical restraint is required, the benzodiazepines midazolam and diazepam have been used extensively for sedation of manatees via intramuscular injection. Due to the extensive subcutaneous fat layer (blubber) of sirenians, specialised 'spinal' needles of 8.75 cm length are generally used for intramuscular injections (Nolan and Walsh 2014). The unique anatomy of sirenians also slows down absorption of injected chemicals such that onset of drug effects is typically 15–20 min with intramuscular injections. Gaseous anaesthesia using isoflurane is possible for maintenance during invasive procedures, but requires specialised management and monitoring of ventilation (Nolan and Walsh 2014).

Blood collection

Venipuncture is usually achieved from the pectoral flukes, through the 'brachial vascular bundle', accessed between the radius and ulna (Nolan and Walsh 2014).

Euthanasia

Euthanasia can be achieved by intramuscular sedation followed by intravenous injection of pentobarbitone. Any animal euthanased with pentobarbitone represents a secondary toxicity risk to wild scavengers and should be disposed of via deep burial. In remote areas where alternatives are unavailable, death by gunshot is the most practical alternative. Euthanasia laws vary among jurisdictions and cultural acceptance of euthanasia is variable.

Infectious pathogens

Faecal pathogens are the only recognised zoonoses associated with dugongs and basic hygiene protocols can easily protect handlers. The few records of dugong deaths from infectious disease are mostly single-case studies (see Owen *et al.* 2012). No major mortality events in dugongs have been definitely attributed to infectious disease (Marsh *et al.* 2011). A wide variety of gastrointestinal parasites has been recorded in wild dugongs (see Marsh *et al.* 2011; Owen *et al.* 2012) but usually these are of little clinical significance.

General operating procedures

Research methods and procedures relevant to studying dugongs are covered in more detail elsewhere in the book and may include aerial survey methods (Chapter 6), observational studies, capture methods, collection of biological samples and marking methods and attachment of various devices (Chapter 12). Several veterinary procedures apply to the study of dugongs.

In addition, researchers should consult AIATSIS (2020).

PINNIPEDS (SEALS AND SEA LIONS)

Rebecca McIntosh, Rachael Gray and Michael J. Lynch

Characteristics

Three families constitute the suborder Pinnipedia – the Phocidae or 'true seals', Otariidae (sea lions and fur seals) and Odobenidae (walrus, confined to Northern Hemisphere waters). The phocids (true seals) have internal ears ('earless') and poor terrestrial locomotion because of their short fore flippers and caudal facing hind flippers, which make little contribution to terrestrial locomotion. The Otariids have external ears and locomote well on land given their ability to tuck their hind flippers underneath them as well as support their weight using their fore flippers.

Biology and behaviour

Pinnipeds are typically top predators but, unlike many ocean predators, they come ashore to breed and rest, making them readily accessible for research. Some species are common to Australian shores (e.g. Australian sea lion, *Neophoca cinerea*, found in South Australia and Western Australia; Australian fur seal, *Arctocephalus pusillus doriferus*, and long-nosed (or New Zealand) fur seal, *A. forsteri*, found in south-east Australia). Other species may visit the Australian coast frequently (e.g. the leopard seal, *Hydrurga leptonyx*; the sub-Antarctic fur seal, *A. tropicalis*; and the southern elephant seal, *Mirounga leonina*). Finally, some species visit the Australian coast only rarely (e.g. the Antarctic fur seal, *A. gazella*).

Southern Hemisphere phocids breed in isolation or in colonies during a synchronised cycle in the austral summer; many breed on fast ice (Weddell seal, *Leptonychotes weddellii*) or in the pack ice (including leopard seals and crabeater seals, *Lobodon carcinophagus*). In contrast, southern elephant seals form large aggregations in breeding colonies on sub-Antarctic islands. Fur seals and sea lions also breed in aggregates or colonies that can number in the thousands, while Australian sea lions can breed in very small groups (< 50 individuals). However, the Australian sea lion breeds every 18 months, each colony breeding at a different time and females exhibiting extreme philopatry, breeding where they were born.

Pinnipeds are predators and exhibit a broad range of foraging strategies including being generalists, benthic or epipelagic, near shore and deep sea; some such as the leopard seal specialise on both ends of the food chain: penguins and krill.

Pinnipeds undergo an annual moult (except for Australian sea lions, moulting approximately every 18 months), which varies from gradual loss of the fur/hair to a catastrophic moult in southern elephant seals where both the fur and epidermis are shed. In general, female Australian pinnipeds breed after the age of 3 years. Most otariids have a lifespan of around 20–26 years and phocids can live to 50 years. Males of sexually dimorphic species (otariids and southern elephant seal) breed after ~10 years of age, once they are large enough to compete with each other for mates. Males of similarly sized species reach full size and breed after the age of seven.

Capture and handling

The varied behaviour and life histories of seal species affect research methods and the animal welfare considerations underlying these methods. With the exception of some Antarctic species, seals have evolved with human predation and typically flee on approach by humans. In large colonies, this tendency can cause dangerous stampedes that can injure or kill vulnerable individuals, such as young pups. Capturing or approaching solitary animals restricts disturbance to individuals rather than groups. Some species are less flighty than others and more robust to approach and capture. For example, the Australian sea lion will protect its pup and stand its ground or even attack researchers in the field. Researchers should minimise the potential disruption of critical social bonds, particularly between mother and pup pairs, and avoid causing disturbance to male mating strategies during the breeding season as doing so can affect a males' lifetime reproductive output. In many species, males are in their breeding prime for a short period or have limited access to mating. The size of the field team should be minimal; groups of animals being approached must have access to an 'escape route'.

Temperature extremes can be problematic for pinnipeds that thermoregulate by behaviour modification (moving into the water when hot). Cold ambient temperatures can result in peripheral vasoconstriction making blood sampling more challenging. However, in terms of animal welfare the restraint of seals in higher latitudes can easily result in overheating. The risk will depend on the ambient temperature, activity of the seal before capture, length of the restraint period and whether effective cooling (e.g. shade and/or water dousing) can be employed. For this reason, it is important that work is undertaken within safe temperature limits with temperature thresholds established for capture. The small body size of pups makes them particularly susceptible to hyperthermia. Early signs of hyperthermia include fine tremors of the head or body and pups who appear unusually quiet or unresponsive. Hyperthermic pups can also exhibit severe seizures. If seizures are observed, all sampling should cease and the pup be placed in a cool location, doused with cold water, kept under observation and safe from conspecifics. Pups can also suffocate or drown from piling on top of each other to avoid capture. Other welfare risks of capture for all age classes include injuries and fatalities from falls from rocks or cliffs (Seguel *et al.* 2014).

It is important to select species, age and size class and individuals appropriate for the research objectives. For example, capture and restraint using a large hoop net should be restricted to animals < 100 kg; therefore, animals of this size are more easily used for research efforts. Furthermore, retrieving and redeploying data loggers are more successful with adult females, since they are the only age class that is expected to return to the colony to feed their pup, making recapture more likely. Unless seals are individually identifiable (e.g. because of specific scars), it is difficult to study seals over their lifetimes and therefore difficult to assess reuse of an individual over time in research programs. Unlike terrestrial mammals where retrapping can be common, seals become flightier and more averse to humans after a capture event, making subsequent attempts more difficult. Consequently, accidental multiple handling is unlikely, but at times such sampling is necessary to understand growth rates, monitor biological variables or responses to intervention and retrieve external devices. Capture stress and the stress of repeat handling must be minimised as a priority. Research design must account for the cumulative lifetime burden of the research for individuals. Gales *et al.* (2009) outline general capture criteria for marine mammals around target and non-target animal welfare and safety.

Small seals or pups are typically captured by hand or net and can be safely restrained manually; a short period of stress occasioned by physical restraint when procedures and sampling are minimally invasive outweighs the risk of potential complications associated with sedation or anaesthesia. Ideally, animals should be approached slowly from behind and downwind where possible to minimise detection. Capture of pups using a purpose designed 'pup bag' or net can be achieved when individuals are sleeping or at rest and restraint within the bag, which has breathing holes to minimise the stress of capture and restraint when required for short periods. Reducing external stimuli by covering the eyes, firm, but gentle restraint, quiet movements and minimising noise impacts can reduce the stress of restraint. Physical restraint of otariids up to ~100 kg is possible with more than three trained people and conical fitted nets; however, restraint becomes more difficult as the size of the seal increases because they are highly mobile and can back out of nets. Phocids of greater size (up to 150–200 kg) can be caught manually in a sausage net plus head bag.

For extended durations of restraint, or invasive procedures, sedation or general anaesthesia is recommended. The use of an amnesiac, such as midazolam, is thought to reduce post-release stress. Specially designed hoop nets or throw nets can be used to capture seals (under ~100 kg) on land followed by intramuscular injection of a sedative (needle or pole syringe) or gas induction via a mask. During chemical immobilisation, the ability of seals to thermoregulate physiologically can be variably impaired depending on the chemical agent used and plane of sedation/anaesthesia. Therefore, the monitoring of body temperature is particularly important during chemical immobilisation.

The use of dart guns is a vital component of seal research, especially for larger, aggressive or flighty species (e.g. McKenzie *et al.* 2013). Many variables affect the success of remote drug delivery, including weather conditions, operator experience, the dart type and needle size, which can affect where drugs are deposited (e.g. subcutaneously into blubber versus intramuscularly – the former resulting in a prolonged time to affect and reduced effect, and darts failing to inject on impact). Additionally, animal factors including mass and poor estimation thereof (accuracy is essential for accurate drug dosage), body condition, age class, and health condition can result in differing individual responses to routine sedation regimes (Baylis *et al.* 2015, Frankfurter *et al.* 2016). The use of acoustic transmitter-equipped remote sedation darts in high-risk situations can make remote sedation in these situations safer, while minimising disturbance to other animals as individual target animals can be better monitored (Frankfurter *et al.* 2016). Risks associated with remote drug delivery include over- and underdosing, limited control of the depth of sedation/anaesthesia, administration of drug to the wrong animal, animals moving to the water after darting with risk of drowning, shelf-life and expense, acquisition of drugs, training and legislation, and safe storage. Managing drug doses and drug combinations that can be specific to a species or age class, with continuous monitoring of vital signs and proper intervention, reduces mortality from anaesthesia (Baylis *et al.* 2015). Recovery from sedation can result in rapid head shaking and lack of body control. Placing padding around rocky substrates in the immediate vicinity of the seal can avoid injury, including tooth damage.

Sampling procedures vary from observational studies (reading tags for mark–recapture–resight surveys and using drones for population census); to minimally invasive procedures (collection of morphometric data, marking, blood and scat collection); to more-invasive procedures (collection of biopsies for DNA studies, flipper and passive integrated transponder (PIT) tagging and attachment of external devices). Highly invasive procedures include branding, insertion of internal data loggers, tooth extraction for ageing, and blubber sampling.

Seals are long lived (20+ years), so long-term research of individuals requires application of an individual mark – the marking method depends on the aims of the research and includes temporary paint marks, 'haircuts' and bleach marks, adhesion of round vinyl (Sarah Michael, pers. comm.) or wooden 'caps' on the fur, flipper tags that can be read for several years, and lifetime marks such as microchips (PIT tags) and brands. Tags in otariids and phocids are applied to the fore flippers (Figure 25.2) and hind flippers respectively; PIT tags are applied subcutaneously on the dorsum just cranial to the tail either under physical or chemical restraint. Flipper tags can tear out or remain attached for a lifetime, but typically become unreadable after several years

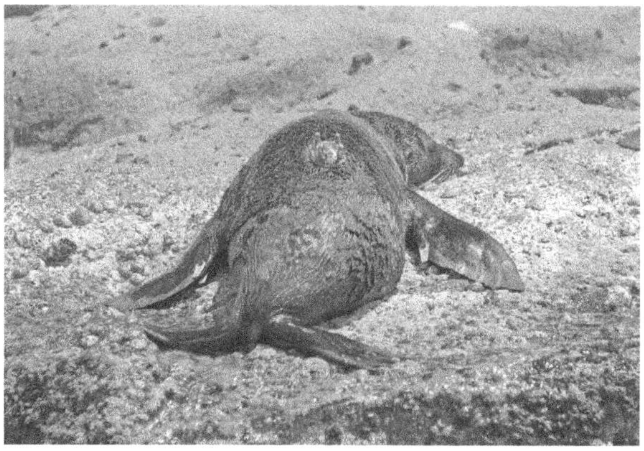

Figure 25.2: Long-nosed fur seal (*Arctocephalus forsteri*) with fore-flipper tags and a back-mounted SPLASH tag (Wildlife Computers). Photo by Vincent Antony.

(Bradshaw *et al.* 2000). Because of these issues and to increase likelihood of resighting, tags are usually placed on both right and left sides. Tag applicators need to be well maintained to ensure they move freely for correct tag application with minimal pain and distress to the animal. Lifetime individual identification can be achieved by PIT tagging, but requires remote tag readers or close-range approach using an antenna (e.g. McIntosh *et al.* 2013). Without external tags, it is impossible to target only PIT-tagged seals, resulting in the close approach of untagged and tagged individuals and potential disturbance.

Cryobranding or hot branding are methods of long-term marking used in the Northern Hemisphere and previously in the Southern Hemisphere; however, hot branding has been banned from use by ministerial decision in Australia and New Zealand because of ethical concerns (McMahon *et al.* 2006; Monamy 2007; Wilkinson *et al.* 2011; Wright *et al.* 2017).

Seals spend most of their time at sea. External tracking devices and internal tags are used to study their aquatic movements and foraging behaviour. Additionally, pinnipeds have been employed as autonomous sampling platforms to capture environmental variables and oceanographic observations (Harcourt *et al.* 2019). The risks and benefits of these techniques have been reviewed (Horning *et al.* 2017; Horning *et al.* 2019) with best practice recommendations developed for their use (Wilson and McMahon 2006; Horning *et al.* 2017).

The main consideration regarding tracking devices, also called tags or data loggers, is that these attachments and/or implants could cause physical pain and suffering resulting in changes in behaviour or survival, although modern methods and procedures have reduced these risks (Field *et al.* 2012). External devices are typically attached on the dorsal midline in the interscapular space using a quick-setting, two-part epoxy glue (Figure 25.2). For larger animals, tracking or camera devices may be glued to the top of the head (Field *et al.* 2012). Epoxy glues get very hot during the setting reaction, while negative effects from this reaction are less likely in cold environments (Field *et al.* 2012); skin burns can occur in warmer climates (R. McIntosh, pers. obs.). Internally implanted tags include subcutaneous heart rate loggers or stomach loggers that record prey acquisition (inserted via a gastroscopy tube into the stomach under anaesthesia) (Horning *et al.* 2017).

Seals have carried instruments of up to 0.6% of their mass and remain apparently unaffected in either the short term (growth rates) or the long term (survival) (McMahon *et al.* 2008). For species that are difficult to recapture to remove trackers, payload recovery devices can be used to remotely dislodge the tracker. Such devices use two components: a bottom platform that is attached to the seal and remains *in situ* until the animal moults, and the upper telemetry device that is ejected from the platform when triggered remotely by the researcher (Wildlife Computers 2020).

VETERINARY CONSIDERATIONS

Sedation and anaesthesia

Special considerations exist for the safe induction and maintenance of anaesthesia in marine mammals, particularly pinnipeds. There are important differences in anaesthetic considerations between these two groups and specific guidelines have been written for phocids (Lynch and Bodley 2014) as well as otariids (Haulena 2014). Due to physiological adaptations to diving and breath holding, and unique anatomical features, pinniped anaesthesia can be very challenging, and anaesthetic complications, including mortalities, can occur.

A range of anaesthetic drugs are used for the chemical immobilisation of seals. If the seal has been captured and restrained in a net, the delivery of the gaseous anaesthetic isoflurane or sevoflurane in oxygen, via a facemask attached to a portable anaesthetic machine, provides for rapid induction of chemical immobilisation (Lian *et al.* 2018). Gaseous agents also have the advantage of more-rapid recovery times compared to many chemical agents delivered by injection (Chapter 16). However, intravenous or intramuscular injections of anaesthetic agents delivered either after restraint or remotely are commonly used for seal immobilisation procedures (Kirkwood *et al.* 2006).

Chemical agents delivered remotely are used to induce a suitable level of sedation or anaesthesia for safe physical restraint. Once physical restraint is possible, additional chemical or gaseous agents can be used to attain a deeper level of immobilisation if required (Figure 25.3). For light to heavy sedation of otariids and phocids, midazolam on its own or in combination with other agents has been employed, for example a combination of medetomidine, butorphanol and midazolam (Katz *et al.* 2019). For anaesthesia, tiletamine–zolazepam has been commonly employed at varying doses, as has midazolam/ketamine

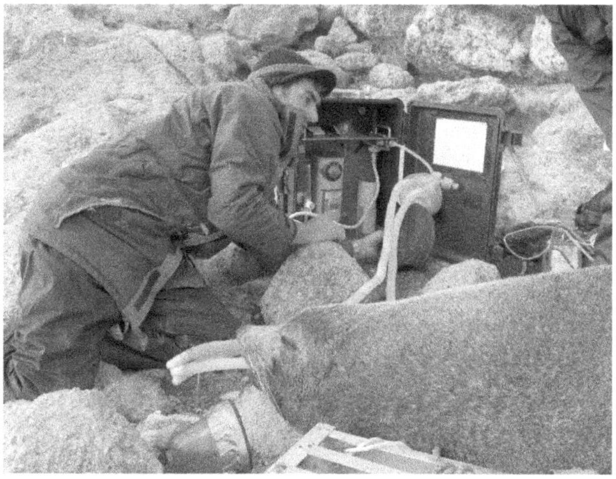

Figure 25.3: A veterinarian administering the gaseous anaesthetic, isoflurane, to an Australian fur seal (*Arctocephalus pusillus doriferus*) before attachment of a transmitter. Photo by John Gibbens.

and medetomidine/midazolam/ketamine combinations, among others.

A commercially available mixture of tiletamine–zolazepam is commonly used for darting seals or, in the case of elephant seals, rapid immobilisation is achieved via intravenous injection of tiletamine–zolazepam into the intervertebral, extradural sinus (Wilson and McMahon 2006; Geschke and Chilvers 2009). Tiletamine–zolazepam has the advantage of a relatively wide safety margin but cannot be fully antagonised (reversed partially or fully), resulting in prolonged recoveries at the higher end of doses. Midazolam alone may be administered as a short-term sedative. Barnes *et al.* (2008) and Bodley (2019 cited in Vogelnest and Woods 2019) provide comprehensive reviews of drug combinations for sedation and anaesthesia of pinnipeds in Australian waters.

Agents or combinations of agents that can be antagonised at the completion of procedures make management of the seal's recovery less problematic. Reversal drugs can assist recovery. However, their success depends largely on the drug combination used for induction of sedation/anaesthesia and reversal is not possible for all drug combinations. Regardless, reversal agents and resuscitation drugs should be on hand whenever possible, particularly for species in which anaesthetic complications are common (e.g. leopard seals). It is highly recommended that one member of the field team with experience in pinniped sedation/anaesthesia is solely dedicated to managing anaesthesia (Bodley 2019 cited in Vogelnest and Woods 2019). Reversal agents commonly used include atipamezole (medetomidine) and flumazenil (midazolam and zolazepam).

The appropriate management of sedated or anaesthetised seals requires a knowledge of the physiological effects of the drugs. Of paramount importance is ensuring that the seal is achieving adequate oxygen exchange by either spontaneous breathing or assisted ventilation. Once anaesthetised, intubation is recommended to control and maintain anaesthesia. The most basic of monitoring is frequent assessment of heart and respiration rates, respiratory effort and mucous membrane colour. A higher level of confidence in the physiological status is achieved using monitoring aids such as capnography (expired air CO_2 concentration) and pulse oximetry (measuring oxygen saturation of the blood; Chapter 16). However, finding suitable attachment sites for monitoring instruments is challenging. Maintaining an open airway is a common issue to manage in anaesthetised pinnipeds and is particularly important in species such as leopard seals where the airway collapses significantly at deeper levels of sedation/anaesthesia.

Blood collection

The brachial vein on the medial aspect of the front flipper is usually the most visible site for venipuncture for otariids; the intervertebral, extradural sinus can be used in phocids. The plantar interdigital veins of the hind flippers can also be used in pinnipeds (Lynch and Bodley 2014).

Euthanasia

Animals in poor health have compromised welfare and an assessment of the likelihood of spontaneous recovery from illness/injury should be made. In the case of severely injured or diseased animals with poor potential to rehabilitate, euthanasia may be required.

The 2020 edition of the American Veterinary Medical Association Guidelines (AVMA 2020) identify recommended euthanasia methods for pinnipeds. The method of euthanasia must result in immediate loss of consciousness, followed by death, with a minimum of pain, discomfort and stress. Methods may vary according to species, location, body size, age and mobility of the animal and according to the availability of drugs and equipment. The safety of handling and degree of restraint must be considered when choosing the method of euthanasia. Euthanasia will most likely involve sedation and/or anaesthesia to render the animal

Table 25.2: Known infectious agents reported in pinnipeds in the Southern Hemisphere.

Adapted from Barnes *et al.* (2008), Ladds (2009), Bodley (2019) and references therein. 'Z' indicates a zoonosis. Species included only when specifically referenced in the literature; probably absent or not investigated/identified in other species.

Category of infection	Infectious agent of disease	Disease in pinnipeds/species
Fungi	*Candida albicans*	Inflammation of mucocutaneous junctions (oral cavity, eye, anus, vulva) (*M. leonina*).
Bacteria	*Streptococcus* spp.	*S. phocae* – peritonitis (*A. forsteri*; R. Gray, pers. comm.) and meningitis and cellulitis (*P. hookeri*[1]); *S. dysgalactiae equisimilis* – meningitis, cellulitis, cystitis (*P. hookeri*[1]); unspecified species in *A. p. doriferus*.
	Campylobacter spp.	Vasculitis, pneumonia (*P. hookeri*); isolated from *A. gazella*.
	Brucella spp. 'Z'	Seropositive (*N. cinerea*, *A. forsteri*, *A. p. doriferus* and all Antarctic phocids); clinical disease not diagnosed.
	Nocardia spp.	Pyogranulomatous lesions (*H. leptonyx*).
	Salmonella spp.	Can be asymptomatic or associated with pneumonia, septicaemia, enteritis, meningoencephalitis; disease reported in *A. p. doriferus* pups and *A. forsteri*.
	Mycobacterium pinnipedii 'Z'	Anorexia, weight loss, respiratory signs including coughing; bronchopneumonia and disseminated disease (*N. cinerea*, *A. p. doriferus*, *A. forsteri*, *A. gazella*, *A. tropicalis*).
	Klebsiella pneumoniae	Neurological signs due to meningitis, subdural haemorrhage, lameness (poly-arthritis), omphalitis (*P. hookeri*).[1]
	Mycoplasma phocacerebrale 'Z'	Oral cavity, no disease; cause of 'seal finger'. *Mycoplasma* sp. implicated in abortion/disease in *A. p. doriferus*.[4]
	Corynebacterium spp.	Pneumonia.
Viruses	Canine distemper virus	Seropositive (*L. carcinophaga*, *Hydrurga leptonyx*); no epizootics.
	Phocine distemper virus (Morbillivirus)	Seropositive (*P. hookeri*, *A. forsteri*); no epizootics.
	Phocine herpesvirus	Seropositive (*L. weddellii*, *L. carcinophagus*); no disease.
Protozoa	*Toxoplasma gondii* 'Z'	Seropositive (*N. cinerea*, S. Lindsay, pers. comm.; *M. leonina*, *L. weddellii*, *L. carcinophaga*, *A. gazella*[2]); pulmonary congestion and peritoneal effusion in an individual *N. cinerea*.
Nematodes (roundworms)	*Dirofilaria immitis* (heartworm)	Disease similar to canines.
	Uncinaria spp. (hookworm)	Intestinal disease, anaemia, weight loss (*N. cinerea*, *P. hookeri*); disease not noted (*A. p. doriferus*, *A. forsteri*).
	Lungworms (*Otostrongylus circumlitus*, *Parafilaroides* spp.)	Respiratory disease when in high numbers (*N. cinerea*, *A. p. doriferus*).
	Contracaecum spp.	Gastric *(M. leonina, A.p. doriferus)* and oesophageal (*A. forsteri*) ulceration
	Anisakis spp.	Incidental finding
Cestodes (tapeworms)	*Diphyllobothrium* spp.	Asymptomatic (*H. leptonyx*); subcutaneous cysts (*A. forsteri*) and granulomatous mastitis (*P. hookeri*) due to plerocercoid cysts of *D. delphini; intestinal infection* (*A.p. doriferus*, *A. forsteri)*
Lice	*Antarctophthirus* spp.	Pruritis (*N. cinerea*, *A.p. doriferus*, *A. forsteri*)[3]; Anaemia (*N. cinerea*, Gray pers. comm.); no disease (*L. weddellii*)
Mites	*Orthohalarachne* spp. *Halarachne miroungae*	Respiratory mites (naso- and oro-pharynx causing irritation and coughing (*N. cinerea*, *A.p. doriferus*); *H. miroungae* in *M. leonina*)

[1] Michael *et al.* (2019); [2] Rengifo-Herreraa *et al.* (2012); [3] McIntosh and Murray (2007); [4] Lynch *et al.* (2011)

unconscious before administration of a chemical terminal agent (Greer *et al.* 2001).

For pinnipeds, intramuscular sedation using tiletamine–zolazepam or medetomidine can be delivered via pole syringe, dart or hand injection (Barnes *et al.* 2008). Once deep sedation has been achieved, an intravenous injection of pentobarbitone can be delivered (refer to the previous section on blood collection). If venipuncture fails, pentobarbitone may be injected into the heart via a long needle. Chest auscultation for cardiac arrest and absence of all reflexes will confirm death. Intraperitoneal injection is also acceptable but delayed absorption can reduce drug efficacy. For both small and large pinnipeds, intracardiac administration is only acceptable in fully anaesthetised, moribund or unconscious individuals. Risks of environmental contamination and secondary poisoning of other animals that might feed on the carcass must be considered when carcasses are disposed of *in situ*; appropriate disposal options are via veterinary clinic or deep burial.

Sometimes, for example when injectable anaesthetics are unavailable and it is inappropriate to capture the animal, gunshot can be an acceptable euthanasia method (Mörner *et al.* 2013). When alternatives are not available, manually applied blunt force trauma to the head can have rapid results but requires experience, expertise and strength. Both the latter options reduce the requirement for drugs and specialised equipment with no risk of secondary toxicity for scavenging animals.

Infectious pathogens

Several reviews of infectious agents and disease in pinnipeds are available. Table 25.2 reports known infectious agents in pinnipeds in the Southern Hemisphere but is not exhaustive.

General operating procedures

A range of research methods and procedures relevant to studying pinnipeds is covered in more detail elsewhere in the book. These methods include observational studies, capture methods, collection of biological samples, and marking methods and attachment of various devices (Chapter 12). A range of veterinary procedures may apply to pinnipeds (Chapter 16).

ACKNOWLEDGMENTS

Special thanks to Professor Robert Harcourt for his review of the cetacean section. Thank you to Geoff Ross and Mandy Watson for their assistance with providing cetacean response documentation.

REFERENCES

AIATSIS (2020) AIATSIS Code of Ethics for Aboriginal and Torres Strait Islander Research. <https://aiatsis.gov.au/sites/default/files/2020-10/aiatsis-code-ethics.pdf>.

Allen SJ, Bejder L, Krützen M (2011) Why do Indo-Pacific bottlenose dolphins (*Tursiops* sp.) carry conch shells (*Turbinella* sp.) in Shark Bay, Western Australia? *Marine Mammal Science* **27**, 449–454. doi:10.1111/j.1748-7692.2010.00409.x

Australian Federal Government (2020). *Cetaceans – Species found in Australian waters, Species Profiles and Threats Database.* Australian Federal Government, Canberra. <http://www.environment.gov.au/marine/marine-species/cetaceans/species-found-Australian-waters>.

AVMA (2020) *AVMA Guidelines for the Euthanasia of Animals: 2020 Edition.* American Veterinary Medical Association, Schaumburg, IL.

Barnes J, Higgins D, Gray R (2008) Pinnipeds. In *Marine Mammal Medicine.* (Eds L Vogelnest and R Woods) pp. 541–589. CSIRO Publishing, Melbourne.

Baylis AMM, Page B, Staniland I, Arnould JPY, McKenzie J (2015) Taking the sting out of darting: risks, restraint drugs and procedures for the chemical restraint of Southern Hemisphere otariids. *Marine Mammal Science* **31**, 322–344. doi:10.1111/mms.12148

Bradshaw CJA, Barker RJ, Davis LS (2000) Modeling tag loss in New Zealand fur seal pups. *Journal of Agricultural Biological & Environmental Statistics* **5**, 475–485. doi:10.2307/1400661

Blyde D, Vogelnest L (2008) Cetaceans. In *Medicine of Australian Mammals.* (Eds L Vogelnest and T Portas) pp. 592–614. CSIRO Publishing, Melbourne.

Blyde D (2019) Cetaceans. In *Current Therapy in Medicine of Australian Mammals.* (Eds L Vogelnest and T Portas) pp. 593–602. CSIRO Publishing, Melbourne.

Blanshard W (2000) Current achievements and future challenges in dugong rehabilitation. Pp 45–58 in ARAZPA / ASZK 2000 Conference Proceedings "Achievements and Challenges "Sea World, Gold Coast Australasian Regional Association of Zoological Parks and Aquaria & Australasian Society of Zoo Keeping.

Bodley KB (2019) Pinnipeds. In *Current Therapy in Medicine of Australian Mammals* (Eds L Vogelnest, Larry and T Portas) pp. 579–591. CSIRO Publishing, Melbourne.

Chittleborough R (1958) The Breeding Cycle of the Female Humpback Whale, Megaptera nodosa (Bonnaterre). *Marine and Freshwater Research* **9**, 1–18. doi:10.1071/MF9580001

Cleguer C, Garrigue C, Marsh H (2020) Dugong (*Dugong dugon*) movements and habitat use in a coral reef lagoonal ecosystem. *Endangered Species Research* **43**, 167–181. doi:10.3354/esr01061

Coughran D, Stiles I, Fuller PJ (2012) Euthanasia of beached humpback whales using explosives. *Journal of Cetacean Research and Management* **12**, 137–144.

Dold C, Ridgway S (2014) Cetaceans. In *Zoo Animal and Wildlife Immobilization and Anaesthesia.* 2nd edn. (Eds G West, D Heard and N Caulkett) pp. 679–691. John Wiley and Sons, Hoboken, NJ.

Field IC, Harcourt RG, Boehme L, de Bruyn PJN, Charrassin J-B, McMahon CR, Bester MN, Fedak MA, Hindell MA (2012) Refining instrument attachment on phocid seals. *Marine Mammal Science* **28**, E325–E332. doi:10.1111/j.1748-7692.2011.00519.x

Flint M, Bonde RK (2017) Assessing welfare of individual sirenians in the wild and in captivity. In *Marine Mammal Welfare* (Ed. A Butterworth) pp. 381–393. Springer, Cham, Switzerland. doi:10.1007/978-3-319-46994-2_21.

Frankfurter G, DeRango E, Johnson S (2016) Use of acoustic transmitter-equipped remote sedation to aid in tracking and capture of entangled California sea lions (*Zalophus californianus*). *Journal of Wildlife Diseases* **52**, 730–733. doi:10.7589/2015-10-274

Fuentes MMPB, Cleguer C, Liebsch N, Bedford G, Amber D, Hankin C, *et al.* (2013) Adapting dugong catching techniques to different cultural and environmental settings. *Marine Mammal Science* **29**, 159–166. doi:10.1111/j.1748-7692.2011.00531.x

Gales NJ, Bowen WD, Johnston DW, Kovacs KM, Littnan CL, Perrin WF, Reynolds JE, III, Thompson PM (2009) Guidelines for the treatment of marine mammals in field research. *Marine Mammal Science* **25**, 725–736. doi:10.1111/j.1748-7692.2008.00279.x

Geschke K, Chilvers BL (2009) Managing big boys: a case study on remote anaesthesia and satellite tracking of adult male New Zealand sea lions (*Phocarctos hookeri*). *Wildlife Research* **36**, 666–674. doi:10.1071/WR09133

Greer LL, Whaley J, Rowles T (2001) Euthanasia. In *Marine Mammal Medicine*. 2nd edn. (Eds LA Dierauf and FMD Gulland) pp. 732–736. CRC Press, Boca Raton, FL.

Hampton JO, Mawson PR, Coughran DK, Vitali SD (2014) Validation of the use of firearms for euthanising stranded cetaceans. *The Journal of Cetacean Research and Management* **14**, 117–123.

Haulena M (2014) Otariid seals. In *Zoo Animal and Wildlife Immobilization and Anaesthesia*. 2nd edn. (Eds G West, D Heard and N Caulkett) pp. 661–72. John Wiley and Sons, Hoboken, NJ.

Harcourt R, Sequeira AMM, Zhang X, Roquet F, Komatsu K, Heupel M, McMahon C, *et al.* (2019) Animal-borne telemetry: an integral component of the ocean observing toolkit. *Frontiers in Marine Science* **6**, 326. doi:10.3389/fmars.2019.00326

Harms CA, McLellan WA, Moore MJ, Barco SG, Clarke EO, Thayer VG, Rowles TK (2014) Low-residue euthanasia of stranded mysticetes. *Journal of Wildlife Diseases* **50**(1), 63–73. doi:10.7589/2013-03-074

Horning M, Andrews R, Bishop A, Boveng P, Costa D, Crocker D, *et al.* (2019) Best practice recommendations for the use of external telemetry devices on pinnipeds. *Animal Biotelemetry* **7**, 20. doi:10.1186/s40317-019-0182-6

Horning M, Haulena M, Tuomi PA, Mellish JE, Goertz CE, Woodie K, Berngartt RK, *et al.* (2017) Best practice recommendations for the use of fully implanted telemetry devices in pinnipeds. *Animal Biotelemetry* **5**, 13. doi:10.1186/s40317-017-0128-9

Jenner KC, Jenner MM, McCabe KA (2001) Geographical and temporal movements of humpback whales in Western Australian waters. *The APPEA Journal* **41**, 749–765. doi:10.1071/AJ00044

Katz H, Reisfeld L, Franco-Trecu V (2019) Chemical immobilization protocols in free-ranging South American fur seal (*Arctocephalus australis*) and adult female South American sea lion (*Otaria byronia*). *Marine Mammal Science* **35**, 327–335. doi:10.1111/mms.12524

Kirkwood R, Lynch M, Gales N, Dann P, Sumner M (2006) At-sea movements and habitat use of adult male Australian fur seals (*Arctocephalus pusillus doriferus*). *Canadian Journal of Zoology* **84**, 1781–1788. doi:10.1139/Z06-164

Ladds P (2009) *Pathology of Australian Native Wildlife*. CSIRO Publishing, Melbourne.

Lanyon J, Noad M, Meager J (2019) Ecology of the marine mammals of Moreton Bay. In *Moreton Bay Quandamooka and Catchment: Past, Present, and Future*. (Eds IR Tibbetts, PC Rothlisberg, DT Neil, TA Homburg, DT Brewer and AH Arthington) pp. 415–429. The Moreton Bay Foundation, Brisbane.

Lanyon JM, Slade RW, Sneath HL, Broderick D, Kirkwood JM, Limpus D, Limpus CJ, Jessop T (2006) A method for capturing dugongs (*Dugong dugon*) in open water. *Aquatic Mammals* **32**, 196–201. doi:10.1578/AM.32.2.2006.196

Lian M, Johnson S, Gelatt T, O'Hara T, Beckman KB, Rea LD (2018) Field anesthesia of juvenile Stellar sea lions (*Eumetopias jubatus*) using inhalation anesthesia. *Marine Mammal Science* **34**, 125–135. doi:10.1111/mms.12445

Lynch M, Bodley K (2014) Phocid seals. In *Zoo Animal and Wildlife Immobilization and Anaesthesia*. 2nd edn. (Eds G West, D Heard and N Caulkett) pp. 647–659. John Wiley and Sons, Hoboken, NJ.

Lynch M, Taylor TK, Duignan PJ, Swingler J, Marenda M, Arnould JP, Kirkwood R (2011) Mycoplasmas in Australian fur seals (*Arctocephalus pusillus doriferus*): identification and association with abortion. *Journal of Veterinary Diagnostic Investigation* **23**, 1123–1130. doi:10.1177/1040638711425699

Marsh H, O'Shea TJ, Reynolds JE, III (2011) *The Ecology and Conservation of Sirenia: Dugongs and Manatees*. Cambridge University Press, Cambridge, UK.

McIntosh RR, Arthur AD, Dennis T, Berris M, Goldsworthy SD, Shaughnessy PD, Teixeira CEP (2013) Survival estimates for the Australian sea lion: negative correlation of sea surface temperature with cohort survival to weaning. *Marine Mammal Science* **29**, 84–108. doi:10.1111/j.1748-7692.2011.00558.x

McIntosh RR, Murray MD (2007) Louse infestations of the Australian sea lion *Neophoca cinerea*. *Australian Mammalogy* **29**, 103–106. doi:10.1071/AM07014

McKenzie J, Page B, Goldsworthy SD, Hindell MA (2013) Behavioral responses of New Zealand fur seals (*Arctophoca australis forsteri*) to darting and the effectiveness of midazolam and tiletamine-zolazepam for remote chemical immobilization. *Marine Mammal Science* **29**, 241–260. doi:10.1111/j.1748-7692.2011.00553.x

McMahon CR, Burton HR, Hoff JVD, Woods R, Bradshaw CJA (2006) Assessing hot-iron and cryo-branding for permanently marking southern elephant seals. *The Journal of Wildlife Management* **70**, 1484–1489. doi:10.2193/0022-541X(2006)70[1484:AHACFP]2.0.CO;2

McMahon CR, Field IC, Bradshaw CJA, White GC, Hindell MA (2008) Tracking and data-logging devices attached to elephant seals do not affect individual mass gain or survival. *Journal of Experimental Marine Biology and Ecology* **360**, 71–77. doi:10.1016/j.jembe.2008.03.012

Meager JJ, Limpus C (2014) Mortality of inshore marine mammals in eastern Australia is predicted by freshwater discharge and air temperature. *PLoS One* **9**, e94849. doi:10.1371/journal.pone.0094849

Michael SA, Hayman DTS, Gray R, Zhang J, Rogers L, Roe WD (2019) Pup mortality in New Zealand sea lions (*Phocarctos hookeri*) at Enderby Island, Auckland Islands, 2013–2018. *PLoS One* **14**, e0225461. doi:10.1371/journal.pone.0225461

Monamy V (2007) Hot iron branding of seals and sea lions: why the ban will remain. *Australian Veterinary Journal* **85**, 485–486. doi:10.1111/j.1751-0813.2007.00239.x

Mörner T, Malmsten J, Bernodt K, Lunneryd SG (2013) A study on the effect of different rifle calibres in euthanisation of grey seals (*Halichoerus grypus*) in seal traps in the Baltic Sea. *Acta Veterinaria Scandinavica* **55**, 79. doi:10.1186/1751-0147-55-79

Nolan EC, Walsh MT (2014) Sirenians (manatees and dugongs). In *Zoo Animal and Wildlife Immobilization and Anaesthesia*. 2nd edn. (Eds G West, D Heard and N Caulkett) pp. 693–702. John Wiley and Sons, Hoboken, NJ.

Owen H, Gillespie A, Wilkie I (2012) Postmortem findings from dugong (*Dugong dugon*) submissions to the University of Queensland: 1997–2010. *Journal of Wildlife Diseases* **48**, 962–970. doi:10.7589/2011-03-080

Paterson R, Paterson P (1984) A study of the past and present status of humpback whales in east Australian waters. *Biological Conservation* **29**, 321–343. doi:10.1016/0006-3207(84)90003-X

Pirotta V, Owen K, Donnelly D, Brasier MJ, Harcourt R (2021) First evidence of bubble-net feeding and the formation of 'super-groups' by the east Australian population of humpback whales during their southward migration. *Aquatic Conservation: Marine and Freshwater Ecosystems* **31**, 2412–2419. doi:10.1002/aqc.3621

Pirotta V, Reynolds W, Ross G, *et al.* (2020) A citizen science approach to long-term monitoring of humpback whales (*Megaptera novaeangliae*) off Sydney, Australia. *Marine Mammal Science* **36**, 472–485. doi:10.1111/mms.12651

Pirotta V, Smith A, Ostrowski M, Russell D, Jonsen ID, Grech A, Harcourt R (2017) An economical custom-built drone for assessing whale health. *Frontiers in Marine Science* **4**, 425. doi:10.3389/fmars.2017.00425

Rengifo-Herrera C, Ortega-Mora LM, Alvarez-García G, Gómez-Bautista M, García-Párraga D, García-Peña FJ, Pedraza-Díaz S (2012) Detection of *Toxoplasma gondii* antibodies in Antarctic pinnipeds. *Veterinary Parasitology* **190**, 259–262. doi:10.1016/j.vetpar.2012.05.020

Seddon JM, Ovenden JR, Sneath HL, Broderick D, Dudgeon CL, Lanyon JM (2014) Fine scale population structure of dugongs (*Dugong dugon*) implies low gene flow along the southern Queensland coastline. *Biological Conservation* **15**, 1381–1392. doi:10.1007/s10592-014-0624-x

Seguel M, Paredes E, Paves H, Gottdenker N (2014) Capture-induced stress cardiomyopathy in South American fur seal pups (*Arctophoca australis gracilis*). *Marine Mammal Science* **30**, 1149–1157. doi:10.1111/mms.12079

Sheppard JK, Preen AR, Marsh H, Lawler IR, Whiting SD, Jones RE (2006) Movement heterogeneity of dugongs, Dugong dugon (Müller), over large spatial scales. *Journal of Experimental Marine Biology and Ecology* **334**, 64–83. doi:10.1016/j.jembe.2006.01.011

Shirihai H, Jarrett B (2006) *Whales, Dolphins and Seals: A Field Guide to the Marine Mammals of the World.* A & C Black, London, UK.

Society of Marine Mammalogy (2020) Ethics. <https://marinemammalscience.org/about-us/ethics/>.

Vogelnest L, Woods R (Eds) (2019) *Current Therapy in Medicine of Australian Mammals.* CSIRO Publishing, Melbourne.

Wilkinson IS, Chilvers BL, Duignan PJ, Pistorius PA (2011) An evaluation of hot-iron branding as a permanent marking method for adult New Zealand sea lions, *Phocarctos hookeri. Wildlife Research* **38**, 51–60. doi:10.1071/WR10077

Wildlife Computers (2020) PRD-PD. <https://wildlifecomputers.com/our-tags/extras/prd-rp/>.

Wilson RP, McMahon CR (2006) Measuring devices on wild animals: what constitutes acceptable practice? *Frontiers in Ecology and the Environment* **4**, 147–154. doi:10.1890/1540-9295(2006)004[0147:MDOWAW]2.0.CO;2

Wright BE, Brown RF, DeLong RL, Gearin PJ, Riemer SD, Laake JL, Scordino JJ (2017) Survival rates of Steller sea lions from Oregon and California. *Journal of Mammalogy* **98**, 885–894. doi:10.1093/jmammal/gyx033

Zeh DR, Heupel MR, Hamann M, Jones R, Limpus C, Marsh H (2018) Evidence of behavioural thermoregulation by dugongs at the high latitude limit to their range in eastern Australia. *Journal of Experimental Marine Biology and Ecology* **508**, 27–34. doi:10.1016/j.jembe.2018.08.004

Zeh DR, Heupel MR, Limpus CJ, Hamann M, Fuentes MMPB, Babcock RC, Pillans RD, Townsend KA, Marsh H (2015) Is acoustic tracking appropriate for air-breathing marine animals? Dugongs as a case study. *Journal of Experimental Marine Biology and Ecology* **464**, 1–10. doi:10.1016/j.jembe.2014.11.013

26 Reptiles

Deborah S. Bower, Ruchira Somaweera, Nick Clemann, Jenna M. Crowe-Riddell, Simon Clulow, Matthew J. Greenlees, Katie Howard, Gerald Kuchling, Donald T. McKnight, Jane Melville, Jason Schaffer, Lin Schwarzkopf, Derek Spielman, Louise Streeting, Eric Vanderduys and Christina N. Zdenek

INTRODUCTION

Reptiles form a paraphyletic taxon (descending from a common evolutionary origin, but excluding some descendants) that, in Australia, includes crocodiles, snakes and lizards, and turtles. The enormous variation among and within the different groups makes summarising their requirements challenging. In Australia, only two crocodylian species are extant, whereas squamates (lizards and snakes) have radiated into > 1000 extant species. Around 31 freshwater turtle species and six marine species occur in Australia. Thirty of the freshwater species are classed as 'side-necked' turtles, a group that is currently only located in Australasia, Africa and South America. Collectively, these reptiles occupy diverse habitats, including the ocean, freshwater, and terrestrial environments. For many species, much remains unknown about their biology, ecology and conservation requirements. Continuing research on this group of animals is critical to address these knowledge gaps.

CROCODILES

Ruchira Somaweera

Characteristics

Two crocodile species occur in Australia. The larger of the two, the saltwater or estuarine crocodile (*Crocodylus porosus*), inhabits possibly all tidal waterways and many adjacent freshwater systems across tropical northern Australia (in Western Australia, Northern Territory and Queensland), and small offshore islands (Webb *et al.* 1983e). Saltwater crocodiles are broad-snouted, have fewer nuchal plates on their necks than other crocodylians, and do not have osteoderms (bony deposits) in the ventral scales. The smaller Australian freshwater or Johnston's river crocodile (*C. johnstoni*) is endemic to tropical mainland northern Australia (in Western Australia, Northern Territory and Queensland). Introduced populations exist as far south as Rockhampton in Queensland (Read *et al.* 2004). They inhabit almost every type of permanent freshwater habitat upstream of tidal influence (Webb and Manolis 2010) and some populations extend into tidal, saline waters (Webb *et al.* 1983d). Males can grow to > 3 m, while females are seldom > 2 m in length. Freshwater crocodiles are a slender-snouted species and have a mean lifespan of ~50 years in the wild (Webb and Manolis 1998). Some isolated populations in higher-elevation rocky escarpments show dwarfism (Britton *et al.* 2013).

Biology and behaviour

Crocodiles are opportunistic feeders and either consume large numbers of small prey or small numbers of large prey, with prey size increasing as body size increases. The frequency of different foods eaten differs significantly with type of habitat, season, and other environmental factors (Somaweera *et al.* 2020). Juvenile saltwater crocodiles feed on crustaceans, amphibians and fish with an increasing percentage of mammals, reptiles and birds included in their diet as they grow (Taylor 1979). In contrast, juvenile and adult freshwater crocodiles largely feed on fish, with insects, crustaceans, amphibians, smaller reptiles, and water birds taken occasionally (Webb *et al.* 1982; Tucker *et al.* 1996). Large mammalian prey (such as wallabies) may be opportunistically taken, especially during the peak dry season (Somaweera *et al.* 2018). Both species will prey on the invasive cane toads (*Rhinella marina*), with some freshwater crocodile populations experiencing significant mortality through direct poisoning after ingestion (Somaweera *et al.* 2013b).

Saltwater crocodiles in non-tidal waterholes in Queensland occupy larger home ranges during the wet season than in the dry season. Males occupy larger home ranges compared to females during the wet season, but similarly sized home ranges during the dry season (Brien *et al.* 2008). Females usually occupy a narrow (< 1 km) length of river, but can travel long distances (> 50 km) to nest (Campbell *et al.* 2013). Juveniles usually stay close to the nest sites where they hatched. Nomadic individuals can travel > 6 km per day during the breeding period. Comparatively little is known about freshwater crocodiles, but they may show a high level of site fidelity. Long-term mark–recapture studies in Queensland show that annual movements from 'home' averaged < 1 km except for those of pubescent males, which are relatively nomadic (Tucker *et al.* 1997). Subadults are generally more nomadic than adults. In the Northern Territory, > 80% of freshwater crocodiles caught over a year were located within 1 km of the pool in which they had been originally marked and released (Webb *et al.* 1983a). Both species show strong homing behaviour, with translocated individuals returning rapidly to their capture locations (Webb *et al.* 1983b; Read *et al.* 2007).

The two species have contrasting nesting strategies. Female saltwater crocodiles mature at ≥ 12 years (~2.5 m in total length) and lay eggs in a mound of vegetation during the annual wet season (October–May). The mean clutch size is around 50 (Webb *et al.* 1983c) and eggs typically hatch after 80–90 days depending on temperature. Some wild females actively defend their nests (Somaweera *et al.* 2013a). Female freshwater crocodiles also sexually mature at ~12 years (~1.5 m in total length), and dig holes to construct nests in a range of diggable substrates on river and lake banks (Somaweera and Shine 2013). Mean clutch size is 13 eggs and incubation normally lasts 75–85 days (Webb and Smith 1984). Females do not guard the nests in the wild, but may return to their nests during the hatching period, assist hatchlings in exiting nests, and transport hatchlings to water (Somaweera and Shine 2012).

Capture and handling

Various methods are used to capture crocodiles (Table 26.1), depending on the species, size, location, habitat type, experience of the researcher, and reason for capture. During capture, the collective safety of both the crocodile and research team is paramount. Individual Australian state and territory authorities regulate methods used to capture crocodiles. These requirements must be incorporated into study designs.

Unlike other reptile groups, crocodiles can experience anaerobic metabolism when struggling during capture, leading to acidosis and death (Bennett *et al.* 1985). When capturing crocodiles, particularly individuals > 4 m, all attempts must be made to limit stress and struggling. Restrained animals must be monitored regularly. When manually handling crocodiles, the body of the animal must be well supported and the head secured firmly.

Care should be taken when collecting and handling eggs. To minimise deposition of human scent, it is advisable to wear rubber boots and latex gloves, and place equipment on plastic drop sheets rather than on the soil surface at nest sites. Eggs can be marked and numbered on the dorsal surface using lead pencils to allow correct replacement and orientation within the clutch cavity.

All crocodiles can inflict serious damage by biting or lashing out with tails. In every capture scenario involving juvenile and adult crocodiles, the head must be controlled and jaws securely tied/tethered to prevent injury to handlers and to the animal. Various equipment can be used to secure jaws. The appropriate choice depends on the size of the animal captured. Rubber bands for animals < 1 m, cable ties, duct tape or ropes/cord for those > 1 m, and one or more snout ropes placed over the top jaw behind the largest teeth, then tied around both jaws after closing them for large animals > 2 m. The diameter of the snout rope should be appropriate to the size of the crocodile, have a spliced loop, and be applied as a noose. This way the rope can be tightened and undone easily and without knots. If large cable ties are being used, it is advisable to attach them to a rope fed through a hollow PVC pipe of at least 1.5 m and then place the loop over the crocodile's snout (so the researcher is not close to the

Table 26.1: Capture methods used for crocodiles based on circumstance and size.

Circumstance	Method	Summary	Size range
Crocodile within reach	Hand capture	Animal grasped behind the neck and constrained using both hands.	< 0.8 m
	Tongs	'Plucking' crocodiles from water using large tongs (e.g. 'Pilstom' tongs).	< 1.2 m
	Hand nets	Animal scooped using hand nets by wading in shallow water or from a boat.	< 1.6 m
	Noosing	Either a self-locking, non-slipping cable or rope tied to a long pole (for large animals) or use of a Ketch-All pole (or alike) for small animals. The noose is ideally secured over upper jaw (for wide snouted species) or neck (for slender snouted species). The latter needs immediate restraining and removal of noose from the neck. Often used from a boat at night combined with a spotlight or wading in shallow water.	1–6 m
	Electric stunning	Delivering an electric charge for ~5 s (depending on size and body condition of the crocodile) via a set of metal forks placed on the skin on the back of the crocodile's neck. Limited to use in smaller and shallow water bodies, but frequently used in captivity.	1–2.4 m
	Skin harpooning	Attaching a barbed detachable harpoon head and line to the skin on the neck or base of tail of a crocodile using a pole. Harpooning is the preferred method of capture for most crocodile management programs in Australia. The harpoon head can also be modified to obtain biopsy samples without having to capture and restrain the crocodile.	> 2 m
	Darting with chemical immobilisers	Use of opioids (e.g. etorphine), dissociative anaesthetics (e.g. ketamine, tiletamine–zolazepam) or other drugs to induce immobilisation. Usually targeted the lateral aspect of the base of the tail behind the hind legs. The effects of most muscle relaxants can be reversed by neostigmine methyl sulphate after restraining/transportation.	> 2 m
Crocodile not within reach, but can be seen	Weighted hooks	Weighted treble hooks attached to a fishing rod and reel casted over the crocodile and rapidly retrieved so the hook is embedded into the epidermal scales of the animal. The barbs of the treble hook should be removed to assist the hook in penetrating the skin.	1.2–3.5 m
	Drone/UAV-based capture	Baited self-locking wire noose attached to an activated payload release mechanism of a UAV and letting the crocodile bite the bait before retrieving the animal and restraining.	2–3 m
Crocodile cannot be seen (passive captures)	Netting	Setting long gill nets across water bodies and retrieving the entangled crocodiles. Nets should be continuously and thoroughly checked for movements and entangled crocodiles should be removed as soon as they are found.	> 0.5 m
	Trapping	Metal, rope and pipe traps used depending on targeted size, location and budget. Traps baited and checked as early as possible in the day to minimise the time a crocodile spends in the trap. Traps set in tidal waters should have adequate flotation so that captured crocodiles do not drown. Traps can also be fitted with radio-alarm devices that indicate when a crocodile has been captured.	2–6 m
	Baited hooks/ snaring	Only used when other capture methods are not possible, appropriate, or there is an urgency for capture. It is crucial that the captured crocodiles have access to shade or permanent water so that they do not overheat, dehydrate or drown after capture. Snares should be checked as often as practicable but, as a minimum, must be checked at first and last light on a daily basis.	1–6 m

crocodile when restraining it). If the mouth is taped closed, a small rope can be fed through the duct tape and attached to a longer rope. The duct tape can be slit right before release and pulled away from the snout using the rope from a safe distance. Regardless of the restraining method, it is crucial to ensure the animal's nostrils are not covered, and the restraints are not too tight, restricting blood flow and causing local cutaneous necrosis. Once jaws are secured, a blindfold (a heavy damp cloth or hessian bag) should be placed over the animal's eyes to reduce stress. Tape can be used on smaller animals, if care is taken to ensure that the eyes have 'sunk' into the animal's skull to prevent any damage before applying tape. Electrical/insulation tape is inappropriate for taping snouts or eyes as it can slip off under wet conditions.

On capture, some individuals regurgitate water or food. To minimise aspiration and prevent this matter flowing back into the trachea and choking the animal, its head should be kept lower than its body so that any regurgitated stomach contents drain out of the mouth immediately. If that position is not possible, then it is advisable to keep the mouth slightly open with a rubber pipe, thick rope or a padded tube placed between the jaws before the crocodile is tied, to allow regurgitated material to drain out.

Depending on project requirements, front and back legs can also be secured ('handcuffed') using bands, duct tape or rope. However, restraining legs in abnormal positions (e.g. pulled too far in a dorsal position) can easily dislocate joints and restraining legs for long periods (> 4 h) can cause severe oedema of the pectoral and pelvic joints. Crocodiles with their legs restrained should be monitored for swelling in the legs at regular intervals and the restraints immediately loosened or removed if swelling is identified.

Animals should be restrained in shady locations away from direct sun, and monitored for exposure to direct sun and biting insects, especially ants. The restrained individual may need to be doused with water to avoid hyperthermia. The time a crocodile is restrained should be minimised. Captured crocodiles can become unconscious and drown after release if not allowed to rest after prolonged physical restraint (Sedgwick 1986). Alternative restraining methods include placing animals in capped round polyvinyl chloride (PVC) pipes with a diameter determined by the size/girth of the crocodile, wrapping in stout cloth sheets, or using immobilising drugs.

Unmarked animals can be marked by scute clipping, PIT tagging, web tagging and plastic tagging (Figure 26.1). Scute clipping is the most common method used in field studies in Australia and involves cutting the raised tail scutes according to a predetermined numbering system. It is suitable for crocodiles of all sizes and the tissue removed from scute clipping can be used for genetic analysis. PIT tags and web tags are suitable for juveniles and adults. PIT tagging involves implanting the tag subcutaneously along the dorsal midline between the posterior margin of the cranial platform and the nuchal scales, or at the base of the tail adjacent to the cloaca. Web tags are small metal tags with a unique identity number 'clipped' to the web skin between digit 1 and 2 in the right front limb. Coloured plastic tags (such as cattle ear tags or anchor fish tags) with unique identity numbers or/and colours can be attached to the nuchal scales or tail scutes of larger adults.

Method of transportation depends on the size of the animal, distance transported and remoteness of area. Hatchlings are best transported in tubs with a wet towel placed on the bottom while juveniles can be placed in individual tubes or PVC pipes appropriate to their size (e.g. Wilson 1994). Larger animals are usually tied to 'carry boards' to prevent excessive struggling during transportation. Carry boards also make loading and unloading animals easier. Large crocodiles can also be transported in custom-built ventilated crates.

General considerations for welfare of crocodiles during transportation include the following:

- All ropes around the body should be locked rather than slip knots that can continually tighten.
- No sharp or abrasive surfaces should be in contact with the crocodile.
- The animal should not be exposed to excessive heating or cooling.
- The head should be lower than the body and facing downwards and/or the mouth slightly open to prevent vomiting and choking.
- The eyes should be covered (large animals) or the crocodile kept in a dark tub/ pipe (small animals).
- The crocodile should be doused with water regularly if transporting it for long durations or under hot conditions.
- Padding should be used between and under containers to reduce vibrations and insulate from heat from the vehicle.

Veterinary considerations

Sedation and anaesthesia

Manual restraint of large crocodylians is dangerous even under controlled conditions and can require many people. Although electrical stunning with a 110 V charge delivered to the back of the neck can be arguably less stressful than manual restraint for large crocodiles (Pfitzer *et al.* 2014), chemical immobilisation is preferred in most contexts. Medetomidine (0.5 mg/kg via intramuscular injection, usually given in the triceps muscle) effectively immobilises juvenile farmed crocodiles of 3–12 kg for at least 40 min. For crocodiles up to two orders of magnitude larger, the doses required can

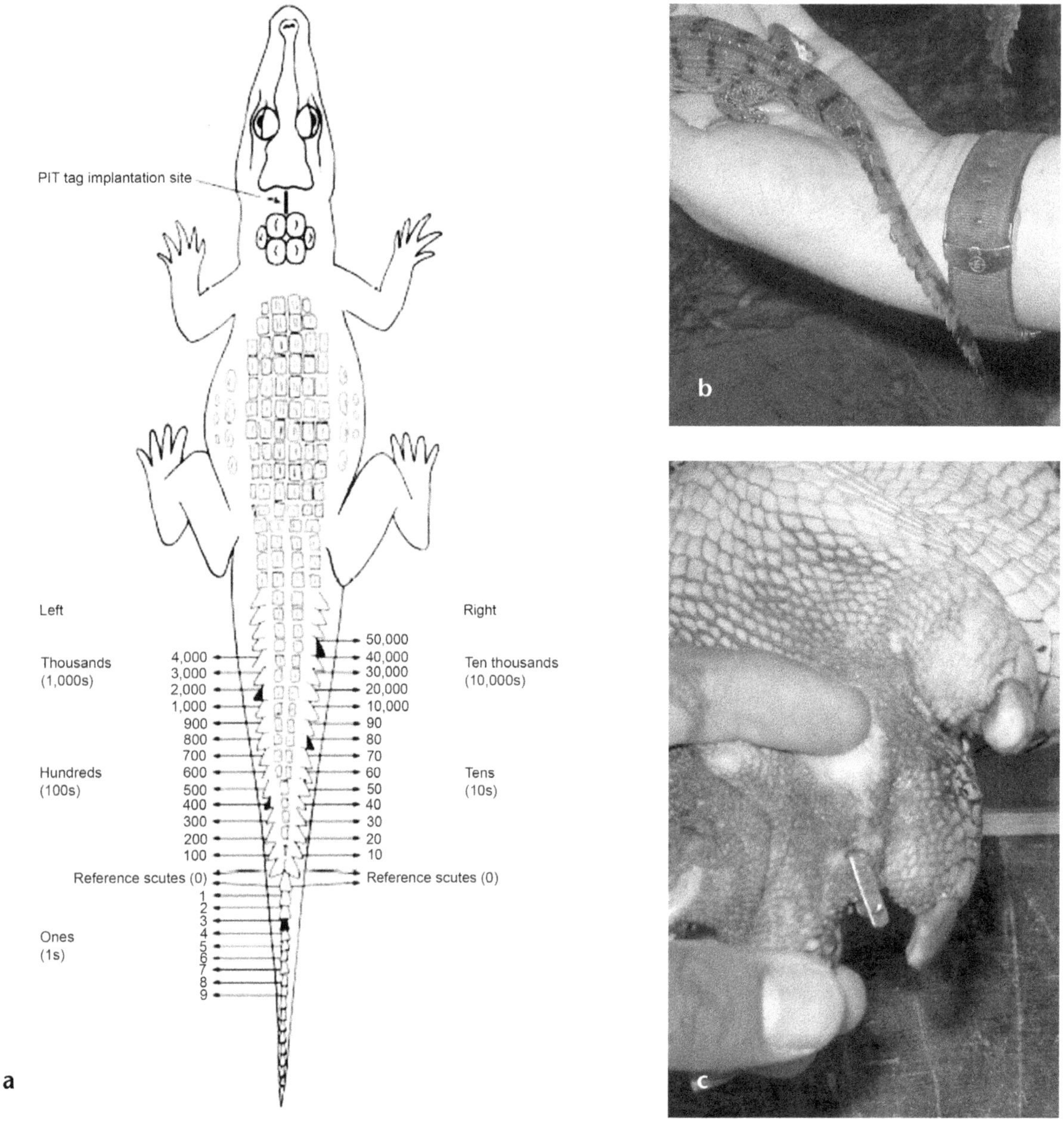

Figure 26.1: Methods for marking crocodiles. (a) Scute clipping system and PIT tag locations. Illustration by Kay (2005). (b) Example of scute clipping on a juvenile crocodile. (c) Example of a metal web tag attached between digits. Photos by Ruchira Somaweera.

be calculated using metabolic scaling for reptiles. Atipamezole should be administered into the opposite triceps muscle to reverse the medetomidine; otherwise medetomidine can affect behaviour for up to 2 days (Olsson 2014). Historically, neuromuscular blockers (e.g. suxamethonium) were used for crocodile immobilisation, but their use for research is not permitted in non-anaesthetised animals in Australia. Inhalant anaesthesia can also be used for crocodiles (Fleming 2014), but because of challenges associated with reptile anaesthesia, this approach is not recommended for minor procedures.

Blood collection

Both large volumes and smaller serial blood samples can be taken from the spinal venous sinus of crocodiles, accessed through the interarcuate space between the atlas and axis (C1 and C2: the first and second cervical vertebrae) by inserting a 22 G needle angled just off the perpendicular in the midline through the craniodorsal

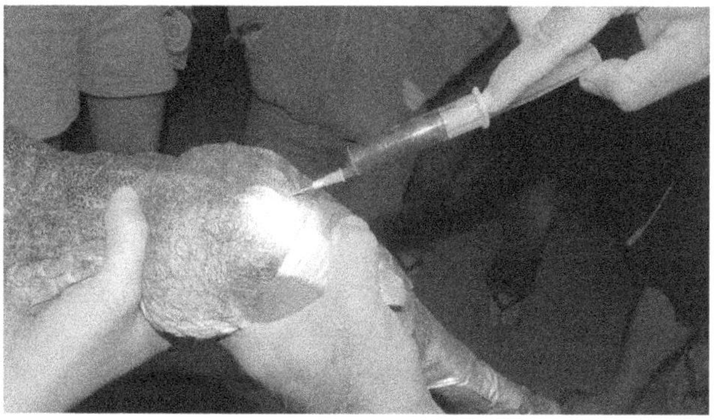

Figure 26.2: Obtaining blood from a freshwater crocodile (*Crocodylus johnstoni*) in the field via the spinal venous sinus. Photo by Ruchira Somaweera.

cervical skin, cranial to the cranial borders of the first cervical osteoderms (see Figure 26.2; Myburgh *et al.* 2014). The needle should be moved slowly towards the vertebral column, taking care to avoid the spinal cord. A blood sample can also be obtained from the caudal tail vein that lies ventral to the tail vertebrae. With the crocodile in dorsal recumbency (abdomen facing up, back to the table or substrate), insert the needle about one-third of the distance from the tail tip to the base of the tail (Myburgh *et al.* 2014).

Euthanasia

Personnel should refer to recommendations from the Veterinary Science Group of the IUCN Crocodile Specialists Group (CSG) (Martelli *et al.* 2020) and relevant codes of practice (Department of Environment and Science 2008; Commonwealth of Australia 2009). Physical euthanasia techniques include destruction of the brain with captive-bolt rifle shot (Huchzermeyer 2003), blunt force trauma and cervical severance, with all followed by pithing if required (Nevarez *et al.* 2014). Chemical euthanasia via pentobarbitone can also be used, but the body must be then disposed in a manner that prevents scavenging (i.e., deep burial). All euthanasia methods must be conducted by appropriately experienced, licensed, and trained personnel. Euthanasia methods that are generally considered to be unacceptable for crocodylians include inhalation of toxic gases, drowning, heating, freezing and exsanguination (Hutton 1992).

Infectious pathogens

Studies on infectious pathogens of wild crocodiles in Australia are scarce and little is known of their zoonotic potential. A precautionary approach regards all crocodiles as potentially harbouring zoonotic pathogens. Pathogens and parasites known from Australian crocodile species are largely based on records from the commercial crocodile farming industry (see Table 26.2). Not all listed pathogens cause diseases, nor will all parasites always cause harm.

General operating procedures

General operating procedures that may be relevant to crocodile research include collection of scats, evaluation of eDNA and other traces (Chapter 4), camera trapping (Chapter 5), a range of research methods for marine and freshwater animals (Chapters 12 and 14, respectively), tracking methods (Chapter 9), and several veterinary procedures (Chapter 16).

SNAKES AND LIZARDS

Deborah S. Bower, Nick Clemann, Jenna M. Crowe-Riddell, Simon Clulow, Matthew Greenlees, Jane Melville, Lin Schwarzkopf, Derek Spielman, Eric Vanderduys and Christina N. Zdenek

Characteristics

Squamates are the most speciose group of Australian reptiles, comprising 852 lizard and 214 snake species (Wilson and Swan 2021); new species are described regularly. Australian squamates are ecologically diverse, ranging enormously in size. For example, the largest Australian snake species is the scrub python (*Simalia kinghorni*) with a mass of around 30 kg and body length of up to 6 m. Australia's largest lizard species, the iconic perentie (*Varanus giganteus*) of arid western and central Australia, can reach a mass of 17 kg. The lizards also include some of Australia's smallest reptile species, with some skinks weighing < 0.2 g. Squamates show extensive variation in reproductive mode (laying eggs, including parthenogenesis; bearing live young; or sometimes both) and habitat preferences. Knowledge of species' biology and ecology ranges from extensive information collected through multi-decadal studies of sleepy lizards (*Tiliqua rugosa*) (Bull *et al.* 2017) to limited information for roughly one-quarter of fossorial blind snake (*Anilios* spp.) species, many of which are known from only a single specimen or location, without photographs of extant species (Vanderduys 2013).

Biology and behaviour

Diets are diverse, ranging from specialist to generalist, with some species, such as the carnivorous perentie, preying primarily on eggs, insects, birds and other reptiles

Table 26.2: Known pathogens and parasites identified in Australian crocodile species.

Pathogen category	Taxa
Virus	Flaviviridae Herpesviridae Poxviridae
Bacteria	Dermatophilaceae, including *Dermatophilus* spp. Enterobacteriaceae, including *Serratia liquefaciem, Salmonella* spp. *Edwardsiella* spp., *Proteus rettgeri, Klebsiella* spp. Mycobacteriacea, including *Mycobacterium intracellulare, M. szulgai* Streptococcaceae, including *Streptococcus agalactiae* Vibrionaceae, including *Aeromonas hydrophila*
Fungi	Nectriaceae, including *Fusarium* spp. Onygenaceae, including *Nannizziopsis crocodili, Chrysosporium* spp. Saccharomycetaceae, including *Candida* spp. Syncephalastraceae, including *Syncephalastrum* spp. Trichocomaceae, including *Penicillium oxalicum, Paecilomyces* spp.
Parasites	Anisakidae, including *Terranova crocodili, Goezia holmesi, Typhlophorus spratti* Ascarididae, including *Brevimulticaecum australiensis, Dujardinascaris blairi* Capillariidae, including *Paratrichosoma crocodylus, Crocodilocapillaria longiovata* Cryptogonimidae, including *Proctocaecum blairi, P. nicolli* Diphyllobothriidae, including *Spirometra erinacei* Exotidendriidae, including *Renivermis crocodyli* Ixodidae, including *Amblyomma* spp. Micropleudidae, including *Micropleura australiensis* Oswaldofilariidae, including *Oswaldofilaria kanbaya* Plagiorchioidea, including *Deurithitrema gingae* Schistosomatidae, including *Griphobilharzia amoena* Sebekidae, including *Alofia* spp., *Leiperia australiensis, Sebekia multiannulata, Selfia* spp. Trichosomoididae, including *Paratrichosoma crocodylus* Trypanosomatidae, including *Leishmania* spp. Unidentified coccidian spp. Unidentified hirudian spp.

(including other goannas; e.g. Macdonald 2007; Rhind *et al.* 2019). Others, such as blind snakes, feed primarily on ant larvae and pupae (Webb and Shine 1993). Within populations, diet can vary spatially and temporally (Goodyear and Pianka 2011; Atkins *et al.* 2018), and in response to environmental factors (Griffiths and Christian 1996). Within species, foraging modes may vary with sex and season (e.g. in sleepy lizards) (Kerr and Bull 2006). Diet may also vary with sex and ontogeny. For example, bearded dragons switch from insectivores to omnivores as they mature, and large males are primarily herbivorous (*Pogona barbata*) (Wotherspoon and Burgin 2016).

Movement patterns vary with body size and shape (Smith and Griffiths 2009), sex (Olsson and Shine 2003), and environmental factors (e.g. drought; fire). Habitat use and occupancy are influenced by natural (e.g. geology, vegetation or fire) and human-driven processes (e.g. conversion of native vegetation to agriculture, weed invasion, grazing and fire). Some species, including certain widespread squamates, will avoid some types of modified environments (e.g. the gecko *Gehyra versicolor* avoids farmland; Hansen *et al.* 2020).

Most squamates are polygynous, polyandrous, or both (Whiting and While 2017), but monogamous pairing does occur. For example, sleepy lizards form monogamous pair bonds that can last > 10 years (Bull 2000; Bull *et al.* 2017). Kin-based relationships occur in at least one radiation of skinks (*Egernia* spp.) with stable family groups that have multiple cohorts (Gardner *et al.* 2016). Communal nesting (Doody *et al.* 2009a; Doody *et al.* 2018) and communal use of shelter and over-winter sites in unrelated individuals not uncommon (e.g. prickly forest skink, *Gnypetoscincus queenslandiae*; Sumner 2006).

Groups can be wholly oviparous (e.g. all Australian dragon species), viviparous (e.g. Arafura file snake, *Acrochordus arafurae*), or have a mixture of reproductive modes (e.g. skinks). In some lizards, different populations and even single clutches can be facultatively oviparous or viviparous (e.g. three-toed skink, *Saiphos equalis*, Laird *et al.* 2019; Bougainville's skink, *Lerista bougainvillii*, Qualls and Shine 1998). Parthenogenesis occurs in several lizard species (Moritz 1984; Adams *et al.* 2003) and snakes (Nussbaum 1980; Allen *et al.* 2018). Primary sex development is determined by temperature or genetic pathways (occasionally both). For example, bearded dragons (*Pogona vitticeps*) can reverse their sex when temperature overrides genetic determination (Holleley *et al.* 2016).

Most squamates have seasonal reproduction, even in tropical regions where nesting follows monsoonal rains (e.g. keelback snake, *Tropidonophis mairii*) (Brown and Shine 2006), but timing varies considerably among species (James and Shine 1985). Mating activity in temperate regions occurs mostly in warmer months, with at least some species also active in winter, such as red-bellied black snakes (*Pseudechis porphyriacus*; Shine 1979). In temperate zones spring mating and birth or hatching in late summer is common, but autumn mating, sperm storage over winter, and spring fertilisation also occur (e.g. Murphy *et al.* 2006). Discrete breeding seasons and diel activity cycles are important considerations for study design.

Capture and handling

Options for capturing (Table 26.3) and marking (Table 26.4) squamates are diverse and depend on the study species, project aims and location.

Restraint methods are species-specific. In general, the firmer the grip, the more a lizard will struggle. A towel or gloves can protect handlers from sharp nails or bites but may reduce the sensitivity of the handler's touch. Large lizards can be placed on a table in a crossed-hands hold (a handler crosses hands over the lizard's body and holds the back of the head with one hand and the tail or pelvis with the other). For many species, tail loss is a risk, so handlers should take care to prevent loss of the tail in species capable of tail autotomy, which is a defensive adaptation that allows the tail to fracture and detach from the body when held by a predator or when the lizard is fearful of attack. Tails will regrow in most cases, but that will require the animal to direct energy to doing so. Some lizard species can be relaxed by gently stroking the pineal

Table 26.3: Summary of common survey and capture techniques for Australian squamates.

Method	Suitable taxa
Artificial cover objects (ACO) (arboreal or terrestrial)	Terrestrial, arboreal and fossorial squamates
Raking	Fossorial squamates
Active searching including spotlighting and road cruising	Terrestrial and arboreal squamates
Passive searching	Surface active terrestrial and arboreal squamates
PVC pipes	Monitors (as a trap), earless dragons (as a burrow)
Cage and Elliott traps	Monitors, skinks, and dragons
Funnel traps	Terrestrial, arboreal, and some fossorial squamates
Pitfall traps	Terrestrial, arboreal, and some fossorial squamates
Sticky traps	Small lizards
Noosing/fishing	Skinks, monitors, and dragons
Fyke nets	Freshwater snakes: colubrid and file snakes
Snorkelling/diving/manta tow	Aquatic snakes, water dragons
Baited remote underwater video stations	Aquatic snakes
Hand nets	Aquatic snakes
Gill/trammel netting nets	Aquatic snakes
Camera trapping	Larger lizards, snakes
Long range photography	Skinks

Table 26.4: Summary of common marking techniques for Australian squamates.

Method	Taxa
Toe clipping	Small to medium-sized skinks
Scale clipping	Colubrid and elapid snakes
Passive integrated transponder (PIT) tags and other small chip devices, such as radio frequency identification (RFID)	All groups*
Photographic identification	Species with adequate and unique markings (e.g. skinks, pygopodids, terrestrial snakes and some sea snakes)
Non-toxic paint, dye, or pens,	All groups
Visual implant elastomer (VIE)	All groups

* Where individuals are large enough

gland on the top of their head or by securing cotton balls over their eyes with self-adhesive tape, which induces a vasovagal (fainting) response. Small lizards can be restrained more easily with a towel in some cases, or anaesthetised (see 'Veterinary considerations').

Because some snake species are venomous, personnel should be confident at handling target species and able to identify the species likely to be encountered. Dangerous reptiles (venomous snakes, large snakes and lizards) require specialised skills and experience, including specific equipment (e.g. snake hook, tongs, snake bag, and sometimes snake tubes and a snake pinner; Figure 26.3). Handlers should have appropriate first aid equipment on hand and an emergency response plan.

Animals must be protected from one another, hydrated, and maintained at a safe temperature during transportation. Non-aquatic squamates can be kept in calico bags for durations that are species-specific. Dehydration can be avoided to some extent by wetting a corner of the bag, while temperature can be kept relatively stable by keeping bags inside insulated containers, such as 'eskies'. Ice bricks can also be added to keep temperatures from rising beyond safe limits, but should be covered by newspaper or cloth. The newspaper or cloth material also acts as a 'cushion' to prevent forceful impact on container walls. Health and safety protocols should be adhered to for venomous snakes. Generally, venomous snakes should be transported individually inside sturdy cloth bags that are placed inside lockable containers with small air holes. The containers should have a label stating the number and species of snake inside, and 'venomous' should be clearly displayed on the container.

Species-specific requirements for temperature, humidity, space, and social interaction should be followed when housing reptiles. Housing should provide access to light and shade. Diurnal desert species require high levels of ultraviolet (UV) light (preferably direct sunlight) particularly during growth, for proper bone formation. A suitable substrate and access to food and water must also be provided.

Food must provide sufficient energy, calcium, vitamins D and A, and fibre. Uneaten food should be removed. Species-specific dietary requirements should be considered. Many species are specialist eaters (e.g. sea snakes are piscivorous (feeding on fish)), and generalist-feeding species are easier to feed and survive better in captivity than specialists (J. M. Crowe-Riddell, pers. obs.).

Veterinary considerations

Sedation and anaesthesia

All reptiles should be restrained appropriately when undertaking procedures, and handlers should be mindful of the potential for tail loss in some species. Reptile anaesthesia is challenging compared to that of mammals or birds, requiring specialised approaches. These challenges are exacerbated under field conditions. In broad terms, gaseous anaesthesia (typically isoflurane) is the mainstay of squamate chemical restraint. Induction chambers are especially useful for venomous snakes while mask induction can be used for varanids. Snakes are usually intubated (Bryant *et al.* 2010). Injectable approaches also have value, especially the use of intramuscular alfaxalone for anaesthetic induction, as well as tiletamine–zolazepam (with the drawback of prolonged recoveries). Safe administration of reptile anaesthesia

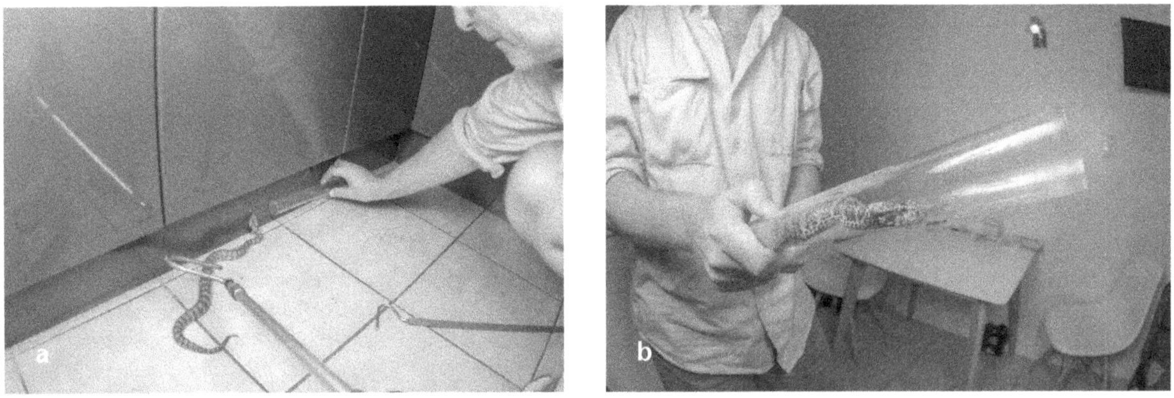

Figure 26.3: A snake restraining tube being used to safely handle a common death adder (*Acanthophis antarcticus*). (a) Working in pairs, one uses a snake hook to encourage the snake to move forward, while the other holds the tube. (b) The snake inside of the restraining tube, which is matched to the size of the snake. Work can then safely proceed on the posterior half of the snake. Photos by Elliot Budd.

requires close attention to maintaining correct temperature and providing mechanical ventilation. For detailed instructions, see Bertelsen (2014).

Blood collection

Caudal vein puncture is recommended for snakes and lizards to obtain small volumes of blood. For snakes, a maximum 'safe' single draw blood volume estimate is 0.6% of the animal's body mass (6 mL per kg). Two of the descriptions below are relatively 'blind' techniques that require aspiration. If unsuccessful on the insertion, personnel should apply gentle or intermittent aspiration throughout a slow needle retraction (Dyer and Cervasio 2008). Snakes should be placed in ventral recumbency with the tail held vertically below (e.g. on a table with the tail over the edge) to enable blood to 'pool' caudally. The belly should face the collector (Lloyd and Morris 1999). The paired hemipenes of male snakes and the paired musk glands of females should be avoided (Dyer and Cervasio 2008).

The ventral coccygeal vein can be accessed by placing the needle on the ventral midline and angling it 45–60° to the plane of the subcaudal scales (Figure 16.3a in Chapter 16). The needle should be inserted and pushed in direction of the head until the needle touches the vertebra. Then it should be withdrawn slowly, but with a slight negative pressure. Snakes < 250 g in mass require a 27 G, 5/8 inch needle with a 1–2 mL syringe; larger snakes require a 25 G needle (Lloyd and Morris 1999). The needle should be inserted into the mid-ventral tail at ~30° towards the feet in a perpendicular line. Blood flow is best when the needle is withdrawn very slightly after contacting the ventral coccygeal vertebral body. Both sexes of some species have large musk glands. If punctured, the sample will be contaminated with musk fluid.

Collection of blood from the heart can be used when a large volume of blood is required. The snake must be anaesthetised and positioned in dorsal recumbency, with the location of the heart determined by watching for the heartbeat. The heart should be stabilised between the finger and thumb and the needle introduced underneath a ventral scale about one or two scales posterior to the heart's location. The needle should be inserted 45° towards the animal's head through its skin and into the apex of the ventricle. Too much negative pressure on the syringe may collapse the ventricles, causing death.

The caudal tail vein is the most clinically useful site for blood collection from lizards. Blood collection can be made from the ventral or lateral part of the tail, anywhere from 20–80% down its length. If approaching from the ventrum, the needle should be positioned along the ventral midline perpendicular to the skin, and inserted while applying a slight negative pressure. If coccygeal vertebrae are encountered, the needle should be withdrawn slightly. If the vein is approached laterally (from the side), the lateral processes of the coccygeal vertebrae should be palpated and the needle inserted through the skin just ventral to these processes. However, lymphatic contamination can be more likely with the lateral approach (Bertelsen 2014).

Euthanasia

Reptile euthanasia is challenging with few recognised best-practice approaches (Warren 2014). Intravenous administration of pentobarbitone (60 mg/kg) is recommended for euthanasia of squamates (Warren 2014), but this method is not always available because it can only be administered by individuals with appropriate qualifications and licences, and can interfere with electrophysiological studies (Keifer and Zheng 2017). If barbiturates are administered via any other route, the animal must be anaesthetised. Any animal euthanased with pentobarbitone represents a secondary toxicity risk to wild scavengers and should be disposed of via deep burial. Alternatively, tricaine methanesulfonate injected into the intracoelomic cavity of reptiles is effective, but requires a buffer to prevent acidity (Conroy *et al.* 2009).

Physical euthanasia methods include blunt force trauma to the head followed by brain destruction and decapitation. Decapitation without pithing is widely considered to be unacceptable. Hypothermia (cooling then freezing) is currently debated as an acceptable method of euthanasia or anaesthesia (before euthanasia) for small-bodied ectotherms (Zulkifli *et al.* 2014; Shine *et al.* 2015; Keifer and Zheng 2017; Lillywhite *et al.* 2017). It has been suggested as an alternative method in the absence of access to Schedule 4 drugs, does not require great technical skill and training, and results in less damage to specimens than physically destructive methods. Despite some practitioners being in favour of this method, hypothermia as an anaesthetic or euthanasia method is currently prohibited by some animal ethics committees (e.g. University of Canberra AEC 2017) and is considered by some to have unacceptable animal welfare outcomes. Debate on this method continues (Lillywhite *et al.* 2017; Shine *et al.* 2019). Prohibitions on this method are based on the belief that ice crystal formation in tissue is likely to be painful

(Close *et al.* 1997; AVMA 2020) and that insufficient evidence is available to suggest cooling and freezing is not painful or distressing (Sharp *et al.* 2011; Galex *et al.* 2020).

Infectious pathogens

A suite of emerging infectious diseases (viruses, bacteria, fungi, eukaryotes) infect squamates, including zoonotic pathogens such as *Salmonella*, vectors (e.g. ticks) and *Borrelia lusitaniae* (Bower *et al.* 2019). Infectious pathogens are diverse. Researchers working with reptiles should consult the latest guidelines on pathogens of note when planning their research. Resources such as Wildlife Health Australia (2021) can assist. In some instances, it may be important to report suspected cases. Particular consideration should be given for the potential to transmit pathogens from captive animals to wild animals. For example, the fungal pathogen *Nannizziopsis barbatae* (yellow fungus disease), which had only been found in captive reptiles, has recently been detected in wild reptiles in Queensland (Wildlife Health Australia 2021).

General operating procedures

Other research methods that may apply to squamates include indirect sampling methods, such as observation (with or without spotlighting), collection of scats and eDNA, assessment of visual signs, including tracks and burrows (Chapter 4), camera trapping, and using conservation detector dogs (Chapter 5). A range of capture methods, including pitfall, cage, funnel, and aluminium box trapping (Chapter 7) may apply. Some species, such as sea snakes, may be captured by hand (Chapter 12). Depending on the species and study objectives, identification methods may include microchipping, tattooing, photographic identification, visible implant elastomer and alphanumeric tags, and toe, scale or tail-tip clipping may apply to squamates (Chapter 8). Various tracking methods may be used to study their movement and habitat use (Chapter 9). Veterinary procedures are detailed in Chapter 16.

TURTLES

Deborah S. Bower, Simon Clulow, Katie Howard, Gerald Kuchling, Donald T. McKnight, Jason Schaffer, Lin Schwarzkopf, Derek Spielman and Louise Streeting

Characteristics

Native turtles in Australia can be grouped into three taxonomic categories: sea turtles, the pig-nosed turtle, and chelids. Six of the world's seven sea turtle species occupy Australian marine waters. The freshwater pig-nosed turtle (*Carettochelys insculpta*) is the sole representative of its family (Carettochelyidae) and primarily occupies freshwater rivers. The remaining ~30 extant species are Australian chelids ('side-necked' turtles) belonging to seven genera (Wilson and Swan 2021) and occur mostly in freshwater habitats.

Biology and behaviour

Turtle diets are diverse varying from generalist omnivores (e.g. *Emydura* spp.), to more specialised carnivores (e.g. *Chelodina* spp. and western swamp turtle, *Pseudemydura umbrina*) and herbivorous turtles (e.g. *Elseya* spp.) (Welsh *et al.* 2017). Diet can also vary within species depending on habitat (Arthur *et al.* 2008), seasonal availability, and ontogeny (Kennett and Tory 1996). Some sympatric species partition resources; for example, the five turtle species occurring in the Daly River have minimal competition because of their varying diets and habitat selection (Micheli-Campbell *et al.* 2017; Welsh *et al.* 2017).

Freshwater turtles generally exhibit site fidelity, with an affinity for discrete areas that contain optimal habitats (Tucker *et al.* 2001), although male *Chelodina expansa* move up to 25 km (Bower *et al.* 2012). Sea turtles can undertake extensive migrations to reach foraging sites or return to natal sites (e.g. juvenile loggerhead sea turtles, *Caretta caretta*, can travel > 13 000 km) (Hays and Scott 2013). Species vary in their use of terrestrial habitat, which generally includes the land necessary for nesting. Aestivation (prolonged seasonal torpor or dormancy) and movement between wetlands are important for several freshwater species.

Social organisation of turtles in Australia is poorly known. Synchronous hatching occurs in the Murray short-necked turtle (*Emydura macquarii*), suggesting that individuals may adjust heart and metabolic rates within the egg (McGlashan *et al.* 2012). Underwater acoustic studies of Australian freshwater turtles have also revealed evidence of communication between turtles, but the extent to which this influences sociality remains unknown (Giles *et al.* 2009; Ferrara *et al.* 2017).

All turtles are oviparous, and almost all bury clutches in nests on land. The northern snake-necked turtle (*Chelodina rugosa*) is the exception, nesting underwater in ephemeral billabongs (Kennett *et al.* 1993). A major threat to turtle populations in Australia is the depredation of nests by the European red fox (*Vulpes vulpes*; Spencer and

Thompson 2005). Individual nests can be protected using mesh or steel cages with openings large enough to allow the emerging hatchlings to exit, but small enough to exclude predators. Nesting areas can sometimes be protected with fencing to exclude predators. Individual turtle species vary in reproductive strategies such as clutch size and nesting frequency (Broderick *et al.* 2003). Sperm storage and multiple paternity occur in at least some species (Pearse and Avise 2001). All sea turtles and the freshwater pig-nosed turtle have temperature-dependent sex determination, whereas other Australian freshwater species tested have genetically determined sexes (Mazzoleni *et al.* 2020).

Freshwater turtle activity occurs mostly in the warmer months (Fielder 2012), but *P. umbrina* is only active during the cooler half of the year. Nesting generally occurs within distinct seasons and may be cued by environmental features (e.g. temperature and rain) (Bowen *et al.* 2005). Aquatic hibernation occurs in some highly aquatic species (Fielder 2012). Some freshwater turtles occupy ephemeral habitats and, when water levels are low, may congregate in pools or aestivate.

Table 26.5: Summary of common survey and capture techniques for Australian turtles.

Method	Taxa
Corralling	Sea turtles
Rodeo	Sea turtles
Muddling	Chelids
Snorkelling	Chelids
Seine netting	Chelids
Fyke nets	Chelids
Gill/trammel nets	Chelids
Turtle traps: collapsible crayfish traps, crab pots, cathedral traps, and hoop nets/drum nets	Chelids
Basking traps	Basking turtles
Dip netting	Pig nose turtles, chelids
Baited remote underwater video (BRUV)	All species where water clarity permits
Drift fences with pitfalls or traps	Chelids

Table 26.6: Summary of common marking techniques for turtles in Australia.

Method	Taxa
Turtle tags	Sea turtles
Notching	Australian chelids, hatchling sea turtles.
Hole punch into marginal scutes via a syringe needle with small pieces of fish line knotted on both ends	Hatchling *Pseudemydura umbrina*
Visible implant elastomer	Chelid hatchlings
Passive integrated transponder (PIT) tags	All turtles
Photograph identification	Sea turtles, *Pseudemydura umbrina*

Capture and handling

Capture and marking

A variety of options exist for capturing (see Table 26.5) and marking turtles (see Table 26.6) and chosen techniques vary with targeted species, study design and activity location.

When using any form of net or trap, it is imperative that steps are taken to prevent turtles from drowning. These steps include placing floats in turtle traps and fyke nets, securing nets to stakes, trees or other structures, continually checking gill/trammel nets, and monitoring the weather closely. Once turtles are captured, they should be firmly held by the posterior plastral lobe or anterior and posterior of the carapace, and quickly transferred to a tub or bag.

Highly aquatic turtles can be held for up to 24 h in secure tubs with a small amount of water (not so much that individuals must tread water) or wet mesh bags. More terrestrial species (e.g. *Chelodina* spp. and *P. umbrina*) can be held in dry cardboard boxes with shredded newspaper (Parker *et al.* 2015). Care should be taken to ensure turtles are protected from crushing, scratching, or biting. Placing a thin rubber mat or cloth over individuals can calm them. Holding tubs should have adequate ventilation and be placed in a cool, shaded area to prevent overheating. Turtles should be transported in a ventilated escape-proof container lined with damp towels to avoid the risk of drowning, injury or stress because of sloshing.

Turtles should be kept individually or else need appropriate spacing and cover to limit aggressive behaviour between individuals. Ideally, turtles should be housed outside with access to light and dark cycles, shade, basking locations, and water for submersion. Water quality (i.e. appropriate salinity and low ammonia) should be maintained through filtration, UV sterilisation, or water exchange. For freshwater turtles, habitat enrichment should be provided (e.g. rocks and logs, aquatic vegetation and cover). Appropriate water temperatures can be maintained using an aquatic heater in cool climates and shading containers during hot weather. Housing should be predator proof. Turtles housed indoors require UVB lighting on a diel schedule. If turtles are to be released into the wild, care should be taken to limit habituation to people and to avoid modifying natural behaviours.

Food should be supplemented with calcium and vitamin D. Uneaten food should be removed. Species-specific requirements (e.g. herbivorous *v.* carnivorous diets) require consideration.

Veterinary considerations

Sedation and anaesthesia

As with other reptiles, chelonian anaesthesia is challenging (Vigani 2014). Consequently, anaesthesia of turtles is not recommended for minor procedures such as the collection of blood samples. When needed, sedation can be achieved through injection of intravenous or intramuscular alfaxalone (Scheelings 2013), or gaseous anaesthesia can be maintained via intubation (Vigani 2014), with specialised monitoring required for body temperature maintenance and ventilation.

Blood collection

The diversity in morphology of chelonians precludes any single recommended venipuncture site for all species (Vigani 2014). The jugular vein is preferred for collection of blood from turtles because larger volumes can be collected with minimal risk of lymph contamination. However, it can be difficult to extract and hold the head. The jugular vein runs along the neck at the level of the tympanic membrane, which is considerably more dorsally located than in mammals. Personnel should extend the head and occlude the jugular vein with a finger or cotton-tipped applicator while another person draws the blood. Turning the head slightly away from the side of the neck to be sampled can make the vein more visible. The intended puncture site should be disinfected. Use a new, single use needle for each animal. The needle should be placed just caudal to the tympanum and inserted towards the head. Firm (not excessive) pressure should be applied to the puncture site (with a finger is fine) after the sample has been collected to minimise haematoma formation. (Vigani 2014). Excessive pressure interferes with flow and reduces platelets forming a clot over the wound, prolonging bleeding and haematoma formation.

To collect blood from the tail vein, personnel should extend the tail and insert a 25 G needle on the dorsal midline 45–90° to the plane of the skin towards the head while exerting slight negative pressure on the needle. If the vertebra is hit, the needle should be withdrawn slightly and redirected cranially or caudally. The site is easily accessible, but only small blood volumes can be collected and samples from the caudal vein tend to be contaminated with lymph (Gottdenker and Jacobson 1995). In uncooperative chelonians, whose head and tail are inaccessible, the subcarapacial vein may be easier to access. This site is formed by the communication of the anterior intercostal vessels and the caudal cervical anastomosis of the left and right jugular veins. A 22–25 G needle should be inserted at the midline, slightly caudal to the area of skin insertion on the ventral aspect of the anterior rim of the carapace. The needle should be pushed in caudo-dorsally with slight negative pressure. If vertebrae are encountered, the needle should be withdrawn slightly and redirected cranially or caudally. Lymph contamination is also possible using this method (Vigani 2014).

Euthanasia

Similarly to squamates, intravenous pentobarbitone (60 mg/kg) is the recommended euthanasia method for turtles (Warren 2014). Pentobarbitone should be administered via the intravenous route unless the turtle is anaesthetised. This method is not always available (access to Schedule 4 drugs is not always possible) (Keifer and Zheng 2017). Any animal euthanased with pentobarbitone represents a secondary toxicity risk to wild scavengers and should be disposed of via deep burial. Captive bolt rifles have recently been trialled for euthanasia of sea turtles (Hing *et al.* 2019). In remote locations, blunt trauma to the head followed by destruction of the brain via pithing may be more appropriate (Work and Balazs 2013). Recent studies suggest that inducing hypothermia may be a feasible euthanasia method (Keifer and Zheng 2017), but, as in other taxa (e.g. amphibians), this method remains contentious and is typically not approved for use.

Infectious pathogens

Infectious disease collapsed Australia's Bellinger River snapping turtle (*Myuchelys georgesi*) population in 2015 (Zhang *et al.* 2018) with substantial resources dedicated to the species' recovery since (e.g. DPI 2015; Chessman *et al.* 2020). This event demonstrates the risks posed to chelonian populations by infectious pathogens. Care should be taken to prevent the transmission of pathogens between catchments or populations, and protocols developed for doing so should consider the specific environment and species being targeted. Avoid the translocation of turtles between catchments. Equipment used for trapping, holding, marking and transporting turtles should be disinfected with chlorine solution (200 mg/L active chlorine) to kill pathogens, or disposed of after use. Some bacteria in freshwater turtles are zoonotic. *Salmonella* spp. are carried by turtles in Australia (Scheelings *et al.* 2011) along with *Mycobacterium* spp., which can be problematic for immunosuppressed humans (Miller *et al.* 1990). *Chlamydia* spp. and *Leptospira* spp. are also associated with freshwater turtles, but to what degree these pathogens occur in Australia is unknown (Oliveira *et al.* 2016; Mitura *et al.* 2017).

General operating procedures

Techniques that may apply to turtle research are provided in more detail elsewhere in the book, including observation, evaluation of tracks and traces, eDNA and burrow/nest evaluations (Chapter 4) and camera trapping (Chapter 5). Marking methods, such as microchipping and shell notching are covered in Chapter 8, and tracking methods in Chapter 9. Citizen science approaches may also apply to turtle research (Chapter 10; also see Santori *et al.* 2018). Capture techniques and a range of marking and tracking methods relevant to marine turtles are provided in Chapter 12 but also apply to freshwater turtles (Doody *et al.* 2009b). Key capture techniques for freshwater species are detailed in Chapter 14. Veterinary procedures, including anaesthesia, sedation, and analgesics are outlined in Chapter 16.

REFERENCES

Adams M, Foster R, Hutchinson MN, Hutchinson RG, Donnellan SC (2003) The Australian scincid lizard *Menetia greyii*: a new instance of widespread vertebrate parthenogenesis. *Evolution* **57**, 2619–2627. doi:10.1111/j.0014-3820.2003.tb01504.x

Allen L, Sanders K, Thomson V (2018) Molecular evidence for the first records of facultative parthenogenesis in elapid snakes. *Royal Society Open Science* **5**, 171901. doi:10.1098/rsos.171901

Arthur KE, Boyle MC, Limpus CJ (2008) Ontogenetic changes in diet and habitat use in green sea turtle (*Chelonia mydas*) life history. *Marine Ecology Progress Series* **362**, 303–311. doi:10.3354/meps07440

Atkins ZS, Clemann N, Schroder M, Chapple DG, Davis NE, Robinson WA, Wainer J, Robert KA (2018) Consistent temporal variation in the diet of an endangered alpine lizard across two south-eastern Australian sky-islands. *Austral Ecology* **43**, 339–351. doi:10.1111/aec.12572

AVMA (2020) *AVMA Guidelines for the Euthanasia of Animals: 2020 Edition*. American Veterinary Medical Association. <https://www.avma.org/sites/default/files/2020-01/2020-Euthanasia-Final-1-17-20.pdf>.

Bennett A, Seymour R, Bradford D (1985) Mass-dependence of anaerobic metabolism and acid-base disturbance during activity in the salt-water crocodile, *Crocodylus porosus*. *The Journal of Experimental Biology* **118**, 161–171. doi:10.1242/jeb.118.1.161

Bertelsen MF (2014) Squamates (snakes and lizards). In *Zoo Animal and Wildlife Immobilization and Anaesthesia*. 2nd edn. (Eds G West, D Heard and N Caulkett) pp. 233–243. John Wiley and Sons, Hoboken, NJ.

Bowen KD, Spencer RJ, Janzen FJ (2005) A comparative study of environmental factors that affect nesting in Australian and North American freshwater turtles. *Journal of Zoology* **267**, 397–404. doi:10.1017/S0952836905007533

Bower DS, Hutchinson M, Georges A (2012) Movement and habitat use of Australia's largest snake-necked turtle: implications for water management. *Journal of Zoology* **287**, 76–80. doi:10.1111/j.1469-7998.2011.00891.x

Bower DS, Brannelly LA, McDonald CA, Webb RJ, Greenspan SE, Vickers M, Gardner MG, Greenlees MJ (2019) A review of the role of parasites in the ecology of reptiles and amphibians. *Austral Ecology* **44**, 433–448. doi:10.1111/aec.12695

Brien ML, Read MA, McCallum HI, Grigg GC (2008) Home range and movements of radio-tracked estuarine crocodiles (*Crocodylus porosus*) within a non-tidal waterhole. *Wildlife Research* **35**, 140–149. doi:10.1071/WR06116

Britton AR, Britton EK, McMahon CR (2013) Impact of a toxic invasive species on freshwater crocodile (*Crocodylus johnstoni*) populations in upstream escarpments. *Wildlife Research* **40**, 312–317. doi:10.1071/WR12215

Broderick AC, Glen F, Godley BJ, Hays GC (2003) Variation in reproductive output of marine turtles. *Journal of Experimental Marine Biology and Ecology* **288**, 95–109. doi:10.1016/S0022-0981(03)00003-0

Brown G, Shine R (2006) Why do most tropical animals reproduce seasonally? Testing hypotheses on an Australian snake. *Ecology* **87**, 133–143. doi:10.1890/04-1882

Bryant GL, Eden P, De Tores P, Warren K (2010) Improved procedure for implanting radiotransmitters in the coelomic cavity of snakes. *Australian Veterinary Journal* **88**, 443–448. doi:10.1111/j.1751-0813.2010.00633.x

Bull CM (2000) Monogamy in lizards. *Behavioural Processes* **51**, 7–20. doi:10.1016/S0376-6357(00)00115-7

Bull CM, Gardner MG, Sih A, Spiegel O, Godfrey SS, Leu ST (2017) Why is social behavior rare in reptiles? Lessons from sleepy lizards. *Advances in the Study of Behavior* **49**, 1–26. doi:10.1016/bs.asb.2017.02.001

Campbell HA, Dwyer RG, Irwin TR, Franklin CE (2013) Home range utilisation and long-range movement of estuarine crocodiles during the breeding and nesting season. *PLoS One* **8**, e62127. doi:10.1371/journal.pone.0062127

Chessman BC, McGilvray G, Ruming S, Jones HA, Petrov K, Fielder DP, Spencer R-J, Georges A (2020) On a razor's edge: status and prospects of the critically endangered Bellinger river snapping turtle, *Myuchelys georgesi*. *Aquatic Conservation* **30**, 586–600. doi:10.1002/aqc.3258

Close B, Banister K, Baumans V, Bernoth E-M, Bromage N, Bunyan J, Erhardt W, Flecknell P, Gregory NC, Hackbarth H, Norton D, Warwick C (1997) Recommendations for euthanasia of experimental animals: Part 2. *Laboratory Animals* **31**, 1–32. doi:10.1258/002367797780600297

Commonwealth of Australia (2009) *Code of Practice on the Humane Treatment of Wild and Farmed Australian Crocodiles*. Natural Resource Management Ministerial Council, Canberra.

Conroy C, Papenfuss T, Parker J, Hahn N (2009) Use of tricaine methanesulfonate (MS222) for euthanasia of reptiles. *Journal of the American Association for Laboratory Animal Science; JAALAS* **48**, 28–32.

Department of Environment and Science (2008) Code of practice for the taking, handling and transportation of crocodiles. The State of Queensland, Department of Environment and Science.

Doody JS, Freedberg S, Keogh JS (2009a) Communal egg-laying in reptiles and amphibians: evolutionary patterns and hypotheses. *The Quarterly Review of Biology* **84**, 229–252. doi:10.1086/605078

Doody JS, Rose J, Mayes P, Ishiyama L (2009b) Telemetry tagging methods for some freshwater reptiles. *Marine & Freshwater Research* **60**, 293–298. doi:10.1071/MF08158

Doody JS, McHenry C, Brown M, Canning G, Vas G, Clulow S (2018) Deep, helical, communal nesting and emergence in the sand monitor: ecology informing paleoecology? *Journal of Zoology* **305**, 88–95. doi:10.1111/jzo.12543

DPI (2015) Bellinger River snapping turtle management program. <https://www.dpi.nsw.gov.au/__data/assets/pdf_file/0006/559113/bellinger-river-snapping-turtle-managment-plan.pdf>.

Dyer SM, Cervasio EL (2008) An overview of restraint and blood collection techniques in exotic pet practice. *The Veterinary Clinics of North America. Exotic Animal Practice* **11**, 423–443. doi:10.1016/j.cvex.2008.03.008

Ferrara CR, Vogt RC, Eisemberg CC, Doody JS (2017) First evidence of the pig-nosed turtle (*Carettochelys insculpta*) vocalizing underwater. *Copeia* **105**, 29–32. doi:10.1643/CE-16-407

Fielder DP (2012) Seasonal and diel dive performance and behavioral ecology of the bimodally respiring freshwater turtle *Myuchelys bellii* of eastern Australia. *Journal of Comparative Physiology. A, Neuroethology, Sensory, Neural, and Behavioral Physiology* **198**, 129–143. doi:10.1007/s00359-011-0694-x

Fleming GJ (2014) Crocodilians (crocodiles, alligators, caiman, and gharial). In *Zoo Animal and Wildlife Immobilization and Anaesthesia.* 2nd edn. (Eds G West, D Heard and N Caulkett) pp. 325–335. John Wiley and Sons, Hoboken, NJ.

Galex IA, Gallant CM, D'Avignon N, Kuchenbrod LM, Fletcher CA, Rogala AR (2020) Evaluation of Effective and Practical Euthanasia Methods for Larval African Clawed Frogs (*Xenopus laevis*). *Journal of the American Association for Laboratory Animal Science; JAALAS* **59**, 269–274. doi:10.30802/AALAS-JAALAS-19-000141

Gardner MG, Pearson SK, Johnston GR, Schwarz MP (2016) Group living in squamate reptiles: a review of evidence for stable aggregations. *Biological Reviews of the Cambridge Philosophical Society* **91**, 925–936. doi:10.1111/brv.12201

Georges A, Thomson S (2010) Diversity of Australasian freshwater turtles, with an annotated synonymy and keys to species. *Zootaxa* **2496**, 1–37. doi:10.11646/zootaxa.2496.1.1

Giles JC, Davis JA, McCauley RD, Kuchling G (2009) Voice of the turtle: the underwater acoustic repertoire of the long-necked freshwater turtle, *Chelodina oblonga. The Journal of the Acoustical Society of America* **126**, 434–443. doi:10.1121/1.3148209

Goodyear SE, Pianka ER (2011) Spatial and temporal variation in diets of sympatric lizards (Genus *Ctenotus*) in the Great Victoria Desert, Western Australia. *Journal of Herpetology* **45**, 265–271. doi:10.1670/10-190.1

Gottdenker NL, Jacobson ER (1995) Effect of venipuncture sites on hematologic and clinical biochemical values in desert tortoises (*Gopherus agassizii*). *American Journal of Veterinary Research* **56**, 19–21.

Griffiths A, Christian K (1996) The effects of fire on the frillneck lizard (*Chlamydosaurus kingii*) in northern Australia. *Australian Journal of Ecology* **21**, 386–398. doi:10.1111/j.1442-9993.1996.tb00625.x

Hansen N, Driscoll D, Michael D, Lindenmayer D (2020) Movement patterns of an arboreal gecko in fragmented agricultural landscapes reveal matrix avoidance. *Animal Conservation* **23**, 48–59. doi:10.1111/acv.12505

Hays GC, Scott R (2013) Global patterns for upper ceilings on migration distance in sea turtles and comparisons with fish, birds and mammals. *Functional Ecology* **27**, 748–756. doi:10.1111/1365-2435.12073

Hing S, Hampton JO, Gibson TJ (2019) Animal welfare and the killing of wildlife by captive bolt in Australia. *Australian Zoologist* **40**, 170–180. doi:10.7882/AZ.2018.035

Holleley CE, Sarre SD, O'Meally D, Georges A (2016) Sex reversal in reptiles: Reproductive oddity or powerful driver of evolutionary change? *Sexual Development: Genetics, Molecular Biology, Evolution, Endocrinology, Embryology, and Pathology of Sex Determination and Differentiation* **10**, 279–287. doi:10.1159/000450972

Huchzermeyer FW (2003) *Crocodiles: Biology, Husbandry and Diseases.* CABI, Cambridge, MA.

Hudson S (1996) Natural toe loss in southeastern Australian skinks: implications for marking lizards by toe-clipping. *Journal of Herpetology* **30**, 106–110.

Hutton JM (1992) Humane killing of crocodilians. In *Crocodiles. Proceedings of the 11th Working Meeting of the IUCN-SSC Crocodile Specialist Group.* pp. 194–196. IUCN, Gland, Switzerland.

James C, Shine R (1985) The seasonal timing of reproduction. *Oecologia* **67**, 464–474. doi:10.1007/BF00790016

Kay WR (2005) Population ecology of *Crocodylus porosus* (Schneider 1801) in the Kimberley region of Western Australia. PhD thesis. The University of Queensland, Australia.

Keifer J, Zheng Z (2017) Cold block of in vitro eyeblink reflexes: evidence supporting the use of hypothermia as an anesthetic in pond turtles. *The Journal of Experimental Biology* **220**, 4370–4373.

Kennett R, Christian K, Pritchard D (1993) Underwater nesting by the tropical fresh-water turtle, *Chelodina rugosa* (Testudinata, Chelidae). *Australian Journal of Zoology* **41**, 47–52. doi:10.1071/ZO9930047

Kennett R, Tory O (1996) Diet of two freshwater turtles, *Chelodina rugosa* and *Elseya dentata* (Testudines: Chelidae) from the wet-dry tropics of northern Australia. *Copeia* 409–419. doi:10.2307/1446857

Kerr GD, Bull CM (2006) Movement patterns in the monogamous sleepy lizard (*Tiliqua rugosa*): effects of gender, drought, time of year and time of day. *Journal of Zoology* **269**, 137–147. doi:10.1111/j.1469-7998.2006.00091.x

Laird MK, Thompson MB, Whittington CM (2019) Facultative oviparity in a viviparous skink (*Saiphos equalis*). *Biology Letters* **15**, 20180827. doi:10.1098/rsbl.2018.0827

Lillywhite HB, Shine R, Jacobson E, Denardo DF, Gordon MS, Navas CA, Wang T, Seymour RS, Storey KB, Heatwole H, Heard D, Brattstrom B, Burghardt GM (2017) Anesthesia and Euthanasia of Amphibians and Reptiles Used in Scientific Research: Should Hypothermia and Freezing Be Prohibited? *Bioscience* **67**, 53–61. doi:10.1093/biosci/biw143

Lloyd M, Morris PJ (1999) Phlebotomy techniques in snakes. *Bulletin of the Association of Reptilian and Amphibian Veterinarians* **9**, 30–33. doi:10.5818/1076-3139.9.4.30

Macdonald S (2007) Observations on the stomach contents of a road-killed perentie, *Varanus giganteus* in Western Queensland. *Biawak* **1**, 21–23.

Martelli P, Shilton C, Manolis C (2020) Humane euthanasia/killing methods for crocodilians – an update. *Crocodile Specialist Group Newsletter* **39**, 6–8.

Mazzoleni S, Augstenová B, Clemente L, Auer M, Fritz U, Praschag P, Protiva T, Velenský P, Kratochvíl L, Rovatsos M (2020) Sex is determined by XX/XY sex chromosomes in Australasian side-necked turtles (Testudines: Chelidae). *Scientific Reports* **10**, 1–11. doi:10.1038/s41598-020-61116-w

McGlashan JK, Spencer R-J, Old JM (2012) Embryonic communication in the nest: metabolic responses of reptilian embryos to developmental rates of siblings. *Proceedings. Biological Sciences* **279**, 1709–1715. doi:10.1098/rspb.2011.2074

Micheli-Campbell MA, Connell MJ, Dwyer RG, Franklin CE, Fry B, Kennard MJ, Tao J, Campbell HA (2017) Identifying critical habitat for freshwater turtles: integrating long-term monitoring tools to enhance conservation and management. *Biodiversity and Conservation* **26**, 1675–1688. doi:10.1007/s10531-017-1325-9

Miller AC, Commens CA, Jaworski R, Packham D (1990) The turtle's revenge: a case of soft tissue *Mycobacterium chelonae* infection. *The Medical Journal of Australia* **153**, 493–495. doi:10.5694/j.1326-5377.1990.tb126158.x

Mitura A, Niemczuk K, Zaręba K, Zając M, Laroucau K, Szymańska-Czerwińska M (2017) Free-living and captive turtles and tortoises as carriers of new *Chlamydia* spp. *PLoS One* **12**, e0185407. doi:10.1371/journal.pone.0185407

Moritz C (1984) The origin and evolution of parthenogenesis in *Heteronotia binoei* (Gekkonidae). *Chromosoma* **89**, 151–162. doi:10.1007/BF00292899

Murphy K, Hudson S, Shea G (2006) Reproductive seasonality of three cold-temperate viviparous skinks from southeastern Australia. *Journal of Herpetology* **40**, 454–464. doi:10.1670/0022-1511(2006)40[454:RSOTCV]2.0.CO;2

Myburgh J, Kirberger RM, Steyl J, Soley JT, Booyse DG, Huchzermeyer FW, Lowers RH, Guillette LJ (2014) The post-occipital spinal venous sinus of the Nile crocodile (*Crocodylus niloticus*): its anatomy and use for blood sample collection and intravenous infusions. *Journal of the South African Veterinary Association* **85**, E1–E10. doi:10.4102/jsava.v85i1.965

Nevarez JG, Strain GM, Da Cunha AF, Beaufrère H (2014) Evaluation of four methods for inducing death during slaughter of American alligators (*Alligator mississippiensis*). *American Journal of Veterinary Research* **75**, 536–543. doi:10.2460/ajvr.75.6.536

Nussbaum RA (1980) The brahminy blind snake (*Ramphotyphlops braminus*) in the Seychelles Archipelago: distribution, variation, and further evidence for parthenogenesis. *Herpetologica* **36**, 215–221.

Oliveira J, Kawanami A, Silva A, Chung D, Werther K (2016) Detection of *Leptospira* spp. in wild *Phrynops geoffroanus* (Geoffroy's side-necked turtle) in urban environment. *Acta Tropica* **164**, 165–168. doi:10.1016/j.actatropica.2016.08.019

Olsson M, Shine R (2003) Female-biased natal and breeding dispersal in an alpine lizard, *Niveoscincus microlepidotus*. *Biological Journal of the Linnean Society. Linnean Society of London* **79**, 277–283. doi:10.1046/j.1095-8312.2003.00116.x

Olsson AR (2014) Anaesthesia of large estuarine crocodiles (*Crocodylus porosus*). In *Proceedings of the 45th Conference of the International Association for Aquatic Animal Medicine*. Gold Coast, Australia.

Parker KA, Adams L, Baling M, Kemp L, Kuchling G, Lloyd B, Parsons S, Ruffell J, Stringer I, Watts C, Dickens MJ (2015) Practical guidelines for planning and implementing fauna translocations. In *Advances in Reintroduction Biology of Australian and New Zealand Fauna*. (Eds DP Armstrong, MW Hayward, D Moro and PJ Seddon) pp. 255–272. CSIRO Publishing, Melbourne.

Pearse D, Avise J (2001) Turtle mating systems: behavior, sperm storage, and genetic paternity. *The Journal of Heredity* **92**, 206–211. doi:10.1093/jhered/92.2.206

Pfitzer S, Ganswindt A, Fosgate GT, Botha PJ, Myburgh JG (2014) Capture of farmed Nile crocodiles (*Crocodylus niloticus*): comparison of physiological parameters after manual capture and after capture with electrical stunning. *The Veterinary Record* **175**, 304. doi:10.1136/vr.102438

Qualls CP, Shine R (1998) Costs of Reproduction in Conspecific Oviparous and Viviparous Lizards, *Lerista bougainvillii*. *Oikos* **82**, 539–551. doi:10.2307/3546374

Read M, Wright B, Enoch C (2004) *Crocodiles in Queensland–an overview, Crocodiles*. Proceedings 17th Working Meeting IUCN-SSC Crocodile Specialist Group. IUCN, Gland, Switzerland.

Read MA, Grigg GC, Irwin SR, Shanahan D, Franklin CE (2007) Satellite tracking reveals long distance coastal travel and homing by translocated estuarine crocodiles, *Crocodylus porosus*. *PLoS One* **2**, e949. doi:10.1371/journal.pone.0000949

Rhind D, Doody JS, Clulow S, Godwin C, Bartek B, Murray C (2019) *Varanus giganteus* (Perentie): diet. *Herpetological Review* **50**, 382.

Santori C, Spencer R-J, Van Dyke JU, Thompson MB (2018) Road mortality of the eastern long-necked turtle (*Chelodina longicollis*) along the Murray River, Australia: an assessment using citizen science. *Australian Journal of Zoology* **66**, 41–49. doi:10.1071/ZO17065

Scheelings TF (2013) Use of intravenous and intramuscular Alfaxalone in Macquarie River Turtles (*Emydura macquarii*). *Journal of Herpetological Medicine and Surgery* **23**(3), 91–94. doi:10.5818/1529-9651-23.3.91

Scheelings TF, Lightfoot D, Holz P (2011) Prevalence of Salmonella in Australian reptiles. *Journal of Wildlife Diseases* **47**, 1–11. doi:10.7589/0090-3558-47.1.1

Sedgwick C (1986) Inhalation anesthesia for captive wild mammals, birds, and reptiles. In *Zoo and Wild Animal Medicine* (Ed. ME Fowler) pp. 52–56. Saunders, WB, Philadelphia, PA.

Sharp T, Lothian A, Munn A, Saunders G (2011) *CAN001 Methods for the Field Euthanasia of Cane Toads*. Department of Primary Industries, Orange.

Shine R (1979) Activity patterns in Australian elapid snakes (Squamata: Serpentes: Elapidae). *Herpetologica* **35**, 1–11.

Shine R, Amiel J, Munn AJ, Stewart M, Vyssotski AL, Lesku JA (2015) Is 'cooling then freezing' a humane way to kill amphibians and reptiles? *Biology Open* **4**, 760–763. doi:10.1242/bio.012179

Shine R, Lesku JA, Lillywhite HB (2019) Assessment of the cooling-then-freezing method for euthanasia of amphibians and reptiles. *Journal of the American Veterinary Medical Association* **255**, 48–50. doi:10.2460/javma.255.1.48

Smith J, Griffiths A (2009) Determinants of home range and activity in two semi-aquatic lizards. *Journal of Zoology* **279**, 349–357. doi:10.1111/j.1469-7998.2009.00623.x

Somaweera R, Shine R (2012) Australian Freshwater Crocodiles (*Crocodylus johnstoni*) Transport Their Hatchlings to the Water. *Journal of Herpetology* **46**, 407–411. doi:10.1670/11-056

Somaweera R, Shine R (2013) Nest-site selection by crocodiles at a rocky site in the Australian tropics: Making the best of a bad lot. *Austral Ecology* **38**, 313–325. doi:10.1111/j.1442-9993.2012.02406.x

Somaweera R, Nifong J, Rosenblatt A, Brien ML, Combrink X, Elsey RM, Grigg G, Magnusson WE, Mazzotti FJ, Pearcy A (2020) The ecological importance of crocodylians: towards evidence-based justification for their conservation. *Biological Reviews of the Cambridge Philosophical Society* **95**, 936–959. doi:10.1111/brv.12594

Somaweera R, Rhind D, Reynolds S, Eisemberg C, Sonneman T, Woods D (2018) Observations of mammalian feeding by Australian freshwater crocodiles (*Crocodylus johnstoni*) in the Kimberley region of Western Australia. *Records of the Western Australian Museum* **33**, 103–107. doi:10.18195/issn.0312-3162.33(1).2018.103-107

Somaweera R, Brien M, Shine R (2013a) The role of predation in shaping crocodylian natural history. *Herpetological Monograph* **27**, 23–51. doi:10.1655/HERPMONOGRAPHS-D-11-00001

Somaweera R, Shine R, Webb J, Dempster T, Letnic M (2013b) Why does vulnerability to toxic invasive cane toads vary among populations of Australian freshwater crocodiles? *Animal Conservation* **16**, 86–96. doi:10.1111/j.1469-1795.2012.00578.x

Somaweera R, Webb JK, Shine R (2011) Determinants of habitat selection by hatchling Australian freshwater crocodiles. *PLoS One* **6**, e28533. doi:10.1371/journal.pone.0028533

Spencer RJ, Thompson M (2005) Experimental analysis of the impact of foxes on freshwater turtle populations. *Conservation Biology* **19**, 845–854. doi:10.1111/j.1523-1739.2005.00487.x

Sumner J (2006) Higher relatedness within groups due to variable subadult dispersal in a rainforest skink, *Gnypetoscincus queenslandiae*. *Austral Ecology* **31**, 441–448. doi:10.1111/j.1442-9993.2006.01599.x

Taylor JA (1979) The foods and feeding habits of subadult *Crocodylus porosus* Schneider in northern Australia. *Wildlife Research* **6**, 347–359. doi:10.1071/WR9790347

Tucker A, Limpus C, Priest T, Cay J, Glen C, Guarino E (2001) Home ranges of Fitzroy River turtles (*Rheodytes leukops*) overlap riffle zones: potential concerns related to river regulation. *Biological Conservation* **102**, 171–181. doi:10.1016/S0006-3207(01)00097-0

Tucker AD, Limpus CJ, McCallum HI, McDonald KR (1996) Ontogenetic Dietary Partitioning by *Crocodylus johnstoni* during the Dry Season. *Copeia* **1996**, 978–988. doi:10.2307/1447661

Tucker AD, Limpus CJ, McCallum HI, McDonald KR (1997) Movements and home ranges of *Crocodylus johnstoni* in the Lynd River, Queensland. *Wildlife Research* **24**, 379–396. doi:10.1071/WR95073

University of Canberra AEC (2017) Standard Operating Procedures (SOPs) for the care and use of animals in laboratory studies, teaching and field research. <https://www.canberra.edu.au/research/archived/ucresearch/ethics/accordion/animal_ethics/animal-ethics-documents/SOP_2017_final.pdf>.

Vanderduys EP (2013) Additional information on *Ramphotyphlops aspina* Couper, Covacevich and Wilson 1998, a poorly known blind snake from the Mitchell Grass Downs of Queensland. *Memoirs of the Queensland Museum - Nature* **56**, 615–619.

Vigani A (2014) Chelonia (tortoises, turtles, and terrapins). In *Zoo Animal and Wildlife Immobilization and Anaesthesia.* 2nd edn. (Eds G West, D Heard and N Caulkett) pp. 365–387. John Wiley and Sons, Hoboken, NJ.

Warren K (2014) Reptile euthanasia – no easy solution? *Pacific Conservation Biology* **20**, 25–27. doi:10.1071/PC140025

Webb G, Manolis C (1998) *Crocodiles of Australia.* Reed Books, Frenchs Forest.

Webb G, Manolis S, Buckworth R (1983a) *Crocodylus johnstoni* in the McKinlay River Area N. T, II.* Dry-Season Habitat Slection and an Estimate of the Total Population Size. *Australian Wildlife Research* **10**, 373–382. doi:10.1071/WR9830373

Webb G, Manolis S, Buckworth R (1983b) *Crocodylus johnstoni* in the McKinlay River Area N. T, IV.* A Demonstration of Homing. *Australian Wildlife Research* **10**, 403–406. doi:10.1071/WR9830403

Webb G, Manolis S, Buckworth R, Sack G (1983c) An examination of *Crocodylus porosus* nests in two northern Australian freshwater swamps, with an analysis of embryo mortality. *Wildlife Research* **10**, 571–605. doi:10.1071/WR9830571

Webb GJW, Manolis SC, Sack GC (1983d) *Crocodylus johnstoni* and Saltwater Crocodiles coexisting in a Tidal River. *Australian Wildlife Research* **10**, 639–650. doi:10.1071/WR9830639

Webb GJW, Sack GC, Buckworth R, Manolis CS (1983e) An Examination of *Crocodylus porosus* Nests in Two Northern Australian Freshwater Swamps, with an Analysis of Embryo Mortality. *Australian Wildlife Research* **10**, 571–605. doi:10.1071/WR9830571

Webb GJW, Manolis SC (2010) Australian freshwater crocodile *Crocodylus johnstoni.* In *Crocodiles. Status Survey and Conservation Action Plan.* 3rd edn. (Eds SC Manolis and C Stevenson) pp. 66–70. Crocodile Specialist Group, Darwin.

Webb GJW, Manolis SC, Buckworth R (1982) *Crocodylus johnstoni* in the McKinlay River Area, N.T. I. variation in the diet, and a new method of assessing the relative importance of prey. *Australian Journal of Zoology* **30**, 877–899. doi:10.1071/ZO9820877

Webb GJW, Smith AMA (1984) Sex ratio and survivorship in the Australian freshwater crocodile *Crocodylus johnstoni. Symposia of the Zoological Society of London* **52**, 319–355.

Webb JK, Shine R (1993) Dietary habits of Australian blindsnakes (Typhlopidae). *Copeia* 762–770. doi:10.2307/1447239

Welsh MA, Doody JS, Georges A (2017) Resource partitioning among five sympatric species of freshwater turtles from the wet–dry tropics of northern Australia. *Wildlife Research* **44**, 219–229. doi:10.1071/WR16202

Whiting M, While G (2017) Sociality in lizards. In *Comparative Social Evolution.* (Eds D Rubenstein and P Abbot) pp. 390–426. Cambridge University Press, Cambridge, UK. doi:10.1017/9781107338319.014

Wildlife Health Australia (2021) 'Ongoing incidents'. <https://wildlifehealthAustralia.com.au/DiseaseIncidents/OngoingIncidents.aspx>.

Wilson DS (1994) A method for the restraint and transport of crocodylians. *Herpetological Review* **25**, 14–15.

Wilson SK, Swan G (2021) *A Complete Guide to the Reptiles of Australia.* 6th edn. Reed New Holland, Sydney.

Work TM, Balazs GH (2013) A simple humane method to euthanize a sea turtle. *Marine Turtle Newsletter* **136**, 5–6.

Wotherspoon D, Burgin S (2016) Sex and ontogenetic dietary shift in Pogona barbata, the Australian eastern bearded dragon. *Australian Journal of Zoology* **64**, 14–20. doi:10.1071/ZO15019

Zhang J, Finlaison DS, Frost MJ, Gestier S, Gu X, Hall J, Jenkins C, Parrish K, Read AJ, Srivastava M (2018) Identification of a novel nidovirus as a potential cause of large scale mortalities in the endangered Bellinger River snapping turtle (*Myuchelys georgesi*). *PLoS One* **13**, e0205209. doi:10.1371/journal.pone.0205209

Zulkifli I, Goh YM, Norbaiyah B, Sazili AQ, Lotfi M, Soleimani AF, Small AH (2014) Changes in blood parameters and electroencephalogram of cattle as affected by different stunning and slaughter methods in cattle. *Animal Production Science* **54**, 187–193. doi:10.1071/AN12128

27 Amphibians

David Hunter, Sam Young, Michael McFadden, Shannon Kelleher and Helen P. Waudby

INTRODUCTION

Over 240 native frog species are recognised in Australia (Cogger 2018). This number is increasing as new species are discovered in remote areas or via molecular techniques. Most (89%) of these species belong to three families (Hylidae, Limnodynastidae and Myobatrachidae), with an additional two families (Ranidae and Microhylidae) constituting the other 11%. Amphibian taxonomy continues to be an important area of research and critical for Australian frog conservation (Gillespie *et al.* 2020). Two exotic amphibian species have become established in Australia. The most well-known is the cane toad (*Rhinella marina*) from Latin America, which was introduced in the 1930s to north-east Queensland as a biological control agent, and spread across northern Australia to the Kimberley, and south to Sydney (Shine 2018). A European amphibian species, the smooth newt (*Lissotriton vulgaris*), has become established in parts of Melbourne (Tingley *et al.* 2015). Periodically, other exotic amphibian species are detected in Australia, but none has become established to date.

Australian frog species richness is greatest in the wet tropics of North Queensland, with up to 49 species occurring in the Daintree River region alone (Cogger 2018). In subtropical areas of south-east Queensland and north-eastern New South Wales, up to 44 species may occur in a region. High species richness also characterises the wet and dry tropics of northern Australia, and from the east coast to mesic areas of eastern Victoria (Cogger 2018). Most of Australia's semi-arid and arid areas also support desert-adapted frog species, many of which can survive extended dry periods by aestivating (prolonged torpor or dormancy during a hot or dry period) underground in a cocoon made from their skin. While drier parts of Australia may not have similarly high species richness, they sometimes support high frog biomass (Predavec and Dickman 1993). The only area of Australia seemingly devoid of any frog species is the Nullarbor Plains of southern Australia (Cogger 2018). Global amphibian diversity has been decimated by the spread of pathogens, particularly the amphibian chytrid fungus (Scheele *et al.* 2019), which causes the fatal disease chytridiomycosis. This chapter reviews key considerations for working with amphibians in Australia and provides general operating procedures for evaluating amphibians for chytrid infection with swabbing.

FROGS AND TOADS

David Hunter, Sam Young, Michael McFadden, Shannon Kelleher and Helen P. Waudby

Characteristics

Australian frogs have a relatively consistent body form, with females being larger than males (male tusked frogs, *Adelotus brevis*, are an exception). Variations in body form are generally related to lifestyle and environment. For example, fossorial species typically have more-rotund bodies and shorter limbs than species occupying riverine or arboreal environments. A notable feature of amphibian physiology is their external skin, which acts as a permeable membrane, allowing liquid and gas exchange, and often serving as a secondary respiratory system to their lungs. Amphibians attain water and rehydrate via their skin instead of drinking. Amphibian skin contains an abundance of mucus glands that produce peptides to help regulate moisture and protect the frog from predation and infection. Consequently, their skin properties can make amphibians particularly sensitive to contaminants and moisture loss during research.

Biology and behaviour

Most Australian frog species rely on free-standing water to complete their life cycles. All species reproduce via external fertilisation where the male fertilises eggs (holding the female in a grip called amplexus) as the female lays them. Frog eggs have a gelatinous membrane that is susceptible to desiccation, and most species have an aquatic tadpole larval stage. However, life-cycle strategies do vary, allowing Australian frogs to adapt to diverse habitats. Several species in the Myobatrachidae family, and the long-snouted frog (*Litoria longirostris*), are terrestrial breeders (lay their eggs on land), although the tadpoles move to an aquatic environment after hatching. Species in the family Microhylidae, and some Myobatrachidae species, do not have a tadpole stage, but hatch as fully formed frogs. The hip-pocket frog (*Assa darlingtoni*) and the possibly extinct gastric brooding frogs (*Rheobatrachus silus* and *R. vitellinus*) have more-unusual life histories. The tadpoles of the hip-pocket frog develop in skin pouches on the side of the male's abdomen, while female gastric brooding frogs swallow their eggs and later regurgitate fully developed frogs (Anstis 2013).

Males typically call during their reproductive season to attract females. Males may also emit threat calls to ward off other males, with some species having two parts to their call (biphasic), which includes both the advertisement and threat call. Frog species generally have different calls (sometimes regional variation also occurs within species), which researchers often use to answer various population- and demographic-based questions. Typically, calling is loudest at night, so studies often target frogs at these times.

The behaviour and population ecology of Australian frogs are diverse. Some species exhibit site fidelity to breeding habitat, while others may be effective colonisers, moving large distances and occupying new areas. Vast differences in fecundity and other demographic traits occur among species. Some species are highly fecund, laying many hundreds or thousands of eggs, and exhibit large fluctuations in population size associated with variable recruitment. Age to sexual maturity and longevity may also vary, with some species exhibiting rapid population turnover, while for others adults may live for multiple breeding seasons.

Adult frogs are generally unspecialised carnivores, usually feeding on small invertebrates, although larger species will also eat small mammals, reptiles and other frogs. Australian frogs prey on live food items that are moving, whereas the introduced cane toad may consume non-living food items like dog food. Tadpoles can have a highly varied diet and feeding behaviour that includes filtering microorganisms, grazing algae, catching and consuming small prey items, or consuming flesh from dead and decaying larger animals. Tadpoles of some species, such as the Baw Baw frog (*Philoria frosti*), do not feed at all as the embryo contains sufficient resources to develop through to metamorphosis.

Capture and handling

Standard hygiene protocols should be followed when working with amphibians in the field (e.g. DPIE 2020). Amphibians are generally small and delicate, so handling should be undertaken with care to avoid damaging joints and bones. Following the discovery that many enigmatic frog declines were a result of the spread of the amphibian chytrid fungus pathogen (Berger *et al.* 1998), it has become standard hygiene practice to wear a new pair of nitrile, latex or vinyl gloves, or use a single-use lightweight plastic bag when handling individual amphibians. All frogs possess skin glands that produce potentially toxic compounds, which evolved as a predator deterrent and can be irritating or dangerous to humans. Consequently, wearing non-powdered gloves and/or washing hands thoroughly after handling is also recommended to protect handlers. Gloves should be rinsed in clean water before handling amphibians, including tadpoles. Some types of disposable gloves appear to be toxic to the tadpoles of some species (e.g. Cashins *et al.* 2008). Vinyl gloves may be most appropriate for tadpole handling (Cashins *et al.* 2008), but they can also be handled using a small net, or clean and disinfected bare hands. Thorough cleaning and disinfecting of hands or handling equipment (with 70% alcohol) instead of the use of gloves may reduce the large amount of waste associated with single-use products. Ideally, hands should be rinsed with clean water after using alcohol-based disinfectants or, if not possible, hands should be allowed to dry before handling amphibians. Amphibians should be released at their point of capture and never transported between sites.

Short-term housing and transportation of amphibians are often required for research involving field-collected animals or translocations. This activity can be a period of high risk to the welfare of individuals if adequate procedures are not maintained. Important considerations include container size and density of individuals per container, temperature, moisture, ventilation and nitrogenous wastes. These issues are alleviated by maintaining amphibians in a cool environment as their activity and metabolic requirements are reduced greatly at lower temperatures. Constant monitoring of temperature is important, particularly during transport. If amphibians are being housed in relatively small containers for > 24 h, containers must be rinsed with clean water each day. Containers should be kept moist, but not wet. Providing moist sphagnum moss can assist with moisture regulation.

Wild-caught or captive-bred amphibians are often the subject of laboratory experiments involving the housing of individuals for extended periods. Husbandry requirements depend on a range of species-specific factors, including developmental stage, length of time in captivity and whether breeding is required. Length of time in captivity is particularly important because a range of detrimental health issues manifest after prolonged exposure to poor husbandry regimes. Frog health in captivity is maintained by consideration of a range of factors, including the provision of appropriate temperature and moisture gradients, nutrition, water quality, shelter and waste management. Management of waste material is important as faecal matter or uneaten food in a moist environment can foul quickly, producing a bacterial environment that is harmful to amphibians. A clean environment can be achieved using automated systems, such as sprayers on a timer and passive drainage, and through regular substrate changes. Waste management and food availability are also key considerations for determining the density of frogs that can be housed in a given area.

Providing the correct quality and quantity of food for amphibians is an important aspect of amphibian health (Ferrie *et al.* 2014). An adequate diet can be provided by combining bought crickets and other invertebrates with calcium and multivitamin supplements (dusted or gut loaded). Providing food two or three times per week is often appropriate for frogs. However, this regime may need to be adjusted based on the species and the age of the individual, as captive frogs are prone to becoming overweight.

One critical husbandry consideration is the provision of sufficient calcium to maintain good health or adequate growth and development. Frogs' capacity to assimilate calcium is usually influenced by ultraviolet B light (UVB) availability, presence of calcium and vitamin D3 in the diet, temperature and water quality. Deficiencies in any one of these factors can have negative health consequences for frogs. These issues are amplified if frogs are reared in captivity from a young age when calcium uptake is crucial for preventing developmental bone abnormalities, such as curvature of the spine and deformed limbs (Tapley *et al.* 2015). UVB lighting specifically produced for reptiles and amphibians, such as fluorescent tubes, are available through pet product suppliers and should be installed so that captive amphibians have access to direct light (Baines *et al.* 2016). As the level of UVB reduces with distance from the tube, the light should typically be placed within ~30 cm of the amphibian and where the light does not have to pass through glass.

Water quality, particularly the removal of copper and chlorine, is critical for frogs (Odum and Zippel 2008). Exposure to metals or chemicals in the water will probably result in ongoing chronic stress that may affect individual fitness. Knowledge of natural water parameters, such as pH and hardness, may be important to determine the level of filtration required. For most species, filtering source water with simple sediment and carbon filtration is sufficient to remove most impurities from the water. However, for certain species that live in purer, high-altitude water bodies, reverse-osmosis filtration may be required.

Husbandry requirements for tadpoles are species-specific; however, several general principles should be considered for most species. Maintaining good water quality is critical; doing so often involves treating the water coming in, and diluting waste and nutrient build up (Mendelson and Altig 2016). This process can be undertaken through regular water changes to dilute and remove excess waste build up or utilising an aquarium filter, which consists of at least mechanical and biological filtration. The volume of water change or filtration required will depend on the density of tadpoles being maintained.

Regular testing of nitrogenous waste (ammonia, nitrites and nitrates) should be undertaken to ensure they are maintained within safe parameters. Water turbulence caused by filtration or water aeration should be monitored closely as pond-dwelling species can tire and become stressed with high levels of water movement. Nutrition is also important. Tadpole diet can be species-specific, although most species can be fed on a combination of good quality fish flakes, algal wafers and frozen or boiled endive or lettuce. Presentation of the food should be reflective of the species needs, with benthic tadpoles requiring food that sinks to the bottom. Care must be taken not to overfeed captive tadpoles as doing so will result in increased ammonia in the tank.

Veterinary considerations

Sedation and anaesthesia

Administering anaesthetics and analgesics can take various forms in amphibians, including via topical application, oral ingestion or injection. The most common form of anaesthetic is bathing in buffered tricaine methanesulfonate (MS-222) (Baitchman and Stetter 2014). Tricaine is acidic and should be mixed in a sodium phosphate-buffered solution to balance the pH. Effective dose and speed of onset vary depending on the species, although adult amphibians are usually induced within 30 min in 0.1% tricaine solution or 1 g/L in buffered solution (Wright 2001a). Once the appropriate anaesthetic plane is achieved, the amphibian should be moved to water free of tricaine. This method often gives enough anaesthesia for blood collection or minor surgical procedures. If the amphibian starts to recover prematurely, it should be returned to the diluted tricaine solution (0.03–0.05%) (Dyer and Cervasio 2008). The recommended concentration to induce anaesthesia for larvae is 0.2 g/L in buffered solution (Wright 2001a).

If alternative chemical restraint is required, isoflurane can be applied topically in a gel form at a dose of 0.025–0.035 mL/g bodyweight, depending on the species. When the animal has lost its withdrawal and righting reflex, the skin should be wiped free of anaesthetic solution with a saline-soaked gauze. The animal will typically remain anaesthetised for 45–80 min (Stetter 2001). Unfortunately, few studies have examined the appropriate use of analgesics in amphibians (Stevens 2011). Of the few studies that have been published, injectable morphine and flunixin have been shown to be effective (Wright 2001b; Coble *et al.* 2011).

Blood collection

If blood collection is required, the most appropriate collection sites are the lingual venous plexus, midline abdominal vein and the heart. The lingual venous plexus lies immediately under the tongue of many frogs and can be accessed in frogs as small as 25 g. The frog's mouth should be opened carefully (using a rubber spatula or mini cotton-tipped applicator) to avoid fracture of mandibular bones. The tongue can be drawn forward to identify the venous plexus on the underside of the tongue and buccal floor as a purple-to-red network of veins. The plexus should be lacerated with a 25–26 G needle and blood collected in a heparinised microhaematocrit tube. Contamination from oral secretions can be minimised by swabbing the site with a dry cotton-tipped applicator before venipuncture (Dyer and Cervasio 2008). The midline ventral abdominal vein runs subcutaneously over the linea alba. A 26–27 G needle with a 0.5–1.0 mL syringe should be inserted craniodorsally into the vein midway between the caudal edge of the sternum and the cranial edge of the pelvis (Dyer and Cervasio 2008). Cardiac puncture can be used only under general anaesthesia. With the amphibian in dorsal recumbency, personnel should identify the cardiac pulse and penetrate the apex of the heart using a 25–27 G needle.

Euthanasia

Amphibians can be euthanased by blunt force trauma to the cranium followed by decapitation or pithing of the brain (AVMA 2020). Decapitation involves severing the individual's neck close to its head with a sharp instrument. The animal must be stunned before decapitation because amphibians tolerate hypoxic and hypotensive conditions, so time to death may be prolonged if they are not rendered insensible first (AVMA 2020). Personnel should wear a full face mask or similar when stunning cane toads because their toxin glands (located just behind the head) may rupture, spraying personnel with toxins (Sharp *et al.* 2011).

Pentobarbitone (60–100 mg/kg) can be injected intravenously (preferred), intracoelomically, and via the subcutaneous lymph spaces or lymph sacs. However, depending on the route, insensibility may not be immediate (AVMA 2020). Any animal euthanased with pentobarbitone represents a secondary toxicity risk to wild scavengers and should be disposed of via deep burial. Anaesthetic agents typically used for fish, such as isoeugenol, may be used to euthanase amphibians by immersing them in the solution to achieve an overdose following the manufacturer's instructions for dosage. However, a study on euthanasia methods for cane toads concluded that the method was inappropriate for that species because individuals showed clear signs of distress (OEH 2014). Frogs can also be euthanased with ventral cutaneous application of benzocaine gel (Chen and Combs 1999). Loss of consciousness is typically rapid (60–90 s) and death usually occurs within 2 min.

Infectious pathogens

Symptoms associated with infectious pathogens can be painful or lethal for many species (Nichols *et al.* 2001) and many pathogens are easily spread via contaminated equipment or footwear if strict protocols are not followed. Consequently, quarantine and biosecurity are important considerations for amphibian research – particularly for projects involving the moving of animals from one area to another. In general, all amphibian research and conservation management programs should adhere to the protocols outlined in Phillott *et al.* (2010) and Murray *et al.* (2011). To limit the possible introduction of novel amphibian pathogens into Australia, the following guidelines have been suggested. First, no exotic amphibians should be imported into Australia for the purpose of research or exhibition. Second, no research, where amphibians may directly or indirectly be returned to the wild, should be undertaken within a facility housing live exotic amphibians, including zoological institutions with exotic amphibians on display and university facilities maintaining the African clawed frog (*Xenopus laevis*). Third, no native Australian species occurring in another country (e.g. bell frogs, *Litoria aurea* and *L. raniformis*, in New Zealand) should be exported live back into Australia.

To minimise the probability of inadvertently spreading a pathogen within Australia, the following protocols should be maintained. First, unless specifically part of a research project, all species taken into captivity should not be returned to the wild. Second, captive components of research associated with reintroduction or translocation programs should be undertaken using a dedicated quarantine facility, and all unintended deaths autopsied to evaluate cause of death.

To minimise the possible spread of pathogens from one field site to another, the following protocols should be maintained. First, all equipment in contact with frogs should either be disposable or disinfected using appropriate chemicals (≥ 70% alcohol or bleach). Second, all equipment and clothing that contacts frogs or moist habitat should be cleaned and dried between each site. Shoes should be disinfected. Third, if undertaking research at a site that is presumed to be pathogen-free, the site should not be visited immediately after visiting other sites.

Mycobacterium marinum poses the most significant zoonotic risk to immunocompromised humans. To reduce infection risks, personnel should wear gloves when cleaning amphibian enclosures and wash their hands after handling amphibians. Disposable powder-free gloves prevent callouses and fingerprint ridges from abrading the sensitive skin of amphibians. After use, gloves should be turned inside out and discarded into hazardous waste containers (Dyer and Cervasio 2008).

General operating procedures

Other research methods and procedures relevant to studying amphibians are covered in more detail elsewhere in the book, including collection of scats for dietary analysis and detection of environmental DNA (Chapter 4), acoustic recorders and call playback (Chapter 5), citizen science and teaching techniques (Chapter 10), hand capture (Chapter 9), trapping methods for tadpoles (Chapter 14), marking by toe clipping, visible implant elastomers and alphanumeric tags (Chapter 8), tracking methods (Chapter 9) and several veterinary procedures (Chapter 16).

SWABBING FOR CHYTRID FUNGUS

Sam Young and David Hunter

Target taxa

This general operating procedure (GOP) applies to wild and captive amphibian species of all stages (larval, juvenile and adult).

Context and scope

This GOP describes the collection of swabs for molecular diagnostic testing for chytrid fungus (*Batrachochytrium dendrobatidis*) infection in amphibians. The emergence and spread of amphibian chytrid fungus has resulted in unprecedented global amphibian declines and extinctions at the population and species level (Skerratt *et al.* 2007). Much remains unknown about the pathogen and the resulting disease; research to improve understanding and mitigate effects of chytridiomycosis on wild amphibian populations continues. Effective sampling regimes and validated diagnostic assays are critical to this research (Hyatt *et al.* 2007).

Infection with chytrid occurs in the superficial keratinised layers of amphibian skin, particularly the ventral abdomen, digits and the pelvic 'drink patch' of juvenile and adult frogs (Berger *et al.* 1998). In larval anurans (frog tadpoles), only the mouthparts are keratinised and susceptible to infection. Infection is most commonly diagnosed by histological examination of formalin-fixed skin sections or mouthparts (Berger *et al.* 1998), and/or detection of fungal DNA by quantitative polymerase chain reaction (PCR) testing of swabs collected from the ventral skin surfaces or mouthparts (Boyle *et al.* 2004; Retallick *et al.* 2006). Epidemiological studies in wild and captive amphibian populations are largely based on quantitative PCR testing of skin and mouthpart swabs collected from live (or dead) amphibians. This molecular testing technique is generally preferred to other methods as it is rapid, has high sensitivity and enables estimation of infection load. With very low infection loads, submerging amphibians in water within collection containers for 24 h, filtering the water and then amplifying DNA using nested PCR may be a more-sensitive diagnostic technique than skin swabbing (Shin *et al.* 2014).

Animal welfare considerations

Swabbing for chytrid requires capture and manual restraint of amphibians. Effects on individual animals should be minor if the procedure is performed efficiently and the amphibian is returned to its natural environment as soon as possible after capture. Wild amphibians should be released at the place of capture immediately after sampling to minimise impacts on social, territorial and reproductive dynamics within local populations and to prevent pathogen spread.

Physiological stress

Physiological stress from capture and handling for swab collection can be minimised by performing the procedure as quickly as possible; the effects of this stress on individual animals are likely to be transient. Substantial physiological stress may occur when wild amphibians are held in a captive environment, and they should only be removed from a field site when necessary. Researchers should carefully consider study design and species selection if captivity is required.

Soft tissue trauma from swab collection

Amphibian skin is relatively fragile, and both the manual restraint and swabbing processes can cause physical damage to the skin and oral cavity. These animals are particularly susceptible to skin irritation from chemicals and other contaminants because of the absorptive capacity of their integument. The effects of physical and chemical trauma can be minimised by the operator wearing moistened gloves (nitrile gloves may be toxic to tadpoles, so vinyl gloves are preferred (see details in 'Frogs and toads'; Cashins *et al.* 2008) and performing the procedure as quickly as possible. Superficial minor skin, oral or mouthpart trauma at swab sites is unavoidable because of the nature of the procedure; adequate operator training will minimise the risk of excessive soft tissue trauma from the restraint and swabbing processes.

Respiratory distress in larval amphibians

Larval amphibians rely on aquatic respiration via gills. Removing them from water to swab their mouthparts can cause progressive respiratory distress over a short time. The impacts of this technique can be minimised by performing the procedure quickly (ideally within 10 to 20 s) and adequate operator training.

Identification techniques for individual amphibians

Individual adult amphibians often require unique identification for monitoring health status over time and recording recapture rates for field studies. Identification techniques may require individual housing, photographic records, tag insertion (passive integrated transponder (PIT), visible implant alphanumeric (VIA), visible implant elastomer (VIE), and toe tipping/clipping (see Chapter 8. If individual identification of captive larval amphibians is required, they can be housed in separate containers and allocated unique identification codes.

Disease transmission

Handling multiple amphibians can increase the risk of disease transmission between individuals. Researchers travelling between different field sites can also increase the risk of disease spread between populations. Researchers should be diligent in following strict hygiene protocols for these procedures by sterilising hands and footwear and changing clothing between field sites, wearing new gloves and sterilising equipment or containers for each amphibian. Phillott *et al.* (2010) review hygiene considerations for amphibian field studies in detail; also, see details in 'Frogs and toads'. Toe tipping or clipping for identification is a surgical procedure (Chapter 8). Disinfectant solutions should be selected based on efficacy and safety (both for amphibians and humans) and should not be allowed to contaminate water bodies.

General procedures

Skin swabbing of post-metamorphic anurans (and salamanders)

Juvenile and adult anurans and salamanders can be captured and restrained in one hand; using the other hand, the ventral skin surfaces can then be swabbed using a dry, sterile fine-tipped swab. The cotton tip of the swab should be rolled gently, but firmly, 20 to 30 times (three to five times per site) over the ventral abdomen and pelvic 'drink patch', the ventral thighs, and the palmar and plantar surfaces (underside) of the toe webbing of all four feet (Figure 27.1; Hyatt *et al.* 2007). Single-use powder-free nitrile or vinyl gloves should be worn and replaced between individuals. A new sterile swab should be used for each individual.

Mouthpart swabbing of larval anurans

Tadpoles can be captured and restrained in one hand and using the other hand their mouthparts swabbed using a rounded, wooden toothpick with a sharply pointed end; the pointed end is scraped and rolled over and between the tooth rows and the keratinised beak of the tadpole (Retallick *et al.* 2006). A new toothpick should be used for each individual. This technique is less sensitive than lethal sampling of mouthparts from tadpoles, and it is recommended that more tadpoles be sampled to estimate prevalence at a confidence level comparable to lethal sampling (Retallick *et al.* 2006). Mouthparts can also be sampled using a dry, sterile fine-tipped swab with the cotton tip inserted into the mouth and twirled several times (Hyatt *et al.* 2007). Single-use powder-free nitrile or vinyl gloves should be worn and replaced between individuals.

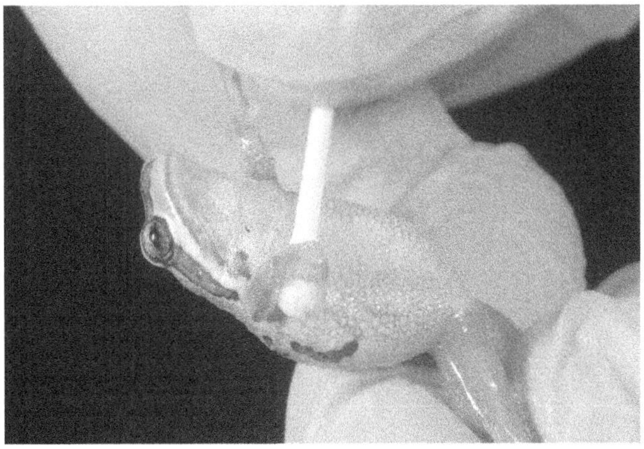

Figure 27.1: Captive bred and reared alpine tree frog (*Litoria verreauxii alpina*) being swabbed for assessing amphibian chytrid fungus infection status before release in Kosciuszko National Park. Photo by David Hunter.

Animal treatment, withdrawal and euthanasia

With the exception of superficial skin or oral cavity trauma during manual restraint and swab collection, the risk of injury through swabbing for chytrid is low. The risk of more-serious injury to amphibians during field capture may be increased during attempted removal of individuals from sites that are difficult to access. Individual amphibians with pre-existing injuries or diseases may be encountered during field capture studies. If medical treatment is required for a minor injury/disease state, the most appropriate *in situ* treatment should be administered by suitably trained and experienced researchers, or veterinary advice should be sought. If euthanasia is required for serious injuries or debilitating disease, suitably trained and experienced researchers should use the most appropriate species-specific technique and/or seek veterinary advice (see the earlier section in this chapter).

Equipment and maintenance

Items required for swabbing amphibians for chytrid include:

- single-use, powder-free nitrile or vinyl gloves
- sterile dry fine-tipped cotton swabs, toothpicks
- identification equipment (e.g. tags, PIT scanner, camera, sterile surgical equipment and disinfectant solution)
- data recording equipment
- holding containers for animals (e.g. single-use lightweight plastic bags, small plastic containers with ventilation holes) and aged tap water or amphibian-specific isotonic electrolyte solution
- materials for dealing with injured and diseased frogs
- field hygiene equipment (disinfectant solution, change of clothes and footwear).

Specific qualifications, experience and training

Researchers capturing and restraining amphibians for chytrid swabbing should be suitably experienced and trained in various aspects of handling, and captive and field research techniques.

Workplace health and safety

The method poses little risk to personnel with most risks related to fieldwork. Personnel should have appropriate operational procedures in place, carry suitable equipment and receive adequate prior training.

Alternative procedures

Molecular testing of skin or mouthpart swabs for chytrid is the most sensitive non-lethal method for detecting infection in live amphibians. The only other method of testing that may be lower in terms of physical impact involves submerging amphibians in water in a small container for up to 24 h and then testing the water. This method does not require restraint of the amphibian for the swabbing process, but does require close confinement in a foreign environment for much longer than the time required to collect the swab. Confinement is likely to cause additional physiological stress and is unlikely to be a suitable test technique for many field studies or certain amphibian species.

REFERENCES

Anstis M (2013) *Tadpoles and Frogs of Australia*. New Holland, Sydney.

AVMA (2020) *AVMA Guidelines for the Euthanasia of Animals: 2020 Edition*. American Veterinary Medical Association, Schaumburg, IL.

Baines F, Chattell J, Dale J, Garrick D, Gill I, Goetz M, Skelton T, Swatman M (2016) How much UV-B does my reptile need? The UV-Tool, a guide to the selection of UV lighting for reptiles and amphibians in captivity. *The Journal of Zoo and Aquarium Research* **4**, 42–63. doi:10.19227/jzar.v4i1.150

Baitchman E, Stetter M (2014) Amphibians. In *Zoo Animal and Wildlife Immobilization and Anaesthesia*. 2nd edn. (Eds G West, D Heard and N Caulkett) pp 303–311. John Wiley and Sons, Hoboken, NJ.

Berger L, Speare R, Daszak P, Green DE, Cunningham AA, Goggin CL, *et al.* (1998) Chytridiomycosis causes amphibian mortality associated with population declines in the rain forests of Australia and Central America. *Proceedings of the National Academy of Sciences of the United States of America* **95**, 9031–9036. doi:10.1073/pnas.95.15.9031

Boyle DG, Boyle DB, Olsen V, Morgan JAT, Hyatt AD (2004) Rapid quantitative detection of chytridiomycosis *(Batrachochytrium dendrobatidis)* in amphibian samples using real-time TaqMan PCR Assay. *Diseases of Aquatic Organisms* **60**, 141–148. doi:10.3354/dao060141

Cashins SD, Alford RA, Skerratt LF (2008) Lethal effect of latex, nitrile, and vinyl gloves on tadpoles. *Herpetological Review* **39**, 298–301.

Chen MH, Combs CA (1999) An alternative anesthesia for amphibians: ventral application of benzocaine. *Herpetological Review* **30**, 34.

Coble DJ, Taylor DK, Mook DM (2011) Analgesic effects of meloxicam, morphine sulfate, flunixin meglumine, and xylazine hydrochloride in African-clawed frogs (*Xenopus laevis*). *Journal of the American Association for Laboratory Animal Science; JAALAS* **50**, 355–360.

Cogger HG (2018) A brief demographic overview of Australia's native amphibians. In *Status of Conservation and Decline of Amphibians: Australia, New Zealand and Pacific Islands*. (Eds H Heatwole and JJL Rowley) pp. 5–13. CSIRO Publishing, Melbourne.

DPIE (2020) *Saving Our Species Hygiene Guidelines: Protocols to Protect Priority Biodiversity Areas in NSW from* Phytophora cinnamomi, *Myrtle Rust, Amphibian Chytrid Fungus and Invasive Plants*. Department of Planning, Industry and Environment, Sydney.

Dyer SM, Cervasio EL (2008) An Overview of Restraint and Blood Collection Techniques in Exotic Pet Practice. *The Veterinary Clinics of North America. Exotic Animal Practice* **11**, 423–443. doi:10.1016/j.cvex.2008.03.008

Ferrie GM, Alford VC, Atkinson J, Baitchman E, Barber D, Blaner WS, *et al.* (2014) Nutrition and health in amphibian husbandry. *Zoo Biology* **33**, 485–501. doi:10.1002/zoo.21180

Gillespie GR, Roberts JD, Hunter D, Hoskin CJ, Alford RA, Heard GW, Hines H, Lemckert F, Newell D, Scheele BC (2020) Status and priority conservation actions for Australian frog species. *Biological Conservation* **247**. doi:10.1016/j.biocon.2020.108543

Hyatt AD, Boyle DG, Boyle DB, Berger L, Obendorf D, Dalton A, *et al.* (2007) Diagnostic assays and sampling protocols for the detection of *Batrachochytrium dendrobatidis*. *Diseases of Aquatic Organisms* **73**, 175–192. doi:10.3354/dao073175

Mendelson III JR, Altig R (2016) Tadpoles, froglets and conservation: a discussion of basic principles of rearing and release procedures. *Amphibian & Reptile Conservation* **10**, 20–27.

Murray K, Skerratt L, Marantelli G, Berger L, Hunter D, Mahony M, Hines H (2011) *Hygiene Protocols for the Control of Diseases in Australian Frogs. A Report for the Australian Government Department of Sustainability, Environment, Water, Population and Communities*. Department of Sustainability, Environment, Water, Population and Communities, Canberra.

Nichols DK, Lamirande EW, Pessier AP, Longcore JE (2001) Experimental transmission of cutaneous chytridiomycosis in Dendrobatid frogs. *Journal of Wildlife Diseases* **37**, 1–11. doi:10.7589/0090-3558-37.1.1

Odum RA, Zippel KC (2008) Amphibian water quality: approaches to an essential environmental parameter. *International Zoo Yearbook* **42**, 40–52. doi:10.1111/j.1748-1090.2008.00053.x

OEH (2014) *Eradicating Cane Toads in NSW outside their Current Range of Distribution: Best Practice Guidelines*. Office of Environment and Heritage, Sydney.

Phillott AD, Speare R, Hines HB, Skerratt LF, Meyer E, McDonald KR, Cashins SD, Mendez D, Berger L (2010) Minimising exposure of amphibians to pathogens during field studies. *Diseases of Aquatic Organisms* **92**, 175–185. doi:10.3354/dao02162

Predavec M, Dickman CR (1993) Ecology of desert frogs: a study from southwestern Queensland. In *Herpetology in Australia*. (Eds D Lunney and D Ayers) pp. 159–169. Surrey Beatty and Sons, Sydney.

Retallick RWR, Miera V, Richards KL, Field KJ, Collins JP (2006) A non-lethal technique for detecting the chytrid fungus *Batrachochytrium dendrobatidis* on tadpoles. *Diseases of Aquatic Organisms* **72**, 77–85. doi:10.3354/dao072077

Scheele BC, *et al.* (2019) Amphibian fungal panzootic causes catastrophic and ongoing loss of biodiversity. *Science* **363**, 1459–1463. doi:10.1126/science.aav0379

Sharp T, Lothian A, Munn A, Saunders G (2011) *CAN001 Methods for the Field Euthanasia of Cane Toads*. Department of Primary Industries, Orange.

Shin J, Bataille A, Kosch TA, Waldman B (2014) Swabbing often fails to detect amphibian chytridiomycosis under conditions of low infection load. *PLoS One* **9**, e111091. doi:10.1371/journal.pone.0111091

Shine R (2018) The impact of an invasive amphibian: the cane toad *Rhinella marina*. In *Status of Conservation and Decline of Amphibians: Australia, New Zealand and Pacific Islands*. (Eds H Heatwole and JJL Rowley) pp. 107–124. CSIRO Publishing, Melbourne.

Skerratt LF, Berger L, Speare R, Cashins S, McDonald KR, Phillott AD, *et al.* (2007) Spread of chytridiomycosis has caused the rapid decline and extinction of frogs. *EcoHealth* **4**, 125–134. doi:10.1007/s10393-007-0093-5

Stevens CW (2011) Analgesia in amphibians: preclinical studies and clinical applications. *The Veterinary Clinics of North America. Exotic Animal Practice* **14**, 33–44. doi:10.1016/j.cvex.2010.09.007

Stetter MD (2001) Fish and amphibian anaesthesia. *The Veterinary Clinics of North America. Exotic Animal Practice* **4**, 69–82. doi:10.1016/S1094-9194(17)30052-X

Tapley B, Rendle M, Baines FM, Goetz M, Bradfield KS, Rood D, Lopez J, Garcia G, Routh A (2014) Meeting ultraviolet B radiation requirements of amphibians in captivity: A case study with mountain chicken frogs (*Leptodactylus fallax*) and general recommendations for pre-release health screening. *Zoo Biology* **34**, 46–52. doi:10.1002/zoo.21170

Tingley R, Weeks AR, Smart AS, van Rooyen AR, Woolnough AP, McCarthy MA (2015) European newts establish in Australia, marking the arrival of a new amphibian order. *Biological Invasions* **17**, 31–37. doi:10.1007/s10530-014-0716-z

Wright KM (2001a). Restraint techniques and euthanasia. In *Amphibian Medicine and Captive Husbandry.* (Eds KM Wright and BR Whitaker) pp. 111–122. Krieger Publishing Company, Malabar, FL.

Wright KM (2001b). Surgical techniques. In *Amphibian Medicine and Captive Husbandry.* (Eds KM Wright and BR Whitaker) pp. 273–283. Krieger Publishing Company, Malabar, FL.

28 Crustaceans

Maggie J. Watson, Katherine E. Doyle and Culum Brown

INTRODUCTION

Crustaceans are a large and diverse arthropod subphylum of almost 67 000 species that range in size from the 3.7 m long Japanese spider crab (*Macrocheira kaempferi*) to a 100 μm long tantulocarid ectoparasite (*Stygotantulus stocki*). Seven classes are currently recognised (see Oakley *et al.* 2013):

- Branchiopoda (brine shrimp, fairy shrimp, water fleas, shield shrimp, clam shrimp)
- Cephalocarida (horseshoe shrimp)
- Hexanauplia (barnacles and copepods, parasitic tantulocarids)
- Ichthyostraca (minute meiobenthic moustache shrimp, tongue worms, fish lice)
- Malacostraca (crabs, lobsters, crayfish, shrimp, prawns, krill, mantis shrimp, woodlice, hooded shrimp, scuds, sandhoppers, amphipods, isopods, tongue-eating louse, tanaids, anapsid cave shrimp)
- Ostacoda (seed shrimp)
- Remipedia (remipedes).

Recent molecular work has shown that crustaceans are paraphyletic, and that some species are more closely related to insects than they are to other crustaceans. Crustaceans are generally distinguished from other arthropods by limbs with two parts and their larval forms (the nauplius). Most crustaceans are free-living aquatic animals, but some are sessile, terrestrial or parasitic. Decapods (crabs, lobsters, crayfish, shrimp and prawns) are important human farmed and fished food sources. Krill and copepods may be the animals with the greatest biomass on the planet, forming the basis for most marine food webs.

In the Northern Territory, New South Wales and Australian Capital Territory, larger crustaceans in the Malocostraca are protected under the relevant animal welfare legislation, but this protection only applies to crustaceans intended for human consumption. In the Northern Territory and New South Wales, welfare legislation only applies to retail sales. In South Australia and Tasmania, crustaceans are not included in the definition of an animal and are therefore exempt from welfare considerations. The legislation is unclear in Queensland as crustaceans are defined as animals, but animal ethics are not required. In Western Australia, only live invertebrates of a 'prescribed kind' are covered under welfare legislation, but 'prescribed' is not defined (RSPCA Australia 2020a). Researchers, therefore, do not appear to need animal ethics permits in these states. Victoria is the only state that currently requires animal ethics permits for crustacean research, but this is restricted to decapods, specifically lobsters, crabs and crayfish. This chapter focuses mostly on larger crustacean species, although mention is made, where appropriate, of other crustaceans.

CRAB, LOBSTER, CRAYFISH AND PRAWNS

Characteristics

Crabs, lobster, crayfish and prawns are the larger species within the class Malocostraca. Only those that are in the order Decapoda are considered in this chapter, and only those within the infraorders Astacidea (true lobsters, reef lobsters and freshwater crayfish), Achelata (spiny, slipper and furry lobsters), Anomura (squat lobsters and hermit crabs), Brachyura (true crabs) and Dendrobranchiata (prawns) as they contain species that are large and found in Australia. True lobsters are only represented by one species in Australia, the Australian scampi, while freshwater crayfish are mostly endemic, and highly endangered, in Australia. Species that are commonly called lobsters in Australia are actually spiny, slipper, furry or squat lobsters. Hermit crabs are speciose and increasingly found in the pet trade. Prawns are another speciose group in Australia that is commercially harvested. True crabs typically have a short 'tail' (abdomen) hidden entirely under the thorax and there are hundreds of species in Australia, so only a few notable species have been mentioned. Note that hermit crabs, king crabs, porcelain crabs, horseshoe crabs and crab lice are not crabs.

The body of a crustacean is composed of three segments – the cephalon or head, the pereon or thorax, and the pleon or abdomen. The head and thorax may be fused to form a cephalothorax, which may have a single large carapace. Each body segment can have a pair of appendages, so the head has a pair of antennae, mandibles and maxillae, the thoracic segments have legs (pereiopods or walking legs, and maxillipeds or feeding legs). The abdomen has pleopods and ends in a telson, often flanked by uropods to form a tail fan. The body cavity has an open circulatory system. Malacostraca use haemocyanin as the oxygen-carrying pigment while copepods, ostracods, barnacles and branchiopods use haemoglobins.

Biology and behaviour

Crustacean groups are found throughout Australian coastal and freshwater environments, and many in both. The malocostracans (e.g. crabs, lobsters, crayfish, shimp, prawns), which are sometimes the focus of animal ethics applications, are abundant in all marine environments and many freshwater and terrestrial habitats.

Most crustaceans have separate sexes and reproduce sexually, although some barnacles, remipedes and horseshoe shrimp are hermaphroditic. Parthenogenesis can occur in branchiopods, ostracods, isopods and at least one population of freshwater crayfish. Crustaceans have several larval forms, the first of which, and the one that characterises this group, is the nauplius, which has three pairs of appendages emerging from the head, and a single naupliar eye. Most crustaceans are free-living aquatic animals, but some are terrestrial (isopod wood lice or slaters), or parasitic (fish lice), tongue-eating louse (Isopoda) and some are sessile (barnacles). Because of the vast array of sizes and habitats, most species of crustaceans require specialised methods for collection and capture (refer to 'Capture and handling' within this chapter).

Capture and handling

Crustaceans are diverse in form, size and habitat, so capture and handling techniques are diverse (for examples see Boxshall *et al.* 2016; Gerken 2016; Larsen 2016; Martin *et al.* 2016; Poly 2016; Porter 2016; Watling 2016; and Yager 2016). Gear type and mesh size, bait type and time of day (many species are nocturnal) are key considerations. Lobsters and crayfish all require specialist gear for collection, especially when fished commercially. Freshwater crayfish can be collected by turning rocks and capturing them by hand, night collection via torchlight, baited hood traps, dip and seine nets, burrow excavation and the use of a yabby pump (Crandall 2016). Crays and lobsters are primarily handled by holding them behind the head and claws.

Successfully housing crustaceans requires detailed knowledge of the biology and behaviour of the species of interest and may vary within taxa. For example, *Cherax* spp. are easily housed in water for extended periods and will feed from bacterial scunge on submerged logs and dogfood, but all other freshwater crayfish species are difficult to retain in captivity and will usually refuse to eat, and die after moulting unless supplied with a source of calcium. Welfare of crustaceans in aquaculture or other aquatic captive settings is directly related to water quality (water sources and preparation, oxygen supply, temperature maintenance, dissolved oxygen, pH, alkalinity, salinity, turbidity, nitrogenous waste levels, filtration and water exchanges). Crustaceans show a range of physiological tolerances, which requires an understanding of natural habitat requirements and biological strategies. In general, the upper lethal temperature limit for most crustaceans ranges from 30 to 40°C. Crustaceans occur at a range of pH values, but most thrive at neutral pH values. Few species live in environments below a pH of 5.5, where toxicity of heavy metals like aluminium also becomes problematic and the ability to absorb calcium carbonate, important for exoskeleton development, is impaired. Oxygen concentrations affect habitat suitability, which is a more-serious problem in warmer waters that can hold less oxygen.

Housing management (tanks, ponds) may require the preparation and provision of refuge habitat. Crustaceans, mainly decapods (e.g. crayfish, lobster and crabs), may require individual shelters to reduce the risk of damage from frequent fighting. In general, supplying hides or shelters for animals provides some protection from conspecifics, predators and bright sunlight, and also provides increased surface area in the holding container. Crustaceans eat plant material (including phytoplankton), animal material (including insects, zooplankton, and small fish) and detritus. Commercially available pellet feed is often used as it reduces the risk of disease introduction. Overfeeding may reduce water quality. Consequently, feeding rates must be tailored to the requirements of the animal and water temperature, with decreased volume or frequency in cooler waters. In ponds, protection from predator incursions should be provided in the form of filters on intake water supply and, where appropriate, bird nets over ponds and hides in the pond. Clear water, in addition to representing a stressor on the animals because of unstable or inappropriate algal growth, also renders the animals more susceptible to predators.

Generally, only the larger species of the Malacostraca (i.e. crabs, lobsters, and crayfish) are marked. Marking techniques include visible implant elastomer (VIE) tags, visible implant alphanumeric (VIA) tags, coded wire tags, passive integrated transponder (PIT) tags, polythene streamers, telson/uropod ablation (clips), cryogenic marking (freeze-branding) and electric cauterisation (heat-branding) (Haddaway *et al.* 2011).

Most crustaceans are delicate and need to be handled with care. Crabs, lobsters and crayfish are equipped with large pinchers, which can injure handlers. Using thick (riggers) gloves is recommended and hessian or carpet can provide immediate protection and keep individual crustaceans separate. Maintaining a proper grip is important while handling larger crustaceans. For most species, grasping the carapace behind the claws will prevent injury to the crustacean and the handler. If large numbers of crustaceans are captured at once, PVC pipes or 2 L plastic bottles with the bottoms cut off can be used as a temporary holding facility. If longer-term housing is required, claws need to be banded with appropriately sized elastic bands (thick rubber bands or marking rings) or cable ties. Incorrect handling of crustaceans may lead to voluntary shedding of appendages (autotomy), such as legs and claws. Autotomy can have a severe impact on survival and social status, so crustaceans should only be handled by the body.

Short-distance transport is possible for most crustaceans using the water or substrate that the animal was captured in. Long-distance or international transport involves more-elaborate preparation. Most countries require collecting permits to import or export organisms across their borders. International law governs the movement of specific taxa across borders, and personnel should consult the most recent Convention on International Trade in Endangered Species of Wild Fauna and Flora (CITES) before collecting in foreign countries (www.cites.org/).

Veterinary considerations

Agents listed in Table 28.1 are effective immobilising agents for aquatic crustaceans, but it is unknown if they provide real anaesthesia or analgesic properties. Some chemicals listed in Table 28.1 may cause autotomy (shedding of appendages). Crustaceans show responses consistent with signs of pain and distress at least as strong as those shown by fish (Elwood 2012). In situations where gross physical manipulations (i.e. surgery, amputation, internal tagging) are necessary, effective anaesthesia or analgesics should be used with group-specific immobilising agents. Simple manipulations (i.e. haemolymph extraction, behavioural manipulations, transportation) do not require anaesthesia or analgesics.

Euthanasia

Most crustaceans should be euthanased with an anaesthetic (see Table 29.3) followed by brain destruction (ANZCCART 2001). Euthanasia may also be achieved via overdose with a general anaesthetic (Table 28.1), electric stunning in a water bath, or placement in ice slurry (< 4°C) for 20 min (RSPCA Australia 2020b). Ice slurries must be salty for marine species and fresh for freshwater species (AVMA 2020). Two-step euthanasia procedures should be used for confirming death, as assessment of invertebrate death is often difficult. The first step should include anaesthesia that results in non-responsiveness (presumed death). Non-responsiveness means no resistance to handling, loss of limb control, no reaction when eyes or mouthparts are touched. The second step includes either physical (pithing (Figure 28.1), freezing or boiling) or chemical (alcohol, formalin) destruction of the brain.

Table 28.1: Common immobilising agents (anaesthetics) for crustaceans.

Ross and Ross (2008).

Group	Immobilisation agent
All Crustacea	Chlorbutanol (between 0.05% and 0.5%) Chloroform (1%) Urethane (1%) 2-phenoxyethanol (1.5%) Ethane disulphonate (2.5 g/L) Ethanol (5–10% solution) Isobutyl alocohol (1.5–7 cm^3/L) Methyl pentynol 5 cm^3/L) Tricaine methanesulfonate (MS-222) (0.5 g/L): note that this concentration does not work on freshwater crayfish, even at high concentration (1 g/L) Cooling to 1–2°C (risks autotomy of appendages)
Malacostraca Crabs, lobsters, crayfish, shrimp, prawns Krill Mantis shrimp Amphipods, sandhoppers and scuds Isopods, tongue-eating louse and woodlice Hooded or comma shrimp Tanaids Anaspid cave shrimp	Crabs: Clove oil in water ranging from 0.5–1.5 ml L^{-1},1–3ml $L^{-1}$and 0.015–0.25 ml L^{-1} Lobster (marine): immersion in isobutyl alcohol at concentrations of 0.5–14.4 cm^3/L Freshwater crayfish: halothane at 0.01–0.1.0% by volume in air (most effective at 0.5%) Sand shrimp: MS222 at 0.5 g/L Japanese tiger prawn: eugenol at 15–200 ppm Macrobrachium clove oil in ethanol at 30–60 mg/L Mantis shrimp: isobutanol by cardiac injection, reliable and effective at 200 µL/kg at temperatures 11–17°C Amphipods: tricaine methanesulfonate (MS-222) at 0.5–1.0 g/L; safety margin is greatest at lower temperature

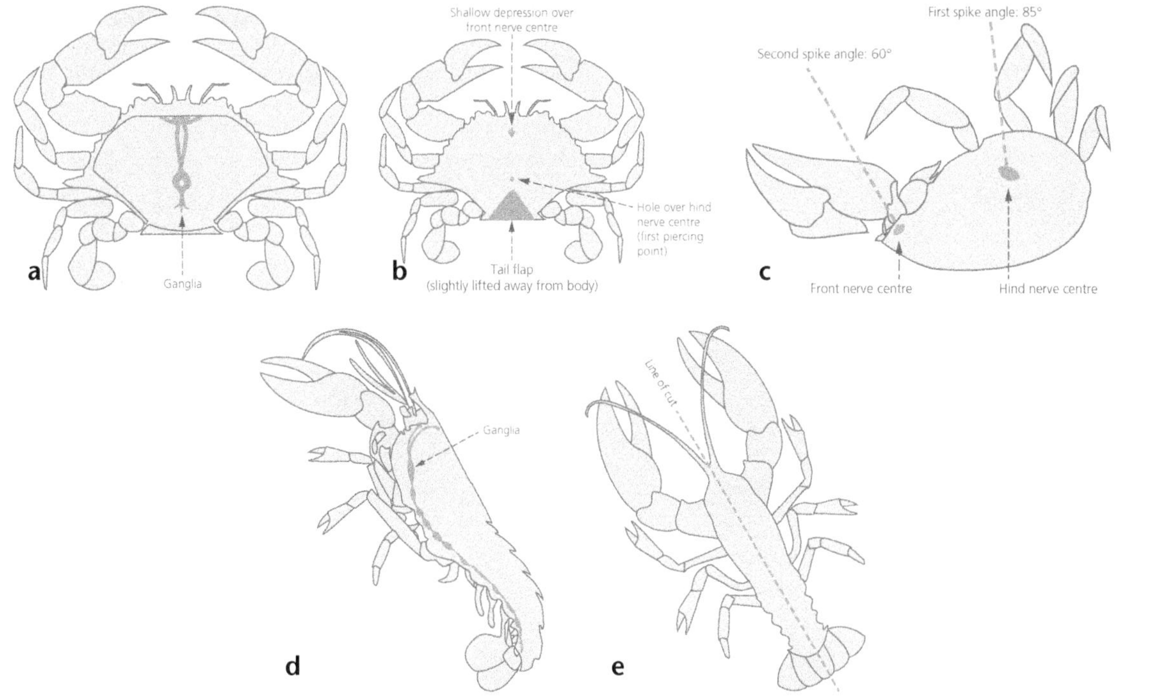

Figure 28.1: Example pithing procedures for crabs: (a) placement of internal ganglia or nerve centres; (b) the underside showing reference points for pithing/spiking; and (c) angles for pithing/spiking. Example pithing procedures for lobsters: (d) placement of multiple internal ganglia or nerve centres; and (e) recommended line of cut). Illustrations provided with permission from RSPCA Australia (2020b).

Table 28.2: Known diseases of crustaceans in Australia.

Edgerton *et al.* (2002); Department of Agriculture (2019).

Disease	Crustaceans affected	Signs
Viral		
White spot syndrome virus, WSSV (white spot disease, WSD)	All decapod crustaceans, prawns, shrimps, lobsters, crabs, freshwater crayfish including *Cherax* spp., *Astacopsis* spp. and *Euastacus* spp., brine shrimp, parasitic and planktonic copepods	Mass mortality, lethargy, cessation of feeding, loose carapace, ectoparasite abandonment, white calcium deposits embedded in shell, colour variation including red, brown or pink body surfaces
Gill-associated virus (mid-crop mortality syndrome or infection with yellowhead virus genotype 2, YHV2)	Prawns (*Penaeus* spp.)	Increase in feeding followed by cessation, reddening of body and appendages, ectoparasite abandonment, pink or yellow gills, organ necrosis, death
Infectious hypodermal and haematopoietic necrosis virus, (IHHNV),infectious hypodermal and haematopoietic necrosis (IHHN), infection with *Penaeus stylirostris* densovirus, PstDNV and runt deformity syndrome, RDS	Prawns and shrimp (*Penaeus* spp., *Artemesia* spp., *Macrobrachium* spp.), crabs (*Hemigrapsus* spp., *Callinectes* spp.)	Reduced food consumption, cannibalism, opaque abdominal muscles, white or buff lesions under carapace, sometimes blue appearance of moribund animals, irregular growth in juveniles and subadults, deformed rostrums or sixth abdominal segment
White tail disease (*Macrobrachium rosenbergii* nodavirus, MrNV)	Prawns and shrimp (*Penaeus* spp., *Macrobrachium* spp.), various penaeid prawns, freshwater crayfish (*Cherax* spp.), brine shrimp (*Artemia* spp.)	Whitish postlarvae, lethargy, mortality
Cherax quadricarinatus bacilliform virus (CqBV)	Freshwater crayfish (*Cherax* spp.)	Lethargy, weakened tails, low virulence
Cherax Giardiavirus-like virus (CGV)	Freshwater crayfish (*Cherax* spp.)	High morbidity in juveniles
Cherax destructor bacilliform virus (CdBV)	Freshwater crayfish (*Cherax* spp.)	Unknown
Systemic rickettsial infection	Freshwater amphipods, marine crabs, isopods, penaeid shrimp, freshwater crayfish	Lethargy, weakened tails
Bacterial and fungal		
Asymptomatic bacteraemia and bacterial septicaemia	All crustaceans	Lethargy, loss of muscle tone, posture abnormalities, often asymptomatic
Bacterial cuticular fouling	Marine aquaculture facilities	Filamentous bacteria on exoskeleton, gills and/or eggs
Burn spot disease (bacterial and fungal agents)	Lobsters, shrimp and prawns, crabs, freshwater crayfish including *Cherax* spp.	Invasion of wounds causing necrosis at the centre
Parasites		
Microsporidian infection	All crustaceans	Lethargy and opacity of musculature turning to chalky white rather than translucent
Ciliate infection	All crustaceans	Lethargy, weakened tails
Digenean infection	Freshwater crayfish	Secondary intermediate host, no disease; occasional encystment
Cestode infection	Freshwater crayfish	Intermediate host, no disease
Nematode infection	All crustaceans	Intermediate host, no disease
Acanthocephalan infection	Freshwater crayfish	Intermediate host, no disease

Disease	Crustaceans affected	Signs
Temnocephalid infection	Freshwater crayfish	Probably symbiont, no disease; often mistaken for leeches
Angiostrongylus cantonensis	All crustaceans	Overseas *Angiostronylus cantonensis* is known to infect a wide range of intermediate hosts, including many crustaceans as intermediate hosts causing no signs to death depending on the load. It is becoming much more widespread in Australia where it is a significant zoonosis, killing one or two infants in some years and occasionally permanently incapacitating adults. If correctly investigated I'm sure it will be found in Australian Crustacea, as well as amphibians and fish. It is known to infect and kill a wide range of Australian mammals and birds.

Many crustaceans have a nerve net with multiple ganglia, which all need to be destroyed appropriately. For example, a longitudinal cut can be used to destroy ganglia in lobsters, as their ganglia tend to lie along the midline Crabs have two main nerve centres (brains); both should be destroyed by pithing. In short, a detailed understanding of the anatomy of the species is necessary to determine the best method for euthanasia. An example from Yue (2008) recommends that crustaceans be placed in an ice slurry for > 20 min followed by rapid destruction of nerve centres in less than 10 s (Figure 28.1). The killing can only be done by a skilled operator and unacceptable methods of killing the animals are specifically spelled out (boiling alive, transverse sectioning of lobsters and cutting crabs into pieces; see Diggles 2019).

Infectious pathogens

Known diseases are mostly described for commercially farmed or harvested species (Department of Agriculture 2019). Wild crustaceans pose some risk to human health in terms of bacterial infection transmitted through cuts while handling. Specifically, crayfish handler's disease (erysipeloid or fish disease), well known in the fishing industry, is caused by various bacteria, including *Erysipelothrix rhusiopathiae* and *Vibrio* spp. and apparently transmitted by lobsters and shellfish. Some of the more-commonly encountered diseases in farmed crustaceans are listed in Table 28.2.

General operating procedures

Standard operating procedures are available for freshwater (Webb *et al.* 2019) and marine crustaceans (Przeslawski and Foster 2018). Capture and observation methods that may be applicable for capturing larger crustaceans (crayfish and lobster) are described in Chapters 12 and 14. General procedures for working with VIE detailed in Chapter 8 may also be useful.

REFERENCES

AVMA (2020) *AVMA Guidelines for the Euthanasia of Animals, 2020 Edition*. American Veterinary Medical Association, Schaumburg, IL.

Boxshall GA, Kihara TC, Huys R (2016) Collecting and processing non-planktonic copepods. *Journal of Crustacean Biology* **36**, 576–583. doi:10.1163/1937240X-00002438

Crandall KA (2016) Collecting and processing freshwater crayfishes. *Journal of Crustacean Biology* **36**, 761–766. doi:10.1163/1937240X-00002466

Department of Agriculture (2019) *Aquatic Animal Diseases Significant to Australia: Identification Field Guide*. 5th edn. Australian Government Department of Agriculture, Canberra.

Diggles BK (2018) Review of some scientific issues related to crustacean welfare. *ICES Journal of Marine Science* **76**, 66–81. doi:10.1093/icesjms/fsy058

Edgerton BF, Evans LH, Stephens FJ, Overstreet RM (2002) Synopsis of freshwater crayfish diseases and commensal organisms. *Aquaculture* **206**, 57–135. doi:10.1016/S0044-8486(01)00865-1

Elwood RW (2011) Pain and suffering in invertebrates? *ILAR Journal* **52**(2), 175–184.

Gerken S (2016) Collecting and processing cumaceans. *Journal of Crustacean Biology* **36**, 833–836. doi:10.1163/1937240X-00002477

Haddaway NR, Mortimer R, Christmas MA, Dunn AM (2011) A review of marking techniques for crustacea and experimental appraisal of electric cauterisation and visible implant elastomer tagging for *Austropotamobius pallipes* and *Pacifastacus leniusculus*. *Freshwater Crayfish* **18**, 55–67. doi:10.5869/fc.2011.v18.55

Larsen K (2016) Collecting and processing tanaids. *Journal of Crustacean Biology* **36**, 589–591. doi:10.1163/1937240X-00002447

Martin JW, Rogers DC, Oleson J (2016) Collecting and processing branchiopods. *Journal of Crustacean Biology* **36**, 396–401. doi:10.1163/1937240X-00002434

Oakley TH, Wolfe JM, Lindgren AR, Zaharoff AK (2013) Phylotranscriptomics to bring the understudied into the fold: monophyletic ostracoda, fossil placement, and pancrustacean phylogeny. *Molecular Biology and Evolution* **30**, 215–233. doi:10.1093/molbev/mss216

Poly WJ (2016) Collecting and processing branchiurans. *Journal of Crustacean Biology* **36**, 855–859. doi:10.1163/1937240X-00002481

Porter ML (2016) Collecting and processing mysids, stygiomysids, lophogastrids. *Journal of Crustacean Biology* **36**, 592–595. doi:10.1163/1937240X-00002443

Przeslawski R, Foster S (Eds) (2018) *Field Manuals for Marine Sampling to Monitor Australian Waters, Version 1*. Report to the National Environmental Science Programme, Marine Biodiversity Hub. doi:10.11636/9781925297669

Reilly JS (Ed) (2001) *Euthanasia of Animals Used for Scientific Purposes*. 2nd edn. Australian & New Zealand Council for the Care of Animals in Research and Teaching (ANZCCART), Adelaide.

Ross LG, Ross B (2008) Anaesthesia of aquatic invertebrates. In *Anaesthetic and Sedative Techniques for Aquatic Animals*. 3rd edn. (Eds L Ross and B Ross) pp. 167–178. Blackwell Publishing, Ames, IA.

RSPCA Australia (Royal Society for the Prevention of Cruelty to Animals) (2020a) *Are crustaceans protected by animal welfare legislation?* RSPCA Australia. <https://kb.rspca.org.au/knowledge-base/are-crustaceans-protected-by-animal-welfare-legislation/>.

RSPCA Australia (Royal Society for the Prevention of Cruelty to Animals) (2020b) *RSPCA humane killing of crustaceans*. RSPCA Australia. <https://kb.rspca.org.au/knowledge-base/what-is-the-most-humane-way-to-kill-crustaceans-for-human-consumption/>.

Watling L (2016) Collecting and processing bathynellaceans, anaspidaceans, spelaeogriphaceans and thermosbaenaceans. *Journal of Crustacean Biology* **36**, 402–404. doi:10.1163/1937240X-00002435

Webb A, Treadwell S, Lakhanpal G, Baker B, Casanelia S, Grace G, Koster W, Lovell D, Morris K, Pettigrove V, Tonkin Z, Vietz G (2019) Standard operating procedures for macroinvertebrates (v1.0). Commonwealth Environmental Water Office. <https://www.environment.gov.au/water/cewo/publications/mer-plan-goulburn-2019>.

Yager J (2016) Collecting and processing remipedes. *Journal of Crustacean Biology* **36**, 405–407. doi:10.1163/1937240X-00002433

Yue S (2008) *The Welfare of Crustaceans at Slaughter. Impacts on Farm Animals 4*. Humane Society of the United States. <https://www.wellbeingintlstudiesrepository.org/hsus_reps_impacts_on_animals/4/>.

29 Cephalopods

Zoë A. Doubleday, Jasmin C. Martino, Jayson M. Semmens and Elise Boultby

INTRODUCTION

In Australia, cephalopods are the only invertebrates included under Australian Code for the Care and Use of Animals for Scientific Purposes (the Code) (NHMRC 2013), where they are defined and protected as an 'animal'. However, the Code does not apply to all research organisations, which affects whether or not cephalopods are protected as an animal. The primary legislative responsibility for animal welfare in Australia is vested in the states and territories (see Chapter 1), so differences in legislation have led to differences in the use of cephalopods for scientific purposes. In animal welfare legislation of the Australian Capital Territory (*Animal Welfare Act 1992*), Queensland (*Animal Care and Protection Act 2001*) and Victoria (*Prevention of Cruelty to Animals Act 1986*), cephalopods fall under the definition of 'animal' in specific circumstances. Cephalopods are not classified as an 'animal' in animal welfare legislation of the other states and territories and so do not fall under the jurisdiction of these acts. Consequently, it is important for researchers to identify the animal welfare framework their organisation adheres to.

SQUID, OCTOPUSES, CUTTLEFISH, SEPIOLIDS AND NAUTILUSES

Characteristics

Cephalopods are a class of exclusively marine molluscs that include squid, octopuses, cuttlefish, sepiolids (bobtail 'squid') and nautiluses. Over 800 species occur worldwide with over 200 species found throughout Australian coastal and oceanic waters, from the tropical north to the cooler south of Tasmania and even Antarctica (Reid 2016). In fact, coastal cephalopods are particularly speciose in Australia, with high levels of endemism in the southern half of the country (Rosa *et al.* 2019). Cephalopods possess a prominent head and 'mantle', containing essential organs, and elongated arms or tentacles, which surround a powerful parrot-like beak. Their locomotion, in part, involves a unique form of jet propulsion, involving a rapid expulsion of water from the mantle cavity through a muscular funnel. Body sizes range from the tiny pygmy squids, reaching only 2 cm long, to the giant and colossal squids, which are the largest invertebrates in the world, reaching up to 18 m.

Biology and behaviour

Cephalopods occupy most marine habitats from equatorial waters to the poles and from shallow coastal waters to the deep sea. They are important predators and key prey for many marine species. Cephalopods support many fisheries worldwide and are becoming an increasingly important source of protein for millions of people (Arkhipkin *et al.* 2015; Sauer *et al.* 2021).

All living cephalopod species, except nautiluses, belong to the subclass Coleoidea. Nautiluses represent an ancient subclass of cephalopods with only five living species; they are distinctly different to coleoids, having an external shell, slow growth and long life spans. In contrast, modern coleoid cephalopods are renowned for their 'live fast, die young' life-history strategy, adaptability (phenotypic plasticity) and intelligence. Their intelligence is supported by well-developed senses, complex centralised nervous systems and large brains (Mather 2012). Coleoids also possess unique camouflaging abilities and can alter the colour (using chromatophores) and texture (using dermal papillae) of their skin to match their environment (Budelmann 2010). In low-light environments, many cephalopod species can produce biologically generated light (bioluminescence) using light organs called photophores. Another distinctive characteristic of coleoid cephalopods is their ability to release dark clouds of ink, which function as a smokescreen or visual decoy to deter or distract predators (Derby 2014). Chemical compounds such as amino acids, which may act as a sensory distraction for predators, can be concurrently released (Derby 2014).

Coleoid cephalopods are generally short-lived and grow rapidly throughout their life cycle (Reid 2016), as well as exhibit flexible reproductive strategies (Rocha *et al.* 2001). These biological characteristics, alongside strong phenotypic plasticity, allow some cephalopods to respond rapidly to changes in the marine environment, potentially bolstering their resilience to future environmental change (Doubleday *et al.* 2016; Reid 2016). In fact, some species are increasing in abundance, potentially driven by climate change and overfishing of predator fish species (Doubleday *et al.* 2016).

Coleoid cephalopods are predatory carnivores and consume a wide variety of prey, such as crustaceans, fish and shellfish, whereas nautiluses are opportunistic scavengers (Reid 2016). Cannibalism is common in cephalopods both within and between species (Ibáñez and Keyl 2010). Squid are generally social and form schools; cuttlefish are mostly solitary, but sometimes form large aggregations (e.g. giant Australian cuttlefish, *Sepia apama*), or swim with several individuals (Boal 2006). Octopuses are generally solitary, although high densities of octopuses have been observed in the wild (Boal 2006).

Capture and handling

Several cephalopod species have been housed successfully in captivity for ecological, biological, human health and robotics research, as well as developmental aquaculture operations (Vidal *et al.* 2014; Gestal *et al.* 2019). However, raising planktonic 'paralarval' stages (i.e. a life-history stage unique to many cephalopod species) remains a key challenge of cephalopod culture because of their husbandry, nutrition and feeding requirements (Budelmann 2010; Vidal *et al.* 2014).

No captive bred cephalopods are available in Australia, but some species are readily sourced from the wild using commercial fishing gear, such as pots, traps and jigged lures, or hand collection via snorkel or SCUBA (Table 29.1). However, animals caught with moving fishing gear, such as trawling, are often too damaged to survive transfer to laboratory aquariums, so these approaches should be avoided where possible (Moltschaniwskyj *et al.* 2007; Fiorito *et al.* 2015). Squid and cuttlefish eggs can be collected from the wild by hand and octopus eggs can be collected using shelter pots. Shelter pots effectively act as an artificial octopus den and many octopus species will inhabit them naturally and lay eggs, particularly when suitable habitat is lacking. For octopus eggs, the brooding mother usually needs to be captured to care for the egg masses. Eggs collected in the very early stages of development may have lower survival rates, and eggs collected in the later stages may hatch prematurely during transportation and handling (Vidal *et al.* 2014). For some sepiolid

Table 29.1: Capture methods used in research for different life history stages of wild cephalopods.

Taxa	Capture method
Squid	Jigged lures with barbless hooks (adults); hand collection by SCUBA or snorkel (eggs from inshore squid species) (Pecl *et al.* 2010; Arkhipkin *et al.* 2015)
Sepiolids	Hand collection by SCUBA (adults) (Pecl *et al.* 2010)
Octopuses	Shelter pots and traps designed for octopuses (adults and eggs); hand collection, crustacean traps (adults) (Pecl *et al.* 2010; Sauer *et al.* 2021)
Cuttlefish	Basket traps (adults), hand collection by SCUBA or snorkel (adults and eggs) (Moltschaniwskyj *et al.* 2007; Payne *et al.* 2013)
Nautiluses	Traps, hand collection by SCUBA (adults) (Dunstan *et al.* 2011)

species, eggs can be sourced from breeding wild-caught adults, which readily mate and lay eggs in aquaria (e.g. Pecl *et al.* 2010).

Cephalopods possess soft delicate skin that can be readily damaged and bruised by physical contact (Moltschaniwskyj *et al.* 2007). When possible, handling should occur under water, using soft nets or buckets, as skin is easily damaged by dry surfaces and should be kept moist (Budelmann 2010). Some octopus species tolerate short periods of air exposure as they naturally inhabit intertidal zones.

The natural habitats, environmental conditions and social behaviour of each species dictate optimal housing conditions (Fiorito *et al.* 2015), as well as optimal temperature and other environmental parameters (e.g. Dupavillon and Gillanders 2009) (Table 29.2). For cephalopods, opaque tanks, which also protect the animals from bright artificial lights, are best for housing. High-quality, well-oxygenated seawater is crucial for all cephalopods, with particular care needed for dissolved nitrogen such as ammonia, nitrate and nitrite, with recommended levels of < 0.1 mg L for ammonia and nitrite and < 20.0 mg L for nitrate (Vidal *et al.* 2014). Consequently, flow-through or recirculation systems that remove nitrogenous wastes are needed (e.g. Pecl *et al.* 2010). In some circumstances, environmental conditions beyond what a species experiences naturally can be changed (i.e. to study human impacts). If undertaking such experiments, conditions should be changed gradually, such as 1°C and 2 parts per thousand (ppt) per day for temperature and salinity respectively (Dupavillon and Gillanders 2009; Semmens *et al.* 2011). Of note, cephalopods are thought to be stenohaline, with salinities below 27 ppt and above 36 ppt considered to be fatal (Vidal *et al.* 2014). However, some cuttlefish and octopus species thrive in hypersaline conditions (above 40 ppt) in the wild in South Australia (Dupavillon and Gillanders 2009; Martino *et al.* 2021).

Healthy cephalopods in captivity should have an appetite, be free of skin lesions and disease and exhibit no unusual behaviour (Vidal *et al.* 2014). In any experiment, individuals should always be monitored for signs of stress

Table 29.2: General guidelines for housing different cephalopod taxa in laboratory aquaria, which can be altered to suit the research being undertaken or the specific requirements of the species or life-history stage.

Taxa	Group rearing	Tank objects or qualities	References
Squid	Yes	No specific substrate or housing needed, but generally require larger tank volumes. Low light conditions and shielding from external disturbances, like sudden changes to light and vibrations, are needed. Round tanks or plastic liner around the sides can help prevent squid from dashing into the sides of the tank. Tank marked with a bold contrasting pattern may minimise collisions for active pelagic species. Artificial substrate may be provided for spawning such as bricks and artificial seagrass.	Budelmann (2010); Pecl *et al.* (2010); Vidal *et al.* (2014); Fiorito *et al.* (2015).
Sepiolids	Possible, but individual housing is preferred	Sandy substrates allow individuals to bury (as per their natural behaviour), but the sand may affect tank hygiene. PVC pipe can provide habitat for spawning.	Moltschaniwskyj *et al.* (2007); Pecl *et al.* (2010).
Octopuses	Species-dependent, but individual housing preferred	Plastic pipes and pots in the tanks provide den-like shelter. Octopus also like shellfish shells. All tank openings need to be securely sealed to prevent escape (i.e. fixed lids or mesh secured with elastic straps).	Semmens *et al.* (2011); Fiorito *et al.* (2015).
Cuttlefish	Possible, but individual housing is preferred	Sandy substrate can be beneficial.	Payne *et al.* (2013); Fiorito *et al.* (2015).
Nautiluses	Yes, at low densities	Texture (such as artificial coral reef) to one tank wall may make it more attractive. Species with known diel vertical migration (e.g. *Nautilus pompilius*) should have a tank of high depth.	Fiorito *et al.* (2015).

while housed (see Fiorito *et al.* 2015 for detailed description of signs and solutions to alleviate stress).

Cephalopods are predatory carnivores and require large quantities of high-quality high-protein feed (Vidal *et al.* 2014). Many captive cephalopods will only eat live feed, which is often a limitation for researchers. However, aquaculture researchers have developed formulated feeds for some species (see Vidal *et al.* 2014 for review). Prey should be of an appropriate size and, where possible, reflect the taxa found in their natural environments. Most octopuses will capture and eat crustaceans, bivalves and gastropod molluscs of appropriate sizes. Squid, sepiolids and cuttlefish will consume fish and crustaceans. Nautiluses require food with high calcium carbonate, such as shrimp with carapace, lobster moult shells or fish heads (Fiorito *et al.* 2015). Uneaten food will quickly decompose and reduce water quality, so tanks should be regularly cleaned of excess food and detritus (Budelmann 2010). Cannibalism can occur in captive cephalopods, particularly if density is high in tanks and individuals in the tank are of different sizes. Naturally solitary cephalopods, such as octopuses, can be kept in separate tanks to avoid cannibalism.

Marking can be difficult in coleoid cephalopods, which lack external shells. Whenever possible, natural markings should be used for identification. However, artificial marking methods have been applied successfully with anaesthesia, including implanted fluorescent elastomer tags (squid and octopuses), subcutaneous dye injection (octopuses) and external tags (all cephalopods) (see Fiorito *et al.* 2015 for more details on procedures and welfare considerations). Chemical markers (such as elemental or isotopic signatures) locked within hard anatomical structures, such as statoliths (ear bones), octopus stylets, cuttlebones or nautilus shells, are also useful to track cephalopods. Chemical markers can be artificial (through injection or immersion) or natural (reflecting environmental conditions that individuals are exposed to; e.g. Pecl *et al.* 2010) and can be used to address ecological or fishery questions by identifying movement and environmental histories.

Cephalopods can be transported in high-quality well-oxygenated seawater and low light conditions; however, the longer the transport duration, the more likely that oxygen depletion and degradation of water quality will affect survival rates (Fiorito *et al.* 2015). Containers, such as plastic buckets or bags, are useful for transportation provided that the animal is covered completely with well-oxygenated water (e.g. Payne *et al.* 2013). Placing octopuses in mesh bags, in either separate containers or a single large container, also works well to prevent interaction and escape. Battery-operated aerators are useful for longer trips, as well as the supply of pure oxygen (see Vidal *et al.* 2014 for detailed shipping and packing methods). Food deprivation may reduce fouling and ammonia accumulation (Fiorito *et al.* 2015), and for large active cephalopods sedation should be considered (Vidal *et al.* 2014). Temperature and salinity of the new tank water should match that of water in the transport container, which can be gradually adjusted to reach desired experimental conditions (see section on housing).

Veterinary considerations

To anaesthetise or sedate cephalopods, individuals should be immersed completely in seawater containing a freshly made anaesthetic solution (Table 29.3).

Animals should be monitored carefully for signs that the anaesthesia is working, including cessation of locomotion, loss of tone of the mantle and arms, and reduced sucker adhesion (Andrews *et al.* 2013; Butler-Struben *et al.* 2018). Respiration should also be monitored to ensure the anaesthetic does not result in death. Relaxation of chromatophores under anaesthetic is also an easily identifiable sign, with cuttlefish and octopuses commonly

Table 29.3: Commonly used anaesthetic or sedative substances for cephalopods.

Andrews *et al.* (2013); Fiorito *et al.* (2015); Butler-Struben *et al.* (2018).

Therapeutic category	Substance	Advantages and disadvantages
Anaesthetic	< 3% ethanol	Not clear if blocks pain perception or is aversive. Variability reported
Anaesthetic	Magnesium chloride ($MgCl_2$)	The most studied and used. Least aversive. Can disturb haemolymph Mg^{2+} levels so not always appropriate
Anaesthetic	Mixture of magnesium chloride and < 3% ethanol	Sufficient for short-term anaesthesia. Limited literature
Anaesthetic/sedative	Clove oil diluted in sea water	Limited literature on efficacy

showing a whole-body paling or yellowing (Butler-Struben *et al.* 2018).

The decision to sedate a cephalopod is dependent on the handling time, the environmental conditions where the handling takes place and the techniques used. Sedation should occur for invasive surgical procedures, and may be necessary for external tagging, tissue biopsies, injections (i.e. for chemical tagging) and measuring biological data from live animals (weight, length, etc.).

Euthanasia

Terminal anaesthetic is the recommended approach for euthanasia or killing of cephalopods. The current recommended method is immersion for at least 15 min in increasing concentrations of magnesium chloride ($MgCl_2$), followed by an adjunct method such as brain destruction after respiratory arrest (AVMA 2020). A range of final concentrations are recommended but should be at least 3.5% (Andrews *et al.* 2013; AVMA 2020). Higher concentrations of $MgCl_2$ (7.5%) may need to be used for species with slow metabolic rates (i.e. cold-water species; Castellanos-Martínez *et al.* 2014), and if an adjunct method cannot be used individuals should be immersed for at least 30 min in $MgCl_2$ (AVMA 2020). Ethanol can also be used as a terminal anaesthetic for cephalopods, alone or in conjunction with $MgCl_2$ (see AVMA 2020 for more details). Specific indicators of death for cephalopods are unknown, but loss of movement and reactivity to stimulus and absence of respiration are recommended indicators for aquatic invertebrates (AVMA 2020). It should be noted that mechanical methods to destroy the brain, such as cutting between the eyes or decapitation, can be difficult and require skill, particularly while at sea (Andrews *et al.* 2013). However, in many circumstances, the only available method to collect wild-caught cephalopods for research is via commercial fishers and terminal anaesthesia is not always a practical option for commercial fishing operations. Terminal anaesthesia is also impractical in many scientific research operations at sea because of rough conditions and limited space or personnel on the vessel. In these circumstances, researchers should discuss practical methods that still prioritise animal welfare, with their institution's animal ethics committee.

Infectious pathogens

As with most wild animals, cephalopods can host a range of bacteria, fungi, viruses and parasites that can pose a risk to handlers. Transmission to humans can arise via accidental ingestion of biological fluids (through handling or dissections) or through bites. Bites of cephalopods can sometimes penetrate human skin with enzymes, venoms, and microorganisms in the saliva exacerbating harmful effects (Fiorito *et al.* 2015). Of note, the bite of the blue-ring octopus (*Hapalochlaena maculosa*) can inject a powerful neurotoxin called tetrodotoxin, which is produced by symbiotic bacteria in salivary glands and can be fatal to humans without medical intervention (Hwang *et al.* 1989).

Limited information is available on the causes and effects of diseases in wild cephalopods, with most knowledge gathered from post-mortem examination of captured or captive animals. For details relating to infectious pathogens known to affect cephalopods refer to Fiorito *et al.* (2015) and Gestal *et al.* (2019). Increased stress from capture and transport, as well as poor aquaria hygiene, may exacerbate bacterial and disease infections (Vidal *et al.* 2014). Lesions and ulcerations on the skin are common for aquarium-held octopuses in high-density tanks. These injuries spread rapidly in the epidermis, enlarging and deepening to affect the dermis and underlying muscle tissue. Unless treated quickly these ulcerations are invariably fatal within 2 to 4 days (Budelmann 2010). Cuttlebone fracture is one of the most common reported pathologies of captive cuttlefish, and possibly related to lower-quality rearing conditions, which can result in fighting or banging against tank walls (Gestal *et al.* 2019). Little research exists for treatments of cephalopod pathogens, although six antibiotics and one antiprotozoal treatment display potential effectiveness (Scimeca 2012; Vidal *et al.* 2014). Disinfection and sterilisation of aquaria systems will also help reduce prevalence of diseases (see Vidal *et al.* 2014 for more details).

General operating procedures

General operating procedures are available in AVMA (2020), Budelmann (2010), Vidal *et al.* (2014) and Fiorito *et al.* (2015). However, some procedures may have been revised since their publication and should be read alongside this chapter. Observation methods that may be applicable cephalopods are detailed in Chapter 12. General procedures for working with VIE detailed in Chapter 8 may also be useful.

REFERENCES

Andrews PL, Darmaillacq A-S, Dennison N, Gleadall IG, Hawkins P, Messenger JB, *et al.* (2013) The identification and management of pain, suffering and distress in cephalopods, including anaesthesia, analgesia and humane killing. *Journal of Experimental Marine Biology and Ecology* **447**, 46–64. doi:10.1016/j.jembe.2013.02.010

Arkhipkin AI, Rodhouse PGK, Pierce GJ, Sauer W, Sakai M, Allcock L, *et al.* (2015) World squid fisheries. *Reviews in Fisheries Science & Aquaculture* **23**, 92–252. doi:10.1080/23308249.2015.1026226

AVMA (2020) *AVMA Guidelines for the Euthanasia of Animals, 2020 Edition*. American Veterinary Medical Association, Schaumburg, IL.

Boal J (2006) Social recognition: a top down view of cephalopod behaviour. *Vie et Milieu* **56**, 69–80.

Budelmann BU (2010) Cephalopoda. In *The UFAW Handbook on the Care and Management of Laboratory and Other Research Animals*. 8th edn. (Eds R Hubrecht, J Kirkwood.) pp. 785–817. Wiley-Blackwell, Chichester, UK.

Butler-Struben HM, Brophy SM, Johnson NA, Crook RJ (2018) *In vivo* recording of reural and behavioral correlates of anesthesia induction, reversal, and euthanasia in cephalopod molluscs. *Frontiers in Physiology* **9**, 109. doi:10.3389/fphys.2018.00109

Castellanos-Martínez S, Prado-Alvarez M, Lobo-da-Cunha A, Azevedo C, Gestal C (2014) Morphologic, cytometric and functional characterization of the common octopus (*Octopus vulgaris*) hemocytes. *Developmental and Comparative Immunology* **44**, 50–58. doi:10.1016/j.dci.2013.11.013

Derby CD (2014) Cephalopod ink: production, chemistry, functions and applications. *Marine Drugs* **12**, 2700–2730. doi:10.3390/md12052700

Doubleday ZA, Prowse TAA, Arkhipkin A, Pierce GJ, Semmens J, Steer M, *et al.* (2016) Global proliferation of cephalopods. *Current Biology* **26**, R406–R407. doi:10.1016/j.cub.2016.04.002

Dunstan A, Bradshaw CJA, Marshall J (2011) Nautilus at risk – estimating population size and demography of *Nautilus pompilius*. *PLoS One* **6**, e16716. doi:10.1371/journal.pone.0016716

Dupavillon JL, Gillanders BM (2009) Impacts of seawater desalination on the giant Australian cuttlefish *Sepia apama* in the upper Spencer Gulf, South Australia. *Marine Environmental Research* **67**, 207–218. doi:10.1016/j.marenvres.2009.02.002

Fiorito G, Affuso A, Basil J, Cole A, de Girolamo P, D'angelo L, *et al.* (2015) Guidelines for the care and welfare of cephalopods in research – a consensus based on an initiative by CephRes, FELASA and the Boyd Group. *Laboratory Animals* **49**, 1–90. doi:10.1177/0023677215580006

Gestal C, Pascual S, Guerra Á, Fiorito G, Vieites JM (Eds) (2019) *Handbook of Pathogens and Diseases in Cephalopods*. Springer, Cham, Switzerland.

Hwang DF, Arakawa O, Saito T, Noguchi T, Simidu U, Tsukamoto K, *et al.* (1989) Tetrodotoxin-producing bacteria from the blue-ringed octopus *Octopus maculosus*. *Marine Biology* **100**, 327–332. doi:10.1007/BF00391147

Ibáñez CM, Keyl F (2010) Cannibalism in cephalopods. *Reviews in Fish Biology and Fisheries* **20**, 123–136. doi:10.1007/s11160-009-9129-y

Martino JM, Steer M, Doubleday ZA (2021) Supporting the sustainable development of Australia's octopus industry: first assessment of an artisanal fishery. *Fisheries Research* **241**, 105999. doi:10.1016/j.fishres.2021.105999

Mather J (2012) Cephalopod intelligence. In *The Oxford Handbook of Comparative Evolutionary Psychology.* (Eds T Shackelford and J Vonk) pp. 118–128. Oxford University Press, New York, NY.

Moltschaniwskyj NA, Hall K, Lipinski MR, Marian JE, Nishiguchi M, Sakai M, *et al.* (2007) Ethical and welfare considerations when using cephalopods as experimental animals. *Reviews in Fish Biology and Fisheries* **17**, 455–476. doi:10.1007/s11160-007-9056-8

NHMRC (2013) *Australian Code for the Care and Use of Animals for Scientific Purposes*. 8th edn. National Health and Medical Research Council, Canberra.

Payne NL, Snelling EP, Semmens JM, Gillanders BM (2013) Mechanisms of population structuring in giant Australian Cuttlefish *Sepia apama*. *PLoS One* **8**, e58694. doi:10.1371/journal.pone.0058694

Pecl GT, Doubleday ZA, Danyushevsky L, Gilbert S, Moltschaniwskyj NA (2010) Transgenerational marking of cephalopods with an enriched barium isotope: a promising tool for empirically estimating post-hatching movement and population connectivity. *ICES Journal of Marine Science* **67**, 1372–1380. doi:10.1093/icesjms/fsq025

Reid A (2016) *Cephalopods of Australia and Sub-Antarctic Territories*. CSIRO Publishing, Melbourne.

Rocha F, Guerra Á, González ÁF (2001) A review of reproductive strategies in cephalopods. *Biological Reviews of the Cambridge Philosophical Society* **76**, 291–304. doi:10.1017/S1464793101005681

Rosa R, Pissarra V, Borges FO, Xavier J, Gleadall IG, Golikov A, *et al.* (2019) Global patterns of species richness in coastal cephalopods. *Frontiers in Marine Science* **6**, 469. doi:10.3389/fmars.2019.00469

Sauer WHH, Gleadall IG, Downey-Breedt N, Doubleday Z, Gillespie G, Haimovici M, *et al.* (2021) World octopus fisheries. *Reviews in Fisheries Science & Aquaculture* **29**, 279–429. doi:10.1080/23308249.2019.1680603

Scimeca JM (2012) Cephalopods. In *Invertebrate Medicine*. (Ed GA Lewbart) pp. 113–125. Wiley-Blackwell, Ames, IA.

Semmens J, Doubleday Z, Hoyle K, Pecl G (2011) A multilevel approach to examining cephalopod growth using *Octopus pallidus* as a model. *The Journal of Experimental Biology* **214**, 2799–2807. doi:10.1242/jeb.051631

Vidal EAG, Villanueva R, Andrade JP, Gleadall IG, Iglesias J, Koueta N, *et al.* (2014) Cephalopod culture: current status of main biological models and research priorities. *Advances in Marine Biology* **67**, 1–98. doi:10.1016/B978-0-12-800287-2.00001-9

30 Marine fishes

Samuel M. Williams, Bonnie J. Holmes, Adam Barnett, Troy Rogers, Lachlan Fetterplace, Heather Middleton, Jonathan Mitchell, Tiffany Sih, David Harasti, Marcus Sheaves, Christopher J. Henderson, Ian R. Tibbetts, Laurie Mitchell, Tyson Martin, Julian Pepperell, Andy Moore, Megan Skelton, Matthew Taylor, Ben L. Gilby, Craig Chargulaf, Fabio Cortesi, Leanne M. Currey-Randall, Sean Tracey, Sheridan Rabbitt and Matthew Campbell

INTRODUCTION

Most marine fishes are members of the largest and most diverse class of vertebrates, the Actinopterygii (ray-finned fishes). Ray-finned fishes account for more than half of all living vertebrate taxa and contain 42 taxonomic orders worldwide. Within Australian waters, marine and freshwater taxa encompass 35 of these orders, all of which are in the infraclass Teleostei (modern bony fishes).

The great diversity of Australian teleosts is reflected in the wide variation in their form, function and habitat. Teleosts have evolved to occupy all aquatic habitats where fishes are found, and now account for over 4000 species that occur in Australian waters. Teleosts have adaptations that allow them to occupy a wide range of environments, including some that are not considered typical aquatic environments, such as mudflats, hot desert springs, subterranean caves, high altitude lakes, polar seas and abyssal depths. In some ecosystems, teleost fishes account for almost the entire food web, from first order consumers (herbivores) through to apex predators. The diversity and complexity of this group also means that many species remain understudied or unknown.

The exact number of species in this grouping is constantly changing as new species are discovered (particularly in sparsely explored environments such as deepwater habitats). Consequently, the taxonomic relationships among species are also somewhat labile. To allow for appropriate consideration of animal ethics for scientific purposes, this chapter focuses on marine teleost families that fall under several broad ecological groupings, and are most commonly interacted with by researchers, teachers and fisheries scientists. This chapter does not consider freshwater fishes, marine eels and several orders of small-bodied fishes (covered in Chapter 32). Consequently, the scope of marine species included here is not intended to be an exhaustive list. While the authors recognise that many families have members that occur in several different marine habitats used in our classification (e.g. gobies, estuarine, benthic and reef-associated fishes), capture, handling and other research-based interactions are often governed by habitat characteristics and the environments they are found in (e.g. capture considerations for small reef-dwelling species versus large pelagic fishes).

ESTUARINE FISHES

Adam Barnett, Marcus Sheaves and Matthew Taylor

Characteristics

Estuarine fishes occurring in Australian waters comprise a diverse group of species and can be characterised by their permanent or partial residence of estuarine systems (representing orders Perciformes, Elopiformes and Mugiliforms). The dynamic nature of estuarine environments, which under the influence of tidal and freshwater flows means that most species have adapted to a wide range of marine, brackish and freshwater environments. For many species these flows are also closely linked to reproductive behaviour and life history. For example, the barramundi (*Lates calcarifer*) lives and breeds in estuaries and shallow coastal waters, but requires brackish conditions of tidal creeks and estuaries for its larvae to develop, and freshwater for the juveniles to mature. Many estuarine species are important to recreational or commercial fisheries in Australia, including species in the families Latidae, Lutjanidae, Sparidae, Serranidae, Haemulidae, Polynemidae, Sciaenidae and Mugilidae.

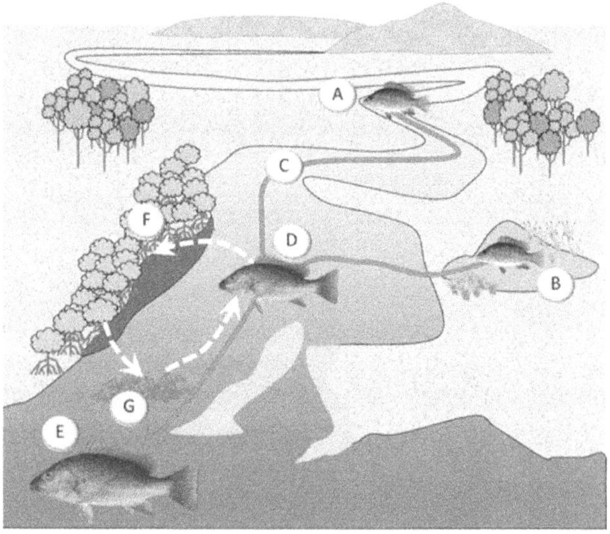

Figure 30.1: Many estuary fish, such as mangrove jack (*Lutjanus argentimaculatus*), undergo many types of migration in estuaries. They use (A) freshwater areas, (B) wetland pools and (C) shallow estuary habitats as early juvenile nurseries. As they reach subadult sizes (D) they spread throughout the estuary, until they move offshore as adults (E). While in the estuary mangrove jack move between many different habitats such as (F) mangroves and (G) seagrass as tidal levels permit to access different habitats and food sources. Illustration by Marcus Sheaves.

Biology and behaviour

The dynamic nature of estuaries, and the variety of ways that fish utilise the resources available there, means that fish occupy them at a range of spatial scales and display a diversity of patterns of movement over a range of temporal schedules. Movements can occur at certain times of the year, between day and night, between high and low tide and to match with particular events such as floods and pulses of food. One class of movements relates to short-term drivers of utilisation. For instance, adult piscivores, such as mulloway (*Argyrosomus japonicas*) move freely in and out of estuaries to access intermittently available prey resources. Another type of utilisation is displayed by life-history migrants, fish such as barramundi, mangrove jack (*Lutjanus argentimaculatus*) and tarpon (*Megalops cyprinoides*). These species use upstream estuarine and freshwater areas as nurseries for early juveniles, moving into deeper estuarine habitats as later stage juveniles and subadults, before migrating to coastal or offshore adult habitats (Russell and Garrett 1985; Russell and McDougall 2005) (Figure 30.1).

A final group are estuary residents. Species such as pikey bream (*Acanthopagrus pacificus*) move within estuaries during the year, as well as undertaking seasonal spawning migrations to estuary mouths or headlands for spawning (Sheaves *et al.* 1999). No matter the class of movement, for most fish life in estuaries requires the occupation of a mosaic of habitats, each providing different requirements of life (Litvin *et al.* 2018). The shallow waters of estuaries and the changes in habitat availability between high and low tide mean that many fish undertake regular movements in phase with the tide. These movements allow them to access rich food resources on intertidal sand and mud flats, mangrove forests and intertidal wetlands, and are instrumental in the translocation of the productivity of these habitats into marine food webs. At a larger scale the stocks of many species extend across state boundaries (e.g. sea mullet, *Mugil cephalus*, and yellowfin bream, *Acanthopagrus australis*, between New South Wales and Queensland; black bream, *A. butcheri*, between New South Wales and Victoria connecting estuaries over large spatial scales).

Estuarine fishes feed on a broad range of prey and display a diversity of foraging behaviours. Generally, they encompass most feeding guilds, including detritovores, herbivores, benthivores, planktivores and omnivores, and as a consequence this group is morphologically and behaviourally diverse. The highly variable nature of estuaries also means that dietary flexibility is a common trait of estuarine fishes. Mugillidae represents some of the most abundant larger-bodied fish taxa in Australian estuaries, and this family is known for preying on a diverse range of detrital and low-trophic level food sources, with sufficient flexibility to support diet switching to cope with competition or changing habitat conditions (Blaber 1977). Gerreidae also feed on a broad range of prey, but rarely forage on anything other than zoobenthos or infauna (Hargreaves *et al.* 2017). With the exception of Scatophagidae (which are primarily herbivorous) and Chanidae (which share similar feeding habits to Mugilidae), most of the other taxa dealt with in the chapter may be considered predatory, feeding on mid-trophic levels and above. Molluscs, polychaetes and crustaceans (such as penaeid prawns) commonly feature in the diets of these species, but some taxa (e.g. sciaenids and latids) may be considered top-level estuarine predators, with larger fish and cephalopods also common prey. Hunting behaviours in these predatory species are poorly understood.

Estuarine fishes display diverse reproductive strategies across multiple spawning habitats, with some species showing specialist traits (such as sequential hermaphroditism, observed in some polynemids and latids). Environmental cues are known to be important in reproduction, such as for inducing gonadal maturation or providing a signal to stimulate a spawning aggregation (e.g. Taylor *et al.* 2014). Spawning events can be episodic, protracted or continual, and this can differ within taxa based on geographical location. Spawning behaviours by adults may select for particular strategies based on advection of eggs and larvae. For example, many coastally spawning species in temperate eastern Australia migrate north to spawn, and to exploit the southward East Australian Current for dispersal towards estuarine nurseries further south. Species that spawn within estuaries may select certain tidal conditions, such as spawning in the ebb tide for dispersal outside the estuary, or flood tide for retention within the estuary.

Capture and handling

Estuarine fishes can be caught using a range of techniques. However, 'hook and line' is considered the main capture method (and least invasive) for estuarine fishes, with some species targeted regularly by recreational fisheries (e.g. barramundi and tarpon). Some estuarine fish species, such as the black jewfish (*Protonibea diacanthus*), are susceptible to barotrauma when caught from depths of greater than 15 m. Physical barotrauma injuries are caused by progressively decreasing pressure as the fish is brought to the surface, and should be taken into account as part of capture and handling practices. Little work has been published on estuarine fish in relation to best catch-and-handling practices and post-release survivorship (Barnett *et al.* 2016). Therefore, in lieu of group-specific protocols, general best practice protocols can be followed (Cooke and Suski 2005; Arlinghaus *et al.* 2007) and those outlined in Chapter 13 should be considered to minimise physiological stress or injury during capture and handling.

Net, trap and finfish trawl methods are also used for some species of estuarine fishes. Net methods are more effective for species from the families Mugilidae, Gerreidae, Chanidae and Scatophagidae than other species such as threadfins (Polynemidae), which are vulnerable to capture by gill netting. If net methods are used, sets should be short, preferably monitored continuously and an appropriate mesh size used to reduce by-catch or damage to the animal. Alternative methods may be better options for some species (e.g. tunnel netting or beach seines), where fish can be scooped out of the enclosure.

External marker tags (conventional tagging), such as coded dart, T-bar, or button/disc tags, can be used for most species in this group (Thorsteinson 2002). For internal identification tags such as coded wire tags, plastic or glass tubing need to be removed from the inside of the fish for identification, and so are mainly used in commercially harvested species (Thorsteinson 2002). Passive integrated transponder (PIT) tagging, where tags are read by scanning the fish with a tag reader, is an internal method that allows fish to be returned to the water after recapture events. Each of these methods aims to provide information on movement, mortality and growth, and fish are required to be recaptured in order to provide movement information. Natural tags such as fin clipping, otolith chemistry, molecular analysis, parasites and biopsies are also regularly used in these species to resolve questions around stock structure, and movement between nursery areas and spawning grounds.

Acoustic telemetry is a widely used method to track estuarine fish. Both external and internal methods can be used for acoustic transmitter attachment. Internal tagging is the preferred method as it avoids fouling issues and limits the risk of losing the tag before the end of battery life. External tagging may be more appropriate for species that do not respond well to implantation procedures (e.g. leading to high mortality), or in short-term studies where the influence of procedures is likely to bias results (e.g. studies on post-release behaviour or short active tracks). The ongoing development of smaller transmitters means that the smaller estuarine fish species and life stages can also be tagged. Loggers and accelerometers that record a range of parameters such as depth, activity, temperature and pitch angle have to be recovered from the fish to access the data, and therefore external attachment methods are preferable. With the development of smaller pop-up satellite archival tags, these methods could feasibly be applied on larger estuarine species such as those in Scianidae and Megalopidae, but are overall less commonly used.

Most work on estuarine fishes is done *in situ* at field locations. However, for some species, particularly those of interest to aquaculture (e.g. barramundi and mulloway), research is also undertaken in captivity. For captive research, fish should be transported to holding facilities in aerated transportation tanks large enough for the fish to swim and maintain orientation without contacting surfaces. Once at the facility, fish are usually held in intensive aquaculture ponds at low to medium densities. Transport, handling and housing methods for fish are covered in detail in Chapter 13.

Veterinary considerations

Therapeutics can be used on bony fishes for various purposes, including fish handling, tagging, post-harvest transportation, diagnostics, surgery/gavage, artificial breeding and euthanasia. When using therapeutics or preparing fish for euthanasia, consideration must be given to the morphology and behaviour of individual species as well as the specific aims of the study. Prior to any application, a literature review for your target species and the method being considered is recommended, as some fish react negatively towards specific therapeutics. Therapeutics used on fishes are dependent on the handling time, size of the fish and the techniques used.

The most common therapeutics delivery method is immersion, where fish are placed in a solution and 'inhale' the drug. Oral or injectable methods are also used in some cases. It is important to understand the interactions of therapeutics with not only the biology of the animal but also abiotic water parameters that may confer an increased toxicity (Neiffer and Stamper 2009).

Sedation and anaesthesia

Whether teleosts feel pain remains a contentious issue (Key 2016). The effects of anaesthetics are largely unknown for most teleosts (Cooke *et al.* 2016). Even between closely related taxa, the effects of anaesthesia may also be vastly different (Readman *et al.* 2017). The effects of anaesthesia can also differ between life-history stages and environmental conditions (Cooke *et al.* 2016). If used, the lightest plane of anaesthesia is recommended (Wargo Rub *et al.* 2014). Consideration must be given to the morphology and behaviour of the species and decisions made on a species-specific basis (Readman *et al.* 2017).

Regardless of research into pain in fish, it is becoming more common for fish to be caught, anaesthetised and released for research purposes (see Chapter 13). Anaesthetics are suggested for use when conducting invasive procedures, or extensive handling, to minimise stress and pain (although not all anaesthetics have analgesic properties), often in conjunction with muscle relaxants such as pancuronium or gallamine. No therapeutics are usually required for external tagging methods or biopsies/fin clips; however, to conduct procedures such as internal acoustic tagging (Pillans *et al.* 2014), anaesthesia is normally used (Mylniczenko *et al.* 2014). For methods such as fin clips or tissue biopsies where therapeutics are not required, handling time should be reduced to minimise stress to the fish. Sedation and non-lethal research methods appropriate for fish are covered in detail in Chapter 13.

Conventional immersion drugs include tricaine methanesulphonate (MS-222), benzocaine, clove oil and clove oil derivatives (i.e. isoeugenol or Aqui-S™). These anaesthetics immobilise fish so that they can be handled for experimental procedures or health checks, then returned to their natural habitat or holding tanks. Additional information on the four levels of anaesthesia can also be found at the New South Wales Department of Primary Industries (see Barker *et al.* 2015) or under 'Procedure for surgically implanting transmitters, including anaesthesia' in Chapter 13.

An alternative to chemical treatment is electroimmobilisation, where electricity is passed through the fish to achieve various levels of anaesthesia dependent on voltage strength. Electroimmobilisation is characterised by fast recovery rates and in many cases has comparable or improved results compared to chemical sedatives (Durhack *et al.* 2020). However, this method has not been widely applied in estuarine fishes and therefore further work is required before it can be considered a recommended approach.

Euthanasia

Euthanasia methods are dependent on the size of the fish and the types of samples being collected. Several euthanasia methods are used for fishes: ice water slurry to euthanase small fish (e.g. Gerreidae); anaesthetic overdose such as clove oil or tricaine methanesulfonate (as for amphibians; Chapter 27); or knocking a fish on the head with a heavy club or spiking the brain, known as the *ike-jime* method (Diggles 2016). Spiking the brain is considered the quickest and most reliable method of killing fish while at sea, minimising pain to the fish. More detailed information on killing for lethal sampling is included in Chapter 13.

Infectious pathogens

Knowledge of zoonotic diseases in estuarine fishes is increasing and this topic has been reviewed in dedicated publications (e.g. Gauthier 2015). There are several pathogenic bacteria that are either indigenous or introduced via the environment or during processing of fish, including *Clostridium botulinum*, *Escherichia coli*, *Listeria monocytogenes* and *Vibrio* spp. Mild illness via ingestion of bacterial toxins or via gastrointestinal infection can occur after ingestion of bacterial cells in food.

General operating procedures

A range of research methods and procedures relevant to studying estuarine fishes are covered in more detail in Chapter 13. Several capture and observation methods described for freshwater species (Chapter 14) may also be useful.

COASTAL FISHES

Troy Rogers, Christopher J. Henderson and Ben L. Gilby

Characteristics

Coastal fishes occurring within Australian waters are a diverse group of species and can be characterised by their permanent or partial residence of coastal ecosystems (representing orders Perciformes, Beloniformes, Albuliformes, Elopiformes and Clupeiformes). The species covered in this chapter includes temperate, subtropical and tropical taxa. The coastal fish families occupy coastal habitats such as large embayments, rocky outcrops, fringing reefs, soft sediments, seagrass, and kelp or algal beds. These habitats are often complex and can occur within close proximity to adjacent estuaries and offshore reefal areas, and as a result play an important role for many permanent residents or temporary occupants. Different coastal habitats are also closely linked to the life history of several species such as *Chrysophrys auratus*, which occupy seagrass in sheltered bays are juveniles, before moving into coastal and offshore rocky reef habitats as adults (Parsons *et al.* 2014). Many coastal fishes are also of high importance to recreational or commercial fisheries in Australia, including species in the families Sillaginidae (sillagos and whitings), Pomatomidae (tailor), Sparidae (breams, seabreams and snappers) and Carangidae (trevallies and jacks).

Biology and behaviour

The movement and habitat association of coastal fishes is associated with seasonal changes in the distribution of food or other resources, reproductive movements, or ontogenetic movements from inshore to offshore ecosystems (Kimirei *et al.* 2013; Potter *et al.* 2015). Many coastal fishes make annual migrations to spawn. For example, yellowfin bream (*Acanthopagrus australis*) migrate to estuary mouths and surf bars annually during winter to spawn (Pollock 1982). Perhaps the textbook example of coastal fish migrations is the ontogenetic migration of fish from inshore wetlands and estuaries to offshore adult and spawning habitats. Here, eggs fertilised on offshore spawning habitats (usually coral or rocky reefs) develop through several pelagic larval stages, before settling on inshore coastal or estuarine nursery habitats and maturing to subadult stages. From here, subadult fish begin a progressive seaward migration through several intermediate habitats (such as inshore reefs) before settling on offshore reefs to spawn and recommence the process. These expansive movements and changes in habitat associations are often associated with changes in sex, colour, behaviour and diet in coastal fishes (Kimirei *et al.* 2013). Within these broader movements, coastal fishes make daily movements between habitat patches or into intertidal areas to maximise opportunities for feeding, and to reduce predation risk (Davis *et al.* 2017). Despite these broad differences, the movement, home range and residency of coastal fishes are usually contingent upon habitat condition, food availability, and life-history stage.

Coastal fishes occupy a diversity of niches in coastal seascapes, meaning that their diet and feeding behaviours are particularly broad (Elliott *et al.* 2007; Kimirei *et al.* 2013). There are, however, several broad functional feeding groups, which are well recognised in the literature (Elliott *et al.* 2007; Potter *et al.* 2015). Zooplanktivores feed predominantly on zooplankton in the water column, and are crucial in bentho-pelagic coupling, and in regulating plankton biomass. Detritivores and herbivores feed on detritus and microphytobenthos, and graze on macrophytes, respectively, and so are crucial trophic links between primary producers and higher coastal predators.

Piscivores feed predominantly on other fishes and regulate prey fish assemblages through predation. Zoobenthivores feed exclusively on benthic invertebrates and are among the most abundant fishes in the coastal zone.

The hunting behaviours of coastal fishes correlate significantly with body shape (Elliott *et al.* 2007). For example, fusiform and sagittiform fishes are long and streamlined (e.g. Carangidae), and are often fast swimmers, so usually feed on motile organisms above the substrate's surface. Compressiform fishes (e.g. Sparidae) are laterally compressed, allowing for quick bursts of speed and rapid turning, and to enter vertical crevices. Anguilliform and taeniform fishes (e.g. Elopidae or Belonidae) are long and thin, enabling these fish to access prey in a variety of crevices and to resist currents.

Given the diverse life histories and behaviours of coastal fishes, reproduction strategies vary significantly (Elliott *et al.* 2007). Coastal fishes are most commonly oviparous (producing eggs that are released into the surrounding environment). Some oviparous fish undertake pelagic broadcast spawning, where male and female gametes are released and mixed in the water column, before being dispersed by currents. These low parental care reproductive strategies are often performed in groups, and mass spawning aggregations can often occur in a variety of coastal ecosystems. Other oviparous fish undertake brooding or nesting behaviours with high parental care, whereby fish produce eggs that settle on substrates (substrate spawners), or adhesive eggs that adhere to substrate or vegetation (vegetation spawners). Alternatively, parents can protect the eggs in a nest (guarders), or within their bodies (e.g. brood pouch or mouth brooders; Elliott *et al.* 2007).

Capture and handling

Many coastal fish species are primarily targeted using baited hook and line or lure fishing techniques, although common commercial gear types include longlines, droplines, hauling nets and fish traps. The gear used should be appropriate for the target species to optimise catchability and reduce unwanted by-catch. For example, circle hooks are recommended when bait fishing as they are more likely to hook the fish in the mouth and reduce the incidence of deep hooking considerably (Grixti *et al.* 2010). Several coastal fish species, such as Australasian snapper (*Chrysophrys auratus*), are susceptible to barotrauma when caught from depths of greater than 15 m; this can cause physical injury (Hughes and Stewart 2013). Similarly, the best way to reduce stress is to decrease fight time by using appropriate gear (e.g. heavier line class, quality equipment and good fishing techniques) and minimise hooking damage by using an appropriate hook type and size. Handling time must be minimised to limit physiological stress (e.g. oxygen exposure) and potential handling injuries (e.g. damage to gills or loss of epidermal mucus), which optimises wellbeing and improves the survival of fish intended for release. Additional handling considerations relevant to coastal fishes are outlined in Chapter 13.

The wide size range of coastal marine fish species means that a variety of natural and artificial tagging methods can be used. Tagging methods typically allow identification of individual fish and include conventional dart tags, archival tags, and acoustic and satellite telemetry. Conventional tagging is the most common artificial tagging method for coastal fishes and can provide information on movement, growth and mortality rates (Gillanders *et al.* 2001; Fowler *et al.* 2002). This method involves inserting the plastic head of the tag through the dorsal fin pterygiphores, near the anterior of the fin, using an applicator needle. An increasingly popular tagging method for coastal fishes is acoustic telemetry, which can provide highly resolved information on movement and post-release survival (Fowler *et al.* 2016; Taylor *et al.* 2018). Acoustic tags should be implanted internally to prevent biofouling and irritating the tagged animal. The tag should be implanted via the ventral surface approximately midway between the pelvic and anal fins (refer to Bradford *et al.* 2009).

Natural tags include fin clips, analysis of parasite assemblages, molecular techniques and the chemical analysis of hard structures. A fin clip is one of the simplest and oldest forms of marking a fish and involves removing a portion of a fin with scissors or a knife. Fin clips can either be used as a natural tag identifier or in molecular studies. Molecular techniques are evolving rapidly and are used increasingly to investigate movement and stock structure of marine fishes. Movement can also be investigated through naturally occurring isotopes and elemental concentrations in the aquatic environment that are retained in hard structures (i.e. otoliths, fin spines and eye lenses). Otolith chemistry has been applied to determine natal origins and investigate movement between nursery areas and spawning grounds (Elsdon *et al.* 2008).

Veterinary considerations

Sedation and anaesthesia

Anaesthetic considerations are similar among bony fish groups (Mylniczenko *et al.* 2014). See 'Estuarine fishes' for a discussion of anaesthetic principles for fish.

Euthanasia

Euthanasia methods are similar among bony fish groups. See 'Estuarine fishes' for a discussion of killing and euthanasia principles for fish. Euthanasia methods are dependent on the size of the fish and the types of samples being collected. For medium to large bodied coastal fish species, the *ikejime* approach (Diggles 2016) is generally regarded as the quickest and most reliable method. For small individual coastal species such as whiting, breaking the neck can be used, while for small bait fish species, an ice slurry is the most common approach to killing.

Infectious pathogens

Knowledge of zoonotic diseases in coastal fishes is increasing and this topic has been reviewed in dedicated publications (e.g. Gauthier 2015). Pathogenic bacteria, histamine-producing bacteria and biotoxins are zoonotic diseases associated with human consumption of coastal fish. There are several pathogenic bacteria that are either indigenous or introduced via the environment or during processing of fish, including *Clostridium botulinum*, *Escherichia coli*, *Listeria monocytogenes* and *Vibrio* spp. Mild illness via ingestion of bacterial toxins or via gastrointestinal infection can occur after ingestion of bacterial cells in food.

General operating procedures

A range of research methods and procedures relevant to studying coastal fishes are covered in more detail in Chapter 13. Several netting and observational methods that apply to freshwater animals may also apply to coastal species (Chapter 14). Veterinary methods that may be relevant are covered in Chapter 16.

BENTHIC AND BURROWING FISHES

Lachlan Fetterplace, Ian R. Tibbetts and Craig Chargulaf.

Characteristics

Benthic fishes live in close association with or within the seabed, including soft sediments and hard substrates from the intertidal shores to the depths of the ocean (representing orders Aulopiformes, Perciformes, Pleuronectiformes and Scorpaeniformes). Benthic fishes typically have adaptations that reflect their benthic environment including secondary loss of the swim bladder (e.g. blennies and flatheads), rendering them negatively buoyant, and, if in euphotic waters, camouflage that allows them to avoid predation or capture prey (e.g. flatfishes and scorpionfishes). Several families present in Australian waters are either economically (e.g. Platycephalidae) or ecologically (e.g. Blenniidae) important.

Biology and behaviour

For the majority of benthic soft sediment–associated fish, adult movement patterns are either unknown or poorly understood. It is often assumed that on this relatively homogenous habitat, fish will be transient and unlikely to have territories (Fetterplace *et al.* 2016). However, the wide range of life histories and morphologies, combined with evidence from a limited number of tracking studies, suggest that movement patterns are highly variable. For example, movements of burrowing species are restricted almost entirely to the burrow and close vicinity. However, bluespotted flathead and dusky flathead both can exhibit intraspecific variation in movement patterns, long-term residency to small areas (18 months+) and long-distance movements (tens to hundreds of kilometres) within the same populations (Fetterplace 2018).

Numerous benthic reef fishes are known to be resident to home reefs or sections of reef. However, home-range size varies considerably between and within species and is dependent on various factors, including time of day, life stage, climate, seasonal conditions and substrate type. Cryptobenthic reef fish often have movements restricted to very small territories. For example, many gobies (Gobiidae) are long-term residents at the scale of individual corals (Munday 2004) and many intertidal gobies, blennies (Blennidae) and triplefins (Tripterygiidae) are highly resident and if displaced are capable of returning to 'their' rockpool (Griffiths 2003). Ontogenetic shifts by juveniles from shallow benthic nursery habitats to offshore benthic habitats are also relatively common (e.g. White and Brown 2013). Many larger benthic species (e.g. members of the Scorpaeniformes and Aulopiformes) are ambush predators that will spend long periods in the same position; however, they are also capable of making larger movements around the reef and are often found moving out onto the soft sediments surrounding reefs or patches between reefs (authors, pers. obs.).

Benthic fish associated with sandy substrates are highly variable in size, and therefore have a variety of diets and hunting mechanisms. Benthic fish range from carnivory to herbivory with species-specific diets including detritivores, corallivores, mucus feeders and planktivores. All foraging types may be prevalent in a single family, such as Blenniidae, whose feeding strategies include omnivory, herbivory, detritivory, molluscivory, corallivory and fish mucus/scale feeders (Hundt *et al.* 2014).

Hunting strategies are usually linked to the morphology and size of the fish: smaller fish, such as Gobiidae, tend to feed on benthic organisms including copepods and nematodes while foraging in the sediment (Chargulaf *et al.* 2011) and larger fish, such as platycephalids, are ambush predators that feed on crustaceans and smaller fish (Coulson *et al.* 2015). Some gobiesocids act as cleaner fish, foraging on parasites from larger fish (Bray 2018).

Benthic marine fishes exhibit a wide diversity of reproductive modes. Some are hermaphrodites (e.g. some gobies and flatheads) others show varying levels of parental care from guarding of eggs laid in shells or burrows (e.g. blennies and gobies) to mouth brooding by males (e.g. jawfishes). Many have a larval stage that provides the benefit of dispersal, while others have direct development with the young hatching as miniature versions of the adults (e.g. handfish). Those that produce large numbers of small eggs (e.g. flatfishes) are less likely to be at risk of local extinction that those with fewer large eggs (e.g. blennies) that either have shorter pelagic dispersal potential or direct development (e.g. handfishes).

Capture and handling

Several families have venomous spines that should be avoided (e.g. flatheads, scorpionfish and stonefishes) by handlers. Capture of small cryptic species, particularly in complex benthic reef habitats, may require specific methods. For example, bilge pumps can be used remove the water from rockpools so that fish can be more easily captured (e.g. Wong *et al.* 2019). For benthic fish that are caught at depth and that will subsequently be returned to the sea alive or kept in captivity, barotrauma effects caused by decompression may complicate capture and handling. In some species, death can occur when fish are brought to the surface even when caught in shallow water (~10 m), while other species are more resilient and may survive when captured in relatively deep water (e.g. many species without swim bladders). Mitigation methods employed include the use of release weights to return fish to the seafloor, seafloor release cages and venting of the swim bladder to release gases (see Butcher *et al.* 2012 and references therein for discussion of the benefits and disadvantages of these methods). Recently, hyperbaric chambers have been used to bring fish to the surface; minimising barotrauma effects and may be a feasible option in some cases (Shepherd *et al.* 2019). Sublethal effects resulting from decompression can also occur (see Pribyl *et al.* 2011).

In Australia, benthic fishes have been marked and tracked relatively infrequently compared to fish inhabiting other habitats. The exceptions are generally either nearshore recreationally valuable species or cryptobenthic coral and rocky reef species tagged in small-scale behavioural studies (e.g. White and Brown 2013). Most benthic fish tracking has used conventional mark–recapture tagging methods or, to a lesser extent, acoustic tagging (fish tagged internally with acoustic tags are often simultaneously tagged with mark–recapture tags).

All mark–recapture methods (e.g. T-bar tags, dart tags, numbered disk tags, plastic tags and elastomers) involve using tags with some form of unique identification (serial number, study identification, unique colour or colour sequence) that will allow the re-identification of a fish if recaptured. The tags are inserted into the dorsal musculature or pterygiophores with a tag 'gun' or manual insertion applicator, or injected subcutaneously in the case of elastomers. In laterally and dorsoventrally compressed species, unconventional placement of tags may be required to avoid puncturing the stomach cavity when inserting the tag. Consequently, tagging flatheads (Platycephalidae, Hoplichthyidae and Bembridae) in the dorsal musculature under the second dorsal fin (and posterior to the anal vent) is recommended and for flounders, soles and halibuts (order Pleuronectiformes), tag placement should be decided based on each species morphology and the size of the fish being tagged. The advantages of mark–recapture tags are that they are minimally invasive, simple to use and quick to apply, but their limitations include low recapture rates and the resulting need to tag large numbers of fish.

Acoustic tagging involves the attachment of tags either externally or internally (see Chapter 13). Tagged individuals can be tracked for long periods with relatively high spatio-temporal resolution. Unlike traditional mark–recapture techniques where only release and recapture locations can be obtained, acoustic tags provide data across multiple time points and fish do not need to be recaptured to collect data. However, acoustic tags need to be within range of a receiver for a position to be recorded. Nevertheless, Australia has an extensive collaborative coastal receiver network with over 1800 receivers, so the chances of detecting tagged fish are relatively high (for a detailed description of the IMOS animal tracking facility network, see Taylor *et al.* 2017).

Veterinary considerations

Sedation and anaesthesia

Anaesthetic considerations are similar among bony fish groups (Mylniczenko *et al.* 2014). See 'Estuarine fishes' for a discussion of anaesthetic principles for fish.

Euthanasia

Euthanasia methods are similar among bony fish groups. See 'Estuarine fishes' for a discussion of killing and euthanasia principles for fish. Euthanasia should be achieved, where possible, by an overdose of anaesthetic drugs. It is best practice to keep fish in solutions up to 10 min after cessation of opercular movement and then follow up with direct destruction of the brain tissues (e.g. pithing, spiking, *ikejimi*) (Diggles 2016). In some cases, where overdose using anaesthetic drugs is not possible or suitable, it may be necessary to use other euthanasia methods (see Chapter 13 for details).

Infectious pathogens

Zoonotic diseases in coastal fishes are associated with human consumption, including pathogenic bacteria, histamine-producing bacteria and biotoxins. There are several pathogenic bacteria that are either indigenous or introduced via the environment or during processing of fish, including *Clostridium botulinum*, *Escherichia coli*, *Listeria monocytogenes* and *Vibrio* spp. Mild to serious illness via ingestion of bacterial toxin or via gastrointestinal infection can occur after ingestion of bacterial cells in food (Gauthier 2015).

General operating procedures

A range of research methods and procedures relevant to studying benthic and burrowing fishes is covered in more detail in Chapter 13. Several netting and observational methods that apply to freshwater animals may also apply to these species (Chapter 14). Veterinary methods that may be relevant are covered in Chapter 16.

CORAL REEF FISHES (ORNAMENTAL)

Heather Middleton, Laurie Mitchell and Fabio Cortesi

Characteristics

Ornamental coral reef fishes comprise over 500 species belonging to 13 families that occur in Australia's tropical and subtropical waters (representing families Malacanthidae, Chaetodontidae, Pomacentridae, Ephippidae, Pomacanthidae, Zanclidae, Acanthuridae, Pempheridae, Plesiopidae, Apogonidae, Pseudochromidae, Balistidae and Opisthognathidae). The coral reefs they inhabit create a wide range of habitats including sand flats, rubble areas, seagrass meadows, silty lagoons, coral stands, algae-covered platforms and coral barriers. These habitats are often in close proximity to each other and provide a variety of ecological niches that many species of coral reef fish have adapted to.

Most ornamental coral fishes are small bodied (~5–10 cm in length), but in particular members of the surgeonfishes (Acanthuridae), batfishes (Ephippidae) and angelfishes (Pomacanthidae) can grow to considerable sizes (> 50 cm). Ornamental coral reef fishes are beloved in the aquarium trade because of their dazzling colours, diverse shapes, and coral-associated lifestyles, which make for attractive aquaria displays. As such, they are an important resource for recreational and commercial aquarium collectors. They are also frequently used in scientific projects looking at a variety of questions ranging from climate change and its impact on the coral reef ecosystem to the neuroethology of marine inhabitants.

Biology and behaviour

Despite their small size, the pelagic larvae of ornamental reef fishes have a well-developed sensory system that they use to orient and actively swim towards the reef for settlement. Many species recognise olfactory cues of natal reefs and will favour returning to these areas at the end of their pelagic phase (Gerlach *et al.* 2007). These behavioural adaptations mean that coral reef fishes exhibit more-restricted larval dispersal and reduced genetic connectivity between populations than would otherwise be expected from passive dispersal via wind and water movements (Gerlach *et al.* 2007).

Post-settlement juveniles and adults are non-migratory across large spatial scales; however, surgeonfishes of the genus *Naso* inhabit inshore waters as juveniles and migrate out to the reef slope as adults. Most other species, however, usually live within relatively confined home ranges in a variety of habitats including live hard and soft coral, coral rubble and sand flats as well as rocky and algae-covered substrates. Intra- and interspecific competition for resources (e.g. food and shelter) mediate spatial distribution and habitat segregation (Bay *et al.* 2001). Many species, most notably members of the damselfish genus *Dischistodus*, are highly aggressive and territorial, and maintain strict hierarchical structures over well-defended algal turf patches. While most species demonstrate a high site fidelity, such as the humbug damselfish, *Dascyllus aruanus*, which can live its entire adult life within a single coral head (Sale 1971), larger animals are known to forage over wider spatial scales. For example, cardinalfishes (Marnane and Bellwood 2002) return to restricted shelter areas and resting sites after searching for food over grounds spanning hundreds of metres.

Ornamental reef fishes, with the exception of the spiny chromis (*Acanthochromis polyacanthus*), have a pelagic larval phase where plankton, primarily comprising copepods and invertebrate larvae and eggs, form their diet (Carassou *et al.* 2009). Adults, however, exhibit highly diverse foraging and feeding habits. For example, within Chaetodontidae alone there exist obligate and facultative corallivores as well as non-coral feeders that consume small invertebrate prey. Many species of ornamental reef fish are herbivorous (e.g. damselfishes and surgeonfishes) and feed on algal turf, while the pinnate batfish (*Platax pinnatus*) feeds mostly on benthic invertebrates and plankton, but will opportunistically feed heavily on the macroalgae *Sargassum* spp. (Bellwood *et al.* 2006). Furthermore, some species, including most cardinalfishes and prettyfins, are nocturnal predators and forage for smaller fish and crustaceans over different areas to their daytime resting sites (Marnane and Bellwood 2002).

Coral reef fishes use one of three fertilisation strategies: demersal spawning, mouthbreeding, or pelagic-broadcast spawning. Demersal spawners include damselfishes (Pomacentridae), tilefishes (*Hoplolatilus* spp. and *Malacanthus* spp.), dottybacks (*Pseudochromis* spp.), prettyfin (*Calloplesiops* sp.) and triggerfishes (Balistidae). Most demersal spawners form pair bonds with spawning carried out within rubble mounds or on solid substrate. Parental care displayed by demersal spawners include the cleaning, aerating and defending of eggs often by both parents, although there can be higher paternal investment in some species (e.g. *Amphiprion* spp.) (Allen 1975).

Mouthbreeders also show parental care by incubating eggs usually within the male's mouth. Although energetically costly, this provides greater protection to offspring. Common mouthbreeders include cardinalfishes (Apogonidae), jawfishes (Opistognathidae) and some prettyfins (*Assessor* spp.). Eggs laid by demersal spawners and mouthbreeders typically hatch at night to avoid predators, and hatching is often encouraged in demersal spawners by the vigorous mouthing and/or fanning of eggs. This disturbance of the eggs is crucial for successful egg hatching in captivity and is often simulated by pumping air bubbles.

Pelagic-broadcast spawners provide no parental care to eggs, and instead synchronise their release of vast clouds of sperm and egg in the water column. Spawning in many reef fish species is closely timed in relation to lunar cycles and/or tidal change. Ornamental reef fishes that are pelagic-broadcast spawners include bullseyes (Pempheridae), surgeonfishes (Acanthuridae), Moorish idol (*Zanclus cornutus*), spadefishes (Ephippidae), angelfishes (Pomacanthidae) and butterflyfishes (Chaetodontidae).

Capture and handling

Capture methods for ornamental reef fish are determined by the life stage of interest and species' mobility. The capture and handling of these taxa differ considerably from other species groups. For pre-settlement pelagic larvae, light traps set at night are an effective way of capturing many animals indiscriminately. Post-settlement larvae, juveniles and adults may be captured using hand or dip-nets; however, more active swimmers can be herded into a barrier net before capture at the net face. In any case, ornamental reef fish can be delicate and easily injured so the size of the net mesh must be appropriate for the size of the fish to prevent gill and fin damage. Occasionally, capture is aided by the use of clove oil solutions (5–10% in ethanol in seawater) to anaesthetise or stun the animal; the use of explosives or poisons, such as sodium cyanide, is prohibited.

Housing and transport of ornamental reef fish are commonly undertaken for wildlife research. Suboptimal transport conditions can increase the stress response of the fish and cause high mortality rates. If fish need to be transported long distances (such as from the field collection site to a laboratory), some general rules should be adhered to:

- *Feeding*: fish should be fasted before transport to reduce the build-up of waste products (e.g. ammonia) or prevent the consumption of solid waste.
- *Air enrichment*: pure oxygen or oxygen-enriched air should be used to fill the packing bags or containers to maintain a high dissolved oxygen level in the water.
- *Insulation*: packing containers and bags should be thermally insulated to prevent large temperature fluctuations.

The housing needs of ornamental reef fish are largely species-specific and require a sound understanding of their biology. Generally, these fish are intolerant of poor water quality; however, optimal physical parameters (including temperature and light intensity), the need for environmental enrichment (including substrates and shelter), and the exhibition of territorial or social behaviours are highly variable among species (Sneddon and Wolfenden 2019). For example, a flowerpot or tile structure serves as an ideal egg-laying surface and shelter for many demersal spawners, particularly in the families Pomacentridae (e.g. *Neopomacentrus* sp., *Chrysiptera* spp., *Amphiprion* spp.) and Pseudochromidae (*Manonichthys* sp. and *Pseudochromis* spp.). Furthermore, captive stress is reduced in the striated surgeonfish *Ctenochaetus striatus* when provided with a moving brush that simulates the tactile stimulation of cleaner fishes (Soares *et al.* 2011); while some damselfishes are highly aggressive and should be transported and housed individually (Wood 2001). For more information on transport, handling and housing see Chapter 13.

As most ornamental reef fish are small-bodied animals, conventional tagging techniques, such as those requiring large acoustic transmitters, are often unfeasible. However, smaller, externally placed transmitters can be successfully used with larger species (e.g. surgeonfishes) to study movement patterns with acoustic telemetry (Claisse *et al.* 2011). T-bar anchor tags are also commonly used for the rapid identification of study animals without appreciable effects on foraging or reproductive behaviours (Berumen and Almany 2009). Large external tags can have a deleterious effect on smaller species, so the tag should be size matched to the animal and appropriate for the life stage. Should a small species or larval fish need tagging, subcutaneous fluorescent and non-fluorescent elastomer tags can be injected into the animal for identification (Hoey and McCormick 2006). Where possible, *in situ* tagging should be favoured to reduce stress and allows the animals to be released into the same area of capture. Doing so is particularly important for species that form pair bonds or have high site fidelity.

Larval recruitment studies often employ chemical markers, such as tetracycline and stable isotope solutions to map dispersal patterns of reef fish. Tetracycline is used to mark egg clutches of demersal spawning species, while stable isotope solutions (e.g. $^{137}BaCl_2$) are injected into ripe females and incorporated into developing eggs (Jones 2015). Both forms of chemical marker can be considered destructive as the chemistry is incorporated into the otoliths of the embryonic fish, which must then be dissected for analysis. As such, these methods are becoming less common and are being replaced by non-lethal genetic approaches.

Veterinary considerations

Sedation and anaesthesia

Anaesthetic considerations are similar among bony fish groups (Mylniczenko *et al.* 2014). See 'Estuarine fishes' for a discussion of anaesthetic principles for fish. Therapeutic agents are routinely used in the handling and care of ornamental reef fish. As for other bony fish groups, common anaesthetics approved for use include tricaine methanesulfonate, benzocaine, clove oil and associated compounds including eugenol and isoeugenol (Javahery *et al.* 2012).

Euthanasia

Euthanasia methods are similar among bony fish groups. See 'Estuarine fishes' for a discussion of killing and euthanasia principles for fish. Consistent with other marine fishes, appropriate euthanasia methods are dependent on the size of the fish and the types of samples being collected. Euthanasia of ornamental fishes can occur using chemical or physical methods, or a combination of both (e.g. Underwood and Anthony 2013). When using chemical compounds, the procedure and chemicals are the same as those used for anaesthesia and sedation, except that the chemicals are administered at a higher concentration or for a longer period to induce a loss of opercular movement (breathing stops) followed by cardiac arrest. When using any chemical compound, it is important that fishes do not experience an osmotic shock causing unnecessary suffering, which can be prevented by using the same water the fish were kept in and ensuring pH and osmolarity remain stable throughout the procedure. Physical methods are also used for killing in some coral reef fishes; see 'Lethal biological sampling' in Chapter 13 for more details.

Infectious pathogens

Reports of zoonotic diseases in Australia from ornamental reef fishes are rare and largely restricted to incidents of a non-lethal skin infection known as 'fish tank granuloma', caused by the bacterium *Mycobacterium marinum* (Weir *et al.* 2012). The condition is caused after water containing the bacteria enters through cuts or broken skin and is therefore most common among aquarists who routinely handle fish or clean tanks. Importantly, the bacterium does not always cause disease in fishes so infection may be transmitted to humans from apparently healthy animals (Weir *et al.* 2012). Some fish species also contain marine biotoxins. Ciguatera poisoning involves a bioaccumulation of ciguatoxins from the dinoflagellate *Gambierdiscus toxicus* in several species of coral reef fish. Other zoonotic diseases are known to occur sporadically (Gauthier 2015).

General operating procedures

A range of research methods and procedures relevant to coral reef fishes are covered in more detail in Chapter 13. Several netting and observational methods that apply to freshwater animals may also apply to these species (Chapter 14). Veterinary methods are covered in Chapter 16.

REEF-ASSOCIATED FISHES

Jonathan Mitchell, Tyson Martin, Leanne M. Currey-Randall and Matthew Campbell

Characteristics

The reef-associated species that occur within Australian waters do not fall within a uniform systematic grouping, with the taxa represented by the reef habitat that they occupy. Reef-associated fishes include taxa from 10 different families of perciform fishes (Caesionidae, Cirrhitidae, Glaucosomatidae, Haemulidae, Labridae, Latridae, Lethrinidae, Lutjanidae, Nemipteridae and Serranidae). Many of these reef-associated fishes in Australia are found in tropical and subtropical waters, with a few species being predominantly found in cooler temperate waters. Several of these families represent some of the most commercially and recreationally important finfishes in Australia, including those from the families Lutjanidae (hussars, jobfishes, snapper), Serranidae (groupers, rockcods and their allies), Lethrinidae (emperors), Latridae, and to a lesser extent the Haemulidae (morwongs) and Glacosomatidae (pearl perches).

Biology and behaviour

Most of the species in this fish group remain relatively resident to particular habitat features in small areas, such as sections of coral reef or pinnacles. For example, several labrid fish species are known to be permanent reef residents (Bryars *et al.* 2012). Haemulidae feed on crustaceans in rubble and sandy substrates adjacent to reef habitats at night, then move to daytime resting sites in complex reef structures (Appeldoorn *et al.* 2009). Research from a large-scale tagging program in Queensland has shown that several species of *Lutjanus* and *Lethrinus* were predominantly recaptured within 1 km of their tagging location, with few moving greater than 20 km (Sumpton *et al.* 2008). Acoustic tracking studies have also further demonstrated high site fidelity of some coral groupers (*Plectropomus* spp.) and redthroat emperor (*Lethrinus miniatus*) (Currey *et al.* 2014).

Some smaller serranids and cirrhitids are also known to be highly site attached, such as the halfbanded seaperch (*Hypoplectrodes maccullochi*), which has a home range as small as 12 m^2 (Kingsford and Carlson 2010). In contrast some larger serranid fish such as the common coral trout (*Plectropomus leopardus*) can have home-range sizes up to 18 km^2 (Zeller 1997) and other species may undertake migratory movements linked to reproduction (e.g. > 100 km). Some lethrinids can also undertake larger scale movements; for example, a tagged redthroat emperor was recorded to travel ~160 km from its original tagging location (Currey *et al.* 2014), and spangled emperor (*Lethrinus nebulosus*) were found to travel over 130 km during return migrations to spawning locations (Babcock *et al.* 2017).

Reef-associated fishes display a wide range of feeding strategies from predatory piscivores to planktivores and algal feeders. Species in the Lutjanidae, Serranidae and Haemulidae families are predominantly predatory, feeding on small fishes, benthic crustaceans, molluscs and annelids. In contrast many species from the families Caesionidae and Labridae are known for being planktivores and algal feeders, respectively.

The reproductive strategy of these fishes generally involves broadcast spawning, which occurs during aggregations for many of these species, and is linked to specific locations and environmental cues such as lunar phase and temperature ranges (Choat 2012). Conversely, some species may form distinct breeding pairs as opposed to large aggregations, including *Pomadasys* spp., or males may defend a harem of females, as in some species of cirrhitid fish. Hermaphroditism is common in some groups such as Labridae, Scaridae, Serranidae and Lethrinidae (De Mitcheson and Liu 2008). Simultaneous hermaphroditism also occurs in some groups, including some species from the genus *Hypoplectrodes*. Reproductive periodicity is highly variable across these fish families, with some species spawning only once per year and others multiple times within the same spawning season.

Capture and handling

Reef fishes are commonly caught in recreational and commercial fisheries using standard line or trap methods, but additional specialised capture, handling and release techniques may be employed to reduce physiological stress on the animals. Other methods, such as trawl and trap, can also be used when capturing larger reef-associated species, but are each associated with different welfare considerations. The gear used should be appropriate for the target species to optimise catchability, reduce unwanted by-catch and minimise stress.

If the aim is to catch fish but not release them, spearfishing can be an effective alternative for many larger reef associates found in shallow water (e.g. those in the families Serranidae, Lutjanidae, Haemulidae, Latridae and Labridae). This technique reduces by-catch compared with line or trap methods considerably. However, careful consideration should be given to the aims of the study, as spears may occasionally damage the fish (e.g. otoliths or stomach contents). Reef-associated fishes require careful handling when captured. Handling considerations related to barotrauma, oxygen exposure and depredation are particularly important for this species group when undertaking research procedures that result in the release of animals.

Tagging programs aim to release tagged animals in good condition so that they may return to their environment with 'normal' physiological and behavioural functioning. Exceptions to this may be in studies where post-release survival may be the focus of the study. The most common devices for marking and tracking reef-associated fishes are dart tags and acoustic tags, which aim to provide information on movement, growth and mortality rates.

Tagging of fish using coded dart tags is done by anchoring a metal or plastic tag head into the dorsal musculature of the fish between pterygiophores. The external placement of these tags ensures that they are minimally invasive and quick to deploy, and can be easily deployed by researchers and recreational fishers, compared to more-complicated procedures required for internal tagging. In contrast, acoustic transmitters are regularly implanted into the body cavity (but can also be deployed externally depending on the animal). In fish, implanting tags in the body cavity is preferred where possible; however, for large animals or those that do not handle capture stress well, external application may be the safest means of deployment.

A range of other marking and tagging methods can be used for studying the movement ecology of fish in this group, including satellite tagging, accelerometers, oxytetracycline marking, crittercams and radio tagging. However, these techniques have so far only been used in a small number of studies. For example, Scott (2019) used accelerometers in *Plectropomus leopardus* to determine how they partition time and energy to regulate foraging and fitness. Natural tagging methods such as fin clips, analysis of parasite assemblages, molecular techniques and the chemical analysis of hard structures requiring lethal or non-lethal approaches, are also often used in research on reef-associated fish species. More information on operational aspects of tagging can be found in Chapter 13.

Veterinary considerations

Sedation and anaesthesia

Anaesthetic considerations are similar among bony fish groups (Mylniczenko *et al.* 2014). See 'Estuarine fishes' for a discussion of anaesthetic principles for fish.

Euthanasia

Euthanasia methods are similar among bony fish groups. See 'Estuarine fishes' for a discussion of euthanasia principles for fish. Euthanasia methods are dependent on the size of the fish and the types of samples being collected. Direct physical destruction of brain tissue via *ikejime* (Diggles 2016) or brain spike results in immediate insensibility (but this method may damage otoliths if these samples are required) and is common practice particularly for samples collected via commercial fishers. Immersion of tropical fish into an ice water slurry is also used by some researchers. More detail on appropriate euthanasia methods can be found under lethal sampling in Chapter 13.

Infectious pathogens

A wide range of diseases are known to affect fish within this broad group, including bacterial infections such as *Streptococcus agalactiae*, which has been documented in wild Queensland grouper (*Epinephelus lanceolatus*) and javelin grunter (*Pomadasys kaakan*) (Bowater *et al.* 2012). *Vibrio parahaemolyticus*, *V. fluvialis* and *Photobacterium* spp. have all been found to infect West Australian dhufish

(*Glaucosoma hebraicum*) (Pironet and Jones 2000). Viruses, including viral encephalopathy and retinopathy (VER), which is caused by a *Betanodavirus*, has been found in a range of serranid and lutjanid species and mainly affects larvae and juveniles (Shetty *et al.* 2012). Reef-associated fish can also be affected by skin melanomas, with up to 15% of *Plectropomus leopardus* sampled at off-shore sites in the Great Barrier Reef displaying melanoma, and prevalence in larger *Epinephelus quoyanus* individuals (> 340 mm total length), thought to be caused by ultraviolet light exposure (Diggles *et al.* 2018; Sweet *et al.* 2012).

Fish in this group are also known to transmit zoonotic diseases to humans. Some zoonotic diseases that occur in this fish group are *Mycobacterium marinum*, *Streptococcus iniae* and *Photobacterium damselae*, which may be transferred to humans via spine puncture or open wounds (Lehane and Rawlln 2000). Ciguatera poisoning is a common condition that can occur in humans as a result of eating infected reef fish, especially from larger individuals from the Serranidae and Labridae families (Fenner *et al.* 1997). The ciguatoxins (biotoxins) that cause this poisoning originate from the dinoflagellate *Gambierdiscus toxicus*, and these toxins are known to bioaccumulate in larger predatory fish.

General operating procedures

A range of research methods and procedures relevant to studying reef-associated fishes are covered in more detail in Chapter 13. Several netting and observational methods that apply to freshwater animals may also apply to these species (Chapter 14). Veterinary methods that may be relevant are covered in Chapter 16.

PELAGIC FISHES

Samuel Williams, Julian Pepperell and Sean Tracey

Characteristics

Pelagic fishes that occur in Australian waters are characterised by their predatory nature, analogous occupancy of open ocean habitat and seasonal migratory behaviour (Pepperell, 2010). Pelagic fishes generally exhibit a thunniform morphological shape, which minimises drag to enable both rapid bursts of speed and long-distance movement or migrations with reduced energy expenditure (Webb and Weihs 1986). Species of pelagic fish include several of the largest ray-finned fishes in the world, including species of ocean sunfishes (Molidae) and billfishes (Istiophoidae), and many smaller species such as the pomfrets (Bramidae) (Pope *et al.* 2010) and other families (Lampridae, Xiphidae, Scombridae, Sphyraenidae, Coryphaenidae, Carangidae, Rachycentridae, Echeneidae, Gempylidae and Luvaridae). Another notable difference among pelagic species is that while the majority of species are permanent residents of the open ocean environment (holoepipelagic), some only spend part of their life in the open ocean (meroepipelagic) (Pepperell 2010). Meroepipelagic fishes include the members of the genera *Scomberomorus*, all of which migrate seasonally throughout the epipelagic environment.

Biology and behaviour

The migratory behaviours of most pelagic fishes mean that they are commonly recognised as having no territories. Some species, such as the mackerels, bonitos, tunas and dolphinfishes, school, while other species, such as the louvar, ocean sunfishes, and moonfishes or opahs, live relatively solitary lives. Movements (migration, post-breeding dispersal) and distribution are highly variable, and dependent on species, climate and seasonal conditions, habitat and prey availability. While seasonal spawning aggregation of many species are relatively predictable, the dispersal from spawning sites can be highly divergent. Some species have been tracked moving across major ocean basins as part of their dispersal pattern, commonly occupying areas beyond national jurisdiction, while the migration of other species occurs along continental shelves.

The broad movement patterns of pelagic fishes have led many of these species to be formally defined under the United Nations Convention on Law of the Sea (UNCLOS) as 'highly migratory'. Management of highly migratory species is undertaken by the relevant regional fisheries management organisation, of which the Commonwealth Government of Australia is a member and regulates fisheries interactions within Australia's Exclusive Economic Zone (EEZ). For species where the majority of the stock (population) distribution occurs within the Australian, EEZ is managed by either the Commonwealth (e.g. blue mackerel, *Scomber australasicus*), the states and territories (e.g. dolphinfish or cobia, *Rachycentron canadum*), or jointly managed (e.g. gemfish, *Rexea solandri*).

Pelagic fishes are nearly all predatory and have developed specialised morphological characteristics to aid their hunting ability, with some species hunting in surface waters, while others forage at depth, or during the night. Open ocean habitats typically lack structural features and nutrients, which drive productivity/food availability, and so pelagic species must be capable of moving large distances over short periods of time to find food (Pepperell 2010).

The majority of pelagic fishes are at the apex of the food web with small bait fishes (i.e. pilchards, sauries and scads), pelagic crustaceans and squid tending to be the primary food source for most pelagic predators (Potier *et al.* 2007). Several of the larger pelagic fish groups have large mouth gapes and employ a foraging method known as ram feeding to engulf their prey, before trapping them in their gill rakers or swallowing them whole (Rooker *et al.* 2007). Some of the species, such as the swordfish and sailfish, will even stun their prey using their bills before engulfing the prey (Domenici *et al.* 2014). There are also several pelagic fishes, such as the wahoo, mackerels, snake mackerels, barracudas and dogtooth tuna, with rows of extremely sharp teeth that are used to bite through prey species. Two species with hunting strategies that are notable exceptions to that typical of pelagic fishes are the remoras of the family Echeneidae (feed on the parasites and remains of food left from their hosts) and the sunfishes (varied diet including jellyfishes, salps, stenophores, and occasionally small crustaceans and fish; Pope *et al.* 2010).

The reproduction strategy of many pelagic fishes involves migration to defined spawning sites. Migrations can cover extremely long distances, such that of billfishes and true tunas (*Thunnus*) whose migrations may cross ocean basins (Bestley *et al.* 2009). Migration often coincides with a seasonal spawning event that can last from weeks to months. Pelagic fishes undertake broadcast spawning. The reproductive strategy involves courtship between male and female fish, before shedding eggs and sperm into the water column where fertilisation takes place. The sporadic nature of broadcast spawning in the marine environment means that spawning sites for many pelagic species often align with prominent oceanic features, such as reef shelves and edges, or oceanic pinnacles or sea mounts, that facilitate entrainment of eggs and sperm into ocean eddies or reef lagoons to maximise the chance of fertilisation (Domeier and Speare 2012). In some of the larger pelagic fishes, mature females may produce hundreds of millions of eggs in a single season. Spawning events for many species are known to involve environmental cues that act as spawning inducers to allow the release of hormones and promote the hydration of eggs (Pepperell 2010; Pope *et al.* 2010).

Capture and handling

The primary methods of capture of most pelagic fishes by researchers are with either standard hook-and-line fishing methods (e.g. trolling, baiting and casting) or longlines. In most cases the capture of these species for research is undertaken in collaboration with recreational, commercial or charter fishers. Standard line fishing methods are the most targeted approach, and can select for fish of different sizes through hook, lure or bait type. For some species that reside over deeper waters, such as pomfrets, swordfish or gemfish, deep set longlines, droplines or trawl methods may be required. However, pelagic fishes are generally larger-bodied species, which may present problems in capturing and handling, and so can often require assistance of skilled fishers to minimise stress to animals (i.e. reduce capture times). When using standard hook and line capture methods, best practice approaches for capture and handling as outlined by Tracey *et al.* (2016) should be considered.

Pelagic fishes are regularly tagged with conventional or electronic tags to provide information on movement and migratory patterns, habitat use, environmental influences, post-release survival and growth information. Most pelagic fish tagging is done either with coded dart tags or pop-up satellite archival tags (PSATs). However, for some smaller or less-mobile species such as dolphinfish, mackerels and cobia, acoustic tags are also commonly used. Other methods such as accelerometers, archival tagging, crittercams and radio tagging are used to a lesser extent.

Coded dart tags (conventional tags) are based on the assumption that fish will be first tagged and released, and then recaptured to provide information about movement or growth (in the latter case, fish would be killed to obtain hard parts when recaught). Dart tagging of pelagic fishes requires numerically coded tags to be inserted into the dorsal musculature or between pterygiophores using a tag applicator/or tag pole (Bradford *et al.* 2009). When tagging with pelagic tags, most fish should be removed from the water before tagging to improve the tag placement. However, tagging of larger fish may need to be undertaken in water (boat-side). During boat-side tagging it is usually best to keep the boat moving slowly forwards to pass water over the gills and to enable better control of the fish.

Pop-up satellite archival tags are externally attached devices that use the same underlying approach as dart tag deployment (i.e. the device attached to a tether and tag anchor head). PSATs are designed to record and store data (e.g. temperate, depth and light level) through the entire time of deployment, allowing for fine-scale information on movement (horizontally and vertically), post-release survival and interaction with the physical environment. These tags also do not require fish to be recaptured, so it is more likely that data will be recovered for study.

Analysis of parasite assemblages, molecular techniques and chemical analysis of hard structures are also commonly used in research on pelagic fishes. These studies incorporate either lethal or non-lethal research approaches and are some of the most commonly applied methods for determining population structure and natal origins, and investigating movement between nursery areas and spawning grounds (for more information see Chapter 13).

Veterinary considerations

Anaesthesia

Anaesthetic considerations are similar among bony fish groups (Mylniczenko *et al.* 2014). See 'Estuarine fishes' for a discussion of anaesthetic principles for fish.

However, pelagic fishes are often large obligate ram ventilators (constant forward movement) and therefore anaesthesia is not always recommended due to problems such as fish jumping out of the anaesthetising tub, anaesthesia killing fish due to unmet oxygen demands, or difficult recovery through impaired oxygen uptake. (Brownscombe *et al.* 2019). See Chapter 13 for information on non-therapeutic techniques for immobilisation in pelagic fishes such as hypnosis (Wells *et al.* 2005).

Euthanasia

Euthanasia methods are similar among bony fish groups. See 'Estuarine fishes' for a discussion of euthanasia principles for fish. Euthanasia of pelagic fishes is recommended using the *ikejime* method (Diggles 2016). This is the quickest and most reliable method of euthanasing fish while at sea and minimises stress and pain to the animal. This method should be considered if physiological impairment occurs during non-lethal research, or when conducting biological research requiring lethal approaches as outlined in Chapter 13. For ageing or sensory work there should be a conscious effort to ensure *ikejime* methods do not damage otoliths or sensory organs.

Infectious pathogens

Zoonotic diseases in pelagic fish are relevant to human consumption, including pathogenic bacteria, histamine-producing bacteria, and biotoxins. Some fishes are also subject to histamine-producing bacteria (e.g. *Morganella morganii*, *Photobacterium phosphoreum*). Fish containing high concentrations of histidine include many scombroid fishes (e.g. tuna and mackerel), sardines, anchovies, dolphinfish and Australian salmon. Ingestion of high concentrations of histamine can result in mild to severe gastrointestinal illness and allergic reactions. Some fish species also contain marine biotoxins. Ciguatera poisoning involves a bioaccumulation of ciguatoxins from the dinoflagellate *Gambierdiscus toxicus* in several species of fish such as the Spanish mackerel, *Scomberomorus commerson*.

General operating procedures

A range of research methods and procedures relevant to studying pelagic fishes are covered in more detail in Chapter 13. Several netting and observational methods that apply to freshwater animals may also apply to these species (Chapter 14). Veterinary methods that may be relevant are covered in Chapter 16.

DEEPWATER FISHES

Tiffany Sih and Andy Moore

Characteristics

Deepwater communities are composed of diverse assemblages of fishes that both captivate and inspire further exploration. Opportunities to sample deep marine ecosystems are rare and deepwater taxa are among the least known of all global habitats, because of the difficulties associated with conducting research at depth. The terms 'deepwater' and 'deep sea' are relative and many of the teleost fishes discussed in this sub-chapter inhabit a depth gradient from mesophotic depths (50–150 m), the approximate depth of the continental shelf edge (~200 m), upper continental slope (200–500 m), down to abyssal (3000–6000 m) or even hadal depths (6000–11 000 m). What unites these diverse piscine groups and habitats is the increased difficulty and logistical constraints in deepwater sampling. Researching deepwater species is restricted by equipment, vessel-based time, associated operational costs and risks. Moreover, deepwater fishes may be scattered or patchily distributed within vast areas of potential habitat and this increases the logistically difficult, often opportunistic, nature of sampling.

Worldwide, deepwater ecosystems are areas of discovery and limited exploration. Over 350 species are discovered in the deep sea (> 500 m) each year in the last three decades and that rate is still increasing (Glover *et al.*

2020). Researchers are still compiling baseline estimates of the relative abundance and basic biological parameters of deepwater fishes. What is known about the biology and ecology of deepwater fishes often comes from research on a few species over a limited spatial extent. However, as more becomes known regarding the unique biology and ecology of deepwater fishes and the fragility of the ecosystems they occupy, so do the unique ethical challenges that arise when sampling these fishes both *in situ* and by extraction, and the need to account for these challenges during research planning and implementation.

Species covered within this chapter (representing 27 family groups from orders Perciformes, Zeiformes, Aulopiformes, Notacanthiformes, Argentiniformes, Aulopiformes, Myctophiformes, Lampridiformes, Gadiformes, Ophidiiformes and Beryciformes) inhabit polar to tropical waters, but depth is arguably the most important feature to understanding the biology and ecology of taxa. While the ecology of deepwater fishes remains poorly understood, a variety of deepwater species are highly important to commercial fisheries in Australia, including species in the families Centrolophidae (trevallas), Zeidae (dories), Merlucciidae (southern hakes), Macrouridae (grenadiers), Trachichthyidae (roughies) and Berycidae (alfonsinos).

Biology and behaviour

Deepwater fish distributions are often confined to discrete depth ranges, though this can vary according to life history stage. Among deepwater fishes there are groups that are more benthic that move very little to conserve energy, and those that are more benthopelagic that use more of the water column. Tapering bodies and eel-like forms such as the notacanthids and halosaurids are generally slow cruisers (Marshall 1965). Deepwater fishes that aggregate near seamounts (e.g. orange roughy and oreodories) can have more robust bodies and exhibit greater metabolic requirements in order to swim against strong currents (Koslow 1997). As deepwater research often extends into the 'high seas' beyond any one nation's jurisdiction, it is important to consider ethical considerations that scientific information is shared, for example genetic data, and future regulations and restrictions do not unfairly benefit certain groups or pose a considerable hindrance to scientific pursuits (Heffernan 2019).

Deepwater fishes exhibit diverse feeding strategies and many nutrient cycles are not fully understood. Some fishes follow the diel vertical migration of plankton and other prey sources and move several hundred metres from the mesopelagic to the epipelagic zones daily (Frost and McCrone 1979). Notacanthids (deepsea spiny eels) and halosaurids (halosaurs) feed on benthic invertebrates. *Bathysaurus* spp. are predators that feed opportunistically on the bottom using 'sit and wait' ambush foraging strategies. Grenadiers are active foragers. In trophic studies from south-east Australia, orange roughy (*Hoplostethus atlanticus*), warty oreodory (*Allocyttus verrucosus*) and serrulate whiptail (*Coryphaenoides serrulatus*) have been identified as benthic omnivores with a diet of mesopelagic fish, squid and crustaceans (Bulman *et al.* 2002). Other macrourids exhibited a range of feeding behaviours, some were benthopelagic omnivores and others fed primarily on benthic invertebrates and pelagic crustaceans (e.g. carid and penaeid prawns). Alepocephalids (slickheads) and the smooth oreodory (*Pseudocyttus maculatus*) fed mostly on pyrosomes (Bulman *et al.* 2002).

Bioluminescence is a predominant trait in deepwater species with over 1500 fishes known to use it in various functions (Martini and Haddock 2017). Some deepwater fishes rely on vision for hunting and finding mates, while the use of vision in other species such as the 'faceless' fish remains unknown. Recent advances also indicate fishes can perceive subtle differences in colour and light at depths where there is no light from the surface and at least 16 species are 'ultra-black' with almost no reflectance (Davis *et al.* 2020).

Reduced resources and encounter rates at deeper depths have necessitated reproductive adaptations such as hermaphroditism (e.g. tripodfishes), extreme sexual dimorphisms (e.g. anglerfishes) and skewed sex ratios in deepwater fishes (Merrett and Haedrich 1997). Ophidioids are highly fecund livebearers and some deepwater fishes are known to form large spawning aggregations seasonally (e.g. orange roughy, and basketwork eels (Williams *et al.* 2021)). It may be important to consider current or anthropogenic effects on populations when designing studies. For instance, the fecundity of orange roughy may vary according to fishing intensity (Koslow *et al.* 1995).

Fishes have diverse roles in deepwater marine ecosystems and the extent of these niches is not yet known. Deepwater research has largely been limited to a small number of fishes in disparate geographic locations. Within the same family, fishes are not uniform in their biology, ecology or behaviour. Some of the characteristics discussed here may assist researchers to select sufficient study methods, however, greater understanding of these factors would enhance each researcher's ability to account for the ethical treatment of deepwater fishes. Future objectives should work towards minimally invasive sampling, but demographic parameters such as age, growth, reproduction and natural mortality (which often require lethal methods of research) are not known for many species. Further, understanding the ecology and behaviour of deepwater fishes (e.g. deepwater foodwebs and movement/migration among populations) would be relevant to designing deepwater fish studies.

Capture and handling

Techniques for studying fishes at depth vary from minimally invasive to extractive techniques. *In situ* methods such as remotely operated vehicles, underwater video stations (e.g. deep BRUVS; Marouchos *et al.* 2011), submersibles (e.g. Starr *et al.* 1996), and towed cameras and acoustics (e.g. Kloser *et al.* 2002; Williams *et al.* 2021) are considered minimally invasive as they enhance the capability to observe deepwater fishes without removing animals from the natural environment. However, the placement, movement and lighting necessary for studying fishes with these methods may have some non-lethal effects on animal welfare.

Deepwater research often requires the physical collection of specimens that cannot be accomplished with less-invasive techniques (Williams *et al.* 2015). Specimens or samples are necessary for species' descriptions (Rocha *et al.* 2014), isotopic studies, genetic population studies, biogeography, phylogenetic and evolutionary investigations (Gaither *et al.* 2016). Deepwater sampling methods will differ according to the type of habitat and depths targeted. Several methods can be used for fishes, including traditional fishery techniques, or smaller scientific sampling bottom or pelagic trawls, benthic sleds, baited cages and baited hooks. In these cases, rapid euthanasia of the fish at the water's surface may be needed.

Sampling method or mesh size will vary depending on the target species, depths and scientific purpose. For fishes that are to be kept alive (e.g. tag and release, telemetry studies and aquarium studies), bringing a specimen with a gas-filled swim bladder to the water's surface rapidly can cause barotrauma. To reduce the effects of rapid ascent, specimens can be brought up in stages or at a slow and steady pace. Purpose-built pressurised chambers have also been used to bring live mesophotic fishes up from ~100 m depths with staged decompression (Shepherd *et al.* 2018). However, many samples are collected from deepwater (> 500 m) trawl shots where ascent is controlled both by the speed of the vessel and the winches. These trawls may take several hours from deployment to retrieval.

Traditional mark–recapture techniques have limited use for most deepwater fish because of their low survival associated with barotrauma. The technique has been used with moderately deepwater fish species (< 500 m; Treble *et al.* 2008). However, passive acoustic tracking and *in situ* underwater tagging equipment has been used to tag deepwater species (Daley *et al.* 2015). Quick recompression of fish through the use of release weights and venting of swim bladders has been shown to increase survivorship after tags have been deployed (Sumpton *et al.* 2010). Internally implanted or ingested acoustic transmitters have been successful for tracking spatial movements of several species of deepwater fishes (Hussey *et al.* 2017). For more information on internal tagging procedures see Chapter 13. Ship-based acoustic monitoring of deepwater fish populations is a non-invasive method of monitoring biomass (e.g. Kloser *et al.* 1996).

Veterinary considerations

Anaesthesia

Anaesthetic considerations are similar among bony fish groups (Mylniczenko *et al.* 2014). See 'Estuarine fishes' for a discussion of anaesthetic principles for fish.

Immersion in anaesthetic or sedatives is generally suitable for deepwater fishes, depending on the specimen end use (Silbernagel and Yochem 2016).

Euthanasia

Euthanasia methods are similar among bony fish groups. See 'Estuarine fishes' for a discussion of euthanasia principles for fish. Lethal sampling for deepwater teleosts is undertaken as part of standard biological and ecological studies. Details on appropriate euthanasia methods are covered in Chapter 13. It should be noted that standard ice slurries used in commercial fisheries operations are unlikely to be useful for deepwater species that live in low temperature waters.

Infectious pathogens

Zoonotic diseases in deepwater fish may be relevant to human consumption, including pathogenic bacteria, histamine-producing bacteria, and biotoxins; however, there is limited study into these for deepwater species.

General operating procedures

A range of research methods and procedures relevant to studying deepwater fishes are covered in more detail in Chapter 13. Veterinary methods that may be relevant are covered in Chapter 16.

SYNGNATHIDS AND SEAMOTHS

David Harasti, Megan Skelton, Sheridan Rabbitt and Ian R. Tibbetts

Characteristics

Australia has one of the highest diversities of syngnathids in the world, with ~127 known species. At least 19 seahorse species, 94 pipefishes, 11 pipehorses and three seadragons occur in Australian waters, compromising ~40% of all species (Martin-Smith and Vincent 2006). Families of these species include the Solenostomidae, Syngnathidae, Aulostomidae, Fistulariidae, Macroramphosidae, Centriscidae from the order Syngnathiformes; and the Pegasidae from the order Gasterosteiformes.

Biology and behaviour

Syngnathids are generally found in shallow coastal habitats (less than 20 m depth) but some species are known to occur at depths of 150 m (Lourie *et al.* 2016). Australian species can be found over a large depth range, with species such as the seahorse *Hippocampus abdominalis* and the pipefish *Urocampus carinirostris* occurring in protected shallow water habitats (< 15 m), while species such as *H. minotaur* and *H. paradoxus* are found in much greater depths (> 60 m) (Kuiter 2009). A single species, the Madura pipefish *Hippichthys heptagonus* occurs in brackish water and the lower reaches of freshwater streams (Thompson and Bray 2020).

Syngnathids occur in a large variety of natural habitats such as sponges, corals, seagrasses, gorgonian sea fans and kelp forests (Kuiter 2009), but they also utilise artificial structures such as bather protection nets, jetty pylons and purpose built artificial habitats. All seahorses and many pygmy pipehorses and pipefishes have prehensile tails, which they use to hold onto their host substrate. Some prehensile species may wrap themselves around objects using their flexible bodies. The longer and more-flexible tail of seahorses may enable enhanced attachment than the prehensile pipefish and pipehorses, which grip with only the distal region of the tail (Neutens *et al.* 2017). Therefore, differences in their ability to grasp structure may facilitate habitat partitioning.

Most syngnathids and seamoths are slow swimmers using a combination of pectoral fins and dorsal fins (seahorses) and caudal fins (non-prehensile pipefishes, seamoths). Studies on *Hippocampus* spp. in Australia have shown that many species have very small home ranges with females generally moving further than the males (Moreau and Vincent 2004) while some *Hippocampus* spp. show strong site attachment (Harasti *et al.* 2014). Seasonal changes in abundance are common with juvenile recruitment in the warmer months often driving seasonal variation in syngnathid density and abundance in many species (Correia *et al.* 2015).

While the largest member of this group in Australia, the flutemouth (*Aulostomus chinensis*) has been identified as a piscivore (Randall 1985), most syngnathids and seamoths have small elongate mouths with a narrow gape, restricting them to a diet of small pelagic or benthic crustaceans (i.e. amphipods and copepods). In captivity they are often maintained on a diet of live brine shrimp (*Artemia* sp.).

Syngnathid males become pregnant and give birth. For the seahorses (*Hippocampus* spp.), the female transfers her eggs to the male's abdominal pouch where they are fertilised with the male becoming pregnant. Male pipefishes and pipehorses carry the eggs on the underside of their body, often held in place by small pouches while the male seadragons carry the eggs on the underside of their tail. Some *Hippocampus* spp. are monogamous and mate continuously during a breeding season and also over subsequent seasons. Once a male gives birth, there is no parental care for the progeny.

Capture and handling

Capture and handling of these taxa vary considerably from that of other marine fishes. If syngnathids need to be collected from the wild for aquarium studies, animals can be placed in plastic sealable bags, containers or small mesh bags, kept in the shade and transferred into a large container of seawater once on land. They should be transported immediately to the aquarium or research facility and placed in water of the same temperature as that of the environment from where they were collected.

Marking of syngnathids is primarily done using visible implant elastomer (VIE), which is recommended as a suitable marking method by the IUCN Seahorse, Pipefish and Seadragon Specialist Group. Visible implant elastomer is a bio-compatible elastomer that creates small coloured tags in a variety of colours. The elastomer is injected just beneath the skin of the syngnathid and sets into a small solid mark. Seahorses are generally given three tags of the same colour into different areas of the body, with the tag locations allowing individual identification. For small individuals, a single tag is inserted and if they are resighted at a larger size, then two more tags can be inserted. Use of VIE in syngnathids has not been found to show any adverse effects in the wild or in aquarium studies, and elastomer tags are known to remain within the animals for up to 5 years following marking (Harasti *et al.* 2012). Injecting the VIE tags with a syringe is quite a delicate process, so only personnel with appropriate training and experience should undertake the procedure.

Large syngnathids may also be tagged with neck collar tags and acoustic transmitters. However, these external tags are large and subject to fouling. Using natural markings to identify individuals has been successful for a few syngnathid species (Correia *et al.* 2014); however, this method is less suitable for those species where natural markings are either difficult to see or change through time. Syngnathids should be tagged *in situ* wherever possible because removal from the water can be very stressful for these taxa. Additionally, because many syngnathids display strong site fidelity (Smith *et al.* 2012), removal from their specific habitat could either lead to separation from a breeding partner or the introduction of the released animal into the small home range of another individual, possibly causing displacement and death of one or the other.

Veterinary considerations

Sedation and anaesthesia

Anaesthetic considerations are similar among bony fish groups (Mylniczenko *et al.* 2014). See 'Estuarine fishes' for a discussion of anaesthetic principles for fish.

The use of sedatives and anaesthetics in syngnathids is considered optional and not deemed a requirement for animals within aquaria that are to be tagged or need to be removed from the water. The majority of studies that involve the use of elastomers for tagging syngnathids have been done without the use of sedatives and no adverse impacts on syngnathid behaviour or physiology have been documented (Sanchez-Camara and Booth 2004). If sedation is required, then isoeugenol is usually used.

Euthanasia

Euthanasia methods are similar among bony fish groups. See 'Estuarine fishes' for a discussion of euthanasia principles for fish. In the event that a syngnathid needs to be euthanased, it is recommended that they be placed in an ice slurry following the methods of Blessing *et al.* (2010).

Infectious pathogens

There is limited information on zoonotic diseases that affect syngnathids. Trematode parasites are known to infect syngnathids, but this is not known to be associated with any risk of transmission to humans.

General operating procedures

A range of research methods and procedures relevant to studying syngnathids and seamoths are covered in more detail in Chapter 13. General procedures for using VIE are detailed in Chapter 8. Several netting and observational methods that apply to freshwater animals may also apply to these species (Chapter 14). Veterinary methods that may be relevant are covered in Chapter 16.

REFERENCES

Allen GR (1975) *The Anemonefishes: their Classification and Biology.* 2nd edn. TFH Publications, Hong Kong.

Appeldoorn RS, Aguilar-Perera A, Bouwmeester BLK, Dennis GD, Hill RL, Merten W, Recksiek CW, Williams SJ (2009) Movement of fishes (Grunts: Haemulidae) across the coral reef seascape: A review of scales, patterns and processes. *Caribbean Journal of Science* **45**, 304–316. doi:10.18475/cjos.v45i2.a16

Arlinghaus R, Cooke SJ, Lyman J, *et al.* (2007) Understanding the complexity of catch-and-release in recreational fishing: an integrative synthesis of global knowledge from historical, ethical, social, and biological perspectives. *Reviews in Fisheries Science* **15**, 75–167. doi:10.1080/10641260601149432

Babcock RC, Pillans RD, Rochester WA (2017) Environmental and individual effects on the behaviour and spawning movements of *Lethrinus nebulosus* on a coral reef. *Marine and Freshwater Research* **68**, 1422–1437. doi:10.1071/MF16194

Barker D, Allan G, Rowland S (2015) *A Guide to Acceptable Procedures and Practices for Aquaculture and Fisheries Research.* NSW Fisheries Animal Care and Ethics Committee, NSW Fisheries, Sydney.

Barnett A, Abrantes KG, Baker R, Diedrich AS, Farr M, Kuilboer A, Mahony T, McLeod I, Moscardo G, Prideaux M, Stoeckl N, van Luyn A, Sheaves M (2016) Sport fisheries, conservation and sustainable livelihoods: a multidisciplinary guide to developing best practice. *Fish and Fisheries* **17**, 696–713. doi:10.1111/faf.12140

Bay L, Jones G, McCormick M (2001) Habitat selection and aggression as determinants of spatial segregation among damselfish on a coral reef. *Coral Reefs* **20**, 289–298.

Bellwood DR, Hughes TP, Hoey AS (2006) Sleeping functional group drives coral-reef recovery. *Current Biology* **16**, 2434–2439.

Berumen ML, Almany GR (2009) External tagging does not affect the feeding behavior of a coral reef fish, *Chaetodon vagabundus* (Pisces: Chaetodontidae). *Environmental Biology of Fishes* **86**, 447.

Bestley S, Gunn JS, Hindell MA (2009) Plasticity in vertical behaviour of migrating juvenile southern bluefin tuna (*Thunnus maccoyii*) in relation to oceanography of the south Indian Ocean. *Fisheries Oceanography* **18**, 237–254. doi:10.1111/j.1365-2419.2009.00509.x

Blaber SJM (1977) The feeding ecology and relative abundance of mullet (Mugilidae) in Natal and Pondoland estuaries. *Biological Journal of the Linnean Society. Linnean Society of London* **9**, 259–275. doi:10.1111/j.1095-8312.1977.tb00269.x

Blessing JJ, Marshall JC, Balcombe S (2010) Humane killing of fishes for scientific research: a comparison of two methods. *Journal of Fish Biology* **76**, 2571–2577. doi:10.1111/j.1095-8649.2010.02633.x

Bowater RO, Forbes-Faulkner J, Anderson IG, Condon K, Robinson B, Kong F, Gilbert GL, Reynolds A, Hyland S, McPherson G, O'Brien J (2012) Natural outbreak of *Streptococcus agalactiae* (GBS) infection in wild giant Queensland grouper *Epinephelus lanceolatus* (Bloch), and other wild fish in northern Queensland, Australia. *Journal of Fish Diseases* **35**, 173–186. doi:10.1111/j.1365-2761.2011.01332.x

Bradford RW, Hobday AJ, Evans K, Lansdell M (2009) CMAR code of practice for tagging marine animals. *CSIRO Marine and Atmospheric Research Paper 028*. CSIRO, Hobart.

Bray DJ (2018) Introduction to Australia's fishes. In *Fishes of Australia*. (Eds DJ Bray and MF Gomon). Museums Victoria and OzFishNet. <https://fishesofAustralia.net.au/home/content/166>.

Brownscombe JW, Lédée EJ, Raby GD, Struthers DP, Gutowsky LF, Nguyen VM, Young N, Stokesbury MJ, Holbrook CM, Brenden TO, Vandergoot CS (2019) Conducting and interpreting fish telemetry studies: considerations for researchers and resource managers. *Reviews in Fish Biology and Fisheries* **29**, 369–400. doi:10.1007/s11160-019-09560-4

Bryars S, Rogers P, Huveneers C, Payne N, Smith I, McDonald B (2012) Small home range in southern Australia's largest resident reef fish, the western blue groper (*Achoerodus gouldii*): implications for adequacy of no-take marine protected areas. *Marine and Freshwater Research* **63**, 552–563. doi:10.1071/MF12016

Bulman C, He X, Koslow J (2002) Trophic ecology of the mid-slope demersal fish community off southern Tasmania, Australia. *Marine and Freshwater Research* **53**, 59–72. doi:10.1071/MF01057

Butcher PA, Broadhurst MK, Hall KC, Cullis BR, Raidal SR (2012) Assessing barotrauma among angled snapper (*Pagrus auratus*) and the utility of release methods. *Fisheries Research* **127–128**, 49–55. doi:10.1016/j.fishres.2012.04.013

Carassou L, Le Borgne R, Ponton D (2009) Diet of pre-settlement larvae of coral-reef fishes: selection of prey types and sizes. *Journal of Fish Biology* **75**, 707–715. doi:10.1111/j.1095-8649.2009.02312.x

Chargulaf C, Krück N, Tibbetts I (2011) Does sympatry affect trophic resource use in congeneric tidepool fishes? A tale of two gobies *Favonigobius lentiginosus* and *Favonigobius exquisitus*. *Journal of Fish Biology* **79**, 1968–1983. doi:10.1111/j.1095-8649.2011.03132.x

Choat JH (2012) Spawning aggregations in reef fishes; ecological and evolutionary processes. In *Reef fish Spawning Aggregations: Biology, Research and Management*. (Eds YS De Mitcheson and PL Colin) pp. 85–116. Springer, Dordrecht, The Netherlands. doi:10.1007/978-94-007-1980-4_4

Claisse JT, Clark TB, Schumacher BD, Mctee SA, Bushnell ME, Callan CK, Laidley CW, Parrish JD (2011) Conventional tagging and acoustic telemetry of a small surgeonfish, *Zebrasoma flavescens*, in a structurally complex coral reef environment. *Environmental Biology of Fishes* **91**, 185–201. doi:10.1007/s10641-011-9771-9

Cooke SJ, Wilson AD, Elvidge CK, Lennox RJ, Jepsen N, Colotelo AH, Brown RS (2016) Ten practical realities for institutional animal care and use committees when evaluating protocols dealing with fish in the field. *Reviews in Fish Biology and Fisheries* **26**, 123–133. doi:10.1007/s11160-015-9413-y

Cooke SJ, Suski CD (2005) Do we need species specific guidelines for catch-and-release recreational angling to effectively conserve diverse fishery resources? *Biodiversity and Conservation* **14**, 1195–1209. doi:10.1007/s10531-004-7845-0

Correia M, Caldwell IR, Koldewey HJ, Andrade JP, Palma J (2015) Seahorse (Hippocampinae) population fluctuations in the ria Formosa lagoon, south Portugal. *Journal of Fish Biology* **87**, 679–690. doi:10.1111/jfb.12748

Correia M, Palma J, Koldewey H, Andrade JP (2014) The use of a non-invasive tool for capture-recapture studies on a seahorse *Hippocampus guttulatus* population. *Journal of Fish Biology* **84**, 872–884. doi:10.1111/jfb.12304

Coulson P, Platell M, Clarke K, Potter I (2015) Dietary variations within a family of ambush predators (*Platycephalidae*) occupying different habitats and environments in the same geographical region. *Journal of Fish Biology* **86**, 1046–1077. doi:10.1111/jfb.12612

Currey LM, Heupel MR, Simpfendorfer CA, Williams AJ (2014) Sedentary or mobile? Variability in space and depth use of an exploited coral reef fish. *Marine Biology* **161**, 2155–2166. doi:10.1007/s00227-014-2497-4

Daley RK, Williams A, Green M, Barker B, Brodie P (2015) Can marine reserves conserve vulnerable sharks in the deep sea? A case study of *Centrophorus zeehaani* (Centrophoridae), examined with acoustic telemetry. *Deep-sea Research. Part II, Topical Studies in Oceanography* **115**, 127–136. doi:10.1016/j.dsr2.2014.05.017

Davis AL, Thomas KN, Goetz FE, Robison BH, Nke Johnsen S, Osborn KJ (2020) Ultra-black camouflage in deep-sea fishes. *Current Biology* **30**, 3470–3476.e3. doi:10.1016/j.cub.2020.06.044

Davis JP, Pitt KA, Olds AD, Harborne AR, Connolly RM (2017) Seagrass corridors and tidal state modify how fish use habitats on intertidal coral reef flats. *Marine Ecology Progress Series* **581**, 135–147. doi:10.3354/meps12311

De Mitcheson YS, Liu M (2008) Functional hermaphroditism in teleosts. *Fish and Fisheries* **9**, 1–43. doi:10.1111/j.1467-2979.2007.00266.x

Diggles BK (2016) Development of resources to promote best practice in the humane dispatch of finfish caught by recreational fishers. *Fisheries Management and Ecology* **23**, 200–207. doi:10.1111/fme.12127

Diggles BK, Ernst I, Wesche S (2018) Emergence of serranid pigment abnormality syndrome (SPAS) in wire netting cod (*Epinephelus quoyanus*) from Heron Island on the southern Great Barrier Reef. *Marine and Freshwater Research* **69**, 1201–1207.

Domeier ML, Speare P (2012) Dispersal of adult black marlin (*Istiompax indica*) from a Great Barrier Reef spawning aggregation. *PLoS One* 7. doi:10.1371/journal.pone.0031629

Domenici P, Wilson ADM, Kurvers RHJM, Marras S, Herbert-Read JE, Steffensen JF, Krause S, Viblanc PE, Couillaud P, Krause J (2014) How sailfish use their bills to capture schooling prey. *Proceedings of the Royal Society B: Biological Sciences* **281**. doi:10.1098/rspb.2014.0444

Durhack TC, Jeffrey JD, Enders EC (2020) In search of an anaesthesia alternative for field-based research. *Aquaculture* **525**. doi:10.1016/j.aquaculture.2020.735285

Elliott M, Whitfield AK, Potter IC, Blaber SJM, Cyrus DP, Nordlie FG, Harrison TD (2007) The guild approach to categorizing estuarine fish assemblages: a global review. *Fish and Fisheries* **8**, 241–268. doi:10.1111/j.1467-2679.2007.00253.x

Elsdon TS, Wells BK, Campana SE, Gillanders BM, Jones CM, Limburg KE, Walther BD (2008) Otolith chemistry to describe movements and life-history parameters of fishes – hypotheses, assumptions, limitations and inferences. *Oceanography and Marine Biology - an Annual Review* **46**, 297–330. doi:10.1201/9781420065756.ch7

Fenner PJ, Lewis RJ, Williamson JA, Williams ML (1997) A Queensland family with ciguatera after eating coral trout. *The Medical Journal of Australia* **166**, 473–475. doi:10.5694/j.1326-5377.1997.tb123219.x

Fetterplace LC (2018) The ecology of temperate soft sediment fishes: implications for fisheries management and marine protected area design. Doctor of Philosophy thesis. The University of Wollongong, Australia.

Fetterplace LC, Davis AR, Neilson JM, Taylor MD, Knott NA (2016) Active acoustic tracking suggests that soft sediment fishes can show site attachment: a preliminary assessment of the movement patterns of the blue-spotted flathead (*Platycephalus caeruleopunctatus*). *Animal Biotelemetry* **4**, 15. doi:10.1186/s40317-016-0107-6

Fowler AJ, Jones GK, McGarvey R (2002) Characteristics and consequences of movement patterns of King George whiting (Perciformes: *Sillaginodes punctata*) in South Australia. *Marine and Freshwater Research* **53**, 1055–1069. doi:10.1071/MF02023

Fowler AM, Smith SM, Booth DJ, Stewart J (2016) Partial migration of grey mullet (*Mugil cephalus*) on Australia's east coast revealed by otolith chemistry. *Marine Environmental Research* **119**, 238–244. doi:10.1016/j.marenvres.2016.06.010

Frost BW, McCrone LE (1979) Vertical distribution, diel vertical migration, and abundance of some mesopelagic fishes in the eastern subarctic Pacific Ocean in summer. *Fishery Bulletin* **76**, 751.

Gaither MR, Bowen BW, Rocha LA, Briggs JC (2016) Fishes that rule the world: circumtropical distributions revisited. *Fish and Fisheries* **17**, 664–679. doi:10.1111/faf.12136

Gauthier DT (2015) Bacterial zoonoses of fishes: a review and appraisal of evidence for linkages between fish and human infections. *Veterinary Journal (London, England)* **203**, 27–35. doi:10.1016/j.tvjl.2014.10.028

Gerlach G, Atema J, Kingsford MJ, Black KP, Miller-Sims V (2007) Smelling home can prevent dispersal of reef fish larvae. *Proceedings of the National Academy of Sciences of the United States of America* **104**, 858–863. doi:10.1073/pnas.0606777104

Gillanders BM, Ferrell DJ, Andrew NL (2001) Estimates of movement and life-history parameters of yellowtail kingfish (*Seriola lalandi*): how useful are data from a cooperative tagging programme? *Marine and Freshwater Research* **52**, 179–192. doi:10.1071/MF99153

Glover AG, Higgs N, Horton T (2020) World Register of Deep-sea species (WoRDSS). Accessed at <http://www.marinespecies.org/deepsea> on 15 July 2020. doi:10.14284/352

Griffiths SP (2003) Rockpool ichthyofaunas of temperate Australia: species composition, residency and biogeographic patterns. *Estuarine, Coastal and Shelf Science* **58**, 173–186. doi:10.1016/S0272-7714(03)00073-8

Grixti D, Conron SD, Ryan K, Versace VL (2010) Circle versus long-shank hooks: comparing hooking locations and recreational catch for juvenile snapper Pagrus auratus and King George whiting Sillaginodes punctata. *Fisheries Research* **106**, 27–31. doi:10.1016/j.fishres.2010.06.013

Harasti D, Martin-Smith K, Gladstone W (2012) Population dynamics and life history of a geographically restricted seahorse, *Hippocampus whitei*. *Journal of Fish Biology* **81**, 1297–1314. doi.org/10.1111/j.1095-8649.2012.03406.x

Harasti D, Martin-Smith K, Gladstone W (2014) Ontogenetic and sex-based differences in habitat preferences and site fidelity of the White's seahorse *Hippocampus whitei*. *Journal of Fish Biology* **85**, 1413–1428. doi:10.1111/jfb.12492

Hargreaves D, Buckland A, Sheaves M (2017) Trophic guild concept: factors affecting within-guild consistency for tropical estuarine fish. *Marine Ecology Progress Series* **564**, 175–186. doi:10.3354/meps11955

Heffernan O (2019) Seabed mining is coming – bringing mineral riches and fears of epic extinctions. *Nature* **571**, 465–468. doi:10.1038/d41586-019-02242

Hoey AS, McCormick MI (2006) Effects of subcutaneous fluorescent tags on the growth and survival of a newly settled coral reef fish, *Pomacentrus amboinensis* (Pomacentridae). *Proceedings of the 10th International Coral Reefs Symposium*, pp. 420–425.

Hughes JM, Stewart J (2013) Assessment of barotrauma and its mitigation measures on the behaviour and survival of snapper (*Chrysophrys auratus*) and mulloway (*Argyrosomus japonicus*). New South Wales Department of Primary Industries, Fisheries Final Report Series No. 138. <https://www.dpi.nsw.gov.au/__data/assets/pdf_file/0007/545749/FFRS-138_Hughes-and-Stewart-2013.pdf>.

Hundt PJ, Nakamura Y, Yamaoka K (2014) Diet of combtooth blennies (Blenniidae) in Kochi and Okinawa, Japan. *Ichthyological Research* **61**, 76–82. doi:10.1007/s10228-013-0366-7

Hussey NE, Hedges KJ, Barkley AN, Treble MA, Peklova I, Webber DM, Ferguson SH, Yurkowski DJ, Kessel ST, Bedard JM, Fisk AT (2017) Movements of a deep-water fish: establishing marine fisheries management boundaries in coastal Arctic waters. *Ecological Applications* **27**, 687–704. doi:10.1002/eap.1485

Javahery S, Nekoubin H, Moradlu AH (2012) Effect of anaesthesia with clove oil in fish. *Fish Physiology and Biochemistry* **38**, 1545–1552. doi:10.1007/s10695-012-9682-5

Jones GP (2015) Mission impossible: unlocking the secrets of coral reef fish dispersal. In *Ecology of Fishes on Coral Reefs*. (Ed. C Mora) pp. 16–27. Cambridge University Press, Cambridge, UK.

Key B (2016) Why fish do not feel pain. *Animal Sentience* **3**, 2016.003. doi:10.51291/2377-7478.1011

Kimirei IA, Nagelkerken I, Trommelen M, Blankers P, Hoytema N, Hoeijmakers D, Huijbers CM, Mgaya YD, Rypel AL (2013) What drives ontogenetic niche shifts of fishes in coral reef ecosystems? *Ecosystems* **16**, 783–796. doi:10.1007/s10021-013-9645-4

Kingsford MJ, Carlson IJ (2010) Patterns of distribution and movement of fishes, *Ophthalmolepis lineolatus* and *Hypoplectrodes maccullochi*, on temperate rocky reefs of south eastern Australia. *Environmental Biology of Fishes* **88**, 105–118. doi:10.1007/s10641-010-9621-1

Kloser R, Koslow J, Williams A (1996) Acoustic assessment of the biomass of a spawning aggregation of orange roughy (*Hoplostethus atlanticus*, Collett) off south-eastern Australia, 1990–93. *Marine and Freshwater Research* **47**, 1015–1024. doi:10.1071/MF9961015

Kloser RJ, Ryan T, Sakov P, Williams A, Koslow JA (2002) Species identification in deep water using multiple acoustic frequencies. *Canadian Journal of Fisheries and Aquatic Sciences* **59**(6), 1065–1077. doi:10.1139/f02-076

Koslow J, Bell J, Virtue P, Smith D (1995) Fecundity and its variability in orange roughy: effects of population density, condition, egg size, and senescence. *Journal of Fish Biology* **47**, 1063–1080. doi:10.1111/j.1095-8649.1995.tb06030.x

Koslow JA (1997) Seamounts and the ecology of deep-sea fisheries: the firm-bodied fishes that feed around seamounts are biologically distinct from their deepwater neighbors – and may be especially vulnerable to overfishing. *American Scientist* **85**, 168–176.

Kuiter RH (2009) *Seahorses and their Relatives*. Aquatic Photographics, Seaford.

Lehane L, Rawlln GT (2000) Topically acquired bacterial zoonoses from fish: a review. *The Medical Journal of Australia* **173**, 256–259. doi:10.5694/j.1326-5377.2000.tb125632.x

Litvin SY, Weinstein MP, Sheaves M, Nagelkerken I (2018) What makes nearshore habitats nurseries for nekton? An emerging view of the nursery role hypothesis. *Estuaries and Coasts* **41**, 1539–1550. doi:10.1007/s12237-018-0383-x

Lourie SA, Pollom RA, Foster SJ (2016) A global revision of the Seahorses Hippocampus Rafinesque 1810 (Actinopterygii: Syngnathiformes): Taxonomy and biogeography with recommendations for further research. *Zootaxa* **4146**, 1–66. doi:10.11646/zootaxa.4146.1.1

Marnane MJ, Bellwood DR (2002) Diet and nocturnal foraging in cardinalfishes (Apogonidae) at One Tree Reef, Great Barrier Reef,

Australia. *Marine Ecology Progress Series* **231**, 261–268. doi:10.3354/meps231261

Marouchos A, Sherlock M, Barker B, Williams A (2011) Development of a stereo deepwater baited remote underwater video system (DeepBRUVS). *OCEANS 2011 IEEE - Spain*, pp. 1–5. doi:10.1109/Oceans-Spain.2011.6003410

Marshall NB (1965) Systematic and biological studies of the macrourid fishes (Anacanthini – Teleostii). *Deep-Sea Research and Oceanographic Abstracts* **12**, 299–322. doi:10.1016/0011-7471(65)90004-5

Martini S, Haddock SHD (2017) Quantification of bioluminescence from the surface to the deep sea demonstrates its predominance as an ecological trait. *Scientific Reports* **7**, 45750. doi:10.1038/srep45750

Martin-Smith KM, Vincent AC (2006) Exploitation and trade of Australian seahorses, pipehorses, sea dragons and pipefishes (family Syngnathidae). *Oryx* **40**, 141–151. doi:10.1017/S003060530600010X

Merrett NR, Haedrich RL (1997) *Deep-sea Demersal Fish and Fisheries*. Chapman & Hall, Melbourne.

Moreau M-A, Vincent ACJ (2004) Social structure and space use in a wild population of the Australian short-headed seahorse *Hippocampus breviceps* Peters, 1869. *Marine and Freshwater Research* **55**, 231–239. doi:10.1071/MF03159

Munday PL (2004) Competitive coexistence of coral-dwelling fishes: the lottery hypothesis revisited. *Ecology* **85**, 623–628. doi:10.1890/03-3100

Mylniczenko ND, Neiffer DL, Clauss TM (2014) Bony fish (lungfish, sturgeon, and teleosts). In *Zoo Animal and Wildlife Immobilization and Anaesthesia*. 2nd edn. (Eds G West, D Heard and N Caulkett) pp. 209–260. John Wiley and Sons, Hoboken, NJ.

Neiffer DL, Stamper MA (2009) Fish sedation, anesthesia, analgesia, and euthanasia: considerations, methods, and types of drugs. *ILAR Journal* **50**, 343–360. doi:10.1093/ilar.50.4.343

Neutens C, Dobbelar B, Claes P, Adriaens D (2017) Prehensile and non-prehensile tails among syngnathid species: what's the difference? *Zoology (Jena, Germany)* **120**, 62–72. doi:10.1016/j.zool.2016.11.002

Parsons DM, Sim-Smith CJ, Cryer M, Francis MP, Hartill B, Jones EG, Le Port A, Lowe M, McKenzie J, Morrison M, Paul LJ, Radford C, Ross PM, Spong KT, Trnski T, Usmar N, Walsh C, Zeldis J (2014) Snapper (*Chrysophrys auratus*): a review of life history and key vulnerabilities in New Zealand. *New Zealand Journal of Marine and Freshwater Research* **48**, 256–283. doi:10.1080/00288330.2014.892013

Pepperell J (2010). *Fishes of the Open Ocean, a Natural History and Illustrated Guide*. UNSW Press and University of Chicago Press.

Pillans RD, Bearham D, Boomer A, Downie R, Patterson TA, Thomson DP, Babcock RC (2014) Multi year observations reveal variability in residence of a tropical demersal fish, *Lethrinus nebulosus*: implications for spatial management. *PLoS One* **9**(9), e105507. doi:10.1371/journal.pone.0105507

Pironet FN, Jones JB (2000) Treatments for ectoparasites and diseases in captive Western Australian dhufish. *Aquaculture International* **8**, 349–361. doi:10.1023/A:1009257011431

Pollock BR (1982) Movements and migrations of yellowfin bream, *Acanthopagrus australis* (Gunther), in Moreton Bay, Queensland as determined by tag recoveries. *Journal of Fish Biology* **20**, 245–252. doi:10.1111/j.1095-8649.1982.tb04705.x

Pope EC, Hays GC, Thys TM, Doyle TK, Sims DW, Queiroz N, Hobson VJ, Kubicek L, Houghton JD (2010) The biology and ecology of the ocean sunfish *Mola mola*: a review of current knowledge and future research perspectives. *Reviews in Fish Biology and Fisheries* **20**, 471–487. doi:10.1007/s11160-009-9155-9

Potier M, Marsac F, Cherel Y, Lucas V, Sabatié R, Maury O, Ménard F (2007) Forage fauna in the diet of three large pelagic fishes (lancetfish, swordfish and yellowfin tuna) in the western equatorial Indian Ocean. *Fisheries Research* **83**, 60–72. doi:10.1016/j.fishres.2006.08.020

Potter IC, Tweedley JR, Elliott M, Whitfield AK (2015) The ways in which fish use estuaries: a refinement and expansion of the guild approach. *Fish and Fisheries* **16**, 230–239. doi:10.1111/faf.12050

Pribyl AL, Kent ML, Parker SJ, Schreck CB (2011) The Response to Forced Decompression in Six Species of Pacific Rockfish. *Transactions of the American Fisheries Society* **140**, 374–383. doi:10.1080/00028487.2011.567858

Randall JE (1985) *Guide to Hawaiian Reef Fishes*. Harrowood Books, Kaneohe, HI.

Readman GD, Owen SF, Knowles TG, Murrell JC (2017) Species specific anaesthetics for fish anaesthesia and euthanasia. *Scientific Reports* **7**, 7102. doi:10.1038/s41598-017-06917-2

Rocha LA, Aleixo A, Allen G, Almeda F, Baldwin CC, Barclay MVL, Bates JM, Bauer AM, Benzoni F, Berns CM (2014) Specimen collection: An essential tool. *Science* **344**, 814–815. doi:10.1126/science.344.6186.814

Rooker JR, Alvarado Bremer JR, Block BA, Dewar H, De Metrio G, Corriero A, Kraus RT, Prince ED, Rodríguez-Marín E, Secor DH (2007) Life history and stock structure of Atlantic bluefin tuna (*Thunnus thynnus*). *Reviews in Fisheries Science* **15**, 265–310. doi:10.1080/10641260701484135

Russell DJ, Garrett RN (1985) Early life history of barramundi, *Lates calcarifer* (Bloch), in north-eastern Queensland. *Marine and Freshwater Research* **36**, 191–201. doi:10.1071/MF9850191

Russell DJ, McDougall AJ (2005) Movement and juvenile recruitment of mangrove jack, *Lutjanus argentimaculatus* (Forsskål), in northern Australia. *Marine and Freshwater Research* **56**, 465–475. doi:10.1071/MF04222

Sale PF (1971) Extremely limited home range in a coral reef fish, *Dascyllus aruanus* (Pisces; Pomacentridae). *Copeia* **1971**, 324–327. doi:10.2307/1442839

Sanchez-Camara J, Booth DJ (2004) Movement, home range and site fidelity of the weedy seadragon *Phyllopteryx taeniolatus* (Teleostei: Syngnathidae). *Environmental Biology of Fishes* **70**(1), 31–41. doi:10.1023/B:EBFI.0000022850.33643.e3

Scott M (2019) Spatial and temporal variation in movement patterns and behaviour of a large, coral reef mesopredator, *Plectropomus leopardus*, on the Great Barrier Reef, Australia. PhD thesis. James Cook University, Australia. doi:10.25903/5d5b2d6435e76

Sheaves MJ, Molony BW, Tobin AJ (1999) Spawning migrations and local movements of a tropical sparid fish. *Marine Biology* **133**, 123–128. doi:10.1007/s002270050450

Shepherd B, Pinheiro HT, Wandell M, Rocha LA (2019) The SubCAS: a pressure chamber for fish. *Frontiers for Young Minds* **7**. doi:10.3389/frym.2019.00040

Shepherd B, Wandell M, Pinheiro HT, Rocha LA (2018) SubCAS: a portable, submersible hyperbaric chamber to collect living mesophotic fishes. *Frontiers in Marine Science* **5**, 187. doi:10.3389/fmars.2018.00187

Shetty M, Maiti B, Santhosh KS, Venugopal MN, Karunasagar I (2012) Betanodavirus of marine and freshwater fish: distribution, genomic organization, diagnosis and control measures. *Indian Journal of Virology* **23**, 114–123. doi:10.1007/s13337-012-0088-x

Silbernagel C, Yochem P (2016) Effectiveness of the anesthetic AQUI-S® 20E in marine finfish and elasmobranchs. *Journal of Wildlife Diseases* **52**, S96–S103. doi:10.7589/52.2S.S96

Smith RE, Grutter AS, Tibbetts IR (2012) Extreme habitat specialisation and population structure of two gorgonian-associated pygmy seahorses. *Marine Ecology Progress Series* **444**, 195–206. doi:10.3354/meps09471

Sneddon L, Wolfenden D (2019) Ornamental Fish (Actinopterygii). In *Companion Animal Care and Welfare: The UFAW Companion Animal*

Handbook. (Ed. J Yeates) pp. 440–466. John Wiley and Sons, Hoboken, NJ.

Soares MC, Oliveira RF, Ros AF, Grutter AS, Bshary R (2011) Tactile stimulation lowers stress in fish. *Nature Communications* **2**, 534. doi:10.1038/ncomms1547

Starr RM, Fox DS, Hixon MA, Tissot BN, Johnson GE, Barss WH (1996) Comparison of submersible-survey and hydroacoustic-survey estimates of fish density on a rocky bank. *Fishery Bulletin* **94**, 113–123.

Sumpton W, Mayer D, Brown I, Sawynok B, McLennan M, Butcher A, Kirkwood J (2008) Investigation of movement and factors influencing post-release survival of line-caught coral reef fish using recreational tag–recapture data. *Fisheries Research* **92**, 189–195. doi:10.1016/j.fishres.2008.01.019

Sumpton WD, Brown IW, Mayer DG, McLennan MF, Mapleston A, Butcher AR, Welch DJ, Kirkwood JM, Sawynok B, Begg GA (2010) Assessing the effects of line capture and barotrauma relief procedures on post-release survival of key tropical reef fish species in Australia using recreational tagging clubs. *Fisheries Management and Ecology* **17**, 77–88. doi:10.1111/j.1365-2400.2009.00722.x

Sweet M, Kirkham N, Bendall M, Currey L, Bythell J, *et al.* (2012) Evidence of Melanoma in Wild Marine Fish Populations. *PLoS One* **7**, e41989. doi:10.1371/journal.pone.0041989

Taylor MD, Babcock RC, Simpfendorfer CA, Crook DA (2017) Where technology meets ecology: acoustic telemetry in contemporary Australian aquatic research and management. *Marine and Freshwater Research* **68**, 1397–1402. doi:10.1071/MF17054

Taylor MD, van der Meulen DE, Brodie S, Cadiou G, Knott NA (2018) Applying acoustic telemetry to understand contaminant exposure and bioaccumulation patterns in mobile fishes. *The Science of the Total Environment* **625**, 344–354. doi:10.1016/j.scitotenv.2017.12.177

Taylor MD, van der Meulen DE, Ives MC, Walsh CT, Reinfelds IV, Gray CA (2014) Shock, stress or signal? Implications of freshwater flows for a top-level estuarine predator. *PLoS One* **9**. doi:10.1371/journal.pone.0095680

Thompson VJ, Bray DJ (2020) *Hippichthys heptagonus* in Fishes of Australia, accessed 5 May 2020. <http://136.154.202.208/home/species/1532>.

Thorsteinson V (2002) Tagging Methods for Stock Assessment and Research in Fisheries. Report of Concerted Action FAIR CT.96.1394 (CATAG). Reykjavik. Marine Research Institute Technical Report 79, p. 179.

Tracey S, Hartmann K, McAllister J, Conron S, Leef M (2016) Capture-induced physiological stress and post-release survival of recreationally-caught Southern Bluefin Tuna. Final report FRDC project 2013–025. Institute for Marine and Antarctic Studies, Hobart.

Treble MA, Campana SE, Wastle RJ, Jones CM, Boje J (2008) Growth analysis and age validation of a deepwater Arctic fish, the Greenland halibut (*Reinhardtius hippoglossoides*). *Canadian Journal of Fisheries and Aquatic Sciences* **65**, 1047–1059. doi:10.1139/F08-030

Underwood W, Anthony R (2013) AVMA Guidelines for the Euthanasia of Animals: 2020 Edition. Retrieved on March, 30(2020), 2020–01, <https://www.avma.org/sites/default/files/2020-01/2020-Euthanasia-Final-1-17-20.pdf>.

Wargo Rub AM, Jepsen N, Liedtke TL, Moser ML, Weber ES, III (2014) Surgical insertion of transmitters and telemetry methods in fisheries research. *American Journal of Veterinary Research* **75**, 402–416. doi:10.2460/ajvr.75.4.402

Webb PW, Weihs D (1986) Functional locomotor morphology of early life history stages of fishes. *Transactions of the American Fisheries Society* **115**, 115–127. doi:10.1577/1548-8659(1986)115<115:FLMOEL>2.0.CO;2

Weir M, Rajić A, Dutil L, Cernicchiaro N, Uhland F, Mercier B, Tuševljak N (2012) Zoonotic bacteria, antimicrobial use and antimicrobial resistance in ornamental fish: a systematic review of the existing research and survey of aquaculture-allied professionals. *Epidemiology and Infection* **140**, 192–206. doi:10.1017/S0950268811001798

Wells RMG, McNeil H, MacDonald JA (2005) Fish hypnosis: induction of an atonic immobility reflex. *Marine and Freshwater Behaviour and Physiology* **38**, 71–78. doi:10.1080/10236240400029341

White GE, Brown C (2013) Site fidelity and homing behaviour in intertidal fishes. *Marine Biology* **160**, 1365–1372. doi:10.1007/s00227-013-2188-6

Williams A, Althaus F, Schlacher TA (2015) Towed camera imagery and benthic sled catches provide different views of seamount benthic diversity. *Limnology and Oceanography, Methods* **13**(2), e10007. doi:10.1002/lom3.10007

Williams A, Osterhage D, Althaus F, Ryan T, Green M, Pogonoski JA (2021) Very large spawning aggregation of a deep-sea eel: magnitude and status. *Journal of Marine Science and Engineering* **9**, 723. doi:10.3390/jmse9070723

Wong MYL, Gordon P, Paijmans KC, Rees MJ (2019) Finding rockpool fishes: a quantitative comparison of non-invasive and invasive methods for assessing abundance, species richness and assemblage structure. *Environmental Biology of Fishes* **102**, 81–94. doi:10.1007/s10641-019-0846-3

Wood E (2001) *Collection of Coral Reef Fish for Aquaria: Global Trade, Conservation Issues and Management Strategies*. Marine Conservation Society, Ross-on-Wye, UK.

Zeller DC (1997) Home range and activity patterns of the coral trout *Plectropomus leopardus* (*Serranidae*). *Marine Ecology Progress Series* **154**, 65–77. doi:10.3354/meps154065

31 Sharks, rays and chimaeras

Bonnie J. Holmes, Samuel M. Williams, Adam Barnett, Kathy A. Townsend, Barbara E. Wueringer, Ross K. Daley, Christine L. Dudgeon, Asia Armstrong, Christopher Henderson, Brittany Finucci, Charlie Huveneers, Paul A. Butcher, Kevin Crook, Jamie Hicks, Cassandra L. Rigby, Christopher Izzo, Michelle A. Treloar, Adrian N. Gutteridge and Stephen M. Taylor

INTRODUCTION

Sharks, rays and chimaeras comprise one of the two major taxonomic classes of contemporary fishes, the chondrichthyes. Chondrichthyans are all jawed vertebrates with paired fins and nares (nostrils), V-shaped denticles and cartilaginous skeletons. The class is divided into two subclasses: the Elasmobranchii (sharks, rays, skates, and sawfish) and the Holocephali (chimaeras). Over 320 species are described in Australia (Last and Stevens 2009), and range considerably in size, form, function and the habitats they occupy. Ecologically important, chondrichthyans occupy many niches in marine, estuarine and freshwater environments. Lethal sampling methods are often used for studying chondrichthyans, and particularly for collecting biological samples that cannot be collected from live animals. Consequently, methods for euthanasia and lethal sampling are provided in more detail in Chapter 13.

FLAT SKATES AND RAYS

Kathy A. Townsend, Asia Armstrong, Kevin Crook, Jamie Hicks and Michelle A. Treloar

Characteristics

Defined by their dorsoventrally flattened, disc-shaped bodies, rays are the largest subgroup in the class Chondrichthyes. The group currently comprises over 633 species from 26 different families worldwide (Last *et al.* 2016). While Rhinopristiformes (guitarfishes and sawfishes) are orders of ray, they are addressed separately because of their conservation status and unique morphological adaptations. The remaining groups are commonly known as flat skates and rays (now referred to as 'rays'). Australia has a high diversity of rays currently consisting of 120 species from three different orders; 54 species are known only from Australian waters. They can be found across a wide range of ecological niches, from freshwater to marine, from water < 50 cm deep through to abyssal depths. Despite their abundance and importance for commercial fisheries and ecotourism, basic ecological data are lacking for most ray species (Last *et al.* 2016).

All rays have a cartilaginous skeleton and dermal denticles of varying size and density. The defensive caudal sting(s) found on the tail of many rays consists of modified denticles (Last *et al.* 2016). While common among the group, not all rays possess a stinging barb. For example, several species from the family Mobulidae and the order Torpediniformes have lost this function over evolutionary time, replacing the need for a defensive stinging barb with size and swimming speed (e.g. Mobulidae) or the ability to generate an electric field (e.g. Torpediniformes) (Last and Stevens 2009).

Biology and behaviour

Many rays and skates have a benthic lifestyle and do not range over large areas. Skates generally use relatively small habitat areas over the short term but may undergo seasonal migrations to mate, give birth, and/or find suitable attachment sites for egg cases (Last *et al.* 2016). Juvenile stingrays (Dasyatidae) often use shallow coastal embayments as nursery areas and can be highly resident to these areas, but may migrate daily between intertidal and subtidal areas with the tide. Mature individuals migrate to deeper waters; however, movements of adult stingrays are largely unknown. Eagle rays (Aetobatidae) and cownose rays (Rhinopteridae) undertake seasonal migrations from temperate areas in the summer to the tropics or subtropics during winter (Ajemian and Powers 2014). Devil rays (Mobulidae) are capable of navigating large distances < 1000 km and making vertical migrations from surface waters down to depths of > 1000 m to feed (Thorrold *et al.* 2014).

Rays generally occupy the middle trophic levels of aquatic food webs, although some (e.g. Gymnuridae, Torpedinidae, Rajidae) may feed at similar levels to top predators (Jacobsen and Bennett 2013). Prey capture and processing appears to have been a strong evolutionary pressure on batoid fishes and has resulted in diverse diets and jaw morphologies (Dean *et al.* 2007). Many rays have evolved jaw articulations and musculature that allow them to process hard-bodied prey internally and eject undigestible items (e.g. bivalve shells) (Kolmann *et al.* 2016). The two largest species of Mobulids have large, terminal mouths and filter plankton from the water column through modified gill plates. All other taxa have ventrally located mouths and are mostly benthic foragers with diets consisting of crustaceans, polychaetes, molluscs and small fish.

Like other chondrichthyans, rays have an internal mode of fertilisation. Rajiformes are oviparous and young develop in egg cases that are deposited on the seafloor by females. All other species bear live young and young are nourished through yolk-sac vivipary or lipid histotrophy, which is unique among the Myliobatiformes. The provision of lipid-rich uterine milk (histotroph) to nourish young is highly efficient and allows embryos to develop and grow more rapidly than from yolk-sac vivipary (Last *et al.* 2016).

Capture and handling

Rays can tire very easily during capture with nets, trawls and hooks, making them vulnerable to predation. Most netting operations can collect large numbers of animals, but rays can be injured and die if left in nets for long periods. Hooks can be used with minimal damage, but dislocation of the jaw can occur in large heavy species, especially when collecting from deep waters.

Prior to handling rays, the location of the defensive caudal sting(s) must be determined, and the tail restrained. Once the tail is controlled the animal can be lifted with an appropriately sized hand net. Small to medium rays without caudal stings (i.e. skates and shovelnose rays) may be handled carefully wearing protective gloves. Nets, lifting harnesses and mechanical lifting devices are recommended for large species. Special consideration needs to be made when handling electric rays, which are susceptible to skin damage because of reduced denticle protection. Their ability to produce a pulse-like current (up to 200 V and 35 A) can injure the handler (Last *et al.* 2016). Rubber gloves and rubber boots are recommended when handling live electric rays to reduce the possibility of electrical shock.

Tank design and life support systems (LSS) should be a primary consideration for keeping rays in captivity. The size of tank required will depend on the species, stocking density, ontogeny and behaviour to provide sufficient space for natural swimming behaviour. Tank drainage and input lines should be considered and located in such a way to prevent injury or entrapment. A seawater source and a recirculation pump are critical for water exchange. If freshwater is used to manufacture artificial seawater or contain freshwater species, it should be analysed for contaminants and filtered or treated before use (Smith *et al.* 2004).

Monitoring and maintaining water quality are imperative as an imbalance of parameters can have detrimental effects. LSS should monitor and control dissolved oxygen, temperature, salinity, pH and nutrient concentrations. Natural or artificial lighting should be used to provide 12 h day/night photoperiods. Captive rays are primarily fed crustaceans, cephalopods or worms distributed *ad libitum* or as a percentage of body mass. Tanks should be cleaned regularly and particularly after feeding to remove biological waste, and to avoid ammonia toxicity and bacterial and fungal infections. Parasites, infections and disease are common in captive rays and can often be treated with medication and freshwater dips (Smith *et al.* 2004).

Many species of chondrichthyans are tagged and released to understand their movement patterns in time and space. These data can be critical in gaining a better understanding of habitat use, seasonal or prey drivers, and discovering other associated oceanographic or ocean chemistry factors that influence movements. Information on movements, growth rates, relative abundance and mortality obtained from tags can also assist in scientific assessments of shark and ray populations. Photographic identification, conventional tagging, acoustic telemetry and satellite tags have been used to study the movements and home ranges for the species in this group.

Tissue samples can be acquired from large pelagic rays for genetic investigations, stable isotope and fatty acid analysis (Couturier *et al.* 2013). Samples can be collected using SCUBA or via free diving using a modified Hawaiian sling spear, resulting in a biopsy (< 5 mm) taken from the animal, and leaving only a small puncture wound. The target area is the dorsal or ventral musculature on the pectoral wing, away from the organs and body cavity of the animal. Alternatively, pig ear notchers can be used to obtain a fin clip from the pelvic region of rays captured in gill or seine nets (Newby *et al.* 2014). Mucus sampling, where a toothbrush is used to remove the mucus from the dermal surface of the ray, is an alternative technique for acquiring genetic samples from rays (Burgess *et al.* 2018). This method is considered minimally invasive, comparative to tissue sampling via fin clips or biopsy, and can be conducted on free swimming or benthic rays.

Veterinary considerations

Tagging and biological sampling are invasive minor procedures often required during research on species within this group. Historically, anaesthetics or sedatives have not been widely used as processing needs to happen rapidly, and chondrichthyans also rarely exhibit a stimulus response to tagging procedures involving dorsal fin or subdermal skin intrusions (e.g. biopsies). Recent publications suggest that, physiologically, chondrichthyans have very few unmyelinated nerve fibres, which differentiates them from mammals in how they perceive pain (Smith and Lewin 2009; Sneddon 2018). For internal tagging procedures, application of a local anaesthesia may be considered based on the species-specific morphology and behaviour of each chondrichthyan (Readman *et al.* 2017).

Anaesthesia

It should be noted that the effects of anaesthetics are largely unknown for most chondrichthyans (Neiffer and Stamper 2009; Cooke *et al.* 2016), although some broad guidelines exist for the group (Mylniczenko *et al.* 2014). For more details on when anaesthetics or sedatives can be safely used in this group, refer to Chapter 13.

Blood collection

Blood collection from rays can be done via caudal, pectoral or cardiac venipuncture, while the ray is under sedation or manual restraint (Phillips *et al.* 2016). In many batoid species, the presence of cartilage, lack of specific landmarks and small vessel size can make blood collection difficult. The mesopterygial vein, which is easily landmarked for several Myliobatiform species, can provide dependable vascular access for blood sampling (Westmoreland *et al.* 2019) (see Chapter 13 for details). Faecal samples for dietary analysis in rays can be obtained opportunistically during in-water activities, or during capture (Poulakis *et al.* 2017).

Euthanasia

Killing and euthanasia of rays is often undertaken for the collection of internal tissues that cannot otherwise be non-lethally sampled in the chondrichthyans. Research may include (but not limited to) reproduction, age and growth, brain form and function, diet, sensory biology, bioaccumulation, biomechanics, homeostasis and taxonomy. General operating procedures outlining the accepted methods for euthanasia can be found in Chapter 13.

Infectious pathogens

Disease in chondrichthyans is not well studied. Water mould is an infectious freshwater, fungus-like microorganism of the class Oomycota, and has been described in freshwater rays, particularly in captivity. Once infected, the teeth and mouth of the ray exhibit a yellow fuzzy appearance, and severe cases can result in excess teeth shedding, lethargy and loss of body condition (Reynolds *et al.* 2017). Continuous exposure to salt (NaCl) at a dosage of 3.0–4.5 mg/L for a minimum of 6 weeks should eliminate water mould (Reynolds *et al.* 2017).

Chondrichthyans do house a significant number of internal and external parasites, although this is also an area of research that is significantly understudied. Parasites including copepod, nematode and cestodes are commonly found in the external surface, gill filaments, digestive tract and flesh of rays. The coccidan parasite *Eimeria southwelli* has been reported in both spotted eagle rays (*Aetobatus narinari*) and cownose rays (*Rhinoptera bonasus*), but is likely to occur in all myliobatid species. The parasite causes coelomic effusion and is lethal in *R. bonasus* (Dove *et al.* 2017).

General operating procedures

A range of research methods and procedures relevant to studying flat skates and rays are covered in more detail in Chapter 13. Netting and observational methods that apply to freshwater animals may also apply to these species (Chapter 14). Veterinary methods that may be relevant are covered in Chapter 16.

GUITARFISH, WEDGEFISH AND SAWFISH

Barbara E. Wueringer, Christopher Henderson and Bonnie J. Holmes

Characteristics

The order Rhinopristiformes comprises five families with 15 extant Australian species (Pristidae, Glaucostegidae, Rhinidae, Rhinobatidae, Trygonorrhinidae). The Rhinopristiformes are often referred to as the shark-like rays, given that their shark-like tail differentiates them morphologically from most other batoids. Moreover, their pectoral fins are not fused into a disk, like in other batoids. While sawfish possess an elongated, saw-like rostrum, the other groups including fiddler rays are characterised by either a flatted acutely pointed head (the *Aptychotrema*, thus the term 'shovelnose'), or by a broadly rounded snout (present in the *Trygonorrhina*, often referred to as 'banjo rays', and also in the bowmouth guitarfish, *Rhina ancylostoma*).

Sawfishes can reach up to 7 m total length (TL), making them the largest of all shark-like rays. Sawfishes are largely benthic, with narrow sawfish (*Anoxypristis cuspidata*) occurring the furthest offshore (Peverell 2005). Once common in tropical and subtropical coastal habitats around the world, they have long been considered the most endangered family of all elasmobranchs (Dulvy *et al.* 2016). However, recent assessments indicate that wedgefishes are now also critically endangered (Kyne *et al.* 2020). The guitarfishes and wedgefishes are shark-like batoids that also inhabit coastal waters.

Biology and behaviour

The home ranges of sawfish are extremely small, considering the animals can grow to very large sizes. While juveniles remain inshore and in estuaries and shallow riverine waters, adult sawfish probably move further offshore into deeper waters (Peverell 2005). Not much is known about their movements in Australian waters. The home ranges of giant guitarfish are also small and driven by the distribution of nearshore habitats (mangroves forests and seagrass meadows); however, they do move further offshore throughout the year (Henderson *et al.* 2018).

Of the fiddler rays, the three species of *Aptychotrema* (shovelnose rays) are spatially distributed between the Australian west coast (*A. vincentiana*), the Timor Sea (*A. timorensis*) and the east coast (*A. rostrata*) without overlap between ranges. The *Trygonorrhina* are similar, with the eastern fiddler ray (*T. fasciata*) restricted to the east coast, and the southern fiddler ray (*T. dumerilii*) inhabiting cooler southern Australian waters. Little is known about species-specific movements and fine scale or seasonal habitat use within these areas.

All Rhinopristiformes consume a range of benthic invertebrates, including prawns, shrimps, crabs, and molluscs (Last *et al.* 2016). Some, including sawfishes, also prey upon small teleosts. Guitarfishes and wedgefishes are important benthic predators that feed on invertebrates and fish in seagrass meadows, mangrove fringes, surf zones and sandy coastal bays. The elongated rostrum of sawfish, the 'saw', is used to detect and stun prey (Wueringer *et al.* 2012). Rhinobatids use their disc to pin prey down.

All Rhinopristiformes are aplacental viviparous. Sawfish give birth to up to 12 live young (Peverell, 2009), while bottlenose wedgefish (*Rhynchobatus Australiae*) have between seven and 19 pups (Kyne *et al.* 2020). The *Trygonorrhina* have small litters of two to six pups, while the *Aptychotrema* litters are slightly larger between four and 18 pups (Bray 2017).

Capture and handling

Sawfish, large guitarfish and wedgefish are most easily captured in bottom-set gill nets. The sawfish's saw, and the acutely pointed head of wedgefish, easily entangle in the mesh. The head shape of bowmouth guitarfish often prevents their entanglement, allowing the animals to move along nets uncaptured (B. Wueringer, pers. obs.). Large wedgefishes and giant guitarfishes (*Glaucostegus typus*) can also be caught using bottom set lines with 2 m long tracers and circle hooks to reduce the likelihood of deep hooking. When groups of smaller sawfish and giant guitarfish are observed resting in shallow waters, they can be caught by cast-netting.

Many procedures used for the shark-like rays are similar to those used for sharks. Shark-like rays do not possess a venomous spine like other batoids, and their oral teeth are small and not as sharp or pointy as shark teeth. Handling procedures should consider the size of the animal and the handler's expertise. Sawfish will use their saw to defend themselves, producing fast lateral swipes. Narrow sawfish are the most susceptible to injury during handling, so any manipulations should be kept minimal.

Smaller animals (< 2 m) can be brought on board a vessel to be tagged/sampled in a cradle. While sawfish can be maintained out of the water for a few minutes without having their gills ventilated, placing them in a cradle with water is preferred. Continuous flow of water over their spiracle/gills will aid respiration but, unlike sharks, no pump mouthpiece is required. In sawfish, and probably other shark-like rays, tonic immobility can be induced by placing the animals with their ventral side facing up (Figure 31.1). However, even when the animal is placed dorsal side up, it is recommended to always secure the base of the saw/rostrum with a secure grip, preventing or reducing the impact of lateral swipes of the rostrum. If done with two hands, doing so will also cover the eyes of the animal, which will reduce stress. In guitarfish and wedgefish a similar grip on the rostrum near the nostrils will also reduce stress, calming them and making them easier and safer to handle.

Larger sawfish or wedgefish are best secured to the side of a vessel, with a rope around the base of the saw/pectoral, with the rope tied to the stern, and a tail rope tied to the bow. This method allows the animals to ventilate their gills in the water, and reduces the likelihood of animal handling personnel to be struck by a swiping saw. The vessel should be oriented into the current, allowing water to flow into the gills. Like other elasmobranchs, sawfish and guitarfish can change their body colouration in response to discomfort, and the appearance of pink blotches on the underside of an animal is a clear indication of stress.

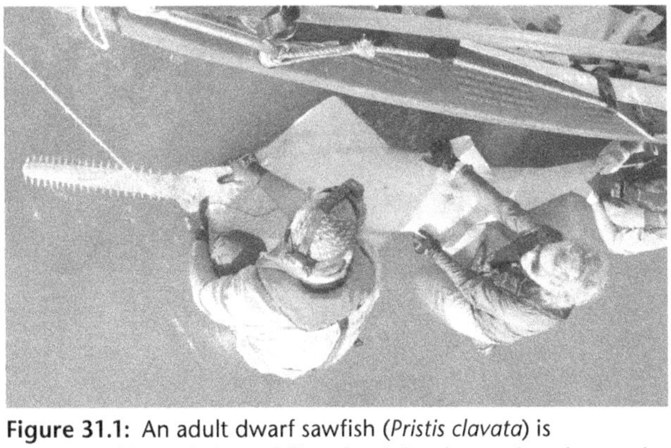

Figure 31.1: An adult dwarf sawfish (*Pristis clavata*) is maintained in tonic immobility after it has been placed ventral side up. The animal is additionally secured with rostrum and tail ropes, and by two people, with a secure grip near the base of the rostrum and on the anal fins, while a blood sample is taken from the caudal vein. Photo supplied by Barbara Wueringer.

Conventional tagging methods, acoustic telemetry and satellite tags have been used to study the movements and home ranges for the species in this group. In sawfishes, satellite tags should not be fin mounted, as these animals can lower their dorsal fins when they move into shallow waters (B. Wueringer, pers. obs.). Previous studies that used this technique resulted in fewer location fixes (Stevens *et al.* 2008) than those conducted with tethered tags that trail behind the first dorsal fin (Guttridge *et al.* 2015). Some researchers prefer dart tags over rototags for mark–recapture studies, because of biofouling (Kyne and Pillans 2014), but in largetooth sawfish (*P. pristis*) rototags have been successfully used in long-term monitoring studies (Lear *et al.* 2019). Fin clips can be obtained from captured animals for genetic studies (Green *et al.* 2018). However, because of the endangered status of many Pristidae, Rhinidae and Rhinobatidae, lethal sampling is mostly prohibited. Conversely, members of the Trygonorrhinidae, like the eastern shovelnose ray (*A. rostrata*), are heavily fished in commercial and recreational fisheries, although corresponding biological studies are in their infancy.

Veterinary considerations

Anaesthesia

The effects of anaesthetics are largely unknown for most chondrichthyans (Neiffer and Stamper 2009; Cooke *et al.* 2016), although some broad guidelines exist for the group (Mylniczenko *et al.* 2014). Recent publications suggest that, physiologically, chondrichthyans have very few unmyelinated nerve fibres, which differentiates them from mammals in how they perceive pain (Smith and Lewin 2009; Sneddon 2018). Historically, anaesthetics or sedatives have not been widely used as processing needs to happen rapidly, and chondrichthyans also rarely exhibit a stimulus response to tagging procedures involving dorsal fin or subdermal skin intrusions (e.g. biopsies). Instead, researchers often secure large elasmobranchs for procedures using tonic immobility, an innate reversible paralysis through dorso-ventral inversion which facilitates a fast recovery (Kessel and Hussey 2015; Williamson *et al.* 2018). For internal tagging procedures, application of a local anaesthesia may be considered based on the species-specific morphology and behaviour of each chondrichthyan (Readman *et al.* 2017).

In controlled captive environments, isoeugenol has been used to sedate pristids at a dosage of 20–25 mL/m^3, raised slowly over a period of 15–20 min (White *et al.* 2017). However, a high variability of response to sedatives has been observed within this taxon, so pristids should be continually monitored for adverse reactions, or the potential for overdose (White *et al.* 2017). For more details on when anaesthetics or sedatives could be safely used in this group, refer to Chapter 13.

Euthanasia

Details of methods of euthanasia can be found in Chapter 13. Due to the conservation status of sawfish, research permits received by researchers may not allow euthanasia in the field, and animals that have been captured in an injured state must instead be returned to the water immediately.

Infectious pathogens

A low number of infectious agents have been identified in chondrichthyans. Largetooth sawfish are euryhaline and can develop fungal infections when housed in freshwater. Saltwater may be preferred for long-term housing (Lyle Squire Jnr, pers. comm.). Pristids can also be affected by sporozoans (parasitic, spore-forming protozoans). These parasites form small white spots on the dorsum and infected pristids can display increased ventilation rates and become anorectic and dehydrated (White *et al.* 2017). The only documented successful treatment for a sporozoan infection is a series of five copper baths, with a 48 h interval between each treatment (White *et al.* 2017). Little information on infectious diseases in other Rhinopristiformes is available.

General operating procedures

Research methods and procedures relevant to studying flat skates and rays are covered in more detail in Chapter 13. Methods that apply to freshwater animals may also apply to these species (Chapter 14). Veterinary methods are covered in Chapter 16.

CHIMAERAS AND DEEP-SEA SHARKS

Ross K. Daley, Brittany Finucci and Cassandra L. Rigby

Characteristics

Chimaeras and deep-sea sharks belong to five orders of chondrichthyans that occur mainly in offshore waters; most are demersal, living mostly within 50 m of the seafloor and a few are pelagic (Last and Stevens 2009). Four of the orders represent sharks: Hexanchiformes (frilled sharks and cowsharks), Pristiophoriformes (sawsharks), Squaliformes (dogfishes and their relatives) and Squatiniformes (angelsharks). The other order included here is the Chimaeriformes (elephantfishes, chimaeras and spookfishes), which differ from sharks in having a single pair of gill openings, a beak-shaped feeding structure, and an upper jaw fused to the cranium. The order Carcharhiniformes also contains Australian deep-sea shark species in the families Scyliorhinidae and Pentanchidae.

Several common factors affect animal survivorship, welfare and stress recovery of these taxa. With the transition to deeper bathomes (seafloor depth zones), the influence of seasonal and geographical differences in light and temperature is reduced. At the same time, the effects of pressure, reduced light, lower temperatures and sparse food increase to extremes. Fortunately, most species are small (< 2 m TL) and easy to handle, reducing stress for both animals and researchers.

Biology and behaviour

For species with strong benthic feeding habitat associations, such as angelsharks and sawsharks, movements associated with feeding may be at a fine scale, such as a single reef patch. Breeding movements tend to be at larger scales. For example, sawsharks spend most of the year offshore, moving inshore to give birth in nurseries during a well-defined breeding season.

The broadnose sevengill shark (*Notorynchus cepedianus*) shows seasonal movement into bays and estuaries with males and females arriving at different times and individuals have fine-scale patterns of habitat use. After departing warmer inshore waters individuals can migrate up to 1800 km into deep water (Barnett *et al.* 2012). In the deeper waters off the continental slope, movement drivers and patterns differ from the shelf. Diel movements have been observed in both gulper sharks and cowsharks with individuals moving into shallower water during the night, then returning to deeper waters during the day. These movements can be either across the sea floor or into the water column. This pattern is associated with the daily vertical migration of nekton near the continental slope (Daley *et al.* 2015).

The bluntnose sixgill shark (*Hexanchus griseus*) shows a remarkable bathymetric range. Immature females move up and down the slope over a wide home territory of between 600 and 1100 m with excursions to depths 1500 m (Carey and Clark 1995). Home territory size is a key consideration for effective conservation in marine protected areas (Daley *et al.* 2019). Effective conservation requires species-specific understanding as even very closely related species can have very different patterns. For example, gulper sharks (*Centrophorus zeehaani*) tracked in Australia showed high residency in a fishery closure area 100 km wide over more than a year. By contrast leafscale gulper sharks (*C. squamosus*) tracked in the Atlantic left a marine protected area and moved more than 1800 km in 80 days (Rodríguez-Cabello and Sánchez 2014).

Each order utilises different strategies to hunt and capture their prey. All chimaeras have a specialised beak-like dentition for capturing and crushing hard-shelled benthic invertebrates such as bivalves and crustaceans. Their diet may also include small fish and some deep-sea chimaeras have a sensory proboscis for finding prey in darkness. Cowsharks are predators of sharks and rays and opportunistically of marine mammals. Sawsharks have an elongate snout with sensory barbels for finding prey near the seafloor. The snout has sensory lateral teeth. Angelsharks, which resemble rays (but have gill openings on the side of the head), feed on crustaceans and molluscs while partially buried in the sand and will ambush passing fish.

Dogfishes and their close relatives eat a range of prey types with different species consuming squid, large demersal fish, small vertical migrating fish, and opportunistically marine mammals. They have similar dentitions consisting of pointed fork-like upper teeth and overlapping knife-like lower teeth. This allows these sharks to feed on larger live prey by twisting their bodies to cut chunks of flesh out of their prey/hosts (Hallett and Daley 2011).

Deep-sea elasmobranchs bear live young; the chimaeras lay eggs. Both have internal fertilisation and are generally long-lived and late maturing, making them particularly vulnerable to human impacts. Most chondrichthyans segregate by sex and size classes for much of the year, either geographically or by depth. This may help to partition food types or protect the young.

Capture and handling

Species-specific considerations for deep-sea chondrichthyans include capture stress as they are brought to the surface from depth, disorientation from light, disturbed buoyancy regulation from changes pressure, and accelerated enzyme reactions from temperature changes. Stress is minimised by eliminating any delays in getting the animals back into the water. To reduce capture stress, demersal hook and set-line capture methods are preferred over nets. Once out of the water, captured chondrichthyans should be treated individually and efficiently. The effects of capture stress can be minimised by limiting soak time to a few hours. Setting at night during winter can reduce temperature shock and light stress. Housing for longer than a few hours can lead to mortality and is likely to prevent safe transport, even at sea. For small chondrichthyans, a medium-sized holding tank (500 L) will allow tags to be fitted to animals while remaining in water. Bubbling oxygen through tank water is not essential as deep-sea chondrichthyans are adapted to low oxygen.

Conventional tagging, acoustic telemetry, archival and satellite tags have been used to study the movements and home ranges for these taxa. The main type of conventional tag for use on deep-sea sharks is a spaghetti dart tag, which is attached at the base of the dorsal fin. Cattle ear tags are alternatively used for gulper sharks and species with very tough skin. Acoustic telemetry has had very limited use on the continental slope because of increased capture stress (additional time out of water to fit tags), high costs and the high risk of loss of deployed acoustic receiver stations required on the seafloor to receive shark tag detections. In gulper sharks because of problems with liver swelling, tags are mainly fitted to the dorsal fin (Figure 31.2), rather than internally. Internal acoustic transmitters can be implanted in the body cavity in other species.

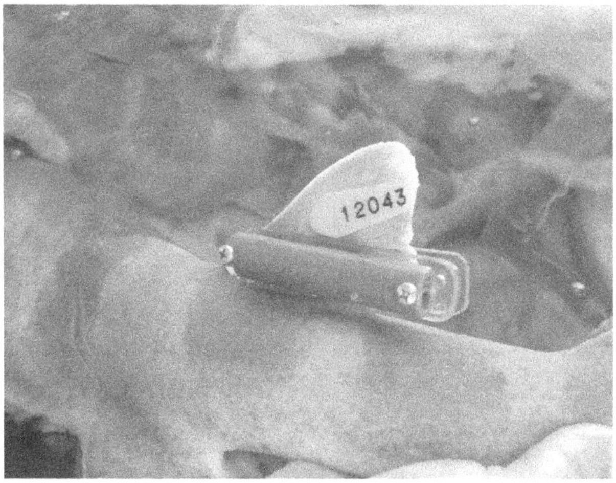

Figure 31.2: Dorsal-fin mounted transmitter and cattle ear tag for sharks with tough skin. Photo by Ross Daley.

Ecological patterns and movements of deep-sea sharks have also been studied using pop-up satellite tags. This method has lower overall costs than passive acoustic tracking in the deepsea because the data are recovered via satellite rather than sending ships to sea to recover receiver moorings. The main limitation of these tags is that transmission location must be estimated using additional environmental data. The availability of environmental data in the deepsea is patchy, leading to uncertainty in position estimates. Biological sampling of deep-sea chondrichthyans may involve fin clips and biopsies, epidermal swabbing, blood sampling and stomach content collection depending on the research program objectives.

Veterinary considerations

Tagging and biological sampling are invasive and require minor medical procedures on species within this group. Historically, anaesthetics or sedatives have not been widely used as processing needs to happen rapidly, and chondrichthyans also rarely exhibit a stimulus response to tagging procedures involving dorsal fin or subdermal skin intrusions (e.g. biopsies). Recent publications suggest that physiologically, chondrichthyans have very few unmyelinated nerve fibres, which differentiates them from mammals in how they perceive pain (Smith and Lewin 2009; Sneddon 2018). For internal tagging procedures, application of a local anaesthesia may be considered based on the species-specific morphology and behaviour of each chondrichthyan (Readman *et al.* 2017).

Anaesthesia

The effects of anaesthetics are largely unknown for most chondrichthyans (Neiffer and Stamper 2009; Cooke *et al.* 2016), although some broad guidelines exist for the group (Mylniczenko *et al.* 2014). For more details on when anaesthetics or sedatives could be safely used in this group, refer to Chapter 13. For deep-sea chondrichthyes, it is also important to consider post-release mortality as they may need to swim significant depths to return to their habitats. Cages have been trialled to reduce predation as sharks are returned to depth, but this resulted in delays that caused mortality because of presumed physiological effects (Daley 2017). Depth sensors fitted to sharks released free at the surface showed low rates of predation during descent.

Euthanasia

Biological research of deep-sea chondrichthyans requires animals to be killed. See Chapter 13 for the accepted methods for killing for this group.

Infectious pathogens

Disease in chondrichthyans is poorly documented, and even more so for deep-sea species. Sharks can accumulate several internal and external parasites, often affecting specific areas of the body (e.g. gills, intestinal tract). At least two species, the Greenland shark (*Somniosus microcephalus*) and the Pacific sleeper shark (*Somniosus pacificus*), have been found to have high infection rates of the parasitic copepod *Ommatokoita elongata* (Benz *et al.* 1998). This parasite attaches to the corneas of the shark and is thought to lead to severe vision impairment and possibly blindness. The same, or a similar copepod species, has also been observed on chimaeras via *in situ* video, but has not been studied further. The parasitic barnacle (*Anelasma squalicola*) infects individuals of the lantern shark family (Etmopteridae), embedding into and feeding off the flesh of its host (Long and Waggoner 1993). Host health is likely to be dependent on parasitic load and attachment; in some cases, infection can lead to reduced vision and impaired feeding and reproductive ability.

Some of the largest and long-lived sharks, including those from the deep sea, can bioaccumulate heavy metals in their tissues, such as mercury, zinc, copper, selenium and cadmium (Pethybridge *et al.* 2010). This can result in human health concerns for consumers of shark meat.

General operating procedures

Research methods and procedures relevant to studying chimaeras and deep-sea sharks are covered in more detail in Chapter 13. Veterinary methods that may be relevant are covered in Chapter 16.

HORN SHARKS AND CARPET SHARKS

Christine L. Dudgeon, Charlie Huveneers and Christopher Izzo

Characteristics

The order Heterodontiformes (horn sharks) comprises a single family and genus, with nine species globally. The order Orectolobiformes (carpet sharks) is largely restricted to the Indo-West Pacific region, with seven families and 42 species globally. Several species are listed as threatened because of high levels of exploitation and naturally low population sizes. In Australia, wobbegongs are fished for local consumption, while the remaining species are not targeted and are only incidentally caught.

The Heterodontiformes are all similar in body form and function. They are small- or medium-sized, having enlarged, blunt heads with a prominent crest (the horn) above each eye, spined dorsal fins, and an anal fin. Their nostrils are connected to small, almost terminal mouths by a groove. They are highly patterned and have rough skin. The Port Jackson shark (*Heterodontus portusjacksoni*) is one of the most-studied species in Australia and has the widest distribution. The other two species are restricted in northern Australia reaching into warm-temperate to subtropical waters (Last and Stevens 2009).

The Orectolobiformes are highly diverse in body form and size. All species have two dorsal fins and relatively short-terminal mouths. The nostrils are flanked by barbels (rudimentary in the whale shark, *Rhincodon typus*) that are tactile sensory organs connected by nasoral grooves to the mouths (Compagno *et al.* 2005a). Most species have ornate body patterning, earning the moniker 'carpet shark'. Body size ranges from > 30 cm TL (barbelthroat catshark, *Cirrhoscyllium expolitum*) to the largest extant fish at > 20 m TL, the whale shark (Compagno *et al.* 2005b). Smaller species have more-restricted distributions. Unresolved species complexes exist in the group e.g. redescription of the genus *Hemiscyllium* (Allen *et al.* 2016). Larger Ginglymostomatidae and Stegostomatidae species are more widely distributed, spanning two oceanic regions. The largest Orectolobid (gulf wobbegong, *Orectolobus halei*), reaching 3 m TL, is an Australian endemic. Whale sharks have a circumglobal distribution in tropical and warm temperate waters and has a pelagic lifestyle, which contrasts with the other benthic and demersal species in the order (Compagno *et al.* 2005a).

Biology and behaviour

Residency and movements of Heterodontidae are mostly known for Port Jackson sharks off New South Wales, and characterised by high levels of philopatry interceded with large-scale migrations (Bass *et al.* 2017). Movement in Orectolobiformes are varied, ranging from strong site fidelity to trans-oceanic movements. Orectolobidae show limited movements and dispersal. Distribution and abundance surveys infer strong site attachment, with high resighting rates of individuals at fixed locations (Lee *et al.* 2014), yet movements of ~230 km have also been detected (Hoenner *et al.* 2018). Populations separated by < 200 km show a high degree of genetic differentiation (Corrigan *et al.* 2008).

Leopard sharks undertake extensive (thousands of kilometres) seasonal movements throughout their subtropical distribution (Dudgeon *et al.* 2013). Aggregations and strong site-fidelity have been observed along coastal sites in eastern Australia during warmer months (Dudgeon *et al.* 2013). Satellite telemetry has revealed whale sharks undertake large-scale movements (Robinson *et al.* 2017) potentially resulting in panmixia (Vignaud *et al.* 2014); however, photographic identification shows little connectivity among aggregations (Norman *et al.* 2017).

Many Heterodontiformes and Orectolobiformes are generalist foragers, feeding on benthic invertebrates (including cephalopods, molluscs, crustaceans and echinoderms) and small fishes. Often nocturnal foragers, they hunt close to the substrate or use their camouflaging pattern to ambush prey (Last and Stevens 2009). Whale sharks feed at or close to the surface, employing suction filter-feeding at seasonally productive areas, such as fish spawning grounds or zooplankton blooms (Rowat and Brooks 2012).

Among Heterodontiformes and Orectolobiformes, two distinct reproductive modes are present. Details on the timing and duration of reproductive cycles are lacking for many species. Available data suggest size at maturity is large (50–80%) relative to maximum size (Last and Stevens 2009). Heterodontidae, Hemiscylliidae, Parascylliidae and leopard sharks (*Stegostoma tigrinum*) are oviparous, producing fertilised eggs protected in tough cases (Walker 2020). Egg morphology is species-specific, and eggs are generally deposited on the substrate. Port Jackson sharks position their spiral eggs in fissures of shallow rocky reefs (Last and Stevens 2009). Numbers of eggs range from 10–16 to 100+ eggs per year, and egg development ranges from 6 months to 12–18 months (Harahush *et al.* 2007). Hatching success is variable, influenced by environmental factors and predators, including cannibalism.

Orectolobidae, Brachaeluridae, the tawny nurse shark (*Nebrius ferrugineus*) and the whale shark possess yolk-sac viviparity; fertilised eggs are contained in an egg envelope *in utero* (Walker 2020). Tawny nurse sharks are the only Orectolobiforme to display uterine cannibalism (Teshima *et al.* 1995). Orectolobidae and Brachaeluridae have biennial or triennial reproductive cycles (Walker 2020). Embryos gestate for 9–12 months before parturition (Huveneers *et al.* 2007). Litters vary among species from 4–18 to 304 pups of various stages of development in the single pregnant whale shark examined (Joung *et al.* 1996). Pupping and egg laying are often seasonal, with timing species- and location-specific.

Capture and handling

Smaller horn and carpet sharks (< 1.6 m TL) can be caught by hand or hand nets. Some medium sharks can be captured by larger hand nets on scuba (including wobbegongs). Leopard sharks can be sedated using the species-specific tonic immobility tail grab (Williamson *et al.* 2018). Line fishing is used to capture most sharks over 1–1.5 m TL (e.g. Orectolobidae and Ginglymostomatidae). More recently, whale sharks have been caught and held in large nets.

Many species in this group are buccal pumpers and can withstand being immobile in aquaria for extended periods. *Hemiscyllium* and *Heterodontus* can withstand hypoxic conditions for several hours (Williamson *et al.* 2018) and can be kept out of the water for a few minutes with no impact to the animal. Larger species that are brought out of the water (e.g. *Stegostoma*) can be placed upside down for tonic immobility and have clean seawater pumped over the gills (Williamson *et al.* 2018). Heterodontiformes and Orectolobiformes (including whale sharks) have been maintained in captivity for extended durations (> 10 years) and have reproduced successfully (Lee *et al.* 2015).

Conventional tagging, acoustic telemetry, archival and satellite tags have been used to study the movements and home ranges for the species in this group. The ornate patterning present on many species in this group facilitates photographic-identification studies, including public contributions to surveys. A range of non-lethal approaches commonly used for research on live horn sharks may include blood draws, fin clipping, cloacal swabbing or gastric lavages, and/or ultrasound.

Veterinary considerations

Anaesthesia

The effects of anaesthetics are largely unknown for most chondrichthyans (Neiffer and Stamper 2009; Cooke *et al.* 2016), although some broad guidelines exist for the group (Mylniczenko *et al.* 2014). For more details on when anaesthetics or sedatives could be safely used in this group, refer to Chapter 13.

Euthanasia

Critical research to understand the life history parameters and population assessments of chondrichthyans often requires lethal sampling (Heupel and Simpfendorfer 2010). Chapter 13 outlines acceptable methods of killing in this group.

Infectious pathogens

Infectious diseases in chondrichthyans are not well studied. Chondrichthyans do house a significant number of internal and external parasites that may be zoonoses, although research in this field is still in its infancy. In a study on captive *S. tigrinum*, metazoan, protozoan and fungal infections were documented in the intestine, liver, kidney, spleen, brain and eyes. The environmental source of infection was traced to the introduction of wild caught specimens to captivity, with some protozoan infections causing mortality (Watson and Janse 2017).

General operating procedures

Research methods and procedures relevant to studying horn and carpet sharks are covered in more detail in Chapter 13. Some methods that apply to freshwater animals may also apply to these species (Chapter 14). Veterinary methods that may be relevant are covered in Chapter 16.

MACKEREL SHARKS

Adam Barnett, Charlie Huveneers and Paul A. Butcher

Characteristics

The order Lamniformes is diverse and includes the only species of sharks to have endothermic capabilities (families Lamnidae and Alopiidae), plankton feeders, the fastest moving sharks, top predators, and deep-sea species. Thirteen species occur within Australian waters (representing families Alopiidae, Cetorhinidae, Lamnidae, Mechachasmidae, Mitsukurinidae, Odontaspididae, Carchariidae and Pseudocarcharhiidae). Some are not often seen, probably because of their preference for pelagic waters, and low abundance. Research in Australia has predominantly focused on white (*Carcharodon carcharias*), shortfin mako (*Isurus oxyrinchus*) and grey nurse (*Carcharias taurus*) sharks, with some research on thresher sharks (Alopiidae). White sharks and grey nurse sharks are protected in Australia. Shortfin makos and to a lesser extent common thresher sharks are targeted by recreational and game fishing. Makos, threshers and porbeagle (*Lamna nasus*) are by-catch species in pelagic longline fisheries.

Lamniformes are generally characterised by cylindrical bodies, large mouths extending beyond the eyes, five pairs of gill slits, two spineless dorsal fins and one anal fin. The diversity in this group is evident in several differing biological and behavioural characteristics between species. Most species in this group are large sharks attaining ~3–12 m TL, and many have a wide geographical distribution. Crocodile sharks (*Pseudocarcharias kamoharai*) are an exception, with size reaching a maximum 1.1–1.2 m TL (Kyne *et al.* 2019). All are highly migratory and move across oceanic, coastal-oceanic and deep-sea habitats. The snout is conical in most species with the exception of the megamouth shark, which has a large bulbous head, and the goblin shark, which has a flat elongated snout. Thresher sharks differ with their distinctive scythe like upper caudal fin lobe, which is equal in length to the rest of its body. The Lamnidae are powerful swimmers. Their heat-exchanging circulatory systems allow them to maintain body temperatures above those of the surrounding water (Last and Stevens 2009).

Biology and behaviour

Many Lamniformes have a circumglobal distribution and are highly mobile. Extensive movements of shortfin makos have been documented in the Pacific Ocean (Francis *et al.* 2019) and Southern Ocean (Rogers *et al.* 2015). White sharks exhibit periodic latitudinal (or longitudinal in southern Australia) movements (Bradford *et al.* 2020), but the seasonal patterns and environmental drivers of white shark distribution are not completely understood (Huveneers *et al.* 2018). Basking sharks can undertake extensive trans-oceanic migrations (Skomal *et al.* 2009). The frequency and function of these migrations are unknown. Extensive seasonal coastal migrations between summer and winter habitats have been documented for grey nurse shark populations in Australia (Otway and Ellis 2011). Distances moved by grey nurse sharks have been reported up to 2500 km (Kneebone *et al.* 2014) and vary with sex and season. Migrations are often punctuated by residency and high site fidelity for varying periods of time. Limited information on the movement of sand tiger, goblin, crocodile and megamouth sharks are available. Megamouth sharks may perform latitudinal, seasonal migrations to buffer changes in water temperature and prey availability (Watanabe and Papastamatiou 2019), but a genetic analysis suggests connectivity across the Pacific Ocean (Liu *et al.* 2018). Crocodile sharks are thought to display vertical migrations, occurring in deeper waters during the day, moving towards the surface at night (Last and Stevens 2009).

Lamniformes have a diverse diet from plankton to marine mammals. Most Lamniformes are considered second order predators feeding a medium to large fishes, while some species (i.e. white shark and mako sharks) also feed on marine mammals. Grey nurse, sand tiger and thresher sharks feed on small mesopelagic teleosts and cephalopods, while crocodile and goblin sharks can also feed on crustaceans. Megamouth and basking sharks are planktivorous species feeding on euphausiid shrimps, copepods and jellyfish.

All species in this group are livebearers (viviparous) without placenta, with nutrients supplied to developing embryos through maternal sources (matrotrophic viviparous) by feeding on other eggs continuously produced by the mother (oophagous) or by intrauterine cannibalism of other embryos (adelphophagous) (Awruch 2015). Very little to no reproductive information is available for some species (e.g. sand tiger and megamouth sharks). In general, litter sizes are small (one to eight pups), but white and shortfin mako sharks may have up to 17 and 25 pups, respectively (Last and Stevens 2009; Awruch 2015). Gestation periods are 10–15 months and neonates are large when born, up to 150 cm TL in some species (Awruch 2015).

Capture and handling

For Lamniformes it is prudent to minimise the time spent out of the water during the capture process (Rogers *et al.* 2015). Additional husbandry operations, such as keeping water flowing over the gills or providing medical grade oxygen through a bilge pump while the animal is secured, are recommended. Doing so maintains oxygen across the gills while the animal is restrained and has been reported to have a sedative effect to keep the shark calm (Bruce and Bradford 2013). For white sharks, the capture and release process does not appear to affect stress levels (Gallagher *et al.* 2019). In general, only grey nurse sharks are kept in captivity successfully (Townsend *et al.* 2015). White sharks have been trialled in aquariums in the USA and Japan, but either failed or were planned, short-term exhibits, with the longest duration in captivity being of 198 days.

Many chondrichthyan species are captured and tagged to understand their movement patterns in time and space (see earlier sub-chapters). These data can be critical in gaining a better understanding of habitat use, seasonal drivers, and associated oceanographic or ocean chemistry factors that influence movements. Tagging studies can also provide detailed information on the movement of dangerous species of sharks, assisting in the implementation of shark mitigation strategies and informing ocean users about the risk of their activities. Biological sampling of live lamnids can include tissue and blood sampling, denticle and cloacal swabbing, and stomach content analyses.

Veterinary considerations

Anaesthesia

The effects of anaesthetics are largely unknown for most chondrichthyans (Neiffer and Stamper 2009; Cooke *et al.* 2016), although some broad guidelines exist for the group (Mylniczenko *et al.* 2014). For more details on when anaesthetics or sedatives could be safely used in this group, refer to Chapter 13.

Euthanasia

Details for procedures relating to these activities can be found in Chapter 13. Lethal sampling of the protected species in this group (white and grey nurse sharks) is not possible – therefore life history information can only be obtained from deceased specimens captured as part of other commercial fishing or shark control operations.

Infectious pathogens

Infectious disease agents found in chondrichthyans are not well studied. There are claims that sharks and rays do not get cancer, which has been attributed to the properties of shark cartilage, but previous studies have documented lesions on over 21 species from nine different families of elasmobranchs (e.g. Huveneers *et al.* 2016; Brunnschweiler *et al.* 2017). Even though these ideas have now been largely debunked, sharks continue to be harvested for their cartilage to use in 'folk' medicine (Ostrander *et al.* 2004).

Chondrichthyans do house a significant number of internal and external parasites, although this is an area of research that is significantly understudied. Parasites including copepods, nematodes and cestodes are commonly found in the external surface, gill filaments, digestive tract and flesh of mackerel sharks. Some parasites have been identified as having zoonotic potential (e.g. *Giardia intestinalis*, identified in thresher sharks (*Alopias vulpinus*) (Lasek-Nesselquist *et al.* 2008). Studies of bacteria cultured from the teeth of white sharks (*Carcharodon carcharias*) detected *Vibrio alginolyticus*, *Vibrio fluvialis*, *Vibrio parahaemolyticus* and other genera, which are common in the marine environment (Buck *et al.* 1984). Any shark bite lacerations may serve as a source of these potentially infectious bacteria to humans and should be treated immediately.

General operating procedures

A range of research methods and procedures relevant to studying mackerel sharks are covered in more detail in Chapter 13. Several netting and observational methods that apply to freshwater animals may also apply to these species (Chapter 14). Veterinary methods that may be relevant are covered in Chapter 16.

GROUND SHARKS

Bonnie J. Holmes, Adrian N. Gutteridge and Stephen M. Taylor

Characteristics

The order Carcharhiniformes, or ground sharks, are the most speciose global shark fauna, with over 10 families and > 282 species described globally. Within Australian waters there are seven families (Scyliorhinidae, Pentanchidae, Pseudotriakidae, Triakidae, Hemigaleidae, Sphyrnidae and Carcharhinidae). These families comprise around 83 primarily coastal species; however, species such as the silky (*Carcharhinus falciformis*), blue (*Prionace glauca*) and oceanic whitetip (*Carcharhinus longimanus*) are predominantly pelagic. The Carcharhiniformes are the most commercially fished of all elasmobranchs, and fisheries management regimes for this group across Australia are significantly varied.

The Carcharhiniformes are very similar in form and function, despite occupying a vast range of different habitats. These similar morphologies can make accurate identification difficult. All Carcharhiniformes have nictitating eyelids, a mouth set behind the front of the eyes, five pairs of gill slits, spineless dorsal fins, and an anal fin (Bray 2015). The Scyliorhinidae (catsharks) are morphologically distinct from the other families by the position of their first dorsal-fin base, which is well behind the pelvic-fin base. The Triakidae (houndsharks) are characterised by a smooth leading edge of upper lobe of caudal fin, and no precaudal pits (Last and Stevens 2009). The Hemigaleidae (weasel sharks) are characterised by concave second dorsal fin margins and the presence of spiracles (Last and Stevens 2009). Compared to all Carcharhiniformes, the Sphyrnidae (hammerhead sharks) are the most easily recognisable because of their hammer-shaped heads. The ground sharks are one of the most ecologically important species to marine ecosystems. This group also comprises three of the four shark species considered most dangerous to humans (Last and Stevens 2009).

Biology and behaviour

Within the pelagic and coastal zones, the whaler sharks (Carcharhinidae) are the most common in warm temperate and tropical seas (Compagno 2005). Several species can also tolerate freshwater and move into those habitats to pup (e.g. the bull shark, *Carcharhinus leucas*). Some species in this group maintain relatively shallow distributions (e.g. the sliteye shark, *Loxodon macrorhinus*), while others have been recorded to depths of > 1000 m (e.g. the tiger shark, *Galeocerdo cuvier*). For many of the understudied species, distributions are understood predominantly through fishery captures, but little has been done to discern whether these species are individually wide-ranging, or whether they are part of subpopulations throughout their distribution. Tracking and genetic population structure work is particularly needed for those species that are commercially exploited and/or most vulnerable to fishing practices.

Small whaler species, including the slit-eye shark and Australian sharpnose shark, often utilise coastal embayments and inshore waters. These smaller sharks are not likely to undergo broad-scale movements although patterns of abundance and habitat use vary both spatially and temporally between species (Simpfendorfer and Milward 1993). Many larger whaler shark species are renowned for their migratory capabilities. Large adult bull sharks have been found to regularly migrate between Victoria and Queensland (> 2000 km) on the Australian east coast (Heupel *et al.* 2015). Tiger sharks also move vast distances between the cool temperate and tropical Indo-Pacific waters (Holmes *et al.* 2014).

Most of the Carcharhiniformes are apex or meso-predators that consume a wide variety of prey. Many have a broad diet and have adapted to hunt a variety of species (generalists); this is particularly advantageous for migrating species that move across a wide range of habitat types. Prey typically includes small teleosts, crustaceans and cephalopods, although the larger carcharhinids will exhibit ontogenetic diet shifts and consume larger marine mammals, turtles, sea snakes, rays, seabirds and other sharks. Some Carcharhiniformes have a specialised diet, such as the Australian weasel shark, which consumes predominantly cephalopods.

All Carcharhiniformes fertilise eggs internally after mating. After fertilisation occurs in the shell gland, oviparous species like the catsharks encapsulate the fertilised embryo and the eggs are deposited on the sea floor. Viviparous species, like most of the whaler sharks, give birth to live young that are supplied nutrition through a yolk-sac placenta from the mother. One exception is the tiger shark, which employs aplacental vivipary (ovoviviparity) – where nutrition is supplied to the pups from individual yolk-filled egg sacs. Pupping usually occurs in the warmer spring to summer months in Australia. Litter sizes vary from < 10 individuals (e.g. graceful shark *Carcharhinus amblyrhynchoides*) to > 100 (e.g. blue shark; Last and Stevens 2009). There is no parental care after the egg laying or live birth of pups. Many species have low reproductive rates, and some of the whalers take several years to reach sexual maturity (e.g. 15 years in dusky sharks *Carcharhinus obscurus*; Romine *et al.* 2009). Some species have long gestation periods (~15–16 months), which results in relatively well-developed young. This life-history strategy is purposed to reduce juvenile mortality rates.

The periodicity of gestations is not well understood for most species in this group. Most of the large, commercially important carcharhinid sharks (e.g. common blacktip shark, *Carcharhinus limbatus*) employ biennial reproductive cycles (Clark and von Schmidt 1965), whereby egg development occurs for approximately one year before copulation to fertilise the eggs. Embryos gestate for around 12 months before parturition. Some of the hammerhead sharks (Sphyrnidae) and the sharpnose sharks (*Rhizoprionodon* spp.) reproduce annually (Taylor *et al.* 2016). Even longer cycles of up to 3 years have been proposed for tiger sharks (Whitney and Crow 2007).

Capture and handling

Species-specific considerations for this group include capture stress in hammerhead sharks, which may produce increased levels of lactate, glucose and partial pressure of carbon dioxide (pCO_2) in the great hammerhead (*Sphyrna mokarran*) (Gallagher *et al.* 2014). These data coincide with other studies on at-vessel mortality rates for great hammerheads, which can be > 90%, indicating that reduced fight times and quick turnaround of biological sampling or tagging while *in situ* is advantageous for this species (Morgan and Burgess 2007). Both scalloped and smooth hammerheads are also vulnerable to mortality events depending on the fishing method used.

Various conventional tagging, acoustic telemetry, archival and satellite tags have been used to study the movements and home ranges for the species in this group (see earlier sub-chapters). Chondrichthyan research often involves a biological sampling component, which can include minimally invasive denticle or cloaca swabs. Portable ultrasound machines are now commonly used in the field to externally look for evidence of pregnancy in wild sharks and rays. Biological sampling for genetic or stable isotope work will involve taking either small fin clips or small biopsies of muscle tissue. Blood is optimally taken using needled syringes to the caudal tail of live sharks, and may be used for reproduction, diet (isotopic niche), nutritional state, health, heavy metals and microplastics research. Some age and growth methods involve researchers giving oxytetracycline (OTC) intraperitoneal injections before release; this produces highly visible marks in vertebral centra and dorsal fin spines of recaptured elasmobranchs when viewed under ultraviolet light (Cailliet and Goldman 2004).

Veterinary considerations

Anaesthesia

The effects of anaesthetics are largely unknown for most chondrichthyans (Neiffer and Stamper 2009; Cooke *et al.* 2016), although some broad guidelines exist for the group (Mylniczenko *et al.* 2014). For more details on when anaesthetics or sedatives could be safely used in this group, refer to Chapter 13.

Euthanasia

Lethal sampling of carcharhiniforms for biological studies includes, but is not limited to, age and growth, reproduction, diet and digestion, parasitology, sensory biology (vision, electroreception, etc.), heavy metal and lipid liver analyses, and taxonomy for voucher specimen collections. Details for procedures relating to the application of methods of killing can be found in Chapter 13.

Infectious pathogens

Carcharhinids are susceptible to a range of internal and external parasites, including over 20 *Huffmanela* species of nematodes (Bullard *et al.* 2012). These nematodes cause scribble-like patterns on the skin caused by adult worms moving in the dermis, which has been reported in *C. plumbeus*, *C. amblyrhynchos* and *R. terraenove* (Dove *et al.* 2017). Other fungal diseases caused by *Fusarium solani* have been reported in hammerheads (*Sphyrna* spp.), which can cause mortality in unborn and post-partum pups as well as their adult hosts (Dove *et al.* 2017). It has been acknowledged that viral diagnoses are also likely to be underrepresented in chondrichthyans.

General operating procedures

A range of research methods and procedures relevant to studying ground sharks are covered in more detail in Chapter 13. Several netting and observational methods that apply to freshwater animals may also apply to these species (Chapter 14). Veterinary methods that may be relevant are covered in Chapter 16.

REFERENCES

Ajemian MJ, Powers SP (2014) Towed-float satellite telemetry tracks large-scale movement and habitat connectivity of myliobatid stingrays. *Environmental Biology of Fishes* **97**, 1067–1081. doi:10.1007/s10641-014-0296-x

Allen GR, Erdmann MV, White WT, Fahmi, Dudgeon CL (2016) Review of the bamboo shark genus *Hemiscyllium* (Orectolobiformes: Hemiscyllidae). *Journal of the Ocean Science Foundation* **23**, 51–97.

Awruch CA (2015) Reproduction strategies. In *Fish Physiology, Physiology of Elasmobranch Fishes: Structure and Interaction with the Environment.* (Eds RE Shadwick, AP Farrel and AJ Brauner) pp. 256–295. Elsevier, Sydney.

Barnett A, Braccini JM, Awruch CA, Ebert DA (2012) An overview of the role of Hexanchiformes in marine ecosystems: biology, ecology and conservation status of a primitive order of modern sharks. *Journal of Fish Biology* **80**, 966–990. doi:10.1111/j.1095-8649.2012.03242.x

Bass NC, Mourier J, Knott NA, Day J, Guttridge T, Brown C (2017) Long-term migration patterns and bisexual philopatry in a benthic shark species. *Marine and Freshwater Research* **68**, 1414–1421. doi:10.1071/MF16122

Benz GW, Lucas Z, Lowry LF (1998) New host and ocean records for the copepod *Ommatokoita elongata* (Siphonostomatoidea: Lernaeopodidae), a parasite of the eyes of sleeper sharks. *The Journal of Parasitology* **84**(6), 1271–1274. doi:10.2307/3284688

Bradford R, Patterson TA, Rogers PJ, McAuley R, Mountford S, Huveneers C, Robbins R, Fox A, Bruce BD (2020) Evidence of diverse movement strategies and habitat use by white sharks, *Carcharodon carcharias*, off southern Australia. *Marine Biology* **167**, 96. doi:10.1007/s00227-020-03712-y

Bray DJ (2015) *Ground Sharks, Carcharhiniformes in Fishes of Australia.* <http://136.154.202.208/Home/order/10>.

Bray DJ (2017) *Class Chondrichthyes in Fishes of Australia.* <https://fishesofAustralia.net.au/home/class/4>.

Brunnschweiler J, Huveneers C, Borucinska J (2017) Multi-year growth progression of a neoplastic lesion on a bull shark (*Carcharhinus leucas*). Matters Select ISSN: 2297-9239. doi:10.19185/matters.201709000002

Bruce BD, Bradford RW (2013) *Protocols for Capturing and Tagging Juvenile White Sharks in Near-shore Waters.* CSIRO, Melbourne.

Buck JD, Spotte S, Gadbaw JJ, Jr (1984) Bacteriology of the teeth from a great white shark: potential medical implications for shark bite victims. *Journal of Clinical Microbiology* **20**, 849–851. doi:10.1128/jcm.20.5.849-851.1984

Bullard SA, Ruiz CF, McElwain A, Murray MJ, Borucinska JD, Benz GW (2012) Huffmanela cf. carcharhinid (Nematoda: Trichosomoididae: Huffmanelinae) from skin of a sandbar shark, *Carcharhinus plumbeus*, in the Pacific Ocean. *The Journal of Parasitology* **98**, 333–340. doi:10.1645/GE-2962.1

Burgess K, Guerrero M, Richardson A, Bennett M, Marshall A (2018) Use of epidermal mucus in elasmobranch stable isotope studies: a pilot study using the giant manta ray (*Manta birostris*). *Marine and Freshwater Research* **69**, 336–342. doi:10.1071/MF16355

Cailliet GM, Goldman KJ (2004) Age determination and validation in Chondrichthyan fishes. In *Biology of Sharks and their Relatives* (Eds JC Carrier, JA Musick and MR Heithaus) pp. 399–447. CRC Press, Boca Raton, FL.

Carey FG, Clark E (1995) Depth telemetry from the sixgill shark, *Hexanchus griseus* at Bermuda. *Environmental Biology of Fishes* **42**, 7–14. doi:10.1007/BF00002345

Clark E, Von Schmidt K (1965) Sharks of the central Gulf coast of Florida. *Bulletin of Marine Science* **15**, 13–83.

Cook SJ, Wilson ADM, Elvidge CK, Lennox RJ, Jepsen N, Colotelo AH, Brown RS (2016) Ten practical realities for institutional animal care and use committees when evaluating protocols dealing with fish in the field. *Reviews in Fish Biology and Fisheries* **26**, 123–133. doi:10.1007/s11160-015-9413-y

Compagno LJV (2005) Checklist of living chondrichthyans. In *Reproductive Biology and Phylogeny of Chondrichthyes: Sharks, Batoids and Chimaeras.* (Ed. WC Hamlett) pp. 503–548. Science Publishers Inc., Enfield, CT.

Compagno LJV, Dando M, Fowler SL (2005a) *Sharks of the World.* Princeton University Press, Princeton and Oxford.

Compagno LJV, Dando M, Fowler SL (2005b) *A Field Guide to the Sharks of the World.* Harper Collins Publishers Ltd, London, UK.

Corrigan S, Huveneers C, Schwartz TS, Harcourt RG, Beheregaray LB (2008) Genetic and reproductive evidence for two species of ornate wobbegong shark *Orectolobus* spp. on the Australian east coast. *Journal of Fish Biology* **73**, 1662–1675. doi:10.1111/j.1095-8649.2008.02039.x

Couturier LIE, Rohner CA, Richardson AJ, Marshall AD, Jaine FRA, Bennett MB, Townsend KA, Weeks SJ, Nichols PD (2013) Stable isotope and signature fatty acid analyses suggest reef manta rays feed on demersal zooplankton. *PLoS One* **8**, e77152. doi:10.1371/journal.pone.0077152

Daley RK (2017) Spatial management strategies for deep-sea sharks. PhD thesis. The University of Tasmania, Australia.

Daley RK, Hobday AJ, Semmens JM (2019) Simulation-based evaluation of reserve network performance for *Centrophorus zeehaani* (Centrophoridae): a protected deep-sea gulper shark. *ICES Journal of Marine Science* **76**, 2318–2328. doi:10.1093/icesjms/fsz087

Daley RK, Williams A, Green M, Barker B, Brodie P (2015) Can marine reserves conserve vulnerable sharks in the deep sea? A case study of *Centrophorus zeehaani* (Centrophoridae), examined with acoustic telemetry. *Deep-sea Research. Part II, Topical Studies in Oceanography* **115**, 127–136. doi:10.1016/j.dsr2.2014.05.017

Dean MN, Bizzarro JJ, Summers AP (2007) The evolution of cranial design, diet, and feeding mechanisms in batoid fishes. *Integrative and Comparative Biology* **47**, 70–81. doi:10.1093/icb/icm034

Dove ADM, Clauss TM, Marancik DP, Camus AC (2017) Emerging diseases of elasmobranchs in aquaria. In *The Elasmobranch Husbandry Manual II: Recent Advances in the Care of Sharks, Rays and their Relatives.* (Eds M Smith, D Warmoults, D Thoney, R Heuter, M Murray and J Ezcurra) pp. 99–112. Ohio Biological Survey, Inc, Ohio State University, Columbus, OH.

Dudgeon CL, Lanyon JM, Semmens JM (2013) Seasonality and site fidelity of the zebra shark, *Stegostoma fasciatum*, in southeast Queensland, Australia. *Animal Behaviour* **85**, 471–481. doi:10.1016/j.anbehav.2012.12.013

Dulvy NK, Davidson LNK, Kyne PM, Simpfendorfer CA, Harrison LR, Carlson JK, Fordham SV (2016) Ghosts of the coast: global extinction risk and conservation of sawfishes. *Aquatic Conservation* **26**, 134–153. doi:10.1002/aqc.2525

Francis MP, Shivji MS, Duffy CA, Rogers PJ, Byrne ME, Wetherbee BM, Tindale SC, Lyon WS, Meyers MM (2019) Oceanic nomad or coastal resident? Behavioural switching in the shortfin mako shark (*Isurus oxyrinchus*). *Marine Biology* **166**, 5. doi:10.1007/s00227-018-3453-5

Gallagher AJ, Meyer L, Pethybridge HR, Huveneers C, Butcher PA (2019) Effects of short-term capture on the physiology of white sharks *Carcharodon carcharias*: amino acids and fatty acids. *Endangered Species Research* **40**, 297–308. doi:10.3354/esr00997

Gallagher AJ, Serafy JE, Cooke SJ, Hammerschlag N (2014) Physiological stress response, reflex impairment, and survival of five sympatric shark species following experimental capture and release. *Marine Ecology Progress Series* **496**, 207–218. doi:10.3354/meps10490

Green ME, D'Anastasi BRD, Hobbs JPA, Feldheim K, McAuley R, Peverell S, Stapley J, Johnson G, Appleyard SA, White WT, Simpfendorfer CA, van Herwerden L (2018) Mixed-marker approach suggests maternal philopatry and sex-biased behaviours of narrow sawfish *Anoxypristis cuspidata. Endangered Species Research* **37**, 45–54. doi:10.3354/esr00912

Guttridge TL, Gulak SJ, Franks BR, Carlson JK, Gruber SH, Gledhill KS, Bond ME, Johnson GJ, Grubbs RD (2015) Occurrence and habitat use of the critically endangered smalltooth sawfish *Pristis pectinata* in the Bahamas. *Journal of Fish Biology* **87**, 1322–1341. doi:10.1111/jfb.12825

Hallett CS, Daley RK (2011) Feeding ecology of the southern lantern shark (*Etmopterus baxteri*) and the brown lanternshark (*E. unicolor*) off southeastern Australia. *ICES Journal of Marine Science* **68**, 157–165. doi:10.1093/icesjms/fsq143

Harahush BK, Fisher ABP, Collin SP (2007) Captive breeding and embryonic development of Chiloscyllium punctatum Muller and Henle, 1838 (Elasmobranchii: Hemiscyllidae). *Journal of Fish Biology* **71**, 1007–1022. doi:10.1111/j.1095-8649.2007.01569.x

Henderson CJ, Stevens T, Gilby BL, Lee SY (2018) Spatial conservation of large mobile elasmobranchs requires an understanding of spatio-temporal seascape utilization. *ICES Journal of Marine Science* **75**, 553–561. doi:10.1093/icesjms/fsx192

Heupel MR, Simpfendorfer CA (2010) Science of slaughter: need for lethal sampling of sharks. *Conservation Biology* **24**, 1212–1218. doi:10.1111/j.1523-1739.2010.01491.x

Heupel MR, Simpfendorfer CA, Espinosa M, Smoothey AF, Tobin A, Peddemors V (2015) Conservation challenges of sharks with continental scale migrations. *Frontiers in Marine Science* **2**, 12. doi:10.3389/fmars.2015.00012

Hoenner X, Huveneers C, Steckenreuter A, Simpfendorfer CA, Tattersall K, Jaine FR, Atkins N, Babcock R, Brodie S, Burgess J, Campbell H, Heupel M, Pasquer B, Proctor R, Taylor MD, Udyawer V, Harcourt RG (2018) Australia's continental-scale acoustic tracking database and its automated quality control process. *Scientific Data* **5**, 170206. doi:10.1038/sdata.2017.206

Holmes BJ, Pepperell JP, Griffiths SP, Jaine FRA, Tibbetts IR, Bennett MB (2014) Tiger shark (*Galeocerdo cuvier*) movement patterns and habitat use determined by satellite tagging in eastern Australian waters. *Marine Biology* **161**, 2645–2658. doi:10.1007/s00227-014-2536-1

Huveneers C, Apps K, Becerril-García EE, Bruce B, Butcher PA, Carlisle AB, Chapple TK, Christiansen HM, Cliff G, Curtis TH, Daly-Engel TS *et al.* (2018) Future research directions on the "elusive" white shark. *Frontiers in Marine Science* **5**, 455. doi:10.3389/fmars.2018.00455

Huveneers C, Klebe S, Bruce B, Robbins R, Borucinska JD, Jones R, Michael MZ (2016) First histological examination of a neoplastic lesion from a free-swimming white shark, *Carcharodon carcharias* L. *Journal of Fish Diseases* **39**, 1269–1273. doi:10.1111/jfd.12458

Huveneers C, Walker TI, Otway NM, Harcourt RG (2007) Reproductive synchrony of three sympatric species of wobbegong shark (genus *Orectolobus*) in New South Wales, Australia: reproductive parameter estimates necessary for population modelling. *Marine and Freshwater Research* **58**, 765–777. doi:10.1071/MF06187

Jacobsen IP, Bennett MB (2013) A comparative analysis of feeding and trophic level ecology in stingrays (Rajiformes; *Myliobatoidei*) and electric rays (Rajiformes: *Torpedinoidei*). *PLoS One* **8**. doi:10.1371/journal.pone.0071348

Joung SJ, Chen CT, Clark E, Uchida S, Huang WYP (1996) The whale shark, *Rhincodon typus*, is a livebearer: 300 embryos found in one 'megamamma' supreme. *Environmental Biology of Fishes* **46**, 219–223. doi:10.1007/BF00004997

Kessel ST, Hussey NE (2015) Tonic immobility as an anaesthetic for elasmobranchs during surgical implantation procedures. *Canadian Journal of Fisheries and Aquatic Sciences* **72**, 1287–1291. doi:10.1139/cjfas-2015-0136

Kneebone J, Chisholm J, Skomal G (2014) Movement patterns of juvenile sand tigers (*Carcharias taurus*) along the east coast of the USA. *Marine Biology* **161**, 1149–1163. doi:10.1007/s00227-014-2407-9

Kolmann MA, Welch KC, Summers AP, Lovejoy NR (2016) Always chew your food: freshwater stingrays use mastication to process tough insect prey. *Proceedings. Biological Sciences* **283**, 20161392. doi:10.1098/rspb.2016.1392

Kyne PM, Jabado RW, Rigby CL, Dharmadi, Gore MA, Pollock CM, Herman KB, Cheok J, Ebert DA, Simpfendorfer CA, Dulvy NK (2020) The thin edge of the wedge: Extremely high extinction risk in wedgefishes and giant guitarfishes. *Aquatic Conservation.* doi:10.1002/aqc.3331

Kyne PM, Pillans RD (2014) *Protocols for Surveying and Tagging Sawfishes and River Sharks.* National Environmental Research Program Marine Biodiversity Hub, Hobart.

Kyne PM, Romanov E, Barreto R, Carlson J, Fernando D, Fordham S, Francis MP, Jabado RW, Liu KM, Marshall A, Pacoureau N, Sherley RB (2019) *Pseudocarcharias kamoharai.* The IUCN Red List of Threatened Species 2019. e.T39337A2900108.

Lasek-Nesselquist E, Bogomolni AL, Gast RJ, Welch DM, Ellis JC, Sogin MC, Moore MJ (2008) Molecular characterization of Giardia intestinalis haplotypes in marine animals: variation and zoonotic potential. *Diseases of Aquatic Organisms* **81**, 39–51. doi:10.3354/dao01931

Last PR, Stevens JD (2009) *Sharks and Rays of Australia.* CSIRO Publishing, Melbourne.

Last PR, White WT, de Carvalho MR, Séret B, Stehmann MFW, Naylor GJP (Eds) (2016) *Rays of the World.* CSIRO Publishing, Melbourne.

Lear KO, Gleiss AC, Whitty JM, Fazeldean T, Albert JR, Green N, Ebner BC, Thorburn DC, Beatty SJ, Morgan DL (2019) Recruitment of a critically endangered sawfish into a riverine nursery depends on natural flow regimes. *Scientific Reports* **9**, 17071. doi:10.1038/s41598-019-53511-9

Lee KA, Huveneers C, Gimenez O, Peddemors V, Harcourt RG (2014) To catch or to sight? A comparison of demographic parameter estimates obtained from mark-recapture and mark-resight models. *Biodiversity and Conservation* **23**, 2781–2800. doi:10.1007/s10531-014-0748-9

Lee KA, Huveneers C, Peddemors V, Boomer A, Harcourt RG (2015) Born to be free? Assessing the viability of releasing captive-bred wobbegongs to restock depleted populations. *Frontiers in Marine Science* **2**. doi:10.3389/fmars.2015.00018

Liu SYV, Joung SJ, Yu CJ, Hsu HH, Tsai WP, Liu KM (2018) Genetic diversity and connectivity of the megamouth shark (*Megachasma pelagios*). *PeerJ* **6**, e4432. doi:10.7717/peerj.4432

Long DJ, Waggoner BM (1993) The ectoparasitic barnacle *Anelasma* (Cirripedia, Thoracica, Lepadomorpha) on the shark *Centroscyllium nigrum* (Chondrichthyes, Squalidae) from the Pacific sub-Antarctic. *Systematic Parasitology* **26**, 133–136. doi:10.1007/BF00009220

Morgan A, Burgess GH (2007) At-vessel fishing mortality for six species of sharks caught in the northwest Atlantic and Gulf of Mexico. *Gulf and Caribbean Research* **19**, 123–129. doi:10.18785/gcr.1902.15

Mylniczenko ND, Clauss T, Stamper MA (2014) Elasmobranchs and holocephalans. In *Zoo Animal and Wildlife Immobilization and Anaesthesia.* 2nd edn. (Eds G West, D Heard and N Caulkett) pp. 261–301. John Wiley and Sons, Hoboken, NJ.

Neiffer DL, Stamper MA (2009) Fish sedation, anesthesia, analgesia, and euthanasia: considerations, methods, and types of drugs. *ILAR Journal* **50**, 343–360. doi:10.1093/ilar.50.4.343

Newby J, Darden T, Shedlock AM (2014) Population genetic structure of spotted eagle rays, *Aetobatus narinari*, off Sarasota, Florida and the Southeastern United States. *Copeia* **2014**, 503–512. doi:10.1643/CG-13-122

Norman BM, Holmberg JA, Arzoumanian Z, Reynolds SD, Wilson RP, Rob D, *et al.* (2017) Undersea constellations: the global biology of an endangered marine megavertebrate further informed through citizen science. *Bioscience* **67**, 1029–1043. doi:10.1093/biosci/bix127

Ostrander GK, Cheng KC, Wolf JC, Wolfe MJ (2004) Shark cartilage, cancer, and the growing threat of pseudoscience. *Cancer Research* **64**, 8485–8491. doi:10.1158/0008-5472.CAN-04-2260

Otway NM, Ellis MT (2011) Pop-up archival satellite tagging of *Carcharias taurus*: movements and depth/temperature-related use of south-eastern Australian waters. *Marine and Freshwater Research* **62**, 607–620. doi:10.1071/MF10139

Pethybridge H, Daley RK, Virtue P, Butler ECV, Cossa D, Nichols PD (2010) Lipid and mercury profiles of 61 mid-trophic species collected off south-eastern Australia. *Marine and Freshwater Research* **61**, 1092–1108. doi:10.1071/MF09237

Peverell SC (2005) Distribution of sawfishes (Pristidae) in the Queensland Gulf of Carpentaria, Australia, with notes on sawfish ecology. *Environmental Biology of Fishes* **73**, 391–402. doi:10.1007/s10641-005-1599-8

Peverell SC (2009) Sawfish (Pristidae) of the Gulf of Carpentaria, Queensland, Australia. MSc thesis. James Cook University, Australia.

Phillips BE, Christiansen EF, Stoskopf MK, Broadhurst H, George R, Harms CA (2016) Comparison of haematology, plasma biochemistry, and blood gas variables between 2 venipuncture sites in southern stingrays (*Dasyatis americana*). *Veterinary Clinical Pathology* **45**, 627–633. doi:10.1111/vcp.12424

Poulakis GR, Urakawa H, Stevens PW, DeAngelo JA, Timmers AA, Grubbs RD, Fisk AT, Olin JA (2017) Sympatric elasmobranchs and faecal samples provide insight into the trophic ecology of the smalltooth sawfish. *Endangered Species Research* **32**, 491–506. doi:10.3354/esr00824

Readman GD, Owen SF, Knowles TG, Murrell JC (2017) Species specific anaesthetics for fish anaesthesia and euthanasia. *Scientific Reports* **7**, 7102. doi:10.1038/s41598-017-06917-2

Reynolds J, Hornbrook E, Stettner G, Terrell R (2017) Husbandry of freshwater stingrays. In *The Elasmobranch Husbandry Manual II:*

Recent Advances in the Care of Sharks, Rays and their Relatives. (Eds M Smith, D Warmoults, DThoney, R Heuter, M Murray and J Ezcurra) pp. 99–112. Ohio State University, Columbus, OH.

Robinson DP, Jaidah MY, Bach SS, Rohner CA, Jabado RW, Ormond R, Pierce SJ (2017) Some like it hot: repeat migration and residency of whale sharks within an extreme natural environment. *PLoS One* **12**, e0185360. doi:10.1371/journal.pone.0185360

Rodríguez-Cabello C, Sánchez F (2014) Is *Centrophorus squamosus* a highly migratory deep-water shark? *Deep-sea Research. Part I, Oceanographic Research Papers* **92**, 1–10. doi:10.1016/j.dsr.2014.06.005

Rogers PJ, Huveneers C, Page B, Goldsworthy SD, Coyne M, Lowther AD, Mitchell JG, Seuront L (2015) Living on the continental shelf edge: habitat use of juvenile shortfin makos *Isurus oxyrinchus* in the Great Australian Bight, southern Australia. *Fisheries Oceanography* **24**, 205–218. doi:10.1111/fog.12103

Romine JG, Musick JA, Burgess GH (2009) Demographic analyses of the dusky shark, *Carcharhinus obscurus*, in the Northwest Atlantic incorporating hooking mortality estimates and revised reproductive parameters. *Environmental Biology of Fishes* **84**, 277–289. doi:10.1007/s10641-008-9435-6

Rowat D, Brooks KS (2012) A review of the biology, fisheries and conservation of the whale shark *Rhincodon typus*. *Journal of Fish Biology* **80**, 1019–1056. doi:10.1111/j.1095-8649.2012.03252.x

Simpfendorfer CA, Milward NE (1993) Utilisation of a tropical bay as a nursery area by sharks of the families Carcharhinidae and Sphyrnidae. *Environmental Biology of Fishes* **37**, 337–345. doi:10.1007/BF00005200

Skomal GB, Zeeman SI, Chisholm JH, Summers EL, Walsh HJ, McMahon KW, Thorrold SR (2009) Transequatorial migrations by basking sharks in the western Atlantic Ocean. *Current Biology* **19**, 1019–1022. doi:10.1016/j.cub.2009.04.019

Smith ESJ, Lewin GR (2009) Nociceptors: a phylogenetic view. *Journal of Comparative Physiology. A, Neuroethology, Sensory, Neural, and Behavioral Physiology* **195**, 1089–1106. doi:10.1007/s00359-009-0482-z

Smith MFL, Marshall A, Correia JP, Rupp J (2004) Elasmobranch Transport Techniques and Equipment. In *The Elasmobranch Husbandry Manual II: Recent Advances in the Care qof Sharks, Rays and their Relatives.* (Eds M Smith, D Warmoults, D Thoney, R Heuter, M Murray and J Ezcurra) pp. 169–182. Ohio State University, Columbus, OH.

Sneddon LU (2018) Comparative physiology of nociception and pain. *Physiology (Bethesda, MD)* **33**, 63–73. doi:10.1152/physiol.00022.2017

Stevens JD, McAuley RB, Simpfendorfer CA, Pillans RD (2008) *Spatial Distribution and Habitat Utilisation of Sawfish (*Pristis *spp) in Relation to Fishing in Northern Australia.* CSIRO, Hobart.

Taylor SM, Harry AV, Bennett MB (2016) Living on the edge: latitudinal variations in the reproductive biology of two coastal species of sharks. *Journal of Fish Biology* **89**, 2399–2418. doi:10.1111/jfb.13126

Teshima K, Kamei Y, Toda M, Uchida S (1995) Reproductive mode of the tawny nurse shark taken from the Yaeyama Islands, Okinawa, Japan with comments on individuals lacking the second dorsal fin. *Bulletin of the Seikai National Fisheries Research Institute* **73**, 1–12.

Thorrold SR, Afonso P, Fontes J, Braun CD, Santos RS, Skomal GB, Berumen ML (2014) Extreme diving behaviour in devil rays links surface waters and the deep ocean. *Nature Communications* **5**, 4274. doi:10.1038/ncomms5274

Townsend R, Stow A, Asmyhr M, Momigliano P (2015) Multiple paternity in captive grey nurse sharks (*Carcharias taurus*): Implications for the captive breeding of this critically endangered species. *Pacific Conservation Biology* **21**, 122–125. doi:10.1071/PC14909

Vignaud TM, Maynard JA, Leblois R, Meekan MG, Vázquez-Juárez R, Ramírez-Macías D, *et al.* (2014) Genetic structure of populations of whale sharks among ocean basins and evidence for their historic rise and recent decline. *Molecular Ecology* **23**, 2590–2601. doi:10.1111/mec.12754

Walker TI (2020) Reproduction of Chondrichthyans. In *Reproduction in Aquatic Animals: From Basic Biology to Aquaculture Technology.* (Eds M Yoshida and JF Asturiano) Springer Publishing, Singapore.

Watanabe YY, Papastamatiou YP (2019) Distribution, body size and biology of the megamouth shark *Megachasma pelagios*. *Journal of Fish Biology* **95**, 992–998. doi:10.1111/jfb.14007

Watson L, Janse M (2017) Reproduction and husbandry of zebra sharks, *Stegostoma fasciatum*, in aquaria. In *The Elasmobranch Husbandry Manual II: Recent Advances in the Care of Sharks, Rays and their Relatives.* (Eds M Smith, D Warmoults, D Thoney, R Heuter, M Murray and J Ezcurra) pp. 99–112. Ohio State University, Columbus, OH.

Westmoreland LS, Archibald KE, Christiansen EF, Broadhurst H, Stoskopf MK (2019) The mesopterygial vein: a reliable venipuncture site for intravascular access in batoids. *Journal of Zoo and Wildlife Medicine* **50**, 369–374. doi:10.1638/2018-0137

White S, Duke K, Squire L, Jr (2017) Husbandry of sawfishes. In *The Elasmobranch Husbandry Manual II: Recent Advances in the Care of Sharks, Rays and their Relatives.* (Eds M Smith, D Warmoults, D Thoney, R Heuter, M Murray and J Ezcurra) pp. 75–85. Ohio State University, Columbus, OH.

Whitney NM, Crow GL (2007) Reproductive biology of the tiger shark (*Galeocerdo cuvier*) in Hawaii. *Marine Biology* **151**, 63–70. doi:10.1007/s00227-006-0476-0

Williamson MJ, Dudgeon CL, Slade R (2018) Tonic immobility in the zebra shark, *Stegostoma fasciatum*, and its use for capture methodology. *Environmental Biology of Fishes* **101**, 741–748. doi:10.1007/s10641-018-0734-2

Wueringer BE, Squire LJ, Kajiura SM, Hart NS, Collin SP (2012) The function of the sawfish's saw. *Current Biology* **22**, 150–151. doi:10.1016/j.cub.2012.01.055

32 Freshwater fishes

Nicole Flint, Brendan C. Ebner, David T. Roberts, David L. Morgan, Scott A. Hardie, Jonathan Marshall and Alison J. King

INTRODUCTION

Australia has relatively few freshwater fish species compared to similarly sized land masses – primarily because of its large and mostly arid land area, and its isolation and extended separation from other land masses. Only three Australian fishes are primary freshwater species (ancient animals remaining from the time of the supercontinent Gondwana): the air-breathing Australian lungfish (*Neoceratodus forsteri*) and two species of saratoga (*Scleropages leichhardti* and *S. jardinii*). Fewer than 300 native freshwater species are currently described, an imprecise estimate as new species are still being discovered in Australia's most remote regions (e.g. Morgan *et al.* 2013; Welsh *et al.* 2014; Shelley *et al.* 2019). Furthermore, Australian freshwater fishes show a very high level of endemism, with ~90% of native species occurring nowhere else. Over 40 introduced fish species have been recorded in Australian freshwater systems.

Like freshwater fishes elsewhere, Australian species occupy a wide range of habitats, ecological and trophic niches, and display many different reproductive and life history strategies. Freshwater fishes occupy streams, rivers, tarns, lakes, palustrine wetlands (ephemeral or permanent), and groundwater systems in underground caves and channels. They are also common in artificial habitats like drains, irrigation channels, ponds, impoundments and constructed wetlands.

Some Australian freshwater fishes require specialised handling techniques because of their morphology, physiology, biology or behaviour. For instance, several fish families include venomous species and can harm researchers if not handled carefully (see 'Venomous fishes' later in this chapter). Some species can be easily damaged, lose scales or have their mucosal layer damaged during certain handling or capture techniques (e.g. *Retropinna* spp.). Additionally, requirements for handling introduced fishes may differ between species and jurisdictions.

Species in the superclass Osteichthyes (bony fishes) that are known to rely on freshwater for all or part of their life cycles are included in this chapter. This chapter has been divided into six sub-chapters; some unavoidable overlap occurs between them for the sake of clarity. For instance, Percichthyidae (perches) is discussed in 'Large-bodied fishes', even though some members of this family are small-bodied. Bony fish species that are mostly marine are discussed in Chapter 30 and Australian Chondrichthyes (sharks, batoids and chimaeras) are discussed in Chapter 31.

SMALL-BODIED FISHES

Scott A. Hardie, David L. Morgan, Nicole Flint and Alison J. King

Characteristics

Many of Australia's freshwater fishes are classified as small-bodied species (< 1 kg). This grouping is diverse in terms of taxonomy, biology, ecology and behaviour. Unlike many large-bodied fishes, small-bodied species typically have no direct commercial or recreational value, although some are considered ornamental and are valuable to the aquarium trade (Ebner *et al.* 2016b). Small-bodied fishes have intrinsic value in freshwater ecosystems, being important trophic components of food webs, where they facilitate carbon and nutrient cycling and provide crucial food resources for larger fishes, waterbirds and other animals, as well as being important in the control of nuisance species, such as mosquitos and midges (Lawrence *et al.* 2016).

Small-bodied fishes include some of the most speciose fish families found in Australian freshwaters, including the Eleotridae, Galaxiidae, Gobiidae and Melanotaeniidae (Unmack *et al.* 2013). Many small-bodied species are considered threatened (Lintermans *et al.* 2020). Small-bodied fishes are often highly susceptible to being injured during capture and handling; it is imperative that researchers evaluate the 'robustness' and sensitivities of their target species before conducting research.

Small-bodied fishes that occur in Australian freshwater environments include the orders Atheriniformes, Beloniformes, Clupeiformes, Elopiformes, Gonorhynciformes, Gobiiformes, Mugiliformes, Perciformes, Pleuronectiformes and Salmoniformes (for distributions and behaviours see Allen *et al.* 2002; Pusey *et al.* 2004; Hammer *et al.* 2007; Morgan *et al.* 2011; Humphries and Walker 2013; Unmack *et al.* 2013; Morgan *et al.* 2014; Faulks *et al.* 2017; Hammer *et al.* 2018; Hammer *et al.* 2019a; Allen *et al.* 2020). While it is difficult to separate 'smaller' from 'larger' fishes at the taxonomic level of family, fish from the families listed here are small even when mature, while families described in 'Large-bodied fishes' include species that reach large sizes, as well as some smaller species. One species in the taxonomic order Syngnathiformes occurs in freshwater (the short-tail pipefish, *Microphis brachyurus*); this order is mostly marine and covered in Chapter 30.

Biology and behaviour

Small-bodied fishes are found in most types of natural (e.g. rivers, lakes and other wetlands) and human-made (e.g. channels, reservoirs and constructed wetlands) aquatic habitats, including marginal areas that do not have sufficient resources to support large-bodied fishes (e.g. drying water holes, small drains and headwater streams). Diel and ontogenetic habitat shifts mean that small-bodied fishes often use different habitats spatially and temporally; these shifts can occur over days relating to feeding activity or across several months associated with different life phases. Some small fishes display schooling behaviour that allows them to move continually through open water and between mesohabitats. However, cryptic and shy behaviour is common, with many species favouring the refuge provided by structurally complex microhabitats like rocky substrata, woody debris and aquatic or overhanging vegetation.

Fish of all size classes move at either small spatial scales (between microhabitats), mesohabitat scales (within and between tributaries or pools that act as permanent or temporary home ranges), or macrohabitat scales, including migration for reproductive purposes (Koehn and Crook 2013). Generally, movements of large-bodied fishes have been more thoroughly studied than those of smaller species because movements of small-bodied fishes are not easily monitored through tagging and tracking, or visual monitoring techniques that are suitable for larger species. This bias may also reflect the higher economic value that is often placed on larger species. However, some small-bodied species are diadromous, undertaking large-scale movements between freshwater and estuarine or marine environments to reproduce, including some populations of the spotted galaxias (*Galaxias truttaceus*; Morgan 2003), the Australian grayling (*Prototroctes maraena*; Koster *et al.* 2013) and all sicydiine gobies (Ebner *et al.* 2011a). Smaller-scale movements (between microhabitats and macrohabitats) are typically associated with feeding activity or in response to changes in habitat conditions, such as periodic or seasonal variation in thermal or flow regimes, and inundation of areas associated with flooding.

The feeding strategies of small-bodied fishes are diverse and include herbivory, omnivory or carnivory. The mouth gape of smaller species restricts their ability to capture and consume large prey. However, their diet can overlap with large-bodied species (especially as juveniles). While some species are known to have defined diel and seasonal feeding patterns, it is common for small-bodied fishes to be opportunistic feeders, with diets reflecting the habitats they occupy.

Many small species undergo habitat (and trophic) shifts during early phases of their development (King *et al.* 2013), and this shift, along with an increase in body size and gape, strongly influences their diet. For example, larvae and juvenile galaxiids are typically pelagic for the first few months of life during which time they consume planktonic items (e.g. zooplankton such as copepods, cladocerans and ostracods), before shifting to benthic, epibenthic or mid-water habitats where they consume larger prey items such as aquatic insect larvae, and small crustaceans and molluscs (Fulton 1982; Morgan 2003). These dietary items are typical of omnivorous and carnivorous small fishes, while diatoms and algae are prominent in the diets of herbivorous and omnivorous feeders. Many small-bodied species feed from the water surface at times, where they consume aquatic (e.g. emerging or adult insects) and terrestrial (e.g. insects, spiders) prey. Piscivory does occur in the feeding strategies of small-bodied fishes, but has received less research attention than in some of the predatory larger-bodied fishes.

Reproductive biology and behaviour, and recruitment strategies of Australian small-bodied freshwater fishes are highly varied (see King *et al.* 2013). As such, a general overview of reproductive strategies of small-bodied fishes is provided. Where possible, researchers should familiarise themselves with the life histories of their target species as this will greatly assist study designs and interpretation of results. Many small-bodied fishes are relatively short lived (< 10 years), with some species being annual or only living for a few years (e.g. smelt, *Retropinna* spp.). Therefore, sexual maturity is often reached at a young age (in their first or second year). Spawning modes vary greatly, including those requiring high parental involvement (e.g. the viviparous garfish, Zenarchopteridae, and mouth-brooding Apogonidae) to low-investment strategies such as depositing eggs on aquatic plants (e.g. rainbowfishes, Melanotaeniidae; Flint *et al.* 2017) or broadcast spawning in the water column (e.g. herrings, Clupeidae; Puckridge and Walker 1990). Spawning timing and the locations used are typically influenced by environmental factors, such as day length (photo period), water temperature, flow and hydraulic conditions and available substrata (King *et al.* 2013). For migratory species, stimuli to induce spawning-related movements are also important (e.g. Koster *et al.* 2013). Some common freshwater fish species are able to breed in either fresh- or saltwater, while diadromous species move between fresh and saltwater environments in order to breed.

Capture and handling

Some small fish must be handled gently and for as little time as possible to avoid damaging their skin, fins, scales if present, and eyes if present (Figure 32.1). Soft dip nets may be used or wet cotton gloves worn to help handle small-bodied fish and reduce abrasive contact. In

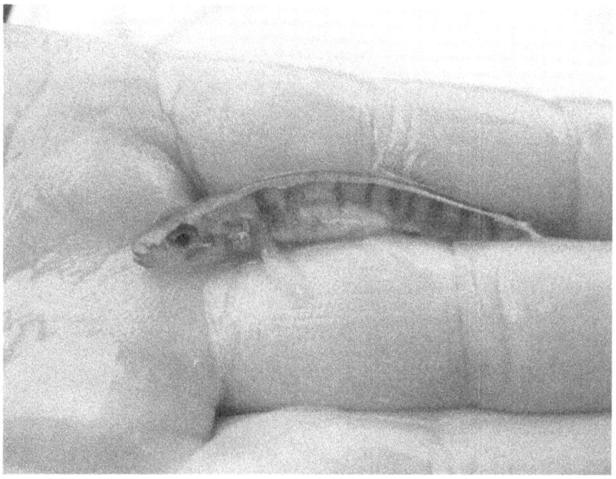

Figure 32.1: Small-bodied fishes such as Arthurs paragalaxias (*Paragalaxias mesotes*), an endemic Tasmanian galaxiid and threatened species, need to be handled very gently to minimise stress and damage. Photo by Kevin Macfarlane.

non-lethal studies, air exposure, or time out of water, is a critical factor for post-release survival (see Chapter 14). While not suitable for all study types, non-invasive methods such as visual monitoring may be preferable for threatened or range-restricted species (Chilcott *et al.* 2013; Ebner *et al.* 2014), although correct identification of small-bodied individuals can be challenging. Netting, trapping and electrofishing are some of the common methods used to capture small-bodied fishes (Chapter 14).

Small tags and transmitters are becoming more readily available, improving research options for tagging and tracking the movements and behaviour of small-bodied fishes. Researchers designing studies that require the tagging of individual fish are encouraged to familiarise themselves with relevant literature. Recently, Allen *et al.* (2020) used visual implant elastomer (VIE) tags (injected into the muscular tissue on the dorsal surface) to estimate population size and migratory movements of the threatened little pygmy perch (*Nannoperca pygmaea*, family Percichthyidae), from refuge pools to an ephemeral tributary for spawning. Other methods for tracking individual fishes include the use of PIT (passive internal transponder) tags and portable or *in situ* readers (e.g. Crook and White 1995; Roussel *et al.* 2000).

Most of the smaller freshwater fishes are relatively easy to house (as demonstrated by the use of many Australian species in the aquarium trade). However, some Australian freshwater fishes or certain life stages can be particularly vulnerable to entrapment or handling. For example, members of the Retropinnidae and some Atherinidae, which are often captured *en masse*, can perish quickly if handled incorrectly or removed from the water. If fish need to be transported, minimising direct handling will provide better outcomes for the fish and researcher. For example, tipping captured fish directly into the water transporter (or even immersing the whole trap in a larger bucket and retaining the water) is preferable to manual handling.

Veterinary considerations

Sedation and anaesthesia

Anaesthetic considerations are similar among bony fish groups (Mylniczenko *et al.* 2014). See 'Estuarine fishes' in Chapter 30 for a discussion of anaesthetic principles for fish. Most small-bodied freshwater fish can be non-invasively handled without a need for anaesthesia; however, it is required for surgical procedures such as implanting internal tags. The use of isoeugenol is often the preferred method of sedation by animal ethics committees, although a variety of anaesthetics are available and can be used for different applications.

Euthanasia

Lethal sampling may be required to gather data including, but not limited to, age and growth, reproduction, diet and digestion, movement history, parasitology and disease diagnosis, sensory biology (e.g. vision, electroreception), toxicant concentrations in tissues, lipid analyses and taxonomy for voucher specimen collections. For the species discussed in this section, euthanasia by immersion in an overdose solution of anaesthetic is common (e.g. isoeugenol, clove oil or tricaine methanesulfonate buffered with sodium bicarbonate) (AVMA 2020). Immersion in an icy slurry may also be considered acceptable for small warm water species (Blessing *et al.* 2010; AVMA 2020). General operating procedures for lethal biological sampling of fish can be found in Chapter 13.

Infectious pathogens

Freshwater fishes are susceptible to a range of pathogens. Furthermore, stress caused by environmental conditions is a key factor driving the vulnerability of fish to disease (Roberts 2012). Infectious diseases are caused by viruses, parasites, bacteria and fungi, while non-infectious diseases can also develop, especially under poor environmental conditions. There are 24 finfish diseases on Australia's National List of Reportable Diseases of Aquatic Animals, including five recorded in Australia. Researchers need to be aware of the diseases that may occur in freshwater fish and their signs, so that they can report any possible infections. Zoonotic diseases are much less likely from handling fish than some other vertebrates, but care should still be taken. The Australian Government has prepared a field guide for the identification of aquatic animal diseases and guidance on reporting (Department of Agriculture, Water and the Environment 2020). The five reportable finfish diseases identified in Australia are (Department of Agriculture, Water and the Environment 2020):

1. Epizootic haemotopoietic necrosis virus (EHNV), characterised by extensive damage to visceral tissue that leads to mortality, was reported in the introduced redfin perch (*Perca fluviatilis*) from Victoria and the upper Murrumbidgee River region (Becker *et al.* 2019). EHNV can be carried on equipment including nets and boats, so care must be taken to disinfect gear between sites in areas where the virus may be present.
2. Viral encephalopathy and retinopathy (VER), caused by a *Betanodavirus*, has been recorded in at least 70 species of fish (mostly marine) globally.
3. Enteric septicaemia of catfish is caused by infection with *Edwardsiella ictaluri* and characterised by swelling or erosion of connective tissue on top of the head (Kelly *et al.* 2018). It is highly infectious among catfish families including the Plotosidae and Ariidae, and also to non-catfish species.
4. Atypical strains of the bacterium *Aeromonas salmonicida* manifest in external lesions and ulceration, and can affect a wide range of fishes in both marine and freshwater environments. Atypical strains have been reported from New South Wales, Queensland, South Australia, Victoria and Tasmania.
5. Infection with *Aphanomyces invadans*, causing epizootic ulcerative syndrome (EUS), also known as red spot disease, ulcerative mycosis or mycotic granulomatosis. Lesions form on the body and can erode to expose muscle, vertebrae or organs. EUS has been reported from New South Wales, Northern Territory, Queensland, Victoria, South Australia and Western Australia.

A range of smaller Australian fish species, including mountain galaxias (*Galaxias olidus*), are known to be susceptible to ENHV. Enteric septicaemia of catfish is also infectious to non-catfish species. Infection with atypical strains of the bacterium *Aeromonas salmonicida* can affect a wide range of fishes in marine and freshwater environments, and has been reported from New South Wales, Queensland, South Australia, Victoria and Tasmania. Infection with *Aphanomyces invadans*, causing EUS or red spot disease, has been recorded in most Australian states. There are more than 100 freshwater and estuarine fishes known to be susceptible, including *Nematalosa erebi* and *Melanotaenia splendida* (Department of Agriculture, Water and the Environment 2020).

Other introduced parasites have been found in Australian freshwater fishes and if found in any fish should be reported to state biosecurity agencies. It is important that these parasites are not transported to other water bodies or holding facilities. Examples include the Asian fish tapeworm (*Schyzocotyle acheilognathi*) which can be lethal to native fishes, the tapeworm (*Ligula intestinalis*) which has varied impacts leading to higher levels of predation and delayed reproductive development (Morgan 2003), and the parasitic copepod (*Lernaea cyprinacea*) which can be lethal to fish (Marina *et al.* 2008).

General operating procedures

A range of research methods relevant to the study of freshwater fishes is detailed in Chapter 14, including netting and other trapping methods, electrofishing and low-impact techniques. Some methods used for studying marine fishes may also apply to freshwater fishes (see Chapter 13), including capture and release methods, lethal and non-lethal biological sampling, internal tagging methods, external tagging and photo identification, and transport, housing and handling methods. General principles for marking animals with PIT tags and VIE are detailed in Chapter 8.

LARGE-BODIED FISHES

Nicole Flint, Scott A. Hardie, Jonathan Marshall and Alison J. King

Characteristics

While small- and large-bodied fishes (see 'Small-bodied fishes') share many similarities, notable differences between these groups include their intrinsic values, pressures and management approaches. Marine and estuarine fishes are much more frequently targeted for consumption by humans; however, several large freshwater fishes support commercial, recreational or Indigenous fisheries as a food source (Harris *et al.* 2013; Forbes *et al.* 2015) and are highly valued by commercial sectors and the community (Ebner *et al.* 2016b). Many large-bodied species are artificially farmed and some are stocked into rivers, lakes and impoundments for the purposes of recreational fishing (Koehn *et al.* 2020); stocking sometimes occurs in areas that are not within the species' natural range (translocation).

Large-bodied fish that occur in Australian freshwater environments include those from the orders Perciformes (larger-bodied families) and Osteoglossiformes (see Allen *et al.* 2002; Pusey *et al.* 2004; Humphries and Walker 2013). Some of the families also include a subset of smaller species (e.g. family Percichthyidae, *Nannoperca* spp. and *Nannatherina balstoni*; and family Terapontidae, *Amniataba* spp., *Hannia greenwayi, Leiopotherapon macrolepis, Synocomistes* spp.). Of course, all large fish also begin life as small fish, so this section should be read in conjunction with 'Small-bodied fishes'. Several families of eels containing freshwater species also grow to large sizes, but may have different handling considerations to other large fishes (see 'Eels').

Biology and behaviour

Large-bodied fishes typically require deeper water to survive and tend to occupy main channels of rivers, lakes and impoundments, although they may also utilise smaller tributaries and shallow areas intermittently for feeding and spawning. Ontogenetic habitat shifts also occur in most species, with smaller (younger) fish occupying different habitats to fully grown adults, including inundated floodplains and shallow pools or riffles (Koehn and Kennard 2013). As adults, some species occupy mid-water habitats (e.g. saratoga, archerfish), while others remain closer to the substrate, riverbanks or structural woody habitat (e.g. barramundi, *Lates calcarifer*; Murray cod, *Maccullochella peelii*). Scour holes created by water flowing around woody structures are favoured by some larger fishes, such as Australian bass (*Percalates novemaculeata*, Borg *et al.* 2007; Koehn and Kennard 2013). Habitat structural complexity and hydraulic conditions in freshwater environments greatly influence fish assemblages (Koehn and Kennard 2013). Another important aspect of fish habitat is water quality. Very high water temperatures, low dissolved oxygen, high conductivity, suboptimal pH, high nutrients and toxicants can render otherwise suitable fish habitats unsuitable.

Movements on varying scales are critical to the ecology of freshwater fishes. Many large-bodied fishes move extensively throughout or at specific times during their life cycles and are reliant on passage between upstream and downstream areas, or between fresh- and saltwater systems. Movements can be impeded by weirs and dry river sections, so it is important that fish passage infrastructure allows for both upstream and downstream movement of large fish (Koehn and Crook 2013).

Movement patterns of many larger freshwater fishes have been studied extensively, and in recent years monitoring technology and techniques have allowed further insights into their behaviour (Koehn and Crook 2013). Murray cod movements have been particularly well documented over many years. While adult Murray cod can exhibit high site fidelity, they can also move extensively on a range of scales, including large-scale upstream movements to spawn (Leigh and Zampatti 2013). Golden perch (*Macquaria ambigua*) are a highly mobile species, with all life stages exhibiting different movement requirements in upstream, downstream and lateral directions (Koehn *et al.* 2020). The movements of some larger fishes, and notably many northern Australian taxa such as southern saratoga (*S. leichardti*), are less well understood (Pusey *et al.* 2004).

Families with predominantly large-bodied species are usually carnivorous or omnivorous, with trophic shifts occurring throughout the growth phase and differences in diet recorded at different capture locations. Murray cod is an apex predator, feeding on decapods and fish (Ebner 2006). The endangered eastern freshwater cod (*Maccullochella ikei*) consumes a range of prey, from small aquatic insects and crustaceans to relatively large terrestrial animals (including mice, rabbits, rats, bandicoot, birds; Butler and Wooden 2012). Adult barramundi are also top predators, feeding mostly on fish (66%) and macrocrustaceans (33%), and cannibalising smaller conspecifics (Pusey *et al.* 2004). Saratoga are aggressive and territorial, and so are probably rarely abundant in a waterway; they have been described as surface feeders, consuming insects, crustaceans, fish and terrestrial plant material (Bishop *et al.* 1990). The diet of spangled perch is dominated by aquatic invertebrates with some aquatic vegetation. Sooty grunter (*Hephaestus fuliginosus*) is similarly omnivorous, but with greater proportions of fish consumed by large size classes (Pusey *et al.* 2004).

Similar to small-bodied fishes, larger fishes display a variety of reproductive strategies. Therefore, researchers should familiarise themselves with the current knowledge of reproduction and life histories of their target species to design studies appropriately (e.g. sampling outside of the breeding periods of threatened species) and also for interpretation of project results. A summary of some aspects of the reproductive strategies of larger-bodied fishes is provided below.

While several of Australia's freshwater fishes display varying levels of parental care towards their young, perhaps the most unusual reproductive behaviour is demonstrated by the forehead brooding nurseryfish (*Kurtus gulliveri*), where the mature male carries the fertilised eggs in a supraoccipital hook (Berra and Wedd 2017). Capture of this species is often difficult and can result in the eggs being accidentally dislodged; careful handling is required when studying this species (see 'Capture and handling' in this sub-chapter).

Barramundi (*L. calcarifer*) are facultative catadromous fish inhabiting tropical and subtropical waterways and are protandrous hermaphrodites, usually beginning to change sex from male to female at around 80 cm in length. While the freshwater residence phase is not required for successful reproduction, and various freshwater–marine migratory contingents exist (Crook *et al.* 2017), it has been theorised that access to freshwater environments provides a fitness advantage for the species through increased growth rates (Roberts *et al.* 2019). The reproductive biology of large fishes with complex life histories is an important consideration when planning research as these species can take a relatively long time to mature and contribute to recruitment.

Female Murray cod migrate upstream to spawn in late winter or early spring, where they deposit large (3–3.5 mm diameter), adhesive eggs onto hard surfaces such as rocks or logs. The number of eggs varies with female size from 10 000 eggs for young fish, to more than 100 000 eggs for large females (Stuart and Koehn 2007). For this reason, large females are particularly important to maintaining populations. Males guard the eggs for up to 2 weeks until they hatch, and hatching larvae drift downstream. The adult fish also move back downstream after spawning, to the same territory that they came from (Koehn *et al.* 2009).

Several Terapontidae species spawn demersal, non-adhesive eggs over sand and mud substrates (e.g. *Amniataba percoides*, *L. unicolor*) and some (e.g. *L. unicolor*, *H. fuliginosus*) have been observed to spawn in aggregations (Pusey *et al.* 2004). Critically endangered silver perch (*Bidyanus bidyanus*) are pelagic spawners and the eggs and larvae drift downstream in a non-uniform manner, with highest egg and larval densities near the shore and low in the water column (Tonkin *et al.* 2007).

The two extant Australian species of saratoga (*S. jardinii* and *S. leichardti*) are ancient primary freshwater fishes that likely originated from the supercontinent Gondwana. Saratoga are mouth brooders; the female incubates small numbers of large (~10 mm diameter) eggs and then guards her young until ~4 weeks after hatching (Pusey *et al.* 2004). While holding a brood in her buccal cavity, the female appears to have a white chin, a sign that alerts researchers to handle these mouth-brooding fish carefully, if captured. Females are not mature until their fourth or fifth year and life span is thought to be at least several years longer than that, possibly decades (Pusey *et al.* 2004).

Capture and handling

Electrofishing is often suitable for capturing large-bodied fish species, but is not useful for all sites or species, and is less effective in turbid, deep, fast-flowing or structurally dense habitats. For example, electrofishing was unsuccessful for capturing nurseryfish (*K. gulliveri*) in northern Australian rivers, as immobilised fish were not visible in turbid water; gill netting was a more-effective method for capturing this species (Berra and Wedd 2017). Purpose-built traps and modified nets (e.g. fykes and gill nets) are also frequently used for capturing large-bodied species.

Handling of very large fishes (e.g. > 80 cm) should take into account their body mass and strength, and their ability to damage smaller fishes if held together temporarily. Capture and containment of very large fishes also require larger equipment. Because of their large body mass, larger fishes need to be supported during capture and handling to avoid tissue damage. 'Lip grippers', which are mechanical devices commonly used by recreational fishers to secure large fish by their jaw (while lifting), can injure fish. A study of barramundi identified damage caused by lip grippers, including holes in the jaw membrane and altered alignment of vertebrae, which had not returned to normal after 3 weeks of observation (Gould and Grace 2009). It is often safer for fish and researchers to avoid lifting very large fish out of the water unless absolutely necessary (e.g. in waters inhabited by crocodiles). If safe to do so, fish can be cradled alongside the boat or bank with gloved hands, in a measuring tube or a fabric sling, to allow for data collection, including species identification and length measurements.

Veterinary considerations

Sedation and anaesthesia

Anaesthetic considerations are similar among bony fish groups (Mylniczenko *et al.* 2014). See 'Estuarine fishes' in Chapter 30) for a discussion of anaesthetic principles for fish. For studies that don't involve extensive fish handling (e.g. fish surveys which identify, measure, weigh and release animals), large fish can be handled without anaesthesia. In other situations, they may need to be immobilised to allow safe handling, for both fish and operator safety. Electro-immobilisation and soluble anaesthetics are commonly used for surgical tagging of large fishes (see 'Venomous fishes' for a description of electroimmobilisation) and in some cases tonic immobility may be an option (see Chapter 13). Poor handling techniques can cause injuries to researchers and fish, especially if the fish have sharp spines on their fins or gill plates or are particularly large. Large fish can suffer injuries and internal damage if their weight is not well supported during handling.

Euthanasia

Lethal sampling may be required to gather data including, but not limited to, age and growth, reproduction, diet and digestion, parasitology and disease diagnosis, sensory biology (vision, electroreception, etc.), toxicant concentrations in tissues, lipid analyses, and taxonomy for voucher specimen collections. This is more accurately described as killing rather than euthanasia, but the same principles apply. Immersion in a hyper-concentrated anaesthetic solution is the preferred method (e.g. isoeugenol, clove oil or tricaine methanesulfonate buffered with sodium bicarbonate) (AVMA 2020). However, some large fish may need to be killed by other means such as by physical methods (AVMA 2020; see also Chapter 13). There are inherent morphological differences of large fish that must be considered. When capturing and handling large fishes, operators need to ensure that sufficient doses of anaesthetics are used for killing (large fish typically require higher doses than smaller fish), and that the fish are handled appropriately.

Infectious pathogens

Freshwater fish diseases are described in 'Small-bodied fishes'. Large Australian fish species including Murray cod (*M. peelii*) and silver perch (*B. bidyanus*) are susceptible to ENHV. Viral encephalopathy and retinopathy have been recorded globally and barramundi (*L. calcarifer*) in Australian aquaculture facilities are now routinely screened for the disease. Enteric septicaemia of catfish is also infectious to non-catfish species including barramundi. Infection with *Aphanomyces invadans*, causing epizootic ulcerative syndrome (EUS) or red spot disease, has been recorded in most Australian states. Freshwater species that are known to be susceptible include golden perch, mouth almighty (*Glossamia aprion*), Murray cod, and saratoga (Department of Agriculture, Water and the Environment 2020).

General operating procedures

See details for 'Small-bodied fishes'.

LAMPREYS AND LUNGFISH

David T. Roberts and David L. Morgan

Characteristics

The only surviving species of the Sarcopterygii, which includes the ancient relic groups of lungfish and coelocanths, extant in Australia is the Australian lungfish (*Neoceratodus forsteri*). The Australian lungfish is endemic to the Mary River and Burnett River in Queensland, but is believed to have been translocated into several other rivers in south-east Queensland (Hughes *et al.* 2015; Bishop *et al.* 2018). The most successful of these introductions being the Brisbane and North Pine River populations.

The lampreys (class Petromyzontida) are one of two surviving groups of jawless fishes (Agnatha) and while some 37 species are present in the Northern Hemisphere, only five species are found in the Southern Hemisphere, three of which occur in Australia (Potter *et al.* 2015; Riva-Rossi et al. 2020). The Southern Hemisphere lampreys belong to either the Geotriidae (two species) or the Mordaciidae (three species) families. The most widely distributed Southern Hemisphere species, the pouched lamprey (*Geotria australis*), is found in the drainages and seas of south-western and south-eastern Australia (including Tasmania), New Zealand and Chile. The other Australian species are both endemic to south-eastern Australia, the short-headed lamprey (*Mordacia mordax*) and the precocious lamprey (*M. praecox*), but of these species only *M. mordax* occurs in Tasmania (Potter *et al.* 2015).

Biology and behaviour

Australian lungfish occur in large slow-flowing rivers, preferring deeper pools and complex structural habitats that provide abundant cover and food sources (Kind 2010). Australian lungfish rarely occupy swiftly flowing water and tend to favour deep water during daylight, venturing into shallow water at night or when spawning within macrophytes (Kind 2010). Relatively little is known about juvenile Australian lungfish habitat requirements, other than an apparent close association with dense macrophytes after hatching. They inhabit artificial impoundments, but are restricted to the shallower depth zones above oxyclines (Roberts *et al.* 2017). While spawning occurs within impoundments, in general they do not provide suitable conditions for recruitment (Roberts *et al.* 2014). The habitats used by lampreys vary with life stage, from a widely ranging oceanic phase, to larvae that bury into the substrate (Potter 1970). The precocious lamprey in contrast completes its life cycle in freshwater habitats. Lamprey larvae generally prefer silty (occasionally sandy) substrates (Potter 1970).

Australian lungfish movements in riverine habitats are restricted to small home ranges, rarely venturing more than a few kilometres, occasionally moving larger distances in flood (Kind 2010). Swimming capabilities are believed to be poor and observations in fishways suggest they are unable to cope with high velocities for long periods (A. Berghuis, pers. comm.). Nothing is known about juvenile movements, although it is believed they remain within the dense macrophyte-dominated habitat of their natal grounds for some time.

The life cycle of the lampreys (*G. australis* and *M. mordax*) is anadromous, and following metamorphosis juveniles migrate to the ocean where they begin their carnivorous (parasitic) journey lasting up to ~2 years. During this period, the juveniles grow and return to freshwaters where their upstream spawning migration begins. Comparatively, precocious lampreys migrate upstream to spawn and their life cycle is completed in freshwater. Little is known about the movements of larvae, but they are likely to locate suitable habitats as water levels rise and fall seasonally, and larvae prefer larger substrate particle sizes as they grow (Dawson *et al.* 2015).

Australian lungfish are considered to be generalist omnivores with a diet dominated by invertebrates (e.g. snails, bivalves and crustaceans) (Tao *et al.* 2020). While copious vegetative matter is observed in faeces, fatty acid analysis suggests little of this is digested or assimilated (Tao *et al.* 2020). Peak foraging activity occurs at night. Pouched lamprey and short-headed lamprey are parasitic as juveniles in their marine phase, but do not eat during their upstream migration phase or as adults (Potter *et al.* 1986). Their distinctive oral disc dentition strongly suggests that they are well adapted for eating flesh (pouched lamprey) or blood (short-headed lamprey) of their hosts when in their parasitic phase (Potter *et al.* 1986). In contrast, the precocious lamprey is non-parasitic. Their larval stages feed on diatoms (Potter 1970).

The Australian lungfish is a slow-growing and long-lived species (Fallon *et al.* 2019) that is believed to mature at ~15 years of age (Kind 2010) and shows no discernible sexual dimorphism. Spawning occurs in small groups over an extended season of up to 5 months from August to December (Kind 2010). Triggers for spawning have been attributed to a combination of day length, water temperature and flow (Espinoza *et al.* 2013). Total fecundity is unknown but is thought to exceed 10 000, with fertilised eggs deposited in small, serially spawned batches of several hundred per spawning event in dense submerged macrophyte beds (Kind 2010). Eggs hatch in 25–30 days and the hatched young are largely immobile until the egg sack is resorbed, when exogenous feeding commences at around 16–26 days post-hatching (Kemp 1981). Spawning and recruitment success is critically dependent on the availability of dense submerged macrophytes.

While all lampreys have a blind larval (ammocoete) stage that is restricted to freshwater habitats, two of the Australian species are anadromous (pouched lamprey and short-headed lamprey), whereby large subadults migrate upstream into rivers from the ocean to mature, and eventually spawn and die. In contrast, the precocious lamprey is potamodromous and completes its life cycle entirely within freshwaters, undertaking short upstream migrations to spawn. The duration of the marine phase of the two anadromous species is unknown, but is believed to last for up to 2 years, while the ammocoete stage varies between the species and lasts for over 4 years in pouched lamprey and over 3 years in short-headed lamprey (Potter 1970; Potter and Hilliard 1986). Manzon *et al.* (2015) provide general information on lamprey metamorphosis, while Potter *et al.* (1980) detail metamorphosis in pouched lamprey.

The function and purpose of the gular pouch in pouched lamprey has been subject to much discussion. It is only relatively recently that the mating and spawning behaviour, gular pouch function (to massage and move eggs around until hatching, supplying oxygen) and tending of nests by pouched lamprey have been described (Baker *et al.* 2017; Paton *et al.* 2020). During sexual maturation, males develop a large gular pouch and their suctorial disc becomes enlarged, and they are frequently aggressive towards each other. According to Baker *et al.* (2017), males seem to pair with the same female during mating. During mating, the male coils around the female and twists and vibrates, leading to the release of eggs and fertilisation. Baker *et al.* (2017) discovered nests of pouched lamprey under boulders after a 15-month (non-feeding) maturation period when mean daily water temperature was ~11°C. Each nest examined contained a male and female pair, which were concealed under boulders with their eggs. The eggs appear as an adhesive coagulated cluster and a single female was found to have a fecundity of over 56 000 eggs (Baker *et al.* 2017). The males tend the eggs until they hatch, ~6 weeks after spawning. The newly hatched larvae have an adhesive caudal region and, rather than burrowing, are attached to boulders for at least 2 weeks while they develop. Some spent fish remain alive for well over a year following spawning.

Capture and handling

The most widely used and accepted technique for effective capture of adult Australian lungfish is boat-mounted electrofishing. The unique morphology, size and general sedentary habit of Australian lungfish makes most other capture techniques, such as netting or trapping, inefficient or impractical. Adults are susceptible to mild electrical fields showing strong positive taxis towards anodes and, with an air-filled lung, they readily rise from depth when immobilised. Juvenile lungfish (< 200 mm in length) are rarely encountered in the wild, but have been collected with electrofishing and nets. Eggs and post-hatch juveniles are primarily collected with nets pushed through shallow macrophyte beds (Espinoza *et al.* 2013).

Adult Australian lungfish are robust and tolerate handling well, including short periods out of the water for processing (since they can breathe air). Adults often measure over 900 mm in length and 7 kg in body weight, so handling and processing considerations are needed to avoid fish and handler injury (see 'Large-bodied fishes'). Adults remain sedate when captured, but can become startled, turning on sudden bursts of activity that risk damaging themselves through cuts, abrasions and scale loss. Handling small numbers of adult fish can be done in holding tanks with water, but for larger numbers, handling and processing are best done without water by shading fish with layers of wet hessian for short periods. This short-term waterless approach also reduces startling from changes in light conditions, cushions large adults from injury when startled, and allows for effective handling during processing.

Back-pack electrofishers are the most efficient technique for capturing lamprey's ammocoete larvae that are buried in the substrate; the electric shock brings them to the substrate's surface. Electrofishing of ammocoete beds also allows an estimation of ammocoete density to be determined. During their upstream migration phase, lampreys are most commonly captured using fyke nets, or by hand when they migrate *en masse* and leave the water to pass barriers (natural and artificial). Electrofishing can also be used to capture over-summering adults and subadults.

Marking of Australian lungfish is best done with implanted tags, such as PIT or acoustic tags (Figure 32.2). External tags are more easily shed or damaged and are less reliable as long-term markers (Brooks and Kind 2002). Chemical marking of scales with dyes like oxytetracycline has been used as a reliable marking technique (Fallon *et al.* 2019). Adult Australian lungfish contain no discernible permanent markings enabling individual identification. Surgical techniques for implanting tags into the body cavity of lungfish require careful consideration, as the abdominal body wall is thick and covered in three large overlapping scales. Consequently, this procedure should be done by experienced personnel to achieve effective incision, suturing and wound closure to ensure tag retention and the best outcome for the fish's welfare.

The very limited visceral space in lampreys means that PIT tags (see Baker *et al.* 2017) or VIE tags are the best options for tagging *Geotria* or *Mordacia* spp. Jellyman and Tsukamoto (2002) attempted to track large pouched lamprey with external radio tags, but tag retention was low. Bice *et al.* (2019) used PIT tags and attached external acoustic tags to monitor lamprey movement in the lower Murray River (primarily pouched *G. australis*) with some success. However, the external tag attachment made tagged fish vulnerable to entanglement in commercial gill nets.

Veterinary considerations

Sedation and anaesthesia

Lungfish and lampreys are susceptible to most commercial fish sedatives. However, when kept in holding vessels they produce considerable quantities of mucus that lessens the effectiveness of sedatives, and regular monitoring and refreshing of water and sedative are needed to maintain effective dose responses. For short-term holding, such as for measuring and PIT tagging, sedation of lungfish may not always be necessary when handled gently and covered, as they remain relatively docile. However, the use of isoeugenol is often the preferred sedative method. In contrast, lampreys are very active and difficult to restrain to measure or tag, so they should be sedated before PIT tag insertion.

Euthanasia

In the event that an Australian lungfish or lamprey requires euthanasia, it is recommended they be given a

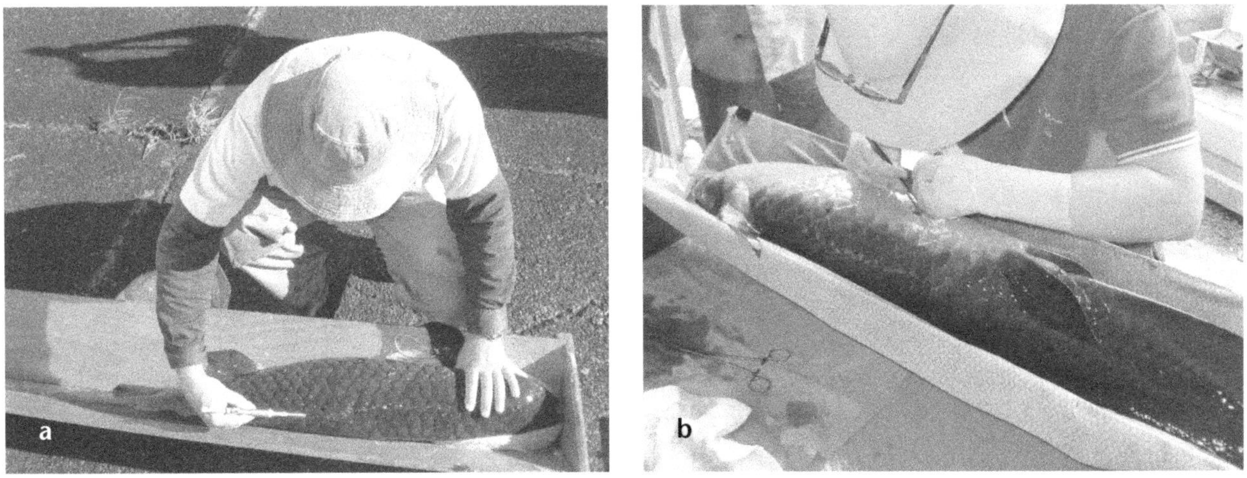

Figure 32.2: Examples of procedures applied to an Australian lungfish (*Neoceratodus forsteri*): (a) PIT tagging and (b) surgical implanting of an acoustic tag by a veterinarian. Photos by David Roberts.

lethal dose of anaesthetic (e.g. isoeugenol) and monitored closely to ensure the dose is effective. A fin-pinch technique is a reliable method for testing reflex response.

Infectious pathogens

Freshwater fish diseases are described in 'Small-bodied fishes'. Limited information is available on specific diseases in lungfish or Australian lamprey species. From personal experience, the incidence of external disease signs in wild Australian lungfish is rare, with occasional observations of losses in body condition or physical damage associated with waterway barrier interaction (e.g. muscle wasting, skin lesions or tissue necrosis). Regular recaptures of fish formerly exhibiting these conditions suggest low rates of disease susceptibility and mortalities associated with minor injury. Captive Australian lungfish have rarely been reported to succumb to disease symptoms (Strike *et al.* 2017). Upstream migrating *G. australis* are susceptible to haemorrhagic septicaemia in wild habitats and in captivity, which can be treated following the methods of Paton *et al.* (2020).

General operating procedures

See details for 'Small-bodied fishes'.

EELS

Brendan C. Ebner

Characteristics

The term 'eel' captures an extraordinary diversity of fishes that are elongate in body shape and comprise many families that are not monophyletic (Nelson *et al.* 2016). Eels that occur in Australian freshwater environments are represented by the orders Anguilliformes (families Anguillidae and Muraenidae) and Synbranchiformes (family Synbranchidae) (for details and distributions see Allen *et al.* 2002; Ebner *et al.* 2011b; Watanabe 2003; Morgan *et al.* 2014; Moore *et al.* 2018; Moore 2019). The genus *Anguilla* comprises several species that are challenging to identify from external features with the taxonomy of the genus evolving (Watanabe 2003). Swamp eel (Synbranchidae) taxonomy is unresolved and species-level identifications in Australia should be treated with caution, with the exception of the unique blind cave eel (*Ophisternon candidum*) (Moore *et al.* 2018; Moore 2019).

Biology and behaviour

Most *Anguilla* species are relatively widespread as a function of a lengthy marine larval phase (Watanabe 2003; Tsukamoto *et al.* 2011). The glass eel phase ceases when young eels migrate into catchments to settle in benthic habitats and bury in the substrate. With ongoing development, juveniles bury less and are increasingly associated with above streambed structure (e.g. undercuts, woody debris, rock interstices) (Pusey *et al.* 2004). Several species occupy streams, rivers and estuaries (e.g. *Anguilla marmorata* and *A. reinhardtii*), while others are associated with essentially lentic waters including swamps (e.g. *A. bicolor*; Hagihara *et al.* 2018).

Freshwater morays (*Gymnothorax polyuranodon*) migrate to and from the ocean as larvae (Tsukamoto *et al.* 2014). Juveniles and adults occupy a den under boulders and cobble (and occasionally in woody debris), which typically has two or three exits (Ebner *et al.* 2016a). The species is highly flexible and strongly laterally compressed, and is typically observed with only the head protruding from the den. In Australia, this species occurs in short, steep, coastal streams in the Wet Tropics bioregion (Ebner *et al.* 2011b, 2016a). The blind cave eel, occupies subterranean caves and groundwater in the Pilbara region of Western Australia. Other swamp eels (*Ophisternon* spp.) inhabit swamps and lowland creeks in northern Australia (e.g. Allen *et al.* 2002).

All species of *Anguilla* undertake large-scale adult migrations to oceanic spawning locations and return to coastal waters as larvae. Crook *et al.* (2014) have shown that maturing southern shortfin eel (*A. australis*) in many cases gradually move lower in the catchment before undertaking oceanic migration. Several species of *Anguilla* are territorial and intraspecific aggression is common based on direct observations and scars on the body (B. C. Ebner, pers. obs.). At some locations individuals actively hunt by day, though *Anguilla* spp. are often most active at night (Jellyman and Sykes 2003; C. Ebner, pers. obs.), rendering them vulnerable to collection by overnight fyke netting. When foraging, freshwater morays typically stay on the benthos and are snakelike in their movement while inspecting interstices for prey. Little is known of movement in swamp eel species in Australia.

As juveniles, *Anguilla* spp. commence feeding on small prey ranging from aquatic and terrestrial insects to crustaceans and fish. All species grow to become top or apex predators feeding primarily on fish, crustaceans and terrestrial insects (Jardine 2016). The freshwater moray is a mesopredator that feeds on benthic crustaceans (mostly prawns, shrimps and crabs) and also worms and benthic fishes (Ebner 2017). This moray actively forages in cobble-boulder habitats by poking its head into interstitial spaces to seek out prey. Synbranchids are carnivorous feeding mostly on zooplankton, aquatic insects, crustaceans and small fishes (Humphreys and Feinberg 1995). *Anguilla* species and freshwater morays have excellent olfactory capabilities. Freshwater morays rely heavily on olfaction and detection of close-range vibrations. *Anguilla* spp. are also capable of visual hunting. Synbranchids are capable of near-range feeding strikes on mobile prey and operate primarily as ambush predators rather than actively pursuing prey (B. C. Ebner, pers. obs.).

Collectively, *Anguilla* species spend most of their lives in freshwater or estuary habitats (Hagihara *et al.* 2018). Then they undertake a rapid transformation to adulthood, including enlargement of the eyes and pigmentation changes just before migrating to group spawn in oceanic waters where they perish soon after (e.g. Hagihara *et al.* 2012). Species and subspecies are associated with major oceanic basins and latitudinal zones more than specific continents (e.g. *A. australis* in the Southern Ocean, *A. bicolor bicolor* in the tropical Indo-Pacific, *A. megastoma* in the tropical central Pacific) (Watanabe 2003).

Unlike most moray species (family Muraenidae), which are marine, the freshwater moray has a marine larval phase and a freshwater or brackish juvenile and adult phase (Ebner *et al.* 2011b, 2016a, 2020; Tsukamoto *et al.* 2014). Published information regarding moray (family Muraenidae) breeding biology is limited (cf. Thresher 1984). The freshwater moray is highly fecund and capable of full oocyte (egg) development in freshwater (B. C. Ebner, unpublished data), and the species is probably capable of catadromy and possibly amphidromy. While there have not been detailed studies of reproduction of Australian synbranchids, some species from outside of Australia are hermaphroditic (Mazzoni *et al.* 2018).

Capture and handling

All eel species discussed in this chapter can be captured by electrofishing; large individuals differ in their susceptibility to being immobilised as a function of their length. Electrofishing is often the only effective method for collecting swamp eels from deep areas within undercut banks and thick tree root complexes. Fyke netting, especially overnight, is effective for collecting *Anguilla* spp. and to some extent freshwater moray; although *Anguilla* spp. can be aggressive towards one another and cause injury and even cannibalism if held for prolonged periods in closed spaces. *Anguilla* spp. and freshwater morays can be collected by hook and line, and lethally sampled by hand-spear or spear-gun, the latter being advantageous in remote areas that must be accessed on foot (e.g. in dense rainforests). However, a bankside chamber for immediately overdosing individuals with anaesthetic is recommended when collecting large individuals by spear, since they can be difficult to kill. Care should be taken during capture, as venomous snakes caught in nets can appear similar to eels on first sight.

Handling, weighing and accurate measuring of eels is best done with temporary sedation. Difficulty with handling eels and efforts to avoid the mucus sloths from some species often lead researchers to release eels quickly; this has undoubtedly led to dubious species-level identifications. Swamp eels are the easiest to handle of the eels mentioned here. Total length can often be estimated on a measuring board without the need for anaesthesia. However, correct identification to species level is currently inhibited by unresolved taxonomy and the few distinguishing external features of swamp eels.

Tagging of eels and telemetry (including archival tags) have been crucial to understanding the life cycles of these animals (e.g. Jellyman and Tsukamoto 2002; Crook *et al.* 2014). However, eels may sloth and self-remove tags, which is problematic from a program design perspective (Baras and Jeandrain 1998).

Transport of eels is best achieved in containers with tight, secure lids to safeguard against their propensity to escape. If multiple individuals are being moved or housed, it is important to separate them and/or grade individuals by size and provide cover to minimise aggression and cannibalism. Freshwater morays of similar sizes can be housed together if adequate space and cover is provided (Ebner 2017).

Veterinary considerations

Sedation and anaesthesia

It can be challenging to achieve even basic length and morphometric measurement of most eels due to their wriggling and twisting behaviour. Therefore, mild anaesthesia is required when performing aquaria trials and studying the ecology of these species in the field. Surgical procedures on eels, including internal tagging, require deep anaesthesia (Ebner 2017; Walsh and Pease 2002). Temporary sedation of eels is commonly achieved by immersion in an anaesthetic, such as clove oil or isoeugenol, or ice slurry, noting that anaesthesia dosages typically need to be two to four times higher than dosage rates that are effective for scaled fishes (Ebner 2017).

Euthanasia

Lethal sampling may be required to gather data including, but not limited to, age and growth, reproduction, diet and digestion, parasitology and disease diagnosis, sensory biology (vision, electroreception, etc.), toxicant concentrations in tissues, lipid analyses, and taxonomy for voucher specimen collections. Killing of *G. polyuranodon*, synbranchids and small individuals of *Anguilla* spp. can be achieved by immersion in a chemical anaesthetic (e.g. clove oil, isoeugenol). Elevated concentrations are required to achieve killing compared with recommended anaesthetic dosages for many scaled fishes. Tightly sealed chambers/buckets with negligible air spaces are needed to remove the opportunity for surface breathing and achieve rapid killing of *Anguilla* spp., particularly large-bodied individuals.

Infectious pathogens

Freshwater fish diseases are described in 'Small-bodied fishes'. There has been limited research into specific diseases of eels. Kennedy (1995) reported a diverse parasite community in *A. reinhardtii* collected from north-eastern Australia. The nematode *Anguillocola australiensis* is common in *A. reinhardtii* but does not appear to have a major pathogenic effect on the host. There has been some preliminary work done on parasites of swamp eels, though not in the Australian context. Infection with atypical strains of the bacterium *Aeromonas salmonicida* can affect a wide range of fishes in both marine and freshwater environments, including eels (*Anguilla* spp.) (Department of Agriculture, Water and the Environment 2020).

General operating procedures

See details for 'Small-bodied fishes'.

VENOMOUS FISHES

Nicole Flint, Jonathan Marshall, David L. Morgan, Alison J. King and Brendan C. Ebner

Characteristics

Australia hosts four families of venomous freshwater fishes. In Australia, there is only one freshwater species in the family Tetrarogidae (bullrout, *Notesthes robusta*); nine in the family Ariidae (forktail catfish); 15 in the family Plotosidae (eel-tailed catfish); and two in the family Scatophagidae (scats) (see Pusey *et al.* 2004; Humphries and Walker 2013). *Urogymnus dalyensis* (freshwater whipray) also has a venomous spine; animal welfare considerations for all marine and freshwater Chrondrichthyes are covered in Chapter 31. All the species listed in this section pose danger to researchers and should be handled with extreme care. It is recommended that researchers who are not familiar with these species seek guidance from practitioners who are experienced in capturing and handling these fishes.

The bullrout is the only Australian freshwater representative of the taxonomic order Scorpaeniformes (scorpionfish), so called for their venomous dorsal, anal and ventral fin spines, which can inflict excruciating pain. The species can grow up to 35 cm in length, although is usually encountered at 15–20 cm or smaller (Pusey *et al.* 2004). Two families of catfish are native to Australia and both contain freshwater species. The taxonomy of Australian Siluriformes is not fully established and new species are still being identified (e.g. Welsh *et al.* 2014). Ariidae are medium- to large-sized catfish, and Australian species range from 30 to 160 cm in maximum length. While the maxillary barbels extending from the mouth are harmless, the dorsal fin and two pectoral fins each have a strong, serrated, venomous spine. Although some species of Plotosidae can reach over 1 m in length, they are commonly encountered at sizes ranging from 10 to 20 cm (Pusey *et al.* 2004). Similar to Ariidae, Plotosidae have maxillary barbels and most possess strong venomous dorsal and pectoral spines, but are easily distinguished from ariids by their flattened tapering caudal fin (soft dorsal, caudal and anal fins are continuous). The exception being the false-spined catfish (*Neosilurus pseudospinosus*), which has a dorsal fin composed of a single non-venomous, flexible cartilaginous ray and four soft rays. The Scatidae are mostly marine, but two species are often found in the lower reaches of northern Australian coastal freshwater systems: spotted scat (*Scatophagus argus*) and striped scat (*Selenotoca multifasciata*). Scats have deep, ovate bodies that are laterally compressed, with a short head and small mouth. Rough spines on the dorsal and anal fins contain cells producing venom (Ghafari *et al.* 2013).

Biology and behaviour

Often found close to the coast, the bullrout is rarely found at elevations greater than 100 m above sea level, and is most frequently encountered in streams with little or no flow and with gravel or rocky substrates (Pusey *et al.* 2004). Submerged vegetation, leaf litter, woody debris and undercut banks are used as cover. Ariidae inhabit a wide range of freshwater habitats. *Neoarius* spp. occur in main channel and off-channel floodplain habitats (Pusey *et al.* 2004) and are common in impounded waters (N. Flint, unpublished data) in tropical and temperate Australia as well as in nearshore marine environments. Plotosids are widely distributed in freshwater habitats, including large rivers, high-velocity streams, shallow lagoons, lakes and impoundments (Pusey *et al.* 2004). For example, Hyrtl's catfish (*Neosilurus hyrtlii*) occurs in habitats ranging from large permanent river channels to intermittent streams, billabongs and floodplain lagoons. The eel-tailed catfish (*Tandanus tandanus*) was naturally ubiquitous within its historical range and can be found in both low- and high-flow waterways, but is declining in south-eastern Australia because of competition with introduced species and altered flow regimes (Clunie and Koehn 2001).

Available movement data suggest that bullrout may be nocturnal (Pusey *et al.* 2004), but as ambush predators they are relatively sedentary on short time scales. The species may be diadromous and thus reliant on connectivity between the freshwater and estuarine reaches of rivers. Similarly, movement records of some Ariidae species suggest a diadromous life cycle (Stuart and Mallen-Cooper 1999) while others are likely to be freshwater only. The available information on Australian species of Plotosidae does not suggest diadromy for any species. However, movements of eel-tailed catfish following high-flow events in subtropical rivers are suggestive of 'home-range shift' behaviour (Burndred *et al.* 2018). Research on the range-restricted freshwater cobbler (*T. bostocki*) (Plotosidae) demonstrates the species undertakes considerable within-river movements and suggests that larger individuals exhibit homing behaviour and site fidelity, possibly to individual pools (Beatty *et al.* 2010; Storer *et al.* 2021). Similar home-ranging patterns have previously been demonstrated for eel-tailed catfish from eastern Australia (Koster *et al.* 2015) and for plotosids in the northern Murray–Darling Basin (Marshall *et al.* 2016). Little information is available on movements of scats, but their reproductive biology (requiring brackish to marine water) suggests some level of diadromy.

The bullrout is an ambush predator that conceals itself amongst aquatic vegetation, feeding on aquatic insects, shrimp and small fishes that swim past (Pusey *et al.* 2004). Ariidae catfishes are opportunistic, feeding on molluscs, shrimp, crabs, insects, fish, vegetation, detritus and even small mammals or birds. Similarly, Plotosidae have an opportunistic diet, feeding on molluscs, crustaceans, insects, worms, fish and small amounts of plants and algae, with some variation between species records (summarised by Pusey *et al.* 2004). Scatophagidae are omnivorous scavengers, feeding on benthic invertebrates and algae (Gupta 2016).

The bullrout is thought to breed in freshwater. However, available movement data (Stuart and Mallen-Cooper 1999) and analysis of otolith chemistry (Miles *et al.* 2009) suggest this species may exhibit complex movements between freshwater and marine environments, indicative of a diadromous life cycle. Records about the biology of the species are few and obscure, and the ecology of larvae is unknown (Pusey *et al.* 2004). Ariidae spawn over spring and summer during the northern Australian wet season. Females spawn relatively few, large eggs (often > 1 cm diameter) and in some species the males incubate the eggs in their mouth. Some species of *Neoarius* and *Sciades* brood both eggs and larvae for 4–8 weeks (species-dependent) until larvae have developed sufficiently to leave their care. Groups of brooding males of *N. midgleyi* have been observed together in deep water (Pusey *et al.* 2004) but little is known of their reproductive behaviour or ecology. Plotosids utilise diverse reproductive strategies. *Neosilurus ater* and *N. hyrtlii* migrate upstream within river channels during flooding to spawn in pairs in shallow riffles, where their demersal eggs lodge in the substrate (Orr and Milward 1984). Both species exhibit colour changes during spawning. *Tandanus tandanus* deposit eggs into nests constructed in the substrate or submerged vegetation, and are guarded and fanned by the male, with larvae hatching after 4–7 days (Burndred *et al.* 2017). Currently, little is known about the reproductive biology of scats; however, increasing aquaculture interests may improve this situation. Embryos are most viable at a salinity of 15 ppt, which is less than the optimal salinity for spawning success of adults (25 ppt) (Su *et al.* 2019), indicating that spawning occurs in marine environments.

Capture and handling

Caution should be exercised when handling species that have venomous spines as they can inflict puncture wounds when handled, causing localised pain which can be severe and persistent. Only experienced practitioners should attempt handling. In particular, bullrout have a sting so severe that urgent medical attention may be warranted and the victim may lose consciousness (Pusey *et al.* 2004). First aid in the field for spine injury includes holding the affected body part in hot water, denaturing the protein toxin (as hot as can be comfortably tolerated, ~45°C) for 20 min, briefly removing and then reimmersing in a cycle for as long as pain persists or until medical care is available (St John Ambulance Australia 2020). Infection also commonly results from the puncture and spine injury, so medical attention is needed as soon as possible.

Catfish are regularly caught using a range of methods, including as non-target species. Their erect spines and rolling movements often cause them to become tangled in mesh nets, sometimes necessitating careful cutting of the net to release them. The rolling and thrashing movements, and erect spines of catfishes and scats, are particularly important to consider when handling the animals. Often, they can be handled with wet fabric gloves or material to cover the spines or the use of hand nets to minimise contact. Bullrout are fairly sedentary and are seldom caught in passive nets, but when captured in nets, they tend to lie still, making them difficult to see in low light conditions (Grant 2014). Care is needed when backpack electrofishing in streams inhabited by bullrout as the erect spines of large, immobilised individuals have been known to pierce waders. Large bullrout are easily and safely held by firmly grasping the upper jaw. Researchers need to take care not to react by catching animals if they flip or move suddenly during handling, or they may receive a spine injury.

A range of internal and external fish tagging methods is described in Chapter 14. Despite the obvious challenges of handling venomous fish, several tagging studies have been undertaken on species described in this section, including freshwater cobbler (*T. bostocki*) (Beatty *et al.* 2010; Storer *et al.* 2021) and salmon catfish (*Neoarius leptaspsis*) (Crook *et al.* 2020). Tag retention rates vary between fish species and with tag type (Butler *et al.* 2009).

Transport and housing requirements for these species are similar to other fishes of the same size (see 'Small-bodied fishes' and 'Large-bodied fishes'), but must be managed carefully because of their venomous spines. Scats are popular aquarium fish (Gupta 2016), and are often captured as juveniles. Scorpionfish and catfish are predatory and will eat any animals smaller than them when housed together.

Veterinary considerations

Sedation and anaesthesia

Chemical anaesthetics can be used for fishes described in this chapter; refer to 'Small-bodied fishes', 'Large-bodied fishes' and Chapter 13. Electronarcosis provides an alternative to the use of chemical anaesthetics, and it has been used for surgical tagging of *T. tandanus* in Australia (Marshall *et al.* 2016). Electronarcosis is implemented using a DC (direct current) power supply with electrodes in a bath with added sea salt to increase conductivity. Fish are placed between the two electrodes on a wet and thus conductive cloth with their head towards the anode. Voltage is increased (mean, 0.54 V/cm; range 0.46–0.57 V/cm; mean, 0.08 A; range, 0.08–0.10 A) until anaesthesia is reached. Regardless of sedation depth, constant opercular motion remains. When surgery is complete, the voltage is turned off (Balazik *et al.* 2013). This method has several advantages, being both effective and time-efficient for conducting invasive procedures. Induction of and recovery from narcosis are virtually instantaneous and, in trials of the technique, plasma cortisol (stress) levels of treated fish were indistinguishable from untreated controls after both 1 and 24 h (Balazik *et al.* 2013). For a detailed review of the technique and its application refer to Reid *et al.* (2019).

Euthanasia

Lethal sampling may be required to gather some biological data. For the species discussed in this sub-chapter, killing by immersion in an overdosed solution of an approved anaesthetic is possible and often preferred by animal ethics committees, and immersion in an icy slurry may also be considered as an acceptable method for small warm-water species (Blessing *et al.* 2010). General operating procedures for killing fishes for scientific purposes can be found in Chapter 13.

Infectious pathogens

Freshwater fish diseases are described in the introductory section of this chapter. Catfish are particularly susceptible to infection with *Edwardsiella ictaluri*, causing the disease enteric septicaemia, characterised by swelling or erosion of connective tissue on top of the head (Kelly *et al.* 2018).

General operating procedures

See details in 'Small-bodied fishes'.

INTRODUCED FISHES

Nicole Flint, Scott A. Hardie and Alison J. King

Characteristics

Introduced fish species (species that are not native to Australia) pose a pervasive threat to Australia's distinct native fish fauna and aquatic ecosystems more broadly. As described in Table 32.1, more than 40 introduced fishes have become established in Australia (Lintermans 2004; Harris 2013; García-Díaz *et al.* 2018) and appear almost impossible to eradicate, although some successful control measures and eradications have occurred at localised scales (e.g. eradication of common carp, *Cyprinus carpio*, from Lake Crescent, central Tasmania; Diggle and Wisniewski 2014). Pathways for introduction include acclimatisation, aquaculture, biocontrol and the ornamental aquarium trade (Lintermans 2004; García-Díaz *et al.* 2018). While historical introductions were deliberately made by acclimatisation societies (e.g. common carp, redfin and Salmonidae species), many of the more recent introductions stem from the ornamental trade (e.g. betta, *Betta*

Table 32.1: Freshwater fish families introduced to Australia.

Researchers are encouraged to investigate local permit and regulatory requirements around the capture of introduced fishes before undertaking studies. Information sources: Arthington *et al.* (1984); Pusey *et al.* (2004); Lintermans (2004); Russell *et al.* (2012); Harris (2013); García-Díaz *et al.* (2018); Hammer *et al.* (2019b); Holmes *et al.* (2020).

Family and number of species currently recorded in Australia	Distribution and relevant notes on ecology
Anabantidae (1 species)	Climbing perch (*A. testudineus*) are not currently well established in Australia but pose a high risk for survival, spread and environmental impacts. They can survive for extended periods out of the water and can travel across land using their pectoral fins.
Cichlidae (19+ species)	A variety of cichlid species have been released in Australian waters. Members of this family occur in Vic, NSW, Qld, WA and NT. Mozambique tilapia (*O. mossambicus*) were first recorded in Australia in 1977. They have become established in northern Australian waterways and caused enormous damage in some river basins through destructive nest-building, aggressive behaviour and an ability to outcompete native fish species. The spotted tilapia (*T. mariae*) has also become established in some waterways in northern Qld. Other introduced cichlids that have been found in Australian waterways include *Aequidens pulcher, A. rivulatus, Archocentrus nigrofasciatus, Thorichthyes meeki, Heros severus, Cichlasoma octofasciatum, C. synspilum, C. trimaculatum, Hemichromis bimaculatus, Amphilophus citrinellus, A. labiatus, Astronotus ocellatus, Geophagus brasiliensis, Tilapia sillii* and *Haplochromis burtoni. Parachromis managuensis* is listed as a Prohibited Animal in Qld. Peacock bass (*Cichla* sp.) were recently sighted in the Pioneer River, Qld and have the potential to become a pest species if established.
Cobitidae (1 species)	Oriental weatherloach (*M. anguillicaudatus*) occur throughout south-eastern Australia in Qld, NSW, Vic and SA. They are tolerant of a wide range of environmental conditions and can survive out of water by gulping air, which also allows them to survive drought by burrowing in mud.
Cyprinidae (8 species)	Common carp (*Cyprinus carpio*) are common in the Murray–Darling Basin and many regions in Australia, posing a serious threat to native fish and habitats, competing for resources and destroying aquatic vegetation. Now distributed from SE Qld, to SE WA, including many coastal river systems of NSW, Vic and SA, and one lake in Tas. They can tolerate poor water quality including severe hypoxia. Other cyprinid species established in Australia include Crucian carp (*Carassius carassius*) in the Murray–Darling Basin, goldfish *C. auratus* throughout most of Australia, roach *Rutilus rutilus* in NSW and Vic, rosy barb *Puntius conchonius* in SE Qld and in one small spring on the south-western tip of WA, Sumatra barb *P. tetrazona* in Qld, tench *Tinca tinca* in Tas, Vic, NSW and SA, and whitecloud mountain minnow *Tanichthys albonubes* in Qld.

(Continued)

Table 32.1: *Continued*

Family and number of species currently recorded in Australia	Distribution and relevant notes on ecology
Cyprinodontidae (1 species)	American flagfish (*Jordanella floridae*) is a small ornamental fish, which was first released in Qld.
Gobiidae (2 species)	Yellowfin goby (*Acanthogobius flavimanus*) and streaked goby (*Acentrogobius pfiaumii*) were introduced accidentally through ballast water in coastal ports and then penetrated freshwater. Currently found in NSW and Vic.
Osphronemidae (2 species)	Betta (*Betta splendens*) and three spot gourami (*Trichopodus trichopterus*) are ornamental fishes that have been introduced through the aquarium trade. Both are highly tolerant of poor water quality including hypoxia and may outcompete native species. Gourami are known from Qld, and a large population of betta has recently been reported from the NT.
Percidae (1 species)	Redfin (*Perca fluviatilis*) was introduced to southern Australia from Europe as an angling fish. Implicated in the decline of Macquarie perch (*Macquaria australasica*) and the local extinction of *Galaxiella munda* in WA. Distributed in many drainages in Tas, Vic, NSW, SA and WA.
Poeciliidae (7 species)	Small-bodied, live-bearing fish including 'mosquitofish' (*Gambusia holbrooki, Phalloceros caudimaculatus, P. harpagos*) and several aquarium fish – mollies (*Poecilia latipinna*), guppies (*P. reticulata*), swordtails (*Xiphophorus hellerii*) and platy (*X. maculatus*). Tend to be very tolerant of environmental degradation and present a serious threat to native species through aggressive behaviours and competition for food and habitat. *Gambusia holbrooki* was introduced in a misguided attempt to control mosquito populations (and were later shown to be no better equipped than many native freshwater fishes). They have been implicated in the decline of nine Australian fish and more than 10 frogs, and are abundant in both coastal and inland drainages of Qld, NT, WA, SA, in a single drainage in Tas, and across Central Australia.
Salmonidae (5 species)	Salmonids, including various species of salmon and trout, were deliberately introduced into Australian rivers and lakes in the 1800s by acclimatisation societies. Many of their populations support recreational fisheries (particularly *Oncorhynchus mykiss, O. tshawytscha, Salmo salar* and *S. trutta*) and are maintained by stocking from hatcheries in some jurisdictions. Salmonids are distributed in cool waters in NSW, Vic, Tas and some regions of Qld. *Salmo trutta* is also found in SA and WA. Salmonids have been implicated in the decline of several frogs and native fish species including galaxiids, pygmy perches and Australian grayling.

splendens, in the Northern Territory, Hammer *et al.* 2019b; jaguar cichlid, *Parachromis managuensis*, in Queensland, Holmes *et al.* 2020), and as reviewed by Harris (2013) and García-Díaz *et al.* (2018).

Introduced fishes have been attributed as the cause of severe ecological damage in some aquatic environments, with impacts including competition and predation on native fishes, habitat engineering and degradation, providing vectors for fish parasites and diseases, and food web alterations (Harris 2013). However, some introduced fishes, particularly salmonids, have recreational value and the fisheries these species support in rivers, lakes and impoundments are managed by state agencies through managed stocking strategies and angler fishing regulations (e.g. size and bag limits; Inland Fisheries Service 2020).

In some jurisdictions, undesirable introduced fishes, which are considered to be restricted or noxious species, cannot be returned to the waterway after being captured and must be killed and disposed of appropriately. Researchers are encouraged to investigate local permit and regulatory requirements around the capture of introduced fishes before undertaking studies.

Biology and behaviour

Like native fishes, introduced fishes vary widely in their biology and behaviour. Many introduced species have life-history traits that allow them to naturalise in

Australian systems, including rapid growth, high fecundity and flexible habitat and feeding requirements. Some are tolerant of variable environmental conditions, including poor water quality, potentially affording them an advantage over native fish species in degraded habitats. Harris (2013) reviews issues with introduced fishes in Australia, their invasion ecology and impacts. This subchapter focuses on several species that are widely distributed and have already had significant impacts on native fishes and habitats.

A characteristic common to many successful invasive freshwater fishes is their ability to inhabit degraded habitats. Common carp have high tolerance to poor water quality, preferring low-flow waterways with aquatic vegetation. They can survive temperature extremes, high salinity and turbidity, and extremely low dissolved oxygen concentrations (Lintermans 2007). Carp can modify aquatic habitats through their destructive feeding as they suck up and stir silt and mud; in some rivers this feeding activity can increase turbidity and reduce light penetration, impacting aquatic vegetation, plankton communities, invertebrates and native fish (Robertson *et al.* 1997; Vilizzi *et al.* 2014). However, Marshall *et al.* (2019) surveyed dryland rivers of south-west Queensland and found no difference in turbidity or in aquatic plant communities (which are naturally sparse in this region) between waterways with and without carp, indicating the impacts of introduced species can vary between regions.

Tilapia (particularly the more-widespread Mozambique tilapia, *O. mossambicus*) can also have negative impacts on Australian freshwater habitats, with males building large circular nests in the substrate, damaging aquatic vegetation and increasing turbidity if tilapia populations are abundant. The species tolerates poor water quality, with a wide temperature tolerance, salinity tolerance and ability to survive under very low dissolved oxygen concentrations through air gulping. Tilapia can occupy many aquatic habitats, but prefer well-vegetated, slow-flowing streams, lakes and impoundments (Russell *et al.* 2012; Harris 2013).

Eastern gambusia (also called plague minnow or mosquitofish, *G. holbrooki*) prefer warm, shallow waters with low flow and are often found around the edge habitats of waterways and among aquatic vegetation (Lintermans 2007). They are tolerant of poor water quality, including extremes in temperature and low dissolved oxygen concentrations. Their ability to tolerate a range of conditions has allowed them to spread throughout much of Australia. Oriental weatherloach (*M. anguillicaudatus*) are nocturnal and demersal, preferring cool, low-flow waterways with sandy or muddy substrates. They can burrow into the substrate to avoid predation or hibernate (Lintermans 2007) and it has been suggested that their burrowing and feeding behaviours can have an impact on water quality (Keller and Lake 2007). They tolerate temperature extremes, high turbidity and low dissolved oxygen concentrations, having the ability to swallow air (Lintermans 2007). Redfin perch are generally pelagic and can occupy a wide variety of habitats. They prefer to inhabit still or slow-flowing waterways with abundant refugia, especially aquatic vegetation, and their distribution in Australia is strongly associated with their inability to withstand temperatures over 31°C (Lintermans 2007).

Through their diets and feeding habits, introduced fishes may prey on and potentially compete with native fishes. Many have generalist diets, giving them a further advantage in Australian waterways. Carp have a highly plastic diet as omnivores and detritivores, consuming small molluscs, crustaceans, insect larvae, fish eggs and larvae as they suck in mud and water (Harris 2013; Vilizzi *et al.* 2014). Eastern gambusia are smaller-bodied fishes that prey on fish eggs and larvae, frog eggs and small invertebrates. Their diet overlaps with native fishes and they pose serious threats to biodiversity through predation and competition (Lintermans 2007; Harris 2013). Tilapia are omnivorous and eventually grow to be large (~40 cm). They demonstrate trophic plasticity, consuming a wide variety of foods and competing with many native species throughout their life phases (Doupé *et al.* 2009, Russell *et al.* 2012). They have also been shown to prey on a range of juvenile Australian freshwater fish species (Doupé *et al.* 2009). Oriental weatherloach have similarly broad dietary preferences, feeding on algae, aquatic insect larvae, crustaceans worms, rotifers and detritus, and competing with small native fishes (Keller and Lake 2007; Lintermans 2007; Harris 2013). Redfin perch (*P. fluviatilis*) are voracious pelagic predators that have been observed hunting both individually or in schools, and feeding on invertebrates and fish from a young age (Morgan *et al.* 2002; Lintermans 2007; Wedderburn and Barnes 2016).

Many introduced fish species are highly fecund, with their ability to rapidly reproduce and spread increasing their invasion potential. For instance, each female common carp (*C. carpio*) can produce up to 2 million eggs over multiple protracted spawning events (Harris 2013). Carp are long lived, surviving to up to 34 years and reaching a maximum size of ~80 cm; they mature at around 3 years of age (Lintermans 2007). Carp congregate in shallow water to spawn and lay their adhesive eggs in clumps on submerged vegetation and woody debris (Lintermans 2007).

Eastern gambusia are small (up to ~6 cm length), sexually dimorphic and viviparous, producing up to ~450 live young each season. Females produce live broods at frequent intervals throughout the 2–9 month breeding season resulting in a high larval survival rate to sexual maturity, which is reached in less than 2 months (Pen and Potter 1991; Lintermans 2007).

Mozambique tilapia increase their chances of reproductive success through maternal care. Large females likely produce 1000–2000 young per year, although in most populations the brood sizes are probably much smaller (e.g. 250 eggs upwards). Males build circular nests (leks) in the substrate and defend large territories, driving other fish away with aggressive behaviour (Russell *et al.* 2012). Females in spawning condition are attracted to the lek where they deposit eggs, which are externally fertilised by the male. She takes the eggs into her mouth to brood for around 20 days and continues to defend the fry once they are mobile and capable of feeding (Russell *et al.* 2012). Young can survive if the mother fish has died, so dead fish must be appropriately disposed of away from the waterway.

The oriental weatherloach matures at ~10 cm and reaches < 20 cm total length. Spawning occurs during summer and females spawn multiple times in a season, laying between 4000 and 8000 eggs onto aquatic vegetation or other substrata (Lintermans 2007). Redfin perch may start to mature at 1 year of age. Females deposit a gelatinous ribbon containing several thousand eggs in sheltered areas amongst aquatic vegetation or on submerged woody debris, which hatch after 1–2 weeks (Lintermans 2007).

Capture and handling

Capture and handling methods for introduced fishes vary by species and are similar to those described for native fishes of a similar size (see 'Small-bodied fishes' and 'Large-bodied fishes'). Electrofishing, netting, trapping and angling can all be effective capture methods, depending on the species of interest. Capture and killing of introduced fishes is sometimes employed as a population control method and in some jurisdictions noxious fish species must be killed. Dead fish should be disposed of away from the waterway.

Veterinary considerations

Sedation and anaesthesia

Like native species, most introduced fishes can be non-invasively handled without a need for anaesthesia, but it is required for surgical procedures. The use of anaesthetics such as isoeugenol is often preferred for smaller fishes, although a variety of anaesthetics is available and can be used for different applications (see 'Small-bodied fishes'). Alternative methods may be required for larger species ('Large-bodied fishes', 'Eels' and 'Venomous fishes' within this chapter).

Euthanasia

Lethal sampling is required as a permit condition in some jurisdictions, due to the deleterious impacts of some introduced species on Australian waterways. For this reason, even when conducting research that does not require lethal sampling, freshwater fish researchers should be prepared and equipped to kill introduced fishes that may be captured. Researchers are encouraged to investigate local permit and regulatory requirements around the capture of introduced fishes before undertaking studies.

For many introduced species, killing by immersion in a hyper-concentrated anaesthetic solution is possible, and immersion in an icy slurry may also be considered as an acceptable method for small, warm-water species (Blessing *et al.* 2010; AVMA 2020). General operating procedures for killing of fishes for scientific purposes can be found in Chapter 13.

Infectious pathogens

Fish diseases present in Australia are described in 'Small-bodied fishes'. As well as being the victim of aquatic diseases, introduced fishes can act as vectors for diseases and parasites (Department of Agriculture, Water and the Environment 2020) and there are numerous records of diseases introduced by ornamental fishes both in Australia and globally.

Redfin perch (*P. fluviatilis*) can spread the viral disease EHNV, which also poses danger to native fish species, including galaxiids (Becker *et al.* 2019; Department of Agriculture, Water and the Environment 2020). As EHNV can be transferred between waterways on sampling gear (e.g. boats, nets), gear needs to be sterilised after use in a waterway where the virus may occur. The introduction of the Mozambique tilapia (*O. mossambicus*) to Australia probably also resulted in the co-introduction of four species of fish parasites (Wilson *et al.* 2019). Globally, cyprinids have been implicated in the spread of parasites and diseases, including parasitic copepods (*Lernaea* spp.) (Rowland and Ingram 1991; Marina *et al.* 2008). Some Australian scientists are currently investigating the potential to release a highly specific cyprinid herpesvirus-3 as a possible biocontrol measure for carp (for discussion on this topic, see relevant emerging literature, e.g. McColl *et al.* 2017; Marshall *et al.* 2018; Kopf *et al.* 2019; National Carp Control Plan 2020).

General operating procedures

See details for 'Small-bodied fishes'.

REFERENCES

Allen GR, Midgley SH, Allen M (2002) *Field Guide to the Freshwater Fishes of Australia*. Western Australian Museum, Perth.

Allen MG, Morgan DL, Close PG, Beatty SJ (2020) Too little but not too late? Biology of a recently discovered and imperiled freshwater fish in a drying temperate region and comparison with sympatric fishes. *Aquatic Conservation* **30**, 1412–1423. doi:10.1002/aqc.3346

Arthington AH, McKay RJ, Russell DJ, Milton DA (1984) Occurrence of the introduced Cichlid *Oreochromis mossambicus* (Peters) in Queensland. *Australian Journal of Marine and Freshwater Research* **35**, 267–272. doi:10.1071/MF9840267

American Veterinary Medical Association (AVMA) (2020) *AVMA Guidelines for the Euthanasia of Animals, 2020 Edition*. AVMA. <https://www.avma.org/sites/default/files/2020-01/2020-Euthanasia-Final-1-17-20.pdf>.

Baker CF, Jellyman DJ, Reeve K, Crow S, Stewart M, Buchinger T, Weiming L (2017) First observations of spawning nests in the pouched lamprey (*Geotria australis*). *Canadian Journal of Fisheries and Aquatic Sciences* **74**, 1603–1611. doi:10.1139/cjfas-2016-0292

Balazik MT, Langford BC, Garman GC, Fine ML, Stewart JK, Latour RJ, McIninch SP (2013) Comparison of MS-222 and electronarcosis as anesthetics on cortisol levels in juvenile Atlantic sturgeon. *Transactions of the American Fisheries Society* **142**, 1640–1643. doi:10.1080/00028487.2013.824924

Baras E, Jeandrain D (1998) Evaluation of surgery procedures for tagging eel *Anguilla anguilla* (L.) with biotelemetry transmitters. *Hydrobiologia* **371**, 107–111. doi:10.1007/978-94-011-5090-3_13

Beatty SJ, Morgan DL, McAleer FJ, Ramsay AR (2010) Groundwater contribution to baseflow maintains habitat connectivity for *Tandanus bostocki* (Teleostei: Plotosidae) in a south-western Australian river. *Ecology Freshwater Fish* **19**, 595–608. doi:10.1111/j.1600-0633.2010.00440.x

Becker JA, Gilligan D, Asmus M, Tweedie A, Whittington RJ (2019) Geographic distribution of Epizootic haemotopoietic necrosis virus (EHNV) in freshwater fish in South Eastern Australia: lost opportunity for a notifiable pathogen to expand its geographic range. *Viruses* **11**, 315–329. doi:10.3390/v11040315

Berra TM, Wedd D (2017) Salinity and spawning of nurseryfish, *Kurtus gulliveri*, in the Adelaide River of northern Australia with notes on electrofishing and photos of a male carrying eggs. *Environmental Biology of Fishes* **100**, 959–967. doi:10.1007/s10641-017-0620-3

Bice CM, Zampatti BP, Koster W (2019) Tracking lamprey spawning migrations in the River Murray. South Australian Research and Development Institute (Aquatic Sciences), Adelaide. SARDI Publication No. F2019/000190-1. SARDI Research Report Series No. 1027.

Bishop KA, Allen SA, Pollard DA, Cook MJ (1980) Ecological studies on the fishes of the Alligator Rivers Region, Northern Territory (Final Report in 3 parts). Report to the Office of the Supervising Scientist, Canberra.

Bishop CR, Hughes JM, Schmidt DJ (2018) Mitogenomic analysis of the Australian lungfish (*Neoceratodus forsteri*) reveals structuring of indigenous riverine populations and late Pleistocene movements between drainage basins. *Conservation Genetics* **19**, 587–597. doi:10.1007/s10592-017-1034-7

Blessing JJ, Marshall JC, Balcombe SR (2010) Humane killing of fishes for scientific research: a comparison of two methods. *Journal of Fish Biology* **76**, 2571–2577. doi:10.1111/j.1095-8649.2010.02633.x

Borg D, Rutherford ID, Stewardson M (2007) The geomorphic and ecological effectiveness of habitat rehabilitation works: continuous measurement of scour and fill around large logs in sand-bed streams. *Geomorphology* **89**, 205–216. doi:10.1016/j.geomorph.2006.07.027

Brooks SG, Kind PK (2002) *Ecology and Demography of the Queensland Lungfish (*Neoceratodus forsteri*) in the Burnett River, Queensland with reference to the Impacts of Walla Weir and Future Water Infrastructure Development*. Department of Primary Industries, Queensland Agency for Food and Fibre Sciences, Brisbane.

Burndred KR, Cockayne BJ, Donaldson JA, Ebner BC (2018) Natural flow events influence the behaviour and movement patterns of eel-tailed catfish (*Tandanus tandanus*) in a subtropical Queensland river. *Australian Journal of Zoology* **66**, 185–194. doi:10.1071/ZO18033

Burndred KR, Cockayne BJ, Lou DC (2017) Early development of eel-tailed catfish, *Tandanus tandanus* (Mitchell) (Teleostei: Plotosidae), with validation of daily otolith increment formation. *Australian Journal of Zoology* **65**, 12–20. doi:10.1071/ZO16069

Butler GL, MacKay B, Rowland SJ, Pease BC (2009) Retention of intra-peritoneal transmitters and post-operative recovery of four Australian native fish species. *Marine and Freshwater Research* **60**, 361–370. doi:10.1071/MF08147

Butler GL, Wooden IJ (2012) Dietary habits of a large, long-lived endangered Australian percichthyid, the eastern freshwater cod *Maccullochella ikei*. *Endangered Species Research* **16**, 199–209. doi:10.3354/esr00406

Chilcott S, Freeman R, Davies PE, Crook DA, Fulton W, Hamr P, Jarvis D, Sanger AC (2013) Extinct habitat, extant species: lessons learned from conservation recovery actions for the Pedder galaxias (*Galaxias pedderensis*) in south-west Tasmania, Australia. *Marine and Freshwater Research* **64**, 864–873. doi:10.1071/MF12257

Clunie P, Koehn J (2001) *Freshwater Catfish: A Resource Document*. Murray–Darling Basin Commission, Canberra.

Crook DA, Buckle DJ, Allsop Q, Baldwin W, Saunders TM, Kyne PM, Woodhead JD, Maas R, Roberts B, Douglas MM (2017) Use of otolith chemistry and acoustic telemetry to elucidate migratory contingents in barramundi *Lates calcarifer*. *Marine and Freshwater Research* **68**, 1554–1566. doi:10.1071/MF16177

Crook DA, Buckle DJ, Morrongiello JR, Allsop QA, Baldwin W, Saunders TM, Douglas MM (2020) Tracking the resource pulse: Movement responses of fish to dynamic floodplain habitat in a tropical river. *Journal of Animal Ecology* **89**, 795–807. doi:10.1111/1365-2656.13146

Crook DA, Macdonald JI, Morrongiello JR, Belcher CA, Lovett D, Walker A, Nicol SJ (2014) Environmental cues and extended estuarine residence in seaward migrating eels (*Anguilla australis*). *Freshwater Biology* **59**, 1710–1720. doi:10.1111/fwb.12376

Crook DA, White RWG (1995) Evaluation of subcutaneously implanted Visual Implant Tags and Coded Wire Tags for marking and benign recovery in a small scaleless fish, *Galaxias truttaceus* (Pisces: Galaxiidae). *Marine and Freshwater Research* **46**, 943–946. doi:10.1071/MF9950943

Dawson HA, Quintella BR, Almeida PR, Treble AJ, Jolley JC (2015) The ecology of larval and metamorphosing lampreys. In: *Lampreys: Biology, Conservation and Control, Volume 1.* (Ed. MF Docker) pp. 75–137. Springer, Dordrecht, The Netherlands.

Department of Agriculture, Water and the Environment (2020) *Aquatic Animal Diseases Significant to Australia: Identification Field Guide.* 5th edn. Commonwealth of Australia, Canberra.

Diggle J, Wisniewski C (2014) The biology, management, control and eradication of carp populations in Tasmania. In Forum Proceedings: Carp Management in Australia – State of Knowledge (Eds W Fulton, K Hall) pp. 47–52. Invasive Animals CRC, Canberra.

Doupé RG, Knott MJ, Schaffer J, Burrows DW (2009) Investigational piscivory of some juvenile Australian freshwater fishes by the introduced Mozambique tilapia *Oreochromis mossambicus. Journal of Fish Biology* **74**, 2386–2400. doi:10.1111/j.1095-8649.2009.02254.x

Ebner B (2006) Murray cod an apex predator in the Murray River, Australia. *Ecology Freshwater Fish* **15**, 510–520. doi:10.1111/j.1600-0633.2006.00191.x

Ebner BC (2017) Growth, maximum daily ration and intraspecific cohabitation of the moray *Gymnothorax polyuranodon* (Pisces: Muraenidae) in a freshwater aquarium. *Cybium* **41**, 93–99.

Ebner BC, Donaldson JA, Courtney R, Fitzpatrick R, Starrs D, Fletcher C, Seymour J (2020) Averting danger under the bridge: video confirms adult Small-toothed moray, tolerate salinity before and during tidal influx. *Pacific Conservation Biology* **26**, 182–189. doi:10.1071/PC19023

Ebner BC, Thuesen PA, Larson H, Keith P (2011a) A review of distribution, field observations and precautionary conservation requirements for sicydiine gobies in Australia. *Cybium* **35**, 397–414.

Ebner BC, Kroll R, Godfrey P, Thuesen PA, Vallance T, Pusey B, Allen G, Rayner TS, Perna CN (2011b) Is the elusive *Gymnothorax polyuranodon* really a freshwater moray? *Journal of Fish Biology* **79**, 70–79. doi:10.1111/j.1095-8649.2011.02987.x

Ebner BC, Starrs D, Morgan DL, Fulton CJ, Donaldson JA, Doody JS, Cousins S, Kennard M, Butler G, Tonkin Z, Beatty S, Broadhurst B, Clear R, Lintermans M, Fletcher CS (2014) Emergence of field-based underwater video for understanding the ecology of freshwater fishes and crustaceans in Australia. *Journal of the Royal Society of Western Australia* **97**, 287–296.

Ebner BC, Donaldson JA, Fulton C, Schaffer J (2016a) Distinct habitat selection by freshwater morays in tropical rainforest streams. *Ecology Freshwater Fish* **25**, 329–335. doi:10.1111/eff.12213

Ebner BC, Morgan DL, Kerezsy A, Hardie S, Beatty SJ, Seymour JE, *et al.* (2016b) Enhancing conservation of Australian freshwater ecosystems: identification of freshwater flagship fishes and relevant target audiences. *Fish and Fisheries* **17**, 1134–1151. doi:10.1111/faf.12161

Espinoza T, Marshall SM, McDougall A (2013) Spawning of the endangered Australian Lungfish (*Neoceratodus forsteri*) in a heavily regulated river: a pulse for life. *River Research and Applications* **29**, 1215–1225. doi:10.1002/rra.2607

Fallon SJ, McDougall AJ, Espinoza T, Roberts DT, Brooks S, Kind PK, Kennard MJ, Bond N, Marshall SM, Schmidt D, Hughes J (2019) Age structure of the Australian lungfish (*Neoceratodus forsteri*). *PLoS One* **14**, e0210168. doi:10.1371/journal.pone.0210168

Faulks LK, Kerezsy A, Unmack PJ, Johnson JB, Hughes JM (2017) Going, going, gone? Loss of genetic diversity in two critically endangered Australian freshwater fishes, *Scaturiginichthys vermeilipinnis* and *Chlamydogobius squamigenus*, from Great Artesian Basin springs at Edgbaston, Queensland, Australia. *Aquatic Conservation* **27**, 39–50. doi:10.1002/aqc.2684

Flint N, Pearson RG, Crossland MR (2017) Reproduction and embryo viability of a range-limited tropical freshwater fish exposed to fluctuating hypoxia. *Marine and Freshwater Research* **69**, 267–276. doi:10.1071/MF16388

Forbes JP, Watts RJ, Robinson WA, Baumgartner LJ, Steffe AS, Murphy JJ (2015) Recreational fishing effort, catch, and harvest for Murray cod and golden perch in the Murrumbidgee River, Australia. *North American Journal of Fisheries Management* **35**, 649–658. doi:10.1080/02755947.2015.1032452

Fulton W (1982) Observations on the ecology of four species of the genus *Paragalaxias* (Pisces: Galaxiidae) from Tasmania. *Australian Journal of Marine and Freshwater Research* **33**, 999–1016. doi:10.1071/MF9820999

García-Díaz P, Kerezsy A, Unmack PJ, Lintermans M, Beatty SJ, Butler GL, *et al.* (2018) Transport pathways shape the biogeography of alien freshwater fishes in Australia. *Diversity & Distributions* **24**, 1405–1415. doi:10.1111/ddi.12777

Grant E (2014) *Grant's Guide to Fishes.* EM Grant Pty Ltd, Redcliffe North.

Gould A, Grace BS (2009) Injuries to barramundi *Lates calcarifer* resulting from lip-gripping devices in the laboratory. *North American Journal of Fisheries Management* **29**, 1418–1424. doi:10.1577/M08-232.1

Ghafari SM, Jamili S, Bagheri KP, Ardakani EM, Fatemi MR, Shahbazzadeh F, Shahbazzadeh D (2013) The first report on some toxic effects of green scat, *Scatophagus argus* an Iranian Persian Gulf venomous fish. *Toxicon* **66**, 82–87. doi:10.1016/j.toxicon.2013.01.025

Gupta S (2016) An overview on morphology, biology, and culture of spotted scat *Scatophagus argus* (Linnaeus 1766). *Reviews in Fisheries Science & Aquaculture* **24**, 203–212. doi:10.1080/23308249.2015.1119800

Hagihara S, Aoyama J, Limbong D, Tsukamoto K (2012) Morphological and physiological changes of female tropical eels, *Anguilla celebesensis* and *Anguilla marmorata*, in relation to downstream migration. *Journal of Fish Biology* **81**, 408–426. doi:10.1111/j.1095-8649.2012.03332.x

Hagihara S, Aoyama J, Limbong D, Tsukamoto K (2018) Interspecific and sexual differences in riverine distribution of tropical eels *Anguilla* spp. *Journal of Fish Biology* **93**, 21–29. doi:10.1111/jfb.13666

Hammer MP, Adams M, Unmack PJ, Walker KF (2007) A rethink on *Retropinna*: conservation implications of new taxa and significant genetic sub-structure in Australian smelts (Pisces: Retropinnidae). *Marine and Freshwater Research* **58**, 327–341. doi:10.1071/MF05258

Hammer MP, Allen GR, Martin KC, Adams M, Ebner BC, Raadik TA, Unmack PJ (2018) Revision of the Australian Wet Tropics endemic rainbowfish genus *Cairnsichthys* (Atheriniformes: Melanotaeniidae), with a description of a new species. *Zootaxa* **4413**. doi:10.11646/zootaxa.4413.2.3.

Hammer MP, Allen GR, Martin KC, Adams M, Unmack PJ (2019a) Two new species of dwarf rainbowfishes (Atheriniformes: Melanotaeniidae) from northern Australia and southern New Guinea. *Zootaxa* **4701**. doi:10.11646/zootaxa.4701.3.1.

Hammer MP, Skarlatos Simoes MN, Needham EW, Wilson DN, Barton MA, Lonza D (2019b) Establishment of Siamese Fighting Fish on the Adelaide River floodplain: the first serious invasive fish in the Northern Territory, Australia. *Biological Invasions* **21**, 2269–2279. doi:10.1007/s10530-019-01981-3

Harris JH (2013) Fishes from elsewhere. In *Ecology of Australian Freshwater Fishes.* (Eds P Humphries and KF Walker) pp. 259–282. CSIRO Publishing, Melbourne.

Harris JH, Bond NR, Closs GP, Gehrke PC, Nicol SJ, Ye Q (2013) Dynamics of populations. In *Ecology of Australian Freshwater Fishes.* (Eds P Humphries and KF Walker) pp. 223–244. CSIRO Publishing, Melbourne.

Holmes BJ, Williams SM, Power TN (2020) Evidence of naturalisation of the invasive jaguar cichlid *Prachromis managuensis* (Gunther, 1897), in Queensland, Australia. *BioInvasions Records* **9**, 146–157. doi:10.3391/bir.2020.9.1.19

Hughes JM, Schmidt DJ, Huey JA, Real KM, Espinoza T, McDougall A, Kind PK, Brooks S, Roberts DT (2015) Extremely low microsatellite diversity but distinct population structure in a long-lived threatened species, the Australian lungfish *Neoceratodus forsteri* (Dipnoi). *PLoS One* **10**, e0121858. doi:10.1371/journal.pone.0121858

Humphreys WF, Feinberg MN (1995) Food of the blind cave fishes of northwestern Australia. *Records of the Western Australian Museum* **17**, 29–33.

Humphries P, Walker KF (2013) *Ecology of Australian Freshwater Fishes*. CSIRO Publishing, Melbourne.

Inland Fisheries Service (2020) Farm dam stocking. Inland Fisheries Service, Tasmanian Government, Hobart. <https://www.ifs.tas.gov.au/forms/farm-dam-stocking>.

Jardine TD (2016) A top predator forages low on species-rich tropical food chains. *Freshwater Science* **35**, 666–675. doi:10.1086/685858

Jellyman D, Tsukamoto K (2002) First use of archival transmitters to track migrating freshwater eels *Anguilla dieffenbachii* at sea. *Marine Ecology Progress Series* **233**, 207–215. doi:10.3354/meps233207

Jellyman DJ, Sykes JR (2003) Diel and seasonal movements of radio-tagged freshwater eels, *Anguilla* spp., in two New Zealand streams. *Environmental Biology of Fishes* **66**, 143–154. doi:10.1023/A:1023691604088

Keller RP, Lake PS (2007) Potential impacts of a recent and rapidly spreading coloniser of Australian freshwaters: oriental weatherloach (*Misgurnus anguillicaudatus*). *Ecology Freshwater Fish* **16**, 124–132. doi:10.1111/j.1600-0633.2006.00204.x

Kelly E, Martin PAJ, Gibson-Kueh S, Morgan DL, Ebner BC, Donaldson J, Buller N, Crook DA, Brooks S, Davis AM, Hammer MP, Foyle L, Hair S, Lymbery AJ (2018) First detection of *Edwardsiella ictaluri* (Proteobacteria: Enterobacteriaceae) in wild Australian catfish. *Journal of Fish Diseases* **41**, 199–208. doi:10.1111/jfd.12696

Kemp A (1981) Rearing of embryos of the Australian lungfish *Neoceratodus forsteri* under laboratory conditions. *Copeia* **1981**, 776–784. doi:10.2307/1444177

Kennedy CR (1995) Richness and diversity of macroparasite communities in tropical eels *Anguilla reinhardtii* in Queensland, Australia. *Parasitology* **111**, 233–245. doi:10.1017/S0031182000064994

Kind PK (2010) The natural history of the Australian Lungfish *Neoceratodus forsteri* (Krefft, 1870). In *Biology of Lungfishes*. (Eds JM Jorgensen and J Joss) pp. 61–96. CRC Press, Enfield, NH.

King AJ, Humphries P, McCasker NG (2013) Reproduction and early life history. In *Ecology of Australian Freshwater Fishes*. (Eds P Humphries and KF Walker) pp. 159–193. CSIRO Publishing, Melbourne.

Koehn JD, Crook DA (2013) Movements and migration. In *Ecology of Australian Freshwater Fishes*. (Eds P Humphries and KF Walker) pp. 159–193. CSIRO Publishing, Melbourne.

Koehn JD, Kennard MJ (2013) Habitats. In *Ecology of Australian Freshwater Fishes*. (Eds P Humphries and KF Walker) pp. 159–193. CSIRO Publishing, Melbourne.

Koehn JD, McKenzie JA, O'Mahony DJ, Nicol SJ, O'Connor JP, O'Connor WG (2009) Movements of Murray cod (*Maccullochella peelii peelii*) in a large Australian lowland river. *Ecology Freshwater Fish* **18**, 594–602. doi:10.1111/j.1600-0633.2009.00375.x

Koehn JD, Raymond SM, Stuart I, Todd CR, Balcombe SR, Zampatti BP, *et al.* (2020) A compendium of ecological knowledge for restoration of freshwater fishes in Australia's Murray–Darling Basin. *Marine and Freshwater Research* **71**, 1391–1463. doi:10.1071/MF20127

Kopf RK, Boutier M, Finlayson CM, Hodges K, Humphries P, King A, Kingsford RT, Marshall J, McGinness HM, Thresher R, Vanderplasschen A (2019) Biocontrol in Australia: can a carp herpesvirus (CyHV-3) deliver safe and effective ecological restoration? *Biological Invasions* **21**, 1857–1870. doi:10.1007/s10530-019-01967-1

Koster WM, Dawson DR, Clunie P, Hames F, McKenzie J, Moloney PD, Crook DA (2015) Movement and habitat use of the freshwater catfish (*Tandanus tandanus*) in a remnant floodplain wetland. *Ecology Freshwater Fish* **24**, 443–455. doi:10.1111/eff.12159

Koster WM, Dawson DR, Crook DA (2013) Downstream spawning migration by the amphidromous Australian grayling (*Prototroctes maraena*) in a coastal river in south-eastern Australia. *Marine and Freshwater Research* **64**, 31–41. doi:10.1071/MF12196

Lawrence C, Rutherford N, Hamilton R, Meredith D (2016) Experimental evidence indicates that native freshwater fish outperform introduced *Gambusia* in mosquito suppression when water temperature is below 25°C. *Hydrobiologia* **766**, 357–364. doi:10.1007/s10750-015-2470-3

Leigh SJ, Zampatti BP (2013) Movement and mortality of Murray cod, *Maccullochella peelii*, during overbank flows in the lower River Murray, Australia. *Australian Journal of Zoology* **61**, 160–169. doi:10.1071/ZO12124

Lintermans M (2004) Human-assisted dispersal of alien freshwater fish in Australia. *New Zealand Journal of Marine and Freshwater Research* **38**, 481–501. doi:10.1080/00288330.2004.9517255

Lintermans M (2007) Fishes of the Murray-Darling Basin: An introductory guide. Murray Darling Basin Authority, Canberra ACT.

Lintermans M, Geyle HM, Beatty S, Brown C, Ebner BC, Freeman R, Hammer MP, Humphreys WF, Kennard MJ, Kern P, Martin K, Morgan DL, Raadik TA, Unmack PJ, Wager R, Woinarski JCZ, Garnett ST (2020) Big trouble for little fish: identifying Australian freshwater fishes in imminent risk of extinction. *Pacific Conservation Biology* **26**, 365–377. doi:10.1071/PC19053

Manzon RG, Youson JH, Holmes JA (2015) Lamprey metamorphosis. In *Lampreys: Biology, Conservation and Control, Volume 1*. (Ed. MF Docker) pp. 139–214. Springer, Dordrecht, The Netherlands.

Marina H, Beatty SJ, Morgan DL, Doupé RG, Lymbery AL (2008) An introduced parasite, *Lernaea cyprinacea*, found on native freshwater fish in the south west of Western Australia. *Journal of the Royal Society of Western Australia* **91**, 149–153.

Marshall JC, Blessing JJ, Clifford SE, Hodges KM, Negus PM, Steward AL (2019) Ecological impacts of invasive carp in Australian dryland rivers. *Aquatic Conservation* **29**, 1870–1889. doi:10.1002/aqc.3206

Marshall JC, Davidson AJ, Kopf RK, Boutier M, Stevenson P, Vanderplasschen A (2018) Biocontrol of invasive carp: risks abound. *Science* **359**, 877. doi:10.1126/science.aar7827

Marshall JC, Menke N, Crook DA, Lobegeiger JS, Balcombe SR, Huey JA, Fawcett JH, Bond NR, Starkey AH, Sternberg D, Linke S, Arthington A (2016) Go with the flow: the movement behaviour of fish from isolated waterhole refugia during connecting flow events in an intermittent dryland river. *Freshwater Biology* **61**, 1242–1258. doi:10.1111/fwb.12707

Mazzoni TS, Lo Nostro FL, Antoneli FN, Quagio-Grassiotto I (2018) Action of the metalloproteinases in gonadal remodeling during sex reversal in the sequential hermaphroditism of the teleostei fish *Synbranchus marmoratus* (Synbranchiformes: Synbranchidae). *Cells* **7**, 34. doi:10.3390/cells7050034

McColl KA, Sheppard AW, Barwick M (2017) Safe and effective biocontrol of common carp. *Nature, Ecology & Evolution* **1**, 0134. doi:/10.1038/s41559-017-0134

Miles NG, West RJ, Norman MD (2009) Does otolith chemistry indicate diadromous lifecycles for five Australian riverine fishes? *Marine and Freshwater Research* **60**, 904–911. doi:10.1071/MF08252

Moore GI (2019) New morphological data and live photographs of the rare subterranean blind cave eel *Ophisternon candidum* (Synbranchidae) from north-western Australia. *Ichthyological Research* **66**, 160–165. doi:10.1007/s10228-018-0647-2

Moore GI, Humphreys WF, Foster R (2018) New populations of the rare subterranean blind cave eel *Ophisternon candidum* (Synbranchidae) reveal recent historical connections throughout north-western Australia. *Marine and Freshwater Research* **69**, 1517–1524. doi:10.1071/MF18006

Morgan DL (2003) Distribution and biology of *Galaxias truttaceus* (Galaxiidae) in south-western Australia, including first evidence of parasitism of fishes in Western Australia by *Ligula intestinalis. Environmental Biology of Fishes* **66**, 155–167. doi:10.1023/A:1023645506913

Morgan DL, Allen GR, Pusey BJ, Burrows DW (2011) A review of the freshwater fishes of the Kimberley region of Western Australia. *Zootaxa* **2816**, 1–65. doi:10.11646/zootaxa.2816.1.1

Morgan DL, Beatty SJ, Adams M (2013) *Nannoperca pygmaea*, a new species of pygmy perch (Teleostei: Percichthyidae) from Western Australia. *Zootaxa* **3637**, 401–411. doi:10.11646/zootaxa.3637.4.1

Morgan DL, Hambleton SJ, Gill HS, Beatty SJ (2002) Distribution, biology and likely impacts of the introduced redfin perch (*Perca fluviatilis*) (Percidae) in Western Australia. *Marine and Freshwater Research* **53**, 1211–1221. doi:10.1080/00288330.2004.9517257

Morgan DL, Unmack PJ, Beatty SJ, Ebner BC, Allen MG, Keleher JJ, Donaldson JA, Murphy J (2014) An overview of the 'freshwater fishes' of Western Australia. *Journal of the Royal Society of Western Australia* **97**, 263–278.

Mylniczenko ND, Neiffer DL, Clauss TM (2014) Bony fish (lungfish, sturgeon, and teleosts). In *Zoo Animal and Wildlife Immobilization and Anaesthesia.* 2nd edn. (Eds G West, D Heard and N Caulkett) pp. 209–260. John Wiley and Sons, Hoboken, NJ.

National Carp Control Plan (2020) *National Carp Control Plan.* Australian Government, Canberra. <https://www.carp.gov.au/>.

Nelson JS, Grande TC, Wilson MV (2016) *Fishes of the World.* John Wiley and Sons.

Orr TM, Milward NE (1984) Reproduction and development of *Neosilurus ater* (Perugia) and *Neosilurus hyrtlii* Steindachner (Teleostei: Plotosidae) in a Tropical Queensland Stream. *Australian Journal of Marine and Freshwater Research* **35**, 187–195. doi:10.1071/MF9840187

Paton KR, Cake MH, Bird DJ, Potter IC (2020) Descriptions of spawning of the pouched lamprey (*Geotria australis*) in tanks and of morphological changes leading up to and following spawning. *Pacific Conservation Biology* **26**, 301–307. doi:10.1071/PC19025

Pen LJ, Potter IC (1991) Reproduction, growth and diet of *Gambusia holbrooki* (Girard) in a temperate Australian river. *Aquatic Conservation* **1**, 159–172. doi:10.1002/aqc.3270010205

Potter IC (1970) The life cycles and ecology of Australian lampreys of the genus *Mordacia. Journal of Zoology* **161**, 487–511. doi:10.1111/j.1469-7998.1970.tb02051.x

Potter IC, Gill HS, Renaud CB, Haoucher D (2015) The taxonomy, phylogeny, and distribution of lampreys. In *Lampreys: Biology, Conservation and Control, Volume 1.* (Ed. MF Docker) pp. 35–73. Springer, Dordrecht, The Netherlands.

Potter IC, Hilliard RW (1986) Growth and average duration of larval life in the Southern Hemisphere lamprey, *Geotria australis* Gray. *Experientia* **42**, 1170–1173. doi:10.1007/BF01941297

Potter IC, Hilliard RW, Bird DJ (1980) Metamorphosis in the Southern Hemisphere lamprey, *Geotria australis. Journal of the Zoological Society of London* **190**, 405–430. doi:10.1111/j.1469-7998.1980.tb01435.x

Potter IC, Hilliard RW, Neira FJ (1986) The biology of Australian lampreys. In *Limnology in Australia.* (Eds P De Dekker and WD Williams). CSIRO, Melbourne.

Puckridge JT, Walker KF (1990) Reproductive Biology and Larval development of a Gizzard Shad, *Nematalosa erebi* (Gunther) (Dorosomatinae: Teleostei), in the River Murray, South Australia. *Australian Journal of Marine and Freshwater Research* **41**, 695–712. doi:10.1071/MF9900695

Pusey B, Kennard M, Arthington A (2004) *Freshwater Fishes of North-Eastern Australia.* CSIRO Publishing, Melbourne.

Pusey BJ, Arthington AH, Read MG (1998) Freshwater fishes of the Burdekin River, Australia: biogeography, history and spatial variation in community structure. *Environmental Biology of Fishes* **53**, 303–318. doi:10.1023/A:1007468417947

Reid CH, Vandergoot CS, Midwood JD, Stevens ED, Bowker J, Cooke SJ (2019) On the electroimmobilization of fishes for research and practice: opportunities, challenges, and research needs. *Fisheries (Bethesda, Md.)* **44**, 576–585. doi:10.1002/fsh.10307

Riva-Rossi C, Barrasso DA, Baker C, Quiroga AP, Baigún C, Basso NG (2020) Revalidation of the Argentinian pouched lamprey *Geotria macrostoma* (Burmeister, 1868) with molecular and morphological evidence. *PLoS One* **15**, e0233792. doi:10.1371/journal.pone.0233792

Roberts BH, Morrongiello JR, King AJ, Morgan DL, Saunders TM, Woodhead J, Crook DA (2019) Migration to freshwater increases growth rates in a facultatively catadromous tropical fish. *Oecologia* **191**, 253–260. doi:10.1007/s00442-019-04460-7

Roberts DT, Mallett S, Kruck NC, Loh W, Tibbetts I (2014) Spawning activity of the Australian lungfish *Neoceratodus forsteri* in an impoundment. *Journal of Fish Biology* **84**, 163–177. doi:10.1111/jfb.12264

Roberts DT, Udyawer V, Franklin C, Dwyer RG, Campbell HA (2017) Using an acoustic telemetry array to assess fish volumetric space use: a case study on impoundments, hypoxia and an air-breathing species (*Neoceratodus forsteri*). *Marine and Freshwater Research* **68**, 1532–1543. doi:10.1071/MF16124

Roberts RJ (2012) *Fish Pathology.* 4th edn. Blackwell Publishing Ltd, Oxford, UK.

Robertson AI, Healey MR, King AJ (1997) Experimental manipulations of the biomass of introduced carp (*Cyprinus carpio*) in billabongs. II. Impacts of benthic properties and processes. *Marine and Freshwater Research* **48**, 445–454. doi:10.1071/MF97032

Roussel J-M, Haro A, Cunjak RA (2000) Field test of a new method for tracking small fishes in shallow rivers using passive integrated transponder (PIT) technology. *Canadian Journal of Fisheries and Aquatic Sciences* **57**, 1326–1329. doi:10.1139/f00-110

Rowland SJ, Ingram BA (1991) *Diseases of Australian Native Freshwater Fishes with Particular Emphasis on the Ectoparasitic and Fungal Diseases of Murray Cod (*Maccullochella peeli*), Golden Perch (*Macquaria ambigua*) and Silver Perch (*Bidyanus bidyanus*).* Fish Bulletin 4. NSW Agriculture & Fisheries, Sydney.

Russell DJ, Thuesen PA, Thomson FE (2012) A review of the biology, ecology, distribution and control of Mozambique tilapia, *Oreochromis mossambicus* (Peters 1852) (Pisces: *Cichlidae*) with particular emphasis on invasive Australian populations. *Reviews in Fish Biology and Fisheries* **22**, 533–554. doi:10.1007/s11160-011-9249-z

Shelley JJ, Dempster T, Le Feuvre MC, Unmack PJ, Laffan SW, Swearer SE (2019) A revision of the bioregionalization of freshwater fish communities in the Australian Monsoonal Tropics. *Ecology and Evolution* **9**, 4568–4588. doi:10.1002/ece3.5059

St John Ambulance Australia (2020) First aid fact sheet: bites and stings quick guide. St John Ambulance Australia Ltd. <https://stjohn.org.au/assets/uploads/fact%20sheets/english/Fact%20sheets_bites%20and%20stings.pdf>.

Storer T, Bannister J, Bennett K, Byrnes E, Crook DA, Morgan DL, Gleiss A, Beatty SJ (2021) Influence of discharge regime on the movement and refuge use of a freshwater fish in a drying temperate region. *Ecohydrology* **14**, e2253. doi:10.1002/eco.2253

Strike TB, Feltrer Y, Flach E, Mcgregor SK, Guillaume S (2017) Investigation and management of an outbreak of multispecies mycobacteriosis in Australian lungfish (*Neoceratodus fosteri*) including the use of triple antibiotic treatment. *Journal of Fish Diseases* **40**, 557–570. doi:10.1111/jfd.12535

Stuart I, Koehn JD (2007) Big cod do breed. *Freshwater Fishing Magazine* **85**, 62–64.

Stuart IG, Mallen-Cooper M (1999) An assessment of the effectiveness of a vertical-slot fishway for non-salmonid fish at a tidal barrier on a large tropical/subtropical river. *Regulated Rivers* **15**, 575–590. doi:10.1002/(SICI)1099-1646(199911/12)15:6<575::AID-RRR562>3.0.CO;2-Q

Su M, Duan Z, Shi H, Zhang J (2019) The effects of salinity on reproductive development and egg and larvae survival in the spotted scat *Scatophagus argus* under controlled conditions. *Aquaculture Research* **50**, 1782–1794. doi:10.1111/are.14056

Tao J, Kennard MJ, Roberts DT, Fry B, Kainz MJ, Chen Y, Bunn SE (2020) Quality and contribution of food sources to Australian lungfish evaluated using fatty acids and stable isotopes. *Aquatic Sciences* **82**, 8. doi:10.1007/s00027-019-0680-x

Thresher RE (1984) *Reproduction in Reef Fishes*. TFH Publications, Hong Kong.

Tonkin Z, King A, Mahoney J, Morrongiello J (2007) Diel and spatial drifting patterns of silver perch *Bidyanus bidyanus* eggs in an Australian lowland river. *Journal of Fish Biology* **70**, 313–317. doi:10.1111/j.1095-8649.2006.01281.x

Tsukamoto K, Chow S, Otake T, Kurogi H, Mochioka N, Miller MJ, Aoyama J, Kimura S, Watanabe S, Yoshinaga T, Shinoda A, Kuroki M, Oya M, Watanabe T, Hata K, Ijiri S, Kazeto Y, Nomura K, Tanaka H (2011) Oceanic spawning ecology of freshwater eels in the western North Pacific. *Nature Communications* **2**, 179. doi:10.1038/ncomms1174

Tsukamoto K, Watanabe S, Kuroki M, Aoyama J, Miller MJ (2014) Freshwater habitat use by a moray eel species, *Gymnothorax polyuranodon*, in Fiji shown by otolith microchemistry. *Environmental Biology of Fishes* **97**, 1377–1385. doi:10.1007/s10641-014-0228-9

Unmack PJ, Allen GR, Johnson JB (2013) Phylogeny and biogeography of rainbowfishes (*Melanotaeniidae*) from Australia and New Guinea. *Molecular Phylogenetics and Evolution* **67**, 15–27. doi:10.1016/j.ympev.2012.12.019

Vilizzi L, Thwaites LA, Smith BB, Nicol JM, Madden CP (2014) Ecological effects of common carp (*Cyprinus carpio*) in a semi-arid floodplain wetland. *Marine and Freshwater Research* **65**, 802–817. doi:10.1071/MF13163

Walsh CT, Pease BC (2002) The use of clove oil as an anaesthetic for the longfinned eel, *Anguilla reinhardtii* (Steindachner). *Aquaculture Research* **33**, 627–635. doi:10.1046/j.1365-2109.2002.00701.x

Watanabe S (2003) Taxonomy of the freshwater eels, genus *Anguilla* Schrank, 1798. In *Eel Biology* (Eds K Aida, K Tsukamoto and K Yamauchi) pp. 3–18. Springer, Tokyo, Japan.

Wedderburn SD, Barnes TC (2016) Piscivory by alien redfin perch (*Perca fluviatilis*) begins earlier than anticipated in two contrasting habitats of Lake Alexandrina, South Australia. *Australian Journal of Zoology* **64**, 1–7. doi:10.1071/ZO15083

Welsh SA, Jerry DR, Burrows DW (2014) A new species of freshwater eel-tailed catfish of the genus *Tandanus* (Teleostei: Plotosidae) from the wet tropics region of Eastern Australia. *Copeia* **2014**, 136–142. doi:10.1643/CI-13-067

Wilson JR, Saunders RJ, Hutson KS (2019) Parasites of the invasive tilapia *Oreochromis mossambicus:* evidence for co-introduction. *Aquatic Invasions* **14**, 332–349. doi:10.3391/ai.2019.14.2.11

33 Perching birds and parrots

Grant C. Palmer, Gisela Kaplan, Daniella Teixeira, Dejan Stojanovic, Andrew Peters and Tegan K. Douglas

INTRODUCTION

Global terrestrial bird assemblages are dominated by the passerines (order Passeriformes), which occupy many of the niches available for birds in terrestrial ecosystems. Australia has played a key role in the evolution and global dispersal of major bird groups, as modern passerines, cockatoos (family Cacatuidae) and parrots (families Psittaculidae and Psittacidae) evolved on the Gondwanan continent, and modern songbirds exclusively in East Gondwana. Together, these taxa dominate species richness and abundance in Australian bird communities, making them a focus of research and monitoring activities.

PASSERINE BIRDS

Grant C. Palmer, Andrew Peters and Gisela Kaplan

Characteristics

Order Passeriformes (passerines) is a diverse group that includes more than half of all bird species on Earth and is represented by ~386 species in Australia (including introduced species). Passerines are typically terrestrial and occupy diverse habitats and niches. They are frequently the most abundant bird taxon in Australian terrestrial habitats and are widely distributed, although many species have restricted distributions.

Despite their taxonomic diversity, passerines are united by several common attributes, including structure of the syrinx, preen gland and sperm (Gill 2007). They share common toe arrangements (three pointing forwards and one backwards) with associated specialised tendons and foot musculature. This facilitates perching, and members of this group are widely referred to as perching birds. Passerines are generally well adapted for flight, with streamlined bodies and specialised wings. Beak shape is typically pointed and relatively narrow. However, considerable variation occurs between species and groups. For example, honeyeater (Meliphagidae) beaks are generally long and curved downward to reach nectar deep within flowers but vary among species based on the type and number of nectar resources used. Some passerine groups, for example fairy-wrens (Maluridae) and fantails (Rhipiduridae), have prominent, long tails. Australian passerines range in size from the tiny weebill (*Smicrornis brevirostris*) (4–8 g) to Albert's lyrebird (*Menura alberti*) (up to 1.2 kg; ABSA 2020). Passerines are usually relatively small birds; however, birds from the broad group of Corvoidea, and some ancient lineages as lyrebirds (Menuridae) or pheasant coucals (*Centropus phasianinus*), are large.

Biology and behaviour

Passerines include species that are largely ground-dwelling (e.g. quail-thrushes, Cinclosomatidae) and aerialists (e.g. swallows and martins, Hirundinidae). They may also be nectarivores (e.g. honeyeaters), insectivores (e.g. robins, Petroicidae), omnivores (e.g. crows and ravens, Corvidae) and granivores (e.g. finches, Estrildidae) that forage at all levels. Passerines are typically diurnal birds (although some may be crepuscular, or partially active at night). Some occupy clearly defined home ranges and can be strongly territorial (e.g. Australian magpie, *Gymnorhina tibicen*; bowerbirds, Ptilonorhynchidae), particularly during the breeding season. Others may be nomadic or migratory.

Passerines display varied and complex mating and social behaviours. Some species are solitary or form year-round pair bonds, others form tight-knit social groups (e.g. white-winged chough, *Corcorax melanorhamphos*; and fairy-wrens) or gather in large flocks. A high proportion of Australian passerines are cooperative breeders, where the breeding pair are assisted in raising their young by helpers (e.g. fairy-wrens; babblers, Pomatostomidae). Other species sometimes form colonies (e.g. noisy miner, *Manorina melanocephala*) in resource-rich areas, which may be defended against other birds. In Australia, the main breeding periods are aligned with periods of maximum plant growth, and typically follow spring and summer in southern temperate regions and the early wet season in more-tropical and monsoonal areas. In arid areas it is highly opportunistic in relation to environmental conditions or events (e.g. breeding booms following significant rainfall). Passerines use a wide variety of nest sites. Most construct nests by arranging plant material, lichens or mud to form a partially or fully enclosed nest, some nest in tree hollows or other cavities, and others on the ground.

Passerines are largely invertebrate feeders, although most take a wide range of foods opportunistically. Some groups and species are omnivores, such as corvids (which may also scavenge food). Highly specialised diets occur less often. For example, the painted honeyeater (*Grantiella picta*) feeds almost exclusively on mistletoe fruits, while some honeyeaters are almost exclusively nectarivorous. Passerines are capable of moving long distances to locate food or in response to changing environmental conditions. Such movement can occur daily or with changes in season or life stages. Movements include altitudinal or nomadic movements, as well as migration (typically intracontinental). Many species are considered sedentary or territorial.

Cooperative behaviour

Cooperative breeding is a social system in animals that involves alloparental care, where young receive care from the parents, as well as additional helpers. Cooperative breeding is particularly prevalent in Australian passerines. Australian magpies, apostlebirds (*Struthidea cinerea*) and white-winged choughs are medium to large passerines that usually live in family groups, a typical feature of cooperatively breeding species. The social structure and behaviour of these birds warrant particular ethical considerations in research. Apostlebirds and white-winged choughs belong to the family of mud-nesters (Corcoracidae), while Australian magpies are grouped among woodswallows (Artamidae). All three species are the only representatives of their genera in Australia, long lived (25–30 years) compared to bird species of similar size, and largely insectivorous ground feeders.

Apostlebirds and white-winged choughs are always cooperative breeders (i.e. have and need helpers at the nest), whereas Australian magpies are occasional cooperative breeders. All three species begin reproducing relatively late in life. Magpies reach sexual maturity around 1 year of age but usually do not breed until aged 4 or 5. Apostlebirds and white-winged choughs breed at a similar age, although they reach sexual maturity at ~4 years of age.

The social cohesion within groups of white-winged choughs and apostlebirds sees members forage, drink, bathe, roost and defend against intruders or predators, as a group. They build nests together, and several females may deposit eggs in one nest, but also share incubation, guarding, feeding and raising of young. Subgroups may consist of two to four birds but the entire group can number around 20 strong. For apostlebird and white-winged chough, offspring of both sexes usually remain within their natal group, assisting the breeding pair for at least 4 years. Magpies, by contrast, tend to evict their offspring before the next breeding season.

All three species are territorial and actively defend their territories. Apostlebirds have sentries and magpies are constantly on the look-out for intruders or dangers. Group cohesion is strong, and individuals are defended if a risk is present. The social ties created by the interdependence of individuals in all three species and their interrelatedness suggest that researchers should be particularly aware of the harm that can be done, even inadvertently, in disrupting social cohesion and even risking the loss of their territory, which depends on group numbers and combined actions.

Capture and handling

Passerine research can often be done with non-invasive approaches, including traditional field surveys incorporating visual and call observation, and acoustic or camera monitoring. Birdwatching is a popular activity and citizen science activities have established substantial databases of location records (e.g. Atlas of Living Australia, BirdLife Australia's Birdata and eBird).

The most common capture method for many passerine birds is mist netting. In Australia, operators of mist nets must be endorsed under the Australian Bird and Bat Banding Scheme (ABBBS), which can only be achieved following extensive tuition from experienced operators. Mist netting poses several risks to birds (see Chapters 7 and 15).

Most passerines can be held safely and temporarily in appropriately sized calico bags. The bag should provide a darkened environment and not allow the bird to flap its wings. When handling birds, it is important to restrict their movement. They should always be gently held so that wings are restrained and positioned naturally against the bird's body, in a closed position. This process is generally practicable for small passerines, as they can be held in one hand, in the bander's (or ringer's) grip (e.g. Figure 33.1).

Marking of passerine birds is typically restricted to leg-banding ('ringing') (Figure 33.1). Metal identification bands with a unique number (issued by the ABBBS) are used. To aid identification of individual, free-flying birds, colour bands may also be used. Colour band combinations are assigned for research purposes as part of a colour-marking authority issued by the ABBBS (see Chapter 15 for additional details on banding and other bird marking methods). Colour bands and other artificial marks (e.g. patagial tags) are useful options for projects that harness citizen science and community engagement in data collection. The need to capture and mark birds for identification of individuals should be carefully considered and may not be necessary in some cases, such as in sexually dimorphic species or species that carry individually identifiable markings (such as Australian magpies). The use of patagial tags must be carefully considered as these are known to cause flight interference, infection, reduced individual health and even mortality in some species (Saunders 1988). Captive trials may be appropriate to demonstrate the suitability of a proposed marking method before being used on free-ranging birds.

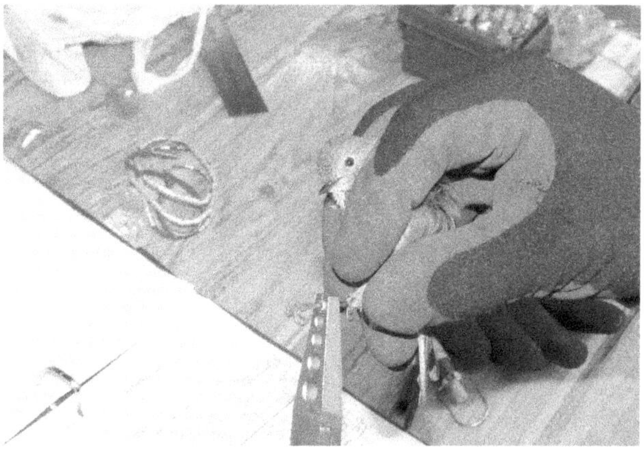

Figure 33.1: Appropriate handling technique for a small passerine, demonstrated here during banding of a brown thornbill (*Acanthiza pusilla*). Photo by Grant Palmer.

As technology advances, transmitters are increasingly used as part of movement studies, even for smaller passerines. A widely adopted standard for passerine birds is that an attached transmitter should weigh < 5% of the bird's body mass (Animal Ethics Infolink 2020), but increasingly lower weight ratios to body weight are encouraged. Factors that must be considered to mitigate negative impacts, include the body mass of the bird relative to the mass of the transmitter, stream-lined transmitters to reduce drag, positioning to minimise impacts on posture and movement, and using colours that are less likely to influence behaviour or increase vulnerability to predation. Appropriate and timely retrieval of transmitters must also be inbuilt into any research, to avoid the negative physiological and behavioural consequences of birds being encumbered indefinitely. Where possible, equipment should be removed from birds once data collection is complete. This process may require recapture or, alternatively, devices may be shed via natural feather moult, material disintegration (e.g. a harness with an inbuilt weak link) or timed-release mechanism (see Chapter 15). The use of transmitters may be unnecessary for species that are largely sedentary, move over relatively small areas, and whose territories can be readily mapped through direct observations.

Passerines are not generally considered to be susceptible to capture myopathy, which has been recorded in several large non-passerine birds. Some small passerines (e.g. thornbills and gerygones, Acanthizidae) are sensitive to any level of respiratory compromise and care should be taken not to restrict respiration while handling them, including through application of pressure to their body. Additionally, small passerines are particularly vulnerable to the effects of heat and cold, the latter of which compounds the effect of compromised respiration. Gaping, panting, closed eyes, drooping head or lethargy are all signs of thermal or respiratory stress. Affected birds should be placed for recovery in a quiet area with adequate shade. Likewise, cold-stressed birds should be placed in a quiet area with adequate warmth. Some passerines (e.g. treecreepers, Climacteridae) are prone to shedding excess feathers during handling and particular care is required for these species.

Passerines can be transported in an enclosed box, with adequate ventilation holes. The box must be appropriate for the size, strength and behaviour of the bird being transported. The box should be secured, so that it does not move during transportation, and must provide protection from direct sunlight, temperature extremes, wind and rain and contain at least one suitably sized perch fixed at a low level so that the bird has something to secure its position on. Transported birds should be monitored frequently.

Interference activities relevant to passerines include call playback and nest inspections. Such activities must be conducted in a manner that minimises distress and will not compromise the wellbeing of adult birds, nestlings or eggs. Passerines typically hatch altricial (i.e. 'undeveloped') young, which are nest bound for a period of time before fledging. In this early phase of life, nestlings are dependent on adult birds for temperature regulation, protection and food. Adult birds may alter their behaviour or abandon nests in response to disturbance, which may increase the nesting vulnerability. Practical and less-obtrusive techniques have been developed, which greatly reduce disturbance at the nest site. Nestling development can be studied by measuring stages of vocal development, using small recording devices placed near the nest. Camera traps can be used for covert observation of eggs, incubation, nestlings and food provisioning.

Call playback is a widely used technique in wildlife research, where an animal call is broadcast to detect the presence of animals via sightings or a call response. However, the physiological responses of birds to call playback are poorly known. Birds can quickly become habituated to call playback and responses to calls may diminish over a short period (Watson *et al.* 2018). For passerines, call playback should be avoided near nesting birds and during the breeding season, and its use limited for species with small population sizes or highly restricted distributions.

Cooperative birds can be well suited to observation-based studies of bird behaviour, as they are often sedentary, active in cohesive groups, and vocal, particularly when maintaining and defending territory. Traditional capture methods, such as walk-in crow traps, are widely used to capture these bird species. Distress calls issued by captured individuals often draw other individuals from the group to the trap site, so it is vital that captured birds are processed and released as quickly as possible to reduce individual and group stress. Recorded territorial calls of the target birds can be effective in luring birds into traps; however, they should be used sparingly to avoid social disruption and undue stress to groups.

Temporarily isolating or removing adults from close-knit social groups of any cooperative breeding species is highly stressful. Such actions may result in attempts of mobbing, or lead to the development of fear and stress, which are difficult to assess, partly because of a behaviour called 'masking behaviour' (i.e. birds that do not appear healthy and confident may become targets for predators). Handling or disturbance of birds should be avoided during their breeding seasons. Birds should not be removed from territories for any extended duration, as transient individuals (typically males) tend to readily occupy 'vacant' territories; this can interfere with or impair social dynamics and breeding success. Competing magpie groups could use the temporary weakness to invade, either to expand or even usurp territory (Kaplan 2018) or, in the case of white-winged choughs, destabilise the group by kidnapping juveniles (Heinsohn 1991). For territorial species, removing any of the adults for > 7 days is discouraged because of the risk such absences present, most notably loss of territory or at least destabilising the group in a way that may lead to territorial invasions. Where this is unavoidable, working outside the breeding season, with subordinate group members, with rehabilitated birds (yet to be released back into the wild) or by removing the entire group may provide less-disruptive alternatives.

Cooperative breeding species typically respond strongly to call playback because of their tight social bonds and territoriality. Care must be taken to avoid unnecessary use that could disrupt social cohesion or territory maintenance. Interestingly, when trapping and handling magpies, if one of the breeding adults needs to be captured, prerecorded territorial calls from the individual can be broadcast at regular intervals during the bird's absence, to maintain territorial stability and prevent neighbourhood takeovers. Carrick (1963) removed a male but broadcast his territorial calls (carolling) and showed that a territory can be maintained for a few weeks by this playback method. Although this is only a temporary measure, it ensures that, for the duration of the research, the captured adult magpie can be safely returned to its own intact social group and territory. However, absences of > 7 days should be avoided and are discouraged during the breeding season.

The use of drones to study these birds requires careful consideration (Vas *et al.* 2015). Australian magpies actively defend their airspace, so using drones to monitor or observe them or their nests may pose a risk. Magpies will readily attack a drone, possibly resulting in injury to the bird. Drone noise, appearance in airspace and hovering are likely to induce stress in a way that seriously interferes with normal behaviour. If drones must be used, only very brief flyovers should be undertaken.

Veterinary considerations

Sedation and anaesthesia

Avian anaesthesia is considerably different to procedures commonly applied to mammals. It is critical to be aware of the unique circulatory and respiratory physiology before contemplating sedating or anaesthetising birds (Zehnder *et al.* 2014). Because of their relatively high metabolic rate, birds generally require much higher doses of common therapeutics in mg/kg than do mammals. In the most general terms, gaseous anaesthesia tends to be used more widely than injectable agents. For passerine birds, inhalant anaesthesia induction is often performed with either a mask or induction chamber. Always consult with an experienced veterinarian when contemplating chemical restraint for birds and refer to an authoritative reference text (Hawkins *et al.* 2014). For many minor research procedures (e.g. banding, blood sampling), chemical restraint is usually not necessary.

Blood collection

For passerine birds, the wing (brachial) vein is generally used for collection of small volumes (50–75 μL) of blood under manual restraint without the need for anaesthesia (Zamora-Vilchis *et al.* 2012).

Euthanasia

The most broadly accepted method for wild passerines involves chemical euthanasia: pentobarbitone via intravenous injection after induction via inhalant anaesthetics. Chemical euthanasia methods require training and must be performed by an experienced investigator or a registered veterinarian. The realities of field research situations often require physical means of euthanasia. One common method for field euthanasia of passerines is the use of inhalant anaesthetic agents in a closed chamber (AVMA 2020). Use of carbon dioxide inhalation is more contentious. Where the capture and handling of large numbers of passerines is expected, materials for this method should be organised in advance of field research. Cervical dislocation, decapitation or concussion are conditionally accepted as a practical and effective method to euthanase smaller passerine birds (< 200 g) and cervical dislocation and decapitation are also conditionally recommended for larger passerines < 3 kg (Reilly 2001; AVMA 2020), where chemical methods of euthanasia are not available. Cervical dislocation or concussion to euthanase birds should only be employed by personnel who are trained and proficient in these methods.

Infectious pathogens

Passerines may occasionally carry zoonoses. Researchers must be alert for signs of disease or other abnormalities in handled birds. The ability to assess feather condition and parasite load, and detect signs of ill-health by examining plumage appearance, gape and throat is required. An awareness of acute signs of disease such as discharge, wheezing, vomiting, diarrhoea or unusual colour in faeces is needed (Contreras *et al.* 2016).

Salmonella spp. are intestinal bacteria that can cause severe disease in people and in passerines, although infection is typically asymptomatic in the latter. It is primarily transmitted through contamination with faecal material. *Campylobacter* spp. are also intestinal bacteria and are similarly transmitted. They can lead to moderate gastrointestinal problems in people but are asymptomatic in passerines. Psittacosis can be a severe, primarily respiratory disease of people and can cause disease or remain asymptomatic in a range of bird species, including passerines. It is caused by the intracellular bacterium *Chlamydia psittaci*, transmitted from birds through ocular, oral or nasal discharges and in faeces.

Diseases of special interest affecting ground foragers, such as the Australian magpie and Australian mudnesters, include aspergillosis (a fungal infection). *Aspergillus* spp. spores are considered ubiquitous in the environment, reaching particularly high levels in organic matter such as soil and litter, where these birds forage. *Aspergillus* spp. spores thrive in organic mulch, resulting in an increase in aspergillosis in magpies in particular. The fungal spores settle in the upper and lower respiratory tracts and infect lungs and air sacs. Coughing and dyspnoea are signs of advanced aspergillosis (Savelieff *et al.* 2018).

Contact between birds through capture and handling poses a risk for the transmission of novel infectious diseases. Spillover of *Trichomonas gallinae* from doves to passerines in Europe and North America has caused significant decline in some species. Hygiene practices to minimise the risk of pathogen transmission or introduction into passerines during research include meticulous cleaning and disinfection of all equipment between field sites, the use of personal protective equipment and frequent hand washing. Any invasive instrument (crop tubes, etc.) must be sterilised between use in individual birds.

PARROTS AND COCKATOOS

Daniella Teixeira, Dejan Stojanovic, Grant Palmer and Andrew Peters

Characteristics

Parrots (order Psittaciformes) are a diverse group of birds comprising three families in Australia. Cockatoos (Cacatuidae) are the largest parrots, characterised by strong beaks, large ceres (a waxy, fleshy covering at the base of the upper beak) and erectile crests. They are typically loud and raucous. Families Psittacidae and Psittaculidae comprise the smaller parrots, lorikeets and rosellas. These species are usually brightly coloured and often travel in large, noisy flocks. Parrots and cockatoos are widely distributed across Australia, occupying rainforests, dry woodlands, grasslands, deserts and urban environments. While many species have adapted to human habitation, several are highly threatened. One mainland species, the paradise parrot (*Psephotus pulcherrimus*) is extinct (Olsen 2007).

Biology and behaviour

Parrots and cockatoos are capable of moving long distances in search of food or other resources. Movements may be seasonal (e.g. altitudinal migration of gang-gang cockatoos, *Callocephalon fimbriatum*, and movement between coastal and island habitats by rock parrots, *Neophema petrophila*), nomadic (e.g. princess parrot, *Polytelis alexandrae*, a desert species) or migratory (Tasmanian blue-winged parrot, *Neophema chrysostoma*, and orange-bellied parrot, *Neophema chrysogaster*). Other species may be sedentary or resident.

Parrots and cockatoos feed mostly on seeds, fruit and nectar. Most parrots and cockatoos are granivorous, with much of their diet comprising seeds, sometimes exclusively. Lorikeets and swift parrots (*Lathamus discolor*) feed principally on nectar, pollen and fruit. Many species of parrot and some cockatoos also eat invertebrates; for example, yellow-tailed black-cockatoos (*Calyptorhynchus funereus*) locate and extract boring insects from tree trunks (Cameron 2007).

Parrots and cockatoos vary widely in their degree of dietary specialisation. The glossy black-cockatoo (*Calyptorhynchus lathami*) is among the most specialised of all parrots, feeding only on the seeds of she-oak trees (*Casuarina* and *Allocasuarina* spp.), and being highly selective in the choice of individual tree to feed on (Cameron and Cunningham 2006). Conversely, many species of cockatoo are generalist feeders, and some have adapted to novel foods. Some species have learned to exploit agricultural crops and for this reason several cockatoo species are considered pests (Cameron 2007).

Parrots and cockatoos are intelligent, and most species are highly social. They often congregate in large flocks, usually to exploit food resources or move through the landscape. Parrots and cockatoos are social learners and young birds acquire critical behaviours and skills during the post-fledging period when they are dependent on their parents and others in their social group. Many species are socially monogamous and form strong pair bonds, but recent studies have revealed that other mating systems (e.g. cooperative polyandry) also exist. Parrots' and cockatoos' food-associated sociality is thought to have driven the evolution of complex vocal repertoires and the rare ability to learn new vocalisations throughout life (Bradbury and Balsby 2016).

Most Australian parrots and cockatoos nest inside tree hollows (typically exploiting existing cavities, but some species excavate their own cavities in decomposing wood). Two extant *Psephotellus* species use termitaria, the *Pezoporus* species are all ground-nesters, and rock parrots nest in rock crevices. Parrot and cockatoo eggs are white, and nestlings are altricial, typically with long nesting periods. Most species produce between two and five eggs, although some produce only one, and breeding success varies widely.

Capture and handling

Monitoring parrots and cockatoos often involves traditional human-observer methods, such as occupancy-style monitoring, distance sampling, flock counts, nest inspections via tree climbing, and individual marking through leg banding. Citizen science is important for many species, including Carnaby's black-cockatoo (*Calyptorynchus latirostris*) and orange-bellied parrots. Bioacoustic sound recorders and camera traps are increasingly used in monitoring (e.g. for nesting swift parrots and red-tailed black-cockatoos, *Calyptorynchus banksii*).

Capture requires specialised training and techniques vary among species and habitats. Nestlings and adults can be captured at the nest. Ground feeders may be captured when foraging or drinking on the ground, using whoosh and mist nets. Care must be taken to avoid being bitten, especially when handling cockatoos with strong beaks. Likewise, captured birds may bite themselves or nearby birds during entanglement, so rapid extrication from nets is crucial. Some species are particularly prone to stress (palm cockatoos, *Probosciger aterrimus*, in particular) and trapping is not recommended. Minimising handling time is crucial to manage capture stress in all individuals.

Dark bird bags are suitable for holding most parrots temporarily. Cardboard boxes may be suitable for short-term transport of small parrots, but larger parrots and cockatoos should always be transported in bird cages or large domestic pet carry cages, as they can chew through cardboard boxes. Birds should be isolated during transport; containers should be dark with minimal visibility to the outside to reduce stress. In all cases, infection control is paramount to avoid transmission of infectious disease among individual birds, such as psittacine beak and feather disease.

Leg-banding is a common method used on a range of parrot and cockatoo species. Other techniques include short-term methods such as tail feather marking (Groom *et al.* 2014) and wing tags (i.e. patagial tags) attached to the patagium (long-term marking) (Davis *et al.* 2017); however, use of patagial tags is not recommended for all species (see Saunders 1988). These methods have been used to monitor individuals in the wild. Tracking studies have also used GPS and satellite devices attached as back or tail mounts (Groom *et al.* 2014; Yeap *et al.* 2017). Attachment may require anaesthesia (but not always), which may necessitate veterinary support (see Chapter 16).

For anything other than short-term housing, parrots and cockatoos should be housed in flight aviaries appropriate for their body and flock size. Large, social species are prone to neurotic behaviour in inadequate captive conditions. For longer-term housing, birds should generally be kept in conditions that maintain sociality. However, social organisation and flock size within aviaries may require careful planning and advice should be sought from experts in parrot and cockatoo husbandry. Enrichment is important to prevent boredom and neurotic behaviour. If birds are to breed in captivity, nest boxes must be provided. Some species (e.g. lorikeets) sleep in boxes when possible.

Interference activities relevant to parrots and cockatoos are similar to passerines considered in this chapter. Nest inspections, including of tree hollows and nest boxes, must be conducted in a manner that minimises distress or risk to wellbeing to adult birds, nestlings and eggs. Disturbance at nest sites presents significant risk of nest abandonment or altered adult bird behaviour, which may increase the vulnerability of eggs and nestlings.

Veterinary considerations

Considerations relating to administration of veterinary chemicals are the same as described previously in 'Passerine birds'.

Sedation and anaesthesia

As for all birds, inhalant gaseous anaesthesia is the preferred approach when available (Hawkins *et al.* 2014). Typically for cockatoos, isoflurane is used, and anaesthetic induction is achieved by using a face mask, followed by endotracheal intubation for anaesthetic maintenance (Le Souëf *et al.* 2013).

Blood collection

Blood samples can be collected via venipuncture of the brachial vein under manual restraint for smaller parrots, as per passerine birds. For larger cockatoos, blood samples are often collected by jugular venipuncture of anaesthetised birds (Le Souëf *et al.* 2013).

Euthanasia

Acceptable methods for euthanasia for parrots and cockatoos follow those described for passerines. Where justified and chemical means of euthanasia are unavailable, accepted mechanical means of euthanasia for most species are cervical dislocation and decapitation (Reilly 2001; AVMA 2020). Blunt trauma is considered an appropriate method, with reservations, for euthanasia of species < 200 g.

Infectious pathogens

Parrots are important carriers of zoonotic diseases (Contreras *et al.* 2016). Psittacine beak and feather disease (PBFD) is a serious disease and a listed Key Threatening Process for parrots. It is widespread in Australia and is the pathogen of most concern for conservation (Raidal and Peters 2018). PBFD has caused fatalities in important captive breeding programs for threatened species. The virus that causes PBFD is environmentally resistant and care needs to be taken to prevent transmission between wild and captive populations, especially where these involve threatened species. Avian chlamydiosis is caused by infection of *Chlamydia psittaci*. While *C. psittaci* is known from wild and captive birds, its prevalence appears to be much higher in captivity (Amery-Gale *et al.* 2020). *Chlamydia psittaci* causes the zoonotic disease psittacosis in humans, although human infection may come from non-avian hosts (Polkinghorne *et al.* 2020). Other diseases known from captive or wild psittacines include avian polyomavirus, psittacine adenovirus and avian poxvirus.

General operating procedures

A range of research methods relevant to the study of passerines, cockatoos and parrots are detailed in other chapters, including acoustic devices and camera traps (Chapter 5), the use of drones (Chapter 6), mist netting (Chapter 7), and citizen science and educational activities (Chapter 10). Avian-specific methods are detailed in Chapter 15, including census and observational techniques, call playback and broadcast surveys, nest and hollow inspections (including handling of eggs and chicks), hand capture and spotlighting, foot snares and noose carpets, methods for capture of individual birds, baited funnel and crow traps, cannon nets, marking methods, telemetry methods and collection of regurgitate, crop contents, scats and pellets. Several veterinary procedures may also be used during passerine research (Chapter 16). Additional standard operating procedures relevant to the birds considered in this chapter are also available (Lowe 1989).

REFERENCES

ABSA (Australian Bird Studies Association) (2020) *Bird in the Hand.* 2nd edn. ABSA. <https://absa.asn.au/pub/bird-in-the-hand-2nd-edn/>.

Animal Ethics Infolink (2020) Radio tracking and GPS tracking. *Animal Research Review Panel Guideline 9.* <http://www.animalethics.org.au/policies-and-guidelines/wildlife-research/radio-tracking>.

AVMA (2020) *AVMA Guidelines for the Euthanasia of Animals, 2020 Edition.* American Veterinary Medical Association, Schaumburg, IL.

Amery-Gale J, Legione AR, Marenda MS, Owens J, Eden PA, Konsak-Ilievski BM, *et al.* (2020) Surveillance for *Chlamydia* spp. with multilocus sequence typing analysis in wild and captive birds in Victoria, Australia. *Journal of Wildlife Diseases* **56**, 16–26. doi:10.7589/2018-11-281

Bradbury JW, Balsby TJS (2016) The functions of vocal learning in parrots. *Behavioral Ecology and Sociobiology* **70**, 293–312. doi:10.1007/s00265-016-2068-4

Cameron M (2007) *Cockatoos.* CSIRO Publishing, Melbourne.

Cameron M, Cunningham R (2006) Habitat selection at multiple spatial scales by foraging glossy black-cockatoos. *Austral Ecology* **31**, 597–607. doi:10.1111/j.1442-9993.2006.01591.x

Carrick R (1963) Ecological significance of territory in the Australian Magpie. *Proceedings of the XIIIth Ornitholgical Congress* **13**, 740–753.

Contreras A, Gomez-Martin A, Paterna A, Tatay-Dualde J, Prats-Van Der Ham M, Corrales JC, *et al.* (2016) Epidemiological role of birds in the transmission and maintenance of zoonoses. *Revue Scientifique et Technique (International Office of Epizootics)* **35**, 845–862. doi:10.20506/rst.35.3.2574

Davis A, Major RE, Taylor CE, Martin JM (2017) Novel Tracking and Reporting Methods for Studying Large Birds in Urban Landscapes. *Wildlife Biology* **2017**, 4. doi:10.2981/wlb.00307

Gill FB (2007) *Ornithology.* 3rd edn. W H Freeman and Company, New York, NY.

Groom C, Warren K, Le Souëf A, Dawson R (2014) Attachment and performance of Argos satellite tracking devices fitted to black cockatoos (*Calyptorhynchus* spp.). *Wildlife Research* **41**, 571–583. doi:10.1071/WR14138

Hawkins MG, Zehnder AM, Pascoe PJ (2014) Cagebirds. In *Zoo Animal and Wildlife Immobilization and Anaesthesia.* 2nd edn. (Eds G West, D Heard and N Caulkett) pp. 399–433. John Wiley and Sons, Hoboken, NJ.

Heinsohn RG (1991) Kidnapping and reciprocity in cooperatively breeding white-winged choughs. *Animal Behaviour* **41**, 1097–1100. doi:10.1016/S0003-3472(05)80652-9

Kaplan G (2018) Development of meaningful vocal signals in a juvenile territorial songbird (*Gymnorhina tibicen*) and the dilemma of vocal taboos concerning neighbours and strangers. *Animals* **8**, 228. doi:10.3390/ani8120228

Le Souëf AT, Holyoake CS, Vitali SD, Warren KS (2013) Hematologic and plasma biochemical reference values for three species of black cockatoos (*Calyptorhynchus* species). *Journal of Avian Medicine and Surgery* **27**, 14–22. doi:10.1647/2010-056.1

Lowe KL (1989) *The Australian Bird Banders Manual.* Australian Bat and Bird Banding Schemes and Australian National Parks and Wildlife Service, Canberra.

Olsen P (2007) *Glimpses of Paradise: The Quest for the Beautiful Parrakeet.* National Library of Australia, Canberra.

Polkinghorne A, Weston K, Branley J (2020) Recent history of psittacosis in Australia: expanding our understanding of the epidemiology of this important globally distributed zoonotic disease. *Internal Medicine Journal* **50**, 246–249. doi:10.1111/imj.14726

Raidal SR, Peters A (2018) Psittacine beak and feather disease: ecology and implications for conservation. *Emu - Austral Ornithology* **118**, 80–93. doi:10.1080/01584197.2017.1387029

Reilly JS (Ed.) (2001) *Euthanasia of Animals Used for Scientific Purposes.* 2nd edn. Australian & New Zealand Council for the Care of Animals in Research and Teaching (ANZCCART), Adelaide.

Saunders DA (1988) Patagial tags: do benefits outweigh risks to the animals? *Australian Wildlife Research* **15**, 565–569. doi:10.1071/WR9880565

Savelieff MG, Pappalardo L, Azmanis P (2018) The current status of avian aspergillosis diagnoses: veterinary practice to novel research avenues. *Veterinary Clinical Pathology* **47**, 342–362. doi:10.1111/vcp.12644

Vas E, Lescroël A, Duriez O, Boguszewski G, Grémillet D (2015) Approaching birds with drones: first experiments and ethical guidelines. *Biology Letters* **11**, 20140754. doi:10.1098/rsbl.2014.0754

Watson DM, Znidersic E, Craig ML (2018) Ethical birding call playback and conservation. *Conservation Biology* **33**, 469–471. doi:10.1111/cobi.13199

Yeap L, Shephard JM, Bouten W, Jackson B, Vaughan-Higgins R, Warren K (2017) Development of a tag-attachment method to enable capture of fine- and landscape-scale movement in black-cockatoos. *Australian Field Ornithology* **34**, 49–55. doi:10.20938/af034049055

Zamora-Vilchis I, Williams SE, Johnson CN (2012) Environmental temperature affects prevalence of blood parasites of birds on an elevation gradient: implications for disease in a warming climate. *PLoS One* 7(6), e39208. doi:10.1371/journal.pone.0039208

Zehnder AM, Hawkins MG, Pascoe PJ (2014) Avian anatomy and physiology. In *Zoo Animal and Wildlife Immobilization and Anaesthesia*. 2nd edn. (Eds G West, D Heard and N Caulkett) pp. 391–398. John Wiley and Sons, Hoboken, NJ.

34 Raptors

Penny D. Olsen

INTRODUCTION

All of Australia's raptors live a predatory lifestyle, and are morphologically and behaviourally similar (Debus 2019). Every species has a hooked beak and strong feet with sharp, curved talons, relatively forward-facing eyes, and plumage in colour combinations of black, brown, grey and/or white. However, they are a diverse group belonging to five families in three distantly related orders (McClure *et al.* 2019). Currently, 24 diurnal raptor and 11 owl species are resident in Australia. These species include diurnal raptors from orders Accipitriformes (families Pandionidae and Accipitridae) and Falconiformes (family Falconidae), and owls from order Strigiformes (families Tytonidae and Strigidae) (Debus 2009). Visiting (itinerant) species, from the north of Australia, include oriental honey-buzzard (*Pernis ptilorhynchus*), Eurasian hobby (*Falco subbuteo*) and northern boobook (*Ninox japonicus*). See the Working List of Australian Birds (version 3; https://www.birdlife.org.au/conservation/science/taxonomy).

EAGLES, KITES, GOSHAWKS, FALCONS AND OWLS

Characteristics

Differences and details in raptors' morphology often relate to hunting techniques. Pacific bazas (*Aviceda subcristata*), for example, feed on insects, small vertebrates and fruit in tree canopies, and have relatively weak feet and bills, and short broad wings for lift rather than speed. Powerful owls (*Ninox strenua*) have massive feet to dispatch arboreal mammals and very concave broad wings for high lift at slow speeds. Australian hobbies (*Falco longipennis*) have scimitar-shaped wings to overtake and catch birds, bats and insects in the air, whereas swamp harriers (*Circus approximans*) have very long and broad wings to keep them aloft at slow speeds while they scan the ground before dropping onto prey. Wings are short and rounded in forest dwellers; long, broad and fingered in soarers; and long and pointed in fast, open country species.

Raptors are often strongly sexually dimorphic. Females are larger than males in diurnal raptors and barn owls (*Tyto* spp.). Males are the larger sex in larger hawk owls (*Ninox* spp.) and females in the smaller hawk owls, including the southern boobook (*Ninox boobook*), morepork (*Ninox novaeseelandiae*) and Christmas Island boobook (*Ninox natalis*). Diurnal raptors range in body mass from ~130 g for male collared sparrowhawks (*Accipiter cirrocephalus*) to ~4 kg for female wedge-tailed eagles (*Aquila audax*). Owls vary in mass from around 150 g for a male Christmas Island boobook, to around 2 kg for a male powerful owl (*Ninox strenua*). Wingspans range from ~60 cm for sparrowhawks to ~2 m for wedge-tailed eagles.

Biology and behaviour

Raptors are highly mobile and, typically, widely dispersed across mainland, coastal and offshore islands of Australia. They are difficult to study when not breeding, so most research has been conducted during the breeding season on individuals near nest sites. Raptors can also be difficult to capture, particularly the more-aerial species, such as Australian hobbies and peregrine falcons (*Falco peregrinus*). Targeted surveys are essential to provide meaningful estimates of abundance or distribution (e.g. Andersen in Bird and Bildstein 2007; DWHEA 2010). Owls are almost unique among raptors in that they can be surveyed using call playback. Owl survey protocols have been developed for a few species, but require further refining and testing (e.g. Wintle *et al.* 2005; Cooke *et al.* 2017).

Most Australian raptors are territorial during the breeding season, if not year-round (the letter-winged kite, *Elanus scriptus*, is a possible exception). Movements (migration, post-breeding dispersal), territory size and home ranges are poorly known, highly variable, and dependent on species, climate and seasonal conditions, habitat and prey availability. Estimated home-range size during the breeding season is as little as 18 ha for some southern boobooks and up to 5000 ha for wedge-tailed eagles (Cherriman 2007). Monitored home-range sizes in powerful owls range from 4770 ha in forest to 137 ha in urban areas (Bradsworth *et al.* 2017). Only the Tasmanian swamp harrier and perhaps the Tasmanian boobook (*Ninox leucopsis*) seem to undertake regular true directional migration, to the Australian mainland in winter. Other species are partially migratory with a variable direction, where some individuals of either sex leave their breeding grounds in autumn/winter to travel to warmer parts of the mainland (e.g. little eagle, *Hieraaetus morphnoides*; nankeen kestrel, *Falco cenchroides*); partly nomadic (e.g. black kite, *Milvus migrans*; barn owl); or irruptive (letter-winged kite, barn owl). The juveniles of all species are dispersive.

Diurnal raptors, as the term suggests, are mostly active by day, although the letter-winged kite is entirely nocturnal. Others, such as Australian hobbies and the brown falcon (*Falco berigora*), are quite crepuscular (active at dawn or dusk). Owls are nocturnal, although hawk owls can also be crepuscular. Hawk owls have large eyes, as do the more nocturnal of the diurnal raptors. Barn owls (tytonids) are highly specialised nocturnal hunters, with enhanced hearing and feathers that dampen flight noise. Raptors are typically solitary or live in loosely associated pairs, and in family groups during the fledgling period. Several species, such as letter-winged kites, black kites and young wedge-tailed eagles, may congregate where food is temporarily plentiful.

All Australian raptors are predatory, some more so than others. Smaller species typically eat more invertebrates than larger species, which primarily prey on vertebrates. All species hunt live prey and a few also feed opportunistically on carrion (e.g. black kite, regularly; wedge-tailed eagle, occasionally), some eat eggs and nestlings (e.g. square-tailed kite, *Lophoictinia isura*; swamp harrier) and one species, the Pacific baza, occasionally eats fruit. Some species are more specialised in their choice of prey and method of hunting than others. For example, black-shouldered kites (*Elanus axillaris*), kestrels and barn owls favour ground-living rodents and drop on them from a hovering position, while eastern ospreys (*Pandion cristatus*) plunge into the sea to catch fish. Some of the falcons fly down aerial birds using high speed dives or rapid level flight. Harriers fly low, quartering the ground, listening for prey hidden among vegetation. The three accipiters sit hidden and wait, making short dashes after prey or using their long legs to snatch it from among vegetation. Species such as brown and little falcons and black and whistling kites may be attracted to disruptions such as grass fires or travelling stock that flush and concentrate prey.

Typically, courting male raptors bring food to the female, and later to the female and chicks. Females contribute more prey to the family as the nestling period progresses. Diet can be studied by observation (directly or via cameras) and by collection of prey remains and from in or under nests or roosts (Bird and Bildstein 2007). Some researchers autoclave the pellets to kill pathogens, but most do not consider it necessary.

With a few exceptions, Australian raptors are monogamous and isolated pairs breed in spring and summer. Letter-winged kites breed in pairs in colonies when their main prey, long-haired rats (*Rattus villosissimus*), are abundant. Some larger species (e.g. powerful owls) with longer nesting periods start breeding in winter. In the tropics, some species avoid breeding in the summer wet season. Most species produce one brood a year at most, although a few continue to breed if climatic conditions are favourable (e.g. elanid kites and barn owls). Clutch size varies with body size, and larger species tend to have fewer eggs than smaller species, at least within taxonomic families. Incubation periods range from 4 weeks in small species to 6 weeks in the largest species (eagles), and the nestling period from 4 weeks to 3 months. Fledglings stay with one or both parents for several months, occasionally, in some species, until the next breeding attempt.

Eastern ospreys and all accipitrids build nests of sticks, but falcons do not build a nest at all, using a tree hollow, ledge or a stick nest built by another species. Owls all nest in tree hollows. Typically, the same site or sites are used each year. Nest sites may be located on the ground (e.g. swamp harriers and eastern grass owls (*Tyto longimembris*) regularly; eastern ospreys occasionally) to, more often, the highest trees and cliff ledges. Artificial structures, such as electricity pylons and ledges on tall buildings, offer nest sites for a few species.

Most raptors flee when their nest is approached. Only a few individuals of certain species, such as peregrine falcons and powerful owls, will defend the nest. It is important not to flush the birds from the nest too suddenly to prevent damage to the eggs or a chick being knocked from the nest (Bird and Bildstein 2007 and references therein). Some raptors, notably wedge-tailed eagles and swamp harriers, are particularly prone to nest desertion from disturbance, especially when starting nesting activity. The risk of desertion tends to decrease as breeding progresses; nest sites are more likely to be deserted than eggs and eggs are more likely to be deserted than chicks. If adults are kept away from the nest, eggs or young chicks may overheat or chill, or be exposed to predators such as currawongs (*Strepera* spp.), ravens (*Corvus* spp.) and other raptors.

Capture and handling

Raptors are strong and flighty, and require specialised capture, handling, housing and transport techniques (see Bird and Bildstein 2007). Cannon netting (Krone and Treu 2018) and net launchers (Domenech *et al.* 2021) are two methods that have been used to capture adult eagles overseas and have recently been successfully used on wedge-tailed eagles (J. Pay, pers. comm.). Many raptors will only respond to live prey (Bird and Bildstein 2007). Trapping for these species may include use of live 'bait' animals, such as mice or pigeons. The lure animal should be protected by a cage, or similar arrangement, and cared for appropriately. Dead animals used to attract scavenging raptors (e.g. wedge-tailed eagles and black kites) can be found opportunistically (e.g. roadkill) or appropriate prey species can be killed. Avoid using carcasses of animals shot with lead-based bullets as bait (Pay *et al.* 2021). Owls can be trapped using call playback as an audio lure, but playback disturbs the birds and is best used sparingly. Nestling birds can be captured by climbing trees containing nests and physically capturing birds by hand before they can fly (Pay *et al.* 2021) – care should be taken not to cause them to leave the nest prematurely.

Cages for housing and transport should be non-abrasive and isolative to keep birds calm and prevent them from breaking or abrading their feathers. A simple sturdy, ventilated cardboard box is adequate for temporary transport in most cases. A raptor's feet present a danger to the handler. Handling can be stress free and painless if the bird is held confidently and correctly, such as around the lower body and upper legs, so that the wings and legs are secured. Larger species will require the handler to use two hands: one around and separating the thighs, the other encircling the wings and tail. Secured in this way, the raptor will rarely struggle and, because of its stiff backbone, is unable reach down far enough to bite. Covering the head with a loose bag or well-fitted falconry hood, although not always necessary, calms the bird. Fresh water and food should be provided if a raptor is held captive. Food should be size appropriate and whole food where possible: laboratory mice or rats, day-old chicks or lean red meat, supplemented with calcium and vitamins as necessary.

In Australia, numbered stainless-steel leg bands, issued by the Australian Bird and Bat Banding Scheme (ABBBS), or riveted-on numbered, aluminium colour bands (made overseas) are used to individually identify wild raptors. Occasionally, plastic coloured bands, glued shut, are used on smaller species, but adults are likely to pick them off. Reflective tape glued to a band can be useful for marking the nestlings of nocturnal species. The relevant leg (left or right) should be carefully recorded. Band numbers (or part thereof) can be read when birds are recovered dead or alive, or with persistence and luck, by observation with telescope or via digital camera photograph. A banding authority is required from the ABBBS, which oversees the recruitment and training of bird banders in Australia and issues and records the use of numbered leg bands and colour bands.

Passive integrated transponder (PIT) tags and microchips, which allow automated collection of data when set up at locations that the raptor approaches closely, are not typically used on wild raptors in Australia, and rarely elsewhere. PIT tags can be attached to leg bands. Microchips have potential for use in identifying captives and have been used widely to mark falconry birds overseas. Microchips (unalterable 134.2 kHz ISO 11784 International Standard–compliant transponders are recommended) are usually fitted by a veterinarian, typically without need for sedation or anaesthesia. They are implanted subcutaneously with a wide gauge needle, on the left side of the keel (sternum), parallel to the keel. The entry wound is sealed with suitable adhesive (methacrylate-based). The direction of the implant is not important if a universal (forward-and-backward reading) scanner is in use.

Telemetric devices allow tracking of the movements and activities of raptors during the non-breeding and breeding seasons (Meyburg and Meyburg 2002; Bird and Bildstein 2007). Typically, satellite trackers are favoured over VHF radio-tracking devices, which are labour intensive. The tracker should be as streamlined and light as possible, and generally weigh no more than 3% of the individual's body mass, and should be removed or designed to drop off after its life or purpose has been achieved (Bird and Bildstein 2007). Several tag-attachment methods have been used, most commonly back harnesses (Brawata *et al.* 2019) and tail mounts. Back harnesses with a weak link detach if the raptor becomes entangled in vegetation; however, if the bird cannot be recaptured, the harness may stay attached beyond the life of the transmitter. Tail-mounted tags, attached to the two central tail feathers, with the tag sitting at the base of the feathers, close to, but not obstructing the oil gland, are quicker to fit and, if recapture isn't possible, drop off with the next moult. Depending on the size of the tag and length of the whip-antennae, tags are usually secured with superglue, TESA® tape and cotton ties.

Veterinary considerations

Considerations relating to administration of veterinary chemicals are the same as described in 'Passerine birds' in Chapter 33.

Analgesia, sedation and anaesthesia

Use of therapeutics for analgesia or chemical restraint (see Chapter 16) is similar to other bird groups, with some special considerations. Consult an authoritative specialised text if considering raptor anaesthesia (Redig *et al.* 2014). When raptors require anaesthesia in veterinary hospitals, mask induction using isoflurane is generally used (Holz 2003). Some injectable approaches have been used (though are not recommended) and these are described in Table 34.1.

Blood collection

For raptor nestlings, < 2 mL of blood can be taken from the brachial vein using a 26 G needle without chemical restraint (Pay *et al.* 2021). For adult raptors, a similar approach can be taken, using the brachial vein with larger gauge needles (25 G) and larger blood volumes (2–4 mL) possible, as practised during live capture of raptors overseas (e.g. Domenech *et al.* 2021).

Euthanasia

Euthanasia by intravenous injection of pentobarbitone is recommended, where available (Reilly 2001). Any animal euthanased with pentobarbitone represents a secondary toxicity risk to wild scavengers and should be disposed of via deep burial. Cervical dislocation or gunshot is acceptable only where circumstances necessitate (e.g. working in a remote area where alternatives are unavailable, or where there is a low chance of survival and/or the level of pain and distress is too great to warrant further suffering).

Table 34.1: Examples of commonly used anaesthetics and sedatives and their doses for raptors.

Gunkel and Marin (2005).

Therapeutic category	Substance	Dosage	Comments
Anaesthetic	Ketamine	20–40 mg/kg IM	Insufficient analgesia may be a problem if used alone for painful procedures. Best used in conjunction with xylazine (~40 mg/kg), which provides 20–30 min of anaesthesia.
Inhalant anaesthetic	Isoflurane or sevoflurane	Induction with 5% isoflurane and maintenance with 2.5% isoflurane	Intubation is only used for procedures > 30 min and for species > 150 g.
Analgesic	Meloxicam	0.3–0.5 mg/kg IM or oral	Non-steroidal anti-inflammatory.
Sedative	Diazepam	0.2–1.0 mg/kg IM, IV	Also useful for treatment of seizures.

Infectious pathogens

Wild raptors appear to be reasonably free of zoonoses (Contreras *et al.* 2016), but knowledge of their infectious agents is relatively poor. Captive birds are more prone to disease, exacerbated by confinement and greater ease of spread. Generally, a veterinarian should advise on disease diagnosis and research.

Bird and Bildstein (2007) provide a comprehensive overview of disease, endoparasites and ectoparasites in raptors. Some of the more commonly encountered diseases and pathogens of raptors and their impact on humans are itemised below.

- The pathogen causing frounce or canker *(Trichomanas gallinae)* is usually caught by raptors when they eat infected pigeons and it can cause death. It is not known to be medically important to humans, but good hygiene is important to prevent spread between birds.
- Psittacosis (due to *Chlamydia psittaci*), a respiratory tract infection occasionally fatal to birds, can be transmitted to humans via aerosolised, contaminated bodily fluids. However, it is uncommon in wild raptors (Spickler 2017) and has rarely been reported in Australian raptors.
- As with wounds from most wild animals, humans can develop painful subcutaneous bacterial infections from raptor claw punctures.

Raptors may contract and spread avian influenza, contracted by hunting or scavenging infected prey. Rare cases of the highly pathogenic avian influenza virus H5N1 (a well-known zoonotic disease) have been reported in raptors, but not in Australia (van den Brand *et al.* 2015). Outbreaks of another type of H5 virus have killed many young white-tailed sea eagles (*Haliaeetus albicilla*) in Germany but are not known from Australia (Krone *et al.* 2018).

General operating procedures

A range of research methods relevant to the study of raptors are detailed in other chapters, including acoustic devices and camera traps (Chapter 5), and citizen science and educational activities (Chapter 10). Avian-specific methods are detailed in Chapter 15, including census and observational techniques, call playback and broadcast surveys, nest and hollow inspections (including handling of eggs and chicks), hand capture and spotlighting, methods for capture of individual birds, baited funnel and crow traps, bal-chatris, marking methods, telemetry methods and collection of regurgitate, crop contents, scats and pellets. Several veterinary procedures may also be used during raptor research (Chapter 16).

ACKNOWLEDGEMENTS

The author wishes to thank Nick Bradsworth, Stephen Debus and Nick Mooney for valuable feedback on early versions of this chapter.

REFERENCES

Bird DM, Bildstein K (Eds) (2007) *Raptor Research and Management Techniques*. Hancock House, Washington, DC.

Bradsworth N, White JG, Isaac B, Cooke R (2017) Species distribution models derived from citizen science data predict the fine scale movements of owls in an urbanizing landscape. *Biological Conservation* **213**, 27–35. doi:10.1016/j.biocon.2017.06.039

Brawata R, Rae S, Gruber B, Reid S, Roberts D (2019) Confirmation of little eagle (*Hieraaetus morphnoides*) migration by satellite telemetry. *Australian Journal of Zoology* **66**, 247–250.

Cherriman SC (2007) Territory size and diet throughout the year of the Wedge-tailed Eagle *Aquila audax* in the Perth region, Western Australia. BSc (Hons) thesis. Curtin University, Australia.

Contreras A, Gomez-Martin A, Paterna A, Tatay-Dualde J, Prats-Van Der Ham M, Corrales JC, *et al.* (2016) Epidemiological role of birds in the transmission and maintenance of zoonoses. *Revue Scientifique et Technique (International Office of Epizootics)* **35**, 845–862. doi:10.20506/rst.35.3.2574

Cooke R, Grant H, Ebsworth I, Rendall AR, Isaac B, White JG (2017) Can owls be used to monitor the impacts of urbanisation? A cautionary tale of variable detection. *Wildlife Research* **44**, 573–581. doi:10.1071/WR16185

Debus S (2009) *The Owls of Australia: A Field Guide to Australian Night Birds*. Envirobook, Canterbury.

Debus S (2019) *Birds of Prey of Australia*. CSIRO Publishing, Melbourne.

Department of Water, Heritage, Environment and the Arts (DWHEA) (2010) *Survey Guidelines for Australia's Threatened Birds: Guidelines for Detecting Birds Listed as Threatened under the* Environment Protection and Biodiversity Conservation Act 1999. Commonwealth of Australia, Canberra.

Domenech R, Shreading A, Ramsey P, McTee M (2021) Widespread lead exposure in golden eagles captured in Montana. *The Journal of Wildlife Management* **85**, 195–201. doi:10.1002/jwmg.21980

Gunkel C, Marin ML (2005) Current techniques in avian anaesthesia. *Seminars in Avian and Exotic Pet Medicine* **14**(4), 263–276. doi:10.1053/j.saep.2005.09.006

Holz PH (2003) Coracoid fractures in wild birds: repair and outcomes. *Australian Veterinary Journal* **81**, 469–471. doi:10.1111/j.1751-0813.2003.tb13362.x

Krone O, Globig A, Ulrich R, Harder T, Schinköthe J, Herrmann C, Gerst S, Conraths FJ, Beer M (2018) White-tailed sea eagle (*Haliaeetus albicilla*) die-off due to infection with highly pathogenic avian influenza virus, subtype H5N8, in Germany. *Viruses* **10**, 478. doi:10.3390/v10090478

Krone O, Treu G (2018) Movement patterns of white-tailed sea eagles near wind turbines. *The Journal of Wildlife Management* **82**, 1367–1375.

Meyburg B-U, Meyburg C (2002) Monitoring raptors by means of satellite telemetry. In *Raptors in the New Millenium*. (Eds R Yosef, ML Millar and D Peplar) pp. 22–32. International Birding and Research Centre, Eilat, Israel.

McClure CJW, Schulwitz SE, Anderson DL, Robinson BW, Mojica EK, Therrien J-F, Oleyar MD, Johnson J (2019) Commentary: defining raptors and birds of prey. *Journal of Raptor Research* **53**, 419–430. doi:10.3356/0892-1016-53.4.419

Pay JM, Katzner TE, Hawkins CE, Koch AJ, Wiersma JM, Brown WE, *et al.* (2021) High frequency of lead exposure in the population of an endangered Australian top predator, the Tasmanian wedge-tailed eagle (*Aquila audax fleayi*). *Environmental Toxicology and Chemistry* **40**, 219–230. doi:10.1002/etc.4914

Redig PT, Willette M, Ponder J (2014) Raptors. In *Zoo Animal and Wildlife Immobilization and Anaesthesia*. 2nd edn. (Eds G West, D Heard and N Caulkett) pp. 459–472. John Wiley and Sons, Hoboken, NJ.

Reilly JS (Ed) (2001) *Euthanasia of Animals Used for Scientific Purposes*. 2nd edn. Australian and New Zealand Council for the Care of Animals in Research and Teaching (ANZCCART), Adelaide.

Spickler AR (2017) *Psittacosis/Avian Chlamydiosis*. Centre for Food Security and Public Health, Iowa State University. <http://www.cfsph.iastate.edu/Factsheets/pdfs/psittacosis.pdf>.

van den Brand JMA, Krone O, Wolf PU, van de Bildt MWG, van Amerongen G, Osterhaus ADME, Kuiken T (2015) Host-specific exposure and fatal neurologic disease in wild raptors from highly pathogenic avian influenza virus H5N1 during the 2006 outbreak in Germany. *Veterinary Research* **46**, 24–35. doi:10.1186/s13567-015-0148-5

Wintle BA, Kavanagh RP, McCarthy MA, Burgman MA (2005) Estimating and dealing with detectability in occupancy surveys for forest owls and arboreal marsupials. *The Journal of Wildlife Management* **69**, 905–917. doi:10.2193/0022-541X(2005)069[0905:EADWDI]2.0.CO;2

35 Aquatic birds

John Porter, Jennifer Spencer, Lisa O'Neill, Kate Brandis and Maggie J. Watson

INTRODUCTION

Aquatic birds or 'waterbirds' encompass a diverse group of species that can be highly mobile and frequent a range of aquatic habitats. In this chapter, wetland birds (including shorebirds) and seabirds are treated separately, based on their habitat use outside of their breeding seasons (i.e. generally seabirds only come to land to breed). However, inevitably some overlap occurs in habitats frequented by these broad groups.

Wetland birds depend on wetlands for most of their life cycles. Many wetland bird families include species that also use shallow inshore waters, including species of egrets, herons, cormorants, gulls, some terns, pelican and shorebirds, but these taxa are grouped with wetland birds rather than treated as seabirds. Seabird species such as albatrosses, petrels, storm-petrels, shearwaters and some terns are entirely pelagic away from their breeding sites, and other seabird species frequent inshore habitats, including frigatebirds, tropicbirds, gannets, and some tern and cormorant species. This chapter does not consider other wetland-dependent bird species such as reed-inhabiting passerines and wetland raptors that can also use wetland habitats.

Waterbirds are abundant, highly visible and iconic wildlife that attract considerable scientific and public interest. Accordingly, recreational bird watching of waterbirds is a popular pastime. Duck hunting, initially for subsistence by Aboriginal and Torres Strait Islander hunters and later for food and sport by European Australians, has a long history in Australia. Shearwaters (muttonbirds) and some petrels were a highly valued food source for Aboriginal and Torres Strait Islander peoples and European Australians on Norfolk and Lord Howe islands, Bass Strait islands and Tasmania. More recently, awareness of wetland values and heightened competition for scarce water resources has led to increased recognition of wetland birds as important indicators of wetland and river health. Similarly, seabird species are highly visible indicators of change in the marine environment.

WETLAND BIRDS

John Porter, Jennifer Spencer and Kate Brandis

Characteristics

Australian wetland birds comprise around 20 families and 93 species, including Australian darter *Anhinga novaehollandiae* (Anhingidae), cormorants (Phalacrocoracidae), Magpie goose *Anseranas semipalmata* (Anseranatidae), ducks, geese and black swans *Cygnus atratus* (Anatidae), herons, egrets and bitterns (Ardeidae), Black-necked stork *Ephippiorhynchus asiaticus* (Ciconiidae), cranes (Gruidae), Australian pelicans *Pelecanus conspicillatus* (Pelicaniidae), grebes (Podicipedidae), crakes, rails and swamphens (Rallidae), ibis and spoonbills (Threskiornithidae), gulls and terns (Laridae) and waders (including Burhinidae, Haematopodidae, Glareolidae, Recurvirostridae, Charadriidae,

Rostratulidae, Jacanidae, Scolopacidae). They range in size considerably with red-necked stints (*Calidris ruficollis*) being one of the smallest wetland birds in Australia, weighing as little as 25–30 g. Each year this shorebird species flies up to 25 000 km between Australia and breeding grounds in Siberia and Alaska, following their annual migratory cycle. At the other extreme are large wetland birds such as the Australian pelican with a wingspan of 2.3–2.6 m and mass ranging from 4.5–6.8 kg. This species is capable of continental scale movements (> 1000 km) and is highly nomadic, with longer-distance movements corresponding to drought or flooding (Roshier *et al.* 2002).

Biology and behaviour

In general, knowledge of biology and behaviour remains poor for many Australian wetland bird species, particularly rare and cryptic species (Kingsford and Norman 2002). Patterns of movement in Australian wetland birds have developed in response to a highly variable climate and river flooding patterns that drive the availability of wetland habitats. This contrasts with their counterparts in the Northern Hemisphere, which are in comparison well studied and where day length and temperature are more-obvious drivers of wetland bird movements (Kingsford and Norman 2002). Some Australian wetland bird species can move large distances. For example, a satellite-tracking study showed that grey teals (*Anas gracilis*) moved nearly 1000 km in 40 h travelling from southern New South Wales to Lake Eyre in central Australia (Roshier *et al.* 2008). Only migratory shorebird species have regular annual movements, migrating between their breeding grounds in the Northern Hemisphere to non-breeding habitat in Australia during austral summer (Lane 1987).

Most wetland bird species depend on aquatic food sources, such as aquatic vegetation, invertebrates, fish and frogs. Their morphology is diverse, varying in size, bill length and shape, and leg length which, when combined with differences in vision and feeding method, allow them as a group to exploit a range of different habitats and food sources (e.g. shoreline foragers, small waders, deep water foragers, larger waders and fish eaters). Diet is typically studied through the collection of faeces and observational studies of prey selection. More-recent advancements in stable isotope technology have allowed differences in diet among species to be studied through collection of feather, blood and tissue samples. Disturbance of feeding and roosting habitats by recreational users, including fishers, walkers and dogs in urban areas, can be a threat to wetland bird species, as it affects birds' ability to feed and rest effectively (Blumstein *et al.* 2003).

Reproductive strategies include colonial and non-colonial nesting. Colonial species can nest in large mixed colonies of egrets, ibises, spoonbills, pelicans, cormorants and herons in some parts of Australia, including the Northern Territory, Lake Eyre and Murray-Darling River basin. These species can form large colonies of tens of thousands of nests in floodplain wetlands when widespread flooding occurs. Loosely colonial species include grebes, swans and magpie geese, and some Australian resident shorebirds, which can form large congregations in suitable habitat. Non-colonial species include waterfowl, crakes, rails and waterhens. While these species do not congregate in large numbers to breed, they are still dependent on wetlands for nesting and feeding.

Most Australian wetland birds breed opportunistically when conditions are suitable, which can be sporadic in ephemeral wetlands, although in more-permanent coastal wetlands some species breed annually. Some species pair for life – for example, Australian wood duck (*Chenonetta jubata*), magpie goose and black swan. Most form single pair bonds, but a magpie goose male may have two females, and comb-crested jacana (*Irediparra gallinacea*) females will form stable unions with more than one male. Some species are also territorial during the breeding season. For example, the nationally endangered Australasian bittern (*Botaurus poiciloptilus*) is thought to maintain large territories that can hold three or four females.

Sexual dimorphism is uncommon in wetland birds, but present in many Australian waterfowl species. The black-necked stork is also one of few stork species to show marked sexual dichromatism in iris colour. Many species develop breeding plumage and change in facial skin colour to indicate breeding status. For example, breeding Eastern great egrets (*Ardea modesta*) develop a blueish-green facial skin colour and long lacy plumes. The difference between non-breeding and breeding plumage can also be quite marked for some species of migratory shorebirds, grebes and terns. Black swans become flightless during moulting, making them more vulnerable to predation, but little information is available on individual moulting patterns for most Australian wetland bird species (Kingsford and Norman 2002).

Responses to disturbance varies greatly among different breeding species. Nearly all wetland birds flee the nest when approached, and only a small number will attempt to protect or divert predators away from young. For nest-based studies of reproductive success it is important to consider total time spent at individual nests or clumps of nests as eggs and chicks can suffer from exposure (overheating or hyperthermia) if adults are kept away as a result of interference by researchers. Disturbance at nests can also make eggs and chicks more vulnerable to predators, including introduced pigs (*Sus scrofa*), red foxes (*Vulpes vulpes*) and ravens (*Corvus* spp.).

Capture and handling

In many wetland birds, taking flight (or fleeing) because of human disturbance is costly and can reduce fitness through disruption to foraging, increased energy expenditure, physiological stress, reduced reproductive output or reduced ability to detect predators (Mayer *et al.* 2019; Wilson *et al.* 2019). The effects increase from relatively passive sampling (e.g. camera traps, static counts from a distance) to active sampling (e.g. counts while moving or pursuing on foot or in a vehicle), up to capture, marking, fitting of tracking devices and release that require direct handling and contact of birds and may induce sufficient stress to cause death (e.g. capture myopathy, abandonment of eggs or chicks) (Wilson *et al.* 2019). Responses to disturbance may also vary depending on a range of other factors, including weather conditions, time of day, season, proximity to conspecifics, timing relative to breeding cycle or moulting, habitat type and location, and varying levels of predation (Mayer *et al.* 2019).

Common capture techniques for wetland birds include corral traps, cage traps, cannon nets, mist nets, snare and noose traps. One of the most widely used capture method for small wetland birds is mist netting, which can be used in terrestrial, shoreline (riparian) or wetland habitats. Decoy models and lure birds are popular and widely used methods to increase trapping success and have been utilised for centuries for hunting wetland birds, especially in the Northern Hemisphere (Bub 1991). Decoy models may range from crude silhouette profiles of birds, to stuffed skins or bodies, to hand-painted realistic models (e.g. duck hunters floating decoys and shorebird decoys) that capitalise on many species' social and flocking instincts to join an apparently unperturbed (safe) group of birds. Decoys (with or without audio playback) have also been effective in attracting some species to nest in particular areas, which is valuable when managing or relocating nesting habitat or restoring habitat (e.g. Roby *et al.* 2002). Relatively few scientific studies of Australian waterbirds have documented methods where live decoys or live lure birds are used (see Bub 1991 for further reading on lure birds).

Birds that feed or congregate close to the edge of the water, such as gulls, waterfowl and shorebirds, are frequently trapped with cannon nets (also known as rocket nets), which are powered by explosive charges. It is a useful technique for capturing large numbers of birds, often of mixed species, but is potentially dangerous and can injure birds and human operators if strict safety protocols are not adhered to (see Fair *et al.* 2010; Standen *et al.* 2018).

Researchers must have a thorough knowledge of the habits and behaviours of the species under study and be experienced in handling each species before attempting to mark wetland birds (see Sharp *et al.* 2007). Permanent marking techniques may increase the likelihood and value of re-sightings, but also potentially increase the risk of injury to the birds, the risk of predation and/or impact breeding success.

Marking methods include metal and coloured leg bands (Figure 35.1), leg flags, neck bands, wing tags and

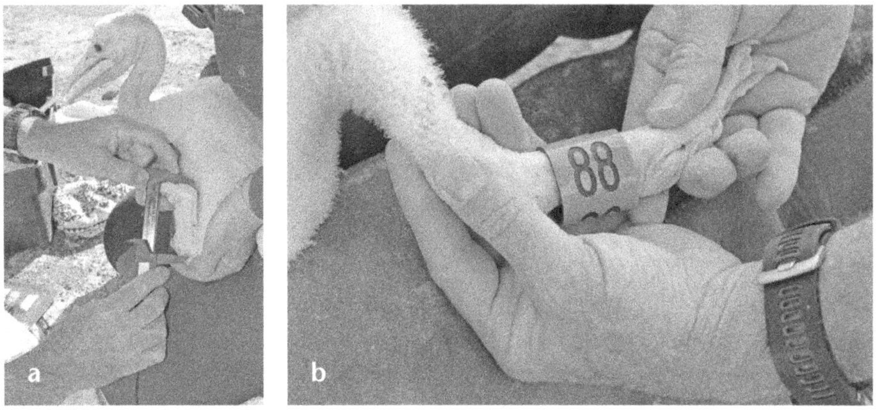

Figure 35.1: (a) Morphometric measurements being taken from a young Australian pelican (*Pelecanus conspicillatus*) chick before banding. (b) Colour band placement on a young pelican banded at Lake Brewster in central New South Wales. Photos by Mal Carnegie/Lake Cowal Foundation.

passive integrated transponder (PIT) tags. A range of band designs and materials that are used for wetland birds include leg bands made of aluminium, aluminium alloys or stainless steel (Fair *et al.* 2010). Coloured bands with unique colour combinations are used to identify banding year or location, individual birds or groups of birds, and leg flags (coloured bands with small extensions) are widely used on migratory shorebirds to enable identification from a distance without requiring re-trapping. Leg flags have allowed researchers to map migratory routes and identify important staging and feeding sites of several shorebird species (Fair *et al.* 2010).

Neck bands consist of rigid plastic or vinyl and are mainly used on long-necked birds, such as swans and geese, as an auxiliary marker to enable long distance identification when birds are swimming. They have been widely used in the Northern Hemisphere for decades, primarily on geese and swans (e.g. Reed *et al.* 2005). Patagial (wing) tags have been used on ducks and gulls in the Northern Hemisphere with some negative effects (Brua 1998); however, Martin and Major (2010) found patagial tags were suitable for Australian white ibis (*Threskiornis molucca*) despite recording some negative effects in smaller birds. Wing tags have had negative impacts on several species, and their continued use is the subject of much debate. Other markers, such as nape tags, nasal saddles and disks, streamers, dye and web markers have been used in the Northern Hemisphere, but their use in Australia remains limited.

PIT tags are lightweight and do not require battery power, enabling large-scale deployment over long periods of time. Since the mid-1980s, PIT tags have allowed investigations into growth rates, movement patterns, breeding and survivorship for many species in a manner more reliable than traditional external marking approaches. They have also been used to mark nests of western sandpipers (*Calidris mauri*), red-necked phalaropes (*Phalaropus lobatus*), dunlin (*C. alpine*), rock sandpipers (*C. ptilocnemis*) and grey plovers (*Pluvialis squatarola*) (Booms and McCaffery 2007).

Four main types of tracking devices are in use today that are relevant to wetland birds: VHF radio tracking, satellite (ARGOS) tracking, light level geolocators (GLS) and global positioning systems (GPS). Locators may be combined with bio-logging sensors that measure various bio-physical parameters (e.g. temperature, immersion, depth, acceleration) and may transmit (via VHF/UHF, GSM mobile phone or satellite communication links) or store and then transmit data on board. Store-on-board designs may require researchers to retrieve the bird and device to access data (with associated recapture and welfare considerations) although they have the advantage of being lighter weight than those that include batteries to transmit data via satellite. Approaches designed to minimise potential effects of devices on individual birds and to improve scientific rigour have advanced substantially, although evaluations of their effects on target animals are not routinely reported. Non-invasive wetland bird tracking techniques are also available. Chemical elements including stable isotopes (e.g ^{13}C, ^{15}N, ^{86}S) have successfully been used to identify movement patterns of bird species since the 1990s (Hobson 1999). This method can be applied to a range of tissue types including moulted feathers. In addition, citizen science programs can provide significant amounts of wetland bird information including phenology, migration routes, stopover points and species distribution data.

Note that the transportation of wild birds away from their site of capture is subject to additional approvals and regulations. The most important issue to consider is careful design of the transport container to minimise stress, prevent injury and escape, and ensure ventilation so birds do not become overheated. Birds can be transported in bird bags (small birds and short trips) or cages for larger birds and longer trips (Fair *et al.* 2010). To reduce stress to the bird it should be kept in a quiet, dark place (e.g. place a cover over the cage while ensuring adequate ventilation is not compromised). If the bird is injured, it can be wrapped with a towel around the wings and held securely to reduce further injury and keep the bird calmer. If multiple birds need to be transported, they should be in individual bags or cages with solid partitioning to ensure adequate ventilation and prevent overcrowding. See advice in Fair *et al.* (2010) for transporting waterbirds and advice on housing captive birds.

Veterinary considerations

Considerations relating to administration of veterinary chemicals is the same as described for 'Passerine birds' in Chapter 33. Also, see Chapter 16 (for veterinary procedures).

Sedation and anaesthesia

Use of therapeutics for analgesia or chemical restraint is similar to other bird groups, with some special considerations, including anatomical features such as long bill and necks and physiological quirks such as apnoea during induction attributed to a 'dive response'. As for all birds, inhalant gaseous anaesthesia is the preferred approach when available. Consult an authoritative specialised text if considering waterbird anaesthesia (Mulcahy 2014).

Blood collection

Blood can be collected from the prominent median metatarsal vein in many wading birds (Figure 16.3b in Chapter 16). For most duck species, the brachial (wing) vein is used (Wille *et al.* 2019). Blood collection is generally done under manual restraint rather than anaesthesia.

Euthanasia

Reilly (2001) provides guidelines for euthanasia of wild birds (see Table 35.1). Most methods require specialised training and occupational health and safety issues should be considered for chemical-based techniques, including inhalant and injectable methods. Generally, chemical methods for euthanasia of wild birds are preferable over physical methods. The American Veterinary Medical Association (AVMA2020) considers the following techniques suitable for wild birds: barbiturates (injected, ideally intravenously), inhalant anaesthetics, carbon dioxide inhalation (this is contentious) and carbon monoxide inhalation. Carbon monoxide is considered an extremely dangerous method for operators and only carbon dioxide is suitable for chicks (Reilly 2001) (Table 35.1).

Euthanasia requirements will vary considerably for different taxa and field situations, and will require consideration before commencement of research. Cervical dislocation is considered a suitable method for euthanasing small- to medium-sized wild birds or chicks (Reilly 2001; AVMA 2020), but this method is not acceptable for birds > 3 kg in size. Shooting in the head is considered acceptable for euthanasia of large birds. However, this method requires specialised training and equipment. Decapitation alone is not considered an acceptable method of euthanasia (Reilly 2001).

Infectious pathogens

Waterbirds can exhibit a range of infectious diseases (see examples in Table 35.2), some of which cause mass mortality events, and may pose a disease risk to humans (Contreras *et al.* 2016). Waterbirds are also susceptible to internal (including tapeworms and flukes) and external (including mites and lice) parasites. Some gull species are known to frequent waste tips, and have a high risk of carrying antibiotic-resistant bacterial strains (see Chapter 16). Researchers should take basic precautions when handling birds and collecting feathers and other samples contaminated with bird faeces. These precautions include hand washing with soap and water, wearing gloves when handling dead birds, not eating, drinking or smoking when handling animals, and washing field clothes and equipment between surveys. Researchers should also use basic first aid for treatment of cuts, bites and scratches from handling birds and inform medical practitioners of their exposure to birds if they develop flu-like symptoms (risk of ornithosis).

SEABIRDS

John Porter, Lisa O'Neill, Jennifer Spencer and Maggie J. Watson

Characteristics

Seabirds are a diverse group that vary considerably in biology, life cycle, and foraging and nesting behaviour. Eleven families and 91 species can inhabit Australian waters:

Table 35.1: Summary of euthanasia techniques for birds.

Reproduced from Reilly (2001).

Techniques	Recommended	Acceptable with reservations	Not acceptable
Inhalant	Carbon dioxide (chicks)	Carbon dioxide (adult birds) Methoxyflurane, halothane, isoflurane (chicks and small/medium adult birds)[b]	Carbon monoxide[b]
Injectable	Pentobarbitone sodium (all birds)[a]		
Physical	None	Cervical dislocation[a] (chicks, small and medium-sized birds only) Shooting[a,b] (large birds only)	Cervical dislocation (large birds)[c] Decapitation[c]

[a] Specialised training required; [b] Occupational health and safety issues; [c] Not recommended

Table 35.2: Summary of diseases to consider when undertaking waterbird research activities and their potential impacts on waterbirds and humans.

Disease	Impact on waterbirds	Potential for transmission to humans
Avian botulism	Paralytic disease is in ducks and shorebirds following consumption of maggots (Type C) from affected carcasses, but can also be recorded in fish-eating waterbirds, such as cormorants, pelicans and gulls, through consumption of infected fish (Type E). Mortalities can range from hundreds to massive die-offs of thousands of birds in affected wetlands.	Type C avian botulism does not affect humans, but it is important not to harvest sick waterbirds. Botulism in humans is usually caused by Type A or B as a result of eating improperly canned foods.
Avian cholera (pasteurellosis)	Can affect waterfowl and cormorants causing massive outbreaks with transmission primarily thought to occur through water.	It is a common pathogen in domestic animals including poultry, cattle, dogs, cats and rodents. Human infections are usually as result from a bite or scratch from a cat or dog which may develop into a serious infection.
Avian influenza (AI or bird flu)	Waterfowl and shorebirds are the primary hosts of influenza A virus (IAV). Some AI viruses circulate in wild bird populations causing no disease or only mild disease (in Australia); however, highly pathogenic strains of AI exist overseas that could be introduced by internationally migratory birds. High mortality rates have been seen overseas.	Rare cases of the highly pathogenic avian influenza virus H5N1 that can infect and cause disease in humans have not been detected in Australia, but are reported in wild birds in parts of Asia. Most human cases are associated with close contact with infected poultry.
Psittacosis	A disease caused by the bacterium *Chlamydia psittaci* carried by birds.	Humans most commonly catch the disease by inhaling dust containing feathers, secretions and droppings from infected birds.
Salmonellosis	The incidence of *Salmonella* species in wild birds tends to be low. Risk can be high in species that forage in human-contaminated environments such as refuse tips or sewage treatment works.	Transmission of salmonella to humans includes direct contact with faeces of infected birds, eating infected meat and contamination of food.
Aspergillosis	A respiratory disease in birds caused by *Aspergillus* fungi. It is common in pet birds, but not commonly reported in free-ranging waterbird species but there has been a lack of surveillance of this disease in waterbirds.	Aspergillus spores are ubiquitous in the environment with little impact on humans. However, they are potentially very dangerous to immunocompromised individuals.
Kunjin virus	This virus has been recorded in Australia and is closely related to West Nile virus.	Mosquitoes can sometimes transmit Kunjin virus from infected birds to people.
Murray Valley encephalitis (MVE)	MVE is commonly spread by mosquitos in freshwater wetlands; infects some wetland bird species including nankeen night-herons (*Nycticorax caledonicus*).	MVE can be transmitted to humans by mosquitos feeding on an infected bird before biting a human. Birds cannot transmit the virus directly to humans.
Herpesvirus	Endemic herpesvirus; strains present in Australia, new strain introduction from elsewhere in Australia could cause mortality. Similarly, exotic herpesvirus (e.g. duck plague) would be a novel strain and could result in significant disease.	Herpesviruses are highly host specific and transmission to humans is rare.
Avian tuberculosis	*Mycobacterium avium* is present in the environment with possible chronic effects with potential long-term population impacts.	In humans, *M. avium* infection typically causes local wound infections with swelling of draining lymph nodes. Infection with this bacterium is extremely rare and is of most risk in severely immunocompromised individuals.

gulls, terns and noddies (Laridae), skuas and jaegers (Stercorariidae), frigatebirds (Fregatidae), tropicbirds (Phaethontidae), cormorants and shags (Phalacrocoracidae), gannets and boobies (Sulidae), albatrosses (Diomedeidae), petrels, shearwaters, fulmars, prions (Procellariidae), storm-petrels (Hydrobatidae), diving-petrels (Pelecanoididae) and penguins (Spheniscidae).

Australian seabirds include very large species, such as the wandering albatross (*Diomedea exulans*), which can reach > 11 kg in body mass with a wingspan of 2.5–3.5 m. Comparatively, storm-petrels weigh only around 40 g, with a wingspan reaching up to 40 cm. The little penguin (*Eudyptula minor*) is the only penguin species that breeds on mainland Australia, and weighs ~1 kg. Several penguin species breed on Australian sub-Antarctic islands but are not considered in this chapter. Many seabirds that use Australian waters are rarely seen from the mainland. Most species range over vast tracts of ocean in the Southern and Northern Hemispheres during their non-breeding periods, and while foraging in their breeding season.

Biology and behaviour

Some seabird species from Australian and southern oceanic waters are famous for the distances they can travel, which can span the hemispheres. Movement patterns vary greatly among pelagic seabirds (species that frequent the open ocean). Some species, such as shearwaters, can be highly gregarious, travelling in dense flocks of hundreds to thousands of birds, while many petrels are solitary while at sea. Typically, pelagic species have long narrow wings adapted to dynamic soaring, which require environments with persistent, continuous winds. Many albatrosses use dynamic soaring to travel enormous distances across the Southern Ocean with minimal energy expenditure. Diving species tend to have shorter wings, although many shearwaters have long wings that suit long-distance movements and diving for prey. Little penguins are typically coastal dwelling but adults can make long trips during their non-breeding season, and some have been found breeding > 1000 km from their original banding site (McCutcheon *et al.* 2011).

Seabirds feed in saltwater, both above and below the ocean surface and are adapted to marine environments. Many species have physiological adaptations to deal with excretion of excess salt, such as salt glands. Prey includes fish, squid, krill, other crustaceans and salps. Some species are opportunistic scavengers, kleptoparasitic, or predators of other seabirds' eggs and chicks. Some terns and gulls will forage inland. Seabirds have four general feeding strategies, including surface feeding (either from the air or while swimming on the water surface), pursuit diving, plunge diving and scavenging from the surface or from other seabirds. For the more-pelagic species, the stage of their breeding cycle influences the length of foraging trips. Adults incubating eggs may forage for different periods and in different places than when foraging for their chicks. Knowledge of foraging patterns is essential to ensure that studies minimise disturbance to individuals who may be incubating an egg or guarding a young chick for many days or weeks without food.

Many Australian seabird species breed on remote islands in colonies that can range from as few as 10 individuals to many thousands of birds. Some species show high site fidelity to individual colonies and even individual nests. Reproductive rates are typically low among long-lived pelagic species, with a single egg laid annually, or less frequently in albatrosses. Some marine terns and gulls can re-lay if the initial egg is lost, though most other seabirds cannot. The total time for individuals to reach maturity is long, ranging from three to 10 years. Most seabirds are socially monogamous and form long-term pair bonds, making mate selection an important process that strongly influences long-term breeding success. The sequence of courtship behaviour varies widely among species, but usually includes displays or calling, territorial defence and selection of nest site.

Most shearwaters, petrels and little penguins are burrow or cavity nesters and can show high fidelity to burrows in nesting colonies. Some petrel and shearwater species nest on the surface of the soil or in crevices. Little penguins have colonies along the coastlines of southern Australia, primarily on offshore islands. Domestic and feral animals, including pigs, cats, dogs, foxes, rabbits, rats and mice, are major threats to seabird nesting sites. Habitat loss and degradation is also a key threat to seabird colonies. Breeding colonies of seabirds on islands in tourist locations, such as the Great Barrier Reef, Philip Island and Christmas Island are also affected by direct disturbance from visitors to islands.

Capture and handling

Most studies of seabirds are completed at breeding colonies. Since most pelagic seabird species attend land solely to breed, the effect of disturbance is most likely to be reflected in breeding success, and in the fitness of the fledgling as it leaves the nest. For example, Adélie penguins (*Pygoscelis adeliae*) experienced reduced breeding success from repeated human approaches and nest checks (Giese 1996).

Capture methods for surface nesting birds are diverse. Capture and marking typically occurs at breeding colonies because it is difficult to capture and assess birds at sea (Ronconi *et al.* 2010), although information on non-breeding foraging ranges and oceanic habits of pelagic seabirds is growing with the increased ease of use, reduced cost and smaller sizes of tracking and bio-logging devices (Yoda *et al.* 2011; Zhang *et al.* 2019).

Most pelagic seabirds are caught at the nest, as doing so is generally the simplest capture method, and is repeatable should recapture of that individual be required. Burrow- or cavity-nesting seabirds can generally be hand captured by carefully reaching into the burrow and extracting eggs or chicks, then quietly returning them to the burrow. (Figure 35.2). A burrow scope (a miniature video camera on a long flexible fibre optic cable) is useful for reducing disturbance and enable improved monitoring. Some surface-nesting seabird species will not leave the nest if approached, and a researcher may be able to capture the bird or assess the nest without risk of it trying to leave. Others are very sensitive to disturbance and require capture by other means. If disturbed during the day, many nocturnal seabirds will not return to the nest until the next night, leaving their egg or chick susceptible to chilling and predation. Many seabirds will regurgitate upon handling, reducing the feed available to the adult while incubating or brooding, or to the chick. Considerations for minimising the impact of capturing seabirds at colonies are provided in detail in Chapter 15.

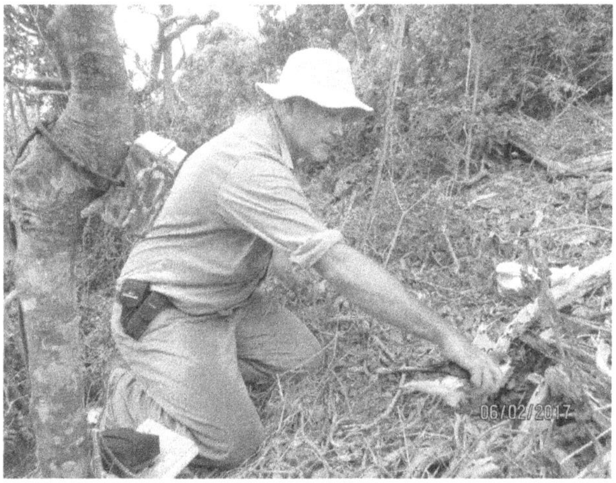

Figure 35.2: Black-winged petrel (*Pterodroma nigripennis*) being released back to its burrow. Photo by Nicholas Carlile, DPIE.

Cage traps, walk-in funnel traps, hand nets and clap traps have been used on surface-nesting seabirds for decades (Bub 1991; Ledwon *et al.* 2015). Traps can sometimes be placed away from nests, reducing the incidence of damage to eggs or chicks. Pull nets and cannon nets have also been used to capture gulls and terns at loafing or resting sites (Bub 1991). Cannon netting is a highly specialised technique (see Chapter 15) and requires specific training and approvals (Fair *et al.* 2010).

At sea, hand-thrown cast nets are potentially useful for capturing surface-feeding species that can be attracted to fishing vessels with lures (oil or offal thrown into the water). However, the technique is ineffective for diving species, is reliant on suitable weather conditions and captured birds must be sufficiently dry before release. Bugoni *et al.* (2008) used a cast net from a fishing boat to capture albatrosses and petrels at sea in the south-western Atlantic Ocean. They captured 500 birds of 13 species, ranging in size from the 30 g Wilson's storm-petrel (*Oceanites oceanicus*) to the 10 kg wandering albatross (*Diomedea exulans*), with no injuries recorded. Net guns have been used to capture petrels, shearwaters and albatrosses (Ronconi *et al.* 2010). Net guns can be fired from boats and from helicopters (Ronconi *et al.* 2010). They are useful for catching birds for whom the breeding site is unknown. Refer to Chapter 7 for more detailed procedures for capture of aquatic birds.

PIT tags have been used to measure land-based activity patterns, foraging activities and breeding in burrow-nesting seabirds. Zangmeister *et al.* (2009) measured incubation failure and nest abandonment by Leach's storm-petrels (*Oceanodroma leucorhoa*) by using PIT tags to record times of birds entering and leaving nesting burrows. Breeding activity of Chatham Island taiko (*Pterodroma magentae*) was monitored by Taylor *et al.* (2012) using PIT tags to record movements of individuals. Foraging little penguins have also been marked (Chiaradia and Kerry 1999) with PIT tags to identify individuals. Birds may be scanned individually when caught, or a detection system may be placed around an individual nest entrance to record that individuals use the nest. The latter is effective for some burrow nesters, but generally not for shearwaters or other prolific burrowers who are prone to digging up and extracting or damaging equipment. PIT tags have also been used as an unobtrusive method to mark nests during breeding surveys, to avoid attracting predators (Booms and McCaffery 2007).

GPS and GLS loggers can provide detailed information on the at-sea behaviour and range of seabirds (e.g. Rayner *et al.* 2016), although use of these loggers is limited to species of a suitable size. GLS loggers are lighter but require the bird to be recaptured for data to be downloaded. A common attachment method for pelagic seabirds is leg-mounted devices, which reduce drag once the leg is tucked up during flight. Adhesive taping to feathers, or other attachment method, on the back or tail can also be used (Zhang *et al.* 2019). A weak link is built into the attachment set-up to allow the device to detach after some time, in case the bird cannot be recaptured.

Transport of seabirds requires well-designed containers that minimise stress and risk of escape, injury or overheating by being appropriately sized, shaded and ventilated. The containers should be water resistant and free draining in case they are inundated during landings and launching vessels from shorelines. Refer to information in wetland bird section for more advice on transporting birds.

Veterinary considerations

Considerations relating to administration of veterinary chemicals is the same as described for 'Passerine birds' (Chapter 33). Procedures for administering veterinary chemicals are detailed in Chapter 16.

Sedation and anaesthesia

Use of therapeutics for analgesia or chemical restraint is similar to other bird groups, with some special considerations. As for all birds, inhalant gaseous anaesthesia is the preferred approach when available. An authoritative specialised text should be consulted if considering seabird anaesthesia (Mulcahy 2014).

Blood collection

Blood can be collected from either the brachial (wing) vein or the jugular (neck) vein. The jugular is preferred because it is larger and there is less chance of a haematoma, which could potentially impact flight. For penguins, which do not have aptera (featherless areas) on the wing or neck, the prominent median metatarsal (leg) vein should be used (Bodley and Schmitt 2014). Blood collection is generally done under manual restraint rather than anaesthesia.

Euthanasia

Refer to more detailed information provided above in the wetland bird section for euthanasia of seabirds. Most euthanasia methods require specialised training and there are occupational health and safety issues to consider for chemical-based techniques, including inhalant and injectable methods. Euthanasia requirements vary considerably between taxa and field situations. When developing research plans for seabird studies it is important to consider arrangements needed to transport seriously injured animals from the field sites to the nearest veterinarian for treatment. Transportation may not be possible for seabird studies in remote areas, such as offshore islands. Consequently, alternative arrangements for treatment or appropriate procedures for euthanasing injured birds should be confirmed before the study starts.

Infectious pathogens

Refer to the wetland bird section above, which identifies zoonoses that may be present in waterbird species and provides recommendations for minimising the risk of transmission to humans (Contreras *et al.* 2016). Additional diseases to be considered for seabirds include pathogens in human-contaminated environments, such as coastal areas contaminated by sewage outfalls, or from seabirds known to scavenge, particularly those that scavenge in urban areas, such as some gull species. Antibiotic-resistant bacterial pathogens have been recorded in such species – see Chapter 16.

General operating procedures

Key research methods relevant to the study of wetland birds and seabirds are detailed in other chapters, including several low-impact and indirect methods such as assessment of tracks and traces, acoustic and camera monitoring (Chapters 4 and 5), aerial methods (Chapter 6), mist netting (Chapter 7), and citizen science and educational activities (Chapter 10). Avian-specific methods are detailed in Chapter 15, including census and observational techniques, call playback and broadcast surveys, nest and hollow inspections (including handling of eggs and chicks), hand capture and spotlighting, methods for capture of individual birds, assessment of colonial birds at breeding colonies, marking methods, telemetry methods and collection of regurgitate, crop contents, scats and pellets. Several veterinary procedures may also be used during waterbird research (Chapter 16).

REFERENCES

AVMA (2020) *AVMA Guidelines for the Euthanasia of Animals, 2020 Edition*. American Veterinary Medical Association, Schaumburg, IL.
Bub H (1991) *Bird Trapping and Bird Banding: A Handbook for Trapping Methods All Over the World*. Cornwell University Press, Ithaca, NY.

Blumstein DT, Anthony LL, Harcourt R, Ross G (2003) Testing a key assumption of wildlife buffer zones: is flight initiation distance a species-specific trait? *Biological Conservation* **110**, 97–100. doi:10.1016/S0006-3207(02)00180-5

Bodley K, Schmitt T (2014) Penguins. In *Zoo Animal and Wildlife Immobilization and Anaesthesia*. 2nd edn. (Eds G West, D Heard and N Caulkett) pp. 435–443. John Wiley and Sons, Hoboken, NJ.

Booms TL, McCaffery BJ (2007) A novel use of passive integrated transponder (PIT) tags as nest markers. *Journal of Field Ornithology* **78**, 83–86. doi:10.1111/j.1557-9263.2006.00088.x

Bugoni L, Neves TS, Peppes FV, Furness RW (2008) An effective method for trapping scavenging seabirds at sea. *Journal of Field Ornithology* **79**, 308–313. doi:10.1111/j.1557-9263.2008.00178.x

Brua RB (1998) Negative effects of patagial tags on ruddy ducks. *Journal of Field Ornithology* **69**, 530–535. https://www.jstor.org/stable/4514356.

Chiaradia AF, Kerry KR (1999) Daily nest attendance and breeding performance in the little penguin *Eudyptula minor* at Phillip Island, Australia. *Marine Ornithology* **27**, 13–20.

Contreras A, Gomez-Martin A, Paterna A, Tatay-Dualde J, Prats-Van Der Ham M, Corrales JC, *et al.* (2016) Epidemiological role of birds in the transmission and maintenance of zoonoses. *Revue Scientifique et Technique (International Office of Epizootics)* **35**, 845–862. doi:10.20506/rst.35.3.2574

Fair J, Paul E, Jones J (2010) *Guidelines to the Use of Wild Birds in Research*. Ornithological Council, Washington, DC.

Giese M (1996) Effects of human activity on Adelie penguin *Pygoscelis adeliae* breeding success. *Biological Conservation* **75**, 157–164. doi:10.1016/0006-3207(95)00060-7

Hobson KA (1999) Tracing origins and migration of wildlife using stable isotopes: a review. *Oecologia* **120**, 314–326. doi:10.1007/s004420050865

Kingsford RT, Norman FI (2002) Australian waterbirds – products of a continent's ecology. *Emu* **102**, 47–69. doi:10.1071/MU01030

Lane B (1987) *Shorebirds in Australia*. Nelson Publishing, Melbourne.

Ledwon M, Betleja J, Neubauer G (2015) An effective method for trapping both parents and chicks of whiskered terns (*Chlidonias hybrida*) and its impact on breeding success. *Waterbirds* **38**, 290–295. doi:10.1675/063.038.0309

Martin JM, Major RE (2010) The use of cattle ear-tags as patagial markers for large birds: a field assessment on adult and nestling Australian white ibis. *Waterbirds* **33**, 264–268. doi:10.1675/063.033.0218

Mayer M, Natusch D, Frank S (2019) Water body type and group size affect the flight initiation distance of European waterbirds. *PLoS One* **14**, e0219845. doi:10.1371/journal.pone.0219845

McCutcheon C, Dann P, Salton M, Renwick L, Hoskins AJ, Gormley AM, Arnould JPY (2011) The foraging range of little penguins (*Eudyptula minor*) during winter. *Emu* **111**, 321–329. doi:10.1071/MU10078

Mulcahy DM (2014) Free-living waterfowl and shorebirds. In *Zoo Animal and Wildlife Immobilization and Anaesthesia*. 2nd edn. (Eds G West, D Heard and N Caulkett) pp. 481–505. John Wiley and Sons, Hoboken, NJ.

Rayner M, Carlile N, Priddel D, Bretagnolle V, Miller M, Phillips RA, Ranjard L, Bury S, Torres LG (2016) Niche partitioning by three Pterodroma petrel species during non-breeding in the equatorial Pacific Ocean. *Marine Ecology Progress Series* **549**, 217–229. doi:10.3354/meps11707

Reed ET, Gauthier G, Pradel R (2005) Effects of neck bands on reproduction and survival of female greater snow geese. *The Journal of Wildlife Management* **69**, 91–100. doi:10.2193/0022-541X(2005)069<0091:EONBOR>2.0.CO;2

Reilly JS (Ed) (2001) *Euthanasia of Animals Used for Scientific Purposes*. 2nd edn. Australian & New Zealand Council for the Care of Animals in Research and Teaching (ANZCCART), Adelaide.

Roby DD, Collis K, Lyons DE, Craig DP, Adkins JY, Myers AM, Suryan RM (2002) Effects of colony relocation on diet and productivity of Caspian terns. *The Journal of Wildlife Management* **66**, 662–673. doi:10.2307/3803132

Ronconi RA, Swaim ZT, Lane HA, Hunnewell RW, Westage AJ, Koopman HN (2010) Modified hoop-net techniques for capturing birds at sea and comparison with other capture methods. *Marine Ornithology* **38**, 23–29.

Roshier DA, Robertson AI, Kingsford RT (2002) Responses of waterbirds to flooding in an arid region of Australia and implications for conservation. *Biological Conservation* **106**, 399–411. doi:10.1016/S0006-3207(01)00268-3

Roshier D, Asmus M, Klaassen M (2008) What drives long-distance movements in the nomadic grey teal *Anas gracilis* in Australia? *The Ibis* **150**, 474–484. doi:10.1111/j.1474-919X.2008.00806.x

Sharp T, Saunders G, Mitchell B (2007) *Marking of Pest Animals used in Research. 2007. Standard Operating Procedures for the Humane Research of Pest Animals in Australia*. NSW Department of Primary Industries, Orange.

Standen R, Jessop R, Minton C (2018) *Cannon-netting Induction Manual*. Australasian Wader Studies Group, Melbourne.

Taylor G, Cockburn S, Palmer D, Liddy P (2012) Breeding activity of Chatham Island taiko (*Pterodroma magentae*) monitored using PIT tag recorders. *New Zealand Journal of Ecology* **36**, 425–432.

Wille M, Lisovski S, Risely A, Ferenczi M, Roshier D, Wong FY, *et al.* (2019) Serologic evidence of exposure to highly pathogenic avian influenza H5 viruses in migratory shorebirds, Australia. *Emerging Infectious Diseases* **25**, 1903. doi:10.3201/eid2510.190699

Wilson RP, Holton M, Wilson VL, Gunner R, Tysse B, Wilson GI, Quintana F, Duarte C, Scantlebury DM (2019) Towards informed metrics for examining the role of human-induced animal responses in tag studies on wild animals. *Integrative Zoology* **14**, 17–29. doi:10.1111/1749-4877.12328

Yoda K, Naito Y, Sato K, Takahashi A, Nishikawa J, Ropert-Coudert Y, Kurita M, Le Maho Y (2011) A new technique for monitoring the behaviour of free-ranging Adelie penguins. *The Journal of Experimental Biology* **204**, 685–690. doi:10.1242/jeb.204.4.685

Zangmeister JL, Haussmann MF, Cerchiara J, Mauck RA (2009) Incubation failure and nest abandonment by Leach's storm-petrels detected using PIT tags and temperature loggers. *Journal of Field Ornithology* **80**, 373–379. doi:10.1111/j.1557-9263.2009.00243.x

Zhang JJ, Rayner M, Vickers S, Landers T, Sagar R, Stewart J, Dunphy B (2019) GPS telemetry for small seabirds: using hidden Markov models to infer foraging behaviour of common diving petrels (*Pelecanoides urinatrix urinatrix*). *Emu* **119**, 126–137. doi:10.1080/01584197.2018.1558997

36 Megapodes, bustard and ratites

Darryl Jones, Mark Ziembicki, Sarah J. Gill and Damian S. Morrant

INTRODUCTION

The three taxa (megapodes, ratites and bustards) included in this chapter are large, terrestrial, ground-dwelling birds with modest or no capacity for flight. Megapodes are reluctant fliers, ratites do not have functional wings and the bustard is Australia's heaviest flying bird. These species include the largest and heaviest birds found in Australia (emu and southern cassowary respectively); the only other large species are associated with aquatic environments and are strong fliers (cranes, storks and pelicans – see Chapter 35). Given their size and strength, the larger of these birds can be difficult and dangerous to capture, handle and treat.

MEGAPODES (BRUSH-TURKEY AND MALLEEFOWL)

Darryl Jones and Sarah J. Gill

Characteristics

The megapodes (Megapodiidae) are also often known as 'mound-builders' because most species construct enormous mounds of organic matter that are employed as incubation sites. There are three Australian species. The first is the Australian brush-turkey (*Alectura lathami*), which is a large black bird (average body mass of 2.3 kg) with a bare red head, yellow throat wattle, and a prominent lateral fan-like tail. It is found along the eastern seaboard from Cape York to central coastal New South Wales. The second is the orange-footed scrubfowl (*Megapodius reinwardt*), which is a medium-sized bird (average body mass of 900 g) that is dark in colour with orange legs and feet, and a distinctive crest at the back of the head. Its distribution is limited to the coastal forests of the tropics and subtropics. The third, the malleefowl (*Leipoa ocellata*) of the southern arid interior of the continent, is a large bird, weighing around 2.5 kg. Its head and neck are buff grey, and its body and tail are dappled brown, black and white. For all three species, males are typically larger than females (Jones and Göth 2008).

The defining characteristic of the family is their use of various sources of environmental heat rather than that provided by contact with an adult's body for the incubation of eggs. These sources include the heat produced by the decomposition of organic matter (the primary source associated with mound-building species), and geothermal heat associated with volcanic activity and solar radiation (Booth and Jones 2002). Species exploiting the latter two sources access their oviposition sites by digging into existing warm substrates and are known as burrow nesters. Each of the three species occurring in Australia are mound builders (Jones and Göth 2008). Despite their remarkable incubation techniques, in most morphological, behavioural and ecological attributes, megapodes closely resemble other galliformes – the chickens, quail and pheasants, the taxonomic grouping to which they belong (Jones *et al.* 1995).

Biology and behaviour

The megapode family consists of 22 extant species (Jones *et al.* 1995). At least another 30 species are known to have existed throughout the islands of Melanesia and Polynesia, most of which appear to have been hunted to extinction during the expansion of humans into this region during the last millennia (Steadman 2006). Today, the remaining species are found throughout the islands to the north of Australia, from Indonesia and the Philippines to Tonga in the south Pacific. Anomalously, an additional species is found in the Nicobar and Andaman islands on the western side of India. It is noteworthy that, apart from Australia and Papua New Guinea, which appear to be the epicentre of speciation, megapodes are found only on islands and are entirely absent from the main land masses west of Wallace's Line, such as Borneo and Java (Jones *et al.* 1995). All megapodes are primarily terrestrial, spending most of the day foraging for invertebrates, seeds, fruit and tubers on the forest floor. In the early evening, they ascend laboriously into the trees to roost, often communally.

By far the most important influence on megapodes' reproductive behaviour revolves around the incubation mound and the way it is used for breeding. Each of the three species exhibit distinctly different activities and social behaviour with respect to mound-related behaviour. The male Australian brush-turkey constructs the mound alone, a process that may take several weeks. Females seeking to inspect the mound or oviposit are usually required to copulate before gaining access (Birks 1997). Males differ greatly in the number of females they attract, from > 12 to none. Females lay single eggs at intervals of several days with the average total being around 12 per season. They typically move between mounds (and the males associated with them), distributing their eggs among several locations. Genetic assessments have shown that most of the eggs deposited in a mound were fertilised by the owner (Birks 1997).

In contrast, malleefowl and scrubfowl are typically monogamous (although trios are known), often with long-lasting pair-bonds (Jones *et al.* 1995). Malleefowl, living in markedly dry environments, are occupied with constructing and maintaining their mounds for many months of the year. The malleefowl's mound consists of an inner core of decomposing leaf litter, which is covered in a deep layer of soil and sand as insulation to prevent heat from escaping. However, each time the bird needs to assess the internal temperature or deposit an egg, a large amount of the outer layer must be removed (Jones and Göth 2008).

The mounds of the orange-footed scrubfowl are among the largest constructions of any animal, being up to 5 m in height and 13 m in diameter (Jones and Göth 2008). However, unlike brush-turkey or malleefowl mounds, which are constructed annually, scrubfowl return to the same site each year and simply add fresh material to one end. Some mounds are known to have been used consecutively for decades and possibly even centuries; hence the enormous sizes reached (Jones *et al.* 1995).

The use of external sources of heat to provide incubation has had profound implications for the parental behaviour of these species. Because eggs are effectively abandoned, and each begins to develop as soon as it is laid, each will develop independently and at separate times. Upon hatching, the chick finds itself deep within a pile of soil and organic material and must spend several days slowly digging its way to the surface. Once it emerges at the top of the incubation mound, it receives no assistance from its parents. In fact, adults do not even recognise the chicks as anything other than some of the other animals that often exploit their mounds. Therefore, the hatchings receive no parental care and immediately start a solitary life (Göth and Vogel 2002). Not unexpectedly, the mortality rate of hatchings is extreme for the first few weeks and typically < 10% survive their first month (Göth and Vogel 2003).

Capture and handling

All megapodes are relatively easy to catch using baited drop traps or larger mesh walk-in traps (Jones 1988). Australian brush-turkeys requiring relocation from suburban areas are routinely captured by placing a mirror at the end of a large wire cage trap, with the bird attempting to attack the image. In places where the birds have become habituated to the presence of people, they can also be snared using a rope noose laid on the ground and the birds attracted with grain (Jones and Everding 1991). These birds are relatively robust and strong, and struggle powerfully when restrained, often flapping their large wings when being handled. Australian brush-turkeys often eject foul-smelling excreta when distressed. They usually become subdued quickly once their heads are covered (Jones 1988).

All species appear to adjust quickly to captivity, but the physical requirements of mound construction can be a major challenge as a large space is required as well as a regular supply of suitable organic material. While pairs of malleefowl and scrubfowl can be housed together, any additional conspecifics will result in attacks on one another (Jones *et al.* 1995). Similarly, brush-turkey males often kill any other conspecifics if the enclosure does not allow escape. For this species, females must be removed quickly following mating or egg laying.

Marking is usually by leg bands or patagial tags (Jones 1990). The latter has been found to be the most reliable method for relatively long-term identification of individuals, although wing tags may be displaced (Göth and Jones 2001). Colour bands may become covered in soil and discoloured, making distinguishing the colours difficult (Jones 1988).

Veterinary considerations

Considerations relating to administration of veterinary chemicals is the same as described for 'Passerine birds' (Chapter 33). Little information is available on therapeutic drug use and dosages in Australian megapodes, so it is often necessary to extrapolate from data available for domestic species, such as the domestic chicken (*Gallus gallus domesticus*) and turkey (*Meleagris gallopavo* f. *domestica*). There is a large difference in the way these domestic animals are treated as a flock versus as individual pets, so it is important to have a detailed understanding of the treatment methods required for a specific situation. Consultation with an avian veterinarian or suitably experienced biologist to determine medication requirements (if any) is recommended before commencing research on these species (see Chapter 16).

Sedation and anaesthesia

Use of therapeutics for analgesia or chemical restraint is similar to other bird groups. It is important to be aware of the unique anatomy and physiology of this group before contemplating sedating or anaesthetising birds (Zehnder *et al.* 2014).

Blood collection

Megapodes have large, easily accessible veins in both their wings and legs (medial metatarsal and brachial veins respectively). Blood can be collected from the brachial vein malleefowl (King *et al.* 1996). Blood collection is generally done under manual restraint rather than anaesthesia.

Euthanasia

Intravenous administration of a lethal dose of pentobarbitone by suitably trained personnel is an acceptable method of euthanasia in a conscious bird (with adequate restraint) (Raidal 1996). Any animal euthanased with pentobarbitone represents a secondary toxicity risk to wild scavengers and should be disposed of via deep burial. Intraperitoneal injection of barbiturate may cause excitation, peritoneal irritation and pain before the bird becomes unconscious, and is not recommended (if it is necessary, ensure the formulation is non-irritant) (Reilly *et al.* 2001). If in a field situation with no access to this drug, cervical dislocation is appropriate for juvenile megapodes (< 3 kg). However, 200 g is considered by some as the upper acceptable weight for cervical dislocation (AVMA 2020). For larger birds, blunt force trauma to the skull, to render unconsciousness, then decapitation is acceptable if performed rapidly by a skilled operator (Reilly *et al.* 2001; AVMA 2020).

Infectious pathogens

Megapodes are not well known as carriers of zoonotic diseases (Contreras *et al.* 2016). Although megapodes carry a remarkable load and diversity of feather lice and mites, none of these ectoparasites are known as risks to humans or indeed any other species (Proctor and Jones 2004). Megapodes also carry ticks (*Ixodes* spp.), sometimes at heavy loads.

AUSTRALIAN BUSTARD

Mark Ziembicki and Darryl Jones

Characteristics

The Australian bustard (*Ardeotis australis*) is the sole Australian member of the Otididae – an Old World family that comprises 25 species in 11 genera, with greatest representation in Africa, and several species in Europe and Asia (Davies 2002). Although considered a separate lineage, the family's origin is with the Gruiformes, placing them in the same order as cranes, crakes and rails. Bustards are characterised by a distinctive robust body shape with long, thin legs and necks, somewhat large heads with stout straight beaks, and small three-toed feet. Several bustard species, including the Australian bustard, show pronounced sexual size dimorphism with males substantially larger and heavier than females. In specimens from Australia's northern savannas, the mean body mass of female bustards was 3.2 kg while males weighed almost twice that at 6.3 kg (Ziembicki 2009, 2010). Differences between the sexes have implications for the capture, handling and marking of individuals.

Biology and behaviour

Although distributed across most of mainland Australia (Garnett *et al.* 2010), the species has suffered a significant decline in many parts of its range, particularly in southern Australia. These declines have been variously attributed to hunting, pesticides, altered fire regimes, habitat alteration, pastoralism, and predation by introduced predators (Davies 2002). Australian bustards have a general preference for open habitats, ranging from open grassland plains to low shrublands, grassy open woodlands and similar artificial habitats including croplands, golf courses and airfields. Throughout its continent-wide distribution, the Australian bustard exhibits complex movement patterns that vary depending on region and climate (Ziembicki and Woinarski 2007). In regions influenced by productive and predictable seasonal conditions, the species is predominantly sedentary or exhibits more-regular migratory patterns when exploiting seasonally fluctuating resources. However, over most of its range and like many birds of Australia's more climatically variable arid and semi-arid regions, bustards have irregular dispersive or nomadic movements in response to variable climatic conditions.

Like most diurnal birds, bustards have a bimodal pattern of activity, being active from first light for several hours, resting in the middle of the day and resuming more activity in the late afternoon until after sunset (Ziembicki 2009, 2010). Both sexes spend most of their time foraging, but during the peak period of breeding, larger mature males spend much of day in elaborate courtship displays. They tend to be loosely gregarious, often forming small groups but with larger aggregations occurring occasionally in resource-rich locations or recently burnt areas.

Bustards have a broad, omnivorous diet that includes a range of fruits, seeds, flowers, plant materials, various invertebrates, and small reptiles, amphibians and mammals (Ziembicki 2009). They are largely opportunistic in their foraging behaviour with their diet related to the relative availability of food types present in their surroundings. Given the notable difference in their physical sizes, there are also relative differences in diet between the sexes with females generally consuming smaller prey items and less food by volume.

The bustard is a long-lived bird with individuals in captivity living for > 30 years. Sexual maturity (observed in captive populations) is not reached in females until 3–5 years, while males may not breed successfully until they are 7–9 years of age (Davies 2002). This sexual bimaturism has resulted from pronounced sexual selection, which favours larger males through female choice. Bustards are primarily polygynous and in preparation for breeding, aggregate in leks with numerous males preforming mating displays. Females select mates with the most desirable characteristics which are usually found among older, larger and more-experienced males. As is typical for this form of mating system, relatively few males receive most of the matings (Davies 2002). The females alone assume responsibility for incubation and care of young. Females lay one or two eggs in a scrape on the ground with incubation lasting ~24 days. The young are nidifugous (leaving the nest soon after hatching) and precocial (they are mobile and able to feed by themselves very soon). Fledging occurs after 30–35 days, although at this stage the young are still only half grown (Davies 2002).

Capture and handling

Several capture methods have been used with varying success for bustards. The most effective technique is the use of a rocket net gun, which relies on approaching an individual to within 10–15 m in an open area (usually discharged from a vehicle) (Ziembicki 2009). A net is propelled over the neck of the bird, which entraps the individual, which can then be restrained. Drop nets have also been used successfully, although the method is more labour intensive, less mobile and relies on bustards visiting a known location. This approach involves positioning a large net above a location predictably used (e.g. water trough used for drinking) and is triggered remotely. Other techniques include corralling birds between nets set up vertically between trees (Alonso 2008) and leg noose traps (Seddon *et al.* 1999; Shaw *et al.* 2014). The latter method has been trialled for Australian bustards, but was unsuccessful (Ziembicki 2009).

Trapping and handling must be conducted efficiently and safely, particularly given the susceptibility of bustards to capture myopathy. Capture myopathy is more prevalent for long-legged birds (Bailey *et al.* 1996; Marco *et al.* 2006; Shaw *et al.* 2014) and, although treatment to some extent is possible, outcomes are highly unpredictable (Rogers *et al.* 2004; Smith *et al.* 2005). Furthermore, while short-term recovery may occur, longer-term effects are poorly understood. Some studies suggest that while individuals may appear to have recovered, some birds may have a reduced capacity to undertake normal behaviours and a decreased tolerance to exercise, and may be more vulnerable to predation (Ward *et al.* 2011).

To minimise the risk of individuals incurring capture myopathy, the time spent handling and restraining an individual should be minimised, and trapping and capture should be avoided during very hot conditions (larger males are more susceptible to heat stress than smaller individuals and females). Placing a hood over the bird's head makes them easier to handle and reduces stress. Animals should be allowed to stand or use a specially designed sling or harness chair rather than having them sit on their legs. These methods have been used to varying degrees of success for waders (Rogers *et al.* 2004) and Ludwig's bustard (*Neotis ludwigii*) (Shaw *et al.* 2014), although the latter still encountered issues with the method.

Leg banding with numbered stainless-steel bands issued by the Australian Bird and Bat Banding Scheme (ABBBS) has been used to individually mark and identify Australian bustards in the field. Patagial tags have also been used with success for Australian bustards and several other bustard species (see Alonso 2008). Neck collars, occasionally used to mark other large bird species including bustards, are not recommended for male bustards as they may interfere with their neck and throat sacs, which are inflated and extended during courtship displays.

Satellite and radiotelemetry units have been used successfully for Australian bustards over extended periods of time. Such units are best fitted as backpacks using a harness made of Teflon^{TM} ribbon, and should be designed with a weak link to allow detachment over time. This is particularly important for juvenile birds or younger males, which will continue to grow. Alternatively, Alonso (2008) has successfully used and recommends the use of clothing elastic bands for great bustards (*Otis tarda*), a large Eurasian species, and provides a thorough review of other marking methods, which may be useful with reference to the capture and handling of Australian bustards.

Small numbers of Australian bustards are kept in captivity in zoos, nature parks and some private collections in Australia. These birds are generally housed individually in large aviaries or outdoor pens and occasionally in small gender-specific groups. However, housing breeding males together, especially during the breeding season, is not recommended because of aggression between males. A captive breeding program at Werribee Zoo successfully used a series of connected pens whereby mature males were confined to individual pens, but the smaller females could move between pens using a suitably sized opening (Fitzherbert 1978).

Veterinary considerations

Limited information exists on the use of therapeutics for Australian bustards. However, sedatives and anaesthetics are routinely used to reduce stress-related complications (such as capture myopathy) for similarly large or long-legged birds including cranes, storks and waders (Carpenter *et al.* 1991). Moderate sedation using midazolam or butorphanol has been used for minor procedures or when individuals are handled for prolonged periods (Ward *et al.* 2011; Maclean and Beaufrere 2014). In the field, ketamine and xylazine have been used successfully as anaesthetics on endangered cranes (Maclean and Beaufrere 2014). Advice from veterinarians is recommended before the use of therapeutics for the Australian bustard (see also Chapters 15 and 16).

Sedation and anaesthesia

Use of therapeutics for analgesia or chemical restraint is similar to other bird groups. It is important to be aware of the unique anatomy and physiology of this group before contemplating sedating or anaesthetising birds (Zehnder *et al.* 2014).

Blood collection

There are few published approaches for venipuncture in the Australian bustard. As for most birds, blood can be collected from the median metatarsal vein or the brachial (wing) vein).

Euthanasia

As for other large bird species (this chapter, and Chapter 34), euthanasia by intravenous injection of barbiturates is recommended.

Infectious pathogens

There is limited published information on the prevalence of infectious pathogens in the Australian bustard, and no published information on the prevalence of zoonotic pathogens (Contreras *et al.* 2016), but other bustard species have been extensively studied. In *Eopoditus* bustards, for example, multiple infectious diseases have been documented including aspergillosis, avian pox and paramyxovirus type 1 virus. Other detected pathogens include *Salmonella* sp., *Pseudomonas* sp., *Trichomonas* sp., intestinal endoparasites, avian leucosis, reovirus, adenovirus, paramyxovirus type 2 and *Chlamydia* sp. (Bailey *et al.* 1996). Among rufous-crested bustards, *Otiditaenia macqueeni*, *Raillietina* sp., *Paronchocerca tonkinensis* and *Allodapa* sp. have been proposed as contributing to high mortality rates in captivity (Nicholls *et al.* 1995).

RATITES (EMU AND CASSOWARY)

Darryl Jones and Damian S. Morrant

Characteristics

Ratites are large flightless birds that are distantly related to New Zealand's kiwis and extinct moas. This taxon includes the rheas of South America, ostrich of Africa, cassowaries of Papua New Guinea and Australia and the emu – clearly a Gondwandic group (Maderspacher 2017). They are distinct from other avian groups by the absence of a keel bone on the sternum. Australian ratites are all extremely large birds and unmistakable in appearance. Three species occur wild in Australia: the southern cassowary (*Casuarius casuarius*), emu (*Dromaius novaehollandiae*) and ostrich (*Struthio camelus*). The largest of ratites found in Australia is the ostrich, standing at ~3 m in height and weighing around 150 kg. Cassowaries can grow to 2 m tall and are heavy birds, weighing between 55–76 kg. Emus average 1.7 m in height and weigh ~45 kg (Davies 2002). Female cassowaries and emus are generally larger than males, while the opposite is true for the ostrich (Tully 2009). They can defend themselves with powerful kicks from their sharply clawed feet. All species are capable of causing serious injury to a human, although cassowaries are certainly the most dangerous (Fowler 2008; Keller 2009).

Biology and behaviour

The southern cassowary is found only in the coastal rainforests of lower North Queensland. The emu is found throughout the continent in diverse habitats, from the interior deserts to the coastal forests. A tiny remnant population of the ostrich is present near Port Augusta in South Australia. These now feral birds originated from a short-lived plume industry in the late 1800s (Davies 2002).

Cassowaries are normally solitary except during when seeking mates. They are generally regarded as sedentary or locally nomadic, moving in response to the availability of rainforest fruiting patterns (Moore 2007). They are usually highly intolerant of conspecifics, although small groups may form during periods of extreme food stress. Cassowaries maintain and defend territories up to ~7 km^2 with females having larger territories that often overlap with those of several males (Mack 1995). Comparatively, emus often undertake long-distance movements, especially individuals living in the more-arid areas. These journeys may involve large numbers of birds in loose aggregations, which often appear to be in response to large rainfall events.

Cassowaries are frugivorous and play a vital role in the maintenance of rainforest tree diversity (Davies 2002). They are the only species that can move large seeds over long distances within their rainforest habitat, with some plant species germinating only after passing through a cassowary's digestive system. Emus are opportunistic omnivores, although they are primarily herbivorous, foraging on a wide variety of seeds, fruits, grains, but also invertebrates when available.

Ratites have a polyandrous mating system with females mating with multiple males, the male being solely responsible for incubating the eggs and raising the chicks (Davies 2002). Males often incubate the eggs of numerous females and are fiercely protective of their broods. These behaviours make parental males especially dangerous and they must be approached with great care during the breeding season. Young ratites chicks are relatively tame around humans, but often become aggressive and potentially dangerous with age (Keller 2009).

Capture and handling

Wild ratites often panic when restrained and capture attempts can cause extreme stress. Their excitable disposition predisposes them to exertional myopathy and secondary trauma during attempts to escape (Tully *et al.* 1996). Handlers may also be injured during capture attempts. Cassowaries and ostriches and, to a lesser but not insignificant extent, emus are large and potentially dangerous (Keller 2009). All can sustain injuries and damage to their beaks (and the casques of cassowaries) when constrained in corrals and pen traps (D. Morrant, pers. obs.). Administering drugs in water sources is typically difficult and unsuccessful (Hammond *et al.* 2002). However, wild cassowaries have been captured by darting whereby opportunistic searches of suitable habitat are undertaken and birds encountered are sedated by blow dart with tiletamine–zolazepam at ~7.5 mg/kg (Campbell *et al.* 2014). Every effort should be taken to minimise disturbance, particularly during the breeding season and at times of population stress (e.g. cyclones and heatwaves). Ostrich research may also require permits related to biosecurity.

Young ratite chicks and juveniles up to 5 kg can be handled by folding their legs and holding their body next to the body of the handler. The legs of heavier animals should not be forced into a folded position. The bird's vent should be directed away from clothing as they often defecate during handling (Fowler 2008). Adult emus may be handled by grasping with one arm around the bird's chest and the other arm over the body to hold the outer leg. The bird should then be lifted quickly, with the legs directed away from the body and other personnel. If the bird is to be held for an extended duration, it should be gently eased to the ground into a sternally recumbent resting position and straddled over the pelvis by one or two handlers. Handlers should avoid applying pressure to the back as this may induce recumbency. The handlers' feet should be placed beside the bird's feet to prevent the bird pushing outward. Birds should not be placed on their backs, unless doing so is essential, and should only be done under anaesthesia (Fowler 2008). Similarly, their powerful legs must be controlled if the birds are to be restrained on their side.

Cassowaries can jump around 1.5 m high, run at 50 km h^{-1}, and kick with both legs simultaneously. Their second toe is tipped with a dagger-like claw that can be as long as 12.5 cm. Chemical tranquilisation is recommended for most procedures. Once the animal is anaesthetised it should be inspected for injuries and placed in sternal recumbency to minimise interference with normal respiration, with the head and neck elevated and supported (Smith 2003; Fowler 2008). Sedated birds should be moved to shaded areas and vital signs should be monitored. Ostriches are much easier to handle if they can be hooded first. However, emus will not tolerate being hooded and this approach is unreliable in cassowaries (Smith 2003; Fowler 2008).

Ratites can be fitted with leg bands for identification (Davies *et al.* 1971).

Individual cassowaries can be identified by noting individual variation in the colour, shape or the presence of scars on their feet, skirts, necks, wattles, beaks and casques. The lack of similar prominent features makes this approach far less reliable in other species. The movements of ratites have been investigated by attaching telemetry devices. For example, cassowaries have been tracked at Moresby Range National Park in Queensland (Campbell *et al.* 2012) and emus in the forests of south-western Australia (Nield *et al.* 2015) by fitting them with neoprene-lined GPS devices attached to canvas cuffs tailored to fit the leg (tarsus) of individual birds and positioned to allow full flexion of the leg.

Veterinary considerations

Sedation and anaesthesia

Guidance on appropriate therapeutics and dosage regimens should be sought in published literature (Smith 2003; Fowler 2008; Siegal-Willott 2014). It is often necessary to use a pole syringe, blow dart or dart rifle (see Chapter 16) to sedate or anaesthetise adult ratites (Cushing and McClean 2010; Campbell *et al.* 2014). Tiletamine–zolazepam at ~7.5 mg/kg via blow dart is effective for wild cassowaries (Campbell *et al.* 2012). If the animal does not appear highly distressed, an intramuscular injection (into the quadriceps) of a sedative or anaesthetic can be administered. A wide range of injectable sedatives and anaesthetics can be used for ratites (Smith 2003). Young birds may be anaesthetised with isoflurane delivered via a face mask (Fowler 2008). Oral diazepam at 1.0 mg/kg has also been used (Smith 2003). Ostriches and emus can experience difficult recoveries after treatment with tiletamine–zolazepam. Negative effects may be minimised by administering diazepam (5.0 mg/kg intravenous) when the bird begins to arouse and struggle during recovery (Fowler 2008).

Blood collection

Blood samples may be taken from the brachial vein underneath the wing, the right jugular vein, or the medial metatarsal vein if the bird has been immobilised.

Euthanasia

Animals should be euthanased by lethal barbiturate overdose, under general anaesthesia delivered via a gas mask or intramuscular sedatives. Any animal euthanased with pentobarbitone represents a secondary toxicity risk to wild scavengers and should be disposed of via deep burial. Where possible, medicines should be administered by a veterinarian or another appropriately trained and legally authorised person. Where chemical euthanasia is not possible, gunshot may be used as a euthanasia method.

Infectious pathogens

Ratites can suffer from a variety of infectious and non-infectious diseases. These have been well documented in ostriches and emus but little is known about diseases of cassowaries (Smith 2003). Many diseases that commonly affect other birds and mammals may be contracted by ratites. Ostriches and emus in other countries contract a host of bacterial and viral pathogens of concern to human health (Contreras *et al.* 2016), including Newcastle disease and avian influenza in ostriches, and eastern and western equine encephalitis in emus, in the USA (Smith 2003). *Mycobacterium avium* has been diagnosed in captive cassowaries but does not appear to be an issue in wild populations (Schultz *et al.* 1996). The disease in humans is similar to tuberculosis, causing fever, lethargy, weight loss, abdominal pain, diarrhoea and pulmonary effects similar to tuberculosis.

General operating procedures

Research methods and procedures relevant to studying megapodes, Australian bustards and ratites are covered in more detail elsewhere in the book. These methods include several low-impact and indirect methods such as assessment of tracks and traces, acoustic and camera monitoring (Chapters 4 and 5), and citizen science and educational activities (Chapter 10). Avian-specific methods are detailed in Chapter 15, including census and observational techniques, call playback and broadcast surveys, nest and hollow inspections (including handling of eggs and chicks), hand capture and spotlighting, methods for capture of individual birds, marking methods, telemetry methods and collection of regurgitate, crop contents, scats and pellets. Several veterinary procedures may also be used during megapode research (Chapter 16).

REFERENCES

Alonso JC (2008) Guidelines for radio-tracking great bustards. *Bustard Studies* **7**, 81–95.

AVMA (American Veterinary Medical Association) (2020) AVMA guidelines for the euthanasia of animals: 2020 edition. AMVA, Schaumburg, USA. <https://www.avma.org/KB/Policies/Document>.

Bailey TA, Nicholls PK, Samour JH, Naldo J, Werney U, Howlett JC (1996) Post-mortem findings in bustards in the United Arab Emirates. *Avian Diseases* **40**, 296–305. doi:10.2307/1592224

Birks S (1997) Paternity in the Australian brush-turkey, *Alectura lathami*, a megapode bird with uniparental care. *Behavioral Ecology* **8**, 560–568. doi:10.1093/beheco/8.5.560

Booth DT, Jones DN (2002) Underground nesting in megapodes. In *Avian Incubation: Behaviour, Environment, and Evolution*. (Ed. DC Deeming) pp. 192–206. Oxford University Press, Oxford, UK.

Campbell HA, Dwyer RG, Fitzgibbons S, Klein CJ, Lauridsen G, McKeown A, *et al.* (2012) Prioritising the protection of habitat utilised by southern cassowaries *Casuarius casuarius johnsonii*. *Endangered Species Research* **17**, 53–61. doi:10.3354/esr00397

Campbell H, Dwyer R, Sullivan S, Mead D, Lauridsen G (2014) Chemical immobilisation and satellite tagging of free-living southern cassowaries. *Australian Veterinary Journal* **92**, 240–245. doi:10.1111/avj.12193

Carpenter JW, Thomas NJ, Reeves S (1991) Capture myopathy in an endangered sandhill crane (*Grus canadensis pulla*). *Journal of Zoo and Wildlife Medicine* **22**, 488–493.

Contreras A, Gomez-Martin A, Paterna A, Tatay-Dualde J, Prats-Van Der Ham M, Corrales JC, *et al.* (2016) Epidemiological role of birds in the transmission and maintenance of zoonoses. *Revue Scientifique et Technique (International Office of Epizootics)* **35**, 845–862. doi:10.20506/rst.35.3.2574

Cushing A, McClean M (2010) Use of thiafentanil-medetomidine for the induction of anesthesia in emus (*Dromaius novaehollandiae*) within a wild animal park. *Journal of Zoo and Wildlife Medicine* **41**, 234–241. doi:10.1638/2009-0143R1.1

Davies SJ, Beck MW, Kruiskamp JP (1971) Results of banding 154 emus in Western Australia. *Wildlife Research* **16**, 77–79. doi:10.1071/CWR9710077

Davies SJJF (2002) *Ratites and Tinamous: Tinamidae, Rheidae, Dromaiidae, Casuariidae, Apterygidae, Struthionidae*. Oxford University Press, Oxford, UK.

Fitzherbert K (1978) Observations on breeding and display in a colony of captive Australian Bustards (*Ardeotis australis*). BSc (Hons) thesis. Monash University, Australia.

Fowler M (2008) *Restraint and Handling of Wild and Domestic Animals*. 3rd edn. John Wiley and Sons, Ames, IO.

Garnett S, Szabo J, Dutson G (2010) *Action Plan for Australian Birds*. CSIRO Publishing, Melbourne.

Göth A, Jones DN (2001) Transmitter attachment and its effect on Australian brush-turkey hatchlings. *Wildlife Research* **28**, 73–78. doi:10.1071/WR99111

Göth A, Vogel U (2002) Chick survival in the megapode *Alectura lathami* (Australian brush-turkey). *Wildlife Research* **29**, 503–511. doi:10.1071/WR01054

Göth A, Vogel U (2003) Juvenile dispersal and habitat selectivity in the megapode *Alectura lathami* (Australian brush-turkey). *Wildlife Research* **30**, 69–74. doi:10.1071/WR01053

Hammond EL, Lymbery AJ, Martin GB, Groth D, Wetherall JD (2002) Microsatellite analysis of genetic diversity in wild and farmed emus (*Dromaius novaehollandiae*). *The Journal of Heredity* **93**, 376–380. doi:10.1093/jhered/93.5.376

Jones DN (1988) Behavioural ecology of reproduction in the Australian Brush-turkey. PhD thesis. Griffith University, Australia.

Jones DN (1990) Male mating tactics in a promiscuous megapode: patterns of incubation mound ownership. *Behavioral Ecology* **1**, 107–115. doi:10.1093/beheco/1.2.107

Jones DN, Dekker RW, Roselaar CS (1995) *The Megapodes*. Oxford University Press, Oxford, UK.

Jones DN, Everding SE (1991) Australian brush-turkeys in a suburban environment: implications for conflict and conservation. *Wildlife Research* **18**, 285–297. doi:10.1071/WR9910285

Jones D, Göth A (2008) *Mound-builders*. CSIRO Publishing, Melbourne.

Keller MD (2009) Behaviour of southern cassowary *Casuarius casuarius* towards intruders. *The Sunbird* **39**, 49–53.

King DR, Kirkpatrick WE, McGrath M (1996) The tolerance of malleefowl *Leipoa ocellata* to 1080. *Emu-Austral Ornithology* **96**, 198–202. doi:10.1071/MU9960198

Maclean RA, Beaufrere H (2014) Gruiformes (Cranes, Limpkins, Rails, Gallinules, Coots, Bustards), In *Fowler's Zoo and Wild Animal Medicine, Volume 8. E-Book*. (Eds. ER Miller and ME Fowler) pp. 155–163. Elsevier Health Sciences.

Mack AL (1995) Distance and non-randomness of seed dispersal by the dwarf cassowary *Casuarius bennetti*. *Ecography* **18**, 286–295. doi:10.1111/j.1600-0587.1995.tb00131.x

Maderspacher F (2017) Evolution: flight of the ratites. *Current Biology* **27**, 110–113. doi:10.1016/j.cub.2016.12.023

Marco I, Mentaberre G, Ponjoan A, Bota G, Mañosa S, Lavín S (2006) Capture myopathy in little bustards after trapping and marking. *Journal of Wildlife Diseases* **42**, 889–891. doi:10.7589/0090-3558-42.4.889

Moore L (2007) Population ecology of the southern cassowary Casuarius casuarius johnsonii, Mission Beach, North Queensland. *Journal of Ornithology* **148**, 357–366. doi:10.1007/s10336-007-0137-1

Nicholls PK, Bailey TA, Gibbons LM, Jones A, Samour JH (1995) Parasitic Infection in a Flock of Rufous-Crested Bustards (*Eupodotis ruficrista*) in the United Arab Emirates. *Journal of Zoo and Wildlife Medicine* **26**, 590–596.

Nield AP, Enright NJ, Ladd PG (2015) Study of seed dispersal by Emu (*Dromaius novaehollandiae*) in the Jarrah (*Eucalyptus marginata*) forests of south-western Australia through satellite telemetry. *Emu-Austral Ornithology* **115**, 29–34. doi:10.1071/MU13113

Proctor HC, Jones DN (2004) Geographical structuring of feather mite assemblages from the Australian brush-turkey (Aves: Megapodiidae). *The Journal of Parasitology* **90**, 60–66. doi:10.1645/GE-57R

Raidal S (1996) Haematology, serum biochemistry and cytology. In *Caged Bird Health* (Eds S Raidal, S Vitali and S Jaensch) pp. 19–22, 24–30. Foundation for Continuing Veterinary Education Proceedings, Murdoch University, Murdoch.

Reilly JS (Ed) (2001) *Euthanasia of Animals Used for Scientific Purposes*. 2nd edn. Australian & New Zealand Council for the Care of Animals in Research and Teaching (ANZCCART), Adelaide.

Rogers DI, Battley PF, Sparrow J, Koolhaas A, Hassell CJ (2004) Treatment of capture myopathy in shorebirds: a successful trial in north-western Australia. *Journal of Field Ornithology* **75**, 157–164. doi:10.1648/0273-8570-75.2.157

Schultz DJ, Hough IJ, Boardman W (1996) Special challenges of maintaining wild animals in captivity in Australia and New Zealand: prevention of infectious and parasitic diseases. *Revue Scientifique et Technique (International Office of Epizootics)* **15**, 289–308. doi:10.20506/rst.15.1.917

Seddon PJ, Launay F, Van Heezik Y, Bowardi M (1999) Methods for live trapping Houbara bustards. *Journal of Field Ornithology* **70**, 169–181.

Shaw JM, Dilley BJ, Davies D, Ryan PG (2014) Trapping and capture myopathy in Ludwig's bustard. *South African Journal of Wildlife Research* **44**, 16–23. doi:10.3957/056.044.0108

Siegal-Willott J (2014) Ratites. In *Zoo Animal and Wildlife Immobilization and Anaesthesia*. 2nd edn. (Eds G West, D Heard and N Caulkett) pp. 445–457. John Wiley and Sons, Hoboken, NJ.

Smith DA (2003) Ratites: Tinamiformes (Tinamous) and Struthioniformes, Rheiiformes, Casuariformes (Ostriches, Emus, Cassowaries and Kiwis). In *Zoo and Wild Animal Medicine* (Eds ME Fowler and RE Miller) pp. 75–82. Saunders, St Louis, MO.

Smith KM, Murray S, Sanchez C (2005) Successful treatment of suspected exertional myopathy in a rhea (*Rhea americana*). *Journal of Zoo and Wildlife Medicine* **36**, 316–320. doi:10.1638/04-050.1

Steadman DW (2006) *Extinction and Biogeography of Tropical Pacific Birds*. University of Chicago Press, Chicago, IL.

Tully TN, Hodgin C, Morris JM, Williams J, Zebreznik B (1996) Exertional myopathy in an emu (*Dromaius novahollandiae*). *Journal of Avian Medicine and Surgery* **10**, 96–100.

Tully TN (2009) Ratites. In *Handbook of Avian Medicine*. 2nd edn. (Eds TN Tully, GM Dorrestein, AK Jones, JE Cooper and WB Saunders) pp. 258–274. Saunders, St Louis, MO.

Ward JM, Gartrell BD, Conklin JR, Battley PF (2011) Midazolam as an adjunctive therapy for capture myopathy in bar-tailed godwits (*Limosa lapponica baueri*) with prognostic indicators. *Journal of Wildlife Diseases* **47**, 925–935. doi:10.7589/0090-3558-47.4.925

Zehnder AM, Hawkins MG, Pascoe PJ (2014) Avian anatomy and physiology. In *Zoo Animal and Wildlife Immobilization and Anaesthesia*. 2nd edn. (Eds G West, D Heard and N Caulkett) pp. 389–398. John Wiley and Sons, Hoboken, NJ.

Ziembicki M (2009) Ecology and movements of the Australian Bustard *Ardeotis australis* in a dynamic landscape. PhD thesis. The University of Adelaide, Australia.

Ziembicki M (2010) *Australian Bustard. Australian Natural History Series*. CSIRO Publishing, Melbourne.

Ziembicki M, Woinarski JCZ (2007) Monitoring continental movement patterns of the Australian bustard *Ardeotis australis* through community-based surveys and remote sensing. *Pacific Conservation Biology* **13**, 128–142. doi:10.1071/PC070128

Index

www.ingramcontent.com/pod-product-compliance
Ingram Content Group UK Ltd.
Pitfield, Milton Keynes, MK11 3LW, UK
UKHW060221061026
15625UKWH00007B/435

9 781486 31344